BRIEF

# Core Concepts in Health

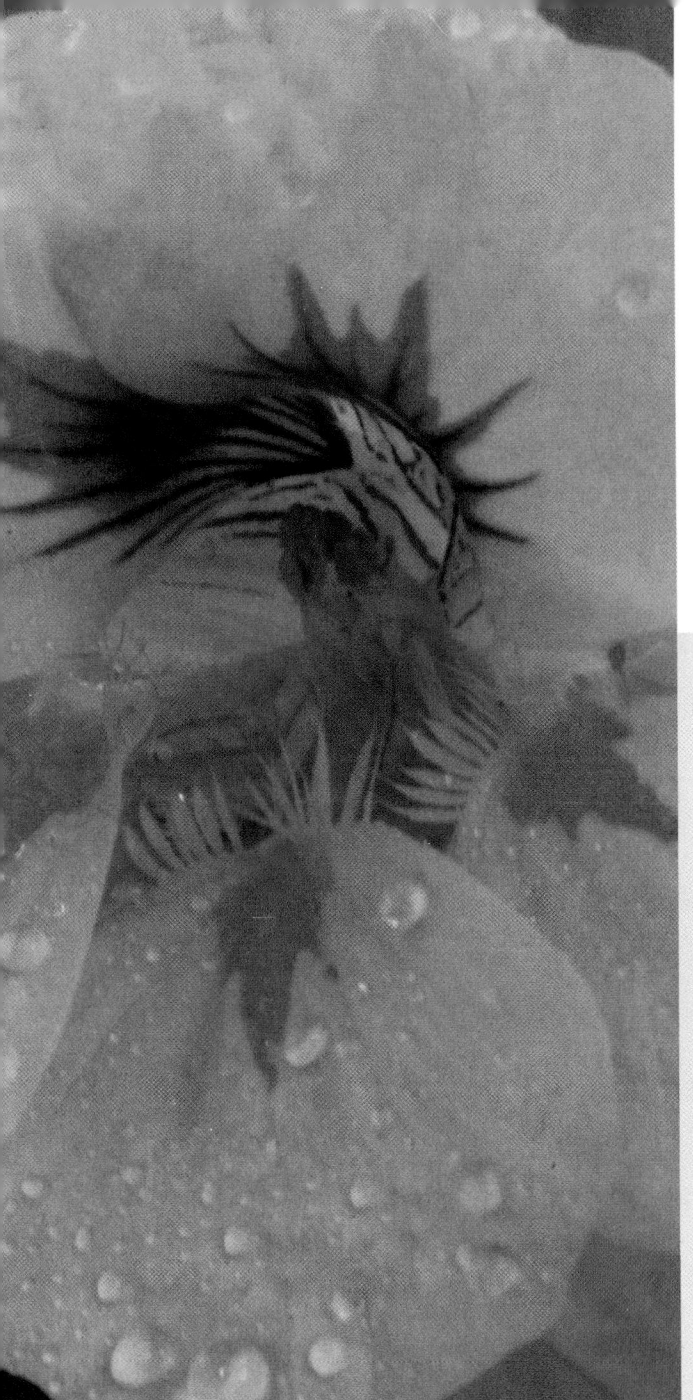

Paul M. Insel
Walton T. Roth
*Stanford University*

Kirstan Price
*Developmental Editor*

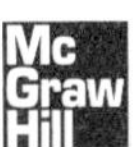


Boston Burr Ridge, IL Dubuque, IA Madison, WI New York
San Francisco St. Louis Bangkok Bogotá Caracas Kuala Lumpur
Lisbon London Madrid Mexico City Milan Montreal New Delhi
Santiago Seoul Singapore Sydney Taipei Toronto

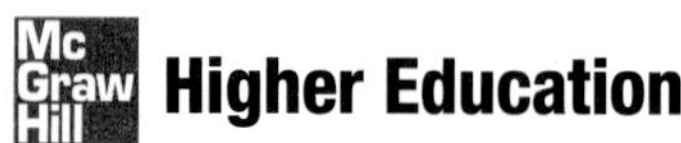

**Higher Education**

Published by McGraw-Hill, an imprint of The McGraw-Hill Companies, Inc., 1221 Avenue of the Americas, New York, NY 10020. 

This book is printed on acid-free paper.

1 2 3 4 5 6 7 8 9 0 VNH/VNH 0 9 8 7 6 5

ISBN 0-07-297235-1

Editor in chief: *Emily Barrosse*
Publisher: *William R. Glass*
Executive editor: *Nicholas R. Barrett*
Director of development: *Kathleen Engelberg*
Executive marketing manager: *Pamela S. Cooper*
Senior developmental editor: *Kirstan A. Price*
Editorial assistant: *Sarah Hill*
Managing editor: *Melissa Williams*
Senior production editor: *Brett Coker*
Manuscript editor: *Darlene Bledsoe*
Art director: *Jeanne M. Schreiber*
Senior design manager and cover designer: *Violeta Díaz*
Text designer: *Mark Ong*
Art manager: *Robin Mouat*
Illustrator(s): *John and Judy Waller, Susan Seed, Kevin Sommerville*
Manager, photo research: *Brian J. Pecko*
Lead production supervisor: *Randy Hurst*
Senior supplements coordinator: *Louis Swaim*
Development editor for technology: *Julia D. Ersery*
Senior media producer: *Lance Gerhart*
Senior media project manager: *Ron Nelms*
Composition: *GTS, Los Angeles*
Printing: *45# Pub Matte Plus by Von Hoffmann Graphics*

Cover: © *Zach Holmes Photography*

**Library of Congress Cataloging-in-Publication Data**

Core concepts in health / [edited by] Paul M. Insel, Walton T. Roth; Kirstan Price, developmental editor.—Brief 10th ed.
p. cm.
Includes bibliographical references and index
ISBN 0-07-297235-1 (alk. paper)
1. Health—Handbooks, manuals, etc. I. Insel, Paul M. II. Roth, Walton T. III. Price, Kirstan.

RA776.C83 2005
613—dc22

The Internet addresses listed in the text were accurate at the time of publication. The inclusion of a website does not indicate an endorsement by the authors or McGraw-Hill, and McGraw-Hill does not guarantee the accuracy of the information presented at these sites.

www.mhhe.com

## *Photo Credits*

**Chapter 1** p. 1, PhotoDisc/Getty Images; p. 10, © Ariel Skelley/Corbis; p. 15, © Michael Newman/PhotoEdit; p. 18, © Jeff Greenberg/PhotoEdit; p. 19, © Steve Mason/Getty Images

**Chapter 2** p. 23, © Tony Freeman/PhotoEdit; p. 27, © Richard Lord/PhotoEdit; p. 33, © AP/Wide World Photos; p. 41, © Joel Gordon

**Chapter 3** p. 45, © Big Cheese Photo/PictureQuest; p. 47, Ryan McVay/Getty Images; p. 51, © Dennis MacDonald/PhotoEdit; p. 61, © Michael Newman/PhotoEdit

**Chapter 4** p. 66, Suza Scalora/Getty Images; p. 67, © Michael Newman/PhotoEdit; p. 75, Ryan McVay/Getty Images; p. 81, Digital Vision/PictureQuest

**Chapter 5** p. 85, Jules Frazier/Getty Images; p. 92, © David Young-Wolff/PhotoEdit; p. 97, © Myrleen Ferguson Cate/PhotoEdit; p. 106, © David Young-Wolff/PhotoEdit

**Chapter 6** p. 114, 117, 124, © Joel Gordon; p. 133L, © Alex Wong/Getty Images; p. 133R, © AP/Wide World Photos

**Chapter 7** p. 140, © Bonnie Kamin; p. 142, © Park Street/PhotoEdit; p. 154, © AP/Wide World Photos; p. 156, © Barbara Stitzer/PhotoEdit

**Chapter 8** p. 164, © Joel Gordon; p. 165, © David Young-Wolff/PhotoEdit; p. 185, © Mark Richards/PhotoEdit; p. 186, © David Young-Wolff/PhotoEdit

**Chapter 9** p. 194, Mitch Hrdlicka/Getty Images; p. 195, © Dana White/PhotoEdit; p. 207, © Royalty-Free/Corbis; p. 211, © David Young-Wolff/PhotoEdit

**Chapter 10** p. 231, © Chris Rogers/PictureQuest; p. 242, Keith Brofsky/Getty Images; p. 249, © David Young-Wolff/PhotoEdit

**Chapter 11** p. 253, © Novastock/PhotoEdit; p. 260, © Cindy Charles/PhotoEdit; p. 269, © AP/Wide World Photos

**Chapter 12** p. 277, © Adamsmith/Superstock; p. 292, © Michael Newman/PhotoEdit; p. 301, © Jilly Wendell/Getty Images/Stone

**Chapter 13** p. 314, © Bill Aron/PhotoEdit; p. 315, © David Young-Wolff/PhotoEdit; p. 338, Ryan McVay/Getty Images; p. 343, © Royalty-Free/Corbis

**Chapter 14** p. 347, © Royalty-Free/Corbis; p. 351, © Amy C. Etra/PhotoEdit; p. 365, © AP/Wide World Photos

**Chapter 15** p. 370, © Michael Newman/PhotoEdit; p. 374, Tomi/PhotoLink/Getty Images; p. 377, Ryan McVay/Getty Images; p. 381, Anthony Saint James/Getty Images

**Chapter 16** p. 393, © Michael Newman/PhotoEdit; p. 399, © Tony Freeman/PhotoEdit; p. 404, © Jonathan Nourok/PhotoEdit; p. 409, © Rachel Epstein/PhotoEdit

**Chapter 17** p. 417, Russell Illig/Getty Images; p. 418, © AP/Wide World Photos; p. 427, © Dennis MacDonald/PhotoEdit

# Brief Contents

**Chapter 1**
Taking Charge of Your Health 1

**Chapter 2**
Stress: The Constant Challenge 23

**Chapter 3**
Psychological Health 45

**Chapter 4**
Intimate Relationships and Communication 66

**Chapter 5**
Sexuality, Pregnancy, and Childbirth 85

**Chapter 6**
Contraception and Abortion 114

**Chapter 7**
The Use and Abuse of Psychoactive Drugs 140

**Chapter 8**
Alcohol and Tobacco 164

**Chapter 9**
Nutrition Basics 194

**Chapter 10**
Exercise for Health and Fitness 231

**Chapter 11**
Weight Management 253

**Chapter 12**
Cardiovascular Disease and Cancer 277

**Chapter 13**
Immunity and Infection 314

**Chapter 14**
The Challenge of Aging 347

**Chapter 15**
Conventional and Complementary Medicine: Skills for the Health Care Consumer 370

**Chapter 16**
Personal Safety: Protecting Yourself from Unintentional Injuries and Violence 393

**Chapter 17**
Environmental Health 417

**Appendix**
Nutritional Content of Popular Items from Fast-Food Restaurants A-1

**Index I-1**

**Study Guide I-15**

# Contents


## 1 Taking Charge of Your Health 1

WELLNESS: THE NEW HEALTH GOAL 1

The Dimensions of Wellness 1
New Opportunities, New Responsibilities 2
National Wellness Goals: The Healthy People Initiative 4
Health Issues for Diverse Populations 5

CHOOSING WELLNESS 10

Factors That Influence Wellness 10
A Wellness Profile 11

HOW DO YOU REACH WELLNESS? 12

Getting Serious About Your Health 13
Building Motivation for Change 13
Enhancing Your Readiness to Change 16
Developing Skills for Change: Creating a Personalized Plan 16
Putting Your Plan into Action 19
Staying with It 19

BEING HEALTHY FOR LIFE 19

*Tips for Today* 20
*Summary* 20
*Take Action* 21
*For More Information* 21
*Selected Bibliography* 22

## 2 Stress: The Constant Challenge 23

WHAT IS STRESS? 24

Physical Responses to Stressors 24
Emotional and Behavioral Responses to Stressor 26

STRESS AND DISEASE 28

The General Adaptation Syndrome 28
Allostatic Load 29
Psychoneuroimmunology 29
Links Between Stress and Specific Conditions 30

COMMON SOURCES OF STRESS 31

Major Life Changes 31
Daily Hassles 31
College Stressors 32
Job-Related Stressors 32
Social Stressors 33

TECHNIQUES FOR MANAGING STRESS 33

Social Support and Communication 34
Exercise 34
Nutrition 35
Sleep 35
Time Management 36
Strive for Greater Spirituality 37
Confide in Yourself Through Writing 37
Cognitive Techniques 37
Relaxation Techniques 38
Counterproductive Coping Strategies 40

CREATING A PERSONAL PLAN FOR MANAGING STRESS 41

Identifying Stressors 41
Designing Your Plan 41
Getting Help 42

*Tips for Today* 42
*Summary* 42
*Behavior Change Strategy: Dealing with Test Anxiety* 43
*Take Action* 43
*For More Information* 43
*Selected Bibliography* 44

## 3 Psychological Health 45

WHAT PSYCHOLOGICAL HEALTH IS NOT 45

DEFINING PSYCHOLOGICAL HEALTH 46

Realism 46
Acceptance 46
Autonomy 47
A Capacity for Intimacy 47
Creativity 47

MEETING LIFE'S CHALLENGES 47

Growing Up Psychologically 47
Achieving Healthy Self-Esteem 48
Being Less Defensive 49
Being Optimistic 50
Maintaining Honest Communication 51

Dealing with Loneliness 51
Dealing with Anger 51

PSYCHOLOGICAL DISORDERS 52

Anxiety Disorders 52
Mood Disorders 55
Schizophrenia 58

GETTING HELP 60

Self-Help 60
Peer Counseling and Support Groups 60
Professional Help 61

*Tips for Today* 62
*Summary* 63
*Behavior Change Strategy: Dealing with Social Anxiety* 63
*Take Action* 64
*For More Information* 64
*Selected Bibliography* 65

4 Intimate Relationships and Communication 66

DEVELOPING INTIMATE RELATIONSHIPS 66

Self-Concept and Self-Esteem 66
Friendship 67
Love, Sex, and Intimacy 68
Challenges in Relationships 69
Successful Relationships 70
Unhealthy Relationships 70
Ending a Relationship 71

COMMUNICATION 71

Nonverbal Communication 71
Communication Skills 71
Gender and Communication 71
Conflict and Conflict Resolution 72

PAIRING AND SINGLEHOOD 74

Choosing a Partner 74
Dating 75
Living Together 75
Same-Sex Partnerships 75
Singlehood 76

MARRIAGE 78

Benefits of Marriage 78
Issues in Marriage 78
The Role of Commitment 78
Separation and Divorce 79

FAMILY LIFE 79

Deciding to Become a Parent 79
Becoming a Parent 80
Parenting 80
Single Parents 81
Stepfamilies 82
Successful Families 82

*Tips for Today* 82
*Summary* 82
*Take Action* 83
*For More Information* 83
*Selected Bibliography* 84

5 Sexuality, Pregnancy, and Childbirth 85

SEXUAL ANATOMY 85

Female Sex Organs 86
Male Sex Organs 86

HORMONES AND THE REPRODUCTIVE LIFE CYCLE 87

Female Sexual Maturation 88
Male Sexual Maturation 91
Aging and Human Sexuality 91

SEXUAL FUNCTIONING 91

Sexual Stimulation 91
The Sexual Response Cycle 92
Sexual Problems 92

SEXUAL BEHAVIOR 94

Sexual Orientation 94
Varieties of Human Sexual Behavior 94
Atypical and Problematic Sexual Behaviors 95
Commercial Sex 95
Responsible Sexual Behavior 96

UNDERSTANDING FERTILITY 97

Conception 97
Infertility 98

PREGNANCY 99

Pregnancy Tests 100
Changes in the Woman's Body 100
Fetal Development 101
The Important of Prenatal Care 103
Complications of Pregnancy and Pregnancy Loss 107

CHILDBIRTH 108

Choices in Childbirth 108
Labor and Delivery 108
The Postpartum Period 110

*Tips for Today* 111
*Summary* 111
*Take Action* 112
*For More Information* 112
*Selected Bibliography* 112

## 6 Contraception and Abortion 114

PRINCIPLES OF CONTRACEPTION 114

REVERSIBLE CONTRACEPTION 115

Oral Contraceptives: The Pill 115
Contraceptive Skin Patch 116
Vaginal Contraceptive Ring 117
Contraceptive Implants 117
Injectable Contraceptives 118
Emergency Contraception 118
Intrauterine Device (IUD) 119
Male Condoms 119
Female Condoms 122
The Diaphragm with Spermicide 123
Lea's Shield 124
The Cervical Cap 124
The Contraceptive Sponge 124
Vaginal Spermicides 125
Abstinence, Fertility Awareness, and Withdrawal 125
Combining Methods 127

PERMANENT CONTRACEPTION: STERILIZATION 127

WHICH CONTRACEPTIVE METHOD IS RIGHT FOR YOU? 129

THE ABORTION ISSUE 131

The History of Abortion in the United States 131
Current Legal Status 131
Moral Considerations 133
Public Opinion 133
Personal Considerations 133
Current Trends 134
Methods of Abortion 135
Complications of Abortion 136

*Tips for Today* 137
*Summary* 137
*Take Action* 138
*For More Information* 138
*Selected Bibliography* 139

## 7 The Use and Abuse of Psychoactive Drugs 140

ADDICTIVE BEHAVIOR 140

What Is Addiction? 141
Characteristics of Addictive Behavior 141
The Development of Addiction 142
Characteristics of People with Addictions 142
Examples of Addictive Behaviors 142

DRUG USE, ABUSE, AND DEPENDENCE 143

Drug Use and Dependence 143
Who Uses Drugs? 144
Why Do People Use Drugs? 146
Risk Factors for Dependence 147
Other Risks of Drug Use 147

HOW DRUGS AFFECT THE BODY 147

Changes in Brain Chemistry 147
Drug Factors 148
User Factors 148
Social Factors 148

REPRESENTATIVE PSYCHOACTIVE DRUGS 149

Opioids 149
Central Nervous System Depressants 149
Central Nervous System Stimulants 152
Marijuana and Other Cannabis Products 154
Hallucinogens 155
Inhalants 156

DRUG USE: THE DECADES AHEAD 156

Drugs, Society, and Families 157
Legalizing Drugs 158
Drug Testing 158
Treatment for Drug Dependence 158
Preventing Drug Abuse 160
The Role of Drugs in Your Life 160

*Tips for Today* 161
*Summary* 161
*Take Action* 161
*Behavior Change Strategy: Changing Your Drug Habits* 162
*For More Information* 162
*Selected Bibliography* 163

## 8 Alcohol and Tobacco 164

THE NATURE OF ALCOHOL 164

The Chemistry of Alcohol 164
Absorption 165
Metabolism and Excretion 165
Alcohol Intake and Blood Alcohol Concentration 166

ALCOHOL AND HEALTH 167

The Immediate Effects of Alcohol 167
Drinking and Driving 169
The Effects of Chronic Use 170
The Effects of Alcohol Use During Pregnancy 171
Possible Health Benefits of Alcohol 171

ALCOHOL ABUSE AND DEPENDENCE 172
Alcohol Abuse 172
Binge Drinking 172
Alcoholism 173
Gender and Ethnic Differences 175
Helping Someone with an Alcohol Problem 177

WHY PEOPLE USE TOBACCO 177
Nicotine Addiction 177
Social and Psychological Factors 179
Why Start in the First Place? 179
Who Uses Tobacco? 179

HEALTH HAZARDS 180
Tobacco Smoke: A Toxic Mix 180
The Immediate Effects of Smoking 181
The Long-Term Effects of Smoking 181
Other Forms of Tobacco Use 184

THE EFFECTS OF SMOKING ON THE NONSMOKER 185
Environmental Tobacco Smoke 185
Smoking and Pregnancy 187
The Cost of Tobacco Use to Society 187

WHAT CAN BE DONE? 187
Action at Many Levels 187
What You Can Do 188

HOW A TOBACCO USER CAN QUIT 188
The Benefits of Quitting 188
Options for Quitting 189
*Tips for Today* 190
*Summary* 190
*Behavior Change Strategy: Kicking the Tobacco Habit* 191
*Take Action* 192
*For More Information* 192
*Selected Bibliography* 193

## 9 Nutrition Basics 194

NUTRITIONAL REQUIREMENTS: COMPONENTS OF A HEALTHY DIET 194
Proteins—The Basis of Body Structure 195
Fats—Essential in Small Amounts 196
Carbohydrates—An Ideal Source of Energy 199
Fiber—A Closer Look 201
Vitamins—Organic Micronutrients 202
Minerals—Inorganic Micronutrients 204
Water—Vital but Often Ignored 204
Other Substances in Food 204

NUTRITIONAL GUIDELINES: PLANNING YOUR DIET 206
Dietary Reference Intakes (DRIs) 206
Dietary Guidelines for Americans 208
USDA's MyPyramid 212
The Vegetarian Alternative 217
Dietary Challenge for Special Population Groups 218

A PERSONAL PLAN: MAKING INFORMED CHOICES ABOUT FOOD 220
Reading Food Labels 220
Reading Dietary Supplement Labels 220
Organic Foods 223
Additives in Food 223
Food Irradiation 223
Genetically Modified Foods 223
Food Allergies and Food Intolerances 224
*Tips for Today* 224
*Summary* 224
*Behavior Change Strategy: Improving Your Diet by Choosing Healthy Beverages* 225
*Take Action* 226
*For More Information* 226
*Selected Bibliography* 227
*Nutrition Resources* 228

## 10 Exercise for Health and Fitness 231

WHAT IS PHYSICAL FITNESS? 232
Cardiorespiratory Endurance 232
Muscular Strength 232
Muscular Endurance 232
Flexibility 232
Body Composition 233

THE BENEFITS OF EXERCISE 233
Improved Cardiorespiratory Functioning 234
More Efficient Metabolism 234
Improved Body Composition 234
Disease Prevention and Management 234
Improved Psychological and Emotional Wellness 234
Improved Immune Function 235
Prevention of Injuries and Low-Back Pain 235
Improved Wellness over the Life Span 235

DESIGNING YOUR EXERCISE PROGRAM 237
Physical Activity and Exercise for Health and Fitness 237
First Steps 240
Cardiorespiratory Endurance Exercises 241
Developing Muscular Strength and Endurance 242

Flexibility Exercises 244
Training in Specific Skills 245
Putting It All Together 245

GETTING STARTED AND STAYING ON TRACK 246

Selecting Instructors, Equipment, and Facilities 246
Eating and Drinking for Exercise 246
Managing Your Fitness Program 248

*Tips for Today* 250
*Summary* 250
*Take Action* 250
*Behavior Change Strategy: Planning a Personal Exercise Program* 251
*For More Information* 251
*Selected Bibliography* 252

## 11 Weight Management 253

BASIC CONCEPTS OF WEIGHT MANAGEMENT 253

Body Composition 254
Energy Balance 255
Evaluating Body Weight and Body Composition 255
Excess Body Fat and Wellness 256
What Is the Right Weight for You? 258

FACTORS CONTRIBUTING TO EXCESS BODY FAT 260

Genetic Factors 260
Metabolism 260
Lifestyle Factors 260
Psychosocial Factors 261

ADOPTING A HEALTHY LIFESTYLE FOR SUCCESSFUL WEIGHT MANAGEMENT 262

Diet and Eating Habits 262
Physical Activity and Exercise 263
Thinking and Emotions 264
Coping Strategies 264

APPROACHES TO OVERCOMING A WEIGHT PROGRAM 265

Doing It Yourself 265
Diet Books 265
Dietary Supplements and Diet Aids 265
Weight-Loss Programs 268
Prescription Drugs 268
Surgery 269

BODY IMAGE 269

Severe Body Image Problems 269
Acceptance and Change 270

EATING DISORDERS 271

Anorexia Nervosa 271
Bulimia Nervosa 271
Binge-Eating Disorder 272
Borderline Disordered Eating 272
Treating Eating Disorders 272
Today's Challenge 273

*Tips for Today* 273
*Summary* 274
*Take Action* 274
*For More Information* 274
*Behavior Change Strategy: A Weight-Management Program* 275
*Selected Bibliography* 276

## 12 Cardiovascular Disease and Cancer 277

THE CARDIOVASCULAR SYSTEM 277

RISKS FACTORS FOR CARDIOVASCULAR DISEASE 278

Major Risk Factors That Can Be Changed 278
Contributing Risk Factors That Can Be Changed 282
Major Risk Factors That Can't Be Changed 283
Possible Risk Factors Currently Being Studied 284

MAJOR FORMS OF CARDIOVASCULAR DISEASE 286

Atherosclerosis 286
Heart Disease and Heart Attack 287
Stroke 289
Congestive Heart Failure 291
Other Forms of Heart Disease 291

PROTECTING YOURSELF AGAINST CARDIOVASCULAR DISEASE 292

Eat Heart-Healthy 292
Exercise Regularly 293
Avoid Tobacco 293
Know and Manage Your Blood Pressure 294
Know and Manage Your Cholesterol Levels 294
Develop Effective Ways to Handle Stress and Anger 294
Manage Other Risk Factors and Medical Conditions 294

WHAT IS CANCER? 294

Benign Versus Malignant Tumors 294
How Cancer Spreads: Metastasis 295
Types of Cancer 295
The Incidence of Cancer 296

COMMON CANCERS 296
Lung Cancer 296
Colon and Rectal Cancer 297
Breast Cancer 297
Prostate Cancer 299
Cancers of the Female Reproductive Tract 300
Skin Cancer 301
Oral Cancer 303
Testicular Cancer 303

THE CAUSES OF CANCER 303
The Role of DNA 303
Dietary Factors 305
Inactivity and Obesity 306
Microbes 306
Carcinogens in the Environment 306

DETECTING, DIAGNOSING, AND TREATING CANCER 308
Detecting Cancer 308
Diagnosing and Treating Cancer 308

PREVENTING CANCER 309
*Tips for Today* 310
*Summary* 310
*Behavior Change Strategy: Modifying Your Diet for Heart Health and Cancer Prevention* 311
*Take Action* 312
*For More Information* 312
*Selected Bibliography* 313

## 13 Immunity and Infection 314

THE CHAIN OF INFECTION 314

THE BODY'S DEFENSE SYSTEM 315
Physical and Chemical Barriers 315
The Immune System 315
Immunization 318
Allergy: The Body's Defense System Gone Haywire 318

THE TROUBLEMAKERS: PATHOGENS AND DISEASE 319
Bacteria 320
Viruses 323
Fungi 326
Protozoa 326
Parasitic Worms 326
Prions 326
Emerging Infectious Diseases 326
Other Immune Disorders: Cancer and Autoimmune Diseases 328

GIVING YOURSELF A FIGHTING CHANCE: HOW TO SUPPORT YOUR IMMUNE SYSTEM 328

SEXUALLY TRANSMITTED DISEASES 328
HIV Infection and AIDS 328
Chlamydia 336
Gonorrhea 337
Pelvic Inflammatory Disease 337
Human Papillomavirus Infection (Genital Warts) 338
Genital Herpes 339
Hepatitis B 340
Syphilis 341

OTHER STDS 341

WHAT YOU CAN DO 342
Education 342
Diagnosis and Treatment 342
Prevention 343
*Tips for Today* 343
*Summary* 344
*Take Action* 345
*For More Information* 345
*Selected Bibliography* 346

## 14 The Challenge of Aging 347

GENERATING VITALITY AS YOU AGE 347
What Happens as You Age? 348
Life-Enhancing Measures: Age-Proofing 348

CONFRONTING THE CHANGES OF AGING 350
Planning for Social Changes 350
Adapting to Physical Changes 351
Handling Psychological and Mental Changes 353

LIFE IN AN AGING AMERICA 355
America's Aging Minority 356
Family and Community Resources for Older Adults 356
Government Aid and Policies 357

WHAT IS DEATH? 357
Defining Death 357
Learning About Death 358
Denying Versus Welcoming Death 358

PLANNING FOR DEATH 358
Making a Will 359
Considering Options for End-of-Life Care 359
Deciding to Prolong Life or Hasten Death 360
Completing an Advance Directive 362
Becoming an Organ Donor 362
Planning a Funeral or Memorial Service 362

COPING WITH DYING 364
The Tasks of Coping 364
Supporting a Dying Person 364

COPING WITH LOSS 364
Experiencing Grief 364
Supporting a Grieving Person 366

COMING TO TERMS WITH DEATH 366
*Tips for Today* 367
*Summary* 367
*Take Action* 367
*For More Information* 368
*Selected Bibliography* 368

## 15 Conventional and Complementary Medicine: Skills for the Health Care Consumer 370

SELF-CARE: MANAGING MEDICAL PROBLEMS 370
Self-Assessment 370
Decision Making: Knowing When to See a Physician 371
Self-Treatment: Many Options 371

PROFESSIONAL MEDICAL AND HEALTH CARE: CHOICES AND CHANGE 373

CONVENTIONAL MEDICINE 373
Premises and Assumptions of Conventional Medicine 373
The Providers of Conventional Medicine 375
Choosing a Primary Care Physician 375
Getting the Most Out of Your Medical Care 377

COMPLEMENTARY AND ALTERNATIVE MEDICINE 380
Alternative Medical Systems 380
Mind-Body Interventions 383
Biological-Based Therapies 383
Manipulative and Body-Based Methods 383
Energy Therapies 385
Evaluating Complementary and Alternative Therapies 386

PAYING FOR HEALTH CARE 388
Health Insurance 388
Choosing a Policy 390
*Tips for Today* 390
*Summary* 390
*Take Action* 391
*For More Information* 391
*Selected Bibliography* 392

## 16 Personal Safety: Protecting Yourself from Unintentional Injuries and Violence 393

UNINTENTIONAL INJURIES 394
Motor Vehicle Injuries 395
Home Injuries 398
Leisure Injuries 400
Work Injuries 400

VIOLENCE AND INTENTIONAL INJURIES 401
Factors Contributing to Violence 401
Assault 403
Homicide 404
Gang-related Violence 404
Hate Crimes 404
School Violence 404
Workplace Violence 405
Terrorism 405
Family and Intimate Violence 405
Sexual Violence 409
What You Can Do About Violence 412

PROVIDING EMERGENCY CARE 412
*Tips for Today* 414
*Summary* 414
*Take Action* 414
*Behavior Change Strategy: Adopting Safer Habits* 415
*For More Information* 415
*Selected Bibliography* 416

## 17 Environmental Health 417

CLASSICAL ENVIRONMENTAL HEALTH CONCERNS 417
Clean Water 418
Waste Disposal 419
Food Inspection 421
Insect and Rodent Control 421

POPULATION GROWTH 421

POLLUTION 422
Air Pollution 422
Chemical Pollution 427
Radiation 429
Noise Pollution 430

HEALING THE ENVIRONMENT 430
*Tips for Today* 431
*Summary* 431
*Take Action* 432
*For More Information* 432
*Selected Bibliography* 433

## APPENDIX


### Nutritional Content of Popular Items from Fast Food Restaurants A-1

### Index I-1

### Study Guide I-15


## BOXES

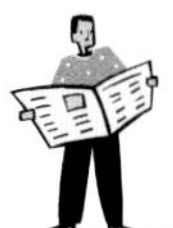

### In the News


Medical Innovations in the Twenty-first Century 12
Coping After Terrorism, Mass Violence, or Natural Disasters 35
Antidepressant Use in Young People 59
Same-Sex Marriage and Civil Unions 77
Reproductive Technology 99
Timeline of Selected Key Abortion Decisions and Legislation 132
Medical Marijuana 155
College Binge Drinking 174
America's Poor Eating Habits 209
Drugs and Supplements for Improved Athletic Performance 245
The Growing American Waistline 254
Putting Cancer Risks in Perspective 307
The Next Influenza Pandemic—When, Not If? 324
Stem Cells 348
Prescription Drug Use and Regulation: Lessons from Vioxx 379
Emergency Preparedness 407
Climate Change: Politics and Science 425


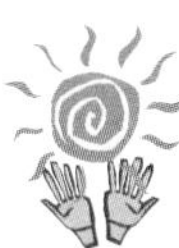

### Mind/Body/Spirit


Ten Warning Signs of Wellness 3
Stress and Your Brain 30
Healthy Connections 36
Paths to Spiritual Wellness 49
Are Intimate Relationships Good for Your Health? 79
Sexual Decision Making 94
Spirituality and Drug Abuse 146
Tobacco Use and Religion: Global Views 178
Exercise and the Mind 235
Exercise, Body Image, and Self-Esteem 264
Anger, Hostility, and Heart Disease 283
Immunity and Stress 329
Help Yourself by Helping Others 352
In Search of a Good Death 360
The Power of Belief: The Placebo Effect 382
Nature and the Human Spirit 418


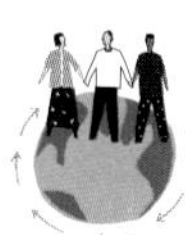

### Dimensions of Diversity


Factors Contributing to Health Disparities Among Ethnic Minorities 9
Diverse Populations, Discrimination, and Stress 34
Ethnicity, Culture, and Psychological Disorders 53
Interfaith and Intrafaith Partnerships 74
Ethnicity and Genetic Diseases 104
Contraceptive Use Among American Women 130
Drug Use and Ethnicity: Risk and Protective Factors 157
Metabolizing Alcohol: Our Bodies Work Differently 166
Exercise for People with Disabilities and Other Special Health Concerns 236
Overweight and Obesity Among U.S. Ethnic Populations 261
Ethnicity and CVD 285
HIV Infection Around the World 330
Día de los Muertos: The Day of the Dead 359
Who Are the Uninsured? 389
Violence and Health: A Global View 406
Poverty and Environmental Health 428


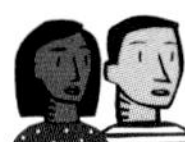

### Gender Matters


Women's Health/Men's Health 7
Women, Men, and Stress 28
Depression, Anxiety, and Gender 57
Gender and Communication 73
Pregnancy Tasks for Fathers 102
Men's Involvement in Contraception 122
Gender Differences in Drug Use and Abuse 145
Gender and Tobacco Use 184
How Different Are the Nutritional Needs of Women and Men? 218
Gender Differences in Muscular Strength 243
Gender, Ethnicity, and Body Image 270
Women and CVD 284
Women Are Hit Hard by STDs 339
Why Do Women Live Longer? 355
Injuries Among Young Men 394
Gender and Environmental Health 429


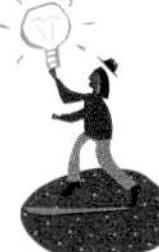

### Critical Consumer


Evaluating Source of Health Information 14
Alternative Remedies for Depression 60
Choosing and Evaluating Mental Health Professionals 62
Dietary Supplements and PMS 90
Buying and Using Over-the-Counter Contraceptives 121
Smoking Cessation Products 189
Using Food Labels 221
Using Dietary Supplement Labels 222
Choosing Exercise Footwear 247
Evaluating Fat and Sugar Substitutes 263
Is Any Diet Best for Weight Loss? 267
Choosing and Using Sunscreens and Sun-Protective Clothing 302
Preventing and Treating the Common Cold 323
Tattoos and Body Piercing 325
Getting an HIV Test 334
Evaluating Health News 376
Avoiding Health Fraud and Quackery 387
Choosing a Bicycle Helmet 398
How to Be a Green Consumer 420


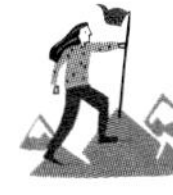

### Take Charge


Motivation Boosters 20
Meditation and the Relaxation Response 39
Breathing for Relaxation 40
Realistic Self-Talk 50
Being a Good Friend 68
Strategies for Enhancing Support in Relationships 70
Guidelines for Effective Communication 72
Online Relationships 76
Communicating About Sexuality 96
Talking with a Partner About Contraception 131
If Someone You Know Has a Drug Problem 159
Dealing with an Alcohol Emergency 168
Drinking Behavior and Responsibility 176
Building Motivation to Quit Smoking 180

Setting Intake Goals for Protein, Fat, and Carbohydrate 199
Choosing More Whole-Grain Foods 201
Eating for Healthy Bones 206
Reducing the Saturated and Trans Fat in Your Diet 212
Food Safety 213
Judging Portion Sizes 216
Eating Strategies for College Students 219
Becoming More Active 238
Determining Your Target Heart Rate Range 242
Strategies for Successful Weight Management 266
If Someone You Know Has an Eating Disorder 273
What to Do in Case of a Heart Attack, Cardiac Arrest, or Stroke 289
Breast Self-Examination 298
Testicle Self-Examination 304
Protecting Yourself Against Tickborne and Mosquitoborne Infections 322
Preventing HIV Infection and Other STDs 366
Talking About Condoms and Safer Sex 344
Tasks for Survivors 363
Coping with Grief 366
Recognizing the Potential for Abusiveness in a Partner 408
Preventing Date Rape 411
Staying Safe on Campus 413
Making Your Letters Count 431

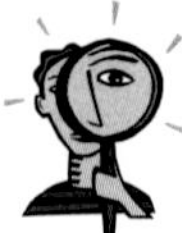

## In Focus

Headaches: A Common Symptom of Stress 31
Shyness 54
Myths About Suicide 58
The Adoption Option 136
Club Drugs 151
Diabetes 259
Alzheimer's Disease 354
Herbal Remedies: Are They Safe? 385
Cellular Phones and Distracted Driving 396
Carpal Tunnel Syndrome 402

## TOPICS OF SPECIAL CONCERN TO WOMEN

Aging among women, 91, 349, 351–355
Alcoholism, patterns among women, 175–177
Alcohol metabolism in women, 166
Alcohol use, special risks for women, 106, 169, 171
Amenorrhea, 258
Anxiety disorders, 52–55
Arthritis, 352
Body composition, 232, 233, 254–257
Body image, negative, 257, 264, 269–271
Breast cancer, 297–299, 309
Breast self-examinations, 298, 309
Cancer and women, 295, 297–299, 300–301, 309
Cardiovascular disease, risk among women, 284
Caregiving for older adults, 356–357
Carpal tunnel syndrome, 402
Causes of death among women, 4, 7, 287, 355, 394
Cervical cancer, 184, 300, 309, 338–339
Communication styles among women, 71–72, 73
Contraception, female methods, 115–119, 121–127, 128–129
Depression, risk among women, 52, 56, 57
Dietary recommendations for women, 105, 199, 202, 207, 213, 216, 218, 228–230
Drug use, rates and special risks for women, 145, 148, 152, 153, 154
Eating disorders, 271–273
Ectopic pregnancy, 107, 336
Environmental health risks, 105–106, 427–428, 429
Family violence, 405–409
Female athlete triad, 258
Financial planning for retirement, 351
Folic acid, 105, 203, 207, 228, 286, 293, 306
Gender roles, 27, 67
Health concerns and status, general, 6, 7
Heart attack risk among women, 284, 287
HIV infection rates and transmission, 331–332, 339
Hormone replacement therapy, 91, 284, 297, 353
Hormones, female, 87–91
Infertility, female, 98–99
Life expectancy of women, 7, 355
Marital status, 78
Menopause, 91, 284, 353
Menstrual cycle, 88–91
Migraine, 31
Muscular strength, development of, 243
Osteoporosis, 91, 184, 206, 234, 236, 353
Ovarian cancer, 300–301
Pap tests and pelvic exams, 116, 300, 309
Parenting, single, by women, 81
Pelvic inflammatory disease, 93, 337–338
Post-traumatic stress disorder, 30, 35, 52, 54–55
Poverty rates among older women, 351, 356
Pregnancy and childbirth, 99–111
Premenstrual syndrome and premenstrual dysphoric disorder, 89–91
Psychological disorders among women, 52
Rape, 409–411
Sexual anatomy, female, 86
Sexual health problems and dysfunctions, female, 92–94
Sexual functioning, female, 91–92
Sexual harassment, 412
Sexually transmitted diseases and pregnancy, 106, 333, 337–342
Sexually transmitted diseases, symptoms and special risks among women, 337–341
Stalking and cyberstalking, 407–408
Sterilization, female, 128–129
Stressors and responses to stress among women, 27–28
Tobacco use, rates and special risks among women, 179, 181, 184, 187
Uterine cancer, 300, 309
Violence against women, 403, 405–412

## TOPICS OF SPECIAL CONCERN TO MEN

Aging among men, 91, 349, 351–355
Alcohol abuse and dependence, patterns among men, 175–177
Alcohol metabolism in men, 166
Body composition, 232, 233, 254–257
Body image, negative, 257, 269–271
Cancer and men, 295, 299–300, 303, 309
Cardiovascular disease risk among men, 283–284, 287
Causes of death among men, 4, 7, 287, 355
Cigars and pipes, 185
Circumcision, 86–87
Cluster headaches, 31
Communication styles among men, 71–72, 73
Contraception, male methods, 119–122, 126–128
Dietary recommendations for men, 199, 202, 216, 218, 228–230
Drug use, rates of, 145
Environmental health risks, 429
Family violence, 405–409
Firearm-related injuries, 394, 400, 403, 406, 412
Gambling, 142–143
Gender roles, 27, 67
Health concerns and status, general, 6, 7

Heart attack risk among men, 283–284, 287
HIV infection rates and transmission, 331–332
Homicide, rates among men, 394, 403, 404
Hormones, male, 87–88, 91, 394
Infertility, male, 98–99
Injuries, rates of, 394
Life expectancy of men, 355
Marital status, 78
Motorcycle and moped injuries, 397
Motor vehicle injuries, 395–397
Muscular strength, development of, 243
Oral cancer, 184–185, 303, 305
Parenting, single, by men, 81
Poverty rates among older men, 356
Pregnancy, men's roles, 102, 107
Prostate cancer, 299–300, 305, 309
Psychological disorders among men, 52, 57, 58–59
Rape, 409–411
Schizophrenia, 53, 58–59
Sexual anatomy, male, 86–87
Sexual health problems and dysfunctions, male, 93–94
Sexual functioning, male, 91–92
Sexual harassment, 412
Sexually transmitted diseases, symptoms and special risks among men, 337–341
Spit tobacco, 184–185, 303
Stalking and cyberstalking, 407–408
Sterilization, male, 128
Stressors and responses to stress among men, 27–28
Suicide, 56, 57, 354–355
Testicular cancer, 93, 301, 303
Testicular self-examination, 304
Tobacco use, rates and special risks among men, 179, 181, 184–185
Violent behavior among men, 403–405
Violent deaths of men, 394–395

*Note: The health issues and conditions listed here include those that disproportionately influence or affect women or men. For more information, see the Index under gender, women, men, and any of the special topics listed here.*

## DIVERSITY TOPICS RELATED TO ETHNICITY

Alcohol use and abuse patterns, 175–177
Alcohol metabolism, 166
Asthma, 319, 428
Body image, 269–271
Cancer, rates and risk, 297, 299, 300, 301, 303
Cardiovascular disease patterns and risks, 284, 285, 287
Contraceptive use, patterns of, 130
Cystic fibrosis, 104
Death, attitudes toward, 358, 359
Diabetes, 8, 257–259
Dietary patterns and considerations, 211, 285, 293
Discrimination and health, 9, 34, 285, 428
Drug use, risk and protective factors, 157
Environmental health, 427, 428
Genetic disorders, 7, 8, 104
Glaucoma, 351
Hate crimes, 404
Health disparities, general, 4–9
Health insurance status, 8, 9, 389
Health status and concerns, general, 8–9
Heart disease, 284, 285
Hemochromatosis, 104
HIV/AIDS rates, 332
Homicide rates, 402, 404
Hypertension, 211, 236, 279–280, 285, 293
Lactose intolerance, 104, 210, 224
Lead poisoning, 427, 428
Marketing, targeted, 179, 192
Metabolic syndrome, 285–286
Osteoporosis, 206, 234, 236, 353
Overweight/obesity, rates and trends, 261
Poverty rates among older adults, 356
Prostate cancer, 299–300, 309
Psychological disorders, symptoms and rates, 53, 56
Sickle cell disease, 104
Single-parent families, 81–82
Smoking rates, 179, 181
Stress and discrimination, 27, 34
Suicide rates, 56, 355
Tay-Sachs disease, 104
Thallasemia, 104
Tobacco use, 179, 181
Violence, rates of, 402, 404

*Note: The health issues and conditions listed here include those that disproportionately influence or affect specific U.S. ethnic groups or for which patterns may appear along ethnic lines. For more information, see the Index under ethnicity, culture, names of specific population groups, and any of the topics listed here.*

# Preface

*Core Concepts in Health* has maintained its leadership in the field of health education for more than 25 years. Since we pioneered the concept of self-responsibility for personal health in 1976, hundreds of thousands of students have used our book to become active, informed participants in their own health care. Each edition of *Core Concepts* has brought improvements and refinements, but the principles underlying the book have remained the same. Our commitment to these principles has never been stronger than it is today, and it is reflected as fully in this Brief Edition as in the tenth edition of *Core Concepts* on which this edition is based. We have prepared the Brief Edition to accommodate instructors whose courses afford too little time for the complete range of topics and the level of detail of the larger edition.

## OUR GOALS

Our goals in writing this book can be stated simply:

- To present scientifically based, accurate, up-to-date information in an accessible format
- To involve students in taking responsibility for their health and well-being
- To instill a sense of competence and personal power in students

The first of these goals means making expert knowledge about health and health care available to the individual. *Core Concepts* brings scientifically based, accurate, up-to-date information to students about topics and issues that concern them—exercise, stress, nutrition, weight management, contraception, intimate relationships, HIV infection, drugs, alcohol, and a multitude of others. Current, complete, and straightforward coverage is balanced with user-friendly features designed to make the text appealing. Written in an engaging, easy-to-read style and presented in a colorful, open format, *Core Concepts* invites the student to read, learn, and remember. Boxes, tables, artwork, photographs, and many other features highlight areas of special interest throughout the book.

Our second goal is to involve students in taking responsibility for their health. *Core Concepts* uses innovative pedagogy and unique interactive features to get students thinking about how the material they're reading relates to their lives. We invite them to examine their emotions about the issues under discussion, to consider their personal values and beliefs, and to analyze their health-related behaviors. Beyond this, for students who want to change behaviors that detract from a healthy lifestyle, we offer guidelines and tools, ranging from samples of health journals and personal contracts to detailed assessments and behavior change strategies.

Perhaps our third goal in writing *Core Concepts in Health* is the most important: to instill a sense of competence and personal power in the students who read the book. Everyone has the ability to monitor, understand, and affect his or her health. Although medical and health professionals possess impressive skills and have access to a huge body of knowledge that benefits everyone in our society, people can help to minimize the amount of professional care they actually require in their lifetime by taking care of themselves—taking charge of their health—from an early age. Our hope is that *Core Concepts* will continue to help young people make this exciting discovery—that they have the power to shape their futures.

## ORGANIZATION AND CONTENT OF THE TENTH EDITION

The Brief Edition of *Core Concepts* focuses on the health issues and concerns of greatest importance to students. The general content of this edition remains essentially the same as the ninth edition, with coverage of behavior change, stress, psychological health, intimate relationships and communication, sexuality, substance use and abuse, nutrition, exercise, weight management, cardiovascular disease, cancer, infectious diseases, aging, consumer health, and environmental health.

Taken together, the chapters of the book provide students with a complete guide to promoting and protecting their health, now and through their entire lives, as individuals, as participants in a health care community and system, and as citizens of a planet that also needs to be protected if it is to continue providing human beings with the means to live healthy lives.

For the tenth edition, all chapters were carefully reviewed, revised, and updated. The latest information from scientific and health-related research is incorporated in the text, and newly emerging topics and issues are discussed. The following list gives a sample of some of the current concerns addressed in the tenth edition:

- 2005 Dietary Guidelines for Americans and the USDA's MyPyramid food guidance system
- Physical activity guidelines from the USDA, Surgeon General, ACSM, and other organizations
- Prescription drug safety issues
- Ecstasy, GHB, and other club drugs
- Health problems associated with overweight and obesity, and popular approaches to weight loss
- HIV/AIDS testing and treatment
- Emergency contraception, the patch, the ring, extended cycle oral contraceptives, and other new contraceptive methods
- Glycemic index and response
- Trans fat labeling requirements
- Pre-diabetes and diabetes
- Food safety issues, including mad cow disease and chemical contamination of fish
- Eating disorders and disordered eating
- Avian influenza, SARS, West Nile virus, and other emerging infections
- Parenting styles, conflict resolution, and interfaith partnerships
- Online relationships
- Dietary supplement safety and labeling
- Emergency preparedness

The tenth edition continues to emphasize the development of total wellness, with expanded coverage of spiritual wellness and the close connections between mind and body. Key topics include paths to spiritual wellness; global religious views on tobacco use; the effects of stress on the brain and the immune system; the use of journal writing and spiritual practices to cope with stress; the advantages of volunteering; and the benefits of close connections with others. Chapter 4 includes information on the benefits of intimate relationships and strategies for building and maintaining healthy interpersonal relationships. Suggested journal writing activities on the Web site that accompanies the book help students to further explore their feelings and values.

*Core Concepts* takes care to address the health issues and concerns of an increasingly diverse student population. Although most health concerns are universal—we all need to eat well, exercise, and manage stress, for example—certain differences among people have important implications for health. These differences can be genetic or cultural, based on factors such as ethnicity, socioeconomic status, and age. Where such differences are important for health, they are discussed in the text or in highlight boxes called Dimensions of Diversity (described in greater detail below). For the tenth edition, coverage of ethnic diversity has been expanded. Diversity topics in the tenth edition include factors underlying health disparities, links between ethnicity and certain genetic diseases, the effects of culture on the expression of psychological disorders, high rates of HIV/AIDS among certain groups, and the relationships among ethnicity, poverty, educational attainment, and such risk factors as smoking, overweight, and exposure to pollutants.

Topics related to gender are also given special attention in the tenth edition of *Core Concepts*. Key gender differences as well as issues of particular importance to women or men are discussed in the text and in new highlight boxes called Gender Matters (described below). New and expanded gender-related topics include differences in such areas as responses to stress, risk of depression and suicide, communication styles, health effects from tobacco and alcohol use, heart attack symptoms, life expectancy, dietary needs, body image, and risk of unintentional injuries and violence.

The health field is dynamic, with new discoveries, advances, trends, and theories reported every week. Ongoing research—on the role of diet in cancer prevention, for example, or on new treatments for HIV infection—continually changes our understanding of the human body and how it works in health and disease. For this reason, no health book can claim to have the final word on every topic. Yet within these limits, *Core Concepts* does present the latest available information and scientific thinking on innumerable topics.

To aid students in keeping up with rapidly advancing knowledge about health issues, *Core Concepts* also includes coverage of the Internet, a key source of up-to-date information. Each chapter includes an annotated list of World Wide Web sites that students can use as a launching point for further exploration of important topics. Chapter 1 includes important information about evaluating health-related Web sites.

**WW** Each chapter in the tenth edition is also closely tied to the Web site developed as a companion to the text. Elements marked with the World Wide Web icon have corresponding links and activities on the *Core Concepts in Health* Online Learning Center (www.mhhe.com/inselbrief10e). The Web site and other online supplements are described below in greater detail.

## FEATURES OF THE TENTH EDITION

This Brief Edition of *Core Concepts in Health* builds on the features that attracted and held our readers' interest in the previous editions. One of the most popular features has always been the **boxes,** which allow us to explore a wide range of current topics in greater detail than is possible in the text itself. The boxes are divided into seven categories, each in a different color and marked with a distinctive icon and label. Refer to the table of contents for a complete list of all the boxes in each category.

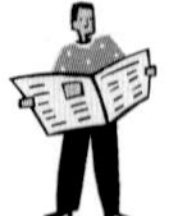

**In the News** boxes focus on current health issues that have recently been highlighted in the media. Most of the In the News boxes are new to the tenth edition; new topics include same-sex marriage, medical innovations, reproductive technology, individual and environmental influences on eating habits, medical marijuana, the next influenza pandemic, problems with antidepressant use in children, and the science and politics of climate change. Each In the News box is accompanied by the World Wide Web icon, indicating that the *Core Concepts* Online Learning Center has links to Internet resources students can use to learn more about the topic of the box.

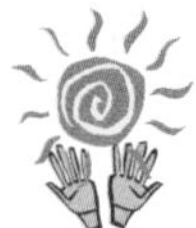

**Mind/Body/Spirit** boxes focus on spiritual wellness and the close connections between people's feelings and states of mind and their physical health. Included in Mind/Body/Spirit boxes are topics such as paths to spiritual wellness, religious views of tobacco use, benefits of being a volunteer, sexual decision making and personal values, the placebo effect, how exercise fosters emotional wellness, and how stress can affect the immune system. Mind/Body/Spirit boxes emphasize that all the dimensions of wellness must be developed for an individual to achieve optimal health and well-being.

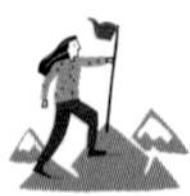

**Take Charge** boxes distill from each chapter the practical advice students need in order to apply information to their own lives. By referring to these boxes, students can easily find ways to foster friendships, for example; to become more physically active; to enhance support in their relationships; to reduce the amount of saturated and trans fats in their diets; to perform deep-breathing exercises for stress reduction; and to help a friend who has a problem with tobacco, drugs, or an eating disorder.

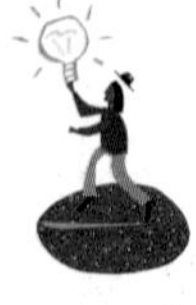

**Critical Consumer** boxes emphasize the key theme of critical thinking by helping students develop and apply critical thinking skills, thereby allowing them to make sound choices related to health and well-being. Critical Consumer boxes provide specific guidelines for evaluating health news and advertising, using food labels to make dietary choices, avoiding quackery, selecting exercise footwear, evaluating dietary supplements, choosing smoking-cessation products, making environmentally friendly shopping choices, and so on.

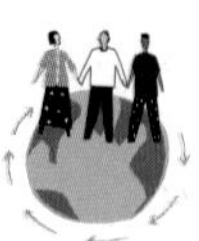

**Dimensions of Diversity** boxes are part of our commitment to reflect and respond to the diversity of the student population. These boxes give students the opportunity to identify any specific health risks that affect them because of who they are as individuals or as members of a group. Most Dimensions of Diversity boxes focus on issues related to U.S. ethnic groups, but some look at other dimensions, including socioeconomic status, age, and ability. Topics covered in these boxes include factors contributing to health disparities among ethnic minorities, diverse populations and stress, ethnic and cultural influences on psychological disorders, risk and protective factors for drug use related to ethnicity, ethnic foods, and exercise for people with special health concerns.

In addition, some Dimensions of Diversity boxes highlight health issues and practices in other parts of the world, allowing students to see what Americans share with people in other societies and how they differ. Students have the opportunity to learn about attitudes toward death in other countries, the pattern of HIV infection around the world, global patterns of violence, and other topics of interest.

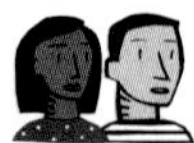

**Gender Matters** boxes, new to the tenth edition, highlight key gender differences related to wellness as well as areas of particular concern to men or women. An overview of key gender-related wellness concerns is provided in Chapter 1. Topics covered in later chapters include gender differences in rates of anxiety, depression, and drug use; in the symptoms and course of heart attack and STDs; and in responses to stress. Other boxes look at pregnancy tasks for fathers and the higher rates of injuries in men.

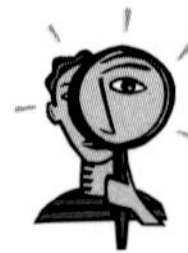

**In Focus** boxes highlight current wellness topics of particular interest. Topics include diabetes, Alzheimer's disease, headaches, carpal tunnel syndrome, and shyness.

In addition to the boxes, many carefully refined features are included in the Brief Tenth Edition of *Core Concepts*. **Vital Statistics** tables and figures highlight important facts and figures in a memorable format that often reveals surprising contrasts and connections. From tables and figures marked with the Vital Statistics label, students can learn about drinking and drug use among college students, alternative medicine use in the United States, world population growth, prevalence of psychological disorders, trends in public opinion about abortion, and a wealth of other information. For students who grasp a subject best when it is displayed graphically, numerically, or in a table, the Vital Statistics feature provides alternative ways of approaching and understanding the text. In addition, for each Vital Statistics table and figure, the *Core*

*Concepts* Online Learning Center has links to sites where students can find the latest statistics and information.

*Core Concepts* features a wealth of attractive and helpful **illustrations.** The anatomical art, which has been prepared by medical illustrators, is both visually appealing and highly informative. These illustrations help students understand such important information as how blood flows through the heart, how alcohol affects the body, and how to use a condom. Other topics illustrated in the tenth edition include diabetes, trends in global temperature, types of stroke, and how exercise affects the body. These lively and abundant illustrations will particularly benefit those students who learn best from visual images.

Chapter-ending **Tips for Today** sections provide brief distillations of the major message of each chapter, followed by suggestions for a few simple things that students can try right away. Tips for Today are designed to encourage students and to build their confidence by giving them easy steps they can take immediately to improve their wellness.

**Take Action,** appearing at the end of every chapter, suggests hands-on exercises and projects that students can undertake to extend and deepen their grasp of the material. Suggested projects include interviews, investigations of campus or community resources, and experimentation with some of the behavior change techniques suggested in the text. Special care has been taken to ensure that the projects are both feasible and worthwhile.

The **Behavior Change Strategies** that conclude many chapters offer specific behavior management/modification plans relating to the chapter's topic. Based on the principles of behavior management that are carefully explained in Chapter 1, these strategies will help students change unhealthy or counterproductive behaviors. Included are strategies for dealing with test anxiety, quitting smoking, planning a personal exercise program, phasing in a healthier diet, and many other practical plans for change.

The **appendix,** "Nutritional Content of Popular Items from Fast-Food Restaurants," provides information on commonly ordered menu items. "Steps for Choking Emergencies" from the Red Cross appears inside the back cover of the text, providing information that can save lives. These guides offer students information they can keep and use for years to come.

Several features from previous editions of *Core Concepts in Health* have been moved to the Online Learning Center. There, you'll find Communicate! exercises, which suggest strategies and activities for improving communication skills to enhance wellness; Journal Entry activities, which help students deepen their understanding of their wellness-related behaviors and become more skilled critical thinkers; and additional information about finding and evaluating Internet resources.

An innovative **built-in Study Guide** is included in the back of the book. Printed on perforated pages for easy removal, the study guide provides sample test questions for each chapter to help students prepare for examinations. Also included are 17 Wellness Worksheets, which provide additional opportunities for self-assessment.

## LEARNING AIDS

Although all the features of *Core Concepts in Health* are designed to facilitate learning, several specific learning aids have been incorporated in the text. Learning objectives labeled **Looking Ahead** appear on the opening page of each chapter, identifying major concepts and helping guide students in their reading and review of the text. Important terms appear in boldface type in the text and are defined in a **running glossary,** helping students handle a large and complex new vocabulary.

**Chapter summaries** offer a concise review and a way to make sure students have grasped the most important concepts in the chapter. **For More Information** sections contain annotated lists of books, newsletters, hotlines, organizations, and Web sites that students can use to extend and broaden their knowledge or pursue subjects of interest to them. Also found at the end of every chapter are **Selected Bibliographies.** A complete **Index** at the end of the book includes references to glossary terms in boldface type.

## TEACHING TOOLS

Available with the Brief Tenth Edition of *Core Concepts in Health* is a comprehensive package of supplementary materials designed to enhance teaching and learning.

### Interactive Instructor's CD-ROM

The **Interactive Instructor's CD-ROM** (ISBN 0-07-297237-8) presents key teaching resources in an easy-to-use format. It is organized by chapter and works in both Windows and Macintosh environments. It includes the following teaching tools:

- The **Course Integrator Guide** includes learning objectives, extended chapter outlines, suggested activities, and lists of additional resources. It also describes all the print and electronic supplements available with the text and shows how to integrate them into lectures and assignments for each chapter. For the tenth edition, the guide was prepared by Cathy Kennedy, Colorado State University.
- The **test bank** includes more than 1500 true-false, multiple choice, and short essay questions; it also

..cludes two 100-question multiple choice tests that cover the content of the entire text. The answer key lists the page number in the text where each answer is found. Contributors to the tenth edition test bank are Phil Kelly, Salem State University; Karen Vail-Smith, East Carolina University; and Kathy McGinnis, San Diego City College. Special thanks also go to our test bank reviewer panel: Phil Kelly; Betty Shepherd, Virginia Western Community College; Charla Blumell, East Carolina University; and Susan Moore, Western Illinois University.

The test bank is available on the Instructor's CD-ROM as Word files and with the EZ Test **computerized testing software.** EZ Test provides a powerful, easy-to-use test maker to create printed quizzes and exams. EZ Test runs on both Windows and Macintosh systems. For secure online testing, exams created in EZ Test can be exported to WebCT, Blackboard, PageOut, and (beginning fall 2005) EZ Test Online. The EZ Test CD is packaged with a Quick Start Guide; once the program is installed, users have access to the complete User's Manual, including multiple Flash tutorials. Additional help is available at www.mhhe.com/eztest.

- The **PowerPoint slides,** expanded for the tenth edition, provide a lecture tool that you can alter or expand to meet the needs of your course. The slides include key lecture points and images from the text and other sources. For the tenth edition, the PowerPoint presentations were created by Andrew Shim, Indiana University of Pennsylvania. As an aid for instructors who wish to create their own presentations, a complete **image bank,** including all the illustrations from the text, is also included on the Instructor's CD-ROM.
- **Transparency masters and handouts**—more than 150 in all—are provided as additional lecture resources. The transparency masters feature tables showing key statistics and data, illustrations from the text and other sources, and key points from the text. Illustrations of many body systems are also provided. The student handouts provide additional information and can be used to extend student knowledge on topics such as prediabetes, glycemic index, yoga for relaxation, and dealing with alcohol emergencies.
- A complete set of **Wellness Worksheets** (ISBN 0-07-297649-7), a student learning aid described below, is also included on the Instructor's CD-ROM

Printed versions of key supplements—the Course Integrator Guide, test bank, transparency masters, handouts, and Wellness Worksheets—are also available (ISBN 0-07-310568-6). The printed supplements are loose-leaf and three-hole-punched, ready to be placed in a binder.

## Video and Other Visual Resources

A variety of visual resources is available for use with *Core Concepts in Health.*

- **Resource Presentation Manager CD-ROM** (ISBN 0-07-310567-8), new for the tenth edition, is a presentation tool with chapter-specific video clips and images designed to engage students and promote critical thinking and dialogue on relevant topics in personal health. The searchable library contains contemporary student interviews, news clips, and historical health videos on body image, depression, stress, genetics, spirituality, and many other topics. Each video clip is accompanied by an Instructor Guide that describes the objective of the clip and gives critical thinking questions to ask before the clip is shown and discussion questions to use for follow-up.
- A set of 80 color **Transparency Acetates** (ISBN 0-07-310562-7) is available as a lecture resource. The acetates are not duplicates the transparency masters on the Instructor's CD-ROM; many are from sources other than the text.

Videos from Films for Humanities are also available.

## Digital Solutions

The *Core Concepts in Health* **Online Learning Center** (www.mhhe.com/inselbrief10e) provides many additional resources for both instructors and students. Instructor tools include downloadable versions of the Course Integrator Guide and all the PowerPoint slides, links to professional resources, and a guide to using the Internet. For students, there are learning objectives, self-quizzes and glossary flashcards for review, interactive Internet activities, and extensive links. The Online Learning Center also includes many tools for wellness behavior change, such as interactive versions of the Wellness Worksheets and a workbook for behavior change. Through the Online Learning Center, students can also access **PowerWeb** (www.dushkin.com/online) resources, including articles on key health topics, self-scoring quizzes, interactive exercises, study tips, and a daily news feed.

The **Online Wellness Workbook** (ISBN 0-07-310566-X), developed in collaboration with Quia™, offers an electronic version of assessments and quizzes compiled from the text and its main supplements. This new online supplement provides students with interactive assessments, self-scoring quizzes, and instant feedback. Benefits for instructors include a gradebook that automatically scores, tracks, and records students' results; it also offers instructors the opportunity to review individual and class performance and customize activities and features for their course. Access to the Quia™ Online Wellness Workbook can be packaged with the text for a small additional fee.

**Classroom Performance System (CPS)** brings interactivity into the classroom or lecture hall. CPS is a wireless response system that gives instructors and students immediate feedback from the entire class. Each student uses a wireless response pad similar to a television remote to respond instantly to polling or quiz questions. Contact your local sales representative for more information about using CPS with *Core Concepts in Health*.

**PageOut** (www.pageout.net) is a free, easy-to-use program that enables instructors to quickly develop Web sites for their courses. PageOut can be used to create a course home page, an instructor home page, an interactive syllabus that can be linked to elements in the Online Learning Center, Web links, online discussion areas, an online gradebook, and much more.

Instructors can combine Online Learning Center resources with popular **course-management systems.** The McGraw-Hill Instructor Advantage program offers access to a complete online teaching Web site called the Knowledge Gateway, toll-free phone support, and unlimited e-mail support directly from WebCT and Blackboard. Instructors who use 500 or more copies of a text can enroll in the Instructor Advantage Plus program, which provides on-campus, hands-on training from a certified platform specialist.

For more information about McGraw-Hill's digital resources, including how to obtain passwords for PageOut and PowerWeb, contact your local representative or visit McGraw-Hill on the Internet (www.mhhe.com/solutions).

## Student Resources Available with Core Concepts in Health

Students who purchase a new copy of *Core Concepts* receive free access to **premium resources on the Online Learning Center.** These premium resources include interactive self-assessments, articles on health and human performance, and a daily news feed. Students who purchase a used copy of the text can purchase access to the premium resources by visiting the Online Learning Center (www.mhhe.com/inselbrief10e).

Many other resources are available to help students learn and apply key concepts; contact your local representative to find out more about packaging any of the following with *Core Concepts in Health*.

- More than 100 **Wellness Worksheets** (ISBN 0-07-297649-7) are available to help students become more involved in their wellness and better prepared to implement successful behavior change. The worksheets include assessment tools, Internet activities, and knowledge-based reviews of key concepts. They are available shrink-wrapped with the text in an easy-to-use pad and in the premium resources section of the Online Learning Center.
- **NutritionCalc Plus** (ISBN 0-07-292126-9) is a dietary analysis program with an easy-to-use interface that allows users to track their nutrient and food group intakes, energy expenditures, and weight control goals. It generates a variety of reports and graphs for analysis, including comparisons with the latest Dietary Reference Intakes (DRIs). The ESHA database includes thousands of ethnic foods, supplements, fast foods, and convenience foods, and users can add their own foods to the food list. NutritionCalc Plus is available on CD-ROM (Windows only) or as an online version.
- **The Daily Fitness and Nutrition Journal** (ISBN 0-07-284432-9) is a handy booklet that guides students in planning and tracking a fitness program. It also helps students assess their current diet and make appropriate changes.
- The **Health and Fitness Pedometer** (ISBN 0-07-320933-3) can be packaged with copies of the text. It allows students to count their daily steps and track their level of physical activity.
- The interactive **HealthQuest CD-ROM** (ISBN 0-07-295117-6) helps students explore and change their wellness behavior. It includes tutorials, assessments, and behavior change guidelines in such key areas as stress, fitness, nutrition, cardiovascular disease, cancer, tobacco, and alcohol.

Additional supplements and many packaging options are available; check with your McGraw-Hill sales representative.

## A NOTE OF THANKS

The efforts of innumerable people have gone into producing this tenth edition of *Core Concepts in Health*. The book has benefited immensely from their thoughtful commentaries, expert knowledge and opinions, and many helpful suggestions. We are deeply grateful for their participation in the project.

### Academic Contributors

Virginia Brooke, Ph.D., University of Texas Medical Branch at Galveston
*The Challenge of Aging*

Theodore C. Dumas, Ph.D., Institute of Neuroscience, University of Oregon
*Stress: The Constant Challenge*

Thomas D. Fahey, Ed.D., California State University, Chico
*Exercise for Health and Fitness*

Samuel Goth, Ph.D., Center for Children's Environmental Health, University of California, Davis
*Immunity and Infection*

Michael R. Hoadley, Ph.D., Assistant Vice-President for Academic Affairs, Center for Academic Technology Support, Eastern Illinois University

ersonal Safety: Protecting Yourself from Unintentional Injuries and Violence*

Paul M. Insel, Ph.D., Stanford University
*Taking Charge of Your Health*

Nancy Kemp, M.D.
*Alcohol and Tobacco; Immunity and Infection*

Charles Ksir, Ph.D., University of Wyoming
*The Use and Abuse of Psychoactive Drugs*

Howard Lee, M.D., M.P.H., Health Officer, Colusa County Department of Health and Human Services
*Cardiovascular Disease and Cancer*

Tova Marx, Ph.D.
*Intimate Relationships and Communication*

Nancy E. Mason, M.D., Department of Gynecology and Obstetrics, Stanford University School of Medicine
*Contraception and Abortion; Sexuality, Pregnancy, and Childbirth*

David Quadagno, Ph.D., Florida State University
*Sexuality, Pregnancy, and Childbirth*

Jacob W. Roth, M.D., Dana Farber Cancer Institute, Harvard University
*The Challenge of Aging*

Walton T. Roth, M.D., Stanford University
*Psychological Health*

James H. Rothenberger, M.P.H., University of Minnesota
*Environmental Health*

Judith Sharlin, Ph.D., R.D., Department of Nutrition, Simmons College
*Weight Management*

David S. Sobel, M.D., M.P.H., Director of Patient Education and Health Promotion, Kaiser Permanente Northern California
*Conventional and Complementary Medicine: Skills for the Health Care Consumer*

Mae V. Tinklenbeg, R.N., N.P., M.S.
*Contraception and Abortion*

Jennifer A. Tremmel, M.D., S.M., Department of Cardiovascular Medicine, Stanford University Medical Center
*Cardiovascular Disease and Cancer*

R. Elaine Turner, Ph.D., R.D., University of Florida
*Nutrition Basics*

Patrick Zickler, Senior Science Writer, Masimax Resources, Inc.
*Alcohol and Tobacco*

## Academic Advisers and Reviewers of the Tenth Edition

Charlene Brown, Western Michigan University

Mary V. Brown, Utah Valley State College

Susan T. Burge, Cuyahoga Community College

Laura Burger, Grossmont College

Karen Camarata, Eastern Kentucky University

Jacquie Cottingham, Confederation College

Paula J. Dahl, Bakersfield College

Kathi Deresinski, Triton College

P. K. Doyle-Baker, University of Calgary

Maqsood M. Faquir, Palm Beach Community College

Kathi Fuller, Western Michigan University

Cathy Hammond, Morehead State University

Mary E. Iten, University of Nebraska at Kearney

Belinda L. Jones, North Carolina Central University

Roland J. Lamarine, California State University, Chico

Teresa A. Lyles, University of Florida

Susan A. Lyman, University of Louisiana at Lafayette

Lori S. Mallory, Johnson County Community College

Tom Pestolesi, Irvine Valley College

Roseann L. Poole, Tallahassee Community College

Donna Jeanne Pugh, Florida Metropolitan University

Bruce M. Ragon, Albany State University

Priscilla Rice, Bucks County Community College

Leah E. Robinson, Bucks County Community College

Stafford C. Rorke, Oakland University

Andrew Shim, Indiana University of Pennsylvania

Carol A. Smith, Elon University

Phillip B. Sparling, Georgia Institute of Technology

Debra Tavasso, East Carolina University

Finally, we would like to thank the members of the *Core Concepts* book team at McGraw-Hill Higher Education. First, we are indebted to Kirstan Price for her dedication and her extraordinary creative energies, which have helped to make this book such a success. Thanks also go to Nick Barrett, executive editor; Julia Ersery, developmental editor for technology; Pam Cooper, senior marketing manager; Sarah Hill, editorial assistant; Lance Gerhart, media producer; Ron Nelms, media project manager; Brett Coker, production editor; Randy Hurst, production supervisor; Violeta Díaz, design manager; Robin Mouat, art manager; Brian Pecko, photo researcher; and Marty Granahan, permissions editor. To all we express our deep appreciation.

*Paul M. Insel*
*Walton T. Roth*

# A Guided Tour of *Core Concepts in Health*

Are you looking for ways to improve your health behaviors and quality of life? Do you need help finding reliable wellness resources online? Would you like to boost your grade? *Core Concepts in Health* can help you do all this and much more!



## BUILT-IN STUDY GUIDE

The built-in Study Guide includes sample test questions to help you prepare for exams and Wellness Worksheets to help you assess your current level of wellness. The Worksheets are marked with a World Wide Web icon to indicate that you can find them in an interactive format on the *Core Concepts in Health Online* Learning Center (www.mhhe.com/inselbrief10e). Look for this Web icon throughout the text to identify elements to have corresponding activities and links on the Online Learning Center. For courses using the Quia™ Online Wellness Workbook, the self-assessments from the text are also available in the Workbook.

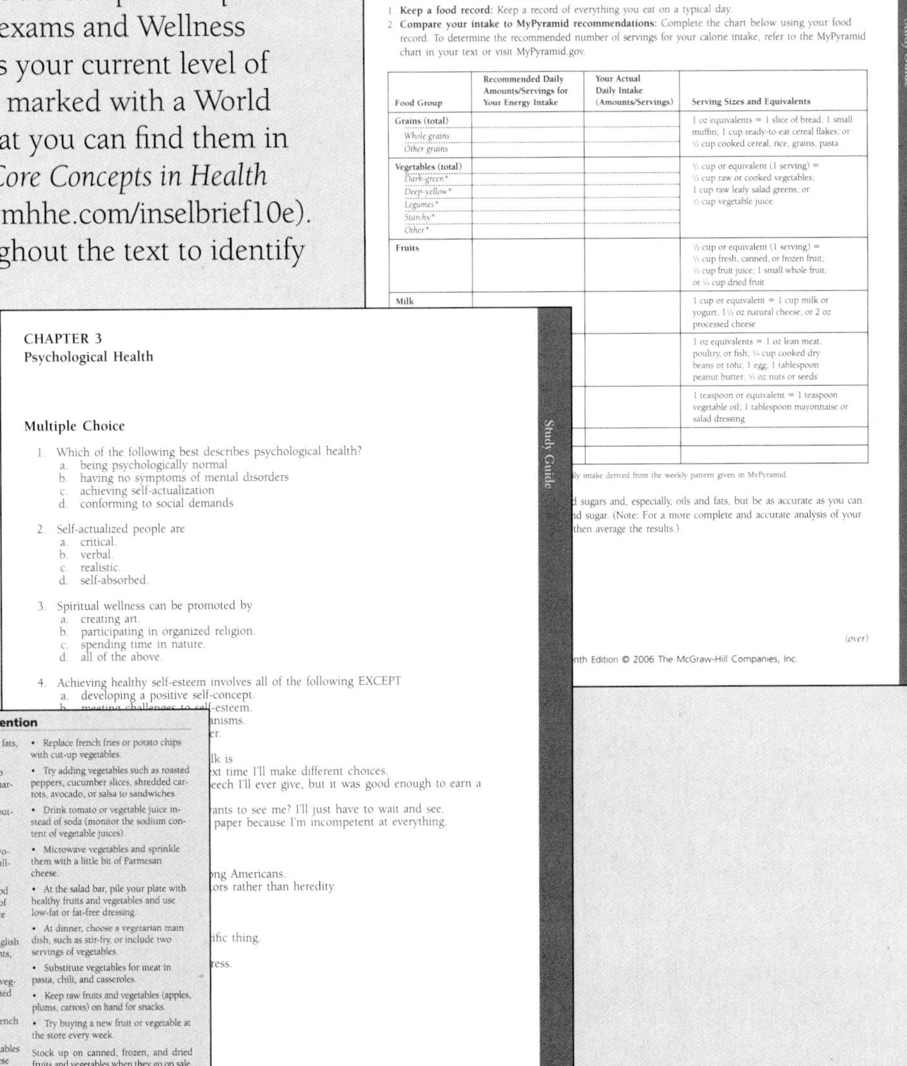

Name ______ Section ______ Date ______

**WELLNESS WORKSHEET S9**

Your Daily Diet Versus MyPyramid Recommendations

1. **Keep a food record:** Keep a record of everything you eat on a typical day.
2. **Compare your intake to MyPyramid recommendations:** Complete the chart below using your food record. To determine the recommended number of servings for your calorie intake, refer to the MyPyramid chart in your text or visit MyPyramid.gov.

| Food Group | Recommended Daily Amounts/Servings for Your Energy Intake | Your Actual Daily Intake (Amounts/Servings) | Serving Sizes and Equivalents |
|---|---|---|---|
| **Grains (total)** | | | 1 oz equivalents = 1 slice of bread; 1 small muffin; 1 cup ready-to-eat cereal flakes; or ½ cup cooked cereal, rice, grains, pasta |
| *Whole grains* | | | |
| *Other grains* | | | |
| **Vegetables (total)** | | | ½ cup or equivalent (1 serving) = ½ cup raw or cooked vegetables; 1 cup raw leafy salad greens; or ½ cup vegetable juice |
| *Dark-green** | | | |
| *Deep-yellow** | | | |
| *Legumes** | | | |
| *Starchy** | | | |
| *Other** | | | |
| **Fruits** | | | ½ cup or equivalent (1 serving) = ½ cup fresh, canned, or frozen fruit; ½ cup fruit juice; 1 small whole fruit; or ¼ cup dried fruit |
| **Milk** | | | 1 cup or equivalent = 1 cup milk or yogurt; 1½ oz natural cheese; or 2 oz processed cheese |
| | | | 1 oz equivalents = 1 oz lean meat, poultry, or fish; ¼ cup cooked dry beans or tofu; 1 egg; 1 tablespoon peanut butter; ½ oz nuts or seeds |
| | | | 1 teaspoon or equivalent = 1 teaspoon vegetable oil; 1 tablespoon mayonnaise or salad dressing |
| | | | |
| | | | |

...ly intake derived from the weekly pattern given in MyPyramid.

...d sugars and, especially, oils and fats, but be as accurate as you can. ...nd sugar. (Note: For a more complete and accurate analysis of your ...then average the results.)

*(over)*

...nth Edition © 2006 The McGraw-Hill Companies, Inc.

Study Guide

CHAPTER 3
Psychological Health

**Multiple Choice**

1. Which of the following best describes psychological health?
   a. being psychologically normal
   b. having no symptoms of mental disorders
   c. achieving self-actualization
   d. conforming to social demands
2. Self-actualized people are
   a. critical.
   b. verbal.
   c. realistic.
   d. self-absorbed.
3. Spiritual wellness can be promoted by
   a. creating art.
   b. participating in organized religion.
   c. spending time in nature.
   d. all of the above.
4. Achieving healthy self-esteem involves all of the following EXCEPT
   a. developing a positive self-concept.
   b. meeting challenges to self-esteem.

...anisms. ...er. ...lk is ...xt time I'll make different choices. ...eech I'll ever give, but it was good enough to earn a ...ants to see me? I'll just have to wait and see. ... paper because I'm incompetent at everything. ...ng Americans. ...ors rather than heredity. ...ific thing. ...ress.

Study Guide

**Modifying Your Diet for Heart Health and Cancer Prevention**

Behavior Change Strategy

Gradually modifying your diet to include less saturated and trans fat and more fruits and vegetables can help you avoid both CVD and cancer in the future. Begin by assessing your current diet. Keep a record in your health journal of everything you eat for a week. At the end of the week, you can evaluate your diet and start taking steps to modify it.

**Reducing Saturated and Trans Fat in Your Diet**

The American Heart Association recommends that no more than 10% of the calories in your diet come from saturated and trans fat. Foods high in these fats include meat, poultry skin, full-fat dairy products, coconut and palm oils, and products made with hydrogenated vegetable oils, such as deep-fried fast food and packaged baked goods. To find out if your diet is within the 10% recommendation, at the end of the week, record the grams of saturated and trans fat next to the foods you've listed in your health journal. This information is available on many food labels, in books, and on the Internet. For fast foods, use the Appendix. Trans fat content can be more difficult to determine. Here are the average values per serving for a few trans fat–rich foods: french fries (large), 5 g; pound cake, 5 g; doughnut, 4 g; fried breaded chicken, 3 g; Danish pastry, 3 g; vegetable shortening, 3 g; sandwich cookies, 2 g; crackers, 2 g; margarine (stick), 2 g; margarine (tub), 1 g.

Once you have the grams of fat listed, add up what you consumed each day. For a 1600-calorie diet, the 10% limit corresponds to 18 grams of saturated and trans fat; for a 2200-calorie diet, it corresponds to 24 grams; and for a 2800-calorie diet, it corresponds to 31 grams. (If you have high cholesterol, you may want to follow the 7% limit set by the NCEP, which corresponds to 12 grams of saturated and trans fat in a 1600-calorie diet, 17 grams in a 2200-calorie diet, and 22 grams in a 2800-calorie diet.) If you're not able to get all the data you need, estimate by looking at the number of servings of food high in saturated or trans fat you consume in a day.

If your diet is higher in these fats than it should be, look at your food record to see if you are choosing high-fat foods more often than you should. To reduce your intake of saturated and trans fats, try making healthy substitutions:

- Vegetable oils or trans fat–free tub margarine rather than butter, stick margarine, or vegetable shortening
- Fruits, vegetables, rice cakes, unbuttered popcorn, or pretzels instead of chips, crackers, or cheese puffs
- Low-fat or fat-free milk, cheese, yogurt, or mayonnaise instead of the full-fat versions
- Fruit or a low-fat sweet (angel food cake, frozen yogurt, sorbet) instead of cakes, cookies, pastries, or regular ice cream
- Whole-grain breads and rolls, English muffins, or bagels instead of croissants, muffins, or coffee cake
- Lean meat, skinless poultry, or a veggie burger instead of ground beef, fried chicken, or lunch meats
- Baked potato or rice instead of french fries or onion rings
- Vegetarian chili or pasta with vegetables instead of pizza or macaroni and cheese

When you do eat high-fat foods, eat smaller portions, and balance your higher-fat choices with low-fat choices over the course of the day.

**Increasing Fruits and Vegetables in Your Diet**

Many fruits and vegetables contain phytochemicals, compounds that help slow, stop, or even reverse the process of cancer. For this reason, the National Cancer Institute (NCI) has developed the "Eat 5 to 9 a Day for Better Health" program to help Americans increase their consumption of fruits and vegetables to health-promoting levels. Take a look at the foods you've listed in your health journal for a week. Have you included five or more fruits and vegetables each day? If not, here are some tips from the NCI:

- Drink 100% juice every morning.
- Add raisins, berries, or sliced fruit to cereal; top bagels with tomato slices.
- Make a fruit smoothie from fresh or frozen fruit and orange juice or low-fat yogurt.
- Have vegetable soup or a salad with your lunch.
- Replace french fries or potato chips with cut-up vegetables.
- Try adding vegetables such as roasted peppers, cucumber slices, shredded carrots, avocado, or salsa to sandwiches.
- Drink tomato or vegetable juice instead of soda (monitor the sodium content of vegetable juices).
- Microwave vegetables and sprinkle them with a little bit of Parmesan cheese.
- At the salad bar, pile your plate with healthy fruits and vegetables and use low-fat or fat-free dressing.
- At dinner, choose a vegetarian main dish, such as stir-fry, or include two servings of vegetables.
- Substitute vegetables for meat in pasta, chili, and casseroles.
- Keep raw fruits and vegetables (apples, plums, carrots) on hand for snacks.
- Try buying a new fruit or vegetable at the store every week.

Stock up on canned, frozen, and dried fruits and vegetables when they go on sale. Buy fresh fruits and vegetables in season; they'll taste best and be less expensive.

Some fruits and vegetables are particularly rich in phytochemicals; choose them as often as you can. They include cruciferous vegetables (e.g., broccoli, cauliflower, cabbage, bok choy, brussels sprouts); citrus fruits (e.g., oranges, lemons, grapefruit); berries (e.g., strawberries, raspberries); dark-green leafy vegetables (e.g., spinach, chard, romaine lettuce); and deep-yellow, orange, and red fruits and vegetables (e.g., carrots, red and yellow bell peppers, winter squash, cantaloupe, apricots).

With a little attention and effort, you can modify your diet now, with steps like these, to help safeguard yourself from CVD and cancer in the future.

SOURCES: American Heart Association. 2000. *An Eating Plan for Healthy Americans: The New 2000 Food Guidelines*. Dallas, Tex.: American Heart Association; Food and Drug Administration. 1999. *Questions and Answers on Trans Fat Proposed Rule* (http://vm.cfsan.fda.gov/~dms/qa-trans.html); Center for Science in the Public Interest. 1997. The sat fat switch. *Nutrition Action Healthletter*, January/February; National Cancer Institute. 2000. *Eat 5 to 9 A Day for Better Health* (http://www.5aday.gov, retrieved March 25, 2005); Welland, D. 1999. Fruits and vegetables: Easy ways to five-a-day. *Environmental Nutrition*, June.

www.mhhe.com/inselbrief10e    Summary 311

## BEHAVIOR CHANGE STRATEGIES

Behavior Change Strategies provide specific behavior change plans for particular areas of wellness. Included are strategies for dealing with test anxiety, developing responsible drinking habits, quitting tobacco use, improving diet, planning a personal exercise program, and many other practical plans for change.

GUIDED TOUR

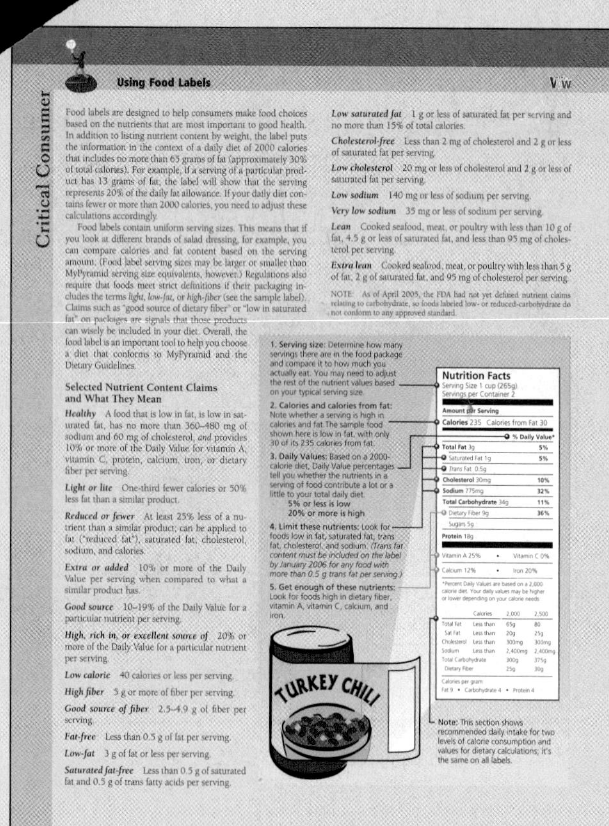

Critical Consumer

## Using Food Labels

V W

Food labels are designed to help consumers make food choices based on the nutrients that are most important to good health. In addition to listing nutrient content by weight, the label puts the information in the context of a daily diet of 2000 calories that includes no more than 65 grams of fat (approximately 30% of total calories). For example, if a serving of a particular product has 13 grams of fat, the label will show that the serving represents 20% of the daily fat allowance. If your daily diet contains fewer or more than 2000 calories, you need to adjust these calculations accordingly.

Food labels contain uniform serving sizes. This means that if you look at different brands of salad dressing, for example, you can compare calories and fat content based on the serving amount. (Food label serving sizes may be larger or smaller than MyPyramid serving size equivalents, however.) Regulations also require that foods meet strict definitions if their packaging includes the terms *light*, *low-fat*, or *high-fiber* (see the sample label). Claims such as "good source of dietary fiber" or "low in saturated fat" on packages are signals that those products can wisely be included in your diet. Overall, the food label is an important tool to help you choose a diet that conforms to MyPyramid and the Dietary Guidelines.

### Selected Nutrient Content Claims and What They Mean

***Healthy*** A food that is low in fat, is low in saturated fat, has no more than 360–480 mg of sodium and 60 mg of cholesterol, *and* provides 10% or more of the Daily Value for vitamin A, vitamin C, protein, calcium, iron, or dietary fiber per serving.

***Light or lite*** One-third fewer calories or 50% less fat than a similar product.

***Reduced or fewer*** At least 25% less of a nutrient than a similar product; can be applied to fat ("reduced fat"), saturated fat, cholesterol, sodium, and calories.

***Extra or added*** 10% or more of the Daily Value per serving when compared to what a similar product has.

***Good source*** 10–19% of the Daily Value for a particular nutrient per serving.

***High, rich in, or excellent source of*** 20% or more of the Daily Value for a particular nutrient per serving.

***Low calorie*** 40 calories or less per serving.

***High fiber*** 5 g or more of fiber per serving.

***Good source of fiber*** 2.5–4.9 g of fiber per serving.

***Fat-free*** Less than 0.5 g of fat per serving.

***Low-fat*** 3 g of fat or less per serving.

***Saturated fat-free*** Less than 0.5 g of saturated fat and 0.5 g of trans fatty acids per serving.

***Low saturated fat*** 1 g or less of saturated fat per serving and no more than 15% of total calories.

***Cholesterol-free*** Less than 2 mg of cholesterol and 2 g or less of saturated fat per serving.

***Low cholesterol*** 20 mg or less of cholesterol and 2 g or less of saturated fat per serving.

***Low sodium*** 140 mg or less of sodium per serving.

***Very low sodium*** 35 mg or less of sodium per serving.

***Lean*** Cooked seafood, meat, or poultry with less than 10 g of fat, 4.5 g or less of saturated fat, and less than 95 mg of cholesterol per serving.

***Extra lean*** Cooked seafood, meat, or poultry with less than 5 g of fat, 2 g of saturated fat, and 95 mg of cholesterol per serving.

NOTE: As of April 2005, the FDA had not yet defined nutrient claims relating to carbohydrate, so foods labeled low- or reduced-carbohydrate do not conform to any approved standard.

**1. Serving size:** Determine how many servings there are in the food package and compare it to how much you actually eat. You may need to adjust the rest of the nutrient values based on your typical serving size.

**2. Calories and calories from fat:** Note whether a serving is high in calories and fat. The sample food shown here is low in fat, with only 30 of its 235 calories from fat.

**3. Daily Values:** Based on a 2000-calorie diet, Daily Value percentages tell you whether the nutrients in a serving of food contribute a lot or a little to your total daily diet.
**5% or less is low**
**20% or more is high**

**4. Limit these nutrients:** Look for foods low in fat, saturated fat, trans fat, cholesterol, and sodium. *(Trans fat content must be included on the label by January 2006 for any food with more than 0.5 g trans fat per serving.)*

**5. Get enough of these nutrients:** Look for foods high in dietary fiber, vitamin A, vitamin C, calcium, and iron.

**Nutrition Facts**
Serving Size 1 cup (265g)
Servings per Container 2

**Amount per Serving**
**Calories** 235 Calories from Fat 30

| | % Daily Value* |
|---|---|
| **Total Fat** 3g | 5% |
| Saturated Fat 1g | 5% |
| *Trans* Fat 0.5g | |
| **Cholesterol** 30mg | 10% |
| **Sodium** 775mg | 32% |
| **Total Carbohydrate** 34g | 11% |
| Dietary Fiber 9g | 36% |
| Sugars 5g | |
| **Protein** 18g | |

Vitamin A 25% • Vitamin C 0%
Calcium 12% • Iron 20%

*Percent Daily Values are based on a 2,000 calorie diet. Your daily values may be higher or lower depending on your calorie needs.

| | Calories | 2,000 | 2,500 |
|---|---|---|---|
| Total Fat | Less than | 65g | 80 |
| Sat Fat | Less than | 20g | 25g |
| Cholesterol | Less than | 300mg | 300mg |
| Sodium | Less than | 2,400mg | 2,400mg |
| Total Carbohydrate | | 300g | 375g |
| Dietary Fiber | | 25g | 30g |

Calories per gram:
Fat 9 • Carbohydrate 4 • Protein 4



**Note:** This section shows recommended daily intake for two levels of calorie consumption and values for dietary calculations; it's the same on all labels.

# CRITICAL CONSUMER BOXES

Critical Consumer boxes are designed to help you develop and apply critical thinking skills so you can make sound choices related to wellness. Included are guidelines for evaluating health news and advertising, popular diets, and food and supplement labels; for choosing smoking cessation products, exercise footwear, and bicycle helments; for making environmentally-friendly shopping choices; and much more.

# TAKE CHARGE BOXES

Take Charge boxes present the practical advice you need to apply information from the text to your own life and to take charge of your health. Take Charge topics include breathing techniques for relaxation; guidelines for dealing with an alcohol emergency; and strategies for judging portion sizes, increasing physical activity, and improving communication.

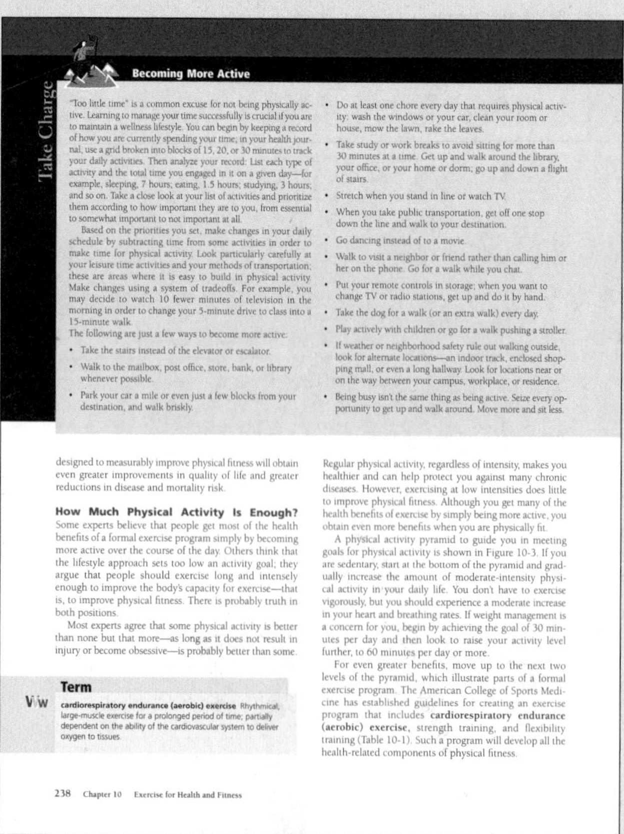

Take Charge

## Becoming More Active

"Too little time" is a common excuse for not being physically active. Learning to manage your time successfully is crucial if you are to maintain a wellness lifestyle. You can begin by keeping a record of how you are currently spending your time; in your health journal, use a grid broken into blocks of 15, 20, or 30 minutes to track your daily activities. Then analyze your record: List each type of activity and the total time you engaged in it on a given day—for example, sleeping, 7 hours; eating, 1.5 hours; studying, 3 hours; and so on. Take a close look at your list of activities and prioritize them according to how important they are to you, from essential to somewhat important to not important at all.

Based on the priorities you set, make changes in your daily schedule by subtracting time from some activities in order to make time for physical activity. Look particularly carefully at your leisure time activities and your methods of transportation; these are areas where it is easy to build in physical activity. Make changes using a system of tradeoffs. For example, you may decide to watch 10 fewer minutes of television in the morning in order to change your 5-minute drive to class into a 15-minute walk.

The following are just a few ways to become more active:

- Take the stairs instead of the elevator or escalator.
- Walk to the mailbox, post office, store, bank, or library whenever possible.
- Park your car a mile or even just a few blocks from your destination, and walk briskly.
- Do at least one chore every day that requires physical activity: wash the windows or your car, clean your room or house, mow the lawn, rake the leaves.
- Take study or work breaks to avoid sitting for more than 30 minutes at a time. Get up and walk around the library, your office, or your home or dorm; go up and down a flight of stairs.
- Stretch when you stand in line or watch TV.
- When you take public transportation, get off one stop down the line and walk to your destination.
- Go dancing instead of to a movie.
- Walk to visit a neighbor or friend rather than calling him or her on the phone. Go for a walk while you chat.
- Put your remote controls in storage; when you want to change TV or radio stations, get up and do it by hand.
- Take the dog for a walk (or an extra walk) every day.
- Play actively with children or go for a walk pushing a stroller.
- If weather or neighborhood safety rule out walking outside, look for alternate locations—an indoor track, enclosed shopping mall, or even a long hallway. Look for locations near or on the way between your campus, workplace, or residence.
- Being busy isn't the same thing as being active. Seize every opportunity to get up and walk around. Move more and sit less.

designed to measurably improve physical fitness will obtain even greater improvements in quality of life and greater reductions in disease and mortality risk.

**How Much Physical Activity Is Enough?** Some experts believe that people get most of the health benefits of a formal exercise program simply by becoming more active over the course of the day. Others think that the lifestyle approach sets too low an activity goal; they argue that people should exercise long and intensely enough to improve the body's capacity for exercise—that is, to improve physical fitness. There is probably truth in both positions.

Most experts agree that some physical activity is better than none but that more—as long as it does not result in injury or become obsessive—is probably better than some.

**Term**

V W **cardiorespiratory endurance (aerobic) exercise** Rhythmical, large-muscle exercise for a prolonged period of time; partially dependent on the ability of the cardiovascular system to deliver oxygen to tissues.

Regular physical activity, regardless of intensity, makes you healthier and can help protect you against many chronic diseases. However, exercising at low intensities does little to improve physical fitness. Although you get many of the health benefits of exercise by simply being more active, you obtain even more benefits when you are physically fit.

A physical activity pyramid to guide you in meeting goals for physical activity is shown in Figure 10-3. If you are sedentary, start at the bottom of the pyramid and gradually increase the amount of moderate-intensity physical activity in your daily life. You don't have to exercise vigorously, but you should experience a moderate increase in your heart and breathing rates. If weight management is a concern for you, begin by achieving the goal of 30 minutes per day and then look to raise your activity level further, to 60 minutes per day or more.

For even greater benefits, move up to the next two levels of the pyramid, which illustrate parts of a formal exercise program. The American College of Sports Medicine has established guidelines for creating an exercise program that includes **cardiorespiratory endurance (aerobic) exercise**, strength training, and flexibility training (Table 10-1). Such a program will develop all the health-related components of physical fitness.

238 Chapter 10 Exercise for Health and Fitness

## MIND/BODY/SPIRIT BOXES

Mind/Body/Spirit boxes focus on the close connections among people's feelings, states of mind, and physical health. Topics include religious views of tobacco use, sexual decision making and personal values, benefits of being a volunteer, exercise and self-esteem, and characteristics of a good death.

Mind/Body/Spirit

**Help Yourself by Helping Others**

Choosing to help others—whether as a volunteer for a community organization or through spontaneous acts of kindness—can enhance emotional, social, spiritual, and physical wellness. In a national survey of volunteers from all fields, helpers reported the following benefits:

- "Helper's high"—physical and emotional sensations such as sudden warmth, a surge of energy, and a feeling of euphoria that occur immediately after helping
- Feelings of increased self-worth, calm, and relaxation
- A perception of greater physical health
- Fewer colds and headaches, improved eating and sleeping habits, and some relief from the pain of chronic diseases such as asthma and arthritis

Just how might helping benefit the health of the helper? By helping others, we may relieve our own distress and guilt over their problems. Helping others can be effective at banishing a bad mood or a case of the blues. Helping may block physical pain because we can pay attention to only a limited number of things at a given time. Helping others can also expand our perspective and enhance our appreciation for our own lives. Helping may benefit physical health by providing a temporary boost to the immune system and by combating stress and hostile feelings linked to the development of chronic diseases.

Helping others doesn't require a huge time commitment or a change of career. To get the most out of helping, keep the following guidelines in mind:

- *Make contact.* Choose an activity that involves personal contact.
- *Help as often as possible.*
- *Volunteer with others.* Working with a group enables you to form bonds with other helpers who can support your interests and efforts.
- *Focus on the process, not the outcome.* We can't always measure or know the results of our actions.
- *Practice random acts of kindness.* Smile, let people go ahead of you in line, pick up litter, and so on.
- *Adopt a pet.* Several studies suggest that pet owners enjoy better health, perhaps by feeling needed or by having a source of unconditional love and affection.
- *Avoid burnout.* Recognize your own limits, pace yourself, and try not to feel guilty or discouraged.

In addition to the benefits for you, volunteering has the added bonus of having a positive impact on the wellness of others. It fosters a sense of community and can provide some practical help for many of the problems facing our society today.

SOURCES: Shmotkin, D., T. Blumstein, and B. Modan. 2003. Beyond keeping active: Concomitants of being a volunteer in old-old age. *Psychological Aging* 18(3): 602–607; adapted with permission from Sobel, D. S., M.D., and R. Ornstein, Ph.D. 1996. *The Healthy Mind, Healthy Body Handbook.* Los Altos, Calif.: DRx.

many people can adjust to it. Some cases of wet AMD can be treated with laser surgery. Both glaucoma and AMD can be detected with regular screening.

Vision can also be affected by conditions that are products of aging. By the time they reach their forties, many people have developed **presbyopia,** a gradual decline in the ability to focus on objects close to them. This occurs because the lens of the eye no longer expands and contracts as readily. **Cataracts,** a clouding of the lens caused by lifelong oxidation damage (a by-product of normal body chemistry), may dim vision by the sixties.

**Arthritis** Half of all people over the age of 65 have some form of arthritis. This degenerative disease causes joint inflammation leading to chronic pain, swelling, and loss of mobility. There are more than 100 different types of arthritis; osteoarthritis (OA) is by far the most common. In a person with OA, the cartilage that caps the bones in joints wears away, forming sharp spurs. It most often affects the hands and weight-bearing joints of the body—knees, ankles, and hips. OA is second only to heart disease in disabling people so that they cannot work; 74% of those it affects are women.

Strategies for reducing the risk of arthritis and, for those who already have OA, for managing it include exercise, weight management, and avoidance of heavy or repetitive muscle use. Exercise lubricates joints and strengthens the muscles around them, protecting them from further damage. Swimming, walking, and tai chi are good low-impact exercises. Maintaining an appropriate weight is important to avoid placing stress on the hips, knees, and ankles.

If joints are severely damaged and activity is limited, surgery to repair or replace joints may be considered, but medication is usually the first treatment. Many people with OA take medication to relieve inflammation and reduce pain. Nonsteroidal anti-inflammatory drugs like ibuprofen can help but can irritate the digestive tract; prescription drugs that relieve pain without damaging the stomach have been found to have other dangerous side effects (see Chapter 15). Acetaminophen can also reduce pain without upsetting the stomach, but exceeding the recommended dosage can cause liver damage. Balancing the benefits and risks of medications is an important consideration for people at any age.

Recent studies suggest that two dietary supplements, glucosamine and chondroitin sulfate, do have a mild anti-inflammatory effect that eases some OA symptoms. Due to potential risks and side effects, a health care provider should be consulted before either compound is taken.

352 Chapter 14 The Challenge of Aging

## GENDER MATTERS

New to the tenth edition, Gender Matters boxes highlight key gender differences related to wellness as well as areas of particular concern to men or women. Topics include gender differences in rates of anxiety, depression, and drug use; in the symptoms and course of heart attack and STDs; in styles of communication; and in responses to stress.

Gender Matters

**Women, Men, and Stress**

**Special Stressors for Men and Women**

Women are more likely than men to find themselves balancing multiple roles—student, employee, parent, spouse, caregiver to aging parents. Women who work outside of the home still do most of the housework, and time-related stress can be severe. All of these stressors can contribute to higher levels of stress-related health problems. Social forces can also undermine opportunities for women and cause stress. Women now make up more than half of the workforce but hold only 5% of the top leadership jobs. On average, women make less money than men with comparable jobs and are more likely to face sexual harassment. Disparity in domestic responsibilities, lack of integration into dominant organization coalitions, and even being considered excessively "nice" can all reduce the chances of being considered for leadership positions. The more women view themselves as fitting the traditional feminine gender stereotype, the less likely they are to report leadership aspirations.

Men who fit a traditional male gender role may feel the need to be active and in charge in all situations. They may have a communication style that is competitive and aggressive, causing stress in many interpersonal situations and limiting their ability to build social support networks. The responsibility to support a family may be felt very keenly among men with a traditional male gender role.

**Physiological Differences and Stress**

Due to hormonal differences, men are considered to be more biologically vulnerable to certain diseases. For example, because of a rise in circulating testosterone levels, from puberty onward, males have higher blood pressure than do age-matched females. Along with other risk factors, including fewer physician visits, the rise in testosterone produces greater wear and tear on the male circulatory system over time, leading to greater risk for cardiovascular disease. A part of the brain responsible for regulating fear and emotional balance, the amygdala, is very sensitive to testosterone. Thus, having more circulating testosterone may predispose men to see social situations as more threatening than a woman would see them, creating more frequent activation of the stress response.

Women, on the other hand, have higher levels of the hormone oxytocin and are more likely to respond to stressors by seeking social support. The tend-and-befriend coping response among women may give them a longevity advantage compared with men by decreasing the risk of stress-related disorders.

**Gender and Stress Among College Students**

Gender role development is a significant source of stress during college for both men and women, but there are gender differences in key stressors and coping strategies. College women are more likely than men to report having roommate conflicts and personal appearance issues. Men have more difficulty relating to and meeting other students, making friends, and dealing with peer pressure. College women report significantly higher emotional resources and ability to give and receive social support than do men. College men more frequently utilize physical coping resources than do women.

change for him than for a woman whose self-image is based on several different roles.

Although both men and women experience the fight-or-flight physiological response to stress, women are more likely to respond behaviorally with a pattern of "tend-and-befriend"—nurturing friends and family and seeking social support and social contacts. Women are more likely to enhance their social networks in ways that reduce stress than to become aggressive or withdraw from difficult situations. See the box "Women, Men, and Stress" for more on gender and stress.

**Past Experiences** Your past experiences significantly influence your response to stressors. For example, if you were unprepared for the first speech you gave in your speech class and performed poorly, you will probably experience greater anxiety in response to future assignments. If you had performed better, your confidence and sense of control would be greater, and you would probably experience less stress with future speeches. Effective behavioral responses, in this case careful preparation and visualizing yourself giving a successful speech, can help overcome the effects of negative past experiences.

**STRESS AND DISEASE**

The role of stress in health and disease is complex, and much remains to be learned. However, evidence suggests that stress—interacting with a person's genetic predisposition, personality, social environment, and health-related behaviors—can increase vulnerability to numerous ailments. Several related theories have been proposed to explain the relationship between stress and disease.

**The General Adaptation Syndrome**

Biologist Hans Selye, working in the 1930s and 1940s, was one of the first scientists to develop a comprehensive theory of stress and disease. Selye coined the term **general adaptation syndrome (GAS)** to describe what he believed was a universal and predictable response pattern to all stressors. He recognized that stressors could be

28 Chapter 2 Stress: The Constant Challenge

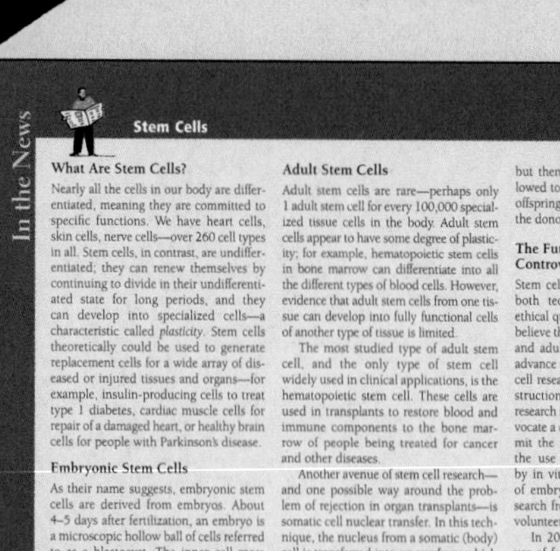

In the News

**Stem Cells**

**What Are Stem Cells?**

Nearly all the cells in our body are differentiated, meaning they are committed to specific functions. We have heart cells, skin cells, nerve cells—over 260 cell types in all. Stem cells, in contrast, are undifferentiated; they can renew themselves by continuing to divide in their undifferentiated state for long periods, and they can develop into specialized cells—a characteristic called *plasticity*. Stem cells theoretically could be used to generate replacement cells for a wide array of diseased or injured tissues and organs—for example, insulin-producing cells to treat type 1 diabetes, cardiac muscle cells for repair of a damaged heart, or healthy brain cells for people with Parkinson's disease.

**Embryonic Stem Cells**

As their name suggests, embryonic stem cells are derived from embryos. About 4–5 days after fertilization, an embryo is a microscopic hollow ball of cells referred to as a blastocyst. The inner cell mass contains about 30 stem cells; researchers can remove these cells and grow them in culture for a fairly long period, producing millions of embryonic stem cells. Currently, most embryonic stem cells used in research are derived from eggs that have been fertilized in vitro and then donated for research purposes; they are not derived from embryos fertilized within a woman's body. Stem cells from embryos are *pluripotent*, that is, they can develop into virtually any cell type.

**Adult Stem Cells**

Adult stem cells are rare—perhaps only 1 adult stem cell for every 100,000 specialized tissue cells in the body. Adult stem cells appear to have some degree of plasticity; for example, hematopoietic stem cells in bone marrow can differentiate into all the different types of blood cells. However, evidence that adult stem cells from one tissue can develop into fully functional cells of another type of tissue is limited.

The most studied type of adult stem cell, and the only type of stem cell widely used in clinical applications, is the hematopoietic stem cell. These cells are used in transplants to restore blood and immune components to the bone marrow of people being treated for cancer and other diseases.

Another avenue of stem cell research—and one possible way around the problem of rejection in organ transplants—is somatic cell nuclear transfer. In this technique, the nucleus from a somatic (body) cell is transferred into an egg from which the nucleus has been removed. The egg is then allowed to develop in the lab into a blastocyst, and the resulting stem cells are removed and cultured. This technique, also known as *therapeutic cloning*, produces a line of stem cells that are genetically matched to the cell donor; using these cells for transplant should eliminate problems with rejection. (This technique is distinct from so-called *reproductive cloning*, in which an embryo is created in the lab using somatic cell transfer but then implanted in a uterus and allowed to develop in order to produce an offspring who is genetically identical to the donor of the original somatic cell.)

**The Future: Potential and Controversy**

Stem cell research is in its infancy, and both technical difficulties and major ethical questions remain. Many scientists believe that research into both embryonic and adult stem cells will be needed to advance the therapeutic potential of stem cell research. However, the use (and destruction) of human embryos for this research is controversial. Some people advocate a complete ban; others would permit the use of existing stem cell lines, the use of "extra" embryos produced by in vitro fertilization, and/or the use of embryos created specifically for research from eggs and sperm donated by volunteers.

In 2001, President Bush banned the use of federal funds for any research related to the creation of new embryonic stem cell lines, thus limiting research to a small number of existing cell lines. Researchers believe that there are problems with this limitation, highlighted by the announcement in 2005 that all existing stem cell lines may have become contaminated with nonhuman compounds via the technique used to maintain them. A number of private institutions and individual states are now providing funds for the creation of new embryonic stem cell lines.

**What Happens as You Age?**

Many of the characteristics associated with aging are not due to aging at all. Rather, they are the result of neglect and abuse of our bodies and minds. These assaults lay the foundation for later problems like arthritis, heart disease, diabetes, hearing loss, and hypertension. We sacrifice our optimal health by smoking, having poor nutrition, overeating, abusing alcohol and drugs, bombarding our ears with excessive noise, and exposing our bodies to too much ultraviolet radiation from the sun. We also jeopardize our bodies through inactivity, and we endure abuse from the toxic chemicals in our environment.

But even with the healthiest behavior and environment, aging inevitably occurs. It results from biochemical processes we don't yet fully understand. Further research may help pinpoint the causes of aging and aid in the development of therapies to repair damage to aging organs (see the box "Stem Cells"). Figure 14-1 shows some of the changes that are a part of aging.

**Life-Enhancing Measures: Age-Proofing**

You can prevent, delay, lessen, or even reverse some of the changes associated with aging through good habits. Simple things you can do daily will make a vast difference to your level of energy and vitality—your overall wellness. The following suggestions have been mentioned throughout this text. But because they are profoundly related to health in later life, we highlight them here.

348 Chapter 14 The Challenge of Aging

## IN THE NEWS BOXES

In the News boxes focus on current health issues that have recently been highlighted in the media, including such topics as same-sex marriage, medical marijuana, prescription drug safety, influenza pandemics, stem cells, and reasons behind poor eating habits among Americans. In the News boxes are marked with the Web icon to indicate that the Online Learning Center has links to Web sites you can use to learn more about In the News topics.

## CORE CONCEPTS IN HEALTH ONLINE LEARNING CENTER

Visit the *Core Concepts in Health* Online Learning Center (www.mhhe.com/inselbrief10e) for resources to help improve your grade and your level of wellness. You'll find chapter objectives and quizzes, flashcards, and many more study aids. You'll also find behavior change tools, Internet activities, and links to reliable wellness-related sites. A password granting access to additional premium online resources is available free with each new copy of the text; these premium resources include interactive self-assessments, articles on health and human performance, and a daily news feed.

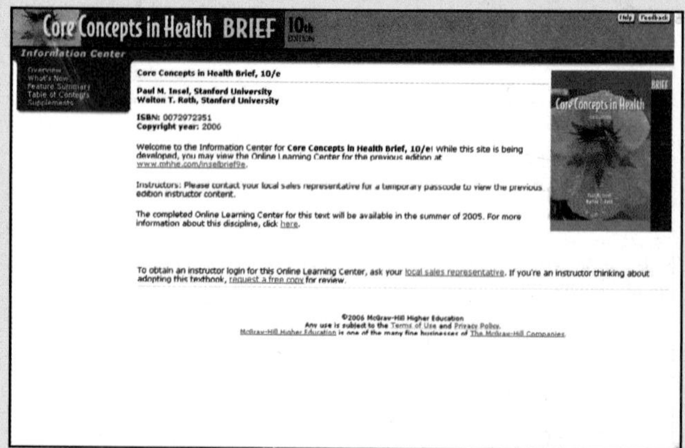

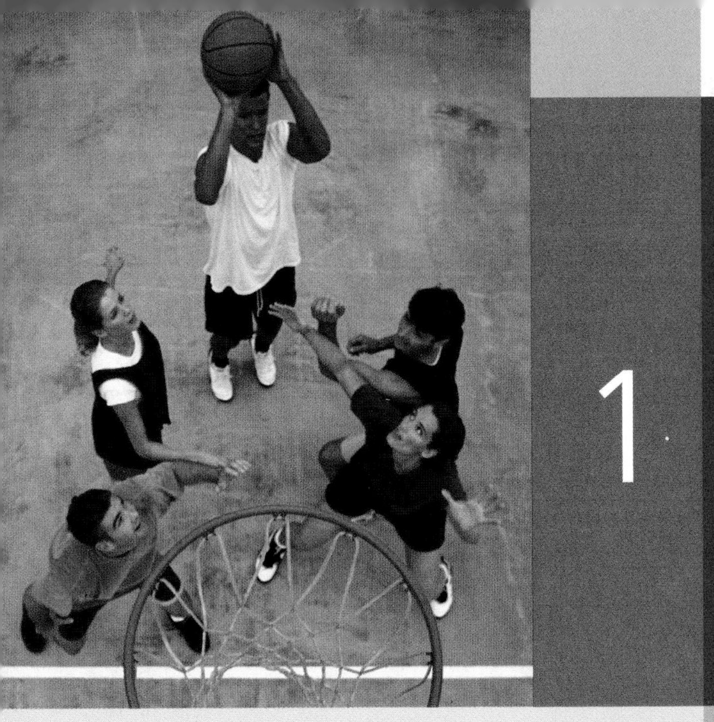

## Looking AHEAD

After reading this chapter, you should be able to

- Describe the six dimensions of wellness and a wellness lifestyle
- Identify major goals of the national Healthy People initiative
- Explain the importance of personal decision making and behavior change in achieving a wellness lifestyle
- Describe the steps in creating a behavior management plan to change a health-related behavior
- Describe the influence of gender, ethnicity, income, disability, family history, and environment on health
- Discuss the available sources of health information and how to think critically about them

# 1 Taking Charge of Your Health

A first-year college student resolves to meet the challenge of making new friends. A long-sedentary senior starts riding her bike to school every day instead of taking the bus. A busy part-time student organizes a group of coworkers to help plant trees in an inner-city neighborhood. What do these people have in common? Each is striving for optimal health and well-being. Not satisfied to be merely free of major illness, these individuals want more. They want to live life actively, energetically, and fully, in a state of optimal personal, interpersonal, and environmental well-being. They have taken charge of their health and are on the path to wellness.

## WELLNESS: THE NEW HEALTH GOAL

**Wellness** is an expanded idea of health. Many people think of health as being just the absence of physical disease. But wellness transcends this concept of health—for example, when individuals with serious illnesses or disabilities rise above their physical or mental limitations to live rich, meaningful, vital lives. Some aspects of health are determined by your genes, your age, and other factors that may be beyond your control. But true wellness is largely determined by the decisions you make about how to live your life. In this book, we will use the terms *health* and *wellness* interchangeably to mean the ability to live life fully—with vitality and meaning.

### The Dimensions of Wellness

No matter what your age or health status, you can optimize your health in each of the following six interrelated dimensions. Wellness in any dimension is not a static goal but a dynamic process of change and growth (Figure 1-1).

**Physical Wellness** Optimal physical health requires eating well, exercising, avoiding harmful habits, making responsible decisions about sex, learning about and recognizing the symptoms of disease, getting regular medical and dental checkups, and taking steps to prevent injuries at home, on the road, and on the job. The habits you develop and the decisions you make today will largely determine not only how many years you will live, but also the quality of your life during those years.

**Emotional Wellness** Optimism, trust, self-esteem, self-acceptance, self-confidence, self-control, satisfying relationships, and an ability to share feelings are just some of the qualities and aspects of emotional wellness. Emotional

**Term**

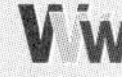

**wellness** Optimal health and vitality, encompassing physical, emotional, intellectual, spiritual, interpersonal and social, and environmental well-being.

**Visit the *Core Concepts in Health* Online Learning Center (www.mhhe.com/inselbrief10e) for study aids and many additional resources.**

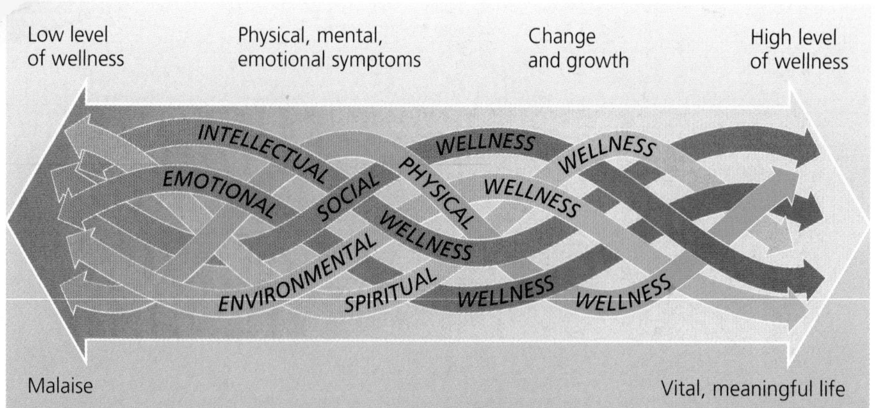


**Figure 1-1 The wellness continuum.** Wellness is composed of six interrelated dimensions, all of which must be developed in order to achieve overall wellness.

health is a dynamic state that fluctuates with your physical, intellectual, spiritual, interpersonal and social, and environmental health. Maintaining emotional wellness requires monitoring and exploring your thoughts and feelings, identifying obstacles to emotional well-being, and finding solutions to emotional problems, with the help of a therapist if necessary.

**Intellectual Wellness** The hallmarks of intellectual health include an openness to new ideas, a capacity to question and think critically, and the motivation to master new skills, as well as a sense of humor, creativity, and curiosity. An active mind is essential to overall wellness, for learning about, evaluating, and storing health-related information. Your mind detects problems, finds solutions, and directs behavior. People who enjoy intellectual wellness never stop learning. They relish new experiences and challenges and actively seek them out.

**Spiritual Wellness** To enjoy spiritual health is to possess a set of guiding beliefs, principles, or values that give meaning and purpose to your life, especially during difficult times. Spiritual wellness involves the capacity for love, compassion, forgiveness, altruism, joy, and fulfillment. It is an antidote to cynicism, anger, fear, anxiety, self-absorption, and pessimism. Spirituality transcends the individual and can be a common bond among people. Organized religions help many people develop spiritual health. Many others find meaning and purpose in their lives on their own—through nature, art, meditation, political action, or good works.

**Interpersonal and Social Wellness** Satisfying relationships are basic to both physical and emotional health. We need to have mutually loving, supportive people in our lives. Developing interpersonal wellness means learning good communication skills, developing the capacity for intimacy, and cultivating a support network of caring friends and/or family members. Social wellness requires participating in and contributing to your community, country, and world.

**Environmental or Planetary Wellness** Increasingly, personal health depends on the health of the planet—from the safety of the food supply to the degree of violence in a society. Other examples of environmental threats to health are ultraviolet radiation in sunlight, air and water pollution, lead in old house paint, and secondhand tobacco smoke in indoor air. Wellness requires learning about and protecting yourself against such hazards—and doing what you can to reduce or eliminate them, either on your own or with others.

The six dimensions of wellness interact continuously, influencing and being influenced by one another. Making a change in one dimension often affects some or all of the others. Maintaining good health is a dynamic process, and increasing your level of wellness in one area of life often influences many others (see the box "Ten Warning Signs of Wellness").

## New Opportunities, New Responsibilities

Wellness is a relatively recent concept. A century ago, people considered themselves lucky just to survive to adulthood. A child born in 1900, for example, could expect to live only about 47 years. Many people died as a result of common **infectious diseases** and poor environmental conditions (unrefrigerated food, poor sanitation, air and water pollution). However, since 1900, the average life span has increased by more than 60%, thanks largely to the development of vaccines and antibiotics to prevent and

### Terms

VW

**infectious disease** A disease that is communicable from one person to another; caused by invading microorganisms such as bacteria and viruses.

**chronic disease** A disease that develops and continues over a long period of time; usually caused by a variety of factors, including lifestyle factors.

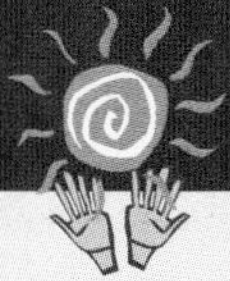



## Ten Warning Signs of Wellness

1. The persistent presence of a support network
2. Chronic positive expectations; the tendency to frame events in a constructive light
3. Episodic outbreaks of joyful, happy experiences
4. A sense of spiritual involvement
5. A tendency to adapt to changing conditions
6. Rapid response and recovery of stress response systems to repeated challenges
7. An increased appetite for physical activity
8. A tendency to identify and communicate feelings
9. Repeated episodes of gratitude and generosity
10. A persistent sense of humor

SOURCE: Ten warning signs of good health. 1996. *Mind/Body Health Newsletter* 5(1).

fight infectious diseases and to public health campaigns to improve environmental conditions (Figure 1-2).

But a different set of diseases has emerged as our major health threat, and heart disease, cancer, and stroke are now the top three causes of death in the United States (Table 1-1). Treating these and other **chronic diseases** has proved enormously expensive and extremely difficult. It has become clear that the best treatment for these diseases is prevention—people having a greater awareness about health and about taking care of their bodies.

The good news is that people do have some control over whether they develop heart disease, cancer, and

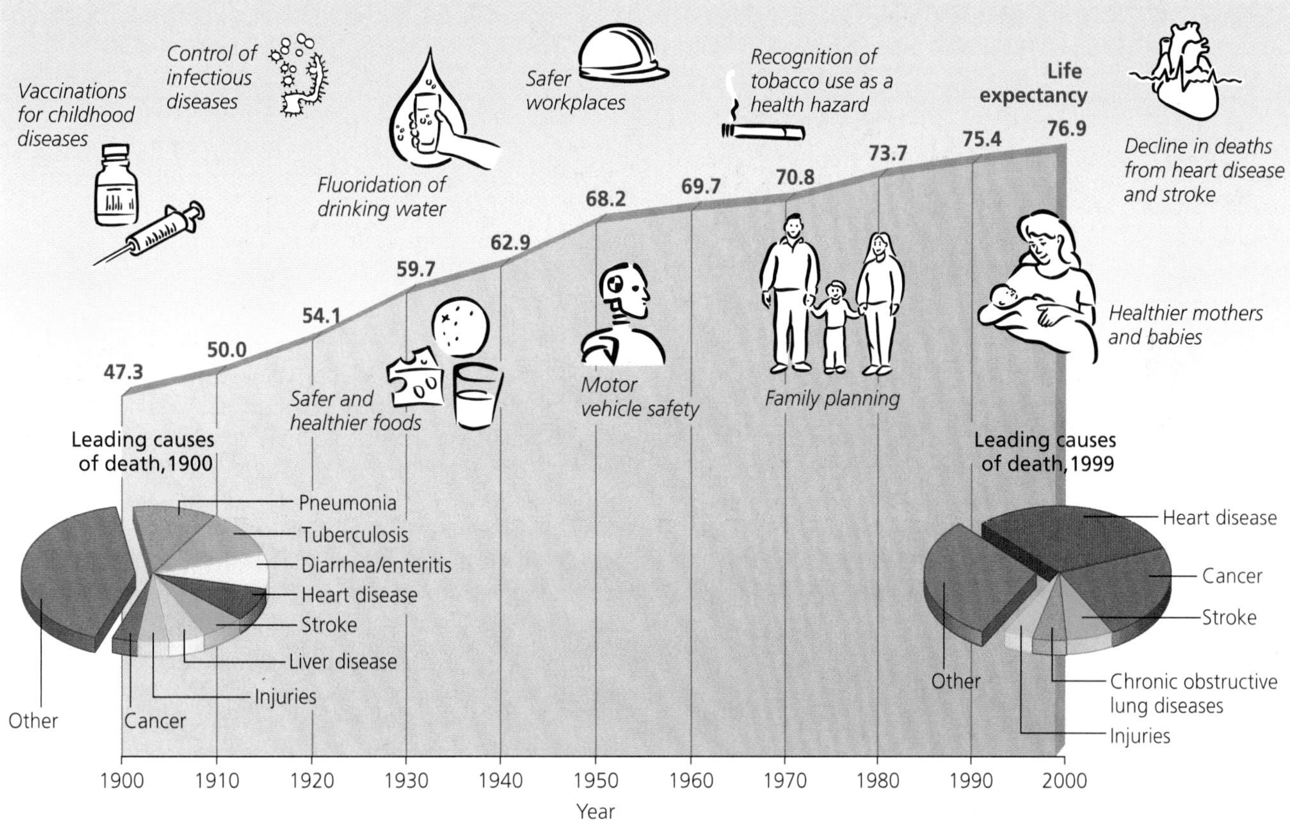


VITAL STATISTICS

**Figure 1-2 Public health achievements of the twentieth century.** During the twentieth century, public health achievements greatly improved the quality of life for Americans, and life expectancy rose from 47 to 77. A dramatic shift in the leading causes of death also occurred, with deaths from infectious diseases declining from over 33% of all deaths to just 2.2%. Heart disease, cancer, and stroke are now responsible for over 50% of all deaths among Americans. SOURCES: National Center for Health Statistics. 2004. *Health, United States, 2004, with Chartbook on Trends in the Health of Americans.* Hyattsville, Md.: National Center for Health Statistics; Centers for Disease Control and Prevention. 1999. Ten great public health achievements—United States, 1900–1999. *Morbidity and Mortality Weekly Report* 48(50): 1141.

VITAL STATISTICS

**Table 1-1 Leading Causes of Death in the United States**

| Rank | Cause of Death | Number of Deaths | Percent of Total Deaths | Female/Male Ratio[a] | Lifestyle Factors |
|---|---|---|---|---|---|
| 1 | Heart disease | 684,462 | 28.0 | 51/49 | D I S A |
| 2 | Cancer[b] | 554,643 | 22.7 | 48/52 | D I S A |
| 3 | Stroke | 157,803 | 6.5 | 61/39 | D I S A |
| 4 | Chronic lower respiratory diseases | 126,128 | 5.2 | 51/49 | S |
| 5 | Unintentional injuries (accidents) | 105,695 | 4.3 | 35/65 | I S A |
| 6 | Diabetes mellitus | 73,965 | 3.0 | 53/47 | D I S |
| 7 | Influenza and pneumonia | 64,847 | 2.7 | 56/44 | S |
| 8 | Alzheimer's disease | 63,343 | 2.6 | 71/29 | |
| 9 | Kidney disease | 42,536 | 1.7 | 52/48 | D I S A |
| 10 | Septicemia (systemic blood infection) | 34,243 | 1.4 | 56/44 | A |
| 11 | Intentional self-harm (suicide) | 30,642 | 1.3 | 20/80 | A |
| 12 | Chronic liver disease and cirrhosis | 27,201 | 1.1 | 36/64 | A |
| 13 | Hypertension (high blood pressure) | 21,841 | 0.9 | 62/38 | D I S A |
| 14 | Parkinson's disease | 17,898 | 0.7 | 47/53 | |
| 15 | Pneumonia due to aspiration | 17,457 | 0.7 | 50/50 | |
| | All causes | 2,443,930 | | | |

*Key*
D Cause of death in which diet plays a part
I Cause of death in which an inactive lifestyle plays a part
S Cause of death in which smoking plays a part
A Cause of death in which excessive alcohol consumption plays a part

[a]Ratio of females to males who died of each cause. For example, about the same number of women and men died of heart disease, but only about half as many women as men died of unintentional injuries and four times as many men as women committed suicide.
[b]Among people under age 85, cancer is the leading cause of death. Decreased rates of smoking have reduced deaths from both heart disease and cancer, but among ex-smokers, heart disease risk declines more quickly and to a greater degree than cancer risk.

*Note:* Although not among the overall top 15 causes of death, homicide (17,096 deaths) and HIV/AIDS (13,544 deaths) are major killers; both are among the 10 leading causes of death among Americans age 15–44 years.

SOURCES: National Center for Health Statistics. 2005. Deaths: Preliminary data for 2003. *National Vital Statistics Report* 53(15); Jemal, A., et al. 2005. Cancer statistics, 2005. *CA: A Cancer Journal for Clinicians* 55(1): 10–30.

other chronic diseases. People make choices every day that either increase or decrease their risks for these diseases—lifestyle choices involving behaviors such as exercise, diet, smoking, and drinking. When researchers look at the lifestyle factors that contribute to death in the United States, it becomes clear that individuals can profoundly influence their own health risks (Table 1-2). Health care professionals can provide information, advice, and encouragement—but the rest is up to each of us.

## National Wellness Goals: The Healthy People Initiative

You may think of health and wellness as personal concerns, goals that you strive for on your own for your own benefit. But the U.S. government also has a vital interest in the health of all Americans. A healthy population is the nation's greatest resource, the source of its vitality, creativity, and wealth. Poor health, in contrast, drains the nation's resources and raises national health care costs. As the embodiment of our society's values, the federal government also has a humane interest in people's health.

The U.S. government's national Healthy People initiative seeks to prevent unnecessary disease and disability and to achieve a better quality of life for all Americans. Healthy People reports, published first in 1980 and revised every decade, set national health goals based on 10-year agendas. Each report includes both broad goals and specific targets in many different areas of wellness. The latest report, *Healthy People 2010,* proposes two broad national goals:

- *Increase quality and years of healthy life.* The life expectancy of Americans has increased significantly in the past century; however, people can expect poor health to limit their activities and cause distress during the last 15% of their lives (Figure 1-3). Health-related quality of life calls for a full range of functional capacity to enable people to work, play, and maintain satisfying relationships.
- *Eliminate health disparities among Americans.* Many health problems today disproportionately affect certain American populations—for example, ethnic minorities, people of low socioeconomic status or educational

VITAL STATISTICS

**Table 1-2 Actual Causes of Death Among Americans**

| | Number of Deaths Per Year | Percent of Total Deaths Per Year |
|---|---|---|
| Tobacco | 435,000 | 18.1 |
| Poor diet/physical inactivity | 365,000 | 15.2 |
| Alcohol consumption | 85,000 | 3.5 |
| Microbial agents | 75,000 | 3.1 |
| Toxic agents | 55,000 | 2.3 |
| Motor vehicles | 43,000 | 1.8 |
| Firearms | 29,000 | 1.2 |
| Sexual behavior | 20,000 | 0.8 |
| Illicit drug use | 17,000 | 0.7 |

*Note:* Actual causes of death are defined as lifestyle and environmental factors that contribute to the leading killers of Americans. Microbial agents include bacterial and viral infections like influenza and pneumonia; toxic agents include environmental pollutants and chemical agents such as asbestos. The number of deaths due to poor diet/inactivity (obesity) is an area of ongoing controversy.

SOURCES: Mokdad, A. H., et al. 2005. Correction: Actual causes of death in the United States, 2000. *Journal of the American Medical Association* 293(3): 293–294. Mokdad, A. H., et al. 2004. Actual causes of death in the United States, 2000. *Journal of the American Medical Association* 291(10): 1238–1245.

attainment, and people with disabilities. *Healthy People 2010* calls for eliminating disparities in health status, health risks, and use of preventive services among all population groups within the next decade.

Giving substance to these broad goals are hundreds of specific objectives—measurable targets for the year 2010—in many different focus areas that relate to wellness, including fitness, nutrition, safety, substance abuse, health care, and chronic and infectious diseases. Examples of health promotion objectives from *Healthy People 2010,* as well as estimates of our progress toward these targets, appear in Table 1-3. *Healthy People 2010* reflects the changing attitude of Americans: an emerging sense of personal responsibility as the key to good health. The primary concerns of *Healthy People 2010* are the principal topics covered in this book. In many ways, personal wellness goals are no different from the national aspirations.

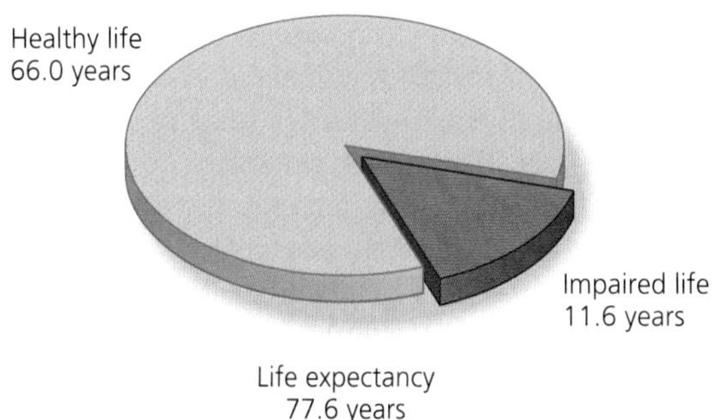


VITAL STATISTICS

**Figure 1-3 Quantity of life versus quality of life.** Years of healthy life as a proportion of life expectancy in the U.S. population.
SOURCES: National Center for Health Statistics. 2005. Deaths: Preliminary data for 2003. *National Vital Statistics Reports* 53(15); National Center for Health Statistics. 2001. *Healthy People 2000 Final Review.* Hyattsville, Md.: Public Health Service.

## Health Issues for Diverse Populations

Americans are a diverse people. Our ancestry is European, African, Asian, Pacific Islander, Latin American, and Native American. We live in cities, suburbs, and rural areas and work at every imaginable occupation. In no other country in the world do so many diverse people live and work together every day. And in no other country are the understanding and tolerance of differences so much a part of the political and cultural ideal. We are at heart a nation of diversity, and, though we often fall short of our goal, we strive for justice and equality among all.

When it comes to health, most differences among people are insignificant; most health issues concern us all equally. We all need to eat well, exercise, manage stress, and cultivate satisfying personal relationships. We need to know how to protect ourselves from heart disease, cancer, sexually transmitted diseases, and injuries. We need to know how to use the health care system.

But some of our differences, as individuals and as members of groups, do have important implications for health. Some of us, for example, have a genetic predisposition for developing certain health problems, such as high cholesterol. Some of us have grown up eating foods that raise our risk of heart disease or obesity. Some of us live in an environment that increases the chance that we will smoke cigarettes or abuse alcohol. These health-related differences among individuals and groups can be biological—determined genetically—or cultural—acquired as patterns of behavior through daily interactions with our families, communities, and society. Many health conditions are a function of biology and culture combined. A person can have a genetic predisposition for a disease, for example, but won't actually develop the disease itself unless certain lifestyle factors are present, such as stress or a poor diet.

When we talk about health issues for diverse populations, we face two related dangers. The first is the danger of stereotyping, of talking about people as groups rather than as individuals. It's certainly true that every person is an individual with a unique genetic endowment and unique life experiences. But many of these influences are shared with others of similar genetic and cultural background. Statements about these group similarities can be

**Table 1-3 Selected *Healthy People 2010* Objectives**

| Objective | Estimate of Current Status (%) | Goal (%) |
|---|---|---|
| Increase the proportion of people age 18 and older who engage regularly in moderate physical activity. | 32 | 50 |
| Increase the proportion of people age 2 and older who consume at least three daily servings of vegetables, with at least one-third being dark-green or orange vegetables. | 3 | 50 |
| Increase the prevalence of healthy weight among all people age 20 and older. | 34 | 60 |
| Reduce the proportion of adults 18 and older who use cigarettes. | 22 | 12 |
| Reduce the proportion of college students reporting binge drinking during the past 2 weeks. | 39 | 20 |
| Increase the proportion of pregnancies that are intended. | 51 | 70 |
| Increase the proportion of adults who take protective measures to reduce the risk of skin cancer (sunscreens, sun-protective clothing, and so on). | 58 | 75 |
| Increase the use of safety belts by motor vehicle occupants. | 75 | 92 |
| Increase the number of residences with a functioning smoke alarm on every floor. | 87 | 100 |
| Increase the proportion of people with health insurance. | 83 | 100 |

SOURCE: National Center for Health Statistics. 2004. *DATA2010: The Healthy People 2010 Database: November 2004 Edition* (http://wonder.cdc.gov/data2010/obj.htm; retrieved February 16, 2005).

useful; for example, they can alert people to areas that may be of special concern for them and their families.

The second danger is that of overgeneralizing, of ignoring the extensive biological and cultural diversity that exists among peoples who are grouped together. Groups labeled Latino or Hispanic, for example, include Mexican Americans, Puerto Ricans, people from South and Central America, and other Spanish-speaking peoples. It's important to keep these considerations in mind whenever you read about culturally diverse populations.

Health-related differences among groups can be identified and described in the context of several different dimensions. Those highlighted in *Healthy People 2010* are gender, ethnicity, income and education, disability, geographic location, and sexual orientation.

**Sex and Gender** Sex and gender profoundly influence wellness. The World Health Organization (WHO) defines **sex** as the biological and physiological characteristics that define men and women; these characteristics are related to chromosomes and their effects on reproductive organs and the functioning of the body. Menstruation in women and the presence of testicles in men are examples of sex-related characteristics. **Gender** is defined as roles, behaviors, activities, and attributes that a given society considers appropriate for men and women. A person's gender is rooted in biology and physiology, but it is shaped by experience and environment—how society responds to individuals based on their sex. Examples of gender-related characteristics that affect wellness include higher rates of smoking and drinking among men and lower earnings among women (compared with men doing similar work).

The effects of sex and gender on wellness can be difficult to separate—but both are important. For example, rates of smoking among American women increased following changes in culturally defined ideas of appropriate behavior for women. This increase in smoking, combined with women's greater biological vulnerability to the cancer-causing agents in tobacco smoke, has led to a substantial increase in the number of deaths from lung cancer among women. See the box "Women's Health/Men's Health" for more on gender differences that impact wellness; throughout the text, boxes labeled Gender Matters focus on key wellness concerns for women and men.

**Ethnicity** Achieving the *Healthy People 2010* goal of eliminating all health disparities will require a national effort to identify and address the underlying causes of ethnic health disparities. Compared with the U.S. population

### Terms

VW

**sex** The biological and physiological characteristics that define men and women.

**gender** The roles, behaviors, activities, and attributes that a given society considers appropriate for men and women.

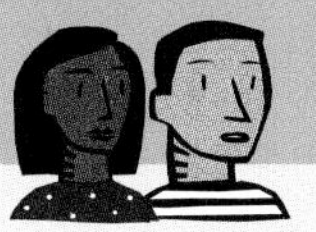

## Women's Health/Men's Health

Men and women have different life expectancies, different reproductive concerns, and different incidences of many diseases. They have different patterns of health-related behaviors, and they respond differently to medications and other medical treatments. The lists below highlight just a few of the many gender differences that can affect wellness.

### Women

- Women live longer than men but have higher rates of disabling health problems like arthritis, osteoporosis, and Alzheimer's disease.
- On average, women are shorter, have a lower proportion of muscle, and tend to have a "pear" body shape, with excess body fat stored in the hips.
- Women score better on tests of verbal fluency, speech production, fine motor skills, and visual and working memory.
- Women experience heart attacks, on average, about 10 years later than men, but they have a poorer 1-year postattack survival rate. Women are more likely to experience atypical heart attack symptoms such as fatigue and difficulty breathing.
- Women are more likely to have a stroke or to die from a stroke, but women are also more likely to recover language ability after a stroke affecting the left side of the brain.
- Women have lower rates of smoking but have a higher risk of lung cancer at a given level of exposure to cigarette smoke.
- Women become more intoxicated at a given level of alcohol intake.
- Women have stronger immune systems and are less susceptible to infection by certain bacteria and viruses, but they are more likely to develop autoimmune diseases like lupus.
- Women are more likely to react to stressors with a response called tend-or-befriend that involves social support; this response may give women a longevity advantage by reducing the risk of stress-related disorders.
- Women are more likely to suffer from depression and to attempt suicide.
- Women are more likely to suffer from migraine headaches and chronic tension headaches.
- Women are more likely to be infected with a sexually transmitted disease (STD) during a heterosexual encounter, and they are more likely to suffer severe and long-term effects from STDs, including chronic infection and infertility.

### Men

- Men have a shorter life expectancy than women, but they have lower rates of disabling health problems.
- On average, men are taller, have a higher proportion of muscle, and tend to have an "apple" body shape, with excess body fat stored in the abdomen.
- Men score better in tests of visual-spatial ability—for example, the ability to imagine the relationships between shapes and objects when rotated in space.
- Men experience heart attacks, on average, about 10 years earlier than women, but they have a better 1-year postattack survival rate. Men are more likely to have classic heart attack symptoms like chest pain.
- Men are less likely to die from a stroke but are also more likely to have permanent loss of language ability following a stroke affecting the left side of the brain.
- Men have higher rates of smoking, spit tobacco use, and alcohol use and abuse.
- Men have higher rates of death from causes linked to intoxication, risk-taking behavior, and firearms: unintentional injuries (car crashes, drowning), homicide, and suicide.
- Men are more likely to be exposed to toxic or cancer-causing chemicals on the job.
- Men have weaker immune systems and are more susceptible to infection by certain bacteria and viruses, but they are less likely to develop autoimmune diseases like lupus.
- Men are more likely to react to stressors with an aggressive or hostile response, a pattern that may increase the risk of stress-related disorders.
- Men have lower rates of depression and are less likely to attempt suicide; however, men are much more likely to succeed at suicide, and many more men than women die each year from suicide.
- Men are more likely to suffer from cluster headaches.
- Men are less likely to be infected with an STD during a heterosexual encounter.

SOURCES: World Health Organization. 2004. *Gender and HIV/AIDS* (http://www.who.int/gender/hiv_aids/en; retrieved August 13, 2004); Entering a new age of gender medicine. 2003. *Consumer Reports on Health,* December; Institute of Medicine. 2001. *Exploring the Biological Contributions to Human Health: Does Sex Matter?* Washington, D.C.: National Academy Press.

as a whole, American ethnic minorities have higher rates of death and disability from many causes. These disparities result from a complex mix of genetic variations, environmental factors, and health behaviors.

Some genetic diseases are concentrated in certain gene pools, the result of each ethnic group's relatively distinct history. Sickle-cell disease is most common among people of African ancestry. Tay-Sachs disease afflicts people of Eastern European Jewish heritage and French Canadian heritage. Cystic fibrosis is more common among Northern Europeans. In addition to biological differences, many cultural differences occur along ethnic lines. Ethnic groups may vary in their traditional diets; their patterns of family and interpersonal relationships; their attitudes toward tobacco, alcohol, and other drugs; and their health beliefs and practices. All of these factors have important implications for wellness.

The federal government collects population and health information on five broad ethnic minority groups in American society; each group has some specific health concerns:

- *Latinos* (13.2% of the total U.S. population) are a diverse group, with roots in Mexico, Puerto Rico, Cuba, and South and Central America; many Latinos are of mixed Spanish and American Indian descent or of mixed Spanish, Indian, and African American descent. Latinos on average have lower rates of heart disease, cancer, and suicide than the general population, but higher rates of infant mortality and a higher overall birth rate; other areas of concern include gallbladder disease and obesity. At current rates, about one in two Latinas will develop diabetes in her lifetime.
- *African Americans* (12.6% of the total U.S. population) have the same leading causes of death as the general population, but they have a higher infant mortality rate and lower rates of suicide and osteoporosis. Areas of special concern for African Americans include high blood pressure, stroke, diabetes, asthma, and obesity. African American men are at significantly higher risk of prostate cancer than men in other groups, and early screening is recommended for them.
- *Asian Americans* (4.5% of the total U.S. population) include people who trace their ancestry to countries in the Far East, Southeast Asia, or the Indian subcontinent, including Japan, China, Vietnam, Laos, Cambodia, Korea, the Philippines, India, and Pakistan. Asian Americans have a lower death rate and a longer life expectancy than the general population. They have lower rates of coronary heart disease and obesity. However, health differences exist among these groups. For example, Southeast Asian men have higher rates of smoking and lung cancer, and Vietnamese American women have higher rates of cervical cancer.
- *American Indians and Alaska Natives* (1.2% of the total U.S. population) typically embrace a tribal identity, such as Sioux, Navaho, or Hopi. American Indians and Alaska Natives have lower death rates from heart disease, stroke, and cancer than the general population, but they have higher rates of early death from causes linked to smoking and alcohol use, including injuries and cirrhosis. Diabetes is a special concern for many groups; for example, the Pimas of Arizona have the highest known prevalence of diabetes of any population in the world.
- *Native Hawaiian and Other Pacific Islander Americans* (0.3% of the total U.S. population) trace their ancestry to the original peoples of Hawaii, Guam, Samoa, and other Pacific Islands. Pacific Islander Americans have a higher overall death rate than the general population and higher rates of some diseases, including diabetes and asthma. High rates of smoking and high prevalence of overweight and obesity are special concerns for this group.

It is often difficult to separate factors related to ethnicity from those associated with socioeconomic status and educational attainment. See the next section and the box "Factors Contributing to Health Disparities Among Ethnic Minorities" for more information.

**Income and Education** Inequalities in income and education underlie many of the health disparities among Americans. Income and education are closely related, and groups with the highest poverty rates and least education have the worst health status. People with low incomes and less education have higher rates of infant mortality, traumatic injury and violent death, and many diseases, including heart disease, diabetes, tuberculosis, and HIV infection. They are more likely to eat poorly, be overweight, smoke, drink, and use drugs. They are exposed to more stressors and have less access to health care services. Poverty and low educational attainment are far more important predictors of poor health than any ethnic factor. However, they are often mixed with other factors in a way that makes it difficult to distinguish what causes what.

**Disability** People with disabilities are those who have activity limitations, need assistance, or perceive themselves as having a disability. About one in five people in the United States has some level of disability, and the rate is rising, especially among younger segments of the population. People with disabilities are more likely to be inactive and overweight. They report more days of depression and fewer days of vitality than people without activity limitations. Many people with disabilities also lack access to health care services.

**Geographic Location** About one in four Americans currently lives in a rural area—a place with fewer than 2500 residents. People living in rural areas are less likely to be physically active, to use safety belts, or to obtain screening tests for preventive health care. They have less access to timely emergency services and much higher rates of injury-related death than people living in urban areas. They are also more likely to lack health insurance.

**Sexual Orientation** The 1–5% of Americans who identify themselves as homosexual or bisexual make up a diverse community with varied health concerns. Their emotional wellness and personal safety are affected by factors relating to personal, family, and social acceptance of their sexual orientation. Gay, lesbian, and bisexual teens are more likely to engage in risky behaviors such as unsafe sex and drug use; they are also more likely to be depressed and to attempt suicide. HIV/AIDS is a major

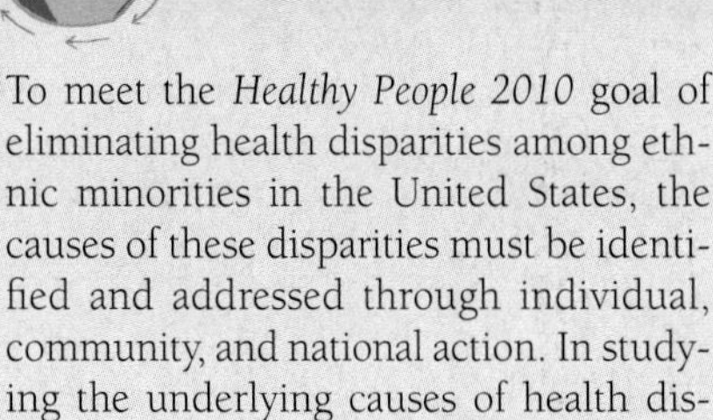

## Factors Contributing to Health Disparities Among Ethnic Minorities

To meet the *Healthy People 2010* goal of eliminating health disparities among ethnic minorities in the United States, the causes of these disparities must be identified and addressed through individual, community, and national action. In studying the underlying causes of health disparities, it is often difficult to separate and assign relative importance to the many potential contributing factors.

### Income and Education

Poverty and low educational attainment are the most important factors underlying health disparities. People with low incomes and less education have higher rates of death from all causes, especially chronic disease and injury, and they are less likely to have preventive health services such as vaccinations and Pap tests. They are more likely to live in an area with a high rate of violence, higher levels of pollutants, and many more environmental stressors. They also have higher rates of unhealthy behaviors such as tobacco and alcohol use, poor diet, and inactivity.

It is important to note that although ethnic disparities in health are significantly reduced when comparing groups with similar incomes and levels of education, they are not eliminated. For example, people living in poverty report worse health than people with higher incomes; but, within the latter group, African Americans and Latinos rate their health as worse than do whites (see figure). Infant mortality rates go down as the education level of mothers goes up; but among mothers who are college graduates, African Americans have significantly higher rates of infant mortality than whites, Latinos, and Asian Americans. These variations point to the complex nature of factors that contribute to health disparities.

### Access to Appropriate Health Care

People with low incomes are less likely to have health insurance and more likely to have problems paying for health care and arranging for transportation and time away from family responsibilities in order to access care. They are also more likely to lack information about available services and appropriate lifestyle choices and preventive care. But disparities persist even at higher income levels; for example, among nonpoor Americans, many more Latinos than whites or African Americans report having no insurance, no usual source of health care, and no health care visits within the past year. Possible contributing factors include the following:

- *Local and regional differences in the availability of high-tech health care and specialists.* Minorities, regardless of income, may be more likely to live in medically underserved areas of the country.
- *Problems with communication and trust.* People whose primary language is not English are more likely to be uninsured and to have trouble communicating with health care providers; they may also have problems interpreting health information from public health education campaigns. Language barriers and lack of culturally competent care may be exacerbated by an underrepresentation of minorities in the health professions.
- *Cultural preferences relating to health care.* Groups may vary in their assessment of when it is appropriate to seek medical care and what types of invasive tests and treatments are acceptable.
- *State and federal laws and programs.* Eligibility for Medicaid (a form of government insurance) varies by state and group. For example, Puerto Ricans are U.S. citizens and Cubans are classified as refugees, so people from these groups are immediately eligible for Medicaid; emigrants from other countries may not be able to access public insurance programs until 5 years after they enter the United States.

### Culture and Lifestyle

As described in the chapter, ethnic groups may vary in health-related behaviors such as diet, tobacco and alcohol use, coping strategies, and health practices—and these behaviors can have important implications for wellness, both positive and negative. For example, African Americans are more likely to report consuming five or more servings of fruits and vegetables per day than people from other ethnic groups. American Indians report high rates of smoking and smoking-related health problems. Cultural background can be an important protective factor, as seen by the fact that low income doesn't affect all groups equally. For example, poverty is strongly

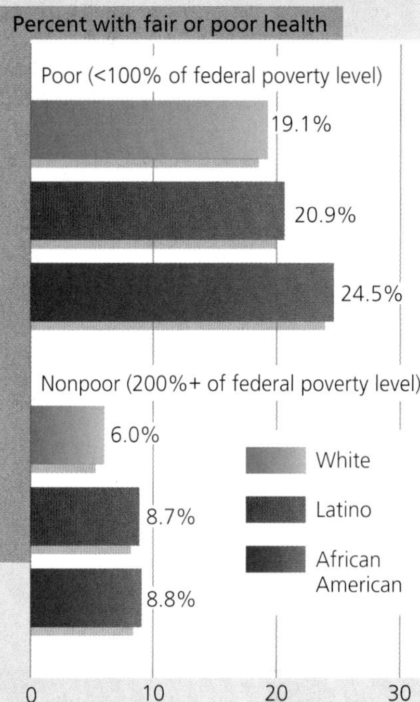


**Self-rated health status.** Respondents were asked to rate their health as excellent, very good, good, fair, or poor. Poverty is strongly associated with negative health status, but disparities persist even among nonpoor Americans.

associated with increased rates of depression; but some groups, including Americans born in Mexico or Puerto Rico, have lower rates of mental disorders at a given level of income and appear to have coping strategies that provide special resilience.

### Discrimination

Racism and discrimination are stressful events that can cause psychological distress and increase the risk of physical and psychological problems. Social discrimination can contribute to lower socioeconomic status and all its associated risks. Bias or discrimination in medical care can directly affect treatment and health outcomes.

SOURCES: National Center for Health Statistics. 2004. *Health, United States, 2004, with Chartbook on Trends in the Health of Americans.* Hyattsville, Md.: National Center for Health Statistics; Centers for Disease Control and Prevention. 2004. REACH 2010 surveillance for health status in minority communities. *MMWR Surveillance Summaries* 53(SS-6); Kaiser Family Foundation. 2003. *Key Facts: Race, Ethnicity, and Medical Care.* Menlo Park, Calif.: Kaiser Family Foundation; U.S. Department of Health and Human Services. 2001. *Mental Health: Culture, Race, and Ethnicity.* Rockville, Md.: U.S. Department of Health and Human Services.

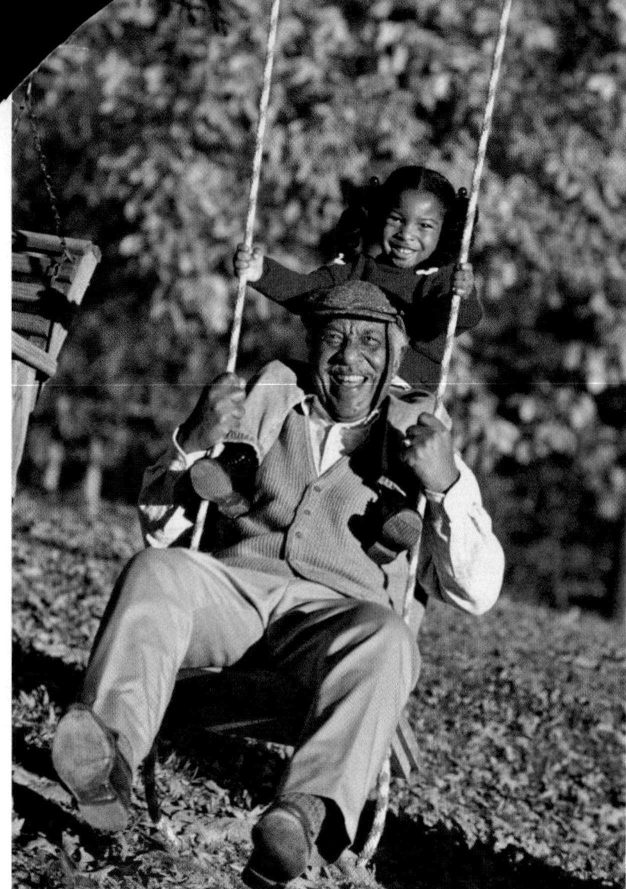

With wellness come health and vitality throughout the life span.

concern for gay men, and gay men and lesbians may have higher rates of substance abuse, depression, and suicide.

These are just some of the differences among people and groups that can influence wellness. Boxes labeled Dimensions of Diversity examine special wellness challenges and solutions of diverse population groups in the United States and around the world.

## CHOOSING WELLNESS

Each of us has the option and the responsibility to decide what kind of future we want—one characterized by zestful living or one marked by symptoms and declining energy. The message of this book is that wellness is something everyone can have. Achieving it requires knowledge, self-awareness, motivation, and effort—but the benefits last a lifetime. Optimal health comes mostly from a healthy lifestyle, patterns of behavior that promote and support your health now and as you get older.

### Factors That Influence Wellness

Our behavior, our family health history, the environment we live in, and whether we have access to adequate health care are all important influences on wellness. These factors, which vary for both individuals and groups, can interact in ways that produce either health or disease. For example, a sedentary lifestyle combined with a genetic predisposition for diabetes can greatly increase a person's risk of developing the disease. If this person also lacks adequate health care, he or she is much more likely to suffer dangerous complications from diabetes and have a lower quality of life. On the flip side, regular physical activity and a healthy diet can delay or prevent the development of the most common form of diabetes.

**Health Habits** Scientific research is continuously revealing new connections between our habits and emotions and the level of health we enjoy. For example, heart disease, the nation's number-one killer, is associated with cigarette smoking, high levels of stress, habitually hostile and suspicious attitudes toward people and the world, a diet high in saturated and trans fat and low in fiber, and a sedentary way of life. Other habits are beneficial. Regular exercise, for example, can help prevent heart disease, high blood pressure, diabetes, osteoporosis, and depression and may reduce the risk of colon cancer, stroke, and back injury. As we learn more about how our actions affect our bodies and minds, we can make informed choices for a healthier life.

**Heredity/Family History** Your **genome** consists of the complete set of genetic material in your cells; it contains about 25,000 genes, half from each of your parents. **Genes** control the production of proteins that serve both as the structural material for your body and as the regulators of all your body's chemical reactions and metabolic processes. The human genome varies only slightly from person to person, and many of these differences do not affect health. However, some differences do have important implications for health, and knowing your family health history can help you determine which conditions may be of special concern for you.

Errors in our genes are responsible for about 3500 clearly hereditary conditions, including sickle-cell disease and cystic fibrosis. Altered genes also play a part in heart disease, cancer, stroke, diabetes, and many other common conditions. However, in these more common and complex disorders, genetic alterations serve only to increase an individual's risk, and the disease itself results from the interaction of many genes with other factors. For example, researchers have identified genes that clearly increase a woman's risk for breast cancer, but these genes explain only a small proportion of cases. In the small number of inherited cases, genetic alterations that increase the risk of cancer are present at birth in the genes of all the cells in the body. In the majority of cases, however, cancer results from genetic changes that occur after birth within particular cells—usually in response to behavioral and environmental factors. Another example of the power of behavior and environment can be seen in the

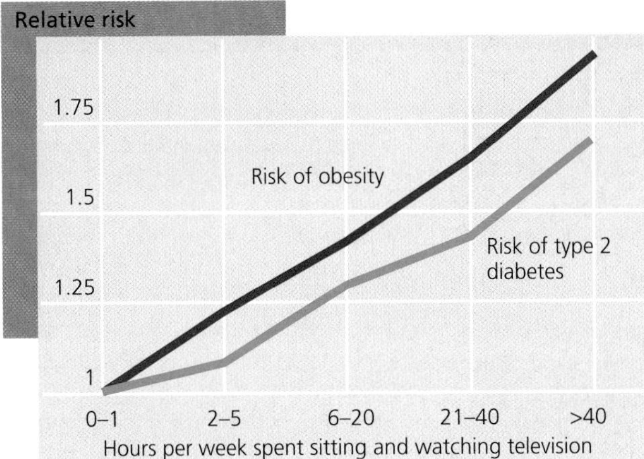


**Figure 1-4 Sedentary lifestyle and risk of obesity and type 2 diabetes.** Heredity and environment can play a role in the development of obesity and diabetes, but health habits are very important.
SOURCE: Hu, F. B., et al. 2003. Television watching and other sedentary behaviors in relation to risk of obesity and type 2 diabetes mellitus in women. *Journal of the American Medical Association* 289(14): 1785–1791. From Thomas D. Fahey, Paul M. Insel, Walton T. Roth, *Fit and Well,* 6th ed., Fig. 1.3a, p. 6. McGraw-Hill, 2004. 

more than 60% increase in the incidence of diabetes that has occurred among Americans since 1990. This huge increase is not due to any sudden change in our genes; it is the result of increasing rates of obesity caused by poor dietary choices and lack of physical activity (Figure 1-4).

**Environment** Your environment includes not only the air you breath and the water you drink but also substances and conditions in your home, workplace, and community. Are you frequently exposed to environmental tobacco smoke or the radiation in sunlight? Do you live in an area with poor air quality or high rates of crime and violence? Has alcohol or drug abuse been a problem in your family? These and other environmental factors all have an impact on wellness.

**Access to Health Care** Adequate health care helps improve both quality and quantity of life through preventive care and the treatment of disease. For example, vaccinations prevent many dangerous infections, and screening tests help identify key risk factors and diseases in their early, treatable stages. Inadequate access to health care is tied to factors such as low income and lack of health insurance. Cost is one of many issues surrounding the development of advanced health-related technologies; see the box "Medical Innovations in the Twenty-First Century" on page 12.

**Health Habits *Can* Make a Difference** In many cases, behavior can tip the balance toward good health, even when heredity or environment is a negative factor. For example, breast cancer can run in families, but it also may be associated with being overweight and inactive. A woman with a family history of breast cancer is less likely to develop and die from the disease if she controls her weight, exercises regularly, performs breast self-exams, and has regular mammograms to help detect the disease in its early, most treatable stage.

Similarly, a young man with a family history of obesity can maintain a normal weight by being careful to balance calorie intake against activities that burn calories. If your life is highly stressful, you can lessen the chances of heart disease and stroke by learning ways to manage and cope with stress. If you live in an area with severe air pollution, you can reduce the risk of lung disease by not smoking. You can also take an active role in improving your environment. Behaviors like these enable you to make a difference in how great an impact heredity and environment will have on your health.

## A Wellness Profile

What does it mean to be healthy today? A basic list of important behaviors and habits includes the following:

- Having a sense of responsibility for your own health and taking an active rather than a passive stance toward your life
- Learning to manage stress in effective ways
- Maintaining high self-esteem and mentally healthy ways of interacting with other people
- Understanding your sexuality and having satisfying intimate relationships
- Avoiding tobacco and other drugs; using alcohol responsibly, if at all
- Eating well, exercising, and maintaining healthy weight
- Knowing the facts about cardiovascular disease, cancer, infections, sexually transmitted diseases, and injuries and using your knowledge to protect yourself against them
- Understanding the health care system and using it intelligently
- Knowing when to treat your illnesses yourself and when to seek help
- Understanding the natural processes of aging and dying and accepting the limits of human existence
- Understanding how the environment affects your health and taking appropriate action to improve it

### Terms

VW

**genome** The complete set of genetic material in an individual's cells.

**gene** The basic unit of heredity; a section of genetic material containing chemical instructions for making a particular protein.

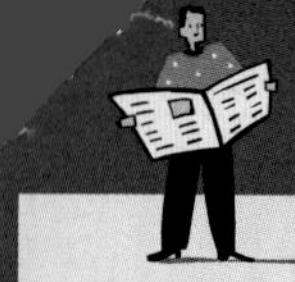

In the News

## Medical Innovations in the Twenty-First Century

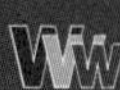

Imagine the following: Each person's DNA has been processed onto computer chips to identify individual disease risks. Vaccines boost the immune system's ability to attack cancerous tumors. Natural hormones stimulate the growth of new blood vessels to bypass clogged arteries feeding the heart. Gene therapies encourage cancer cells to self-destruct or protect nerves from damage following a stroke. Cows are genetically engineered to produce beneficial drugs in their milk. Genetically modified bacteria absorb toxic chemical spills. Science fiction? Not at all! These and many other health-promoting innovations are currently being studied and tested.

### Stem Cells

Many chronic diseases could be cured if damaged cells could be restored. Stem cells are undifferentiated cells that can develop into any type of cell in the body. Stem cells are already being used to replace cancerous cells destroyed in the treatment of leukemia and other cancers, and scientists hope to develop many more therapies. For example, stem cells could potentially be used to replace damaged neurons in people with Parkinson's disease or spinal cord injuries and damaged insulin-producing cells in people with diabetes. See Chapter 19 for more on stem cells and their potential uses.

### Gene Therapy

The manipulation of gene expression in human cells, known as gene therapy, is a potential treatment or cure for genetic diseases and cancer. For gene therapy to succeed, new genes must be delivered to defective cells without disturbing the overall functioning of the cells. In the treatment of cancer, gene therapy would "turn off" the genes responsible for causing the cells to divide rapidly and become malignant.

### Bioengineering

Can we build new organs in the laboratory? Can artificial materials stand in for the body's natural molecules in tissue repair? Bioengineers are developing biodegradeable compounds that can serve as scaffolding for human tissues grown in the laboratory. Stem cells created from a cell donor could be placed on scaffolding and induced to differentiate into specific organ tissue, such as kidney or liver tissue. Once the new organ begins to develop, it could be transplanted into the original cell donor, where it could grow to full size with no danger of organ rejection.

### Ethical Questions, Potential Limits, and Unforeseen Consequences

Although full of promise, the development of innovative medical technologies brings up many potentially troubling issues. For example, the use of human embryos to obtain stem cells is highly controversial. Serious, unforeseen side effects occurred in early gene therapy trials. The expense of developing these technologies and providing them to a growing population is another concern: Cost already limits access to even relatively inexpensive medications and treatments. Privacy and discrimination are other issues: If genetic testing can identify years in advance who is likely to get sick and who is not, employers and health insurance companies could save millions of dollars by not hiring or enrolling people whose genes show them to be at increased risk for disease.

Other questions relate to potential uses of tools for altering the genome. Do we have enough information to know how knocking out "bad" genes will affect our species? For example, the gene alteration that causes sickle-cell disease must be present in both copies of the gene for a person to develop the disease; people who inherit only one copy of the altered gene from their parents have an increased resistance to malaria. If the gene for sickle-cell disease were eliminated, would many more people succumb to malaria? Researchers have found similar links in the genetic mutation that causes cystic fibrosis and protection from cholera and in the genetic mutation that causes Tay-Sachs disease and protection from tuberculosis. Tinkering with the genome could have unknown negative effects.

### Wellness in the Information Age

Perhaps the most important technological advance is the information revolution. A growing number of informative and interactive technologies can help you learn about healthy lifestyle behaviors and preventive medicine as well as aid you in changing your unhealthy habits. The availability of these tools gives each individual the responsibility of making the best use of new information to optimize health. Only you can enhance your ability to make choices that promote wellness in an era of innovation and technological change.

Incorporating these behaviors into your daily life may seem like a tall order, and in a sense it is the work of a lifetime. But the habits you establish now are crucial: They tend to set lifelong patterns. Some behaviors do more than set up patterns—they produce permanent changes in your health. If you become addicted to drugs or alcohol at age 20, for example, you may be able to kick the habit, but you will always face the struggle of a recovering addict. If you contract gonorrhea, you may discover later that your reproductive organs were damaged without your realizing it, making you infertile or sterile. If you ruin your knees doing the wrong exercises or hurt your back in an automobile crash, you won't have them to count on when you're older. Some things just can't be reversed or corrected.

## HOW DO YOU REACH WELLNESS?

Your life may not resemble the one described by the wellness profile at all. You probably have a number of healthy habits and some others that place your health at risk. Taking big steps toward wellness may at first seem like too much work, but as you make progress, it gets easier.

At first you'll be rewarded with a greater sense of control over your life, a feeling of empowerment, higher self-esteem, and more joy. These benefits will encourage you to make further improvements. Over time, you'll come to know what wellness feels like—more energy; greater vitality; deeper feelings of curiosity, interest, and enjoyment; and a higher quality of life.

## Getting Serious About Your Health

Before you can start changing a health-related behavior, you have to know that the behavior is problematic and that you *can* change it. To make good decisions, you need information about yourself and about relevant topics and issues, including what resources are available to help you change your behavior.

**Examining Your Current Health Habits** Have you considered how your current lifestyle is affecting your health today and how it will affect your health in the future? Do you know which of your current habits enhance your health and which detract from it? Begin your journey toward wellness with self-assessment: Think about your own behavior and talk with friends and family members about what they've noticed about your lifestyle and your health.

Many people start to consider changing a behavior when they get help from others. An observation from a friend, family member, or physician can help you see yourself as others do and may get you thinking about your behavior in a new way. Landmark events can also get you thinking about behavior change. A birthday, the birth of a child, or the death of someone close to you can be powerful motivators for thinking seriously about behaviors that affect wellness. New information can also help you get started. As you read this text, you may find yourself reevaluating some of your health-related behaviors. This could be a great opportunity to make healthful changes that will stay with you for the rest of your life.

**Choosing a Target Behavior** To maximize your chances of success, don't try to change all your problem behaviors at once—to quit smoking, give up high-fat foods, start jogging, avoid drugs, get more sleep. Working on even one behavior change will make high demands on your energy. Concentrate on one behavior that you want to change, your **target behavior**, and work on it systematically. Start with something simple, like snacking on candy between afternoon classes or always driving to a particular class instead of walking or biking.

**Obtaining Information About Your Target Behavior** Once you've chosen a target behavior, you need to find out more about it. You need to know its risks and benefits for you—both now and in the future. How is your target behavior affecting your level of wellness today? For what diseases or conditions does this behavior place you at risk? What effect would changing your behavior have on your health?

As a starting point, use material from this text and from the resources listed in the For More Information section at the end of each chapter. See the box "Evaluating Sources of Health Information" for tips on becoming a critical consumer of health information from a wide variety of sources.

**Finding Outside Help** Have you identified a particularly challenging target behavior, such as alcohol addiction, excessive overeating, or depression, that interferes with your ability to function or places you at a serious health risk? Outside help is often needed for changing behaviors or conditions that may be too deeply rooted or too serious for a self-management approach. If this is the case, don't be stopped by the seriousness of the problem—there are many resources available to help you solve it. On campus, the student health center or campus counseling center may be a source of assistance. Many communities offer a variety of services through adult education, health departments, and private agencies. Consult the yellow pages, your physician, your local health department, or the United Way; the last often sponsors local referral services.

## Building Motivation for Change

Knowledge is a necessary ingredient for behavior change, but it isn't usually enough to make people act. Millions of people smoke or have sedentary lifestyles, for example, even though they know it's bad for their health. To succeed at behavior change, you need strong motivation.

**Examining the Pros and Cons of Change** Health behaviors have short-term and long-term benefits and costs associated with them. For example, in the short term, an inactive lifestyle allows for more time to watch TV and hang out with friends but leaves a person less able to participate in recreational activities. Over the long term, it increases the risk of heart disease, cancer, stroke, and premature death. For successful behavior change, you must believe that the benefits of changing outweigh the costs.

Do a careful analysis of the short-term and long-term benefits and costs of continuing your current (target) behavior and of changing to a new, healthier behavior. Focus on the effects that are most meaningful to you, including those that are tied to your personal identity and values. For example, if you see yourself as an active

**Term**

**target behavior** An isolated behavior selected as the object of a behavior change plan.

Vw

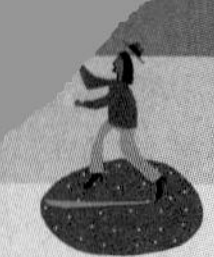

Critical Consumer

## Evaluating Sources of Health Information

V W

### General Strategies

A key first step in sharpening your critical thinking skills is to look carefully at your sources of health information. Critical thinking involves knowing where and how to find relevant information, how to separate fact from opinion, how to recognize faulty reasoning, how to evaluate information, and how to assess the credibility of sources.

- *Go to the original source.* Media reports often simplify the results of medical research. Find out for yourself what a study really reported, and determine whether it was based on good science. What type of study was it? Was it published in a recognized medical journal? Was it an animal study, or did it involve people? Did the study include a large number of people? What did the authors of the study actually report in their findings? (You'll find additional strategies for evaluating research studies in Chapter 21.)
- *Watch for misleading language.* Reports that feature "breakthroughs" or "dramatic proof" are probably hype. Some studies will find that a behavior "contributes to" or is "associated with" an outcome; this does not imply a proven cause-and-effect relationship. Information may also be distorted by an author's point of view.
- *Distinguish between research reports and public health advice.* If a study finds a link between a particular vitamin and cancer, that should not necessarily lead you to change your behavior. But if the Surgeon General or the American Cancer Society advises you to eat less saturated fat or quit smoking, you can assume that many studies point in this direction and that this is advice you should follow.
- *Remember that anecdotes are not facts.* Sometimes we do get helpful health information from our friends and family. But just because your cousin Bertha lost 10 pounds on Dr. Amazing's new protein diet doesn't mean it's a safe, effective way for you to lose weight. Before you make a big change in your lifestyle, verify the information with your physician, this text, or other reliable sources.
- *Be skeptical, and use your common sense.* If a report seems too good to be true, it probably is. Be especially wary of information contained in advertisements. The goal of an ad is to sell you something, to create a feeling of need for a product where no real need exists. Evaluate "scientific" claims carefully, and beware of quackery (see Chapter 15).
- *Make choices that are right for you.* Your roommate swears by swimming; you prefer aerobics. Your sister takes a yoga class to help her manage stress; your brother unwinds by walking in the woods. Friends and family members can be a great source of ideas and inspiration, but each of us needs to find a wellness lifestyle that works for us.

### Internet Resources

Evaluating health information from online sources poses special challenges; when reviewing a health-related Web site, ask the following questions:

- *What is the source of the information? Who is the author or sponsor of the Web page?* Web sites maintained by government agencies, professional associations, or established academic or medical institutions are likely to present trustworthy information. Many other sites post accurate information, but it is important to look at the qualifications of the people who are behind the site. (Check the home page or click on an "about us" or "who we are" link.)
- *How often is the site updated?* Look for sites that are updated frequently. Also check the "last modified" date of any specific Web page on a site.
- *What is the purpose of the page? Does the site promote particular products or procedures? Are there obvious reasons for bias?* Be wary of information from sites that sell specific products, use testimonials as evidence, appear to have a social or political agenda, or ask for money.
- *What do other sources say about a topic?* Be cautious of claims or information that appears at only one site or comes from a chat room or bulletin board.
- *Does the site conform to any set of guidelines or criteria for quality and accuracy?* Look for sites that identify themselves as conforming to some code or set of principles, such as those set forth by the Health on the Net Foundation or the American Medical Association. These codes include criteria such as use of information from respected sources and disclosure of the site's sponsors.

person who is a good role model for others, then adopting behaviors such as regular physical activity and adequate sleep would support your personal identity. If you value independence and control over your life, then quitting smoking would be consistent with your values and goals. To complete your analysis, ask friends and family members about the effects of your behavior on them. For example, a younger sister may tell you that your smoking habit influenced her decision to take up smoking.

Pay special attention to the short-term benefits of behavior change, as these can be an important motivating force. Although some people are motivated by long-term goals, such as avoiding a disease that may hit them in 30 years, most are more likely to be moved to action by shorter-term, more personal goals. Feeling better, doing better in school, improving at a sport, reducing stress, and increasing self-esteem are common short-term benefits of health behavior change.

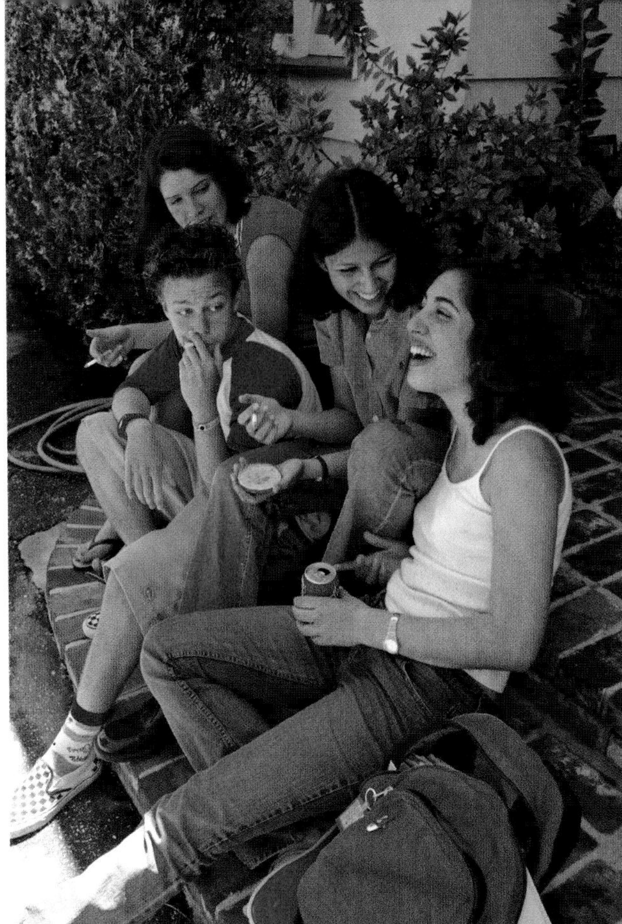

Changing powerful, long-standing habits requires motivation, commitment, and a belief that we are in control of our own behavior. To quit smoking, these young people must overcome a habit that is supported by their addiction to nicotine and by their social environment.

**Boosting Self-Efficacy** When you start thinking about changing a health behavior, a big factor in your eventual success is whether you have confidence in yourself and in your ability to change. **Self-efficacy** refers to your belief in your ability to successfully take action and perform a specific task. Strategies for boosting self-efficacy include developing an internal locus of control, using visualization and self-talk, and obtaining encouragement from supportive people.

**LOCUS OF CONTROL** Who do you believe is controlling your life? Is it your parents, friends, or school? Is it "fate"? Or is it you? **Locus of control** refers to the figurative "place" a person designates as the source of responsibility for the events in his or her life. People who believe they are in control of their own lives are said to have an internal locus of control. Those who believe that factors beyond their control—heredity, friends and family, the environment, fate, luck, or other outside forces—are more important in determining the events of their lives are said to have an external locus of control. Most people are not purely "internalizers" or "externalizers"; their locus of control changes in response to the situation.

For lifestyle management, an internal locus of control is an advantage because it reinforces motivation and commitment. For example, if you believe you can take action to reduce your hereditary risk of breast cancer, you will be motivated to follow guidelines for early detection of the disease. If you find yourself attributing too much influence to outside forces, gather more information about your target behavior. Make a list of all the ways that behavior change will improve your health. If you recognize and accept that you are in charge of your life, you're well on your way to wellness.

**VISUALIZATION AND SELF-TALK** One of the best ways to boost your confidence and self-efficacy is to visualize yourself successfully engaging in a new, healthier behavior. Imagine yourself turning down cigarettes, going for a regular after-dinner walk, or choosing healthier snacks. Also visualize yourself enjoying all the short-term and long-term benefits that behavior change will bring. Create a new self-image: What will you and your life be like when you become a nonsmoker, a regular exerciser, or a healthy eater?

You can also use self-talk, the internal dialogue you carry on with yourself, to increase your confidence in your ability to change. Counter any self-defeating patterns of thought with more positive or realistic thoughts: "Behavior change is difficult, but if I work at it, I will succeed," or "I am a strong, capable person, and I can maintain my commitment to change." Refer to Chapter 3 for more on self-talk.

**ROLE MODELS AND OTHER SUPPORTIVE INDIVIDUALS** Social support can also make a big difference in your level of motivation and your chances of success. Perhaps you know people who have reached the goal you are striving for; they could be role models or mentors for you, providing information and support for your efforts. Talk to them about how they did it. What were the most difficult parts of changing their behavior? What strategies worked for them? Gain strength from their experiences, and tell yourself, "If they can do it, so can I."

In addition, find a buddy who wants to make the same changes you do and who can take an active role in your behavior change program. For example, an exercise buddy can provide companionship and encouragement for times when you might be tempted to skip that morning jog. Or you and a friend can watch to be sure that you both have only one alcoholic beverage at a party. If necessary, look beyond your current social network at possible new sources of help, such as a support group.

**Terms**

Vw

**self-efficacy** The belief in one's ability to take action and perform a specific behavior.

**locus of control** The figurative "place" a person designates as the source of responsibility for the events in his or her life.

**Identifying and Overcoming Key Barriers to Change** Have you tried and failed to change your target behavior in the past? Don't let past failures discourage you; they can be a great source of information you can use to boost your chances of future success. Make a list of the problems and challenges you faced in your previous behavior change attempts; to this add the short-term costs of behavior change that you identified in your analysis of the pros and cons of change. Once you've listed these key barriers to change, develop a practical plan for overcoming each one. For example, if one of your key barriers for physical activity is that you believe you can't make time for a 40-minute workout, look for ways to incorporate shorter bouts of physical activity into your daily routine.

Self-talk can also help overcome barriers. Make behavior change a priority in your life, and plan to commit the necessary time and effort. Ask yourself: How much time and energy will behavior change *really* require? Isn't the effort worth all the short- and long-term benefits?

## Enhancing Your Readiness to Change

The transtheoretical, or "stages of change," model, developed by psychologists James Prochaska and Carlo DiClemente, has been shown to be an effective approach to lifestyle self-management. According to this model, you move through six well-defined stages as you work to change your target behavior. Try to identify your current stage, and then adopt appropriate strategies to move forward in the cycle of change.

**Precontemplation: No Intention of Changing Behavior** If you are in this stage, try raising your consciousness of your target behavior and its effects on you and those around you. Obtain accurate information about your behavior, and ask yourself what has prevented you from changing in the past. Enlist friends and family members to help you become more aware of your behavior and your reasons for continuing an unhealthy habit. Also find out more about the campus and community resources available to help you with behavior change.

**Contemplation: Intending to Take Action Within 6 Months** Begin keeping a written record of your target behavior—to help you learn more about it and to use when you begin to plan the specifics of your behavior change program. Work on your analysis of the pros and cons of change: Expand your list of the benefits, and problem-solve to overcome the key barriers on your list of the costs of changing. To be successful, you must believe that the benefits of change outweigh the costs. Engage your emotions and boost self-efficacy through visualization, self-talk, and the support of other people.

**Preparation: Planning to Take Action Within a Month** At this stage, your next step is to create a specific plan for change that includes a start date, realistic goals, rewards, and information on exactly how you will go about changing your behavior (see the next section of the chapter).

**Action: Outwardly Changing Behavior** This stage requires the greatest commitment of time and energy to keep from reverting to old, unhealthy patterns of behavior. You'll need to use all the plans and strategies that you developed during earlier stages.

**Maintenance: Successful Change for 6 or More Months** To guard against slips and relapses, continue with all the positive strategies you used in earlier stages.

**Termination** People at this stage have exited the cycle of change and are no longer tempted to lapse back into their old behavior. They have a new self-image and total self-efficacy with regard to their target behavior. This stage applies to some behaviors, such as addictions, but may not be appropriate for others.

Lapses are a natural part of the process at all stages of change. Many people lapse and must recycle through earlier stages, although most don't go back to the first stage. If you lapse, use what you learn about yourself and the process of change to help you in your next attempt at behavior change.

## Developing Skills for Change: Creating a Personalized Plan

Once you are committed to making a change, it's time to put together a detailed plan of action. Your key to success is a well-thought-out plan that sets goals, anticipates problems, and includes rewards.

### 1. Monitor Your Behavior and Gather Data

Begin by keeping careful records of the behavior you wish to change (your target behavior) and the circumstances surrounding it. Keep these records in a health journal, a notebook in which you write the details of your behavior along with observations and comments. Note exactly what the activity was, when and where it happened, what you were doing, and what your feelings were at the time (see the sample in Figure 1-5). Keep your journal for a week or two to get some solid information about the behavior you want to change.

### 2. Analyze the Data and Identify Patterns

After you have collected data on the behavior, analyze the data to identify patterns. When are you hungriest? When are you most likely to overeat? What events seem to trigger your appetite? Perhaps you are especially hungry at midmorning or when you put off eating dinner until 9:00. Perhaps you overindulge in food and drink when you go

| Date November 5 | | | | Day M TU W TH F SA SU | | | | | | |
|---|---|---|---|---|---|---|---|---|---|---|
| *Time of day* | *M/S* | *Food eaten* | *Cals.* | *H* | *Where did you eat?* | *What else were you doing?* | *How did someone else influence you?* | *What made you want to eat what you did?* | *Emotions and feelings?* | *Thoughts and concerns?* |
| 7:30 | M | 1 C Crispix cereal<br>1/2 C skim milk<br>coffee, black<br>1 C orange juice | 110<br>40<br>—<br>120 | 3 | home | reading newspaper | alone | I always eat cereal in the morning | a little keyed up & worried | thinking about quiz in class today |
| 10:30 | S | 1 apple | 90 | 1 | hall outside classroom | studying | alone | felt tired & wanted to wake up | tired | worried about next class |
| 12:30 | M | 1 C chili<br>1 roll<br>1 pat butter<br>1 orange<br>2 oatmeal cookies<br>1 soda | 290<br>120<br>35<br>60<br>120<br>150 | 2 | campus food court | talking | eating w/ friends; we decided to eat at the food court | wanted to be part of group | excited and happy | interested in hearing everyone's plans for the weekend |
| | M/S = Meal or snack | | | | H = Hunger rating (0–3) | | | | | |

**Figure 1-5 Sample health journal entries.**

to a particular restaurant or when you're with certain friends. Be sure to note the connections between your feelings and external cues such as time of day, location, situation, and the actions of people around you. Do you always think of having a cigarette when you read the newspaper? Do you always bite your fingernails when you're studying?

**3. Set Realistic, Specific Goals** Don't set an impossibly difficult overall goal for your program—going from a sedentary lifestyle to running a marathon within 2 months, for example. Working toward more realistic, achievable goals will greatly increase your chances of success. Your goal should also be specific and measurable, something you can easily track. Instead of a vague general goal such as improving eating habits or being more physically active, set a specific target—eating eight servings of fruits and vegetables each day or walking or biking for 30 minutes at least 5 days per week.

Whatever your ultimate goal, it's a good idea to break it down into a few small steps. Your plan will seem less overwhelming and more manageable, increasing the chances that you'll stick to it. You'll also build in more opportunities to reward yourself (discussed in step 4), as well as milestones you can use to measure your progress. If you plan to lose 15 pounds, for example, you'll find it easier to take off 5 pounds at a time. If you want to start an exercise program, begin by taking 10- to 15-minute walks a few times per week. Take the easier steps first and work up to the harder steps. With each small success, you'll build your confidence and self-efficacy.

**4. Devise a Strategy or Plan of Action** Next, you need to develop specific strategies and techniques that will support your day-to-day efforts at behavior change.

**OBTAIN INFORMATION AND SUPPLIES** Identify campus and community resources that can provide practical help—for example, a stop-smoking course or a walking club. Take any necessary preparatory steps, such as signing up for a stress-management workshop or purchasing walking shoes, nicotine replacement patches, or a special calendar to track your progress.

**MODIFY YOUR ENVIRONMENT** You can be more effective in changing behavior if you control the environmental cues that provoke it. This might mean not having cigarettes or certain foods or drinks in the house, not going to parties where you're tempted to overindulge, or not spending time with particular people, at least for a while. If you always get a candy bar at a certain vending machine, change your route so you don't pass by it. If you always end up taking a coffee break and chatting with friends when you go to the library to study, choose a different place to study, such as your room.

You can change the cues in your environment so they trigger the new, target behavior instead of the old one. Tape a picture of a cyclist speeding down a hill on your TV screen. Leave your exercise shoes in plain view. Put a chart of your progress in a special place at home to make your goals highly visible and inspire you to keep going. When you're trying to change an ingrained habit, small cues can play an important part in keeping you on track.

**REWARD YOURSELF** Another very powerful way to affect your target behavior is to set up a reward system that will reinforce your efforts. Most people find it difficult to change long-standing habits for rewards they can't see right away. Giving yourself instant, real rewards for good

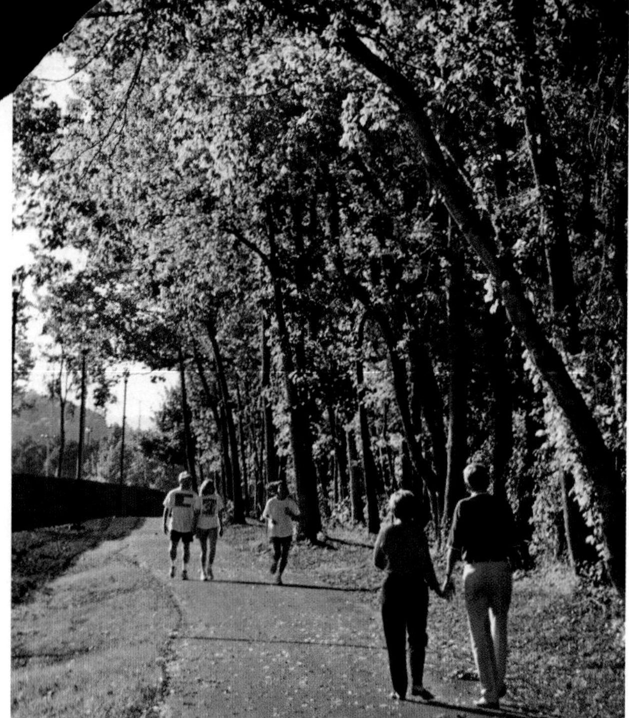

A beautiful day and a spectacular setting contribute to making exercise a satisfying and pleasurable experience. Choosing the right activity and doing it the right way are important elements in a successful health behavior change program.

behavior along the way will help you stick with a plan to change your behavior.

Make a list of your activities and favorite events to use as rewards. They should be special, inexpensive, and preferably unrelated to food or alcohol. Depending on what you like to do, you might treat yourself to a concert, a ball game, a new CD, a long-distance phone call to a friend, a day off from studying to take a long hike in the woods—whatever is rewarding to you. Don't forget to reward yourself for good behavior that is consistent and persistent—such as simply sticking with your program week after week.

**INVOLVE THE PEOPLE AROUND YOU** Rewards and support can also come from family and friends. Tell them about your plan, and ask for their help. Encourage them to be active, interested participants. Ask them to support you when you set aside time to go running or avoid second helpings at Thanksgiving dinner. To help friends and family members who will be involved in your program respond appropriately, you may want to create a specific list of dos and don'ts.

**PLAN AHEAD FOR CHALLENGING SITUATIONS** Take time out now to list situations and people that have the potential to derail your program and to develop possible coping mechanisms. For example, if you think that you'll have trouble exercising during finals week, schedule short bouts of physical activity as stress-reducing study breaks. If a visit to a friend who smokes is likely to tempt you to lapse, plan to bring nicotine patches, chewing gum, and a copy of your behavior change contract to strengthen your resolve.

My Personal Contract for Eating Three Servings of Fruit per Day

I agree to increase my consumption of fruit from one serving per week to three servings per day. I will begin my program on 10/5 and plan to reach my final goal by 12/7. I have divided my program into three parts, with three separate goals. For each step in my program, I will give myself the reward listed.

1. I will begin to have a serving of fruit with breakfast on 10/5.
   (Reward: baseball game)
2. I will begin to have a serving of fruit with lunch on 10/26.
   (Reward: music CD)
3. I will begin to substitute fruit juice for soda for one snack each day on 11/16.
   (Reward: concert)

My plan for increasing fruit consumption includes the following strategies:

1. Keeping my refrigerator stocked with easy-to-carry fruit and fruit juice.
2. Packing fruit in my book backpack every day.
3. Placing reminders to buy, carry, and eat fruit in my room, backpack, and wallet.
4. Buying lunch at a place that serves fruit or fruit juice.

I understand that it is important for me to make a strong personal effort to make the change in my behavior. I sign this contract as an indication of my personal commitment to reach my goal.

Michael Cook 9/28

Witness: Katie Lim 9/28

**Figure 1-6 A sample behavior change contract.**

**5. Make a Commitment by Signing a Personal Contract** A serious personal contract—one that commits your word—can result in a higher chance of follow-through than will a casual, offhand promise. Your contract can help prevent procrastination by specifying the important dates and can also serve as a reminder of your personal commitment to change. Your contract should include a statement of your goal and your commitment to reaching it. Include details of your plan: the date you'll begin, the steps you'll use to measure your progress, the concrete strategies you've developed for promoting change, and the date you expect to reach your final goal. Have someone—preferably someone who will be actively helping you with your program—sign your contract as a witness.

**A Sample Behavior Change Plan** Let's take the example of Michael, who wants to improve his diet. By monitoring his eating habits in his health journal for several weeks, he gets a good sense of his typical diet—what he eats and where he eats it. Through self-assessment and investigation, he discovers that he currently consumes only about one serving of fruit per week, much less than the recommended three to five servings per day. He also finds out that fruit is a major source of fiber, vitamins, minerals, and other substances important for good health. He sets the target of eating three servings of fruit per day as the overall goal for his behavior change plan. Then Michael develops a specific plan for change that involves several changes in his behavior and his environment, which he describes in a contract that commits him to reaching his goal (Figure 1-6). Once Michael has signed his contract, he's ready to take action.

You can apply the general behavior change planning framework presented in this chapter to any target behavior. Additional examples of behavior change plans are presented in the Behavior Change Strategy sections that appear at the end of many chapters.

### Putting Your Plan into Action

The starting date has arrived, and you are ready to put your plan into action. This stage requires commitment, the resolve to stick with the plan no matter what temptations you encounter. Remember all the good reasons you have for making the change—and remember that *you* are the boss. Use all your strategies to make your plan work. Make sure your environment is change-friendly, and obtain as much support and encouragement from others as possible. Use your health journal to keep track of how well you are doing in achieving your ultimate goal and give yourself regular rewards. And don't forget to give yourself a pat on the back—congratulate yourself, notice how much better you look or feel, and feel good about how far you've come and how you've gained control of your behavior.

### Staying with It

As you continue with your program, don't be surprised when you run up against obstacles; they're inevitable. In fact, it's a good idea to expect problems and give yourself time to step back, see how you're doing, and make some changes before going on again. If you find your program is grinding to a halt, try to identify what is blocking your progress and revise your plan if necessary. Consider whether the people around you are supportive, and evaluate your own levels of motivation and commitment (see the box "Motivation Boosters"). High levels of stress can also derail a behavior change program. If stress is a problem for you, consider making stress management your highest priority for behavior change (see Chapter 2).

## BEING HEALTHY FOR LIFE

Your first few behavior change projects may never go beyond the planning stage. Those that do may not all succeed. But as you taste success by beginning to see progress and changes, you'll start to experience new and surprising positive feelings about yourself. You'll probably find that you're less likely to buckle under stress. You may accomplish things you never thought possible—winning a race, climbing a mountain, quitting smoking. Being healthy takes extra effort, but the paybacks in energy and vitality are priceless.

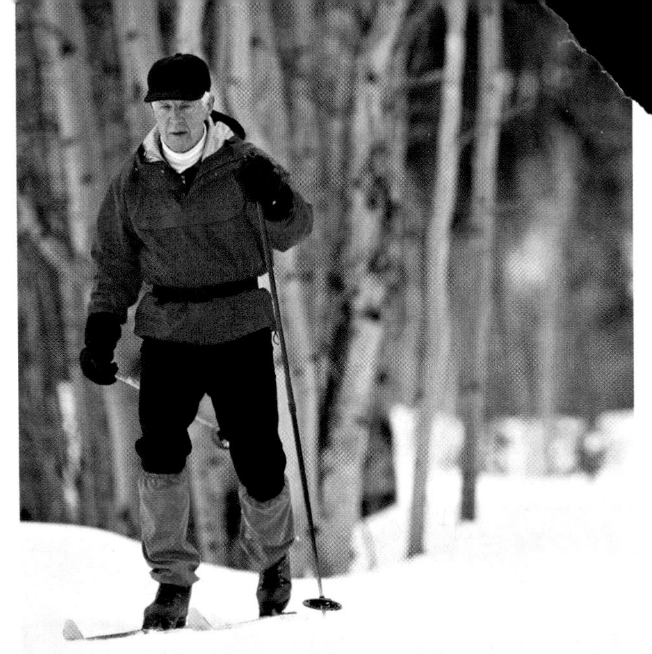
This retiree spends leisure time cross-country skiing. If you want to enjoy vigor and health in *your* middle and old age, begin now to make the choices that will give you lifelong vitality.

Once you've started, don't stop. Remember that maintaining good health is an ongoing process. Tackle one area at a time, but make a careful inventory of your health strengths and weaknesses and lay out a long-range plan. Take on the easier problems first, and then use what you have learned to attack more difficult areas. Keep informed about the latest health news and trends; research is constantly providing new information that directly affects daily choices and habits.

You can't completely control every aspect of your health. At least three other factors—heredity, health care, and environment—play important roles in your wellbeing. But you can make a difference—you can help create an environment around you that supports wellness for everyone. You can help support nonsmoking areas in public places. You can speak up in favor of more nutritious foods and better physical fitness facilities. You can include nonalcoholic drinks at your parties. You can also work on larger environmental challenges: air and water pollution, traffic congestion, overcrowding and overpopulation, and many others.

In your lifetime, you can choose to take an active role in the movement toward increased awareness, greater individual responsibility and control, healthier lifestyles, and a healthier planet. Your choices and actions will have

Take Charge

## Motivation Boosters

Changing behavior takes motivation. But how do you get motivated? The following strategies may help:

- Write down the potential benefits of the change. If you want to lose weight, your list might include increased ease of movement, energy, and self-confidence.
- Now write down the costs of not changing.
- Frequently visualize yourself achieving your goal and enjoying its benefits. If you want to manage time more effectively, picture yourself as a confident, organized person who systematically tackles important tasks and sets aside time each day for relaxation, exercise, and friends.
- Discount obstacles to change. Counter thoughts such as "I'll never have time to shop for and prepare healthy foods" with thoughts such as "Lots of other people have done it and so can I."
- Bombard yourself with propaganda. Subscribe to a self-improvement magazine. Take a class dealing with the change you want to make. Read books and watch talk shows on the subject. Post motivational phrases or pictures on your refrigerator or over your desk. Listen to motivational tapes in the car. Talk to people who have already made the change you want to make.
- Build up your confidence. Remind yourself of other goals you've achieved. At the end of each day, mentally review your good decisions and actions. See yourself as a capable person, in charge of your health.
- Create choices. You will be more likely to exercise every day if you have two or three types of exercise to choose from, and more likely to quit smoking if you've identified more than one way to distract yourself when you crave a cigarette. Get ideas from people who have been successful, and adapt some of their strategies to suit you.
- If you slip, keep trying. Research suggests that four out of five people will experience some degree of backsliding when they try to change a behavior. Only one in four succeeds the first time around. If you retain your commitment to change even when you lapse, you still are farther along the path to change than before you made the commitment. Try again. And again, if necessary.

a tremendous impact on your present and future wellness. The door is open, and the time is now—you simply have to begin.

Tips for Today

You are in charge of your health! Many of the decisions you make every day have an impact on the quality of your life, both now and in the future. By making positive choices, large and small, you help ensure a lifetime of wellness.

*Right now you can*

- Go for a 15-minute walk.
- Have an orange, a nectarine, or a plum for a snack.
- Call a friend and arrange a time to catch up with each other.
- Start thinking about whether you have a health behavior you'd like to change. If you do, consider the elements of a behavior change strategy. For example,
  - Begin a mental list of the pros and cons of the behavior.
  - Think of one or two rewards that will be meaningful to you as you reach interim goals.
  - Think of someone who will support you in your attempts to make a behavior change—either someone who might want to make the same change you're contemplating or someone you can trust to provide you with encouragement. Talk to that person about your plan, get feedback, and ask for support.

## SUMMARY

- Wellness is the ability to live life fully, with vitality and meaning. Wellness is dynamic and multidimensional; it incorporates physical, emotional, intellectual, spiritual, interpersonal and social, and environmental dimensions.
- As chronic diseases have become the leading cause of death in the United States, people have recognized that they have greater control over, and greater responsibility for, their health than ever before.
- The Healthy People initiative seeks to achieve a better quality of life for all Americans. The broad goals of the *Healthy People 2010* report are to increase quality and years of healthy life and to eliminate health disparities among Americans.
- Health-related differences among people that have implications for wellness can be described in the context of gender, ethnicity, income and education, disability, geographic location, and sexual orientation.
- Although heredity, environment, and health care all play roles in wellness and disease, behavior can mitigate their effects.
- To make lifestyle changes, you need information about yourself, your health habits, and resources available to help you change.
- You can increase your motivation for behavior change by examining the benefits and costs of change, boosting self-efficacy, and identifying and overcoming key barriers to change.

- The "stages of change" model describes six stages that people move through as they try to change their behavior: precontemplation, contemplation, preparation, action, maintenance, and termination.
- A specific plan for change can be developed by (1) monitoring behavior by keeping a journal; (2) analyzing the recorded data; (3) setting specific goals; (4) devising strategies for modifying the environment, rewarding yourself, and involving others; and (5) making a personal contract.
- Although we cannot control every aspect of our health, we can make a difference in helping create an environment that supports wellness for everyone.

## Take Action

1. **Start a health journal.** Use a daily planner or PDA as your health journal throughout the course; use it to track your behavior, your emotions, and other factors related to wellness. As a first journal activity, create lists of the positive lifestyle behaviors that enhance your well-being and the behaviors that detract from wellness. Use these lists as the basis for self-evaluation as you proceed through the book. (Visit the Online Learning Center for health journal activities for each chapter.)

2. **Interview older family members.** Ask older members of your family (parents or grandparents) what they recall about patterns of health and disease when they were young. Did any of their friends or relatives die at an early age or of a disease that can now be treated? How have health concerns changed during their lifetime?

3. **Find a wellness role model.** Choose someone you consider to have embraced a wellness lifestyle. How is that person's overall health reflected in each of the dimensions of wellness? What can you borrow from her or his experiences and strategies for success in building a wellness lifestyle?

4. **Locate community resources.** Your school and community may present challenges to making healthy lifestyle choices, but they also have resources that can help you. Find out what local resources are "on your side" and can support your efforts at change; examples include free fitness facilities, stress-management workshops, and stop-smoking programs. As you become more aware of local resources and issues, you may also begin to identify ways that you could become involved to improve your community and its ability to promote wellness for all.

## For More Information

### Books

Komaroff, A. L., ed. 2005. *Harvard Medical School Family Health Guide.* New York: Free Press. *Provides consumer-oriented advice for the prevention and treatment of common health concerns.*

Prochaska, J. O., J. C. Norcross, and C. C. DiClemente. 1994. *Changing for Good: The Revolutionary Program That Explains the Six Stages of Change and Teaches You How to Free Yourself from Bad Habits.* New York: Morrow. *Outlines the authors' model of behavior change and offers suggestions and advice for each stage of change.*

Smith, P. B., M. MacFarlane, and E. Kalnitsky. 2002. *The Complete Idiot's Guide to Wellness.* Indianapolis, Ind.: Alpha Books. *A concise guide to healthy habits, including physical activity, nutrition, and stress management.*

### Newsletters

*Consumer Reports on Health* (800-234-2188; http://www.ConsumerReportsonHealth.org)

*Harvard Health Letter* (800-829-9045; http://www.health.harvard.edu)

*Harvard Men's Health Watch; Harvard Women's Health Watch* (877-649-9457)

*Mayo Clinic Health Letter* (866-516-4974)

*University of California at Berkeley Wellness Letter* (800-829-9170; http://www.wellnessletter.com)

### VW Organizations, Hotlines, and Web Sites

The Internet addresses (also called uniform resource locators, or URLs) listed here were accurate at the time of publication. Up-to-date links to these and many other wellness-oriented Web sites are provided on the links page of the *Core Concepts in Health* Web site (www.mhhe.com/inselbrief10e).

*Centers for Disease Control and Prevention.* Through phone, fax, and the Internet, the CDC provides a wide variety of health information.

800-311-3435
http://www.cdc.gov

Many other government Web sites provide access to health-related materials:

Agency for Healthcare Research and Quality: http://www.ahrq.gov/consumer
FirstGov for Consumers: Health: http://www.consumer.gov/health.htm
National Institutes of Health: http://www.nih.gov
National Library of Medicine, MedlinePlus: http://www.medlineplus.gov
Office of Minority Health Resource Center: http://www.omhrc.gov

*Go Ask Alice.* Sponsored by the Columbia University Health Service, this site provides answers to student questions about stress, sexuality, fitness, and many other wellness topics.

http://www.goaskalice.columbia.edu

*Healthfinder.* A gateway to online publications, Web sites, support and self-help groups, and agencies and organizations that produce reliable health information.

http://www.healthfinder.gov

*Healthy People 2010.* Provides information on Healthy People objectives and priority areas.

http://www.healthypeople.gov

*MedlinePlus: Evaluating Health Information.* Provides background information and links to sites with guidelines for finding and evaluating health information from the Web.
http://www.nlm.nih.gov/medlineplus/evaluatinghealthinformation.html

*National Health Information Center (NHIC).* Puts consumers in touch with the organizations that are best able to provide answers to health-related questions.
800-336-4797
http://www.health.gov/nhic

*National Women's Health Information Center.* Provides information and answers to frequently asked questions.
800-994-WOMAN
http://www.4woman.gov

*NOAH: New York Online Access to Health.* Provides consumer health information in both English and Spanish.
http://www.noah-health.org

*Student Counseling Virtual Pamphlet Collection.* Provides links to more than 400 pamphlets produced by different student counseling centers on a variety of wellness topics.
http://counseling.uchicago.edu/vpc

*World Health Organization (WHO).* Provides information about health topics and issues affecting people around the world.
http://www.who.int

The following are just a few of the many sites that provide consumer-oriented information on a variety of health issues:
*FamilyDoctor.Org:* http://familydoctor.org
*InteliHealth:* http://www.intelihealth.com
*MayoClinic.Com:* http://mayoclinic.com
*WebMD:* http://webmd.com

The following sites provide daily health news updates:
*CNN Health:* http://www.cnn.com/health
*MedlinePlus News:* http://www.nlm.nih.gov/medlineplus/newsbydate.html
*Yahoo Health News:* http://dailynews.yahoo.com/h/hl

## Selected Bibliography


American Cancer Society. 2005. *Cancer Facts and Figures—2005.* Atlanta: American Cancer Society.

American Heart Association. 2005. *2005 Heart and Stroke Statistical Update.* Dallas: American Heart Association.

Calle, E. E., et al. 2003. Overweight, obesity, and mortality from cancer in a prospectively studied cohort of U.S. adults. *New England Journal of Medicine* 348(17): 1625–1638.

Cauley, J. A., et al. 2005. Longitudinal study of changes in hip bone mineral density in Caucasian and African American women. *Journal of the American Geriatrics Society* 53(2): 183–189.

Centers for Disease Control and Prevention. 2005. Racial/ethnic and socioeconomic disparities in multiple risk factors for heart disease and stroke, United States, 2003. *Morbidity and Mortality Weekly Report* 54(5): 113–117.

Centers for Disease Control and Prevention. 1999. Achievements in public health, 1900–1999: Tobacco use, United States. *Morbidity and Mortality Weekly Report* 48(43): 986–993.

Centers for Disease Control and Prevention. 2004. REACH 2010 surveillance for health status in minority communities. *MMWR Surveillance Summaries* 53(SS-6).

Centers for Disease Control and Prevention, Division of Nutrition and Physical Activity. 1999. *Promoting Physical Activity: A Guide for Community Action.* Champaign, Ill.: Human Kinetics.

Glanz, K., F. M. Lewis, and B. K. Rimer, eds. 2002. *Health Behavior and Health Education: Theory, Research, and Practice,* 3rd ed. San Francisco: Jossey-Bass.

Institute of Medicine. 2001. *Exploring the Biological Contributions to Human Health: Does Sex Matter?* Washington, D.C.: National Academy Press.

International Human Genome Sequencing Consortium. 2004. Finishing the euchromatic sequence of the human genome. *Nature* 431: 931–945.

Jemal, A., et al. 2005. Cancer statistics, 2005. *CA: A Cancer Journal for Clinicians* 55(1): 10–30.

Kaiser Family Foundation. 2003. *Key Facts: Race, Ethnicity, and Medical Care.* Menlo Park, Calif.: Kaiser Family Foundation.

Martin, G., and J. Pear. 2003. *Behaviour Modification: What It Is and How to Do It,* 7th ed. Upper Saddle River, N.J.: Prentice-Hall.

Mokdad, A. H., et al. 2003. Prevalence of obesity, diabetes, and obesity-related health risk factors, 2001. *Journal of the American Medical Association* 289(1): 76–79.

Mokdad, A. H., et al. 2004. Actual causes of death in the United States, 2000. *Journal of the American Medical Association* 291(10): 1238–1245.

Mokdad, A. H., et al. 2005. Correction: Actual causes of death in the United States, 2000. *Journal of the American Medical Association* 293(3): 293–294.

Muller, A. 2002. Education, income inequality, and mortality: A multiple regression analysis. *British Medical Journal* 324(7328): 23–25.

National Cancer Institute. 2004. *Cancer Facts: Cancer Clusters* (http://cis.nci.nih.gov/fact/3_58.htm; retrieved October 23, 2004).

National Center for Health Statistics. 2004. *Health, United States, 2004, with Chartbook on Trends in the Health of Americans.* Hyattsville, Md.: National Center for Health Statistics.

National Center for Health Statistics. 2004. Health behaviors of adults: United States, 1999–2001. *Vital and Health Statistics* 10(219).

Slater, M. D., and D. E. Zimmerman. 2002. Characteristics of health-related Web sites identified by common Internet portals. *Journal of the American Medical Association* 288(3): 316–317.

Steenland, K., et al. 2003. Deaths due to injuries among employed adults: The effects of socioeconomic class. *Epidemiology* 14(1): 74–79.

U.S. Census Bureau. 2005. *We the People: Women and Men in the United States.* Washington, D.C.: U.S. Census Bureau.

U.S. Department of Health and Human Services. 2000. *Healthy People 2010,* 2nd ed. Washington, D.C.: DHHS.

World Health Organization. 2004. *Why Gender and Health?* (http://www.who.int/gender/genderandhealth/en; retrieved August 13, 2004).

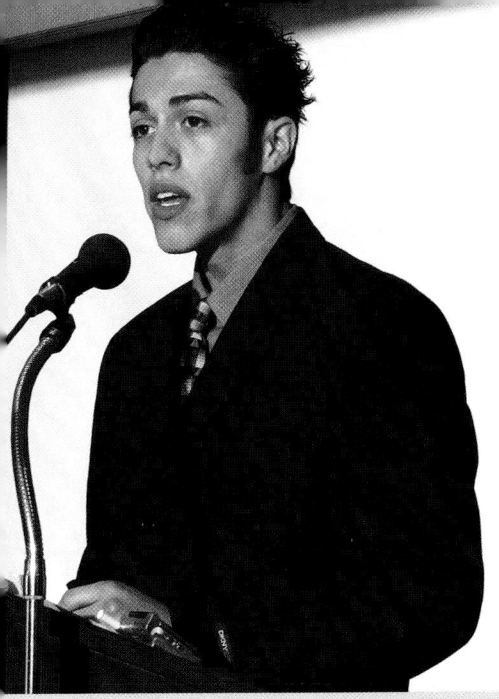

**Looking AHEAD**

After reading this chapter, you should be able to

- Explain what stress is and how people react to it—physically, emotionally, and behaviorally
- Describe the relationship between stress and disease
- List common sources of stress
- Describe techniques for preventing and managing stress
- Put together a step-by-step plan for successfully managing the stress in your life

2

# Stress: The Constant Challenge

Everybody talks about stress. People say they're "overstressed" or "stressed out." They may blame stress for headaches or ulcers, and they may try to combat stress with aerobics classes—or drugs. But what is stress? And why is it important to manage it wisely?

Most people associate stress with negative events: the death of a close relative or friend, financial problems, or other unpleasant life changes that create nervous tension. But stress isn't merely nervous tension. And it isn't something to be avoided at all costs (Figure 2-1). Consider this list of common stressful situations or events: interviewing for a job, running in a race, being accepted to college, going out on a date, watching a basketball game, and getting a promotion.

Obviously, stress doesn't arise just from unpleasant situations. Stress can also be associated with physical challenges and the achievement of personal goals. Physical and psychological stress-producing factors can be pleasant or unpleasant. What is crucial is how you respond, whether in positive, life-enhancing ways or in negative, counterproductive ways.

As a college student, you may be in one of the most stressful periods of your life. You may be on your own for the first time, or you may be juggling the demands of college with the responsibilities of a job, a family, or both. Financial pressures may be intense. Housing and transportation may be sources of additional hassles. You're also meeting new people, engaging in new activities, learning new information and skills, and setting a new course for your life. Good and bad, all these changes and challenges are likely to have a powerful effect on you, both physically and psychologically. Respond ineffectively to stress, and eventually it will take a toll on your sense of wellness.

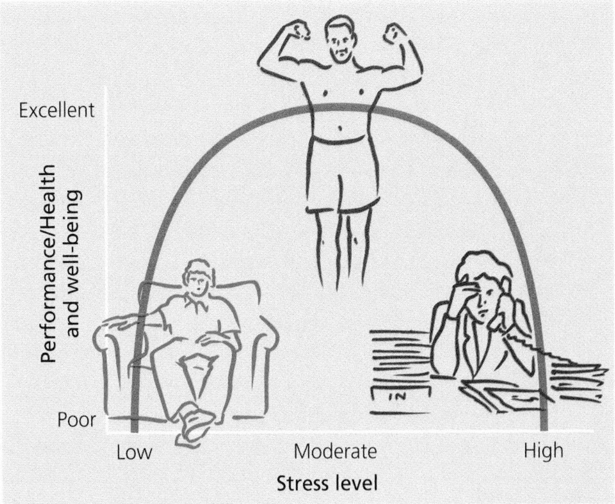


**Figure 2-1 Stress level, performance, and well-being.** A moderate level of stress challenges individuals in a way that promotes optimal performance and well-being. Too little stress, and people are not challenged enough to improve; too much stress, and the challenges become stressors that can impair physical and emotional health.

**Visit the *Core Concepts in Health* Online Learning Center (www.mhhe.com/inselbrief10e) for study aids and many additional resources.**

Learn effective responses, however, and you will enhance your health and gain a feeling of control over your life.

## WHAT IS STRESS?

Just what is stress, if such vastly different situations can cause it? In common usage, "stress" refers to two different things: situations that trigger physical and emotional reactions *and* the reactions themselves. In this text, we'll use the more precise term **stressor** for situations that trigger physical and emotional reactions and the term **stress response** for those reactions. A date and a final exam, then, are stressors; sweaty palms and a pounding heart are symptoms of the stress response. We'll use the term **stress** to describe the general physical and emotional state that accompanies the stress response. A person on a date or taking a final exam experiences stress.

### Terms

VW

**stressor** Any physical or psychological event or condition that produces stress.

**stress response** The physiological changes associated with stress.

**stress** The collective physiological and emotional responses to any stimulus that disturbs an individual's homeostasis.

**autonomic nervous system** The branch of the peripheral nervous system that, largely without conscious thought, controls basic body processes; consists of the sympathetic and parasympathetic divisions.

**parasympathetic division** A division of the autonomic system that moderates the excitatory effect of the sympathetic division, slowing metabolism and restoring energy supplies.

**sympathetic division** A division of the autonomic nervous system that reacts to danger or other challenges by almost instantly accelerating body processes.

**norepinephrine** A neurotransmitter released by the sympathetic nervous system onto target tissues to increase their function in the face of increased activity; when released in the brain, it causes arousal (increased attention, awareness, and alertness); also called *noradrenaline*.

**endocrine system** The system of glands, tissues, and cells that secrete hormones into the bloodstream to influence metabolism and other body processes.

**hormone** A chemical messenger produced in the body and transported by the bloodstream to target cells or organs for specific regulation of their activities.

**hypothalamus** A part of the brain that activates, controls, and integrates the autonomic mechanisms, endocrine activities, and many body functions.

**pituitary gland** The "master gland," closely linked with the hypothalamus, that controls other endocrine glands and secretes hormones that regulate growth, maturation, and reproduction.

**adrenocorticotropic hormone (ACTH)** A hormone, formed in the pituitary gland, that stimulates the outer layer of the adrenal gland to secrete its hormones.

**adrenal glands** Two glands, one lying atop each kidney, whose outer layer (cortex) produces steroid hormones such as cortisol and whose inner core (medulla) produces the hormones epinephrine and norepinephrine.

**cortisol** A steroid hormone secreted by the cortex (outer layer) of the adrenal gland; also called *hydrocortisone*.

**epinephrine** A hormone secreted by the medulla (inner core) of the adrenal gland that affects the functioning of organs involved in responding to a stressor; also called *adrenaline*.

**endorphins** Brain secretions that have pain-inhibiting effects.

**fight-or-flight reaction** A defense reaction that prepares an individual for conflict or escape by triggering hormonal, cardiovascular, metabolic, and other changes.

### Physical Responses to Stressors

Imagine that you are waiting to cross a street, perhaps daydreaming about a movie you saw last week. The light turns green and you step off the curb. Almost before you see it, you feel a car speeding toward you. With just a fraction of a second to spare, you leap safely out of harm's way. In that split second of danger and in the moments following it, you have experienced a predictable series of physical reactions. Your body has gone from a relaxed state to one prepared for physical action to cope with a threat to your life. Two major control systems in your body are responsible for your physical response to stressors: the nervous system and the endocrine system.

**Actions of the Nervous System** The nervous system consists primarily of the brain, spinal cord, and nerves. Part of the nervous system is under voluntary control: commanding your arm to reach for a chocolate, for instance. The part that is not under conscious supervision, such as what controls the digestion of the chocolate, is known as the **autonomic nervous system.** In addition to digestion, it controls heart rate, breathing, blood pressure, and hundreds of other functions you normally take for granted.

The autonomic nervous system consists of two divisions. The **parasympathetic division** is in control when you are relaxed; it aids in digesting food, storing energy, and promoting growth. In contrast, the **sympathetic division** is activated during arousal or when there is an emergency, such as severe pain, anger, or fear. Sympathetic nerves use the neurotransmitter **norepinephrine** to exert their actions on nearly every organ, sweat gland, blood vessel, and muscle to enable your body to handle an emergency. In general, it commands your body to stop storing energy and instead to mobilize all energy resources to respond to the crisis.

**Actions of the Endocrine System** One important target of the sympathetic nervous system is the **endocrine system.** This system of glands, tissues, and cells helps control body functions by releasing **hormones** and other chemical messengers into the bloodstream. Chemicals released into the blood are relatively free to travel throughout the body. The sites of action for circulating stress hormones are determined by specialized receptors in target

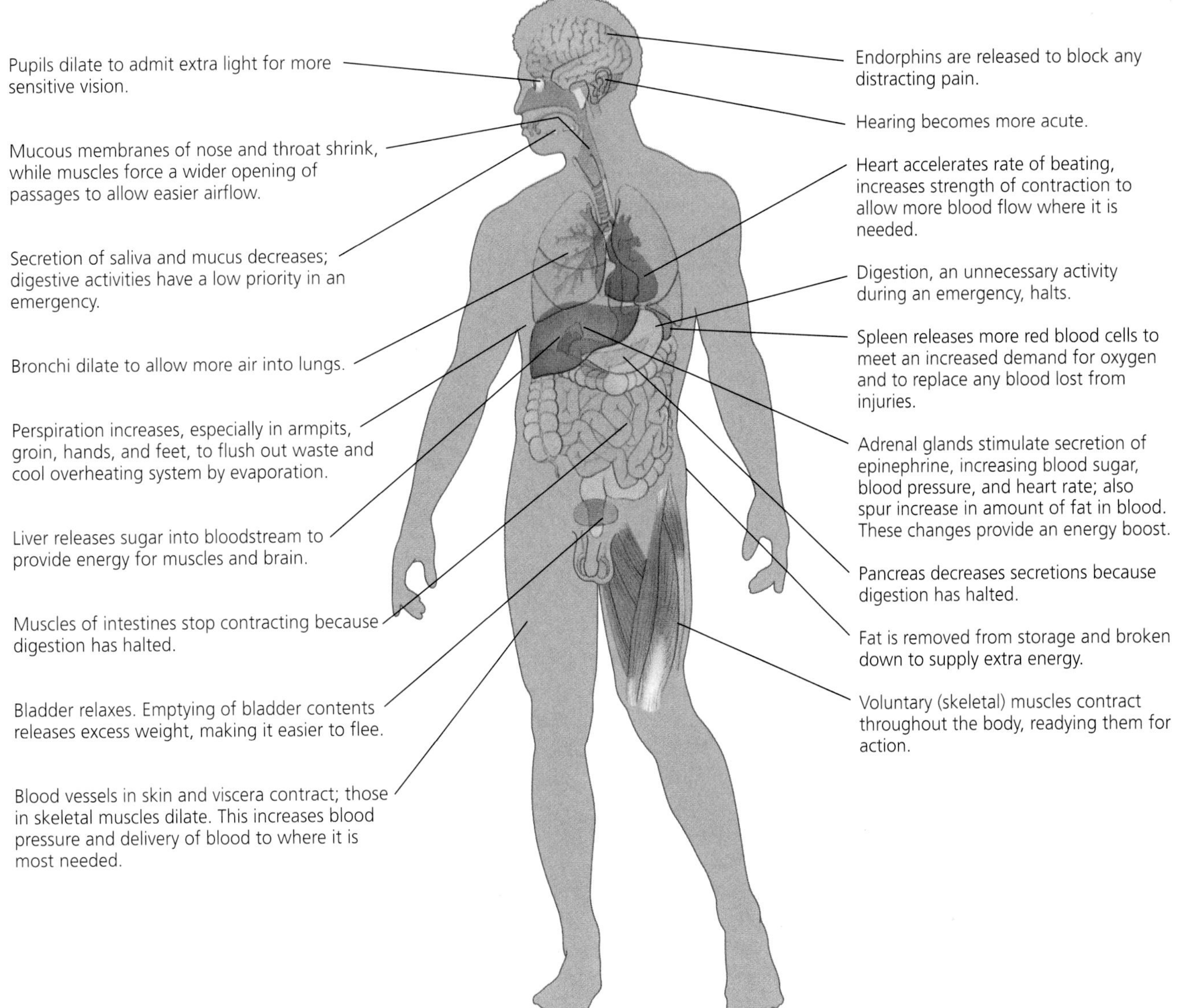


**Figure 2-2 The fight-or-flight reaction.** In response to a stressor, the autonomic nervous system and the endocrine system cause physical changes that prepare the body to deal with an emergency.

tissues. Thus, stress hormones will act only on those organs that have stress hormone receptors.

**The Two Systems Together** How do both systems work together in an emergency? Let's go back to your close call with that car. Both reflexive and higher cognitive areas in your brain quickly make the decision that a large object traveling toward you at a high rate of speed is a threat and requires immediate action. A neurochemical message is promptly sent to the **hypothalamus,** a hormonal control center in the brain, that its services are needed, and it releases a chemical wake-up call to the nearby **pituitary gland.** In turn, the pituitary gland releases **adrenocorticotropic hormone (ACTH)** into the bloodstream. When ACTH reaches the **adrenal glands,** located just above the kidneys, it stimulates them to release **cortisol** and other key hormones into the bloodstream. Simultaneously, sympathetic nerves instruct your adrenal glands to release the hormone **epinephrine,** or adrenaline, which in turn triggers a series of profound changes throughout your body (Figure 2-2). For example, your hearing and vision become more acute. Bronchi dilate to allow more air into your lungs. Your heart rate accelerates and blood pressure increases to ensure that your blood—and the oxygen, nutrients, and hormones it carries—will be rapidly distributed where needed. Your liver releases extra sugar into your bloodstream to provide an energy boost for your muscles and brain. **Endorphins** are released to relieve pain in case of injury.

It was Sir Walter Cannon who first called these almost-instantaneous physical changes, collectively, the **fight-or-flight reaction.** These changes give you the heightened reflexes and strength you need to dodge the car or deal with other stressors. Although these physical changes may vary in intensity, the same basic set of physical reactions occurs in response to any type of stressor, positive or negative.

**The Return to Homeostasis** Once a stressful situation ends, the parasympathetic division of your autonomic nervous system takes command and halts the reaction. It initiates the adjustments necessary to restore **homeostasis,** a state in which blood pressure, heart rate, hormone levels, and other vital functions are maintained within a narrow range of normal. Your parasympathetic nervous system calms your body down, slowing a rapid heartbeat, drying sweaty palms, and returning breathing to normal. Gradually, your body resumes its normal "housekeeping" functions, such as digestion and temperature regulation. Damage that may have been sustained during the fight-or-flight reaction is repaired. The day after you narrowly dodge the car, you wake up feeling fine. In this way, your body can grow, repair itself, and acquire reserves of energy. When the next crisis comes, you'll be ready to respond—instantly—again.

**The Fight-or-Flight Reaction in Modern Life** The fight-or-flight reaction is a part of our biological heritage, a survival mechanism that has served humankind well. It enables our bodies to quickly prepare to escape from an injury or to engage in a physical battle. In modern life, however, the fight-or-flight reaction is often absurdly inappropriate. Many of the stressors we face in everyday life do not require a physical response—for example, an exam, a mess left by a roommate, or a red traffic light. The fight-or-flight reaction prepares the body for physical action regardless of whether such action is a necessary or appropriate response to a particular stressor.

## Emotional and Behavioral Responses to Stressors

The physical response to a stressor may vary in intensity from person to person and situation to situation, but we all experience a similar set of physical changes—the fight-or-flight reaction. However, there is a great deal of variation in how people view potential stressors and in how people respond to them.

**Effective and Ineffective Responses** Common emotional responses to stressors include anxiety, depression, fear, or exhilaration. Although emotional responses are determined in part by inborn personality, we often can moderate or learn to control them. Coping techniques are discussed later in the chapter.

Our behavioral responses—controlled by the **somatic nervous system,** which manages our conscious actions—are under our control. Effective behavioral responses can promote wellness and enable us to function at our best. Ineffective behavioral responses can impair wellness and can even become stressors themselves. Depending on the stressor involved, effective behavioral responses may include talking, laughing, exercising, meditating, learning time-management skills, or finding a more compatible roommate. Inappropriate behavioral responses include overeating, substance abuse, or expressing hostility. Emotional and behavioral responses to stressors depend on a complex set of factors that include personality, cultural background, gender, and past experiences.

**Personality and Stress** In any stressful situation, some people seem nervous and irritable whereas others remain calm and composed. **Personality,** the sum of behavioral, cognitive, and emotional tendencies, clearly affects how an individual perceives and reacts to stressors. To investigate the links among personality, stress, and overall wellness, researchers have looked at different constellations of characteristics, or "personality types."

**TYPE A, B, AND C PERSONALITIES** In the 1960s, researchers began separating people into two basic personality types, Type A and Type B. Type A individuals tended to be more controlling, schedule driven, competitive, and even hostile. Type B individuals were less hurried, more contemplative, and more tolerant of others.

These personality designations received much attention as a result of the findings of Meyer Friedman and Ray Rosenman, who showed that Type A individuals were more likely to have heart disease (they studied middle-age Caucasian males almost exclusively). However, later studies show that most Type A individuals are quite healthy and perhaps even more successful at surviving heart disease than Type B individuals of the same age and stage of disease; it may be that Type A people follow their medication and therapy schedules more exactly and tend to be more competitive against the disease. The only aspects of Type A personality that remain associated with a greater risk for heart disease in women and men of all ethnicities are anger, cynicism, and hostility (see Chapter 12 for more on the link between hostility and heart disease).

In terms of stress, Type A people may have a higher perceived stress level and greater coping difficulties, especially in social situations. They may react more explosively to stressors and become upset by events that others would consider only mild annoyances. Type B individuals,

### Terms

Vw

**homeostasis** A state of stability and consistency in an individual's physiological functioning.

**somatic nervous system** The branch of the peripheral nervous system that governs motor functions and sensory information; largely under our conscious control.

**personality** The sum of behavioral, cognitive, and emotional tendencies.

on the other hand, tend to be less frustrated by the flow of daily events and the actions of others.

Research into personality traits and cancer examined a Type C personality, characterized by difficulty expressing emotions, anger suppression, feelings of hopelessness and despair, and an exaggerated stress response to minor cognitive stressors. People who consistently show these traits have lower levels of immune cells important in fighting cancer as well as lower cancer survival rates. The heightened stress response associated with a Type C personality may be directly related to impaired immune function. Studies of Type A and C personalities suggest that it is beneficial to express your emotions but that consistent or exaggerated arousal or hostility toward others is unhealthy.

**HARDINESS** Researchers have also looked at personality traits that seem to enable people to deal more successfully with stress. Psychologist Suzanne Kobasa examined "hardiness," a particular form of optimism. She found that people with a hardy personality view potential stressors as challenges and opportunities for growth and learning, rather than as burdens. Hardy people tend to perceive fewer situations as stressful, and their reaction to stressors tends to be less intense. They are committed to their activities, have a sense of inner purpose, and feel at least partly in control of events in their lives. People with a hardy personality typically have an internal locus of control, which helps them cope with stress in a more positive way and put setbacks in proper perspective.

**Can a Person Develop a Stress-Resistant Personality?** It is unlikely that you can change your basic personality. However, you can change your typical behaviors and patterns of thinking and develop positive techniques for coping with stressors. Strategies for successful stress management are described later in the chapter. For starters, though, try a few of the following:

- Build greater social support through meaningful relationships.
- Take advantage of opportunities to participate in and contribute to your family and community in productive ways.
- Set slightly higher expectations for yourself with clear boundaries and expectations that are fair and consistent.
- Build life skills such as decision making, effective communication, and stress and conflict management.
- Do not try to control the outcome of every situation (for example, a team competition or a loved one's illness). Know your limitations and trust others.

**Cultural Background** Young adults from all over the world seek higher education at American colleges and universities. The vast majority of students come away from their undergraduate experience with a greater appreciation for other groups and cultures. However, when they are ignored, misunderstood, or disrespected, cultural differences in values, lifestyles, and what is considered to be acceptable behavior can be a source of stress and can lead to stereotyping, prejudice, discrimination, harassment, and even assault. The way you cope with stress and the way you interact with people of other cultures are influenced by the family and culture in which you were raised. Try to avoid the assumption that your way of life is the best or only way. If you take the time to learn about and from other cultures, you will become more aware of the potential strengths and weaknesses of your own culture. You will also reduce the likelihood of cultural differences becoming a source of stress for you.

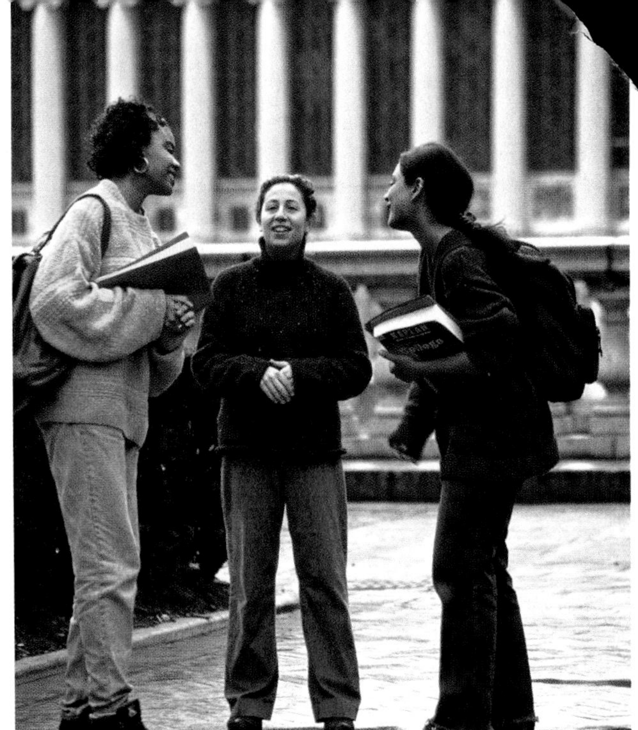

A person's emotional and behavioral responses to stressors depend on many different factors, including personality, gender, and cultural background. Research suggests that women are more likely than men to respond to stressors by seeking social support.

**Gender** Like cultural background, our gender role—the activities, abilities, and behaviors our culture expects of us based on whether we're male or female—also affects our experience of stress. Some behavioral responses to stressors, such as crying or openly expressing anger, may be deemed more appropriate for one gender than the other. Strict adherence to gender roles can place limits on how a person responds to stress and can itself become a source of stress. Adherence to traditional gender roles can also affect the perception of a potential stressor. For example, if a man derives most of his sense of self-worth from his work, retirement may be a more stressful life

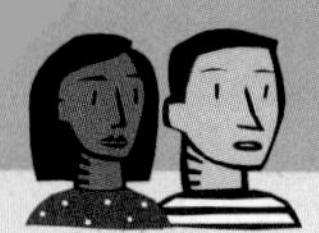

Gender Matters

## Women, Men, and Stress

### Special Stressors for Men and Women

Women are more likely than men to find themselves balancing multiple roles—student, employee, parent, spouse, caregiver to aging parents. Women who work outside of the home still do most of the housework, and time-related stress can be severe. All of these stressors can contribute to higher levels of stress-related health problems. Social forces can also undermine opportunities for women and cause stress. Women now make up more than half of the workforce but hold only 5% of the top leadership jobs. On average, women make less money than men with comparable jobs and are more likely to face sexual harassment. Disparity in domestic responsibilities, lack of integration into dominant organization coalitions, and even being considered excessively "nice" can all reduce the chances of being considered for leadership positions. The more women view themselves as fitting the traditional feminine gender stereotype, the less likely they are to report leadership aspirations.

Men who fit a traditional male gender role may feel the need to be active and in charge in all situations. They may have a communication style that is competitive and aggressive, causing stress in many interpersonal situations and limiting their ability to build social support networks. The responsibility to support a family may be felt very keenly among men with a traditional male gender role.

### Physiological Differences and Stress

Due to hormonal differences, men are considered to be more biologically vulnerable to certain diseases. For example, because of a rise in circulating testosterone levels, from puberty onward, males have higher blood pressure than do age-matched females. Along with other risk factors, including fewer physician visits, the rise in testosterone produces greater wear and tear on the male circulatory system over time, leading to greater risk for cardiovascular disease. A part of the brain responsible for regulating fear and emotional balance, the amygdala, is very sensitive to testosterone. Thus, having more circulating testosterone may predispose men to see social situations as more threatening than a woman would see them, creating more frequent activation of the stress response.

Women, on the other hand, have higher levels of the hormone oxytocin and are more likely to respond to stressors by seeking social support. The tend-and-befriend coping response among women may give them a longevity advantage compared with men by decreasing the risk of stress-related disorders.

### Gender and Stress Among College Students

Gender role development is a significant source of stress during college for both men and women, but there are gender differences in key stressors and coping strategies. College women are more likely than men to report having roommate conflicts and personal appearance issues. Men have more difficulty relating to and meeting other students, making friends, and dealing with peer pressure. College women report significantly higher emotional resources and ability to give and receive social support than do men. College men more frequently utilize physical coping resources than do women.

change for him than for a woman whose self-image is based on several different roles.

Although both men and women experience the fight-or-flight physiological response to stress, women are more likely to respond behaviorally with a pattern of "tend-and-befriend"—nurturing friends and family and seeking social support and social contacts. Women are more likely to enhance their social networks in ways that reduce stress than to become aggressive or withdraw from difficult situations. See the box "Women, Men, and Stress" for more on gender and stress.

**Past Experiences** Your past experiences significantly influence your response to stressors. For example, if you were unprepared for the first speech you gave in your speech class and performed poorly, you will probably experience greater anxiety in response to future assignments. If you had performed better, your confidence and sense of control would be greater, and you would probably experience less stress with future speeches. Effective behavioral responses, in this case careful preparation and visualizing yourself giving a successful speech, can help overcome the effects of negative past experiences.

## STRESS AND DISEASE

The role of stress in health and disease is complex, and much remains to be learned. However, evidence suggests that stress—interacting with a person's genetic predisposition, personality, social environment, and health-related behaviors—can increase vulnerability to numerous ailments. Several related theories have been proposed to explain the relationship between stress and disease.

### The General Adaptation Syndrome

Biologist Hans Selye, working in the 1930s and 1940s, was one of the first scientists to develop a comprehensive theory of stress and disease. Selye coined the term **general adaptation syndrome (GAS)** to describe what he believed was a universal and predictable response pattern to all stressors. He recognized that stressors could be

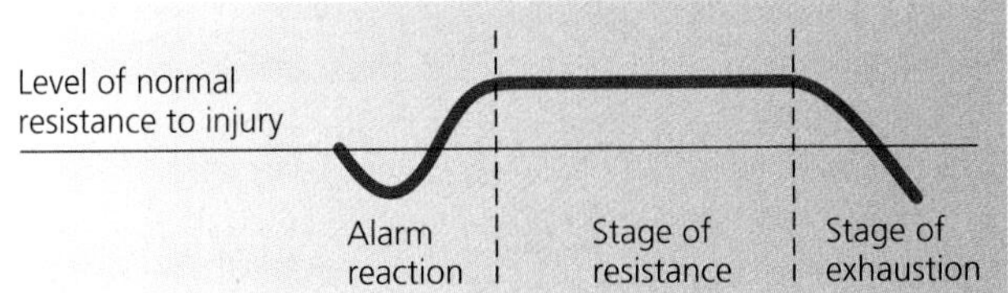


**Figure 2-3 The general adaptation syndrome.** Selye observed a predictable sequence of responses to stress. During the alarm phase, a lower resistance to injury is evident. With continued stress, resistance to injury is actually enhanced. With prolonged exposure to repeated stressors, exhaustion sets in, with a return of low resistance levels seen during acute stress.

pleasant, such as attending a party, or unpleasant, such as getting a flat tire or a bad grade. He called stress triggered by a pleasant stressor **eustress** and stress triggered by an unpleasant stressor **distress.** The sequence of physical responses associated with GAS is the same for both eustress and distress and occurs in three stages: alarm, resistance, and exhaustion (Figure 2-3).

**Alarm** This stage includes the complex sequence of events brought on by the activation of the sympathetic nervous system and the endocrine system—the fight-or-flight reaction. During this stage, the body is more susceptible to disease or injury because it is geared up to deal with a crisis. A person in this phase may experience headaches, indigestion, anxiety, and disrupted sleeping and eating patterns.

**Resistance** With continued stress, Selye theorized, the body developed a new level of homeostasis in which it was more resistant to disease and injury than it normally would be. During the resistance stage, a person can cope with normal life and added stress.

**Exhaustion** As you might imagine, both the mobilization of forces during the alarm reaction and the maintenance of homeostasis during the resistance stage require a considerable amount of energy. If a stressor persists or if several stressors occur in succession, general exhaustion results. This is not the sort of exhaustion people complain of after a long, busy day. It's a life-threatening type of physiological exhaustion characterized by symptoms such as distorted perceptions and disorganized thinking.

## Allostatic Load

While Selye's model of GAS is still viewed as a key contribution to modern stress theory, some aspects of it are now discounted. For example, increased susceptibility to disease after repeated or prolonged stress is now thought to be due to the effects of the stress response itself rather than to a depletion of resources (Selye's exhaustion stage). In particular, long-term overexposure to stress hormones such as cortisol has been linked with health problems.

The long-term wear and tear of the stress response is called the *allostatic load.* An individual's allostatic load is dependent on many factors, including genetics, life experiences, and emotional and behavioral responses to stressors. A high allostatic load may be due to frequent stressors, poor adaptation to common stressors, an inability to shut down the stress response, or imbalances in the stress response of different body systems. A high allostatic load is linked with heart disease, hypertension, obesity, and reduced brain and immune system functioning (see the box "Stress and Your Brain"). In other words, when your allostatic load exceeds your ability to cope, you are more likely to get sick.

## Psychoneuroimmunology

One of the most fruitful areas of current research into the relationship between stress and disease is **psychoneuroimmunology (PNI).** PNI is the study of the interactions among the nervous system, the endocrine system, and the immune system. The underlying premise of PNI is that stress, through the actions of the nervous and endocrine systems, impairs the immune system and thereby affects health.

Researchers have discovered a complex network of nerve and chemical connections between the nervous and endocrine systems and the immune system. In general, increased levels of cortisol are linked to a decreased number of immune system cells, or lymphocytes. Epinephrine and norepinephrine appear to promote the release of lymphocytes but at the same time reduce their efficiency. Interestingly, scientists have identified hormone-like substances called neuropeptides that appear to translate stressful emotions into biochemical events, some of which impact the immune system, providing a physical link between emotions and immune function. Different types of stress may affect immunity in different ways. For instance, during acute stress, there are typically no overall significant immune changes. However, chronic stressors such as caregiving or unemployment have negative effects on almost all functional measures of immunity.

Mood, personality, behavior, and immune functioning are intertwined. For example, people who are generally

### Terms

Vw

**general adaptation syndrome (GAS)** A pattern of stress responses consisting of three stages: alarm, resistance, and exhaustion.

**eustress** Stress resulting from a pleasant stressor.

**distress** Stress resulting from an unpleasant stressor.

**psychoneuroimmunology (PNI)** The study of the interactions among the brain, the endocrine system, and the immune system.

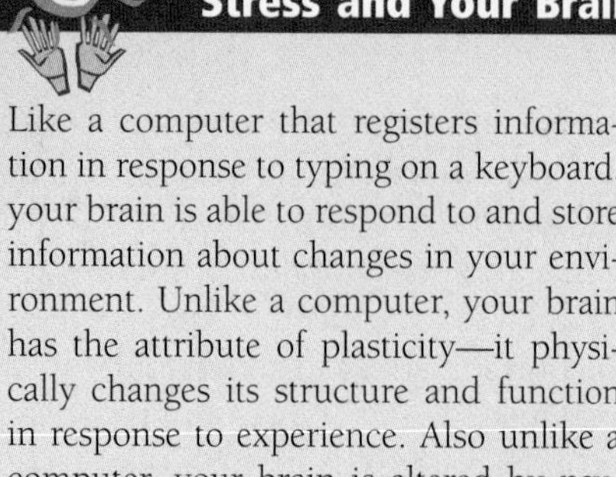


## Stress and Your Brain

Like a computer that registers information in response to typing on a keyboard, your brain is able to respond to and store information about changes in your environment. Unlike a computer, your brain has the attribute of plasticity—it physically changes its structure and function in response to experience. Also unlike a computer, your brain is altered by psychological stress. Moderate stress enhances the ability to acquire information and remember daily events, while high levels of acute stress can impair learning. For example, people can often remember minute details following a fender bender but can't recall the events surrounding a major car crash. Thus, it is good to be a little bit nervous before an exam—but not highly anxious.

The effects of stress on brain form and function are apparent in a structure called the hippocampus, which is involved in learning and memory. High levels of chronic stress cause brain cells (neurons) in the hippocampus to shrink in size or die, thus impairing learning and memory. Exciting new research in neuroscience has revealed that the hippocampus actually grows new neurons during adulthood. However, stress acts to reduce new cell birth in the hippocampus, reducing the replacement of lost neurons. Together, these effects of stress result in fewer neurons and fewer connections between neurons in the hippocampus, thus decreasing the capacity for information processing. People who are depressed or who suffer from post-traumatic stress disorder have higher levels of stress hormones in their bloodstream and smaller hippocampi than others. Even in the absence of a serious disorder, it is thought that the accumulation of stress effects across the life span can contribute to brain aging. Thus, the way you cope with stress can affect the way your brain works both immediately and over the long term.

pessimistic may neglect the basics of health care, become passive when ill, and fail to engage in health-promoting behaviors. Optimism, successful coping, and positive problem solving, on the other hand, may positively influence immunity. The pattern of interaction between the stress and immune responses allows for regulation of energy mobilization and redirection that is necessary to fight attackers both within and without.

## Links Between Stress and Specific Conditions

Although much remains to be learned, it is clear that people who have unresolved chronic stress in their lives or who handle stressors poorly are at risk for a wide range of health problems. In the short term, the problem might be just a cold, a stiff neck, or a stomachache. Over the long term, the problems can be more severe—cardiovascular disease (CVD), high blood pressure, impaired immune function, or accelerated aging.

**Cardiovascular Disease** During the stress response, heart rate increases and blood vessels constrict, causing blood pressure to rise. Chronic high blood pressure is a major cause of *atherosclerosis,* a disease in which the lining of the blood vessels becomes damaged and caked with fatty deposits. These deposits can block arteries, causing heart attacks and strokes.

Certain types of emotional responses may increase a person's risk of CVD. So-called hot reactors, people who exhibit extreme increases in heart rate and blood pressure in response to emotional stressors, may face an increased risk of cardiovascular problems. As described earlier in the section on Type A personality, people who tend to react to situations with anger and hostility are more likely to have heart attacks than are people with a less explosive, more trusting personality.

### Altered Functioning of the Immune System

Sometimes you seem to get sick when you can least afford it—during exam week, when you're going on vacation, or when you have a big job interview. As research in PNI suggests, this is more than mere coincidence. Some of the health problems linked to stress-related changes in immune function include vulnerability to colds and other infections, asthma and allergy attacks, increased risk of cancer, and flare-ups of chronic diseases such as herpes.

**Other Health Problems** Many other health problems may be caused or worsened by uncontrolled stress:

- Digestive problems such as stomachaches, diarrhea, constipation, irritable bowel syndrome, and ulcers.
- Tension headaches and migraines (see the box "Headaches: A Common Symptom of Stress").
- Insomnia and fatigue.
- Injuries, including on-the-job injuries caused by repetitive strain.
- Menstrual irregularities, impotence, and pregnancy complications.
- Type 2 diabetes.
- Psychological problems, including depression, anxiety, eating disorders, and post-traumatic stress disorder (PTSD), which afflicts people who have suffered or witnessed severe trauma.

In Focus

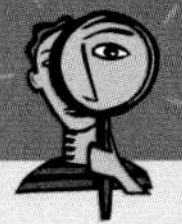

## Headaches: A Common Symptom of Stress

Are you among the more than 45 million Americans who have chronic, recurrent headaches? Headaches come in various types but are often grouped into three major categories: tension headaches, migraines, and cluster headaches. Other types of headaches have underlying organic causes, such as sinus congestion or infection.

### Tension Headaches

Approximately 90% of all headaches are tension headaches, characterized by a dull, steady pain, usually on both sides of the head. It may feel as though a band of pressure is tightening around the head, and the pain may extend to the neck and shoulders. Acute tension headaches may last from hours to days, while chronic tension headaches may occur almost every day for months or even years. Psychological stress, poor posture, and immobility are the leading causes of tension headaches. There is no cure, but the pain can sometimes be relieved with over-the-counter painkillers and with therapies such as massage, relaxation, hot or cold showers, and rest.

If your headaches are frequent, keep a diary with details about the events surrounding each one. Are your headaches associated with late nights, academic deadlines, or long periods spent sitting at a computer? If you can identify the stressors that are consistently associated with your headaches, you can begin to gain more control over the situation. If you suffer persistent tension headaches, you should consult your physician.

### Migraines

Migraines typically progress through a series of stages lasting from several minutes to several days. They may produce a variety of symptoms, including throbbing pain that starts on one side of the head and may spread; heightened sensitivity to light; visual disturbances such as flashing lights; nausea; and fatigue. About 70% of migraine sufferers are women, and migraine headaches may have a genetic component. Research suggests that people who get migraines may have abnormally excitable nerve cells in their brains. When triggered, these nerve cells send a wave of electrical activity throughout the brain, which in turn causes migraine symptoms. Potential triggers include menstruation, stress, fatigue, atmospheric changes, specific sounds or odors, and certain foods. The frequency of attacks varies from a few in a lifetime to several per week.

Keeping a headache journal can help a migraine sufferer identify headache triggers—the first step to avoiding them. In addition, many new treatments can help reduce the frequency, severity, and duration of migraines.

### Cluster Headaches

Cluster headaches are extremely severe headaches that cause intense pain in and around one eye. They usually occur in clusters of one to three headaches each day over a period of weeks or months, alternating with periods of remission in which no headaches occur. About 90% of people with cluster headaches are male. There is no known cause or cure for cluster headaches, but a number of treatments are available. During cluster periods, it is important to refrain from smoking cigarettes and drinking alcohol, because these activities can trigger attacks.

## COMMON SOURCES OF STRESS

We are surrounded by stressors—at home, at school, on the job, and within ourselves. Being able to recognize potential sources of stress is an important step in successfully managing the stress in our lives.

### Major Life Changes

Any major change in your life that requires adjustment and accommodation can be a source of stress. Early adulthood and the college years are typically associated with many significant changes, such as moving out of the family home, establishing new relationships, setting educational and career goals, and developing a sense of identity and purpose. Even changes typically thought of as positive—graduation, job promotion, marriage—can be stressful. For older students, the collection of major life changes may be different but just as powerful—the challenge of balancing school, work, and family responsibilities; parenting teenagers; relationship stress; and providing care for aging parents.

Clusters of major life changes may be linked to the development of health problems in some people. Research indicates that some life changes, particularly those that are perceived negatively, can affect health. However, personality and coping skills are important moderating influences. People with a strong support network and a stress-resistant personality are less likely to become ill in response to major life changes than people with fewer internal and external resources.

### Daily Hassles

Have you done any of the following in the past week?

- Misplaced your keys, wallet, or an assignment
- Had an argument with a troublesome neighbor, coworker, or customer
- Waited in a long line, or been stuck in traffic or had another problem with transportation
- Worried about money
- Been upset about the weather

While major life changes are undoubtedly stressful, they seldom occur regularly. Psychologist Richard Lazarus has proposed that minor problems—life's daily hassles—can be an even greater source of stress because they occur much more often. People who perceive hassles negatively are likely to experience a moderate stress response every time they are faced with one. Over time, this can take a significant toll on health. Researchers have found that for some people daily hassles contribute to a general decrease in overall wellness.

## College Stressors

College is a time of major life changes and abundant minor hassles. You will be learning new information and skills and making major decisions about your future. You may be away from home for the first time, or you may be adding extra responsibilities to a life already filled with job and family.

**Academic Stressors** Exams, grades, and choosing a major are among the many academic stressors faced by college students. In addition to an increased workload compared to that in high school, many students are unpleasantly surprised by the more rigorous evaluation of their work in college. Higher-quality efforts are expected of college students, so earning good grades takes more effort and dedication. Careful planning and preparation can help make academic stressors more predictable and manageable. Students close to graduation may find themselves faced with the need to plan for life after college—a potentially daunting task. Remember that you'll have many opportunities to change career paths in the future and that the training and life experience gained from one path can often be transferred to other endeavors.

**Interpersonal Stressors** The college years often involve potential stressors such as establishing new relationships and balancing multiple roles—student, employee, friend, spouse, parent, and so on. You'll have the opportunity to meet new people and make new friends at the start of every term and in every new class and activity. Social engagements may be exhilarating for some and painful for others. Viewed as an exciting challenge or an odious necessity, interacting with others involves attention, on-the-spot decision making, and energy expenditure—and it's stressful. Be yourself, go with the flow, and try not to be overly concerned with being liked by everyone you meet.

**Time-Related Pressures** Do you accept too many responsibilities or manage your time poorly? Time pressures are a problem for most students, but they may be particularly acute for those who also have job and family responsibilities. Most people do have enough time to fulfill all of their responsibilities but fail to manage their time or their priorities effectively. For these people, it's important to make a plan and *stick to it*. Effective time management strategies are described in the next section.

**Financial Concerns** As young adults leave home and become independent, financial responsibilities such as paying tuition, taking out loans, and managing living expenses are likely to arise. To complicate matters, tuition rates and competition for scholarships are at all-time highs, outpacing increases in family income. As college has become less affordable, more students are borrowing—and are borrowing more—to pay for college. Most students work full-time during the summer and part-time during the school year in order to meet their financial needs; some work full-time and support a family during the school year, creating additional time pressures. A student loan repayment looming over your head can also create substantial worries. A budget is as important as effective time management for successfully dealing with college stress. Create a financial plan for each month or term so you can put your mind more at ease and concentrate on your studies.

**Stressors Among Nontraditional Students** About 70% of undergraduates meet at least one of the defining criteria of nontraditional students: individuals who, in addition to attending college, may be married, a parent, a caretaker for an older family member, a full-time worker, and/or retraining for a new career. Nontraditional students must often contend with the stress of increased responsibilities compared with traditional students, who are typically younger and have fewer demands on their time. Interestingly, nontraditional students have been shown to have higher class attendance, less worry about academic performance, and greater enjoyment of homework; they are more likely to report concern about family responsibilities. Traditional students report being more concerned with social and peer relationships.

Greater social support, especially from family and friends, is a stress buffer for married students and is related to better academic adjustment, personal and social adjustment, and commitment to college. However, married college students express greater marital distress than married couples not attending college. Married graduate students report more satisfaction with their educational programs but less satisfaction with their social and extracurricular activities, whereas commuting couples report less satisfaction with the time they are able to spend with their spouses compared with noncommuting couples. Time pressures may be especially severe for nontraditional students, so time-management strategies may be of particular importance.

## Job-Related Stressors

More than one-third of Americans report that they always feel rushed, and nearly half say they would give up a day's pay for a day off. Tight schedules and overtime contribute to time-related pressures. Worries about job performance, salary, and job security are a source of stress for some people. Interactions with bosses, coworkers, and customers can also contribute to stress. High levels of job stress are also common for people who are left out of important decisions relating to their jobs. When workers are given the opportunity to shape how their jobs are performed, job satisfaction goes up and stress levels go down.

If job-related (or college-related) stress is severe or chronic, the result can be **burnout**, a state of physical, mental, and emotional exhaustion. Burnout occurs most often in highly motivated and driven individuals who feel that their work is not recognized or that they are not accomplishing their goals. People in the helping professions—teachers, social workers, caregivers, police officers, and so on—are also prone to burnout. For some who suffer from burnout, a vacation or leave of absence may be appropriate. For others, a reduced work schedule, better communication with superiors, or a change in job goals may be necessary.

Surveys indicate that as many as 40% of U.S. workers rate their jobs as "very or extremely stressful," and 25% say they are often or very often "burned out by their work." Problems at work are more strongly associated with health complaints than with any other life stressor—more so than even financial problems or family problems. Some 32.9 million working days are lost annually from people taking time off because of illness. Health care expenditures are nearly 50% greater for workers who report high levels of stress.

### Social Stressors

Social networks that affect stress may be real or virtual; each type can help boost your ability to deal with the stress in your life or can itself become a stressor.

**Real Social Networks** Although social support is a key buffer against stress, your interactions with others can themselves be a source of stress. As mentioned earlier, the college years are often a time of great change in interpersonal relationships. The community and society in which you live can also be major sources of stress. Social stressors include prejudice and discrimination. You may feel stress as you try to relate to people of other ethnic or socioeconomic groups. As a member of a particular ethnic group, you may feel pressure to assimilate into mainstream society. If English is not your first language, you face the added burden of conducting many daily activities in a language with which you may not be completely comfortable. All of these pressures can become significant sources of stress. (See the box "Diverse Populations, Discrimination, and Stress" on p. 34 for more information.)

**Virtual Social Networks** New technologies that instantaneously bring information to our fingertips can potentially be time-savers, and telecommuting can ease the time pressures on people who find it necessary to work from home. However, increased electronic interactivity can also impinge on our personal space, waste time, and cause stress. If you are experiencing information overload, learn to use multimedia devices wisely. Give out your phone number only when absolutely necessary. Schedule times when you completely sever your electronic ties. Consider the financial savings that may arise from less frequent cell phone use.

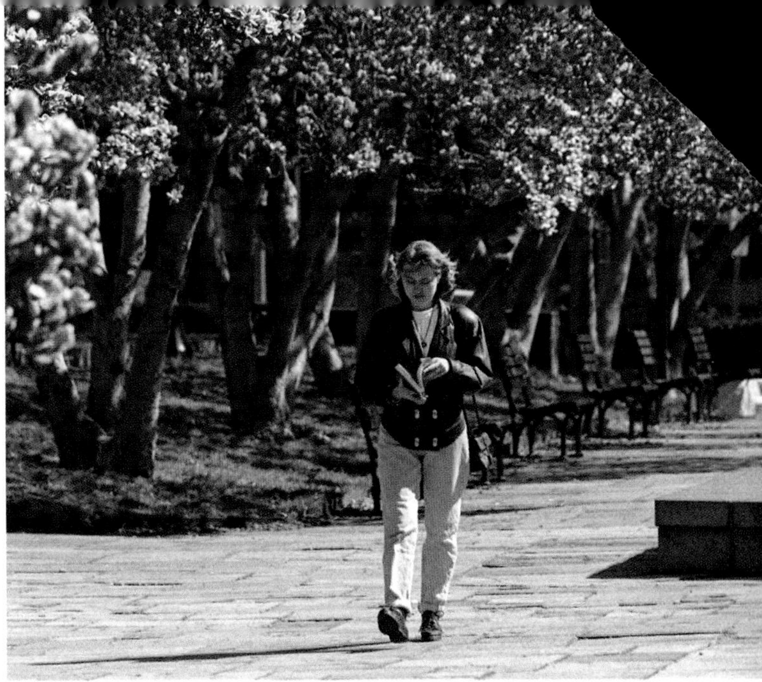

To help prevent excess stress, take time away from your computer, cell phone, and other electronic devices. If your break time can include physical activity in a pleasant environment, you'll further reduce stress and improve overall wellness.

Other stressors are found in the environment and in ourselves. Environmental stressors—external conditions or events that cause stress—include loud noises, unpleasant smells, natural disasters, and acts of violence (see the box "Coping After Terrorism, Mass Violence, or Natural Disasters" on p. 35). Internal stressors can occur as we put pressure on ourselves to reach personal goals and evaluate our progress and performance. Physical and emotional states such as illness and exhaustion are other examples of internal stressors.

## TECHNIQUES FOR MANAGING STRESS

What can you do about all this stress? A great deal. And the effort is well worth the time: People who manage stress effectively not only are healthier but also have more time to enjoy life and accomplish their goals.

**Term**

**burnout** A state of physical, mental, and emotional exhaustion. VW

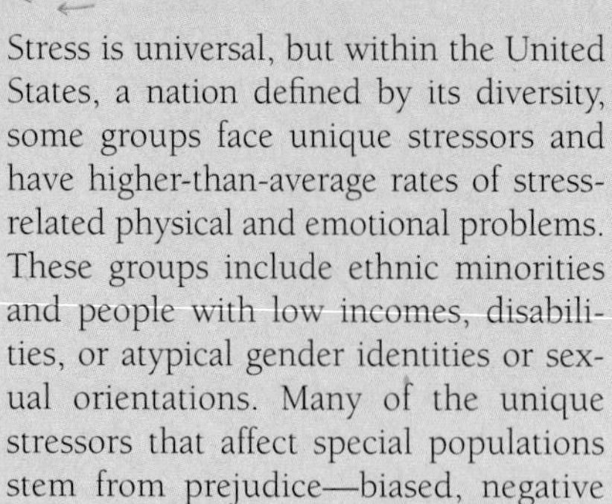


## Diverse Populations, Discrimination, and Stress

Stress is universal, but within the United States, a nation defined by its diversity, some groups face unique stressors and have higher-than-average rates of stress-related physical and emotional problems. These groups include ethnic minorities and people with low incomes, disabilities, or atypical gender identities or sexual orientations. Many of the unique stressors that affect special populations stem from prejudice—biased, negative attitudes toward a group of people.

Discrimination occurs when people act according to their prejudices; it can be blatant or subtle. Blatant examples of discrimination are not common, but they are major stressors akin to significant life changes. Examples include a swastika painted on a Jewish studies house, the defacement of a sculpture honoring the achievements of a gay artist, and bullying of poor children because they wear the same clothes to school each day. Subtler acts may occur much more frequently. For example, an African American student in a mostly white college town feels that shopkeepers are keeping an eye on him; a male-to-female transgendered individual believes she has been "clocked" (discovered) and treated with less respect by her professors and peers; a student using a wheelchair has difficulty with narrow aisles and high counters at local stores; and an obese executive is asked to purchase two seats on his business flights. Some of these social stressors are unique to certain groups, and it may be difficult for other people to understand how serious such stressors can be.

Recent immigrants to the United States must begin new lives in a new society; the stress associated with this process is called *acculturation stress.* Successful integration into a new society can occur in an open society where immigrants are free to retain any aspect of their cultural heritage and their native social customs and beliefs are valued. If there is great pressure to assimilate, minority immigrant groups may become disconnected from both their own culture and that of the host culture; marginalized groups can be targets of significant discrimination, even violence. Different immigrant groups experience variations in accultural stressors. For example, language barriers and limited formal education may make employment more difficult for some groups. In other groups, intense pressure is put on immigrant children to do well in school and enter high-paying professions to boost the honor and position of the family; these high expectations can be a source of stress, guilt, and alienation from the family.

Minorities often face additional job- and school-related stressors because of stereotypes and discrimination. They make less money than whites in comparable jobs and with comparable levels of education, and they may find it more difficult to achieve leadership positions. Many ethnic minorities must develop basic skills that natives of the host nation take for granted; for example, learning to speak English, balancing ancestral and American cultures, and finding employment sufficient to pay for basic necessities. All these types of stressors can contribute to higher levels of stress-related health problems among minorities.

On a positive note, many people who experience hardship, disability, or prejudice develop effective, goal-directed coping skills and are successful at overcoming obstacles and managing the increased stress they face. Resiliency, hopeful expectations for the future, and spiritual wellness all support successful coping.

## Social Support and Communication

People need people. Sharing fears, frustrations, and joys not only makes life richer but also seems to contribute to the well-being of body and mind. Allow yourself time to nourish and maintain a network of people at home, at work, at school, or in your community that you can count on for emotional support, feedback, and nurturance. Consider becoming a volunteer to help build your social support system and enhance your spiritual wellness. Communication skills, discussed in detail in Chapter 4, can be critical in forming and maintaining intimate relationships. To evaluate your current social support system and to find strategies for strengthening your social ties, refer to the box "Healthy Connections" on page 36.

## Exercise

Exercise helps maintain a healthy body and mind and even stimulates the birth of new brain cells. One study found that just a brisk 10-minute walk leaves people feeling more relaxed and energetic for up to 2 hours. Researchers have also found that people who exercise regularly react with milder physical stress responses before, during, and after exposure to stressors. People who took three brisk 45-minute walks a week for 3 months reported that they perceived fewer daily hassles. Their sense of wellness also increased.

If you experience stress and do not physically exert yourself, you are not completing the energy cycle. Physical activity allows you to expend the nervous energy you have built up and trains your body to more readily achieve homeostasis following future disturbances in normal functioning. It's not hard to incorporate light to moderate exercise into your day. Walk to class or bike to the store instead of driving. Use the stairs instead of the elevator. Take a walk with a friend instead of getting a cup of coffee. Go bowling, play tennis, or roller-skate instead of seeing a movie. Make a habit of taking a brisk after-dinner stroll. Plan hikes and easy bike outings for the weekends.

In the News

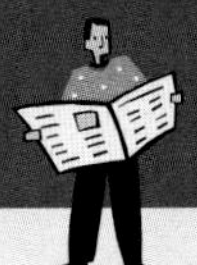

## Coping After Terrorism, Mass Violence, or Natural Disasters

Mass violence occurs somewhat frequently in big cities—for example, when a deeply disturbed person gains access to guns or explosives. Certain areas of the country are also prone to natural disasters like hurricanes, flooding, and earthquakes. Less frequent in the United States are terrorist events such as those that occurred in Oklahoma in April 1995 or in Manhattan in February 1993 and September 2001. Not only do many people suffer direct physical harm during such events, but larger numbers of survivors, witnesses, and emergency personnel experience long-term psychological distress. While most recover, some develop post-traumatic stress disorder (PTSD), a more serious condition.

Cognitive, emotional, and behavioral reactions to trauma are highly variable, and it is normal for an individual to experience a variety of responses. Reactions may include disbelief and shock, fear, anger and resentment, anxiety about the future, difficulty concentrating or making decisions, mood swings, irritability, sadness and depression, panic, guilt, apathy, feelings of isolation or powerlessness, and many of the symptoms of excess stress. Reactions may occur immediately or may be delayed until weeks or months after the event.

Signs of PTSD include reexperiencing the trauma in dreams and intrusive thoughts, feeling generally numb or detached from life, and feeling jumpy or hypervigilant. Following the September 11, 2001, attacks in New York, risk factors for PTSD included being a young adult (age 18–29), being female, having little social support, being close to the site of the attacks or involved in the rescue efforts, and watching a large amount of television coverage. The severity of a person's reaction is not necessarily proportional to the degree of objective loss; in some cases, for example, a person who watches events unfold in the media may experience a more negative or a longer-lasting reaction than someone more directly involved. See Chapter 3 for more on PTSD.

Taking positive steps can help you cope with difficult emotions. Consider the following strategies:

- Immediately after such an event, it is okay to break from your daily routine to evaluate your situation and mourn for others. It is important to share your experiences and feelings with empathetic listeners. Be a supportive listener yourself, and reassure children of their safety.
- Take a break from media coverage. Try to refrain from developing nightmare scenarios for the future or generalizing the situation to all aspects of your life. Instead, find ways to help yourself and others. Donating money, blood, food, clothes, or time can ease difficult emotions and give you a greater sense of control. (In the aftermath of the September 11 attacks, such active coping strategies were shown to be related to lower rates of acute stress and PTSD.) For some people, forming political opinions provides a frame of reference through which to respond to terrorism, and voting can be a coping response because it is another way for people to exert some control over their futures.
- As time passes, maintain your schedule at home, school, and work. Continue to take care of your mind and body. Choose a healthy diet, exercise regularly, get plenty of sleep, and practice relaxation techniques. Try to avoid negative coping techniques such as using alcohol or other drugs.

Everyone copes with and recovers from tragedy differently. If you feel overwhelmed by your emotions even weeks or months after the event, seek professional help.

## Nutrition

A healthy diet will give you an energy bank to draw on whenever you experience stress. Eating wisely also will enhance your feelings of self-control and self-esteem. Learning the principles of sound nutrition is easy, and sensible eating habits rapidly become second nature when practiced regularly. One special nutrition tip for stress management: Avoid or limit caffeine. (For more on sound nutrition, see Chapter 9.)

## Sleep

Lack of sleep can be both a cause and an effect of excess stress. Without sufficient sleep, our mental and physical processes steadily deteriorate. We get headaches, feel irritable, are unable to concentrate, forget things, and may be more susceptible to weight gain and illness. Fatigue and sleep deprivation are major factors in many fatal car, truck, and train crashes. Extreme sleep deprivation can lead to hallucinations and other psychotic symptoms as well as to a significant increase in heart attack risk. Adequate sleep, on the other hand, improves mood, fosters feelings of competence and self-worth, and supports optimal mental and emotional functioning. If you are sleep-deprived, sleeping extra hours may significantly improve your daytime alertness and mental abilities.

Sleep requirements vary considerably among individuals; some adults need only 5 hours of sleep, while others need 9 hours or more to feel fully refreshed and alert. Nearly everyone, at some time in life, has trouble falling asleep or staying asleep—a condition known as insomnia. Strategies for overcoming insomnia include going to bed at the same time every night and getting up at the same time every morning; avoiding tobacco, caffeine in the later part of the day, and alcohol before bedtime; exercising every day, but not too close to bedtime; using your bed only for sleeping, not for eating, reading, or watching TV; and relaxing and having a light snack before you go to bed.

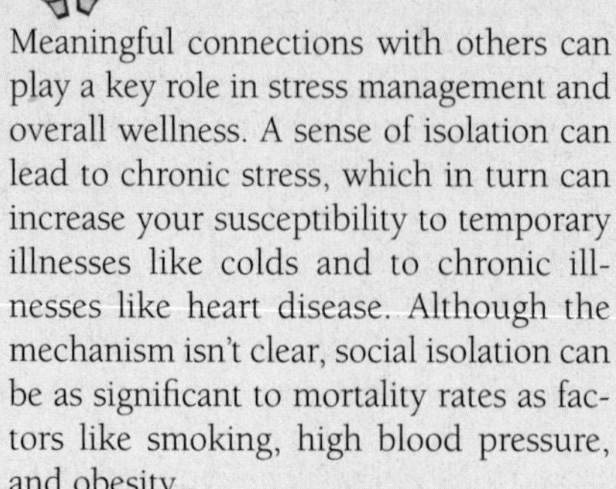

## Healthy Connections

Meaningful connections with others can play a key role in stress management and overall wellness. A sense of isolation can lead to chronic stress, which in turn can increase your susceptibility to temporary illnesses like colds and to chronic illnesses like heart disease. Although the mechanism isn't clear, social isolation can be as significant to mortality rates as factors like smoking, high blood pressure, and obesity.

There is no single best pattern of social support that works for everyone. However, research suggests that having a variety of types of relationships may be important for wellness. To help determine whether your social network measures up, answer true or false to each of the following statements.

1. If I needed an emergency loan of $100, there is someone I could get it from.
2. There is someone who takes pride in my accomplishments.
3. I often meet or talk with family or friends.
4. Most people I know think highly of me.
5. If I needed an early morning ride to the airport, there's no one I would feel comfortable asking to take me.
6. I feel there is no one with whom I can share my most private worries and fears.
7. Most of my friends are more successful making changes in their life than I am.
8. I would have a hard time finding someone to go with me on a day trip to the beach or country.

To calculate your score, add the number of true answers to questions 1–4 and the number of false answers to questions 5–8. If your score is 4 or more, you should have enough support to protect your health. If your score is 3 or less, you may need to reach out. There are a variety of things you can do to strengthen your social ties:

- *Foster friendships.* Keep in regular contact with your friends. Offer respect, trust, and acceptance, and provide help and support in times of need. Express appreciation for your friends.
- *Keep your family ties strong.* Stay in touch with the family members you feel close to. Participate in family activities and celebrations. If your family doesn't function well as a support system for its members, create a second "family" of people with whom you have built meaningful ties.
- *Get involved with a group.* Do volunteer work, take a class, attend a lecture series, join a religious group. These types of activities can give you a sense of security, a place to talk about your feelings or concerns, and a way to build new friendships. Choose activities that are meaningful to you and that include direct involvement with other people.
- *Build your communication skills.* The more you share your feelings with others, the closer the bonds between you will become. When others are speaking, be a considerate and attentive listener. (Chapters 3 and 4 include more information on effective communication.)

Individual relationships change over the course of your life, but it's never too late to build friendships or become more involved in your community. Your investment of time and energy in your social network will pay off—in a brighter outlook now, and in better health and well-being for the future.

SOURCE: Friends can be good medicine. 1998. As found in the Mind/Body Newsletter 7(1): 3–6. Center for the Advancement of Health; Quiz from Japenga, A. 1995. A Family of Friends. *Health,* November/December, 1994. Adapted with permission. Copyright © 2001 Health® magazine. For subscriptions please call 800-274-2522.

## Time Management

A surprising number of the stressors in most people's lives relate to time. Many people never seem to have enough time, and they always seem to feel overwhelmed by the pace of their lives. Others have too much time on their hands and are often bored. Learning to manage your time successfully is crucial to coping with the stressors you face every day. Three common factors that negatively impact time management for college students are perfectionism, overcommitment, and procrastination. If these or time-related stressors are a problem for you, try some or all of the following strategies for managing your time more productively and creatively:

- *Set priorities.* Divide your tasks into three groups: essential, important, and trivial. Focus on the first two. Ignore the third.
- *Schedule tasks for peak efficiency.* You've undoubtedly noticed you're most productive at certain times of the day (or night). Schedule as many of your tasks for those hours as you can, and stick to your schedule.
- *Set realistic goals, and write them down.* Attainable goals spur you on. Impossible goals, by definition, cause frustration and failure. Fully commit yourself to achieving your goals by putting them in writing.
- *Budget enough time.* For each project you undertake, calculate how long it will take to complete. Then tack on another 10–15%, or even 25%, as a buffer against mistakes, interruptions, or unanticipated problems.
- *Break down long-term goals into short-term ones.* Instead of waiting for or relying on large blocks of time, use short amounts of time to start a project or keep it moving.
- *Visualize the achievement of your goals.* By mentally rehearsing your performance of a task, you will be able to reach your goal more smoothly.

• *Keep track of the tasks you put off.* Analyze the reasons why you procrastinate. If the task is difficult or unpleasant, look for ways to make it easier or more fun. If you hate cleaning up your room, break the work into 10-minute tasks and do a little at a time. If you find the readings for one of your classes particularly difficult, choose an especially nice setting for your reading and then reward yourself each time you complete a section or chapter.

• *Consider doing your least favorite tasks first.* Once you have the most unpleasant tasks out of the way, you can have fun with the projects you enjoy more.

• *Consolidate tasks when possible.* For example, try walking to the store so that you run your errands and exercise in the same block of time.

• *Identify quick transitional tasks.* Keep a list of 5-minute tasks you can do while waiting or between other tasks, such as watering your plants, doing the dishes, or checking a homework assignment.

• *Delegate responsibility.* Asking for help when you have too much to do is no cop-out; it's good time management. Just don't delegate to others the jobs you know you should do yourself, such as researching a paper.

• *Say no when necessary.* If the demands made on you don't seem reasonable, say no—tactfully, but without guilt or apology.

• *Give yourself a break.* Allow time for play—free, unstructured time when you ignore the clock. Don't consider this a waste of time. Play renews you and enables you to work more efficiently.

• *Stop thinking or talking about what you're going to do, and just do it!* Sometimes the best solution for procrastination is to stop waiting for the right moment and just get started. You will probably find that things are not as bad as you feared, and your momentum will keep you going.

## Strive for Greater Spirituality

Spirituality involves a high level of faith and commitment with respect to a well-defined worldview or belief system that gives a sense of meaning and purpose to existence. Spirituality also provides an ethical path to personal fulfillment that includes connectedness with self, others, and a higher power or larger reality. Overall, there appears to be a positive relationship between spirituality and adaptive coping, suggesting that aspects of spirituality and spiritual practices can play a significant role as a personal resource for coping. Spirituality can be enhanced through many activities, including participation in organized religion, spending time in nature or working on environmental issues, helping others through volunteer work, and engaging in personal spiritual practices such as prayer or meditation.

## Confide in Yourself Through Writing

Keeping a diary is analogous to confiding in others, except that you are confiding in yourself. This form of coping with severe stress may be especially helpful for those who are shy or introverted and find it difficult to open up to others. Although writing about traumatic and stressful events may have a short-term negative effect on mood, over the long term, stress is reduced and positive changes in health occur. A key to promoting beneficial results with respect to health and well-being through journaling is to write about one's emotional responses to a stressful event. Set aside a special time each day or week to journal your feelings about stressful events in your life.

## Cognitive Techniques

Some stressors arise in our own minds. Ideas, beliefs, perceptions, and patterns of thinking can add to our stress level. Each of the techniques described below can help you change unhealthy thought patterns to ones that will help you cope with stress. As with any skill, mastering these techniques takes practice and patience.

**Think and Act Constructively** Worrying, someone once said, is like shoveling smoke. Think back to the worries you had last week. How many of them were needless? Think about things you *can* control. Try to stand aside from the problem, consider the positive steps you can take to solve it, and then carry them out.

**Take Control** A situation often feels more stressful if you feel you're not in control of it. Time may seem to be slipping away before a big exam, for example. Unexpected obstacles may appear in your path, throwing you off course. When you feel your environment is controlling you instead of the other way around, take charge! Concentrate on what is possible to control, and set realistic goals. Be confident of your ability to succeed.

**Problem-Solve** When you find yourself stewing over a problem, take a moment to sit down with a piece of paper and go through a formal process of problem solving. Within a few minutes you can generate a plan:

1. Define the problem in one or two sentences.
2. Identify the causes of the problem.
3. Consider alternative solutions; don't just stop with the most obvious one.
4. Weigh positive and negative consequences for each alternative.
5. Make a decision—choose a solution.
6. Make a list of what you will need to do to act on your decision.

7. Begin to carry out your list; if you're unable to do that, temporarily turn to other things.
8. Evaluate the outcome and revise your approach if necessary.

**Modify Your Expectations** Expectations are exhausting and restricting. The fewer expectations you have, the more you can live spontaneously and joyfully. The more you expect from others, the more often you will feel let down. And trying to meet the expectations others have of you is often futile.

**Maintain Positivity** If you catch your mind beating up on you—"Late for class again! You can't even cope with college! How do you expect to ever hold down a professional job?"—change your inner dialogue. Talk to yourself as you would to a child you love: "You're a smart, capable person. You've solved other problems; you'll handle this one. Tomorrow you'll simply schedule things so you get to class with a few minutes to spare." (Chapter 3 has more information on self-talk.)

**Cultivate Your Sense of Humor** When it comes to stress, laughter may be the best medicine. Even a fleeting smile produces changes in your autonomic nervous system that can lift your spirits. And a few minutes of belly laughing can be as invigorating as brisk exercise. Hearty laughter elevates your heart rate, aids digestion, eases pain, and triggers the release of endorphins and other pleasurable and stimulating chemicals in the brain. After a good laugh, your muscles go slack; your pulse and blood pressure dip below normal. You are relaxed. Cultivate the ability to laugh at yourself, and you'll have a handy and instantly effective stress reliever.

- Keep a humor journal. Write down funny things that you and others say, including unintentional slips of the tongue. Collect funny and clever sayings that make you smile.
- Look at newspaper and magazine cartoons. Cut out those you find particularly funny and add them to your humor journal.
- Collect some funny props—clown noses, "arrow" headbands, Groucho glasses—that you can put on the next time you feel stressed or anxious. Or simply try making funny faces in front of a mirror.
- Watch funny films and television programs. In a study of college students, those who watched an episode of *Seinfeld* prior to giving an impromptu speech were less anxious and had a lower heart rate than those who didn't watch the program.

**Go with the Flow** Remember that the branch that bends in the storm doesn't break. Try to flow with your life, accepting the things you can't change. Be forgiving of faults, your own and those of others. Instead of anticipating happiness at some indefinite point in the future, realize that pleasure is integral to being alive. You can create it every day of your life. View challenges as an opportunity to learn and grow. Be flexible.

## Relaxation Techniques

First identified and described by Herbert Benson of the Harvard Medical School, the **relaxation response** is a physiological state characterized by a feeling of warmth and quiet mental alertness. This is the opposite of the fight-or-flight reaction. When the relaxation response is triggered by a relaxation technique, heart rate, breathing, and metabolism slow down. Blood pressure and oxygen consumption decrease. At the same time, blood flow to the brain and skin increases, and brain waves shift from an alert beta rhythm to a relaxed alpha rhythm. Practiced regularly, relaxation techniques can counteract the debilitating effects of stress. If one technique doesn't seem to work well enough for you after you've given it a good try, try another one.

**Progressive Relaxation** Unlike most of the others, this simple method requires no imagination, willpower, or self-suggestion. You simply tense, and then relax, the muscles in your body, group by group. The technique, also known as deep muscle relaxation, helps you become aware of the muscle tension that occurs when you're under stress. When you consciously relax those muscles, other systems of the body get the message and ease up on the stress response.

Start, for example, with your right fist. Inhale as you tense it. Exhale as you relax it. Repeat. Next, contract and relax your right upper arm. Repeat. Do the same with your left arm. Then, beginning at your forehead and ending at your feet, contract and relax your other muscle groups. Repeat each contraction at least once, breathing in as you tense, breathing out as you relax. To speed up the process, tense and relax more muscles at one time—both arms simultaneously, for instance. With practice, you'll be able to relax very quickly and effectively by clenching and releasing only your fists.

**Visualization** Also known as using imagery, **visualization** lets you daydream without guilt. Next time you feel stressed, close your eyes. Imagine yourself floating on a cloud, sitting on a mountaintop, or lying in a meadow. What do you see and hear? Is it cold out? Or damp? What do you smell? What do you taste? Involve all your senses. Your body will respond as if your imagery were real. An alternative: Close your eyes and imagine a deep purple light filling your body. Now change the color into a soothing gold. As the color lightens, so should your distress.

Visualization can also be used to rehearse for an upcoming event and enhance performance. By experiencing

Take Charge

## Meditation and the Relaxation Response

Dr. Herbert Benson developed a simple, practical technique for eliciting the relaxation response.

### The Basic Technique

1. Pick a word, phrase, or object to focus on. If you like, you can choose a word or phrase that has a deep meaning for you, but any word or phrase will work. Some meditators prefer to focus on their breathing.
2. Take a comfortable position in a quiet environment, and close your eyes if you're not focusing on an object.
3. Relax your muscles.
4. Breathe slowly and naturally. If you're using a focus word or phrase, silently repeat it each time you exhale. If you're using an object, focus on it as you breathe.
5. Keep a passive attitude. Disregard thoughts that drift in.
6. Continue for 10–20 minutes, once or twice a day.
7. After you've finished, sit quietly for a few minutes with your eyes first closed and then open. Then stand up.

### Suggestions

- Allow relaxation to occur at its own pace; don't try to force it. Don't be surprised if you can't tune out your mind for more than a few seconds at a time; it's not a reason for anger or frustration. The more you ignore the intrusions, the easier doing so will become.
- If you want to time your session, peek at a watch or clock occasionally, but don't set a jarring alarm.
- The technique works best on an empty stomach, before a meal or about 2 hours after eating. Avoid times of day when you're tired—unless you want to fall asleep.
- Although you'll feel refreshed even after the first session, it may take a month or more to get noticeable results. Be patient. Eventually the relaxation response will become so natural that it will occur spontaneously, or on demand, when you sit quietly for a few moments.

an event ahead of time in your mind, you can practice coping with any difficulties that may arise. Think positively, and you can "psych yourself up" for a successful experience.

**Meditation** The need to periodically stop our incessant mental chatter is so great that, from ancient times, hundreds of forms of **meditation** have developed in cultures all over the world. Meditation is a way of telling the mind to be quiet for a while. Because meditation has been at the core of many Eastern religions and philosophies, it has acquired an "Eastern" mystique that has caused some people to shy away from it. Yet meditation requires no special knowledge or background. Whatever philosophical, religious, or emotional reasons may be given for meditation, its power derives from its ability to elicit the relaxation response. Regular practice of this quiet awareness will subtly carry over into your daily life, encouraging physical and emotional balance no matter what confronts you. For a step-by-step description of a basic meditation technique, see the box "Meditation and the Relaxation Response."

Another form of meditation, known as *mindfulness meditation*, involves paying attention to physical sensations, perceptions, thoughts, and imagery. Instead of focusing on a word or object to quiet the mind, you observe thoughts that do occur without evaluating or judging them. Development of this ability requires regular practice but may eventually result in a more objective view of one's perceptions.

**Deep Breathing** Your breathing pattern is closely tied to your stress level. Deep, slow breathing is associated with relaxation. Rapid, shallow, often irregular breathing occurs during the stress response. With practice, you can learn to slow and quiet your breathing pattern, thereby also quieting your mind and relaxing your body. Breathing techniques can be used for on-the-spot tension relief as well as for long-term stress reduction. The primary goal of many breathing exercises is to change your breathing pattern from chest breathing to diaphragmatic ("belly") breathing; refer to the box "Breathing for Relaxation."

**Hatha Yoga** *Yoga* is an ancient Sanskrit word referring to the union of mind, body, and soul.

A session of hatha yoga, the most common yoga style practiced in the United States, typically involves a series of *postures* (asanas), held for a few seconds to several minutes, that stretch and relax different parts of the

### Terms

VW

**relaxation response** A physiological state characterized by a feeling of warmth and quiet mental alertness.

**visualization** A technique for promoting relaxation or improving performance that involves creating or re-creating vivid mental pictures of a place or an experience; also called *imagery*.

**meditation** A technique for quieting the mind by focusing on a particular word, object (such as a candle flame), or process (such as breathing).

Take Charge

## Breathing for Relaxation

### Diaphragmatic Breathing

1. Lie on your back with your body relaxed.
2. Place one hand on your chest and one on your abdomen. (You will use your hands to monitor the depth and location of your breathing.)
3. Inhale slowly and deeply through your nose into your abdomen. Your abdomen should push up as far as is comfortable. Your chest should expand only a little and only in conjunction with the movement of your abdomen.
4. Exhale gently through your mouth.
5. Continue diaphragmatic breathing for about 5–10 minutes per session. Focus on the sound and feel of your breathing.

### Breathing In Relaxation, Breathing Out Tension

1. Assume a comfortable position, lying on your back or sitting in a chair.
2. Inhale slowly and deeply into your abdomen. Imagine the inhaled, warm air flowing to all parts of your body. Say to yourself, "Breathe in relaxation."
3. Exhale from your abdomen. Imagine tension flowing out of your body. Say to yourself, "Breathe out tension."
4. Pause before you inhale.
5. Continue for 5–10 minutes or until no tension remains in your body.

### Chest Expansion

1. Sit in a comfortable chair, or stand.
2. Inhale slowly and deeply into your abdomen as you raise your arms out to the sides. Pull your shoulders and arms back and lift your chin slightly so that your chest opens up.
3. Exhale gradually as you lower your arms and chin, and return to the starting position.
4. Repeat 5–10 times or until your breathing is deep and regular and your body feels relaxed and energized.

### Quick Tension Release

1. Inhale into your abdomen slowly and deeply as you count slowly to four.
2. Exhale slowly as you again count slowly to four. As you exhale, concentrate on relaxing your face, neck, shoulders, and chest.
3. Repeat several times. With each exhalation, feel more tension leaving your body.

SOURCES: Stop stress with a deep breath. 1996. *Health*, October, 53; Breathing for health and relaxation. 1995. *Mental Medicine Update* 4(2): 3–6; When you're stressed, catch your breath. 1995. *Mayo Clinic Health Letter*; December, 5.

body. The emphasis is on breathing, stretching, and balance. There are hundreds of different *asanas*, and they must be performed correctly in order to be beneficial. For this reason, qualified instruction is recommended, particularly for beginners.

**Taijiquan** A martial art that developed in China, taijiquan is a system of self-defense that incorporates philosophical concepts from Taoism and Confucianism. Taijiquan, often called "tai chi," is considered the gentlest of the martial arts. Instead of using quick and powerful movements, taijiquan consists of a series of slow, fluid, elegant movements, which reinforce the idea of moving *with* rather than *against* the stressors of everyday life. The practice of taijiquan promotes relaxation and concentration as well as the development of body awareness, balance, muscular strength, and flexibility. It usually takes some time and practice to reap the stress-management benefits of taijiquan, and, as with yoga, it's best to begin with some qualified instruction.

**Listening to Music** Listening to music is another method of inducing relaxation. It has been shown to influence pulse, blood pressure, and the electrical activity of muscles. To experience the stress-management benefits of music yourself, set aside a time to listen. Choose music that you enjoy and that makes you feel relaxed.

Other relaxation techniques include biofeedback, massage, hypnosis and self-hypnosis, and autogenic training. To learn more about these and other techniques for inducing the relaxation response, refer to For More Information at the end of the chapter.

## Counterproductive Coping Strategies

College is a time when you'll learn to adapt to new and challenging situations and gain skills that will last a lifetime. It is also a time when many people develop habits, in response to stress, that are counterproductive and unhealthy and that may also last well beyond graduation.

- *Tobacco:* The nicotine in cigarettes and other tobacco products can make you feel relaxed and even increase your ability to concentrate, but it is highly addictive. Smoking causes cancer, heart disease, impotence, and many other health problems and is the leading preventable cause of death in the United States.

Taijiquan is among the many techniques for inducing the relaxation response. In addition to helping these men manage stress, regular practice of taijiquan will also improve their balance and increase their muscular strength and flexibility.

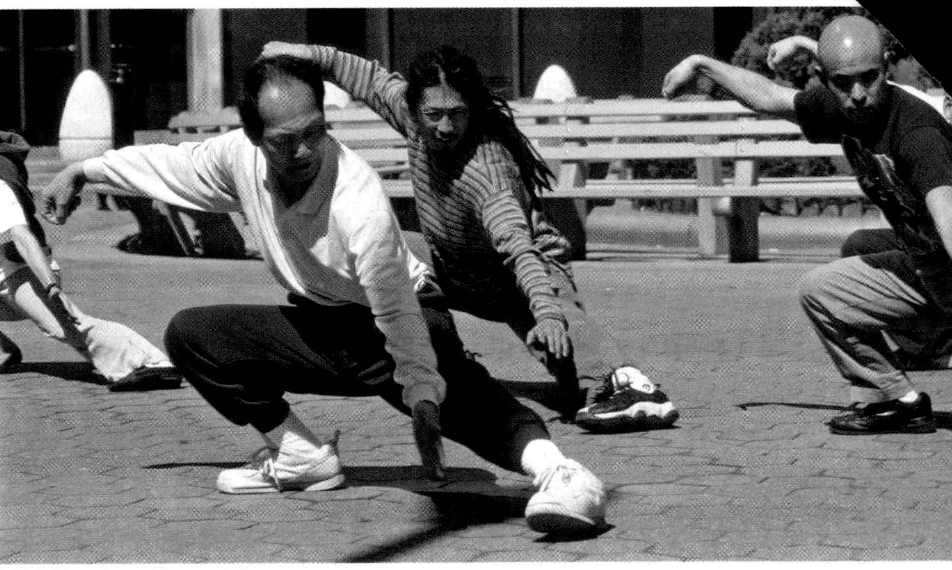

• *Alcohol:* Having a few drinks might make you feel temporarily at ease, and drinking until you're intoxicated may help you forget your current stressors. However, using alcohol to deal with stress places you at risk for all the short- and long-term problems associated with alcohol abuse. It also does nothing to address the causes of stress in your life.

• *Other drugs:* Altering your body chemistry in order to cope with stress is a strategy that has many pitfalls and does not directly address your stressors. For example, caffeine raises cortisol levels and blood pressure and disrupts sleep. Marijuana can elicit panic attacks with repeated use, and it may enhance the stress response. Stimulants such as amphetamine can also activate the stress response.

• *Binge eating:* The feelings of satiation and sedation that follow eating produce a relaxed state that reduces stress. However, regular use of eating as a means of coping with stress may lead to binge eating, a risk behavior associated with weight gain and serious eating disorders. Refer to later chapters for more information on these unhealthy coping strategies: tobacco and alcohol (Chapter 8), drug use (Chapter 7), poor nutrition (Chapter 9), and eating disorders (Chapter 11).

## CREATING A PERSONAL PLAN FOR MANAGING STRESS

What are the most important sources of stress in your life? Are you coping successfully with these stressors? No single strategy or program for managing stress will work for everyone, but you can use the principles of behavior management described in Chapter 1 to tailor a plan specifically to your needs.

### Identifying Stressors

Before you can learn to manage the stressors in your life, you have to identify them. A strategy many experts recommend is keeping a stress journal for a week or two. Keep a log of your daily activities, and assign a rating to your stress level for every hour. Each time you feel or express a stress response, record the time and the circumstances in your journal. Note what you were doing at the time, what you were thinking or feeling, and the outcome of your response.

After keeping your journal for a few weeks, you should be able to identify your key stressors and spot patterns in how you respond to them. Take note of the people, places, events, and patterns of thought and behavior that cause you the most stress. You may notice, for example, that mornings are usually the most stressful part of your day. Or you may discover that when you're angry at your roommate, you're apt to respond with behaviors that only make matters worse. Once you've outlined the general pattern of stress in your life, you may want to focus on a particularly problematic stressor or on an inappropriate behavioral response you've identified. Keep a stress log for another week or two that focuses just on the early morning hours, for example, or just on your arguments with your roommate. The more information you gather, the easier it will be to develop effective strategies for coping with the stressors in your life.

### Designing Your Plan

Now that you've identified the key stressors in your life, it's time to choose the techniques that will work best for you and create an action plan for change. Finding a buddy to work with you can make the process more fun and increase your chances of success. Some experts recommend drawing up a formal contract with yourself.

Whether or not you complete a contract, it's important to design rewards into your plan. You might treat yourself to a special breakfast in a favorite restaurant on the weekend (as long as you eat a nutritious breakfast every weekday morning). If you practice your relaxation techniques faithfully, you might reward yourself with a long bath or an hour of pleasure reading at the end of the day. It's also important to evaluate your plan regularly and redesign it as your needs change. Under times of increased stress, for example, you might want to focus on good eating, exercise, and relaxation habits. Over time, your new stress-management skills will become almost automatic. You'll feel better, accomplish more, and reduce your risk of disease.

## Getting Help

If the techniques discussed so far don't provide you with enough relief from the stress in your life, you might want to read more about specific areas you wish to work on, consult a peer counselor, join a support group, or participate in a few psychotherapy sessions. Excellent self-help guides can be found in bookstores or the library. Additional resources are listed in the For More Information section at the end of the chapter.

Your student health center or student affairs office can tell you whether your campus has a peer counseling program. Such programs are usually staffed by volunteer students with special training that emphasizes maintaining confidentiality. Peer counselors can guide you to other campus or community resources or can simply provide understanding. Short-term phychotherapy is another useful option.

**Tips for Today**

Some stress is unavoidable in life. How you respond to it is what determines whether you become "stressed out" or maintain your serenity. For the stress you can't avoid, develop a range of stress-management techniques and strategies.

*Right now you can*

- Sit in a comfortable chair and practice deep breathing for 5–10 minutes.
- Visualize a relaxing, peaceful place and imagine yourself experiencing it as vividly as possible; you might "feel" a gentle breeze on your skin or "hear" the soothing sound of a waterfall. Stay there as long as you can.
- Stand up and do some stretching exercises, such as gently rolling your head from side to side, stretching your arms out in front of your body and over your head, and slowly bending over and letting your arms hang toward the floor.
- Get out your date book and schedule what you'll be doing the rest of today and tomorrow. Pencil in a short walk and a conversation with a friend. Plan to go to bed 15 minutes earlier than usual.

## SUMMARY

- When confronted with a stressor, the body undergoes a set of physical changes known as the fight-or-flight reaction. The sympathetic nervous system and endocrine system act on many targets in the body to prepare it for action—even if the situation does not require physical action.
- Emotional and behavioral responses to stressors vary among individuals. Ineffective responses increase stress but can be moderated or changed.
- Factors that influence emotional and behavioral responses to stressors include personality, cultural background, gender, and past experiences.
- The general adaptation syndrome (GAS) has three stages: alarm, resistance, and exhaustion.
- A high allostatic load characterized by prolonged or repeated exposure to stress hormones can increase a person's risk of health problems.
- Psychoneuroimmunology (PNI) looks at how the physiological changes of the stress response affect the immune system and thereby increase the risk of illness.
- Health problems linked to stress include cardiovascular disease, colds and other infections, asthma and allergies, cancer, flare-ups of chronic diseases, and psychological problems.
- A cluster of major life events that require adjustment and accommodation can lead to increased stress and an increased risk of health problems. Minor daily hassles increase stress if they are perceived negatively.
- Sources of stress associated with college may be academic, interpersonal, time-related, or financial pressures.
- Job-related stress is common, particularly for employees who have little control over decisions relating to their jobs. If stress is severe or prolonged, burnout may occur.
- New and changing relationships, prejudice, and discrimination are examples of interpersonal and social stressors.
- Social support, exercise, nutrition, sleep, and time management are wellness behaviors that reduce stress and increase energy.
- Cognitive techniques for managing stress involve developing new and healthy patterns of thinking, such as practicing problem solving, monitoring self-talk, and cultivating a sense of humor.
- The relaxation response is the opposite of the fight-or-flight reaction. Techniques that trigger it, including progressive relaxation, imagery, meditation, deep breathing, hatha yoga, taijiquan, and listening to music. Counterproductive coping strategies include smoking, drinking, and unhealthy eating.
- A successful individualized plan for coping with stress begins with the use of a stress journal or log to identify and study stressors and inappropriate behavioral responses. Completing a contract and recruiting a buddy can help your stress-management plan succeed.

## Behavior Change Strategy

### Dealing with Test Anxiety

Are you a person who doesn't perform as well as you should on tests? Do you find that anxiety interferes with your ability to study effectively before the test and to think clearly in the test situation? If so, you may be experiencing test anxiety—an ineffective response to a stressful situation that can be replaced with more effective responses. If test anxiety is a problem for you, try some of the following strategies:

- Before the test, find out everything you can about it—its format, the material to be covered, the grading criteria. Ask the instructor for practice materials. Study in advance; don't just cram the night before. Avoid all-nighters.
- Devise a study plan. This might include forming a study group with one or more classmates or outlining what you will study, when, where, and for how long. Generate your own questions and answer them.
- In the actual test situation, sit away from possible distractions, listen carefully to instructions, and ask for clarification if you don't understand a direction.
- During the test, answer the easiest questions first. If you don't know an answer and there is no penalty for incorrect answers, guess. If there are several questions you have difficulty answering, review the ones you have already handled. Figure out approximately how much time you have to cover each question.
- For math problems, try to estimate the answer before doing the precise calculations.
- For true-false questions, look for qualifiers such as *always* and *never.* Such questions are likely to be false.
- For essay questions, look for key words in the question that indicate what the instructor is looking for in the answer. Develop a brief outline of your answer, sketching out what you will cover. Stick to your outline, and keep track of the time you're spending on your answer. Don't get caught with unanswered questions when time is up.
- Remain calm and focused throughout the test. Don't let negative thoughts rattle you. Avoid worrying about past performance, how others are doing, or the negative consequences of a poor test grade. If you start to become nervous, take some deep breaths and relax your muscles completely for a minute or so.

The best way to counter test anxiety is with successful test-taking experiences. The more times you succeed, the more your test anxiety will recede. If you find that these methods aren't sufficient to get your anxiety under control, you may want to seek professional help.

## Take Action

1. **Interview friends or family members.** Choose someone who seems to deal particularly well with stress. Interview that person about his or her methods for managing stress. What strategies does he or she use? What can you learn from that person that can be applied to your own life?

2. **Check out local services.** Investigate the services available in your community—such as peer counseling, support groups, and time-management classes—to help people deal with stress. If possible, visit or gather information on one or more of them. Write a description and evaluation of their services, including your personal reactions.

3. **Try a stress-management technique.** Reread the techniques described in this chapter, and choose one to try for a week. After a trial period, evaluate the effectiveness of the strategy you chose. Did your stress level decrease during the week? Were you better able to deal with daily hassles and any more severe stressors that you encountered?

4. **Reach out to others by becoming a volunteer.** Whether or not you realize it, you likely have more physical, emotional, and intellectual resources than you need. Transfer some of these resources to people who would benefit greatly from just a few hours of your time and effort. In doing so, you may find that you also benefit in terms of greater self-esteem and appreciation for your own support system and the opportunities you have for a positive future. Look for an opportunity to volunteer to help others in your community.

## For More Information

### Books

Blonna, R. 2005. *Coping with Stress in a Changing World.* 3rd ed. New York: McGraw-Hill. *A comprehensive guide to stress management that includes separate chapters on college stressors and spirituality.*

Kabat-Zinn, J. 2005. *Coming to Our Senses: Healing Ourselves and the World Through Mindfulness.* New York: Hyperion. *Explores the connections among mindfulness, health, and our physical and spiritual well-being.*

Pennebaker, J. W. 2004. *Writing to Heal: A Guided Journal for Recovering from Trauma and Emotional Upheaval.* Oakland, Calif.: New Harbinger Press. *Provides information about using journaling to cope with stress.*

Sapolsky, R. M. 2004. *Why Zebras Don't Get Ulcers.* 3rd ed. New York: Owl Books. *Describes the links between stress and disease in addition to strategies for stress management.*

### WW Organizations and Web Sites

*American Psychological Association.* Provides information on stress management and psychological disorders.
800-374-2721; 800-964-2000 (referrals)
http://www.apa.org; http://helping.apa.org

*Association for Applied Psychophysiology and Biofeedback.* Provides information about biofeedback and referrals to certified biofeedback practitioners.

800-477-8892

http://www.aapb.org

*Harvard Mind-Body Medical Institute.* Provides information about stress-management and relaxation techniques.

http://www.mbmi.org

*Interactive Budgeting Worksheet.* An interactive calculator designed to help students balance income and expenses.

http://www.ed.gov/offices/OSFAP/DirectLoan/BudgetCalc/budget.html

*Medical Basis for Stress.* Includes information on recognizing stress and on the physiological basis of stress, self-assessments for stress levels, and techniques for managing stress.

http://www.teachhealth.com

*National Institute for Occupational Safety and Health (NIOSH).* Provides information and links on job stress.

http://www.cdc.gov/niosh/topics/stress

*National Institute of Mental Health (NIMH).* Publishes informative brochures about stress and stress management as well as other aspects of mental health.

866-615-6464

http://www.nimh.nih.gov

*National Sleep Foundation.* Provides information about sleep and how to overcome problems such as insomnia and jet lag.

http://www.sleepfoundation.org

*Student Counseling Virtual Pamphlet Collection.* Links to online pamphlets from student counseling centers at colleges and universities across the country; topics include stress, sleep, and time management.

http://counseling.uchicago.edu/vpc

See also the listings for Chapters 1 and 3.

## Selected Bibliography

American Psychological Association. 2005. *Learning to Deal with Stress* (http://helping.apa.org/articles/article.php?id=71; retrieved February 17, 2005).

American Psychological Association. 2005. *Managing Traumatic Stress: Tips for Recovering from Natural Disasters* (http://helping.apa.org/articles/article.php?id=69; retrieved February 17, 2005).

Baker, S. R. 2003. A prospective longitudinal investigation of social problem-solving appraisals on adjustment to university, stress, health, and academic motivation and performance. *Personality and Individual Differences* 35(3): 569–591.

Bhattacharya, G., and S. L. Schoppelrey. 2004. Preimmigration beliefs of life success, postimmigration experiences, and acculturative stress: South Asian immigrants in the United States. *Journal of Immigrant Health* 6(2): 83–92.

Bouchard T. J. Jr., and M. McGue. 2003. Genetic and environmental influences on human psychological differences *Journal of Neurobiology* 54(1): 4–45.

Constantine, M. G., S. Okazaki, and S. O. Utsey. 2004. Self-concealment, social self-efficacy, acculturative stress, and depression in African, Asian, and Latin American international college students. *American Journal of Orthopsychiatry* 74(3): 230–241.

Cooper, A. E. 2003. An investigation of the relationships among spirituality, prayer and meditation, and aspects of stress and coping. *Dissertation Abstracts International: Section B: The Sciences and Engineering* 64(3-B): 1484.

Grossman, P., et al. 2004. Mindfulness-based stress reduction and health benefits: A meta analysis. *Journal of Psychosomatic Research* 57(1): 35–43.

Liverant, G. I., S. G. Hofmann, and B. T. Litz. 2004. Coping and anxiety in college students after the September 11th terrorist attacks. *Anxiety, Stress and Coping: An International Journal* 17(2): 127–139.

Longest, M. Q. 2003. Non-reactive, homeostatic, and positive resiliency: Relationships and predictors. *Dissertation Abstracts International: Section B: The Sciences and Engineering* 64(2-B).

Meehan, D.-C.-M., and C. Negy. 2003. Undergraduate students' adaptation to college: Does being married make a difference? *Journal of College Student Development* 44: 670–689.

Meier-Ewert, H. K., et al. 2004. Effect of sleep loss on C-reactive protein, an inflammatory marker of cardiovascular risk. *Journal of the American College of Cardiology* 43: 678–683.

Melamed, S., et al. 2004. Association of fear of terror with low-grade inflammation among apparently healthy employed adults. *Psychosomatic Medicine* 66(4): 484–491.

National Mental Health Association. 2001. *Coping with Disaster: Tips for College Students* (http://www.nmha.org/reassurance/collegetips.cfm).

Pickering, T. G. 2003. Effects of stress and behavioral interventions in hypertension—Men are from Mars, women are from Venus: Stress, pets, and oxytocin. *Journal of Clinical Hypertension* 5(1): 86–8.

Ridley, M. 2003. *Nature Via Nurture.* New York: HarperCollins.

Sax, L. J., et al. 2004. *The American Freshman: National Norms for Fall 2003.* Los Angeles: UCLA Higher Education Research Institute.

Schlenger, W. E., et al. 2002. Psychological reactions to terrorist attacks. Findings from the National Study of Americans' Reactions to September 11. *Journal of the American Medical Association* 288(5): 581–588.

Segerstrom, S. C., and G. E. Miller. 2004. Psychological stress and the human immune system: A meta-analytic study of 30 years of inquiry. *Psychological Bulletin* 130: 601–630.

Smyth, J., and R. Helm. 2003. Focused expressive writing as self-help for stress and trauma. *Journal of Clinical Psychology* 59(2): 227–235.

Steptoe, A., et al. 2003. Influence of socioeconomic status and job control on plasma fibrinogen responses to acute mental stress. *Psychosomatic Medicine* 65(1): 137–144.

Steptoe, A., et al. 2004. Loneliness and neuroendocrine, cardiovascular, and inflammatory stress responses in middle-aged men and women. *Psychoneuroendocrinology* 29(5): 593–611.

Vorona, R. D., et al. 2005. Overweight and obese patients in a primary care population report less sleep than patients with a normal body mass index. *Archives of Internal Medicine* 165(1): 25–30.

Wetter, D. W., et al. 2004. Prevalence and predictors of transitions in smoking behavior among college students. *Health Psychology* 23(2): 168–177.

Wittstein, I. S., et al. 2005. Neurohumoral features of myocardial stunning due to sudden emotional stress. *New England Journal of Medicine* 352(6): 539–548.

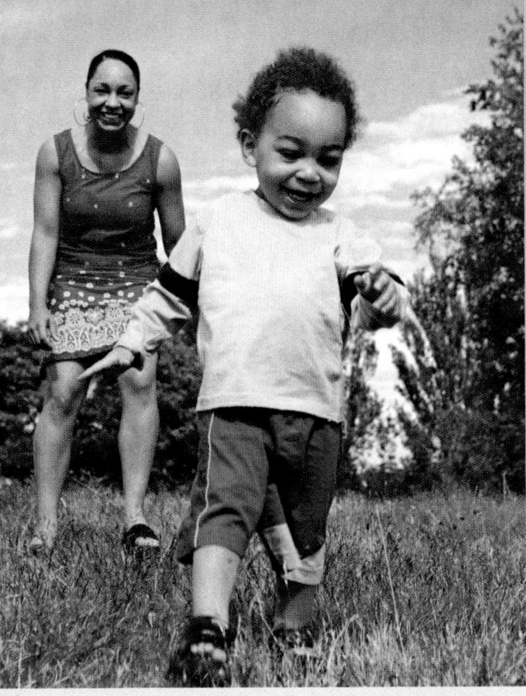

3

## Looking AHEAD

After reading this chapter, you should be able to

- Describe what it means to be psychologically healthy
- Explain how to develop and maintain a positive self-concept and healthy self-esteem
- Discuss the importance to psychological health of an optimistic outlook, good communication skills, and constructive approaches to dealing with loneliness and anger
- Describe common psychological disorders and list the warning signs of suicide
- Explain the different approaches and types of help available for psychological problems

# Psychological Health

What exactly is psychological health? Many people over the centuries have expressed opinions about the nature of psychological (or mental) health. Some even claim that there is no such thing, that psychological health is just a myth. We disagree. We think there is such a thing as psychological health just as there is physical health—and the two are closely interrelated. Just as your body can work well or poorly, giving you pleasure or pain, your mind can also work well or poorly, resulting in happiness or unhappiness. Psychological health is a crucial component of overall wellness. (We are using "mental health" and "psychological health" interchangeably.) If you feel pain and unhappiness rather than pleasure and happiness or if you sense that you could be functioning at a higher level, there may be ways you can help yourself—either on your own or with the aid of a professional. This chapter will explain how.

## WHAT PSYCHOLOGICAL HEALTH IS NOT

Psychological health is not the same as psychological **normality.** Being mentally normal simply means being close to average. You can define normal body temperature because a few degrees above or below this temperature always means physical sickness. But your ideas and attitudes can vary tremendously without your losing efficiency or feeling emotional distress. And psychological diversity is valuable; living in a society of people with varied ideas and lifestyles makes life interesting and challenging.

Conforming to social demands is not necessarily a mark of psychological health. If you don't question what's going on around you, you're not fulfilling your potential as a thinking, questioning human being. Never seeking help for personal problems does not mean you are psychologically healthy, any more than seeking help proves you are mentally ill. Unhappy people may not want to seek professional help because they don't want to reveal their problems to others, may fear what their friends might think, or may not know whom to ask for help. People who are severely disturbed psychologically or emotionally may not even realize they need help, or they may become so suspicious of other people that they can only be treated without their consent.

We cannot say people are "mentally ill" or "mentally healthy" on the basis of symptoms alone. Life constantly presents problems. Time and life inevitably alter the environment as well as our minds and bodies, and changes present problems. The symptom of anxiety, for example,

**Term**

**normality** The psychological characteristics attributed to the majority of people in a population at a given time.

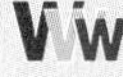

Visit the *Core Concepts in Health* Online Learning Center (www.mhhe.com/inselbrief10e) for study aids and many additional resources.

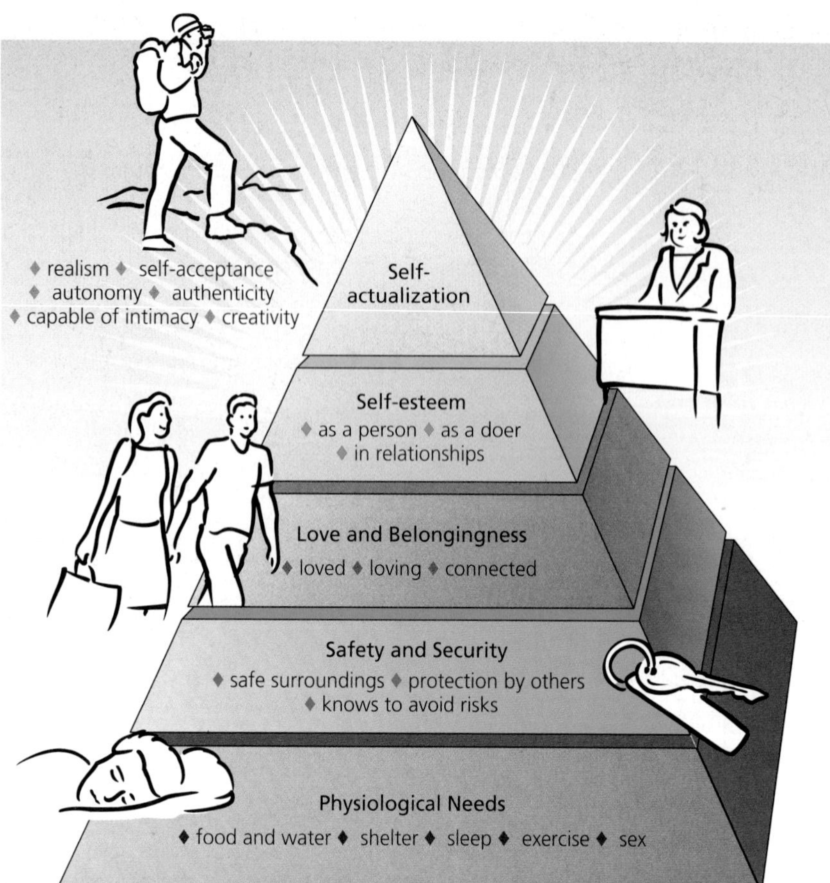


**Figure 3-1 Maslow's hierarchy of needs.** People focus first on the needs at the bottom of the hierarchy because unless basic physiological needs are fulfilled, other needs have little meaning. Once urgent needs are satisfied, people can focus on higher motives. Those who make it to the top of the needs hierarchy achieve self-actualization—they have grown to fulfill much of their human potential and are able to act and make choices unfettered by unfulfilled needs at lower levels. SOURCE: Maslow, A. 1970. *Motivation and Personality,* 2nd ed. New York: Harper & Row.

can help us face a problem and solve it before it gets too big. Someone who shows no anxiety may be refusing to recognize problems or do anything about them. A person who is anxious for good reason is likely to be judged more psychologically healthy in the long run than someone who is inappropriately calm. Finally, we cannot judge psychological health from the way people look. All too often, a person who seems to be OK and even happy suddenly takes his or her own life.

## DEFINING PSYCHOLOGICAL HEALTH

It is even harder to say what psychological health *is* than what it is *not.* Psychological health can be defined either negatively as the absence of sickness or positively as the presence of wellness. A positive definition—psychological health as the presence of wellness—is a more ambitious outlook, one that encourages us to fulfill our own potential. During the 1960s, Abraham Maslow eloquently described an ideal of mental health in his book *Toward a Psychology of Being.* He stated that there is a *hierarchy of needs,* listed here in order of decreasing urgency: physiological needs, safety, being loved, maintaining self-esteem, and self-actualization (Figure 3-1). When urgent needs like the need for food, water, shelter, sleep, and safety are satisfied, less urgent needs take priority. According to Maslow, people who live at their fullest have achieved **self-actualization;** he thought they had fulfilled a good measure of their human potential and share certain qualities.

### Realism

Self-actualized people are able to deal with the world as it is and not demand that it be otherwise. If you are realistic, you know the difference between what is and what you want. You also know what you can change and what you cannot. Unrealistic people often spend a great deal of time and energy trying to force the world and other people into their ideal picture. Realistic people accept evidence that contradicts what they want to believe, and if it is important evidence they modify their beliefs.

### Acceptance

Psychologically healthy people can largely accept themselves and others. Self-acceptance means having a positive **self-concept**, or *self-image,* or appropriately high **self-esteem.** Such people have a positive but realistic mental image of themselves and positive feelings about who they are, what they are capable of, and what roles they play. People who feel good about themselves are likely to live up to their positive self-image and enjoy successes that in turn reinforce these good feelings. A good self-concept is based on a realistic view of personal worth—it does not mean being egocentric or "stuck on yourself." Being able to tolerate our own imperfections and still feel positive about ourselves helps us tolerate the imperfections of others.

### Autonomy

Psychologically healthy people are able to direct themselves, acting independently of their social environment. **Autonomy** is more than freedom from physical control by something outside the self. Many people, for example, shrink from expressing their feelings because they fear disapproval and rejection. They respond only to what they feel as outside pressure. Such behavior is **other-directed.** In contrast, **inner-directed** people find guidance from within, from their own values and feelings. They are not afraid to be themselves. Psychologically free people act because they choose to, not because they are driven or pressured. They have an internal locus of control and a high level of self-efficacy (see Chapter 1).

Autonomy can give healthy people certain childlike qualities. Very small children have a quality of being "real." They respond in a genuine, spontaneous way to whatever happens, without pretenses. Being genuine means not having to plan words or actions to get approval or make an impression. It means being aware of feelings and being willing to express them—being unself-consciously oneself. This quality is sometimes called **authenticity.**

### A Capacity for Intimacy

Healthy people are capable of physical and emotional intimacy. They can expose their feelings and thoughts to other people. They are open to the pleasure of intimate physical contact and to the risks and satisfactions of being close to others in a caring, sensitive way.

### Creativity

Psychologically healthy people are creative and have a continuing fresh appreciation for what goes on around them. They are not necessarily great poets, artists, or musicians, but they do live their everyday lives in creative ways: "A first-rate soup is more creative than a second-rate painting." Creative people seem to see more and to be open to new experiences; they don't fear the unknown or need to minimize or avoid uncertainty.

How did Maslow's group achieve their exemplary psychological health, and (more important) how can *we* attain it? Maslow himself did not answer that question, but it undoubtedly helps to have been treated with respect, love, and understanding as a child, to have experienced stability, and to have achieved a sense of mastery. As adults, since we cannot redo the past, we must concentrate on meeting current challenges in ways that will lead to long-term mental wellness. We must not consider ourselves failures if we do not become self-actualized in every way or at every moment. Self-actualization is an ideal to strive for even if we never or only occasionally attain it to the fullest degree.

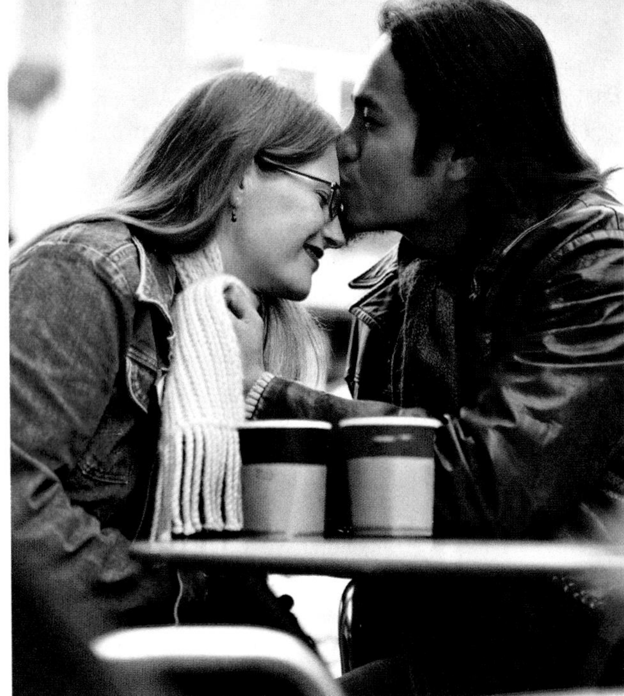

Self-actualized people respond in a genuine, spontaneous way to what happens around them. They are capable of maintaining close interpersonal relationships.

## MEETING LIFE'S CHALLENGES

Life is full of challenges—large and small. Everyone, regardless of heredity and family influences, must learn to cope successfully with new situations and new people.

### Growing Up Psychologically

Along the path from birth to old age, we are confronted with a series of challenges. How we respond influences the development of our personality and identity.

#### Terms

**self-actualization** The highest level of growth in Maslow's hierarchy.

**self-concept** The ideas, feelings, and perceptions one has about oneself; also called *self-image*.

**self-esteem** Satisfaction and confidence in oneself; the valuing of oneself as a person.

**autonomy** Independence; the sense of being self-directed.

**other-directed** Guided in behavior by the values and expectations of others.

**inner-directed** Guided in behavior by an inner set of rules and values.

**authenticity** Genuineness.

Vw

**Developing an Adult Identity** A primary task beginning in adolescence is the development of an adult identity: a unified sense of self, characterized by attitudes, beliefs, and ways of acting that are genuinely one's own. People with adult identities know who they are, what they are capable of, what roles they play, and their place among their peers. They have a sense of their own uniqueness but also appreciate what they have in common with others. They view themselves realistically and can assess their strengths and weaknesses without relying on the opinions of others. Achieving an identity also means that one can form intimate relationships with others while maintaining a strong sense of self.

Our identities evolve as we interact with the world and make choices about what we'd like to do and whom we'd like to model ourselves after. Developing an adult identity is particularly challenging in a heterogeneous, secular, and relatively affluent society like ours, in which many roles are possible, many choices are tolerated, and ample time is allowed for experimenting and making up one's mind.

Early identities are often modeled after parents—or the opposite of parents, in rebellion against what they represent. Later, peers, rock stars, sports heroes, and religious figures are added to the list of possible models. Early identities are rarely permanent, but at some point, most of us adopt a more stable, individual identity that ties together the experiences of childhood and the expectations and aspirations of adulthood.

How far have you gotten in developing your adult identity? Write down a list of characteristics you think a friend who knows you well would use to describe you. Rank them from the most to the least important. Your list might include elements such as gender, socioeconomic status, ethnic and/or religious identification, choice of college or major, parents' occupations, interests and talents, attitudes toward drugs and alcohol, style of dress, the kinds of people with whom you typically associate, your expected role in society, and aspects of your personality. Which elements of your identity do you feel are permanent, and which do you think may change over time? Are there any characteristics missing from your list that you'd like to add?

**Developing Intimacy** Learning to live intimately with others and finding a productive role for yourself in society are other tasks of adulthood—to be able to love and work. People with established identities can form intimate relationships and sexual unions characterized by sharing, open communication, long-term commitment, and love. Those who lack a firm sense of self may have difficulty establishing relationships because they feel overwhelmed by closeness and the needs of another person.

**Developing Values and Purpose in Your Life** Values are criteria for judging what is good and bad; they underlie our moral decisions and behavior. As adults we need to assess how far we have evolved morally and what values we actually have adopted, either explicitly or implicitly. Without an awareness of our personal values, our lives may be hurriedly driven forward by immediate desires and the passing demands of others. But are we doing things according to our principles? What are we striving for with our actions? Living according to values means considering your options carefully before making a choice, choosing between options without succumbing to outside pressures that oppose your values, and making a choice and acting on it rather than doing nothing. Your actions and how you justify them proclaim to others what you stand for.

For more on developing meaning and purpose in your life, see the box "Paths to Spiritual Wellness."

## Achieving Healthy Self-Esteem

Having a healthy level of self-esteem means regarding your self, which includes all aspects of your identity, as good, competent, and worthy of love.

**Developing a Positive Self-Concept** Ideally, a positive self-concept begins in childhood, based on experiences both within the family and outside it. Children need to develop a sense of being loved and being able to give love and to accomplish their goals. If they feel rejected or neglected by their parents, they may fail to develop feelings of self-worth. They may grow to have a negative concept of themselves.

Other components of self-concept are integration and stability. An integrated self-concept is one that you have made for yourself—not someone else's image of you or a mask that doesn't quite fit. Stability depends on the integration of the self and its freedom from contradictions. People who have gotten mixed messages about themselves from parents and friends may have contradictory self-images, which defy integration and make them vulnerable to shifting levels of self-esteem. At times they regard themselves as entirely good, capable, and lovable—an ideal self—and at other times they see themselves as entirely bad, incompetent, and unworthy of love. At neither extreme do such people see themselves or others realistically, and their relationships with other people are filled with misunderstandings and ultimately with conflict.

**Meeting Challenges to Self-Esteem** As an adult, you sometimes run into situations that challenge your self-concept: People you care about may tell you they don't love you or feel loved by you, or your attempts to accomplish a goal may end in failure. You can react to such challenges in several ways. The best approach is to acknowledge that something has gone wrong and try again, adjusting your goals to your abilities without radically revising your self-concept. Less productive responses are denying that anything went wrong and blaming someone else. The worst

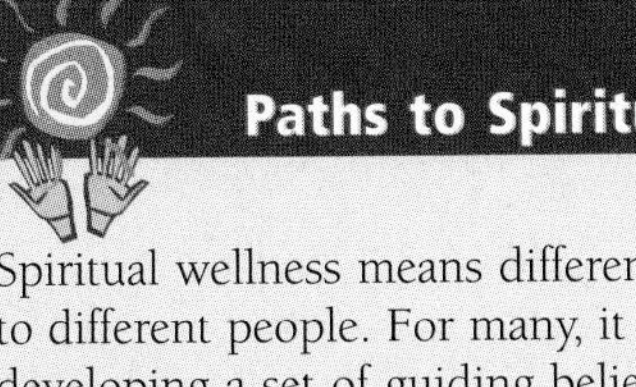

Mind/Body/Spirit

## Paths to Spiritual Wellness

Spiritual wellness means different things to different people. For many, it involves developing a set of guiding beliefs, principles, or values that give meaning and purpose to life. It helps people achieve a sense of wholeness within themselves and in their relationships with others. Spiritual wellness influences people on an individual level, as well as on a community level, where it can bond people together through compassion, love, forgiveness, and self-sacrifice. For some, spirituality includes a belief in a higher power. Regardless of how it is defined, the development of spiritual wellness is critical for overall health and well-being. Its development is closely tied to the other components of wellness, particularly psychological health.

There are many paths to spiritual wellness. One of the most common in our society is organized religion. Some people object to the notion that organized religion can contribute to psychological health and overall wellness, asserting that it reinforces people's tendency to deny real difficulties and to accept what can and should be changed. Freud criticized religion as wishful thinking; Marx called it an opiate to make the poor accept social injustice. However, many elements of religious belief and practice can promote psychological health.

Organized religion usually involves its members in a community where social and material support is available. Religious organizations offer a social network to those who might otherwise be isolated. The major religions provide paths for transforming the self in ways that can lead to greater happiness and serenity and reduce feelings of anxiety and hopelessness. In Christianity, salvation follows turning away from the selfish ego to God's sovereignty and grace, where a joy is found that frees the believer from anxious self-concern and despair. Islam is the word for a kind of self-surrender leading to peace with God. Buddhism teaches how to detach oneself from selfish desire, leading to compassion for the suffering of others and freedom from fear-engendering illusions. Judaism emphasizes the social and ethical redemption the Jewish community can experience if it follows the laws of God. Religions teach specific techniques for achieving these transformations of the self: prayer, both in groups and in private; meditation; the performance of rituals and ceremonies symbolizing religious truths; and good works and service to others. Christianity's faith and works are perhaps analogous to the cognitive and behavioral components of a program of behavior change.

Spiritual wellness does not require participation in organized religion. Many people find meaning and purpose in other ways. By spending time in nature or working on environmental issues, people can experience continuity with the natural world. Spiritual wellness can come through helping others in one's community or by promoting human rights, peace and harmony among people, and opportunities for human development on a global level. Other people develop spiritual wellness through art or through their personal relationships.

Particularly in the second half of life, people seem to have an urge to view their activities and consciousness from a transcendent perspective. Perhaps it is the approach of death that makes older people tend to take less interest in material possessions and to devote more time to interpersonal and altruistic pursuits. At every age, however, people seem to feel better if they have beliefs about the ultimate purpose of life and their own place in the universe.

reaction is to develop a lasting negative self-concept in which you feel bad, unloved, and ineffective—in other words, to become demoralized.

One method for fighting demoralization is to recognize and test your negative thoughts and assumptions about yourself and others. The first step is to note exactly when an unpleasant emotion—feeling worthless, wanting to give up, feeling depressed—occurs or gets worse, to identify the events or daydreams that trigger that emotion, and to observe whatever thoughts come into your head just before or during the emotional experience. It is helpful to keep a daily journal about such events.

At first, it may be hard to figure out a rational response until hours or days after the event that upset you. But once you get used to noticing the way your mind works, you may be able to catch yourself thinking negatively and change the thought process before it goes too far. This approach is not the same as positive thinking—substituting a positive thought for a negative one. Instead, you simply try to make your thoughts as logical and accurate as possible; see the box "Realistic Self-Talk" on page 50.

### Being Less Defensive

Sometimes our wishes come into conflict with people around us or with our conscience, and we become frustrated and anxious. If we cannot resolve the conflict by changing the external situation, we try to resolve the conflict internally by rearranging our thoughts and feelings. These psychological **defense mechanisms** allow us to protect ourselves against unacceptable thoughts or comfort ourselves when under pressure. Common defense mechanisms include repression, denial, rationalization, daydreaming, and humor. The drawback of many of these coping mechanisms is that although they succeed temporarily, they don't help find solutions to the underlying problem or conflict.

**Term**

**defense mechanism** A mental mechanism for coping with conflict or anxiety.

Vw

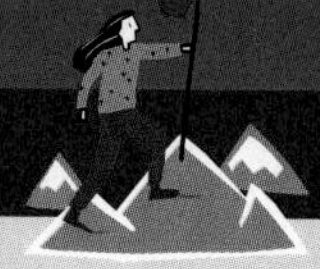

Take Charge

## Realistic Self-Talk

Do your patterns of thinking make events seem worse than they truly are? Do negative beliefs about yourself become self-fulfilling prophecies? Substituting realistic self-talk for negative self-talk can help you build and maintain self-esteem and cope better with the challenges in your life. Here are some examples of common types of **cognitive distortions,** along with suggestions for more accurate and rational responses.

| Cognitive Distortion | Negative Self-Talk | Realistic Self-Talk |
|---|---|---|
| Focusing on negatives | School is so discouraging—nothing but one hassle after another. | School is pretty challenging and has its difficulties, but there certainly are rewards. It's really a mixture of good and bad. |
| Expecting the worst | Why would my boss want to meet with me this afternoon if not to fire me? | I wonder why my boss wants to meet with me. I guess I'll just have to wait and see. |
| Overgeneralizing | (After getting a poor grade on a paper) Just as I thought—I'm incompetent at everything. | I'll start working on the next paper earlier. That way, if I run into problems, I'll have time to consult with the TA. |
| Minimizing | I won the speech contest, but none of the other speakers was very good. I wouldn't have done as well against stiffer competition. | It may not have been the best speech I'll ever give, but it was good enough to win the contest. I'm really improving as a speaker. |
| Blaming others | I wouldn't have eaten so much last night if my friends hadn't insisted on going to that restaurant. | I overdid it last night. Next time I'll make different choices. |
| Expecting perfection | I should have scored 100% on this test. I can't believe I missed that one problem through a careless mistake. | Too bad I missed one problem through carelessness, but overall I did very well on this test. Next time I'll be more careful. |
| Believing you're the cause of everything | Sarah seems so depressed today. I wish I hadn't had that argument with her yesterday; it must have really upset her. | I wish I had handled the argument better, and in the future I'll try to. But I don't know if Sarah's behavior is related to what I said or even if she's depressed. In any case, I'm not responsible for how Sarah feels or acts; only she can take responsibility for that. |
| Thinking in black and white | I've got to score 10 points in the game today. Otherwise, I don't belong on the team. | I'm a good player or else I wouldn't be on the team. I'll play my best—that's all I can do. |
| Magnifying events | They went to a movie without me. I thought we were friends, but I guess I was wrong. | I'm disappointed they didn't ask me to the movie, but it doesn't mean our friendship is over. It's not that big a deal. |

SOURCE: Adapted from Schafer, W. 1995. *Stress Management for Wellness,* 3rd ed. Copyright © 1996. Reprinted with permission of Wadsworth, a division of Thomson Learning: www.thomsonrights.com. Fax 800-730-2215.

Recognizing your favorite defense mechanisms can be difficult, because they've probably become habits, occurring unconsciously. But we each have some inkling about how our mind operates. Try to look at yourself as an objective, outside observer would and analyze your thoughts and behavior in a psychologically stressful situation from the past. Having insight into what strategies you typically use can lead to new, less defensive and more effective ways of coping in the future.

## Being Optimistic

Many psychologists believe that pessimism is not just a symptom of everyday depression but an important root cause as well. Pessimists not only expect repeated failure and rejection but also perversely accept it as deserved. Pessimists do not see themselves as capable of success, and they irrationally dismiss any evidence of their own accomplishments. This negative point of view is learned, typically at a young age from parents and other authority figures. But as an optimist would tell you, that means it also has the potential to be unlearned.

### Terms

VW

**cognitive distortion** A pattern of thinking that makes events seem worse than they are.

**assertiveness** Expression that is forceful but not hostile.

Pessimists must first recognize and then dispute the false, negative predictions they generate about themselves. Learning to be optimistic is easier and more lasting than, for example, learning to eat less. Unlike refusing foods you love, disputing your own negative thoughts is fun—because doing so makes you feel better immediately.

## Maintaining Honest Communication

Another important area of psychological functioning is communicating honestly with others. It can be very frustrating for us and for people around us if we cannot express what we want and feel. Others can hardly respond to our needs if they don't know what those needs are. We must recognize what we want to communicate and then express it clearly. For example, how do you feel about going to the party instead of to the movie? Do you care if your roommate talks on the phone late into the night? Some people know what they want others to do but don't state it clearly because they fear denial of the request, which they interpret as personal rejection. Such people might benefit from **assertiveness** training: learning to insist on their rights and to bargain for what they want. Assertiveness includes being able to say no or yes depending on the situation.

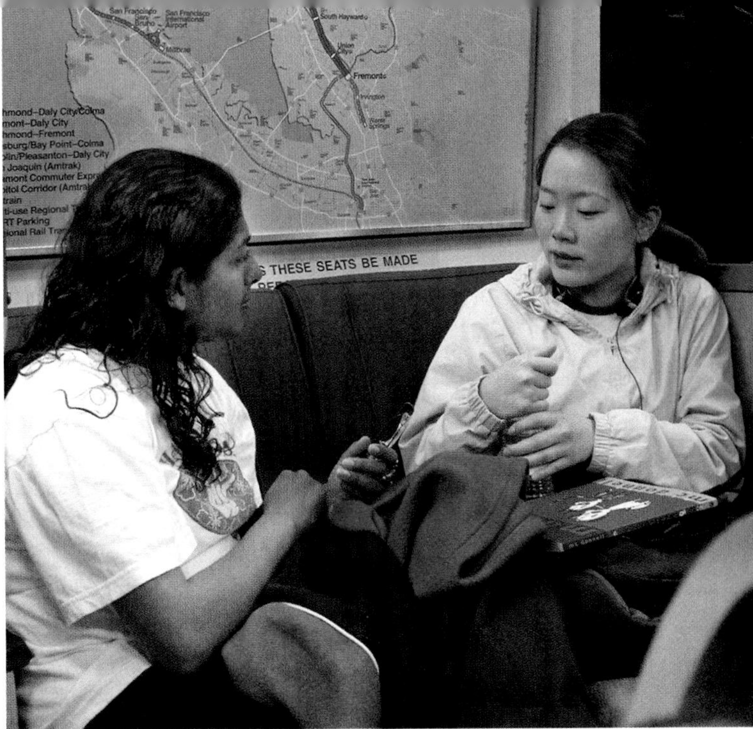


Communication is an important element in any interpersonal relationship. As these women express their thoughts and feelings to each other and listen attentively in response, they enhance their relationship, which in turn supports their psychological well-being.

## Dealing with Loneliness

The right balance between being alone and being with others is often hard to achieve. Some people are motivated to socialize by a fear of being alone—not the best reason to spend time with others. If you discover how to be happy by yourself, you'll be better able to cope with periods when you're forced to be alone. Unhappiness with being alone may come from interpreting it as a sign of rejection—that others are not interested in spending time with you. Before you conclude that, be sure that you give others a real chance to get to know you. Examine your patterns of thinking: You may harbor unrealistic expectations about other people—for example, that everyone you meet must like you and, if they don't, you must be terribly flawed.

If you decide that you're not spending enough time with people, take action to change the situation. College life provides many opportunities to meet people. In addition to classes and dorms, there are organizations of all kinds—hiking clubs, religious groups, advocacy groups, and so on—that offer a chance to meet others who share your interests.

## Dealing with Anger

Popular wisdom has said that you should express your anger rather than suppress it. Letting out your anger was thought to be beneficial for both psychological and physical health. However, recent studies have questioned this idea by showing that people who are overtly hostile seem to be at higher risk for heart attacks. Furthermore, angry words or actions won't contribute to psychological wellness if they damage important personal or professional relationships or produce feelings of guilt or loss of control. Perhaps the best way to resolve this contradiction is to look at the expression of anger in each situation and distinguish between a gratuitous expression of anger and a reasonable level of self-assertiveness.

**Managing Your Own Anger** If you feel explosive anger coming on, consider the following two strategies to head it off. First, try to *reframe* what you're thinking at that moment. You'll be less angry at another person if there is a possibility that his or her behavior was not intentionally directed against you. Did the man who cut into your lane on the freeway do it deliberately to spite you, or did he simply fail to see you? Look for possible mitigating factors that would make you less likely to blame him: Maybe he's late for a job interview. If you're angry because you've just been criticized, avoid mentally replaying scenes from the past when you received similar unjust criticisms. Think about what is happening now, and try to act differently than in the past—less defensively and more analytically. Why am I taking it personally? Why am I acting like a jerk just because she did?

Second, until you're able to change your thinking, try to *distract* yourself. Use the old trick of counting to 10 before you respond, or start concentrating on your breathing. If needed, take a longer cooling-off period by leaving the situation until your anger has subsided. This does not mean that you should permanently avoid the issues and people who make you angry. When you've had a chance to think more clearly about the matter, return to it.

**Dealing with Anger in Other People** If someone you're with becomes very angry, respond "asymmetrically" by reacting not with anger but with calm. Try to validate the other person by acknowledging that he or she has some reason to be angry. This does not mean apologizing, if you don't think you're to blame, or accepting verbal abuse, which is always inappropriate. Try to focus on solving the problem by allowing the individual to explain why he or she is so angry and what can be done to alleviate the situation. Finally, if the person cannot be calmed, it may be best to disengage, at least temporarily. After a time-out, a rational problem-solving approach may become more successful.

## PSYCHOLOGICAL DISORDERS

All of us have felt anxious at times, and in dealing with the anxiety we may have avoided doing something that we wanted to do or should have done. Most of us have had periods of feeling down when we became pessimistic, less energetic, and less able to enjoy life. Many of us have been bothered at times by irrational thoughts or odd feelings. Such feelings and thoughts can be normal responses to the ordinary challenges of life, but when emotions or irrational thoughts start to interfere with daily activities and rob us of our peace of mind, they can be considered symptoms of a psychological disorder (Table 3-1).

Psychological disorders are generally the result of many factors. Genetic differences, which underlie differences in how the brain processes information and experience, are known to play an important role, especially in bipolar disorder and schizophrenia. Learning and life events are important, too: Identical twins often don't have the same psychological disorders in spite of having identical genes. Some people have been exposed to more traumatic events than others, leading either to greater vulnerability to future traumas or, conversely, the development of better coping skills.

VITAL STATISTICS

**Table 3-1 Lifetime Prevalence of Selected Psychological Disorders Among Americans**

| Disorder | Men (%) | Women (%) |
|---|---|---|
| Anxiety disorders | | |
| Simple phobia | 6.7 | 15.7 |
| Social phobia | 11.1 | 15.5 |
| Panic disorder | 2.0 | 5.0 |
| Generalized anxiety disorder | 3.6 | 6.6 |
| Obsessive-compulsive disorder | 1.7 | 2.8 |
| Post-traumatic stress disorder | 5.0 | 10.4 |
| Mood disorders | | |
| Major depressive episode | 12.0 | 20.4 |
| Manic episode | 1.6 | 1.7 |
| Schizophrenia and related disorders | 1.0 | 0.5 |

SOURCES: Kessler, R. C., et al. 2003. The epidemiology of major depressive disorder: Results from the National Comorbidity Survey Replication (NCS-R). *Journal of the American Medical Association* 289(23): 3095–3105. U.S. Department of Health and Human Services. 1999. *Mental Health: A Report of the Surgeon General.* Rockville, Md.: DHHS; Weissman, M. M. 1998. Cross-national epidemiology of obsessive-compulsive disorder. *CNS Spectrums* 3(5 Suppl. 1): 6–9; Kessler, R. C., et al. 1995. Posttraumatic stress disorder in the National Comorbidity Survey. *Archives of General Psychiatry* 52(12): 1048–1060; Kessler, R. C., et al. 1994; Lifetime and 12-month prevalence of DSM-III-R psychiatric disorders in the United States. *Archives of General Psychiatry* 51(1): 8–19.

Furthermore, what your parents, peers, and others have taught you strongly influences your level of self-esteem and how you deal with frightening or depressing life events (see the box "Ethnicity, Culture, and Psychological Disorders").

### Anxiety Disorders

Fear is a basic and useful emotion. It provides motivation for self-protection and for learning to cope with new or potentially dangerous environmental or social situations. Only when fear is out of proportion to real danger can it be considered a problem. **Anxiety** is another word for fear, especially a feeling of fear that is not in response to any definite threat. Only when anxiety is experienced almost daily or in life situations that recur and cannot be avoided can anxiety be called a disorder.

**Simple Phobia** The most common and most understandable anxiety disorder, **simple**, or **specific, phobia** is a fear of something definite like lightning or a particular animal or location. Examples of commonly feared animals are snakes, spiders, and dogs; frightening locations are often high places or enclosed spaces. Sometimes, but not always, these fears originate in bad experiences, such as being bitten by a snake.

### Terms

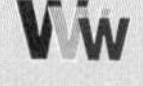

**anxiety** A feeling of fear that is not directed toward any definite threat.

**simple (specific) phobia** A persistent and excessive fear of a specific object, activity, or situation.

**social phobia** An excessive fear of performing in public; speaking in public is the most common example.

**panic disorder** A syndrome of severe anxiety attacks accompanied by physical symptoms.

**agoraphobia** An anxiety disorder characterized by fear of being alone away from help and avoidance of many different places and situations; in extreme cases, a fear of leaving home. From the Greek for "fear of the public market."

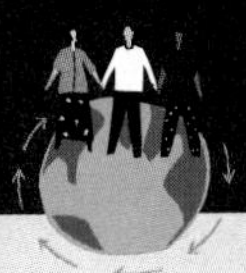

Dimensions of Diversity

## Ethnicity, Culture, and Psychological Disorders

Psychological disorders differ in incidence and symptoms across cultures and ethnic groups around the world. This variability is usually attributable to cultural differences—factors such as how symptoms are interpreted and communicated, whether treatment is sought, and whether a social stigma is attached to a particular symptom or disorder. Cultural differences relating to acculturation, ethnic identity, coping styles, social support, racism, and spirituality can increase the risk for, or provide protection from, psychological disorders.

### Expression of Symptoms

People from different cultures or groups may manifest or describe symptoms differently. Consider the following examples:

- In Japan, where showing respect and consideration for others is highly valued, people with social phobia may be more distressed about the imagined harm to others by their social clumsiness than at their own embarrassment.
- Older African Americans may express depression in atypical ways—for example, denying depression by taking on a multitude of extra tasks.
- Somatization, the indirect reporting of psychological distress through nonspecific physical symptoms, occurs across ethnic groups but is more prevalent among some, including African Americans, Puerto Ricans, and Chinese Americans.
- Schizophrenia may manifest with different delusions depending on the local culture.

### Attitudes Toward Symptoms, Diseases, and Treatment

An important cultural factor is whether a group regards symptoms of a psychological disorder as a social, moral, or health problem. It is relatively easy for Americans of northern European descent to regard an emotional problem as psychological in nature and to therefore accept a psychological treatment like therapy. For other groups, symptoms of psychological distress may be viewed as a spiritual problem, best dealt with by seeking guidance from religious figures.

Attitudes about disease influence whether patients will comply with professional treatment. For example, researchers looking at multiethnic clinics found that Southeast Asians were more likely than other groups to have no detectable blood levels of their prescribed antidepressant medication. The explanation for this, based on cultural norms, is that the patients' respect for the authority of the physician made them reluctant to admit that they did not agree with the doctor's recommendations and had not followed them.

People from some groups may have little hesitation about communicating intimate, personal problems to professional care providers. However, for others, particularly men and members of certain ethnic groups, loss of emotional control may be seen as a weakness. For all groups, culturally competent care is important to avoid misdiagnosis and inappropriate or ineffective treatment.

### Genetic/Biological Risk Factors

Biology can also play a role in the differences seen among patients of different ethnic groups. There is accumulating evidence that genetic differences between ethnic groups can explain some differences in drug metabolism. For example, psychotropic drugs are broken down in the body by a specific enzyme known as CYP2C19. Reduction of the activity of this enzyme is caused by two mutations, one of which appears to be found only in Asian populations. People in whom the action of this enzyme is reduced are called poor metabolizers, who as a result are very sensitive to medications that are broken down by it. The percentage of poor metabolizers among Asians is about 20%; among Latinos, about 5%; and among whites, 3%. Asian patients thus tend to have more adverse reactions to the doses of drugs standardized principally on white patients in the United States.

SOURCES: Kleinman, A. 2004. Culture and depression. *New England Journal of Medicine* 351(10): 951–953; Kirmayer, L. J. 2001. Cultural variations in the clinical presentation of depression and anxiety: Implications for diagnosis and treatment. *Journal of Clinical Psychiatry* 62 (Suppl. 13): 22–28; Lin, K. M. 2001. Biological differences in depression and anxiety across races and ethnic groups. *Journal of Clinical Psychiatry* 62 (Suppl. 13): 13–19; Baker, F. M. 2001. Diagnosing depression in African Americans. *Community Mental Health Journal* 37(1): 31–38; U.S. Department of Health and Human Services. 2001. *Mental Health: Culture, Race, and Ethnicity—A Supplement to Mental Health: A Report of the Surgeon General*. Rockville, Md.: U.S. Department of Health and Human Services.

**Social Phobia** People with **social phobia** fear humiliation or embarrassment while being observed by others. Fear of speaking in public is perhaps the most common phobia of this kind. Extremely shy people can have social fears that extend to almost all social situations (see the box "Shyness" on p. 54).

**Panic Disorder** People with **panic disorder** experience sudden unexpected surges in anxiety, accompanied by symptoms such as rapid and strong heartbeat, shortness of breath, loss of physical equilibrium, and a feeling of losing mental control. Such attacks usually begin in one's early twenties and can lead to a fear of being in crowds or closed places or of driving or flying. Sufferers fear that a panic attack will occur in a situation from which escape is difficult (such as while in an elevator), where the attack could be incapacitating and result in a dangerous or embarrassing loss of control (such as while driving a car or shopping), or where no medical help would be available if needed (such as when a person is alone away from home). Fears such as these lead to avoidance of situations that might cause trouble. The fears and avoidance may spread to a large variety of situations until a person is virtually housebound, a condition called **agoraphobia.**

In Focus

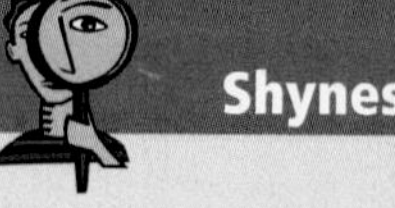

## Shyness

Shyness is a form of social anxiety, a fear of what others will think of one's behavior or appearance. Physical signs include a rapid heartbeat, a nervous stomach, sweating, cold and clammy hands, blushing, dry mouth, a lump in the throat, and trembling muscles. Shy people are often excessively self-critical, and they engage in very negative self-talk. The accompanying feelings of self-consciousness, embarrassment, and unworthiness can be overwhelming.

To avoid situations that make them anxious, shy people may refrain from making eye contact or speaking up in public. They may shun social gatherings. They may avoid college courses or job promotions that demand more interpersonal interaction or public speaking. Shyness is not the same thing as being introverted. Introverts prefer solitude to society. Shy people often long to be more outgoing, but their own negative thoughts prevent them from enjoying the social interaction they desire. The consequences of severe shyness can include social isolation, loneliness, and lost personal and professional opportunities. Very shy people also have higher than average rates of other anxiety and mood disorders and of substance abuse.

Shyness is very common, with 40–50% of Americans describing themselves as shy. However, only about 7–13% of adults are so shy that their condition interferes seriously with work, school, daily life, or interpersonal relationships. Shyness is often hidden, and most shy people manage to appear reasonably outgoing, even though they suffer the physical and emotional symptoms of their anxiety. Many shy people do better in structured rather than spontaneous settings.

What causes people to be shy? Research indicates that for some the trait may be partly inherited. But for shyness, as for many health concerns, biology is not destiny. Many shy children outgrow their shyness, just as others acquire it later in life. Clearly, other factors are involved. The type of attachment between a child and his or her caregiver is important, as are parenting styles. Shyness is more common in cultures where children's failures are attributed to their own actions but successes are attributed to other people or events. People's experiences during critical developmental transitions, such as starting school and entering adolescence, have also been linked to shyness. For adults, the precipitating factor may be an event such as divorce or the loss of a job.

Recent surveys indicate that shyness rates may be rising in the United States. With the advent of technologies such as ATM machines, video games, voice mail, faxes, and e-mail, the opportunities for face-to-face interaction are diminishing. Electronic media can be a wonderful way for shy people to communicate, but they can also allow them to hide from all social interaction. In fact, one study found that greater use of the Internet was associated with a decline in participants' communication with family members, a reduction in the size of their social circles, and an increase in levels of depression and loneliness. It remains to be seen whether the first generation to have cradle-to-grave access to home computers, faxes, and the Internet will experience higher rates of shyness.

Shyness is often undiagnosed, but help is available. Shyness classes, assertiveness training groups, and public speaking clinics are available (see the Behavior Change Strategy at the end of the chapter). For the seriously shy, effective treatments include cognitive-behavioral therapy and antidepressant drugs.

If you're shy, try to remember that shyness is widespread and that there are worse fates. Some degree of shyness has an upside. Shy people tend to be gentle, supportive, kind, and sensitive; they are often exceptional listeners. People who think carefully before they speak or act are less likely to hurt the feelings of others. Shyness may also facilitate cooperation. For any group or society to functon well, a variety of roles is required, and there is a place for quieter, more reflective individuals.

SOURCES: Furmark, T. 2002. Social phobia. *Acta Psychiatrica Scandinavica* 105(2): 84–93; Carducci, B. J. 1999. *Shyness: A Bold New Approach.* New York: Perennial; Kraut, R., et al. 1998. Internet paradox: A social technology that reduces social involvement and psychological well-being? *American Psychologist* 53(9): 1017–1031.

**Generalized Anxiety Disorder** A basic reaction to future threats is to worry about them. **Generalized anxiety disorder (GAD)** is a diagnosis given to people whose worries have taken on a life of their own, pushing out other thoughts and refusing banishment by any effort of will. The topics of the worrying are ordinary concerns: Will I be able to pass the exam next Friday? Where will I get money to get my car fixed? Is my boyfriend really interested in me? Furthermore, the worrying is not completely unjustified—after all, thinking about problems can result in solving them. But the end result is a persistent feeling of nervousness, often accompanied by depression, which impairs one's ability to enjoy life and to get things done.

**Obsessive-Compulsive Disorder** The diagnosis of **obsessive-compulsive disorder (OCD)** is given to people with obsessions or compulsions or both. **Obsessions** are recurrent, unwanted thoughts or impulses. Unlike the worries of GAD, they are not ordinary concerns but improbable fears such as of suddenly committing an antisocial act or of having been contaminated by germs. **Compulsions** are repetitive, difficult-to-resist actions usually associated with obsessions. A common compulsion is hand washing, associated with an obsessive fear of contamination by dirt. Other compulsions are counting and repeatedly checking whether something has been done—for example, whether a door has been locked or a stove turned off. People with OCD feel anxious, out of control, and embarrassed. Their rituals can occupy much of their time and make them inefficient at work and difficult to live with.

**Post-Traumatic Stress Disorder** People who suffer from **post-traumatic stress disorder (PTSD)** are reacting to severely traumatic events (events that produce a sense of terror and helplessness) such as physical violence to oneself or loved ones. Trauma occurs in personal assaults (rape, military combat), natural disasters (floods, earthquakes), and tragedies like fires and airplane or car crashes. Symptoms include reexperiencing the trauma in dreams and in intrusive memories, trying to avoid anything associated with the trauma, and numbing of feelings. Sleep disturbances and other symptoms of anxiety and depression also commonly occur. Such symptoms can last months or even years.

The general rule for treating PTSD in the immediate aftermath of a traumatic event has been to allow the victim to cope with what happened and to heal by avoiding thinking about it. However, if symptoms persist for weeks or months, and if daily functioning and interpersonal relationships are disrupted, then professional help is indicated.

**Treating Anxiety Disorders** Therapies for anxiety disorders range from medication to psychological interventions concentrating on a person's thoughts and behavior.

## Mood Disorders

We all experience ups and downs in our mood in response to daily events. These temporary mood changes typically don't affect our overall emotional state or level of wellness. A person with a mood disorder, however, experiences emotional disturbances that are intense and persistent enough to affect normal functioning.

**Depression** The most common mood disorder, **depression** has forms and degrees. It usually involves demoralization and can include the following:

- A feeling of sadness and hopelessness
- Loss of pleasure in doing usual activities
- Poor appetite and weight loss
- Insomnia or disturbed sleep
- Restlessness or, alternatively, fatigue
- Thoughts of worthlessness and guilt
- Trouble concentrating or making decisions
- Thoughts of death or suicide

Not all these features are present in every depressive episode. Sometimes instead of poor appetite and insomnia, the opposite occurs—eating too much and sleeping too long. Amazingly, people can have most of the symptoms of depression without feeling sad or hopeless or in a depressed mood, although they usually do experience a loss of interest or pleasure in things.

In major depression, symptoms are often severe; a diagnosis of *dysthymic disorder* may be applied to people who experience persistent symptoms of mild or moderate depression for two years or longer. In some cases, depression is a clear-cut reaction to specific events, such as the loss of a loved one or failing in school or work, whereas in other cases no trigger event is obvious.

**RECOGNIZING THE WARNING SIGNS OF SUICIDE** One of the principal dangers of severe depression is suicide. Although a suicide attempt can occur unpredictably and unaccompanied by depression, the chances are greater if symptoms are numerous and severe. Additional warning signs of suicide include the following:

- Expressing the wish to be dead or revealing contemplated methods
- Increasing social withdrawal and isolation
- A sudden, inexplicable lightening of mood (which can mean the person has finally decided to commit suicide)

Certain risk factors increase the likelihood of suicide:

- A history of previous attempts
- A suicide by a family member or friend
- Readily available means, such as guns or pills
- A history of substance abuse or eating disorders
- Serious medical problems

In the United States, men have much higher suicide rates than women, and whites and Native Americans have higher rates than other groups; white men over age 65 have the highest suicide rate (Figure 3-2). Women attempt three times as many suicides as men, yet men succeed at more than three times the rate of women (see the box "Depression, Anxiety, and Gender" on p. 57). Worldwide, someone commits suicide every 40 seconds.

**HELPING YOURSELF OR A FRIEND** If you are severely depressed or know someone who is, expert help from a mental health professional is essential. Don't try to do it all yourself. If you suspect one of your friends is suicidally depressed, try to get him or her to see a professional.

### Terms

Vw

**generalized anxiety disorder (GAD)** An anxiety disorder characterized by excessive, uncontrollable worry about all kinds of things and anxiety in many situations.

**obsessive-compulsive disorder (OCD)** An anxiety disorder characterized by uncontrollable, recurring thoughts and the performing of senseless rituals.

**obsession** A recurrent, irrational, unwanted thought or impulse.

**compulsion** An irrational, repetitive, forced action, usually associated with an obsession.

**post-traumatic stress disorder (PTSD)** An anxiety disorder characterized by reliving traumatic events through dreams, flashbacks, and hallucinations.

**depression** A mood disorder characterized by loss of interest, sadness, hopelessness, loss of appetite, disturbed sleep, and other physical symptoms.

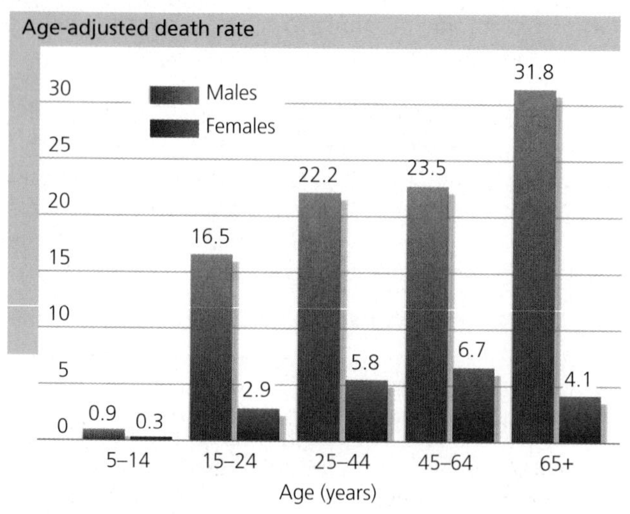


(a) Suicide rate by age and gender

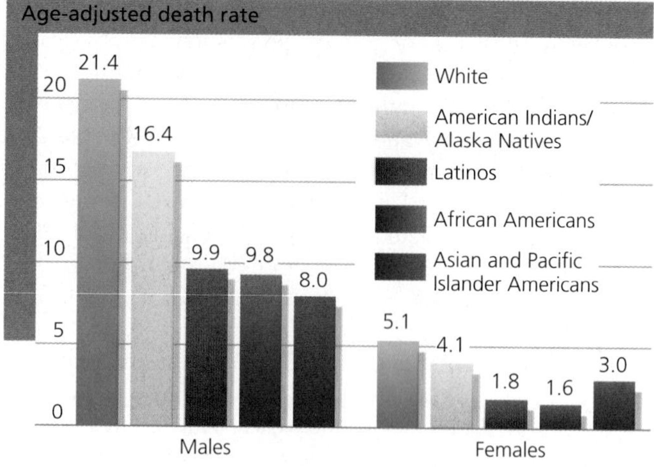


(b) Suicide rate by ethnicity and gender (all ages)

VITAL STATISTICS

**Figure 3-2 Rates of suicide in the United States by ethnicity and gender.** Rates are higher among men than women at all ages and are higher among whites compared to other groups. White men over age 65 have the highest rate of suicide. SOURCE: National Center for Health Statistics. 2004. *Health, United States, 2004.* Hyattsville, Md.: National Center for Health Statistics.

Don't be afraid to discuss the possibility of suicide with people you fear are suicidal. You won't give them an idea they haven't already thought of (see the box "Myths About Suicide" on p. 58). Asking direct questions is the best way to determine whether someone seriously intends to commit suicide. Encourage your friend to talk and to take positive steps to improve his or her situation. If you feel there is an immediate danger of suicide, ensure that the person is not left alone, especially when he or she is emotionally upset and more likely to act impulsively. If you must leave your friend alone, have your friend promise not to do anything to harm himself or herself without first calling you. Get qualified help as soon as possible.

If your friend refuses help, you might try to contact your friend's relatives and tell them that you are worried. If the depressed person is a college student, you may need to let someone in your health service or college administration know your concerns. Finally, most communities have emergency help available, often in the form of a hotline telephone counseling service run by a suicide prevention agency (check the yellow pages).

**TREATING DEPRESSION** Although treatments are highly effective, only about 35% of people who suffer from depression currently seek treatment. Treatment for depression depends on its severity and on whether the depressed person is suicidal. The best initial treatment for moderate to severe depression is a combination of drug therapy and psychotherapy. Combining drug therapy with psychotherapy may be particularly important for people whose condition is linked to psychosocial factors, including high levels of stress, a history of abuse, or relationship problems.

Antidepressants work by affecting the activity of key neurotransmitters in the brain, including serotonin. The view of depression as based in brain chemistry and treatable with medication has been important in lessening the stigma attached to the condition, leading more people to seek treatment. Antidepressants are now among the most widely prescribed drugs in the United States (Table 3-2). All prescription antidepressants have received approval from the U.S. Food and Drug Administration as being safe and more effective than a placebo. However, as with all pharmacological therapies, these drugs may cause side effects, and wide use of antidepressants has raised many questions (see the box "Antidepressant Use in Young People" on p. 59).

Antidepressants may take several weeks to begin working; therefore, if suicidal impulses are strong, hospitalization for a week or so may be necessary. **Electroconvulsive therapy (ECT)** is effective for severe depression when other approaches have failed.

The popular over-the-counter herb St. John's wort may also affect serotonin levels, but because it is a dietary supplement it is not subject to the same type of testing and regulation as prescription medications (see the box "Alternative Remedies for Depression" on p. 60 for more information). Anyone who may be suffering from depression should seek a medical evaluation rather than self-treating with supplements.

One type of depression is treated in a unique way—by having sufferers sit with eyes open in front of a bright light source for an hour or so early every morning. These patients have **seasonal affective disorder (SAD),** in which depression worsens during winter months as the number

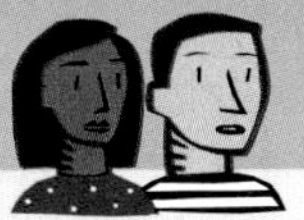

Gender Matters

## Depression, Anxiety, and Gender

### Anxiety Disorders

Panic disorder is more than twice as common in women as in men, whereas obsessive-compulsive disorder occurs in men and women at about the same rate. In population surveys, social anxiety disorder is more common in women than in men, but men are more likely to seek treatment for it—perhaps because men are more likely to find it a barrier to success in white-collar jobs. In some surveys, PTSD is more common in women, but the incidence of PTSD depends on the incidence of traumatic events, which varies in different environments. Men are more often exposed to military combat, and women to rape. Trauma from motor vehicles crashes is a fairly common cause of PTSD in both sexes.

### Depression and Suicide

Over their lifetimes, about 20% of women and 12% of men have serious depression. When women are depressed, they are more likely than men to experience guilt, anxiety, increased appetite and weight gain, and increased sleep. When women take antidepressants, they may need a lower dose than men; at the same dosage, blood levels of medication tend to be higher in women. An issue for women who may become pregnant is whether antidepressants can harm a fetus or newborn. The best evidence indicates that the most frequently prescribed types of antidepressants do not cause birth defects, although some studies have reported withdrawal symptoms in some newborns whose mothers used certain antidepressants.

Although suicidal behavior is strongly associated with depression, and depression is more prevalent in women, in the United States, many more men than women commit suicide. Until age 9, boys and girls have the same suicide rates; from 10 to 14 the boys' rate is twice as high; from 15 to 19, four times as high; and from 20 to 24, six times as high. Overall, about three times as many women as men attempt suicide, but women's attempts are less likely to be lethal. In the United States, 60% of male suicides involve firearms.

### Factors Underlying Gender Differences

Why women have more problems with anxiety and depression than men is a matter of debate. Some experts think much of the difference is due to reporting bias: Women are more willing to admit to experiencing negative emotions, being stressed, or having difficulty coping. Women may also be more likely to seek treatment at a given level of symptoms.

Other experts point to biologically based sex differences, particularly in the level and action of hormones. Greater anxiety and depression in women compared with men is most pronounced between puberty and menopause, when female hormones are most active. However, this period of life is also the time in which women's social roles and expectations may be the most different from those of men. Women may put more emphasis on relationships in determining self-esteem, so the deterioration of a relationship is a cause of depression that can hit women harder than men. In addition, culturally determined gender roles are more likely to place women in situations where they have less control over key life decisions, and lack of autonomy is associated with depression.

The higher suicide rate among young men may relate to gender norms and expectations that men assert independence and physical prowess—sometimes expressed in risky, dangerous, and potentially self-destructive behavior. Such behavior, often involving drugs and alcohol and resulting in motor vehicle crashes, occurs more often in young people who later commit suicide. Even when suicidal intention is never expressed, suicidal impulses are often suspected of contributing to sudden deaths in this age group.

SOURCES: Sanz, E. J., et al. 2005. Selective serotonin reuptake inhibitors in pregnant women and neonatal withdrawal syndrome. *Lancet* 365(9458): 482–487. Kessler, R. C. 2003. Epidemiology of women and depression. *Journal of Affective Disorders* 74: 5–13; World Health Organization. 2002. *Gender and Mental Health.* Geneva: World Health Organization; Pigott, T. A. 1999. Gender differences in the epidemiology and treatment of anxiety disorders. *Journal of Clinical Psychiatry* 60 (Suppl. 18): 4–15; Langhin-richsen-Rohling, J., et al. 1998. Gender differences in the suicide-related behaviors of adolescents and young adults. *Sex Roles: A Journal of Research* 39(11–12): 839–854.

of hours of daylight diminishes and then improves with the lengthening of daylight in the spring and summer. Seasonal depression is more common among people who live at higher latitudes, where there are fewer hours of light in winter. Light therapy may work by extending the perceived length of the day and thus convincing the brain that it is summertime even during the winter months.

**Mania and Bipolar Disorder** People who experience **mania,** a less common feature of mood disorders, are restless, have a lot of energy, need little sleep, and often talk nonstop. They may devote themselves to fantastic projects and spend more money than they can afford. Many manic people swing between manic and depressive states, a syndrome called **bipolar disorder** because of the two opposite poles of mood. Tranquilizers are used to treat individual manic episodes, while special drugs such as the salt lithium carbonate taken daily can prevent future mood swings.

### Terms

VW

**electroconvulsive therapy (ECT)** The use of electric shock to induce brief, generalized seizures; used in the treatment of selected psychological disorders.

**seasonal affective disorder (SAD)** A mood disorder characterized by seasonal depression, usually occurring in winter, when there is less daylight.

**mania** A mood disorder characterized by excessive elation, irritability, talkativeness, inflated self-esteem, and expansiveness.

**bipolar disorder** A mental illness characterized by alternating periods of depression and mania.

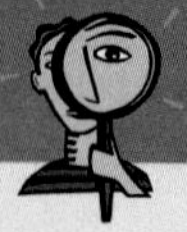

In Focus

## Myths About Suicide

***Myth*** People who really intend to kill themselves do not let anyone know about it.
***Fact*** This belief can be an excuse for doing nothing when someone says he or she might commit suicide. In fact, most people who eventually commit suicide *have* talked about doing it.

***Myth*** People who made a suicide attempt but survived did not really intend to die.
***Fact*** This may be true for certain people, but people who seriously want to end their life may fail because they misjudge what it takes. Even a pharmacist may misjudge the lethal dose of a drug.

***Myth*** People who succeed in suicide really wanted to die.
***Fact*** We cannot be sure of that either. Some people are only trying to make a dramatic gesture or plea for help but miscalculate.

***Myth*** People who really want to kill themselves will do it regardless of any attempts to prevent them.
***Fact*** Few people are single-minded about suicide even at the moment of attempting it. People who are quite determined to take their life today may change their mind completely tomorrow.

***Myth*** Suicide is proof of mental illness.
***Fact*** Many suicides are committed by people who do not meet ordinary criteria for mental illness, although people with depression, schizophrenia, and other psychological disorders have a much higher than average suicide rate.

***Myth*** People inherit suicidal tendencies.
***Fact*** Certain kinds of depression that lead to suicide do have a genetic component. But many examples of suicide running in a family can be explained by factors such as psychologically identifying with a family member who committed suicide, often a parent.

***Myth*** All suicides are irrational.
***Fact*** By some standards all suicides may seem "irrational." But many people find it at least understandable that someone might want to commit suicide, for example, when approaching the end of a terminal illness or when facing a long prison term.

## Schizophrenia

**Schizophrenia** can be severe and debilitating or quite mild and hardly noticeable. Although people are capable of diagnosing their own depression, they usually don't diagnose their own schizophrenia, because they often can't see that anything is wrong. This disorder is not rare; in fact, 1 in every 100 people has a schizophrenic episode sometime in his or her lifetime, most commonly

**Table 3-2 Selected Categories and Examples of Drugs Used in the Treatment of Psychological Disorders**

| Antidepressants (used to treat depression, panic disorder, anxiety) | Mood Stabilizers (used to treat bipolar disorder, types of schizophrenia) | Anxiolytics and hypnotics (used to treat anxiety, insomnia) | Antipsychotics (used to treat schizophrenia, mania) |
|---|---|---|---|
| Selective serotonin reuptake inhibitors (SSRIs)<br>Prozac (fluoxetine)<br>Paxil (paroxetine)<br>Zoloft (sertraline)<br>Luvox (fluvoxamine)<br>Celexa (citalopram)<br>Lexapro (escitalopram)<br>Tricyclics<br>Aventyl (nortriptyline)<br>Elavil (amitriptyline)<br>Monomine oxidase inhibitor (MOI)<br>Nardil (phenelzine)<br>Others<br>Effexor (venlafaxine)<br>Welbutrin (buproprion)<br>Serzone (nefazodone),<br>Remeron (mirtazapine). | Lithium carbonate<br>Depakote (valproic acid)<br>Tegretol (carbamazepine)<br>Lamictil (lamotrigine) | Benzodiazepines<br>Valium (diazepam)<br>Librium (chlordiazepoxide)<br>Xanax (alprazolam)<br>Ativan (lorazepam)<br>Dalmane (flurazepam)<br>Restoril (temazepam)<br>Others<br>Sonata (zaleplon)<br>Ambien (zolpidem) | Older type<br>Haldol (haloperidol)<br>Prolixin (fluphenazine)<br>Newer type<br>Clozaril (clozapine)<br>Zyprexa (olanzapine)<br>Risperdal (risperidone)<br>Seroquel (quetiapine)<br>Geodon (ziprasodone) |

In the News

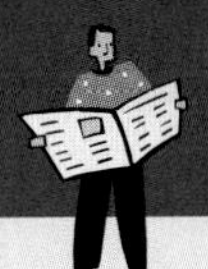

## Antidepressant Use in Young People

WW

In 2004, an FDA advisory committee voted in favor of recommending a warning label for antidepressants on the basis of evidence that their use increases the risk of suicidal thinking and behavior in children and adolescents. The committee based its conclusions on published and unpublished data from trials sponsored by pharmaceutical companies. Controversy immediately followed: Parents wondered why it had taken so long to come to this conclusion, because most of the data had been around for years. Had drug companies ignored indications that their best-selling drugs were not safe? Had physicians deceived themselves and patients' families into thinking that drug treatments worked better than they really did?

### Effectiveness

Drug treatment for depression is considered part of a success story in which people take seriously symptoms of depression and hints of suicidal thinking in children and teens. Over the last decade, the suicide rate among adolescents has fallen. Many factors have likely contributed to the decline, including stricter gun laws that make it harder for young people to gain access to guns. Drug treatment has also been considered a key factor in the decline in suicide rates.

To date, only one drug—fluoxetine (Prozac)—has been approved for use specifically in children and teens. Studies have found that fluoxetine causes a greater improvement than a placebo, but the combination of drug therapy and cognitive-behavioral therapy is more beneficial than either treatment alone. The placebo effect, in which people improve while taking pills containing inactive compounds, is significant in studies of depression and can exceed 30%—meaning a third of people receiving a placebo experience an improvement in their symptoms.

Many antidepressants other than fluoxetine, especially other SSRIs, are also prescribed to young people, but these other drugs haven't been shown to be effective for that age group. Unpublished research data indicates that some SSRIs are *not* effective in children and teens or are only slightly more effective than a placebo. These findings underscore the need for the publication of all research findings—not just positive ones—so that physicians and patients can make informed decisions.

### Safety

All medications have potential risks and side effects. The problem associated with SSRIs that caused the FDA to act is the possibility that they increase the risk of suicide in some young people, particularly in the period immediately following the start of medication use. When study results were pooled, researchers found that in the short term, about 2–3% of users have an increased risk of suicidal thoughts and actions beyond the risk inherent from depression itself.

Researchers aren't exactly sure what causes this effect. Antidepressants are not immediately effective, and one theory is that SSRIs reverse the lethargy associated with depression more quickly than they relieve the depression itself, giving users the energy to contemplate suicide in the interim. It is thought that antidepressants work differently on the developing brains of young people than on the brains of adults, so there may be as yet unidentified effects.

In October 2004, the FDA published a guide to using antidepressants in children and teens. It emphasizes that young people who take antidepressants should be monitored closely, especially when starting a new medication or changing the dosage of a drug. Depression is a serious illness that can increase the risk of suicide, and mental health professionals and patients must balance the risks of doing nothing against the potential risks and benefits of different treatments.

SOURCES: Food and Drug Administration. 2004. *FDA Proposed Medication Guide: About Using Antidepressants in Children or Teenagers* (http://www.fda.gov/cder/drug/antidepressants/SSRIMedicationGuide.htm; retrieved November 5, 2004); Newman, T. B. 2004. Treating depression in children: A black-box warning for antidressants in children? *New England Journal of Medicine* 351(16): 1595–1598; Brent, D. A. 2004. Treating depression in children: Antidepressants and pediatric depression—the risk of doing nothing. *New England Journal of Medicine* 351(16): 1598–1601; Treatment for Adolescents with Depression Study (TADS) Team. 2004. Fluoxetine, cognitive-behavioral therapy, and their combination for adolescents with depression. *Journal of the American Medical Association* 292(7): 807–820.

starting in adolescence. Some general characteristics of schizophrenia include the following:

- *Disorganized thoughts.* Thoughts may be expressed in a vague or confusing way.
- *Inappropriate emotions.* Emotions may be either absent or strong but inappropriate.
- *Delusions.* People with delusions—firmly held false beliefs—may think that their minds are controlled by outside forces, that people can read their minds, that they are great personages like Jesus Christ or the president of the United States, or that they are being persecuted by a group such as the CIA.
- *Auditory hallucinations.* Schizophrenic people may hear voices when no one is present.
- *Deteriorating social and work functioning.* Social withdrawal and increasingly poor performance at school or work may be so gradual that they are hardly noticed at first.

A schizophrenic person needs help from a mental health professional. Suicide is a risk in schizophrenia, and expert treatment can reduce that risk and minimize the social consequences of the illness by shortening the

**Term**

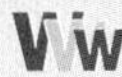

**schizophrenia** A psychological disorder that involves a disturbance in thinking and in perceiving reality.

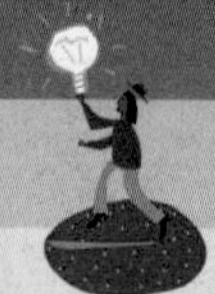

Critical Consumer

## Alternative Remedies for Depression

Mainstream therapies for depression include medications accepted as safe and effective by government regulatory agencies, certain psychotherapies, and light therapy in the case of seasonal affective disorder. Yet, in surveys, 20% of people in the United States who suffer from depression report using unconventional therapies such as acupuncture, body movement therapy, homeopathy, qigong, faith healing, or herbs or other "natural" substances. With the exception of one herb, St. John's wort *(Hypericum perforatum)*, these therapies have not been shown to be effective in double-blind placebo-controlled trials. Such trials are the only scientific way to show that a treatment has healing power beyond that of a **placebo.**

St. John's wort, a flowering plant that grows as a weed in the United States, has been reputed to have curative properties since the time of Hippocrates in ancient Greece. Modern pharmacological studies confirm that its active ingredients produce a number of biochemical and physiological changes in animals, although it's still unclear exactly how these changes might affect depression. Data from a number of studies suggest that St. John's wort could benefit people with mild to moderate depression. But concerns have been raised about the adequacy of those trials, and consumers are left without a definitive answer on the effectiveness of St. John's wort.

An advantage of St. John's wort is that it causes fewer adverse effects than conventional antidepressants. In data from three studies including about 600 depressed patients, the herb produced no more adverse effects than did the placebo. There was no evidence of sedation, gastrointestinal disturbances, or other side effects associated with other antidepressants. However, the safety of St. John's wort in pregnancy has not been established, and it may interact with, and reduce the effectiveness of, certain medications, including oral contraceptives and some medications for treating heart disease, depression, HIV infections, and seizures.

One reason for the popularity of an herb for depression is that it doesn't require a prescription or any kind of contact with a physician or a therapist; for those who are not members of a generous health care plan, an herbal remedy may also be less expensive than a prescription antidepressant. On the other hand, people suffering from depression *should* seek professional advice and not try to get along entirely with self-diagnosis and self-help. If you are depressed enough to contemplate taking St. John's wort, you need to make an appointment to talk to a professional about your depression.

Bear in mind that St. John's wort does not work for everyone, and no expert advocates it for severe depression. Also, because herbal products are classified as dietary supplements, they are not scrutinized by the regulatory agencies that oversee prescription drugs. Thus, consumers have no guarantee that the product contains the herbs and dosages listed on the label (see Chapters 9 and 16 for more on dietary supplements).

SOURCES: Trautmann-Sponsel, R. D., and A. Dienel. 2004. Safety of Hypericum extract in mildly to moderately depressed outpatients: A review based on data from three randomized, placebo-controlled trials. *Journal of Affective Disorders* 82(2): 303–307; Lecrubier, Y., et al. 2002. Efficacy of St. John's wort extract WS 5570 in major depression: A double-blind, placebo-controlled trial. *American Journal of Psychiatry* 159: 1361–1366; Hypericum Depression Trial Study Group. 2002. Effect of *Hypericum perforatum* (St. John's wort) in major depressive disorder: A randomized controlled trial. *Journal of the American Medical Association* 287: 1807–1814; Shelton, R. C., et al. 2001. Effectiveness of St. John's Wort in major depression. *Journal of the American Medical Association* 285 (15): 1978–1986.

period when symptoms are active. The key element in treatment is regular medication.

## GETTING HELP

Knowing when self-help or professional help is required for mental health problems is usually not as difficult as knowing how to start or which professional to choose.

### Self-Help

If you have a personal problem to solve, a smart way to begin is by finding out what you can do on your own. Some problems are specifically addressed in this book. Behavioral and some cognitive approaches involve becoming more aware of self-defeating actions and ideas and combating them in some way: by being more assertive; by communicating honestly; by raising your self-esteem by counteracting thoughts, people, and actions that undermine it; and by confronting, rather than avoiding, the things you fear. Get more information by seeing what books are available in the psychology or self-help sections of libraries and bookstores. But be selective. Watch out for self-help books making fantastic claims that deviate from mainstream approaches.

Some people find it helpful to express their feelings in a journal. Grappling with a painful experience in this way provides an emotional release and can help you develop more constructive ways of dealing with similar situations in the future. Using a journal this way can improve physical as well as emotional wellness.

For some people, religious belief and practice may promote psychological health. Religious organizations provide a social network and a supportive community, and religious practices, such as prayer and meditation, offer a path for personal change and transformation.

### Peer Counseling and Support Groups

Sharing your concerns with others is another helpful way of dealing with psychological health challenges.

Just being able to share what's troubling you with an accepting, empathetic person can bring relief. Comparing notes with people who have problems similar to yours can give you new ideas about coping. Many colleges offer peer counseling through a health center or through the psychology or education department. Peer counseling is usually done by volunteer students who have received special training that emphasizes confidentiality. Peer counselors may steer you toward an appropriate campus or community resource or simply offer a sympathetic ear.

Many self-help groups work on the principle of bringing together people with similar problems to share their experiences and support one another. Support groups are typically organized around a specific problem, such as eating disorders or substance abuse. Self-help groups may be listed in the phone book or the campus newspaper.

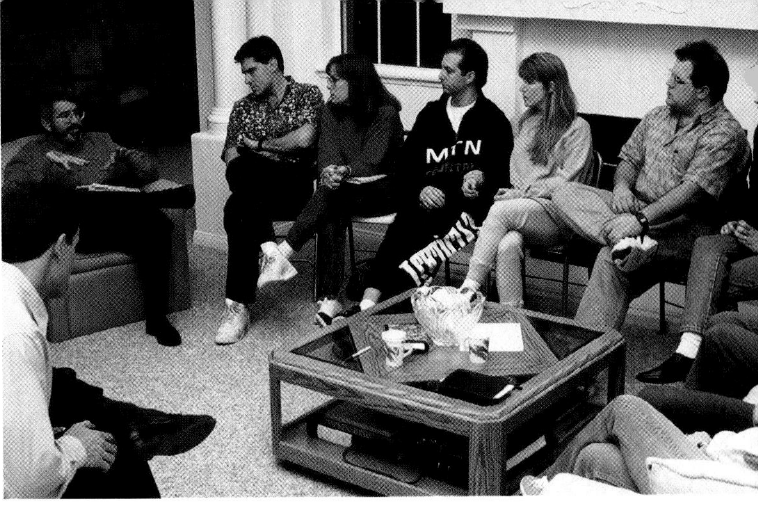

Group therapy is just one of many different approaches to psychological counseling. If you have concerns you would like to discuss with a mental health professional, shop around to find the approach that works for you.

## Professional Help

Sometimes self-help or talking to nonprofessionals is not enough. More objective, more expert, or more discreet help is needed. Many people have trouble accepting the need for professional help, and often those who most need help are the most unwilling to get it. You may someday find yourself having to overcome your own reluctance, or that of a friend, about seeking help.

### Determining the Need for Professional Help

In some cases, professional help is optional. Some people are interested in improving their psychological health in a general way by going into individual or group therapy to learn more about themselves and how to interact with others. Interpersonal friction among family members or between partners often falls in the middle between necessary and optional. Successful help with such problems can mean the difference between a painful divorce and a satisfying relationship.

It's sometimes difficult to determine whether someone needs professional help, but it is important to be aware of behaviors that may indicate a serious problem:

- If depression, anxiety, or other emotional problems begin to interfere seriously with school or work performance or in getting along with others
- If suicide is attempted or is seriously considered (refer to the warning signs earlier in the chapter)
- If symptoms such as hallucinations, delusions, incoherent speech, or loss of memory occur
- If alcohol or drugs are used to the extent that they impair normal functioning during much of the week, if finding or taking drugs occupies much of the week, or if reducing their dosage leads to psychological or physiological withdrawal symptoms

**Choosing a Mental Health Professional** Mental health workers belong to several different professions and have different roles. Psychiatrists are medical doctors. They are experts in deciding whether a medical disease lies behind psychological symptoms, and they are usually involved in treatment if medication or hospitalization is required. Clinical psychologists typically hold a Ph.D. degree; they are often experts in behavioral and cognitive therapies. Other mental health workers include social workers, licensed counselors, and clergy with special training in pastoral counseling. In hospitals and clinics, various mental health professionals may join together in treatment teams. For more on finding appropriate help, see the box "Choosing and Evaluating Mental Health Professionals."

**Types of Psychotherapy** There are a variety of psychotherapy approaches:

- *Behavioral therapy* focuses on current behavior patterns. The goal is to help people replace unhealthy, dysfunctional behaviors with more positive behaviors. Shaping one's environment is a key part of therapy. This approach is often used to treat phobias and other anxiety disorders. For example, a person might be exposed to a feared object or situation in gradual stages.
- *Cognitive therapy* emphasizes the effect of ideas on behavior and feeling. People in cognitive therapy are taught to notice their unrealistic thoughts and to substitute more realistic ones. Cognitive and behavioral therapies are

**Term**

**placebo** A chemically inactive substance that a patient believes is an effective medical therapy for his or her condition. To help evaluate a therapy, medical researchers compare the effects of a particular therapy with the effects of a placebo. The "placebo effect" occurs when a patient responds to a placebo as if it were an active drug.

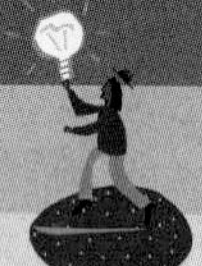

Critical Consumer

## Choosing and Evaluating Mental Health Professionals

V W

College students are usually in a good position to find convenient, affordable mental health care. Larger schools typically have both health services that employ psychiatrists and psychologists and counseling centers staffed by professionals and student peer counselors. Resources in the community may include a school of medicine, a hospital, and a variety of professionals who work independently. It's a good idea to get recommendations from physicians, clergy, friends who have been in therapy, or community agencies rather than pick a name at random.

Financial considerations are also important. Find out how much different services will cost and what your health insurance will cover. If you're not adequately covered by a health plan, don't let that stop you from getting help; investigate low-cost alternatives on campus and in your community. The cost of treatment is linked to how many therapy sessions will be needed, which in turn depends on the type of therapy and the nature of the problem. Psychological therapies focusing on specific problems may require eight or ten sessions at weekly intervals. Therapies aiming for psychological awareness and personality change can last months or years.

Deciding whether a therapist is right for you will require meeting the therapist in person. Before or during your first meeting, find out about the therapist's background and training:

- Does she or he have a degree from an appropriate professional school and a state license to practice?
- Has she or he had experience treating people with problems similar to yours?
- How much will therapy cost?

You have a right to know the answers to these questions and should not hesitate to ask them. After your initial meeting, evaluate your impressions:

- Does the therapist seem like a warm, intelligent person who would be able to help you and interested in doing so?
- Are you comfortable with the personality, values, and beliefs of the therapist?
- Is he or she willing to talk about the techniques in use? Do these techniques make sense to you?

If you answer yes to these questions, this therapist may be satisfactory for you. If you feel uncomfortable—and you're not in need of emergency care—it's worthwhile to set up one-time consultations with one or two others before you make up your mind. Take the time to find someone who feels right for you.

Later in your treatment, evaluate your progress:

- Are you being helped by the treatment?
- If you are displeased, is it because you aren't making progress, or because therapy is raising difficult, painful issues you don't want to deal with?
- Can you express dissatisfaction to your therapist? Such feedback can improve your treatment.

If you're convinced your therapy isn't working or is harmful, thank your therapist for her or his efforts, and find another.

frequently combined. For example, treatment for social anxiety might include gradual exposure to a feared situation like a party along with practice in identifying and changing unrealistic negative self-talk.

- *Psychodynamic and interpersonal therapies* emphasize the role of the past and of unconscious thoughts in shaping present behavior. Uncovering feelings and building self-awareness are common therapy goals. Interpersonal therapy focuses specifically on the improving current relationship skills.
- *Humanistic therapy* focuses on immediate feelings and the potential for future growth. Like psychodynamic therapy, there is a focus on the self and the search for self-awareness. The goal is often personal growth rather than overcoming a specific psychological disorder, and the therapist acts as a guide to self-exploration.

Although these types of therapies may be described as distinctive orientations, most therapists offer a variety of approaches. Combining several approaches or combining psychotherapy with drug treatment is very common in the treatment of psychological disorders.

### Tips for Today

Life inevitably brings change and challenge—they are a part of growth and development. Most of life's psychological challenges can be met with self-help and everyday skills—introspection and insight, honest communication, support from family and friends. Sometimes a psychological problem poses a greater challenge than we can handle on our own; for these situations, professional help is available.

*Right now you can*

- Consider the areas in your life where you can be creative (one of the qualities associated with self-actualization), whether in music, art, Web page design, party planning, or whatever you truly enjoy. With the knowledge that allowing your creative side to flourish is a valuable use of your time, plan a way to spend an hour or more on this activity this week.
- Sit down and write 100 positive adjectives that describe you (friendly, loyal, athletic, smart, musical, sensitive, and so on). If you can't think of 100 right now, write as many as you can and keep thinking about it over the next day or two until you reach 100.

- Take a serious look at how you've been feeling the past few weeks. If you have any feelings that are especially difficult to deal with, begin to think about how you can get help with them. Consider consulting the self-help section at the bookstore, talking to a trustworthy friend or peer counselor, or making an appointment with a staff person at the campus counseling center.

## SUMMARY

- Psychological health encompasses more than a single particular state of normality. Psychological diversity is valuable among groups of people.
- Defining psychological health as the presence of wellness means that to be healthy you must strive to fulfill your potential.
- Self-actualized people have high self-esteem and are realistic, inner-directed, authentic, capable of emotional intimacy, and creative.
- Crucial parts of psychological wellness include developing an adult identity, establishing intimate relationships, developing values and purpose in life, and achieving healthy self-esteem.
- A pessimistic outlook can be damaging; it can be overcome by developing more realistic self-talk.
- Honest communication requires recognizing what needs to be said and saying it clearly.
- People may be lonely if they haven't developed ways to be happy on their own or if they interpret being alone as a sign of rejection. Lonely people can take action to expand their social contacts.
- Dealing successfully with anger involves distinguishing between a reasonable level of assertiveness and gratuitous expressions of anger, heading off rage, and responding to the anger of others.
- People with psychological disorders have symptoms severe enough to interfere with daily living.
- Anxiety is a fear that is not directed toward any definite threat. Anxiety disorders include simple phobias, social phobias, panic disorder, generalized anxiety disorder,

Behavior Change Strategy

### Dealing with Social Anxiety

Shyness is often the result of both high anxiety levels and lack of key social skills. To help overcome shyness, you need to learn to manage your fear of social situations and to develop social skills such as appropriate eye contact, initiating topics in conversations, and maintaining the flow of conversations. To reduce your anxiety in social situations, try some of the following strategies:

- Refocus your attention away from the stress reaction you're experiencing and toward the social task at hand. Your nervousness is much less visible than you think.
- Allow a warm-up period for new situations. Realize that you will feel more nervous at first, and take steps to relax and become more comfortable. Refer to the suggestions for deep breathing and other relaxation techniques in Chapter 2.
- If possible, take breaks during anxiety-producing situations. For example, if you're at a party, take a moment to visit the restroom or step outside. Alternate between speaking with good friends and striking up conversations with new acquaintances.
- Practice realistic self-talk. Replace your self-critical thoughts with more supportive ones: "No one else is perfect, and I don't have to be either." "It would have been good if I had a funny story to tell, but the conversation was interesting anyway."

Starting and maintaining conversations can be difficult for shy people, who may feel overwhelmed by their physical stress reaction. If small talk is a problem for you, try the following strategies:

- Introduce yourself early in the conversation. If you tend to forget names, repeat your new acquaintance's name to help fix it in your mind ("Nice to meet you, Amelia").
- Ask questions, and look for shared topics of interest. Simple, open-ended questions like "How's your presentation coming along?" or "How do you know our host?" encourage others to carry the conversation for a while and help bring forth a variety of subjects.
- Take turns talking, and elaborate on your answers. Simple yes and no answers don't move the conversation along. Try to relate something in your life—a course you're taking or a hobby you have—to something in the other person's life. Match self-disclosure with self-disclosure.
- Have something to say. Expand your mind and become knowledgeable about current events and local or campus news. If you have specialized knowledge about a topic, practice discussing it in ways that both beginners and experts can understand and appreciate.
- If you get stuck for something to say, try giving a compliment ("Great presentation!" or "I love your earrings.") or performing a social grace (pass the chips or get someone a drink).
- Be an active listener. Reward the other person with your full attention and with regular responses. Make frequent eye contact and maintain a relaxed but alert posture.

At first, your new behaviors will likely make you anxious. Don't give up—things *will* get easier. Create lots of opportunities to practice your new behaviors. Eventually, you'll be able to sustain social interactions with comfort and enjoyment. If you find that social anxiety is a major problem for you and self-help techniques don't seem to work, consider looking into a shyness clinic or treatment program on your campus.

SOURCES: Carducci, B. J. 1999. *Shyness: A Bold New Approach*. New York: Perennial; University of Texas at Dallas, Student Counseling Center, 2000. *Overcoming Social Anxiety* (http://www.utdallas.edu/student/slife/counseling/anxiety.html; retrieved August 31, 2000).

obsessive-compulsive disorder, and post-traumatic stress disorder.

- Depression is a common mood disorder; loss of interest or pleasure in things seems to be its most universal symptom. Severe depression carries a high risk of suicide, and suicidally depressed people need professional help.
- Symptoms of mania include exalted moods with unrealistically high self-esteem, little need for sleep, and rapid speech. Mood swings between mania and depression characterize bipolar disorder.
- Schizophrenia is characterized by disorganized thoughts, inappropriate emotions, delusions, auditory hallucinations, and deteriorating social and work performance.
- Help is available in a variety of forms, including self-help, peer counseling, support groups, and therapy with a mental health professional. For serious problems, professional help may be the most appropriate.

## Take Action

1. **Become a peer counselor.** Many colleges and communities have peer counseling programs, hotline services (for both general problems and specific issues such as rape, suicide, and drug abuse), and other kinds of emergency counseling services. Some programs are staffed by trained volunteers. Investigate such programs in your school (through the health clinic or student services) or community (look in the yellow pages), and consider volunteering for one of them. The training and experience can help you understand both yourself and others.

2. **Consider assertiveness training.** Being assertive rather than passive or aggressive is a valuable skill that everyone can learn. To improve your ability to assert yourself appropriately, sign up for a workshop or class in assertiveness training on your campus or in your community.

3. **Support your spiritual side.** Turn off your phone, remove your watch, and spend some quiet time alone with your thoughts and feelings. Engage in an activity that contributes to your sense of spiritual well-being. Examples might include spending time in nature; experiencing art, architecture, or music; expressing your creativity; or engaging in a personal spiritual practice such as prayer, meditation, or yoga.

## For More Information

### Books


Antony, M. M. 2004. *10 Simple Solutions to Shyness: How to Overcome Shyness, Social Anxiety & Fear of Public Speaking.* Oakland, Calif.: New Harbinger. *Practical suggestions for fears of interacting with people you don't know.*

Bourne, E. J., and L. Garano. 2003. *Coping with Anxiety: Simple Ways to Relieve Anxiety, Fear, and Worry.* Oakland, Calif.: New Harbinger. *Provides concrete suggestions for dealing with anxieties.*

Flach, F. 2003. *Resilience: The Power to Bounce Back When the Going Gets Tough.* Rev. ed. Long Island City, N.Y.: Hatherleigh Press. *Provides practical suggestions for personal growth in the face of stress and change.*

Klein, D. F., and P. H. Wender. 2005. *Understanding Depression.* 2nd ed. New York: Oxford University Press. *Includes information on symptoms, diagnosis, and a variety of treatments.*

Miklowitz, D. J. 2002. *The Bipolar Disorder Survival Guide: What You and Your Family Need to Know.* New York: Guilford Press. *Covers the origins, symptoms, and treatments for bipolar (or manic-depressive) disorder.*

Nasar, S. 2001. *A Beautiful Mind: The Life of Mathematical Genius and Nobel Laureate John Nash.* Carmichael, Calif.: Touchstone Books. *The story of how schizophrenia affected the life of a renowned mathematician.*

Rubin-Deutsch, J. 2003. *Why Can't I Ever Be Good Enough? Escaping the Limits of Your Childhood Roles.* Oakland, Calif.: New Harbinger. *Presents strategies for transforming unhealthy patterns of thought and interaction from childhood into more healthy adult roles.*


### WW Organizations, Hotlines, and Web Sites

*American Association of Suicidology.* Provides information about suicide and resources for people in crisis.
http://www.suicidology.org

*American Psychiatric Association (APA).* Provides public information by pamphlet or online about a variety of topics, including depression, anxiety, eating disorders, and psychiatric medications.
888-357-7924; 703-907-7300
http://www.psych.org

*American Psychological Association Consumer HelpCenter.* Provides information about common challenges to psychological health and about how to obtain professional help.
800-964-2000
http://helping.apa.org

*Anxiety Disorders Association of America (ADAA).* Provides information and resources related to anxiety disorders, including listings of support groups.
http://www.adaa.org

*Depression and Bipolar Support Alliance (DBSA).* Provides educational materials and information about support groups and other resources.
800-826-3632
http://www.dbsalliance.org

*Internet Mental Health.* An encyclopedia of mental health information, including medical diagnostic criteria.
http://www.mentalhealth.com

*NAMI (National Alliance for the Mentally Ill).* Provides information and support for people who are affected by mental illness.
800-950-NAMI (Help Line)
http://www.nami.org

*National Hopeline Network.* 24-hour hotline for people who are thinking about suicide or know someone who is; calls are routed to local crisis centers.
800-SUICIDE

*National Institute of Mental Health (NIMH).* Provides helpful information about anxiety, depression, eating disorders, and other challenges to psychological health.

866-615-6464; 301-443-4513
http://www.nimh.nih.gov

*National Mental Health Association.* Provides consumer information on a variety of issues, including how to find help.
800-969-NMHA
http://www.nmha.org

*National Mental Health Information Center.* A one-stop source for information and resources relating to mental health.
800-789-2647
http://www.mentalhealth.org

*Psych Central: Dr. John Grohol's Mental Health Page.* A guide to psychology, support, and mental health issues, resources, and people on the Internet.
http://psychcentral.com

*Student Counseling Virtual Pamphlet Collection.* Provides links to more than 400 pamphlets produced by different student counseling centers; topics range from depression and anxiety to time management and assertiveness.
http://counseling.uchicago.edu/vpc

*Surgeon General: Reports.* Provides the text of reports from the U.S. Surgeon General, including the 1999 report on mental health and the 2001 supplement to the report that focuses on culture and ethnicity.
http://www.surgeongeneral.gov/library/reports.htm

*World Health Organization: 2001 World Health Report.* Focuses on mental health and documents that mental health problems are a major cause of disability in both developed and developing countries; provides suggestions about what can be done about this.
http://www.who.int/whr/2001/en

The following sites include interactive online assessments for various psychological problems:

*Depression-screening.org:* http://www.depression-screening.org
*Freedom from Fear:* http://www.freedomfromfear.com

## Selected Bibliography


American Psychiatric Association. 2000. *Diagnostic and Statistical Manual of Mental Disorders*, 4th ed., Text Revision (*DSM-IV-TR*). Washington, D.C.: American Psychiatric Association Press.

Benton, S. A., et al. 2003. Changes in counseling center client problems across 13 years. *Professional Psychology: Research and Practice* 34(1): 66–72.

Biederman, J., et al. 2001. Further evidence of association between behavioral inhibition and social anxiety in children. *American Journal of Psychiatry* 158(10): 1673–1679.

Brenes, G. A., et al. 2002. Do optimism and pessimism predict physical functioning? *Journal of Behavioral Medicine* 25(3): 219–231.

Cutler, J. L., et al. 2004. Comparing cognitive behavior therapy, interpersonal psychotherapy, and psychodynamic psychotherapy. *American Journal of Psychiatry* 161(9): 1567–1573.

Danner, D. D., D. A. Snowdon, and W. W. Friesen. 2001. Positive emotions in early life and longevity: Findings from the nun study. *Journal of Personality and Social Psychology* 80(5): 804–813.

Dervic, K., et al. 2004. Religious affiliation and suicide attempt. *American Journal of Psychiatry* 161(12): 2303–2308.

Food and Drug Administration. 2005. Safeguards for children taking antidepressants strengthened, *FDA Consumer*, January/February.

Gunnell, D., P. K. Magnusson, and F. Rasmussen. 2005. Low intelligence test scores in 18-year-old men and risk of suicide: Cohort study. *British Medical Journal* 330(7484): 167.

Hershel, J., J. A. Kaye, and S. S. Jick. 2004. Antidepressants and the risk of suicidal behaviors. *Journal of the American Medical Association* 292(3): 338–343.

Kendler, K. S., J. Myers, and C. A. Prescott. 2005. Sex differences in the relationship between social support and risk for major depression: A longitudinal study of opposite-sex twin pairs. *American Journal of Psychiatry* 162(2): 250–256.

Koh, K. B., C. H. Kim, and J. K. Park. 2002. Predominance of anger in depressive disorders compared with anxiety disorders and somatoform disorders. *Journal of Clinical Psychiatry* 63(6): 488–492.

Lewis, C. 2003. The lowdown on depression. *FDA Consumer*, January/February.

Licinio, J., and M. L. Wong. 2005. Opinion: Depression, antidepressants and suicidality: A critical appraisal. *Nature Reviews: Drug Discovery* 4(2): 165–171.

Maruta, T., et al. 2000. Optimists vs. pessimists: Survival rate among medical patients over a 30-year period. *Mayo Clinic Proceedings* 75(2): 140–143.

Messias, E., et al. 2004. Summer birth and deficit schizophrenia: A pooled analysis from 6 countries. *Archives of General Psychiatry* 61(10): 985–989.

Miller, M., D. Azrael, and D. Hemenway. 2002. Household firearm ownership and suicide rates in the United States. *Epidemiology* 13(5): 517–524.

Mufson, L., et al. 2004. A randomized effectiveness trial of interpersonal psychotherapy for depressed adolescents. *Archives of General Psychiatry* 61(6): 577–584.

Nathan, P. E., and J. M. Gorman, eds. 2002. *A Guide to Treatments That Work*, 2nd ed. Oxford: Oxford University Press.

Pampallona, S., et al. 2004. Combined pharmacotherapy and psychological treatment for depression: A systematic review. *Archives of General Psychiatry* 61(7): 714–719.

Pini, S., et al. 2001. Insight into illness in schizophrenia, schizo-affective disorder, and mood disorders with psychotic features. *American Journal of Psychiatry* 158(1): 122–125.

Qin, P., E. Agerbo, and P. M. Bo. 2002. Suicide risk in relation to family history of completed suicide and psychiatric disorders. *Lancet* 360(9340): 1126.

Rothwell, J. D. 2004. *In the Company of Others: An Introduction to Communication*, 2nd ed. New York: McGraw-Hill.

Schatzberg, A. F., J. O. Cole, and C. DeBattista. 2002. *Manual of Clinical Psychopharmacology*, 4th ed. Washington, D.C.: American Psychiatric Association.

Simon, O. R., et al. 2002. Characteristics of impulsive suicide attempts and attempters. *Suicide and Life-Threatening Behavior* 32(1 Suppl): 49–59.

Snow, V., S. Lascher, and C. Mottur-Pilson. 2000. Pharmacological treatment of acute major depression and dysthymia. *Annals of Internal Medicine* 132(9): 738–742.

Swanson, J. W., et al. 2002. The social-environmental context of violent behavior in persons treated for severe mental illness. *American Journal of Public Health* 92(9): 1523–1531.

Szegedi, A., et al. 2005. Acute treatment of moderate to severe depression with hypericum extract WS 5570 (St John's wort): Randomised controlled double blind non-inferiority trial versus paroxetine. *British Medical Journal*, February 11 epub.

Tsai, S. Y., et al. 2002. Risk factors for completed suicide in bipolar disorder. *Journal of Clinical Psychiatry* 63(6): 469–476.

Vaillant, G. E. 1977. *Adaptation to Life*. Boston: Little, Brown.

Walsh, B. T., et al. 2002. Placebo response in studies of major depression. *Journal of the American Medical Association* 287(14): 1840–1847.

Walsh, E., and T. Fahy. 2002. Violence in society. *British Medical Journal* 325(7363): 507–508.

World Health Organization. 2002. *World Report on Violence and Health*. Geneva: World Health Organization.

Zhang, X., et al. 2005. Loss-of-function mutation in tryptophan hydroxylase-2 identified in unipolar major depression. *Neuron* 45(1): 11–16.

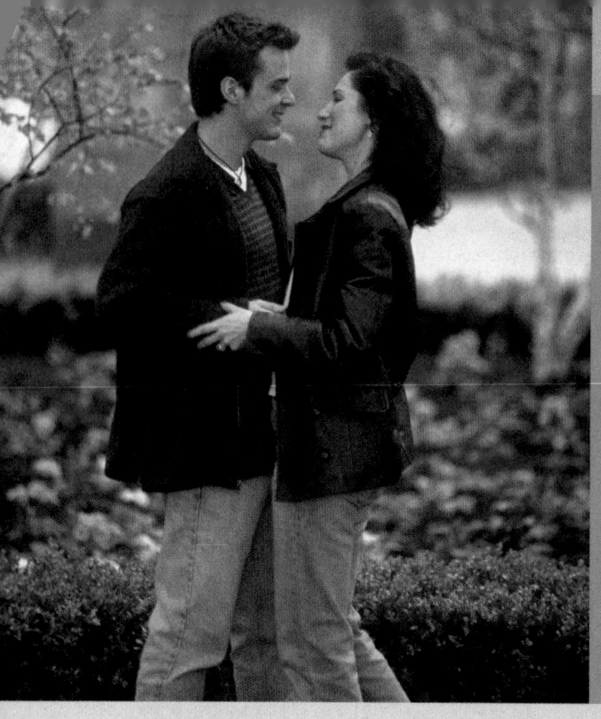

## Looking AHEAD

After reading this chapter, you should be able to

- Explain the qualities that help people develop intimate relationships
- Describe different types of love relationships and the stages they often go through
- Describe common challenges of forming and maintaining intimate relationships
- Explain some elements of healthy and productive communication
- Discuss relationship options available to adults today
- List some characteristics of successful families and some potential problems families face
- Explain some of the joys and challenges of being a parent

4

# Intimate Relationships and Communication

Human beings need social relationships; we cannot thrive as solitary creatures. Nor could the human species survive if adults didn't cherish and support each other, if we didn't form strong mutual attachments with our infants, and if we didn't create families in which to raise children. Simply put, people need people.

Although people are held together in relationships by a variety of factors, the foundation of many relationships is love. Love in its many forms—romantic, passionate, platonic, parental—is the wellspring from which much of life's meaning and delight flows. In our culture, it binds us together as partners, parents, children, and friends. People devote tremendous energy to seeking mates, nurturing intimate relationships, keeping up friendships, maintaining marriages—all for the pleasure of loving and being loved.

Many human needs are satisfied in intimate relationships: the need for approval and affirmation, for companionship, for meaningful ties and a sense of belonging, for sexual satisfaction. Many of society's needs are fulfilled by relationships, too—most notably, the need to nurture and socialize children. Overall, healthy intimate relationships are an important contributor to the well-being of both individuals and society.

## DEVELOPING INTIMATE RELATIONSHIPS

People who develop successful intimate relationships believe in themselves and in the people around them. They are willing to give of themselves—to share their ideas, feelings, time, needs—and to accept what others want to give them.

### Self-Concept and Self-Esteem

The principal element that we all bring to our relationships is our *selves.* To have successful relationships, we must first accept and feel good about ourselves. A positive self-concept and a healthy level of self-esteem help us love and respect others. How and where do we acquire a positive sense of self?

As discussed in Chapter 3, the roots of our identity and sense of self can be found in childhood, in the relationships we had with our parents and other family members. As adults, we probably have a sense that we're basically lovable, worthwhile people and that we can trust others if, as babies and children, we felt loved, valued, and respected; if adults responded to our needs in a reasonably

**WW Visit the *Core Concepts in Health* Online Learning Center (www.mhhe.com/inselbrief10e) for study aids and many additional resources.**

appropriate way; and if they gave us the freedom to explore and develop a sense of being separate individuals.

Our personal identity isn't fixed or frozen. According to psychologist Erik Erikson, it continues to develop as we encounter and resolve various crises at each stage of life. The fundamental tasks of early childhood are the development of trust during infancy and of autonomy during toddlerhood. From these experiences and interactions we construct our first ideas about who we are.

Another thing we learn in early childhood is **gender role**—the activities, abilities, and characteristics our culture deems appropriate for us based on whether we're male or female. In our society, men have traditionally been expected to work and provide for their families; to be aggressive, competitive, and power-oriented; and to use thinking and logic to solve problems. Women have been expected to take care of home and children; to be cooperative, supportive, and nurturing; and to approach life emotionally and intuitively. Although much more egalitarian gender roles are emerging in our society, the stereotypes we absorb in childhood tend to be deeply ingrained.

Our ways of relating to others may also be rooted in childhood. Some researchers have suggested that our adult styles of loving may be based on the style of **attachment** we established in infancy with our mother, father, or other primary caregiver. According to this view, people who are secure in their intimate relationships probably had a secure, trusting, mutually satisfying attachment to their mother, father, or other parenting figure. As adults, they find it relatively easy to get close to others. They don't worry about being abandoned or having someone get too close to them. They feel that other people like them and are generally well intentioned.

Even if people's earliest experiences and relationships were less than ideal, however, they can still establish satisfying relationships in adulthood. People can be resilient and flexible. They have the capacity to change their ideas, beliefs, and behavior patterns. They can learn ways to raise their self-esteem; they can become more trusting, accepting, and appreciative of others; and they can acquire the communication and conflict-resolution skills for maintaining successful relationships. Although it helps to have a good start in life, it may be even more important to begin again, right from where you are.

## Friendship

The first relationships we form outside the family are friendships. With members of either the same or the other sex, friendships give people the opportunity to share themselves and discover others. The friendships we form in childhood are important in our development; through them we learn about tolerance, sharing, and trust. Friendships usually include the following characteristics:

- *Companionship.* Friends are relaxed and happy in each other's company. They typically have common values and interests and make plans to spend time together.
- *Respect.* Friends have a basic respect for each other's humanity and individuality. Good friends respect each other's feelings and opinions and work to resolve their differences without demeaning or insulting each other. They are also honest with each other (see the box "Being a Good Friend" on p. 68).
- *Acceptance.* Friends feel free to be themselves and express their feelings spontaneously without fear of ridicule or criticism.
- *Help.* Sharing time, energy, and even material goods is important to friendship. Friends know they can rely on each other in times of need.
- *Trust.* Friends are secure in the knowledge that they will not intentionally hurt each other.
- *Loyalty.* Friends can count on each other. They stand up for each other in both word and deed.

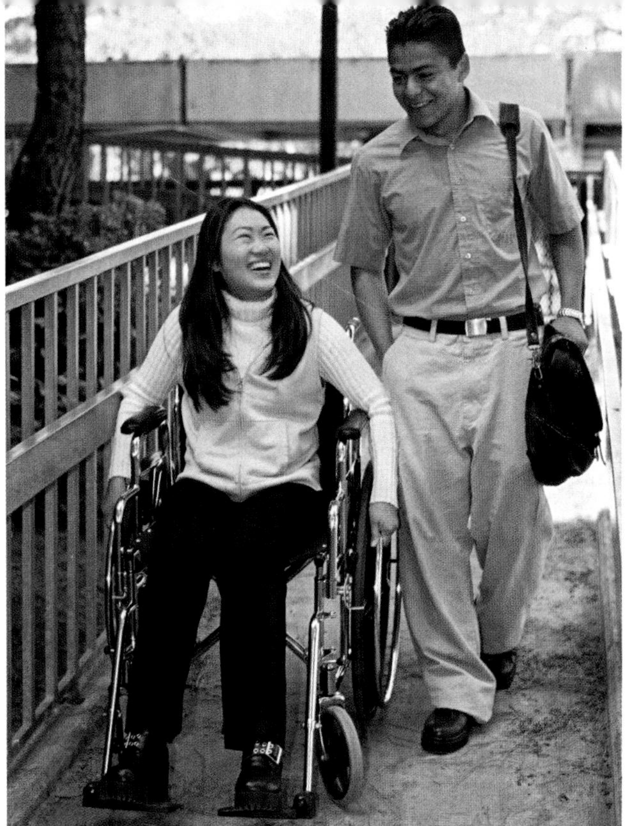

Close relationships without a sexual component are more common than those with sexual activity. Friendship satisfies our need for affection, affirmation, sharing, and companionship.

### Terms

**gender role** A culturally expected pattern of behavior and attitudes determined by whether a person is male or female.

**attachment** The emotional tie between an infant and his or her caregiver or between two people in an intimate relationship.

Vw

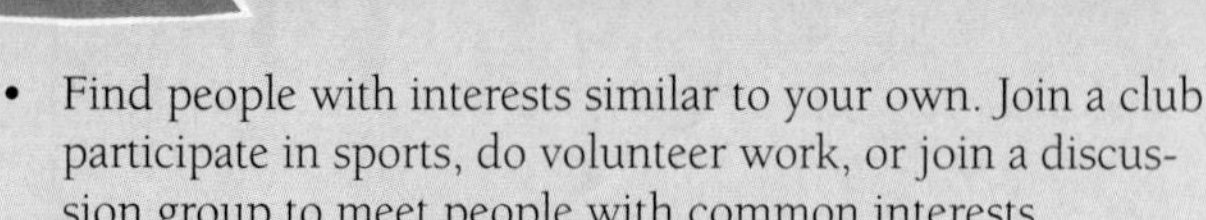

Take Charge

## Being a Good Friend

- Find people with interests similar to your own. Join a club, participate in sports, do volunteer work, or join a discussion group to meet people with common interests.
- Be a good listener. Take a genuine interest in people. Solicit their opinions, and take time to listen to their problems and ideas.
- Take risks. If you meet someone interesting, ask him or her to join you for a meal or an event you would both enjoy.
- Be trustworthy. Honor all confidences, and don't talk about your friend behind his or her back.
- Tell your friend about yourself. Self-disclosure—letting your friend know about your real concerns and joys—signals trust.
- Be supportive and kind. Be there when your friend is going through a rough time. Don't criticize your friend or offer unsolicited advice.
- Develop your capacity for intimacy. Intimate relationships are genuine, spontaneous, and caring.
- Don't expect perfection. Like any relationship, your friendship may go through difficult times. Talk through conflicts as they arise.

- *Mutuality.* Friends retain their individual identities, but close friendships are characterized by a sense of mutuality—"what affects you affects me." Friends share the ups and downs in each other's lives.
- *Reciprocity.* Friendships are reciprocal. There is give-and-take between friends and the feeling that both share joys and burdens more or less equally over time.

Friendships are usually considered both stabler and longer lasting than intimate partnerships. Friends are often more accepting and less critical than lovers, probably because their expectations are different. Like love relationships, friendships bind society together, providing people with emotional support and buffering them from stress.

## Love, Sex, and Intimacy

Love is one of the most basic and profound human emotions. It is a powerful force in all our intimate relationships. Love encompasses opposites: affection and anger, excitement and boredom, stability and change, bonds and freedom. Love does not give us perfect happiness, but it does give our lives meaning.

For most people, love, sex, and commitment are closely linked ideals in intimate relationships. Love reflects the positive factors that draw people together and sustain them in a relationship. It includes trust, caring, respect, loyalty, interest in the other, and concern for the other's well-being. Sex brings excitement and passion to the relationship. It intensifies the relationship and adds fascination and pleasure. Commitment, the determination to continue, reflects the stable factors that help maintain the relationship. Responsibility, reliability, and faithfulness are characteristics of commitment. Although love, sex, and commitment are related, they are not necessarily connected. One can exist without the others. Despite the various "faces" of love, sex, and commitment, most of us long for a special relationship that contains them all.

Other elements can be identified as features of love, such as euphoria, preoccupation with the loved one, idealization of the loved one, and so on, but these tend to be temporary. These characteristics may include **infatuation,** which will fade or deepen into something more substantial. As relationships progress, the central aspects of love and commitment take on more importance.

Another way of looking at love has been proposed by psychologist Robert Sternberg. He sees love as being composed of intimacy, passion, and commitment (Figure 4-1). Intimacy refers to the feelings of warmth and closeness we

**Term**

VW **infatuation** An idealizing, obsessive attraction, characterized by a high degree of physical arousal.

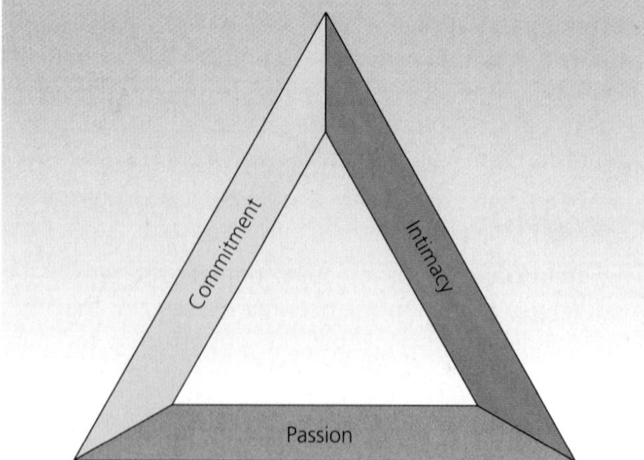


**Figure 4-1 The love triangle.** SOURCE: Sternberg, R., and M. Barnes. 1988. *The Psychology of Love.* New Haven: Yale University Press, p. 37. Copyright © 1998. Reprinted with permission.

have with someone we love. Passion refers to romance, attraction, and sexuality. Commitment refers to both the short-term decision that you love someone and the long-term commitment to be in the relationship. According to Sternberg, these three elements can be enlarged, diminished, or combined in different ways. Each combination gives a different kind of love.

Men and women tend to have different views of the relationship between love (or intimacy) and sex (or passion). Numerous studies have found that men can separate love from sex rather easily, although many men find that their most erotic sexual experiences occur in the context of a love relationship. Women generally view sex from the point of view of a relationship.

**The Pleasure and Pain of Love** The experience of intense love has confused and tormented lovers throughout history. They live in a tumultuous state of excitement, subject to wildly fluctuating feelings of joy and despair. They lose their appetite, can't sleep, and can think of nothing but the loved one. Is this happiness? Misery? Or both?

The contradictory nature of passionate love can be understood by recognizing that human emotions have two components: physiological arousal and an emotional explanation for the arousal. Love is just one of many emotions accompanied by physiological arousal; numerous unpleasant ones can also generate arousal, such as fear, rejection, frustration, and challenge. Although experiences like attraction and sexual desire are pleasant, extreme excitement is similar to fear and is unpleasant. For this reason, passionate love may be too intense to enjoy. Over time, the physical intensity and excitement tend to diminish. When this happens, pleasure may actually increase.

**The Transformation of Love** At first, love is likely to be characterized by high levels of passion and rapidly increasing intimacy. After a while, passion decreases as we become habituated to it and to the person. Sometimes intimacy continues to grow at a deeper, less conscious level; at other times, the couple may drift apart. Commitment isn't necessarily diminished or altered by time. It grows more slowly and is maintained as long as we judge the relationship to be successful. If the relationship begins to deteriorate, the level of commitment usually decreases.

The disappearance of romance or passionate love is often experienced as a crisis in a relationship. If a more lasting love fails to emerge, the relationship will likely break up, and each person will search for another who will once again ignite his or her passion. Love does not necessarily have to be intensely passionate. When intensity diminishes, partners often discover a more enduring love. They can now move from absorption in each other to a relationship that includes external goals and projects, friends, and family. In this kind of intimate, more secure love, satisfaction comes not just from the relationship itself but also from achieving other creative goals, such as work or child rearing. The key to successful relationships is in transforming passion into an intimate love, based on closeness, caring, and the promise of a shared future.

## Challenges in Relationships

Many people believe that love naturally makes an intimate relationship easy to begin and maintain, but, in fact, obstacles and challenges often occur. Even in the best of circumstances, there are times when a loving relationship will be tested. Individuals bring to a relationship diverse needs and wants, some of which emerge only at times of change or stress.

**Honesty and Openness** It's usually best to be yourself from the start of a relationship to give both you and your potential partner a chance to find out if you are comfortable with each other's beliefs, interests, and lifestyles. Getting close to another person by sharing thoughts and feelings is emotionally risky, but it is necessary for a relationship to deepen. Take your time, and self-disclose at a slow but steady rate. Over time, you and your partner will learn more about each other and feel more comfortable sharing.

**Unequal or Premature Commitment** Sometimes one person in an intimate partnership becomes more serious about the relationship than the other partner. In this situation, it can be very difficult to maintain a friendship without hurting the other person. Sometimes a couple makes a premature commitment, and then one of the partners has second thoughts and wants to break off the relationship. Sometimes both partners begin to realize that something is wrong, but each is afraid to tell the other. Most such problems can be dealt with only by honest and sensitive communication.

**Unrealistic Expectations** Each partner brings hopes and expectations to a relationship, some of which may be unrealistic, unfair, and, ultimately, very damaging to the relationship. Common expectations that can hurt a relationship include expecting your partner to change; assuming that your partner has all the same opinions, priorities, interests, and goals as you; and believing that a relationship will fulfill all of your personal, financial, intellectual, and social needs.

**Competitiveness** If one partner always feels the strong need to compete and win, it can detract from the sense of connectedness, interdependence, equality, and mutuality between partners. The same can be said for a perfectionistic need to be right in every instance—to "win" every argument. If competitiveness is a problem for you, ask yourself if your need to win is more important than your partner's feelings or the future of your relationship.

Take Charge

## Strategies for Enhancing Support in Relationships

- *Be aware of the importance of support.* Time and energy spent on support will help both you and your partner deal with stress and create a positive atmosphere that will help when differences or conflicts do occur.
- *Learn to ask for help from your partner.* Try different ways of asking for help and support from your partner and make note of which approaches work best for your relationship.
- *Help your partner the way she or he would like to be helped.* Some people prefer empathy and emotional support, whereas others like more practical help with problems.
- *Avoid negativity, especially when being asked for help.* Asking for help puts a person in a vulnerable position. If your partner asks for your aid, be gracious and supportive; don't use phrases like "I told you so" or "You should have just. . . ." Otherwise, your partner may learn not to ask for your help or support at all.
- *Make positive attributions.* If you're unsure about the reasons for your partner's behavior, give her or him the benefit of the doubt. For example, if your partner arrives for a date 30 minutes late and in a bad mood, assume it's because she or he had a bad day rather than attributing it to a character flaw or relationship problem. Offer appropriate support.
- *Help yourself.* Develop coping strategies for times your partner won't be available. These might include things you can do for yourself, such as going for a walk, or other people you can turn to for support.
- *Keep relationship problems separate.* Avoid bringing up relationship problems when you are offering or asking for help.

SOURCE: Plante, T., and K. Sullivan. 2000. *Getting Together and Staying Together: The Stanford Course on Intimate Relationships.* Bloomington, Ind.: 1stBooks Library, now Author House. Reprinted with permission of the author.

Try engaging in noncompetitive activities or in an activity where you are a beginner and your partner excels. Accept that your partner may hold different views on issues than you do—and that those views may be just as valid and important to your partner as your own views are to you.

### Balancing Time Spent Together and Apart

You may enjoy time together with your partner, but you may also want to spend time alone or with other friends. If time apart is interpreted as rejection or lack of commitment, it can damage a relationship. It's important to talk with your partner about what time apart means and to share your feelings about what you expect from the relationship in terms of time together. Differences in expectations about time spent together can mirror differences in ideas about emotional closeness. Any romantic relationship involves giving up some degree of autonomy in order to develop an identity as a couple. It's important to remember that every individual is unique and has different needs for distance and closeness in a relationship. In addition, traditional gender roles tend to teach women to be caretakers of relationships and men to be independent and self-reliant.

**Jealousy** Jealousy is the angry, painful response to a partner's real, imagined, or likely involvement with a third person. Some people think that the existence of jealousy proves the existence of love, but jealousy is actually a more accurate yardstick for measuring insecurity or possessiveness. In its irrational and extreme forms, jealousy can destroy a relationship by its insistent demands and attempts at control. Jealousy is a factor in precipitating violence in dating relationships, and abusive spouses often use jealousy to justify their violence. (Problems with control and violence in relationships are discusssed in Chapter 16.) When jealousy occurs in a relationship, it's important for the partners to communicate clearly with each other about their feelings.

## Successful Relationships

A true intimate relationship is characterized by a conscious sense of connectedness to another person. It emerges after a period of deep sharing, and it reflects a warm, caring, and trusting concern between partners (see the box "Strategies for Enhancing Support in Relationships"). Successful relationships result in a heightened sense of self-worth for both partners. To build a successful relationship, you need to be able to communicate your needs and wants clearly, listen to your partner, negotiate, and compromise. These skills are described in detail in the next section of the chapter.

## Unhealthy Relationships

Many of the strategies in this chapter suggest ways to make a relationship healthier and to enjoy greater intimacy. Equally important, however, is being able to recognize when a relationship is unhealthy. Relatively extreme examples of unhealthy relationships are those that are physically or emotionally abusive or that involve codependency; strategies for recognizing and addressing these problems are presented in Chapters 16 and 7, respectively.

Even relationships that are not abusive or codependent may still be unhealthy. If your relationship lacks love and respect and places little value on the time you and your partner have spent together, it may be time to get professional help or to end the partnership. Further, if your relationship is characterized by communication styles that include criticism, contempt, defensiveness, and withdrawal the relationship may not be salvageable. Spiritual leaders suggest that relationships are unhealthy when you feel that your sense of spontaneity, your potential for inner growth and joy, and your connection to your spiritual life is deadened. There are negative physical and mental consequences of being in an unhappy relationship; and although breaking up is painful and difficult, it is ultimately better than living in a toxic relationship.

### Ending a Relationship

Even when a couple starts out with the best of intentions, an intimate relationship may not last. Ending an intimate relationship is usually difficult and painful. If you are involved in a breakup, following these guidelines may help make the ending easier:

- Give the relationship a fair chance before breaking up.
- Be fair and honest, tactful and compassionate.
- If you are the rejected person, give yourself time to resolve your anger and pain.
- Recognize the value in the experience.

Use the recovery period following a breakup for self-renewal. Redirect more of your attention to yourself, and reconnect with people and areas of your life that may have been neglected as a result of the relationship. Time will help heal the pain of the loss of the relationship.

## COMMUNICATION

The key to developing and maintaining any type of intimate relationship is good communication.

### Nonverbal Communication

As much as 65% of face-to-face communication is nonverbal. Even when we're silent, we're communicating. We send messages when we look at someone or look away, lean forward or sit back, smile or frown. Especially important forms of nonverbal communication are touch, eye contact, and proximity. If someone we're talking to touches our hand or arm, looks into our eyes, and leans toward us when we talk, we get the message that the person is interested in us and cares about what we're saying. If a person keeps looking around the room while we're talking or takes a step backward, we get the impression the person is uninterested or wants to end the conversation.

The ability to interpret nonverbal messages correctly is important to the success of relationships. It's also important, when sending messages, to make sure our body language agrees with our words. When our verbal and nonverbal messages don't correspond, we send a mixed message.

### Communication Skills

Three keys to good communication in relationships are self-disclosure, listening, and feedback.

- *Self-disclosure* involves revealing personal information that we ordinarily wouldn't reveal because of the risk involved. It usually increases feelings of closeness and moves the relationship to a deeper level of intimacy. Friends often disclose the most to each other, sharing feelings, experiences, hopes, and disappointments; married couples sometimes share less because they think they already know everything about each other.
- *Listening,* the second key of good communication, is a rare skill. Good listening skills require that we spend more time and energy trying to fully understand another person's "story" and less time judging, evaluating, blaming, advising, analyzing, or trying to control. Empathy, warmth, respect, and genuineness are qualities of skillful listeners. Attentive listening encourages friends or partners to share more and, in turn, to be attentive listeners.
- *Feedback,* a constructive response to another's self-disclosure, is the third key to good communication. Giving positive feedback means acknowledging that the friend's or partner's feelings are valid—no matter how upsetting or troubling—and offering self-disclosure in response. Self-disclosure and feedback can open the door to change, whereas other responses block communication and change. (For tips on improving your skills, see the box "Guidelines for Effective Communication.")

### Gender and Communication

Some of the difficulties people encounter in relationships can be traced to common gender role differences in communication. Men and women generally approach conversation and communication differently. Men tend to use conversation in a *competitive* way, perhaps hoping to establish dominance in relationships. When male conversations are over, men often find themselves in a one-up or a one-down position. Women tend to use conversation in a more *affiliative* way, perhaps hoping to establish friendships. They negotiate various degrees of closeness, seeking to give and receive support. Men tend to talk more—though without disclosing more—and listen less. Women tend to use good listening skills such as eye contact, frequent nodding, focused attention, and asking relevant questions.

Even when a man and a woman are talking about the same subject, their unconscious goals may be very different. The woman may be looking for understanding and closeness, while the man may be trying to demonstrate

Take Charge

## Guidelines for Effective Communication

### Getting Started

- When you want to have a serious discussion with your partner, find a time when you will not be interrupted or rushed and a place that is private.
- Face your partner and maintain eye contact. Use nonverbal feedback to show that you are interested and involved in the communication process.

### Being an Effective Speaker

- State your concern or issue as clearly as you can.
- Use "I" statements—statements about how *you* feel—rather than statements beginning with "You," which tell another person how you think he or she feels. When you use "I" statements, you are taking responsibility for your feelings. "You" statements are often blaming or accusatory and will probably get a defensive or resentful response. The statement "I feel unloved," for example, sends a clearer, less blaming message than the statement "You don't love me."
- Focus on a specific behavior rather than on the whole person. Be specific about the behavior you like or don't like. Avoid generalizations beginning with "You always" or "You never." Such statements make people feel defensive.
- Make constructive requests. Opening your request with "I would like" keeps the focus on your needs rather than your partner's supposed deficiencies.
- Avoid blaming, accusing, and belittling. Even if you are right, you have little to gain by putting your partner down. When people feel criticized or attacked, they are less able to think rationally or solve problems constructively.
- Ask for action ahead of time. Tell your partner what you would like to have happen in the future; don't wait for him or her to blow it and then express anger or disappointment.

### Being an Effective Listener

- Provide appropriate nonverbal feedback (nodding, smiling, making eye contact, and so on).
- Don't interrupt.
- Develop the skill of reflective listening. Don't judge, evaluate, analyze, or offer solutions (unless asked to do so). Your partner may just need to have you there in order to sort out feelings. By jumping in right away to "fix" the problem, you may actually be cutting off communication.
- Don't give unsolicited advice. Giving advice implies that you know more about what a person needs to do than he or she does; therefore, it often evokes anger or resentment.
- Clarify your understanding of what your partner is saying by restating it in your own words and asking if your understanding is correct.
- Be sure you are really listening, not off somewhere in your mind rehearsing your reply. Try to tune in to your partner's feelings as well as the words.
- Let your partner know that you value what he or she is saying and want to understand. Respect for the other person is the cornerstone of effective communication.

his competence by giving advice and solving problems. Both styles are valid; the problem comes when differences in style result in poor communication and misunderstanding (see the box "Gender and Communication").

Sometimes communication is not the problem in a relationship—the partners understand each other all too well. The problem is that they're unable or unwilling to change or compromise. Although good communication can't salvage a bad relationship, it does enable couples to see their differences and make more informed decisions.

## Conflict and Conflict Resolution

Conflict is natural in intimate relationships. No matter how close two people become, they still remain separate individuals with their own needs, desires, past experiences, and ways of seeing the world. In fact, the closer the relationship, the more differences and the more opportunities for conflict there will be. Conflict itself isn't dangerous to a relationship; in fact, it may indicate that the relationship is growing. But if it isn't handled in a constructive way, it will damage—and ultimately destroy—the relationship.

Conflict is often accompanied by anger—a natural emotion, but one that can be difficult to handle. If we express anger, we run the risk of creating distrust, fear, and distance; if we act it out without thinking things through, we can cause the conflict to escalate; if we suppress anger, it turns into resentment and hostility. The best way to handle anger in a relationship is to recognize it as a symptom of something that requires attention and needs to be changed. When angry, partners should back off until they calm down and then come back to the issue later and try to resolve it rationally. Negotiation will help dissipate the anger so the conflict can be resolved.

Although the sources of conflict for couples change over time, they often revolve around the basic tasks of living together: dividing the housework, handling money, spending time together, and so on. Sexual interaction is also a source of disagreement for many couples.

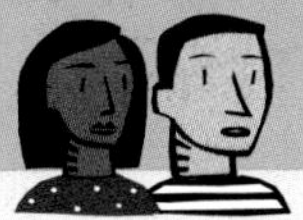

## Gender and Communication

Women and men view and approach relationships differently. One manifestation of these differences that tends to create difficulty in intimate relationships and communication is that women are generally more comfortable with emotion than are men. This difference has been traced in part to socialization and in part to biology.

From an early age, parents, teachers, and society send different messages to girls and boys regarding emotion. Boys learn to suppress and bury their feelings, especially fear and other emotions that make them feel vulnerable. Girls are encouraged to express and talk about their feelings.

In addition to socialization differences, research now shows that men have a more intense physiological response to certain emotions. In discussions around conflict, a man's blood pressure and heart rate rise higher and remain elevated longer. When anyone is physiologically or emotionally overwhelmed ("flooded"), productive communication is impossible.

A common pattern that arises between men and women is called "confront-withdraw." A woman approaches her male partner because she is upset and wants to talk about it. The man tries to calm her down, provides solutions he sees as rational, and/or withdraws. This response may make his partner even more upset and demanding, which causes the man to further shut down. In order to enjoy intimacy, men and women must work to better understand one another and develop a more compatible communication style.

### Advice for Men

- When your partner raises an emotional topic, be aware of uncomfortable feelings and the desire to retreat.
- Do not run away (physically or emotionally)! Telling her to "calm down" will likely create the opposite response.
- Find a way to stay connected. This is the only way to deescalate the conflict.
- Empathize: Listen to what she is saying, and even if you disagree, communicate to her that you understand how she is feeling and where she is coming from. Often when a person feels genuinely heard, that is enough.
- Try not to think of her comments as personal attacks; instead, continue to empathize.
- You may need to calm yourself. Try taking long deep breaths, telling yourself that your partner needs to air her feelings, and remembering that she, too, wants the conflict to end.
- In some cases, a 20-minute break—during which you soothe yourself rather than think upsetting thoughts—can be helpful.

### Advice for Women

- Try to be calm when approaching conflict; practice similar relaxation techniques to those described in "Advice for Men."
- Try to speak in ways that will not provoke defensiveness; complain rather than criticize, be specific, and use "I" statements.
- Try not to be critical of your partner's responses or his attempts to communicate.
- Be aware if he is withdrawing, and, if appropriate, help him to relax by using methods you have discussed previously. For example, reassure him that you love him, and put the argument in perspective. Be careful not to be condescending about this.

SOURCE: Gottman, J. 1994. *Why Marriages Succeed or Fail . . . and How You Can Make Yours Last*. New York: Simon & Schuster.

Some basic strategies are generally useful in successfully negotiating with a partner:

1. *Clarify the issue.* Take responsibility for thinking through your feelings and discovering what's really bothering you. Agree that one partner will speak first and have the chance to speak fully while the other listens. Then reverse the roles. Try to understand the other partner's position fully by repeating what you've heard and asking questions to clarify or elicit more information. Agree to talk only about the topic at hand and not get distracted by other issues. Sum up what your partner has said.

2. *Find out what each person wants.* Ask your partner to express his or her desires. Don't assume you know what your partner wants and speak for him or her. Clarify and summarize.

3. *Identify various alternatives for getting each person what he or she wants.* Practice brainstorming to generate a variety of options.

4. *Decide how to negotiate.* Work out some agreements or plans for change; for example, one partner will do one task and the other will do another task, or one partner will do a task in exchange for something he or she wants. Find a solution that satisfies both partners.

5. *Solidify the agreements.* Go over the plan verbally and write it down, if necessary, to ensure that you both understand and agree to it.

6. *Review and renegotiate.* Decide on a time frame for trying out the new plan, and set a time to discuss how it's working. Make adjustments as needed.

To resolve conflicts, partners have to feel safe in voicing disagreements. They have to trust that the discussion won't get out of control, that they won't be abandoned by the other, and that the partner won't take advantage of their vulnerability. Partners should follow some basic ground rules when they argue, such as avoiding ultimatums and resisting the urge to give the silent treatment. When you do argue, maintain a spirit of goodwill and avoid being harshly critical or contemptuous. If you and your partner find that you argue again and again over the same issue, it may be

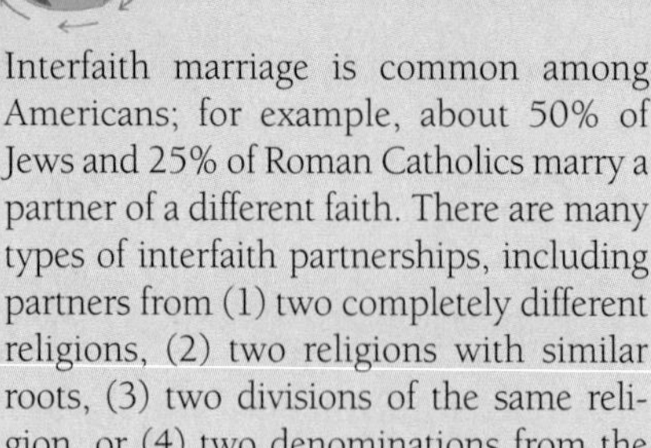


### Interfaith and Intrafaith Partnerships

Interfaith marriage is common among Americans; for example, about 50% of Jews and 25% of Roman Catholics marry a partner of a different faith. There are many types of interfaith partnerships, including partners from (1) two completely different religions, (2) two religions with similar roots, (3) two divisions of the same religion, or (4) two denominations from the same religious division. The latter two are often called intrafaith partnerships.

Marrying someone of a different faith can broaden the partners' worldview and enrich their lives; however, it can also be a potential stressor and a challenge to a relationship. There is no specifically correct way to address religious diversity in a partnership, but the following are some potential approaches.

***Withdrawal:*** In some couples, both partners withdraw from their respective religions. Religious differences may be minimized, but the withdrawal may not last. If a partner was observant prior to the relationship, it is likely that she or he will want to become involved again.

***Conversion:*** In many intrafaith couples, one partner converts to the religion of the other. Religious differences are decreased, but problems can occur if the partner who converts develops resentment, has difficulties with her or his family of origin, misses the old religion, or experiences feelings of guilt or betrayal.

***Compromise:*** Some couples convert together to a new religion, possibly to a religion or denomination at a "midpoint" between their two religions. The couple may find a happy medium that is satisfying to both. However, both may experience the problems associated with conversion.

***Multifaith:*** Some couples join both religions. They may alternate places of worship weekly or make other creative arrangements. The advantage of this pattern is that both partners maintain their religions and learn more about each other. Problems may arise if the religions have conflicting values or practices.

***Ecumenical:*** In some relationships, partners merge their religions. They may combine the "best" of each or observe only the areas where the religions intersect. They may get the best of both worlds and/or discover that their religions have more in common than they thought. In some cases, however, the original religious institutions may condemn compromise.

***Diversity:*** In some couples, each partner chooses to follow his or her own religion. If both partners are very religious, they do not then have to give up an important part of their lives. However, some partners consider this approach undesirable because it means more time spent apart.

***Do Nothing:*** Some couples find no need to address religious differences because neither partner is observant or committed to a religion to an extent that it is a relationship challenge. They address specific issues if and when they arise.

To maintain a successful partnership, couples should communicate about religious issues before getting married or having children. Discuss the importance of your respective religions and your religious needs. Consider ways that you can honor each other's religious traditions. Learn to discuss issues relating to religion and spirituality in ways to bring you closer together.

SOURCES: Robinson, B. A. 2003. *Inter-Faith Marriages: Overview* (http://www.religioustolerance.org/ifm_menu.htm; retrieved November 4, 2004); Robinson, B. A. 1999. *How Inter-Faith and Intra-Faith Couples Handle Religious Differences* (http://www.religioustolerance.org/ifm_diff.htm; retrieved November 4, 2004).

better to stop trying to resolve that problem and instead come to accept the differences between you.

## PAIRING AND SINGLEHOOD

Although most people eventually marry or commit to a partner, everyone spends some time as a single person, and nearly all make some attempt, consciously or unconsciously, to find a partner. Intimate relationships are as important for singles as for couples.

### Choosing a Partner

Most men and women select partners for long-term relationships through a fairly predictable process, although they may not be consciously aware of it. Most people pair with someone who lives in the same geographic area and who is similar in ethnic and socioeconomic background, educational level, lifestyle, physical attractiveness, and other traits. In simple terms, people select partners like themselves.

First attraction is based on easily observable characteristics: looks, dress, social status, and reciprocated interest. Once the euphoria of romantic love winds down, personality traits and behaviors become more significant factors in how the partners view each other. Through sharing and self-disclosure, they gradually gain a deeper knowledge of each other. The emphasis shifts to basic values, such as religious beliefs, political affiliation, sexual attitudes, and future aspirations regarding career, family, and children. If they are compatible, many people gradually discover deeper, more enduring forms of love.

Perhaps the most important question for potential mates is, How much do we have in common? Although differences add interest to a relationship, similarities increase the chances of a relationship's success. If there are major differences, partners should ask first, How accepting of differences are we? and then, How well do we communicate? Areas in, which differences can affect the relationship include values, religion, ethnicity, attitudes toward sexuality and gender roles, socioeconomic status, familiarity with the other's culture, and interactions with the extended family (see the box "Interfaith and Intrafaith Partnerships").

## Dating

Most Americans find romantic partners through some form of dating. They narrow the field through a process of getting to know each other. Traditionally, in the male-female dating pattern, the man took the lead, initiating the date, while the woman waited to be called. In this pattern, casual dating might evolve into steady or exclusive dating, then engagement, and finally marriage.

For many young people today, traditional dating has given way to a more casual form of getting together in groups. People go out in groups, rather than strictly as couples, and each person pays his or her way. A man and woman may begin to spend more time together, but often in the group context. If sexual involvement develops, it is more likely to be based on friendship, respect, and common interests than on expectations related to gender roles. In this model, mate selection may progress from getting together to living together to marriage.

Although the American cultural norm is personal choice in courtship and mate selection, the popularity of dating services and online matchmaking suggests that many people do want help finding a suitable partner (see the box "Online Relationships" on p. 76).

## Living Together

According to the U.S. Bureau of the Census, about 4 million heterosexual couples and an estimated 1.5 million gay and lesbian couples are currently living together; 11% of unmarried partners are same-sex couples. Living together, or **cohabitation**, is one of the most rapid and dramatic social changes that has ever occurred in our society. It seems to be gaining acceptance as part of the normal mate-selection process. By age 30, about half of all men and women will have cohabited.

Living together provides many of the benefits of marriage: companionship; a setting for an enjoyable and meaningful relationship; the opportunity to develop greater intimacy through learning, compromising, and sharing; a satisfying sex life; and a way to save on living costs. Living together also has certain advantages over marriage. For one thing, it can give the partners a greater sense of autonomy and partners may find it easier to keep their identity and more of their independence. Cohabitation doesn't incur the same obligations as marriage. If things don't work out, the partners may find it easier to leave a relationship that hasn't been legally sanctioned.

But living together has some liabilities, too. In most cases, the legal protections of marriage are absent, such as health insurance benefits and property and inheritance rights. These considerations can be particularly serious if the couple has children. Since social acceptance of cohabitation is not universal, couples may feel

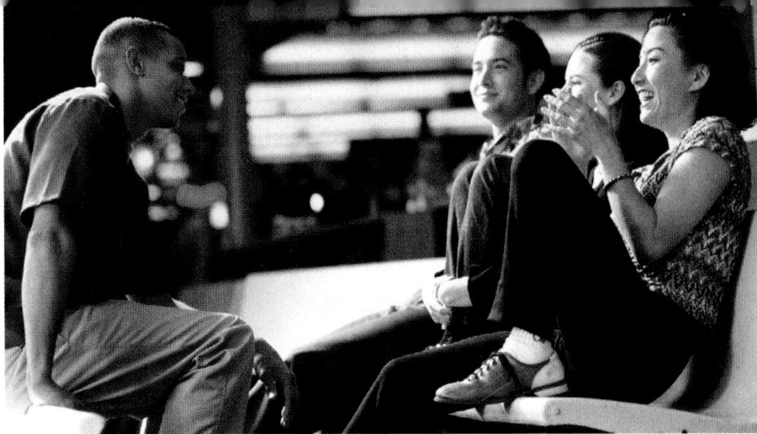

For many college students today, group activities have replaced dating as a way to meet and get to know potential partners.

family pressure to marry or otherwise change their living arrangements, especially if they have young children.

Although many people choose cohabitation as a kind of trial marriage, unmarried partnerships tend to be less stable than marriages. There is little evidence that cohabitation before marriage leads to happier or longer-lasting marriages; in fact, some studies have found slightly less marital satisfaction and slightly higher divorce rates among couples who had previously cohabited.

## Same-Sex Partnerships

Regardless of **sexual orientation,** most people look for love in a close, satisfying, committed relationship. A person whose sexual orientation is lesbian, gay, or bisexual (LGB) may be involved in a **homosexual** (same-sex) relationship. Same-sex couples have many similarities with **heterosexual** couples (those who seek members of the opposite sex). According to one study, most gay men and lesbians have experienced at least one long-term relationship with a single partner. Like any intimate relationship, same-sex partnerships provide intimacy, passion, and security.

### Terms

VW

**cohabitation** Living together in a sexual relationship without being married.

**sexual orientation** A consistent pattern of emotional and sexual attraction based on biological sex; it exists along a continuum that ranges from exclusive heterosexuality (attraction to people of the other sex) through bisexuality (attraction to people of both sexes) to exclusive homosexuality (attraction to people of one's own sex).

**homosexual** Emotional and sexual attraction to people of one's own sex.

**heterosexual** Emotional and sexual attraction to people of the other sex.

Take Charge

## Online Relationships

More and more people today are looking to the Internet to find friends and partners, and an estimated 22 million singles have tried online dating. Communicating with others in cyberspace allows people to be themselves in a relaxed atmosphere, to try out other personas, and to confide in others in a private and less vulnerable way. If your goal is to communicate with someone about a common interest, e-mail, newsgroups, listservs, blogs (online journals), and chat rooms are all good options. For those out of college, living in big cities, not interested in bar scenes, and/or looking to expand beyond their local network of friends, the Internet provides a rich resource for making connections.

There are drawbacks to meeting partners online, however. People can misrepresent themselves, pretending to be very different—older or younger or even of a different sex—than they really are. Investing time and emotional resources in an unrealistic romance can be painful. There have also been a few instances in which online romances have become dangerous or even deadly (see Chapter 16 for information on cyberstalking). When choosing partners online, you are also reducing an important and powerful source of information: chemistry and in-person intuition. You will therefore need to trust your instincts regarding the process of the relationship and use common sense. If you decide to pursue an online relationship, here are some strategies that can help you maximize your experience and keep you safe:

- To increase your chances of meeting people interested in you as a person, avoid sexually orientated Web sites.
- Know what you are looking for as well as what you have to offer someone else. Find out the other person's situation and intentions.
- To start, you can answer someone else's ad, letting them know what you found interesting about their post. Or you can write an ad of your own—something unique that represents some of your interests and personality.
- Many Web sites have a place to put a photo, and if you are serious about the pursuit of a partner, you may find that you get many more responses when you post a photo. However, if this does not feel comfortable, remember that it isn't necessary and that you can always choose to add one later.
- Until you know enough about a cyberfriend, don't give out personal information, including your real full name, school, or place of employment. Consider setting up a second e-mail account for dating-related e-mails.
- Before deciding whether to meet an online friend in person, schedule a phone conversation or a series of phone conversations. Take the relationship at a pace that feels comfortable for you.
- Don't agree to meet someone face-to-face unless you feel completely comfortable about it. Always meet initially in a very public place—a museum, a coffee shop, or a restaurant. Bring along a friend to further increase your safety, or let a friend know where you will be.

Finally, take care that your pursuit of online relationships does not interfere with your other interpersonal relationships and social activities. Don't use the Internet to escape from real-life problems or important personal issues. As described in Chapter 3, extensive use of the Internet is associated with greater loneliness, less communication with family members, and fewer social contacts. To maximize your emotional and interpersonal wellness, use the Internet to widen your circle of friends, not shrink it.

One difference between heterosexual and homosexual couples is that same-sex partnerships tend to be more egalitarian (equal) and less organized around traditional gender roles. Same-sex couples put greater emphasis on partnership than on role assignment. Domestic tasks are shared or split, and both partners usually support themselves financially.

Another difference between heterosexual and homosexual relationships is that same-sex partners often have to deal with societal hostility or ambivalence toward their relationship, in contrast to the societal approval and rights given to heterosexual couples (see the box "Same-Sex Marriage and Civil Unions"). *Homophobia,* fear or hatred of homosexuals, can be obvious, as in the case of violence or discrimination, or more subtle, such as how same-sex couples are portrayed in the media. Due to the impact of societal disapproval, community resources and support may be more important for same-sex couples as a source of identity and social support than they are for heterosexuals.

## Singlehood

Despite the prevalence and popularity of marriage, a significant proportion of adults in our society are unmarried—more than 98 million single individuals. They are a diverse group, encompassing young people who have not married yet but plan to in the future, people who are living together (gay or heterosexual), divorced and widowed people, and those who would like to marry but haven't found a mate (Figure 4-2).

Several factors contribute to the growing number of single people. One is the changing view of singlehood, which is increasingly being viewed as a legitimate alternative to marriage. Education and career are delaying the age at which young people are marrying. The median age for marriage is now 26.8 years for men and 25.1 years for women. More young people are living with their parents as they complete their education, seek jobs, or strive for financial independence. Many other single

In the News

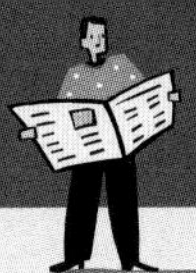

## Same-Sex Marriage and Civil Unions

Marriage is often viewed primarily as a social or religious institution, but it is in fact an institution defined by state and federal statutes that confer legal and economic rights and responsibilities. According to the U.S. General Accountability Office, there are more than 1000 federal laws in which a distinction is based on marriage. Marital status affects Social Security, federal tax status, inheritance, medical decision making and hospital visitation, child custody, and many other benefits.

In 2000, Vermont became the first state to offer the option of civil union to couples for whom legal marriage is not an option. A civil union is a legal status parallel to marriage—but it is valid only within the issuing state. Currently, the only state in which a same-sex couple can legally marry is Massachusetts, where officials began granting marriage licenses to same-sex couples in May 2004. San Francisco also began issuing licenses to same-sex couples in early 2004, but the California Supreme Court eventually ruled that the city had bypassed state law, and the court voided the more than 4000 same-sex marriages performed there. (Internationally, the Netherlands, Belgium, and certain provinces in Canada have legalized same-sex marriage; many other European countries offer civil unions.)

In the cases of Vermont and Massachusetts, state supreme courts ruled that under the states' constitutions, same-sex couples are entitled to the same benefits and protections as married couples. San Francisco officials acted based on their interpretation of the California state constitution's prohibition against discrimination, and the legal case over that constitutional question is still pending.

Other states and the federal government have passed laws and amendments to ban same-sex marriage. A federal law called the Defense of Marriage Act (DOMA), signed by President Clinton in 1996, defines marriage as the legal union between one man and one woman and refuses federal recognition of same-sex marriages. It also allows states to refuse to recognize same-sex marriages and civil unions performed in other states or countries. As of November 2004, more than 40 states had enacted their own mini-DOMAs and/or passed state constitutional amendments banning same-sex marriage and, in some cases, civil unions.

In 2004, President Bush endorsed an amendment to the U.S. Constitution, the "Federal Marriage Amendment," that would permanently ban same-sex marriage and prevent expected future legal challenges to federal and state DOMAs. Under the proposed amendment, states would still be allowed to grant civil unions. The amendment was defeated in Congress in fall 2004, but future action on it is likely.

What cases are made for and against civil union and same-sex marriage? Opponents put forth numerous arguments, including that the purpose of marriage is to procreate, that the Bible forbids same-sex unions, that homosexuals are seeking special rights, that it's bad for children and families, and that the majority of the population opposes such unions. The primary argument, however, is that same-sex marriage undermines the sanctity and validity of marriage as it is traditionally understood and thus undermines society. Rules and restrictions on who can marry preserve the value of the institution of marriage, according to this view. The underlying assumption of this position is that homosexual behavior is a choice and that people can change their orientation.

Proponents of civil unions and same-sex marriage believe that sexual orientation is outside the control of the individual and results from genetic and environmental factors that create an unchangeable orientation. The issue of same-sex union is then seen as one of basic civil rights, in which a group is being denied rights—to publicly express their commitment to one another, to provide security for their children, and to receive the legal and economic benefits afforded to married heterosexual couples—on the basis of something as unalterable as skin color.

To the argument that marriage has a traditional meaning in our society, proponents respond that, on the contrary, marriage is an evolving institution that changes as society changes. Prior to 1967, marriage between whites and African Americans was prohibited in parts of the United States; before the Civil War, African Americans were not allowed to marry at all. These and other trends, according to this view, are leading people to broaden their definition of marriage and to see same-sex marriage as just another variation.

Both opponents and proponents of same-sex marriage point out that marriage is healthy for both men and women and is the main social institution promoting family values; both sides see this assertion as supportive of their position. What remains to be seen is how society in general is going to view same-sex marriage in the future—as a furthering of American values or as an attack on them.

people live together without being married. High divorce rates mean more singles, and people who have experienced divorce in their families may have more negative attitudes about marriage and more positive attitudes about singlehood.

Being single doesn't mean not having close relationships, however. Single people may date, enjoy active and fulfilling social lives, and have a variety of sexual experiences and relationships. Other advantages of being single include more opportunities for personal and career development without concern for family obligations and more freedom and control in making life choices. Disadvantages include loneliness and a lack of companionship, as well as economic hardships (mainly for single women). Single men and women alike experience some discrimination and often are pressured to get married.

Nearly everyone has at least one episode of being single in adult life. How enjoyable and valuable this single time is depends on several factors, including how deliberately the person has chosen it; how satisfied the

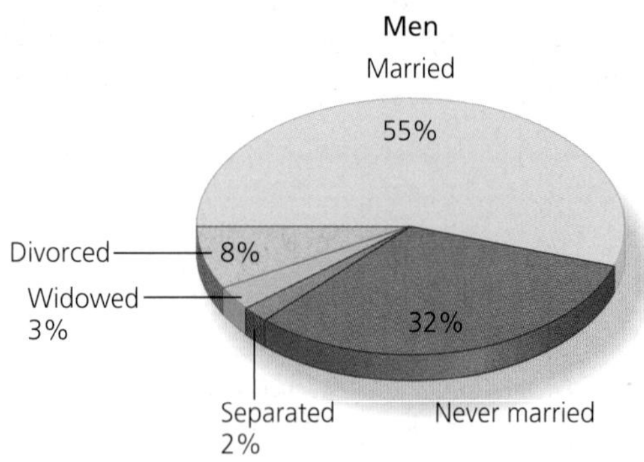


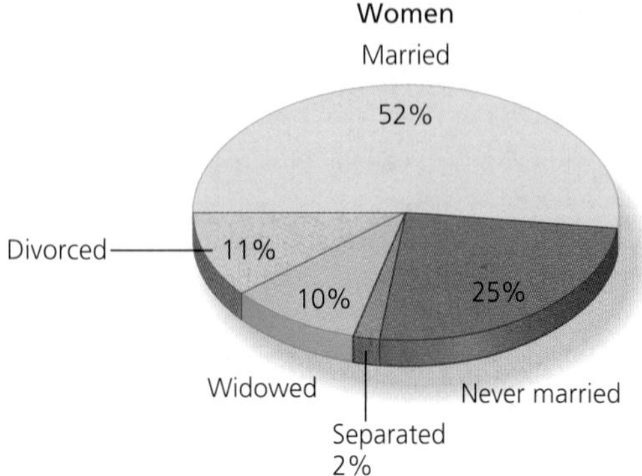


VITAL STATISTICS

**Figure 4-2 Marital status of the U.S. population age 15 years and older.** SOURCE: U.S. Bureau of the Census. 2004. *Marital Status of People 15 Years and Over* (http://www.census.gov/population/www/socdemo/hh-fam/cps2003.html; retrieved November 5, 2004).

person is with his or her social relationships, standard of living, and job; how comfortable the person feels when alone; and how resourceful and energetic the person is about creating an interesting and fulfilling life.

## MARRIAGE

About 95% of all Americans marry at some time in their life. Marriage continues to remain popular because it satisfies several basic needs. There are many important social, moral, economic, and political aspects of marriage, all of which have changed over the years. In the past, people married mainly for practical reasons, such as raising children or forming an economic unit. Today, people marry more for personal, emotional reasons. This shift places a greater burden on marriage to fulfill certain expectations that are sometimes unreasonably high. People may assume that all their emotional needs will be met by their partner; they may think that fascination and passion will always remain at high levels; they may simply expect to "live happily ever after." When people enter marriage with such preconceptions, it may be harder for them to appreciate the benefits that marriage really offers.

### Benefits of Marriage

The primary functions and benefits of marriage are those of any intimate relationship: affection, personal affirmation, companionship, sexual fulfillment, and emotional growth. Marriage also provides a setting in which to raise children, although an increasing number of couples choose to remain childless, and people can also choose to raise children without being married. Marriage is also important for providing for the future. By committing themselves to the relationship, people establish themselves with lifelong companions as well as some insurance for their later years (see the box "Are Intimate Relationships Good for Your Health?").

### Issues in Marriage

Although we might like to believe otherwise, love is not enough to make a successful marriage. Couples have to be strong and successful in their relationship before getting married, because relationship problems will be magnified rather than solved by marriage. The following relationship characteristics appear to be the best predictors of a happy marriage:

- The partners have realistic expectations about their relationship.
- Each feels good about the personality of the other.
- They communicate well.
- They have effective ways of resolving conflicts.
- They agree on religious/ethical values.
- They have an egalitarian role relationship.
- They have a good balance of individual versus joint interests and leisure activities.

Once married, couples must face many adjustment tasks. In addition to providing each other with emotional support, they have to negotiate and establish marital roles, establish domestic and career priorities, handle their finances, make sexual adjustments, manage boundaries and relationships with their extended family, and participate in the larger community. Marital roles and responsibilities have undergone profound changes in recent years. Although women still take most of the responsibility for home and children even when they work and although men still suffer more job-related stress and health problems than women do, the trend is toward an equalization of responsibilities.

### The Role of Commitment

Coping with all these challenges requires that couples be committed to remaining in the relationship through its inevitable ups and downs. They will need to be tolerant of each other's imperfections and keep their perspective and sense of humor. Commitment is based on conscious

Mind/Body/Spirit

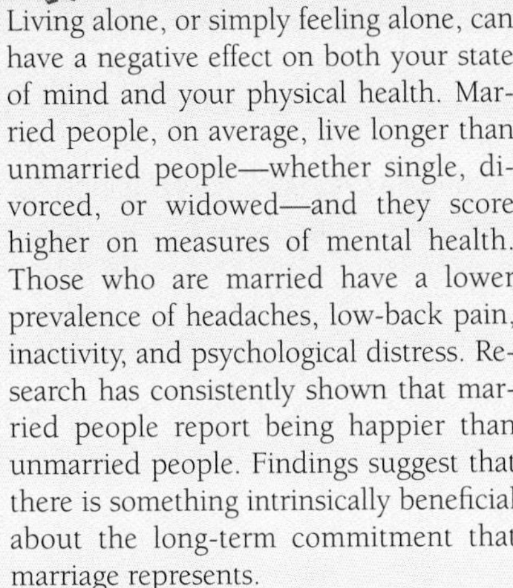

### Are Intimate Relationships Good for Your Health?

Living alone, or simply feeling alone, can have a negative effect on both your state of mind and your physical health. Married people, on average, live longer than unmarried people—whether single, divorced, or widowed—and they score higher on measures of mental health. Those who are married have a lower prevalence of headaches, low-back pain, inactivity, and psychological distress. Research has consistently shown that married people report being happier than unmarried people. Findings suggest that there is something intrinsically beneficial about the long-term commitment that marriage represents.

People with strong social ties are less likely to become ill and tend to recover more quickly if they do. The benefits of intimate relationships have been demonstrated for a range of conditions: People with strong social support are less likely to catch colds. They recover better from heart attacks and live longer with heart disease. Among men with prostate cancer, those who are married live significantly longer than those who are single, divorced, or widowed. Women in satisfying marriages are less likely to develop risk factors associated with cardiovascular diseases than unmarried women or women in unhappy marriages.

What is it about social relationships that support wellness? Part of the answer may be that people who get married are happier people long before they get married. But regarding physical health, friends and partners may encourage and reinforce healthy habits, such as exercising, eating right, and seeing a physician when needed. In times of illness, a loving partner can provide both practical help and emotional support. Feeling loved, esteemed, and valued brings comfort at a time of vulnerability, reduces anxiety, and mitigates the damaging effects of stress and risks of social isolation.

Although good relationships may help the sick get better, bad relationships may have the opposite effect. The impact of relationship quality on the course of illness may be partly explained by effects of the immune system: A study of married couples whose fighting went beyond normal conflict and into criticism and name-calling found them to have weaker immune responses than couples whose arguments were more civil. (The immune effects were particularly strong among the wives, leading some researchers to postulate that women may be more aware of and affected by relationship problems.) High marital stress is linked with risky lifestyle choices and behaviors and nonadherence to medical regimens. Similarly, unhappy marriages are associated with risk factors for heart disease, such as depression, hostility, and anger.

Marriage, of course, isn't the only support system available. Whether married, in a committed partnership, or single, if you have supportive people in your life, you are likely to enjoy better physical and emotional health than if you feel isolated and alone. So when you start planning lifestyle changes to improve your health and well-being, don't forget to nurture your relationships with family and friends. Relationships are powerful medicine.

choice rather than on feelings, which, by their very nature, are transitory. Commitment is a promise of a shared future, a promise to be together, come what may. Committed partners put effort and energy into the relationship, no matter how they feel. They take time to attend to their partner, give compliments, and deal with conflict when necessary. To many people, commitment is a more important goal than living together or marriage.

### Separation and Divorce

People marrying today have a 50–55% chance of divorcing. The high rate of divorce in the United States reflects our extremely high expectations for emotional fulfillment and satisfaction in marriage. It also indicates that we no longer believe in the permanence of marriage.

The process of divorce usually begins with an emotional separation. Often one partner is unhappy and looks beyond the relationship for other forms of validation. Dissatisfaction increases until the unhappy partner decides he or she can no longer stay. Physical separation follows, although it may take some time for the relationship to be over emotionally.

Except for the death of a spouse or family member, divorce is the greatest stress-producing event in life. Both men and women experience turmoil, depression, and lowered self-esteem during and after divorce. People experience separation distress and loneliness for about a year and then begin a recovery period of 1–3 years. During this time they gradually construct a postdivorce identity, along with a new pattern of life. Children are especially vulnerable to the trauma of divorce, and sometimes counseling is appropriate to help them adjust to the changes in their lives.

## FAMILY LIFE

American families are very different today than they were even a few decades ago. Currently, about half of all families are based on a first marriage; almost one-third are headed by a single parent; the remainder are remarriages or involve some other arrangement. Despite the tremendous variation apparent in American families, certain patterns can still be discerned.

### Deciding to Become a Parent

Many factors must be taken into account when you are considering parenthood. Following are some questions to ask yourself and some issues to consider when making this decision. Some issues are relevant to both men and women; others apply only to women.

- *Your physical health and your age.* Are you in reasonably good health? If not, can you improve your health by changing your lifestyle, perhaps by modifying your diet or giving up cigarettes, alcohol, or drugs? Are you overweight? Do you have physical conditions, such as diabetes or high blood pressure, that will require extra care and medical attention during pregnancy?
- *Your financial circumstances.* Can you afford a child? Will your health insurance cover the costs of pregnancy, delivery, and medical attention for mother and baby before and after the birth? Depending on a variety of factors, the annual cost of raising a child averages about $9500.
- *Your relationship with your partner.* Are you in a stable relationship, and do both of you want a child? Are your views compatible on issues such as child-rearing goals, the distribution of responsibility for the child, and work and housework obligations?
- *Your educational, career, and child care plans.* Have you completed as much of your education as you want right now? Have you established yourself in a career, if that is something you want to do? Have you investigated parental leave and company-sponsored child care?
- *Your emotional readiness for parenthood.* Do you have the emotional discipline and stamina to care for and nurture an infant? Are you prepared to have a helpless baby completely dependent on you all day and all night? Are you willing to change your lifestyle to provide the best conditions for a baby's development?
- *Your social support system.* Do you have a network of family and friends who will help you with the baby? Are there community resources you can call on for additional assistance? A family's social support system is one of the most important factors affecting its ability to adjust to a baby and cope with new responsibilities.
- *Your personal qualities, attitudes toward children, and aptitude for parenting.* Do you like infants, young children, and adolescents? Do you think time with children is time well spent? Do you have safe ways of handling anger, frustration, and impatience?

## Becoming a Parent

Few new parents have any preparation for the job of parenting, yet they have to assume that role literally overnight. They have to learn quickly how to hold a baby, how to change it, how to feed it, how to interpret its cries. No wonder the birth of the first child is one of the most stressful transitions for any couple.

Even couples with an egalitarian relationship before their first child is born find that their marital roles become more traditional with the arrival of the new baby. The father becomes the principal provider and protector, and the mother becomes the primary nurturer. Most research indicates that mothers make greater changes in their lives than fathers do. Although men today spend more time caring for their infants than ever before, women still take the ultimate responsibility for seeing that the baby is fed, clean, and comfortable. In addition, women are usually the ones who make job changes; they may quit working or reduce their hours in order to stay home with the baby for several months or more, or they may try to juggle the multiple roles of mother, homemaker, and employee and feel guilty that they never have enough time to do justice to any of these roles.

## Parenting

Sometimes being a parent is a source of unparalleled pleasure and pride—the first smile (at you), the first word, the first home run. But at other times parenting can seem like an overwhelming responsibility. How can you be sure you're not making some mistake that will stunt your child's physical, psychological, or emotional growth?

**Parenting Styles** Most parents worry about their ability to raise a healthy, responsible, and well-adjusted child. Some had parents who were good role models, whereas others want to do things differently than their own parents did. Parents may wonder about the long-term impact of each decision they make on their child's well-being and personality. According to parenting experts, no one action or decision (within limits) will determine a child's personality or development; instead, what is most important is the *parenting style,* or overall approach to parenting. Most parents use a blend of the following four general styles but tend toward one style.

**AUTHORITARIAN** Authoritarian parents give orders and expect them to be obeyed, giving very little warmth or consideration to their children's special needs. They maintain a structured environment where the rules are explicit and set without input or discussion with the child. Children of authoritarian parents rate low on social competence, self-esteem, intellectual curiosity, spontaneity, and initiative. They perform fairly well in school and do not exhibit a lot of problem behavior; however, they have higher levels of depression.

**AUTHORITATIVE** Authoritative parents set clear boundaries and expectations, but they are also loving, supportive, and attuned to their children's needs. They are firm in their decisions but allow for a give-and-take in discussions with the intent of fostering independent thinking. Both authoritarian and authoritative parents hold their children to high expectations. The difference is that authoritarian parents expect their children to follow their commands without question or comment and authoritative parents are more likely to

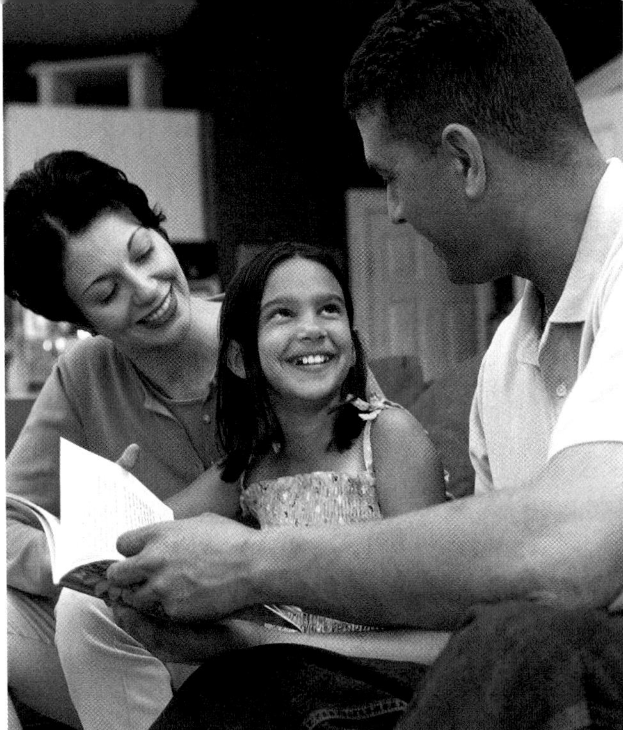

Setting clear boundaries, holding children to high expectations, and responding with warmth to children's needs are all positive parenting strategies.

explain their reasoning and allow children to express themselves. Children of authoritative parents are the most well adjusted and rate particularly high in social competence.

**PERMISSIVE (OR INDULGENT)** Permissive parents do not expect their children to act maturely but instead allow them to follow their own impulses. They are very warm, patient, and accepting, and they are focused on not stifling their child's innate creativity. They use little discipline and are often nontraditional. Children of permissive parents have difficulty with impulse-control, are immature, perform more poorly in school, have more problem behaviors, and take less responsibility for their actions. They also have higher self-esteem, better social skills, and lower levels of depression.

**UNINVOLVED** Uninvolved parents require little from their children and respond with little attention, frequency, or effort. In extreme cases, this style might reach the level of child neglect. Children of uninvolved parents perform worse in all areas measured compared with children of parents using the other styles.

Research across all ethnic groups has found that authoritative parenting has distinct advantages for children and that uninvolved parenting leads to the worst outcomes. Providing a balance of firm limits and clear structure along with high levels of warmth, nurturance, and respect for the child's own special needs and temperament as well as her or his growing independence is the best predictor for raising a healthy child.

**Parenting and the Family Life Cycle** At each stage of the family life cycle, the relationship between parents and children changes. The parents' primary responsibility to a small, helpless baby is to ensure its physical well-being around the clock. As babies grow into toddlers and begin to crawl and walk and talk, they begin to be able to take care of some of their own physical needs. For parents, the challenge at this stage is to strike a balance between giving children the freedom to explore and setting limits that will keep the children safe and secure. As children grow toward adolescence, parents need to give them increasing independence and gradually be willing to let them risk success or failure on their own.

Marital satisfaction for most couples tends to decline somewhat while the children are in school. Reasons include the financial and emotional pressures of a growing family and the increased job and community responsibilities of parents in their thirties, forties, and fifties. Once the last child has left home, marital satisfaction usually increases because the couple have time to enjoy each other once more.

## Single Parents

According to the U.S. Bureau of the Census, about 28% of all children under 18 live with only one parent. In 2003, about 55% of all African American children were living with single parents, as were 30% of Latino children. In single-parent families that are the result of divorce, the mother usually has custody of the children, but about 20% of single-parent families are headed by fathers.

Economic difficulties are the primary problem for single mothers, especially for unmarried mothers who have not finished high school and have difficulty finding work. Divorced mothers usually experience a sharp drop in income the first few years on their own, but if they have job skills or education they usually can eventually support themselves and their children adequately. Other problems for single mothers are the often-conflicting demands of playing both father and mother and the difficulty of satisfying their own needs for adult companionship and affection.

Financial pressures are also a complaint of single fathers, but they do not experience them to the extent that single mothers do. Because they are likely to have less practice than mothers in juggling parental and professional roles, they may worry that they do not spend enough time with their children. Because single fatherhood is not as common as single motherhood, however, the men who choose it are likely to be stable, established, and strongly motivated to be with their children.

Research about the effect on children of growing up in a single-parent family is inconclusive. Evidence seems to indicate that these children tend to have less success in school and in their careers than children from two-parent families, but these effects may be associated more strongly with low educational attainment of the single parent than with the absence of the second parent. Two-parent families are not necessarily better if one of the parents spends little time relating to the children or is physically or emotionally abusive.

## Stepfamilies

Single parenthood is usually a transitional stage: About three out of four divorced women and about four out of five divorced men will ultimately remarry. Rates are lower for widowed men and women, but overall, almost half the marriages in the United States are remarriages for the husband, the wife, or both. If either partner brings children from a previous marriage into the new family unit, a stepfamily (or "blended family") is formed.

Stepfamilies are significantly different from primary families and should not be expected to duplicate the emotions and relationships of a primary family. Research has shown that healthy stepfamilies are less cohesive and more adaptable than healthy primary families; they have a greater capacity to allow for individual differences and accept that biologically related family members will have emotionally closer relationships. Stepfamilies gradually gain more of a sense of being a family as they build a history of shared daily experiences and major life events.

## Successful Families

Family life can be extremely challenging. A strong family is not a family without problems; it's a family that copes successfully with stress and crisis. Many families move through life without a clear direction. Successful families are intentionally more connected—members share experiences and meanings. An excellent way to build strong family ties is to develop family rituals and routines—organized, repeated activities that have meaning for family members. Some of the most common routines identified in research studies are dinnertime, a regular bedtime, and household chores; common rituals include birthdays, Christmas and other holidays, and Sunday activities. You may want to consider incorporating a regular family mealtime into your family routine, as it allows parents and children to develop closer relationships and leads to better parenting, healthier children, and better school performance.

Although there is tremendous variation in American families, researchers have proposed that six major qualities or themes appear in strong families:

1. *Commitment.* The family is very important to its members; sexual fidelity between partners is included in commitment.
2. *Appreciation.* Family members care about one another and express their appreciation. The home is a positive place for family members.
3. *Communication.* Family members spend time listening to one another and enjoying one another's company. They talk about disagreements and attempt to solve problems.
4. *Time together.* Family members do things together, often simple activities that don't cost money.
5. *Spiritual wellness.* The family promotes sharing, love, and compassion for other human beings.
6. *Coping with stress and crisis.* When faced with illness, death, marital conflict, or other crises, family members pull together, seek help, and use other coping strategies to meet the challenge.

It may surprise some people that members of strong families are often seen at counseling centers. They know that the smartest thing to do in some situations is to get help. Many resources are available for individuals and families seeking counseling; people can turn to physicians, clergy, marriage and family counselors, psychologists, or other trained professionals.

Families—and intimate relationships of all kinds—are essential to our overall wellness. A fulfilling life nearly always involves other people. Whether we're single or married, young or old, heterosexual or gay, we continue to need meaningful relationships throughout life.

**Tips for Today**

The fabric of human life is woven from relationships with other people. A wellness lifestyle includes ample time for nourishing relationships with friends, family, and intimate partners. Good communication is the key to keeping all these relationships on track.

*Right now you can*

- Seek out an acquaintance or a new friend and arrange a coffee date to get to know the person a little better.
- Call a parent, sibling, or someone else you love and let him or her know how important the relationship is to you. (Don't wait for a special occasion or a crisis!)
- Think about the last time you experienced conflict with a family member or partner. Identify some ways you might handle such situations better in the future. For example,
  - Be a better listener.
  - Communicate your feelings more clearly.
  - Avoid criticizing or blaming.
  - Be more willing to overlook minor differences.

## SUMMARY

- Successful relationships begin with a positive sense of self and reasonably high self-esteem. Personal identity, gender roles, and styles of attachment are all rooted in childhood experiences.
- The characteristics of friendship include companionship, respect, acceptance, help, trust, loyalty, and reciprocity.

- Love, sex, and commitment are closely linked ideals in intimate relationships. Love includes trust, caring, respect, and loyalty.
- Common challenges in relationships relate to issues of self-disclosure, commitment, expectations, competitiveness, balancing time spent together and apart, and jealousy. Partners in successful relationships have strong communication skills and support each other in difficult times.
- The keys to good communication in relationships are self-disclosure, listening, and feedback. Conflict is inevitable in intimate relationships; partners need to have constructive ways to negotiate their differences.
- Most Americans find partners through dating or getting together in groups. Cohabitation is a growing social pattern that allows partners to get to know each other intimately without being married.
- Gay and lesbian partnerships are similar to heterosexual partnerships, with some differences.
- Marriage fulfills many functions for individuals and society. It can provide people with affection, affirmation, and sexual fulfillment; a context for child rearing; and the promise of lifelong companionship.
- Love isn't enough to ensure a successful marriage. Partners have to be realistic, feel good about each other, have communication and conflict-resolution skills, share values, and have a balance of individual and joint interests.
- When problems can't be worked out, people often separate and divorce. Divorce is traumatic for all involved, especially children, but the negative effects are usually balanced in time by positive ones.
- Factors couples should consider when deciding whether to have children include physical health; financial circumstances; relationship between partners; educational, career, and child care plans; and emotional and social readiness for parenthood.
- Four general parenting styles are authoritarian, authoritative, permissive, and uninvolved; the authoritative style is usually associated with the best outcomes.
- At each stage of the family life cycle, relationships change. Marital satisfaction may be lower during the child-rearing years and higher later.
- Many families today are single-parent families or stepfamilies.
- Important qualities of successful families include commitment to the family, appreciation of family members, communication, time spent together, spiritual wellness, and effective methods of dealing with stress.

## Take Action

1. **Survey your friends.** Take an informal survey among your friends of what they find attractive in a member of the other sex and what they look for in a romantic partner. Are there substantial differences between people's responses? Do men and women look for different things?

2. **Find out how times have changed.** Ask your parents what their experiences of dating and courtship were like. How are they different from your experiences? What do your parents think of current customs?

3. **Reach out to others in your community.** Consider volunteering in your community to help promote successful families. Investigate opportunities such as youth-mentoring organizations like Big Brothers Big Sisters. Positive one-on-one relationships with youth have significant positive effects on you, the child you mentor, and the community as a whole.

## For More Information

For resources in your area, check your campus directory for a counseling center or peer counseling program, or check the agencies listed in the Mental Health section of the phone book.

### Books

Brooks, J. B. 2004. *The Process of Parenting,* 6th ed. New York: McGraw-Hill. *Demonstrates how parents and caregivers can translate their love and concern for children into effective parenting behavior.*

DeGenova, M. K., and F. P. Rice. 2005. *Intimate Relationships, Marriages, and Families,* 6th ed. New York: McGraw-Hill. *A comprehensive introduction to relationships.*

Gottman, J., and J. Declaire. 2002. *The Relationship Cure: A Five-Step Guide to Strengthening Your Marriage, Family, and Friendships.* New York: Three Rivers Press. *Provides research-based tools for improving communication and relationships.*

Olson, D., and J. DeFrain. 2006. *Marriages and Families: Intimacy, Diversity, and Strengths,* 5th ed. New York: McGraw-Hill. *A comprehensive introduction to relationships and families.*

### Organizations and Web Sites

*American Association for Marriage and Family Therapy.* Provides information on a variety of relationship issues and referrals to therapists.

202-452-0109
http://www.aamft.org

*Association for Couples in Marriage Enrichment (ACME).* An organization that promotes activities to strengthen marriage; a resource for books, tapes, and other materials.

800-634-8325
http://www.bettermarriages.org

*Family Education Network.* Provides information about education, safety, health, and other family-related issues.

http://www.familyeducation.com

*Go Ask Alice.* Professional and peer educators provide answers to questions on many topics relating to interpersonal relationships and communication.

http://www.goaskalice.columbia.edu

*Life Innovations.* Provides materials for premarital counseling and marital enrichment.

800-331-1661

http://www.lifeinnovation.com

*Parents Without Partners (PWP).* Provides educational programs, literature, and support groups for single parents and their children. Call for a referral to a local chapter.

800-637-7974

http://www.parentswithoutpartners.org

*Student Counseling Virtual Pamphlet Collection.* Provides links to pamphlets produced by different student counseling centers; topics include relationships, sexual orientation, and assertiveness.

http://counseling.uchicago.edu/vpc

*United States Census Bureau.* Provides current statistics on births, marriages, and living arrangements.

http://www.census.gov

*Whole Family Center.* Provides information on all types of family relationships; the site includes an online magazine and examples of real-life dramas for teens, couples, and parents.

http://www.wholefamily.com

*Yahoo/Lesbians, Gays, and Bisexuals.* A Web site and search engine that contains many links to information and support for lesbians and gays.

http://dir.yahoo.com/society_and_culture/cultures_and_groups

See also the listings for Chapters 3 and 5.

## Selected Bibliography


Associated Press. 2004. *Voters in 11 States Reject Gay Marriage* (http://www.nytimes.com/aponline/national/AP-ELN-Gay-Marriage.html; retrieved November 3, 2004).

Bauserman, R. 2002. Child adjustment in joint-custody versus sole-custody arrangements: A meta-analytic review. *Journal of Family Psychology* 16(1): 91–102.

Bookwala, J. 2005. The role of marital quality in physical health during the mature years. *Journal of Aging and Health* 17(1): 85–104.

Centers for Disease Control and Prevention. 2004. Marital status and health: United States, 1999–2002. *Advance Data from Vital and Health Statistics,* No. 351.

Columbia University Health Education Program. 2002. *Go Ask Alice: Looking for Love Online* (http://www.goaskalice.columbia.edu/1185.html; retrieved February 17, 2003).

Darling, N. 1999. *Parenting Style and Its Correlates* (http://www.athealth.com/Practitioner/ceduc/parentingstyles.html; retrieved November 3, 2004).

Denton, W. H., et al. 2001. Cardiovascular reactivity and initiate/avoid patterns of marital communication: A test of Gottman's psychophysiologic model of marital interaction. *Journal of Behavioral Medicine* 24(5): 401–421.

Fiese, B. H., et al. 2002. A review of 50 years of research on naturally occurring family routines and rituals: Cause for celebration? *Journal of Family Psychology* 16(4): 381–390.

Gallo, L. C., et al. 2003. Marital status and quality in middle-aged women: Associations with levels and trajectories of cardiovascular risk factors. *Health Psychology* 22(5): 453–463.

Goodman, R. F., and A. Gurian. 2001. *Parenting Styles/Children's Temperaments: The Match* (http://www.Aboutourkids.org; retrieved October 14, 2004).

Harris, C. R. 2002. Sexual and romantic jealousy in heterosexual and homosexual adults. *Psychological Science* 13(1): 7–12.

Heller, P. E., and B. Wood. 2000. The influence of religious and ethnic differences on marital intimacy: Intermarriage versus intramarriage. *Journal of Marital and Family Therapy* 26(2): 241–252.

Human Rights Campaign. 2004. *Statewide Marriage Laws* (http://www.hrc.org; retrieved November 3, 2004).

Lucas, R. E. 2003. Reexaming adaptation and the set point model of happiness: Reactions to changes in marital status. *Journal of Personality and Social Psychology* 84(3): 537–539.

Marech, R. 2005. The battle over same-sex marriage: One year later both sides claim victory, but courts will decide. *San Francisco Chronicle,* February 12.

McKinney, L. C., and L. S. Newman. 2002. Anticipating responses to one's own misdeeds: Repressive coping and the prediction of others' reactions to inconsiderate behavior. *Journal of Social and Clinical Psychology* 21(4): 427–440.

Mookadam, F., and H. M. Arthur. 2004. Social support and its relationship to morbidity and mortality after acute myocardial infarction: Systematic overview. *Archives of Internal Medicine* 164(14): 1514–1518.

Murray, S. L., et al. 2003. Once hurt, twice hurtful: How perceived regard regulates daily marital interactions. *Journal of Personality and Social Psychology* 84(1): 126–147.

Najib, A., et al. 2004. Regional brain activity in women grieving a romantic relationship breakup. *American Journal of Psychiatry* 161(12): 2245–2256.

National Center for Health Statistics. 2002. *Cohabitation, Marriage, Divorce, and Remarriage in the United States.* Vital and Health Statistics, Series 23, Number 22.

Olson, D., and J. DeFrain. 2006. *Marriages and Families,* 5th ed. New York: McGraw-Hill.

Online NewsHour. 2004. *The Battle Over Same-Sex Marriage: Expert Debate* (http://www.pbs.org/newshour/bb/law/gay_marriage/q3.html; retrieved November 1, 2004).

Strong, B., et al. 2005. *Human Sexuality: Diversity in Contemporary America,* 5th ed. New York: McGraw-Hill.

Suler, J. 1997. *The Final Showdown Between In-Person and Cyberspace Relationships* (http://www1.rider.edu/users/suler/psycyber/showdown.html; retrieved August 28, 2000).

Tower, R. B., S. V. Kasl, and A. S. Darefsky. 2002. Types of marital closeness and mortality risk in older couples. *Psychosomatic Medicine* 64(4): 644–659.

Wainright, J. L., S. T. Russell, and C. J. Patterson. 2004. Psychosocial adjustment, school outcomes, and romantic relationships of adolescents with same-sex parents. *Child Development* 75(6): 1886–1898.

Whisman, M. A., L. A. Uebelacker, and L. M. Weinstock. 2004. Psychopathology and marital satisfaction: the importance of evaluating both partners. *Journal of Consulting and Clinical Psychology* 72(5): 830–838.

White, L., and J. G. Gilbreth. 2001. When children have two fathers: Effects of relationships with stepfathers and noncustodial fathers on adolescent outcomes. *Journal of Marriage and the Family* 63(1): 155–167.

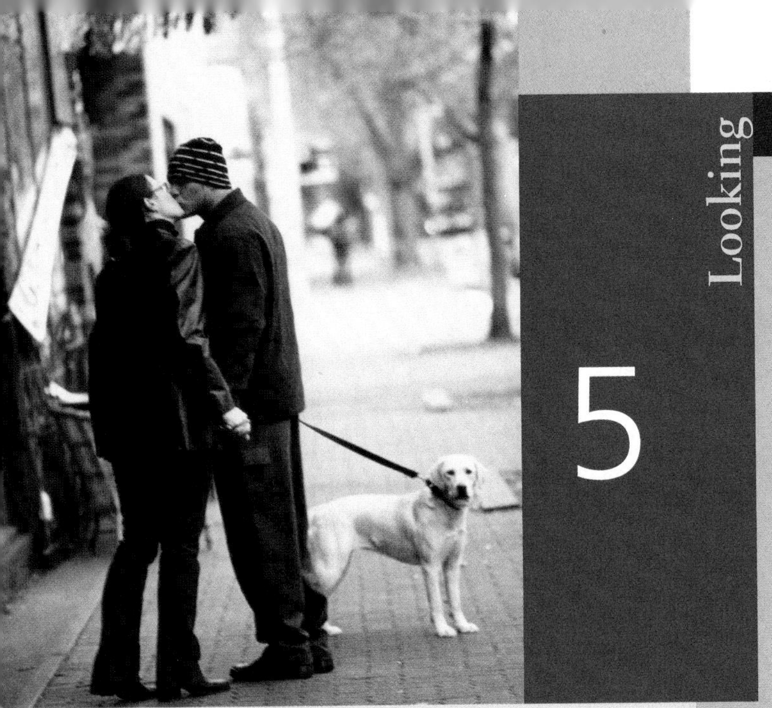

5

## Looking AHEAD

After reading this chapter, you should be able to

- Describe the structure and function of the female and male sex organs
- Explain the changes in sexual functioning that occur across the life span and the various ways human sexuality can be expressed
- Describe guidelines for safe, responsible sexual behavior
- Describe the physical and emotional changes a pregnant woman typically experiences, and discuss the stages of fetal development
- List the important components of good prenatal care
- Describe the process of labor and delivery

# Sexuality, Pregnancy, and Childbirth

Humans are sexual beings. Sexual activity is the source of our most intense physical pleasures, a central ingredient in many of our intimate emotional relationships, and, of course, the key to the reproduction of our species.

**Sexuality** is more than just sexual behavior. It includes biological sex (being biologically male or female), gender (masculine and feminine behaviors), sexual anatomy and physiology, sexual functioning and practices, and social and sexual interactions with others. Our individual sense of identity is powerfully influenced by our sexuality. We think of ourselves in very fundamental ways as male or female; as heterosexual or homosexual; as single, attached, married, or divorced. Sexuality is a complex, interacting group of inborn, biological characteristics and acquired behaviors people learn in the course of growing up in a particular family, community, and society.

Decisions about sexuality have far-reaching consequences. Understanding the basic facts about sexuality, pregnancy, and childbirth will help you make intelligent, informed decisions that are right for you.

## SEXUAL ANATOMY

In spite of their different appearances, the sex organs of men and women arise from the same structures and fulfill similar functions. Each person has a pair of **gonads**; ovaries are the female gonads, and testes are the male gonads. The gonads produce **germ cells** and sex hormones. The germ cells are ova (eggs) in females and sperm in males. Ova and sperm are the basic units of reproduction; their union results in the creation of a new life.

### Terms

**sexuality** A dimension of personality shaped by biological, psychosocial, and cultural forces and concerning all aspects of sexual behavior.

**gonads** The primary reproductive organs that produce germ cells and sex hormones; the ovaries and testes.

**germ cells** Sperm and ova (eggs).

Vw

**Vw Visit the *Core Concepts in Health* Online Learning Center (www.mhhe.com/inselbrief10e) for study aids and many additional resources.**

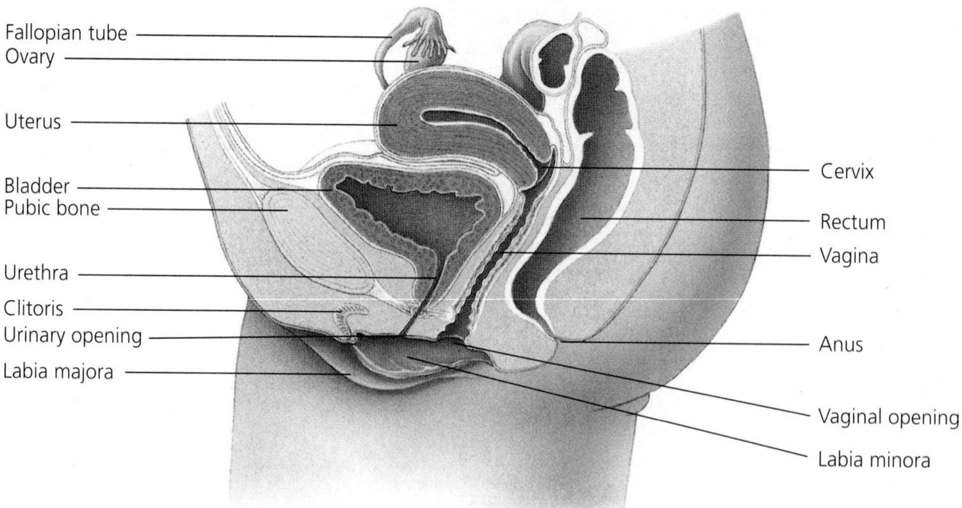


**Figure 5-1 The female sex organs.**

## Female Sex Organs

The external sex organs, or genitals, of the female are called the **vulva** (Figure 5-1). The mons pubis, a rounded mass of fatty tissue over the pubic bone, becomes covered with hair during puberty (biological maturation). Below it are two paired folds of skin called the labia majora (major lips) and the labia minora (minor lips). Enclosed within are the clitoris, the opening of the urethra, and the opening of the vagina. The **clitoris** is highly sensitive to touch and plays an important role in female sexual arousal and orgasm.

The female urethra leads directly from the urinary bladder to its opening between the clitoris and the opening of the vagina; it conducts urine from the bladder to the outside of the body. Unlike the male urethra, it is independent of the genitals.

The vaginal opening is partially covered by the hymen. This membrane can be stretched or torn during athletic activity or when a woman has sexual intercourse for the first time. The idea that an intact hymen is the sign of a virgin is a myth. The **vagina** is the passage that leads to the internal reproductive organs. It is the female structure for heterosexual sexual intercourse and also serves as the birth canal. Its soft, flexible walls are normally in contact with each other.

Projecting into the upper part of the vagina is the **cervix,** the neck of the uterus. Inside the pear-shaped **uterus,** which slants forward above the bladder, the fertilized egg is implanted and grows into a *fetus*. A pair of *fallopian tubes* (or *oviducts*) extend from the top of the uterus. The end of each oviduct surrounds an **ovary** and guides the mature ovum down into the uterus after the egg bursts from its follicle on the surface of the ovary.

## Male Sex Organs

A man's external sex organs, or genitals, are the penis and the scrotum (Figure 5-2). The **penis** consists of spongy tissue that becomes engorged with blood during sexual excitement, causing the organ to enlarge and become erect. The **scrotum** is a pouch that contains a pair of **testes.** The purpose of the scrotum is to maintain the testes at a temperature approximately 5°F below that of the rest of the body. The process of sperm production is extremely heat-sensitive. In hot temperatures the muscles in the scrotum relax, and the testes move away from the heat of the body. Through the entire length of the penis runs the urethra, which can carry both urine and *semen,* the sperm-carrying fluid, to the opening at the tip of the glans. Although urine and semen share a common passage, they are prevented from mixing together by muscles that control their entry into the urethra.

The testes contain tightly packed seminiferous tubules within which sperm are produced. These tubules end in a maze of ducts that flow into a single storage tube called the *epididymis,* on the surface of each testis. This tube leads to the *vas deferens,* a tube that rises into the abdominal cavity. Inside the prostate gland, the two vasa deferentia join the ducts of the two *seminal vesicles,* whose secretions provide nutrients to semen. The *prostate gland* produces some of the fluid in semen that nourishes and transports sperm. The tubes of the seminal vesicle and the vas deferens on each side lead to the *ejaculatory duct,* which joins the urethra. The *Cowper's glands* (bulbourethral glands) are two small structures flanking the urethra. During sexual arousal, these glands secrete a clear, mucuslike fluid that appears at the tip of the penis. The exact purpose of preejaculatory fluid is not known, but in some men, it may contain sperm, so withdrawal of the penis before ejaculation is not a reliable form of contraception.

**Circumcision** The smooth, rounded tip of the penis is the highly sensitive **glans,** an important component in

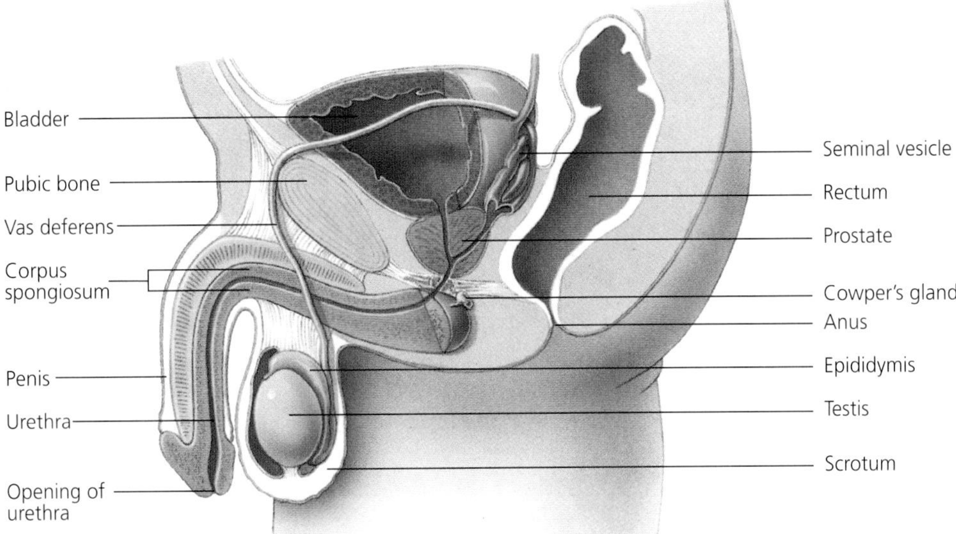


**Figure 5-2 The male sex organs.**

sexual arousal. The glans is partially covered by the foreskin, or prepuce, a retractable fold of skin that is removed by **circumcision** in about 60–70% of newborn males in the United States. Circumcision is performed for cultural, religious, and hygienic reasons, and rates of circumcision vary widely among different groups. Worldwide, the rate is about 20%. Most Europeans, Asians, South and Central Americans, and Africans do not perform circumcision; Jews and Muslims are the major groups who circumcise for religious reasons.

The pros and cons of this simple procedure have been widely debated. Citing research findings, proponents argue that it promotes cleanliness and reduces the risk of urinary tract infections (UTIs) in newborns and the risk of sexually transmitted diseases (STDs), including HIV, later in life. STD education and the practice of abstinence or low-risk sexual behaviors have a far greater impact on the transmission of STDs than does circumcision.

Opponents of circumcision state that it is an unnecessary surgical procedure that causes pain and puts a baby at risk for complications. They also argue that, by removing the foreskin, circumcision exposes the glans of the penis to constant irritation by clothing, thereby reducing its sensitivity; research into this issue has been inconclusive. Two studies of adult men who were circumsized for medical reasons found an increase in sexual activity and sexual satisfaction, but in the larger of the two studies, reduced erectile function and decreased penile sensitivity were also reported.

In part because the overall risk of infant UTIs is low, the American Academy of Pediatrics (AAP) takes the position (opposed by some physicians) that although circumcision has potential medical benefits, the research is not sufficient to recommend the procedure routinely. When circumcision is performed, the AAP recommends that painkilling medication be provided.

## HORMONES AND THE REPRODUCTIVE LIFE CYCLE

Many cultural and personal factors help shape the expression of your sexuality. But biology also plays an important role, particularly through the action of *hormones*, chemical messengers that are secreted directly into the bloodstream by the **endocrine glands.** The sex hormones produced by the ovaries or testes have a major influence on the

### Terms

VW

**vulva** The external female genitals, or sex organs.

**clitoris** The highly sensitive female genital structure.

**vagina** The passage leading from the female genitals to the internal reproductive organs; the birth canal.

**cervix** The end of the uterus opening toward the vagina.

**uterus** The hollow, thick-walled, muscular organ in which the fertilized egg develops; the womb.

**ovary** One of two female reproductive glands that produce ova (eggs) and sex hormones; ovaries are the female gonads.

**penis** The male genital structure consisting of spongy tissue that becomes engorged with blood during sexual excitement.

**scrotum** The loose sac of skin and muscle fibers that contains the testes.

**testis** One of two male gonads, the site of sperm production; plural, *testes.* Also called *testicle.*

**glans** The rounded head of the penis or the clitoris.

**circumcision** Surgical removal of the foreskin of the penis.

**endocrine glands** Glands that produce hormones.

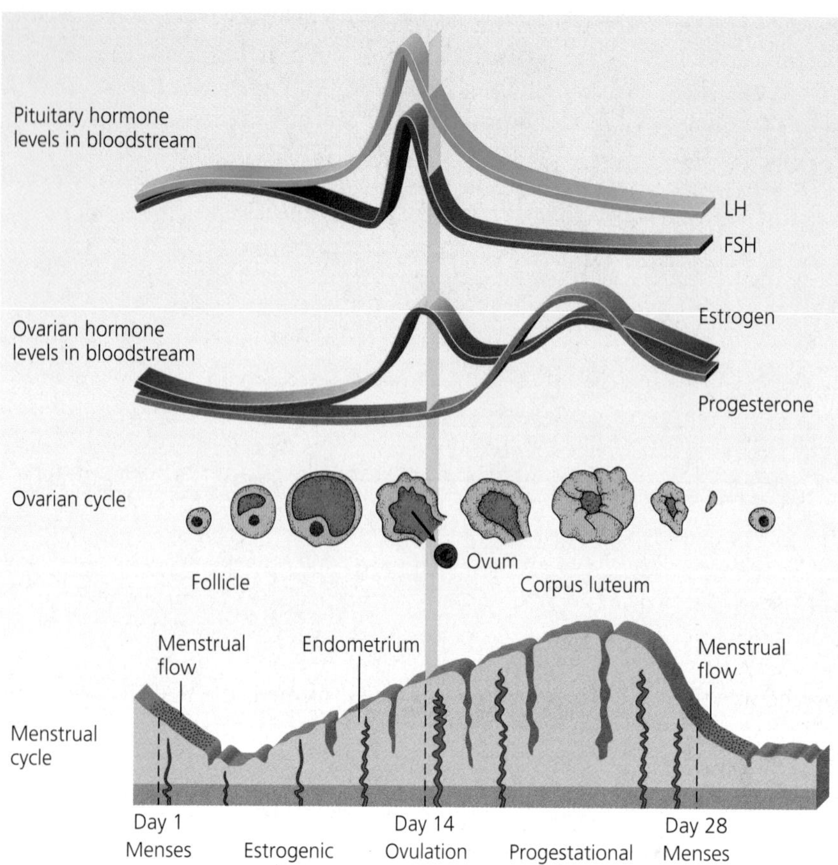


**Figure 5-3 The menstrual cycle.** The anterior pituitary releases FSH and LH, which stimulate the ovarian follicle to develop and release a mature egg. The ovarian follicle releases estrogen and progesterone, which stimulate the endometrium to continue to develop so that it will be ready to receive and nourish a fertilized egg. Unless pregnancy occurs, ovarian hormone levels fall and the endometrium sloughs off (menses).

development and function of the reproductive system throughout life. The sex hormones made by the testes are called **androgens,** the most important of which is *testosterone*. The female sex hormones, produced by the ovaries, belong to two groups: **estrogens** and **progestins,** the most important of which is *progesterone*. The cortex of the **adrenal glands** also produces androgens in both males and females.

The hormones produced by the testes, the ovaries, and the adrenal glands are regulated by the hormones of the **pituitary gland,** located at the base of the brain. This gland in turn is controlled by hormones produced by the **hypothalamus** in the brain. Sex hormones exert their primary developmental influences first in the embryo stage and later during adolescence.

## Female Sexual Maturation

Although humans are fully sexually differentiated at birth, the differences between males and females are accentuated at **puberty,** the period during which the reproductive system matures, secondary sex characteristics develop, and the bodies of males and females come to appear more distinctive. The changes of puberty are induced by **testosterone** in the male and estrogen and **progesterone** in the female.

**Physical Changes** The first sign of puberty in girls is breast development, followed by a rounding of the hips and buttocks. As the breasts develop, hair appears in the pubic region and later in the underarms. Shortly after the onset of breast development, girls show an increase in growth rate. Breast development usually begins between ages 8 and 13, and the time of rapid body growth occurs between ages 9 and 15.

**The Menstrual Cycle** A major landmark of puberty for young women is the onset of the **menstrual cycle,** the monthly ovarian cycle that leads to menstruation (loss of blood and tissue lining the uterus) in the absence of pregnancy. The timing of *menarche,* or the first *menstrual period,* occurs at about the age of 12.1–12.7 years in the United States, but it may also normally start several years earlier or later.

The menstrual cycle consists of four phases: (1) menses, (2) the estrogenic phase, (3) ovulation, and (4) the progestational phase (Figure 5-3). The day of the onset of bleeding is considered to be day 1 of the cycle. For the purposes of our discussion, a cycle of 28 days will be used; however, normal cycles vary in length.

During menses, characterized by the menstrual flow, blood levels of hormones from the ovaries and the anterior pituitary gland are relatively low. This phase of the cycle usually lasts from day 1 to about day 5.

The estrogenic phase begins when the menstrual flow ceases and the anterior pituitary begins to produce increasing amounts of follicle-stimulating hormone (FSH) and luteinizing hormone (LH). Under the influence of FSH, an egg-containing ovarian *follicle* begins to mature, producing increasingly higher amounts of estrogens. Stimulated by estrogen, the *endometrium,* the uterine lining, thickens with large numbers of blood vessels and uterine glands.

A surge of a potent estrogen called *estradiol* from the follicle causes the anterior pituitary to release a large burst of LH and a smaller amount of FSH. The high concentration of LH stimulates the developing follicle to release its ovum. This event is known as *ovulation.* After ovulation, the follicle is transformed into the **corpus luteum,** which produces progesterone and estrogen. Ovulation usually occurs about 14 days prior to the onset of menstrual flow.

During the progestational phase of the cycle, the amount of progesterone secreted from the corpus luteum increases and remains high until the onset of the next menses. Under the influence of estrogen and progesterone, the endometrium continues to develop, readying itself to receive and nourish a fertilized ovum. When pregnancy occurs, the fertilized egg produces the hormone human chorionic gonadotropin (HCG), which maintains the corpus luteum. Thus, levels of ovarian hormones remain high and the uterine lining is preserved, preventing menses.

If pregnancy does not occur, the corpus luteum degenerates, and estrogen and progesterone levels gradually fall. Below certain hormonal levels, the endometrium can no longer be maintained, and it begins to slough off, initiating menses. As the levels of ovarian hormones fall, a rise in LH and FSH occurs, and a new cycle begins.

**MENSTRUAL PROBLEMS** Menstruation is a normal biological process, but it may cause physical or psychological problems. *Dysmenorrhea* is characterized by cramps in the lower abdomen, backache, vomiting, nausea, a bloated feeling, diarrhea, and loss of appetite. Some of these symptoms can be attributed to uterine muscular contractions caused by chemicals called *prostaglandins.* Any drug that blocks the effects of prostaglandins, such as aspirin or ibuprofen, will usually alleviate some of the symptoms of dysmenorrhea.

Many women experience transient physical and emotional symptoms prior to the onset of their menstrual flow. Depending on their severity, these symptoms may be categorized along a continuum: **premenstrual tension, premenstrual syndrome (PMS),** and **premenstrual dysphoric disorder (PMDD).** Premenstrual tension symptoms are mild and may include negative mood changes and physical symptoms such as abdominal cramping and backache. More severe symptoms are classified as PMS; very severe symptoms that cause impairment in social functioning and work-related activities are classified as PMDD. All three conditions share a definite pattern: Symptoms appear prior to the onset of menses and disappear within a few days after the start of menstruation. As many as 75% of women report some discomfort prior to the onset of menses, 20–50% of women experience PMS symptoms, and 3–10% meet the criteria for PMDD.

Symptoms associated with PMS and PMDD include physical changes such as breast tenderness, water retention (bloating), headache, and fatigue; insomnia or excessive sleep; appetite changes and food cravings; irritability, anger, and increased interpersonal conflict; mood swings;

## Terms

**androgens** Male sex hormones produced by the testes in males and by the adrenal glands in both sexes.

**estrogens** A class of female sex hormones, produced by the ovaries, that bring about sexual maturation at puberty and maintain reproductive functions.

**progestins** A class of female sex hormones, produced by the ovaries, that sustain reproductive functions.

**adrenal glands** Endocrine glands, located over the kidneys, that produce androgens (among other hormones).

**pituitary gland** An endocrine gland at the base of the brain that produces follicle-stimulating hormone (FSH) and luteinizing hormone (LH), among others.

**hypothalamus** A region of the brain above the pituitary gland whose hormones control the secretions of the pituitary; also involved in the nervous control of sexual functions.

**puberty** The period of biological maturation during adolescence.

**testosterone** The most important androgen (male sex hormone); stimulates an embryo to develop into a male and induces the development of male secondary sex characteristics during puberty.

**progesterone** The most important progestin (female sex hormone); induces the development of female secondary sex characteristics during puberty, regulates the menstrual cycle, and sustains pregnancy.

**menstrual cycle** The monthly ovarian cycle, regulated by pituitary and ovarian hormones; in the absence of pregnancy, menstruation occurs.

**corpus luteum** The part of the ovarian follicle left after ovulation, which secretes estrogen and progesterone during the second half of the menstrual cycle.

**premenstrual tension** Mild physical and emotional changes associated with the time before the onset of menses; symptoms can include abdominal cramping and backache.

**premenstrual syndrome (PMS)** A disorder characterized by physical discomfort, psychological distress, and behavioral changes that begin after ovulation and cease when menstruation begins.

**premenstrual dysphoric disorder (PMDD)** Severe form of PMS, characterized by symptoms serious enough to interfere with work or school or with social activities and relationships.

Vw

Critical Consumer

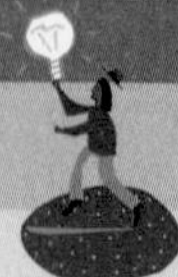

## Dietary Supplements and PMS

VW

Many dietary supplements have been promoted for relief of the symptoms of PMS; those described below are among the most commonly advocated compounds. Only one, calcium, has been shown to provide relief in rigorous clinical studies; several others show promise, but more research is needed.

- *Calcium.* Blood calcium levels are lower during the premenstrual period, and careful research studies have shown calcium supplements to be effective at relieving symptoms of PMS. (A large study showed that 48% of women taking calcium experienced relief, compared to 30% taking a placebo. Although this rate is lower than that for women taking prescription medications such as SSRIs, calcium does offer relief for some women.) The amount of calcium taken by women in these studies, 1000–1200 mg per day, is within accepted safety limits for calcium intake and may also be beneficial for building and maintaining bone density.

- *Magnesium.* Levels of magnesium in certain body cells are lower in women with PMS, and magnesium is involved in neurotransmitter activity. Some small studies have found magnesium to be effective in relieving PMS symptoms; however, a more recent study found that the only effect was a decrease in fluid retention. Magnesium supplements can cause side effects, including diarrhea, in some people and so should be used with caution.

- *Vitamin B-6.* Vitamin B-6 plays an important role in the synthesis of neurotransmitters, so taking supplements of vitamin B-6 may help reduce mood-related symptoms of PMS. Doses in the accepted range of 50–100 mg per day may produce a very mild benefit. Care should be taken, however, because long-term use of high doses of vitamin B-6 can cause permanent nerve damage.

- *Vitamin E.* Although the mechanism is unclear, one study found that vitamin E supplements may improve PMS symptoms.

- *Carbohydrates.* Some women with PMS report craving carbohydrate-rich foods, a change in diet that may actually improve the mood-related symptoms of PMS. Increased intake of carbohydrates may increase blood levels of tryptophan, an amino acid the body uses to produce the neurotransmitter serotonin. Although some dietary supplements containing mixtures of carbohydrates have been marketed for PMS symptoms, it is unclear whether these are any more effective than changing the diet to include more carbohydrate-rich fruits, vegetables, and grains.

SOURCES: American Academy of Family Physicians. 2004. *PMS: What You Can Do to Ease Your Symptoms* (http://familydoctor.org/141.xml; retrieved November 8, 2004); Elliot, H. 2002. Premenstrual dysphoric disorder: A guide for the treating physician. *North Carolina Medical Journal* 63: 72–75; Bendich, A. 2000. Review: The potential for dietary supplements to reduce premenstrual syndrome (PMS) symptoms. *Journal of the American College of Nutrition* 19(1): 3–12.

depression and sadness; anxiety and tearfulness; inability to concentrate; social withdrawal; and the sense that one is out of control or overwhelmed. The key to diagnosing PMS and PMDD is to keep a daily diary of symptoms over several menstrual cycles. PMDD is distinguished from PMS by the severity of symptoms, which in PMDD interfere significantly with work or school and with usual social activities and relationships.

Despite many research studies, the causes of PMS and PMDD are still unknown, and there are no completely effective therapies. Selective serotonin reuptake inhibitors (SSRIs), including Sarafem, Zoloft, Paxil, and Celexa, are the first-line treatment for PMDD. Until recently, women using SSRIs took the medication throughout the entire menstrual cycle, but it has now been shown that taking the medication during just the progestational phase of the cycle is similarly effective. Other drug treatments include estrogen, certain oral contraceptives, diuretics to minimize water retention, and drugs such as aspirin, ibuprofen, and more potent prescription prostaglandin inhibitors that block the effects of prostaglandins. A number of vitamins, minerals, and other dietary supplements have also been studied for PMS relief; see the box "Dietary Supplements and PMS" for more information.

Certain lifestyle changes are often recommended to help prevent or minimize symptoms of PMS and PMDD:

- *Limit salt intake.* Salt promotes water retention and bloating. Avoid salty foods.
- *Exercise.* Women who exercise experience fewer symptoms both before and after their menstrual periods.
- *Don't use alcohol or tobacco.* Alcohol and tobacco may aggravate certain symptoms of PMS and PMDD.
- *Eat a nutritious diet.* Choose a low-fat diet rich in complex carbohydrates from vegetables, fruits, and whole-grain breads, cereals, and pasta. Obtain an adequate calcium intake from calcium-rich foods and, if needed, supplements. Minimize your intake of sugar and caffeine, and avoid chocolate, which is rich in both.
- *Relax.* Stress reduction is always beneficial, and stressful events can trigger PMS symptoms. Try relaxation techniques during the premenstrual time.

If symptoms persist, keep a daily diary to track both the types of symptoms you experience and their severity. See your physician for an evaluation and to learn more about treatments that are available only with a prescription.

### Male Sexual Maturation

Reproductive maturation of boys occurs about 2 years later than that of girls; it usually begins at about age 10 or 11. Physical changes include enlargement of the testes, development of pubic hair, growth of the penis, the onset of ejaculation (usually at about age 11 or 12), deepening of the voice, the appearance of facial hair, and a period of rapid growth.

### Aging and Human Sexuality

Changes in hormone production and sexual functioning occur as we age. As a woman approaches age 50, her ovaries gradually cease to function and she enters **menopause,** the cessation of menstruation. For some women, the associated drop in hormone production causes symptoms that are troublesome. The most common physical symptom of menopause is hot flashes, sensations of warmth rising to the face from the upper chest, with or without perspiration and chills. Other symptoms include headaches, dizziness, palpitations, and joint pains. Osteoporosis—decreasing bone density—can develop, making older women more vulnerable to fractures. Some menopausal women become moody, even markedly depressed, and they may also experience fatigue, irritability, and forgetfulness.

To alleviate the symptoms of menopause and reduce the risk of heart disease and osteoporosis, millions of women have been prescribed hormone replacement therapy (HRT), a regimen of hormones that includes estrogen and progesterone. In the summer of 2002, an ongoing study of HRT involving more than 16,000 women was halted because the women taking HRT for long periods suffered more strokes, heart attacks, and blood clots and had a higher incidence of breast cancer than women in the study taking a placebo. The risks for such health problems were small but significant enough to halt the study. The positive findings from this study were a reduction in hip fractures and a reduced risk of colon cancer among the women taking HRT. As a result of these findings, women taking HRT were advised to consult their health care providers about their personal risks and benefits.

In men, testosterone production gradually decreases with age. This drop is associated with a loss of energy, depressed mood, decreased sex drive, erectile dysfunction, decreased muscle mass and osteoporosis. As men get older, they depend more on direct physical stimulation for sexual arousal. They take longer to achieve an erection and find it more difficult to maintain; orgasmic contractions are less intense.

As women and men age, sexual activity can continue to be a source of pleasure and satisfaction for them. A recent survey found that nearly half of all Americans age 60 or older engage in sexual activity at least once a month.

## SEXUAL FUNCTIONING

In this section, we discuss sexual physiology—how the sex organs function during sexual activity—and problems that can occur with sexual functioning.

### Sexual Stimulation

Sexual excitement can come from many sources, both physical and psychological. Although physical stimuli have an obvious and direct effect, some people believe psychological stimuli—thoughts, fantasies, desires, perceptions—are even more powerfully erotic.

**Physical Stimulation** Physical stimulation comes through the senses: We are aroused by things we see, hear, taste, smell, and feel. The most obvious and effective physical stimulation is touching. Even though culturally defined practices vary and individual people have different preferences, most sexual encounters eventually involve some form of touching with hands, lips, and body surfaces. Kissing, caressing, fondling, and hugging are as much a part of sexual encounters as they are of expressing affection.

The most intense form of stimulation by touching involves the genitals. The clitoris and the glans of the penis are particularly sensitive to such stimulation. Other highly responsive areas include the vaginal opening, the nipples, the breasts, the insides of the thighs, the buttocks, the anal region, the scrotum, the lips, and the earlobes. Such sexually sensitive areas, or **erogenous zones,** are especially susceptible to sexual arousal for most people, most of the time. Often, though, what determines the response is not *what* is touched but how, for how long, and by whom. Under the right circumstances, touching any part of the body can cause sexual arousal.

**Psychological Stimulation** Sexual arousal also has an important psychological component, regardless of the nature of the physical stimulation. Fantasies, ideas, memories of past experiences, and mood can all generate sexual excitement. Arousal is also powerfully influenced by emotions. How you feel about a person and how the person feels about you matter tremendously in how sexually responsive you are likely to be. Even the most direct

**Terms**

**menopause** The cessation of menstruation, occurring gradually around age 50.

**erogenous zone** Any region of the body highly responsive to sexual stimulation.

VIW

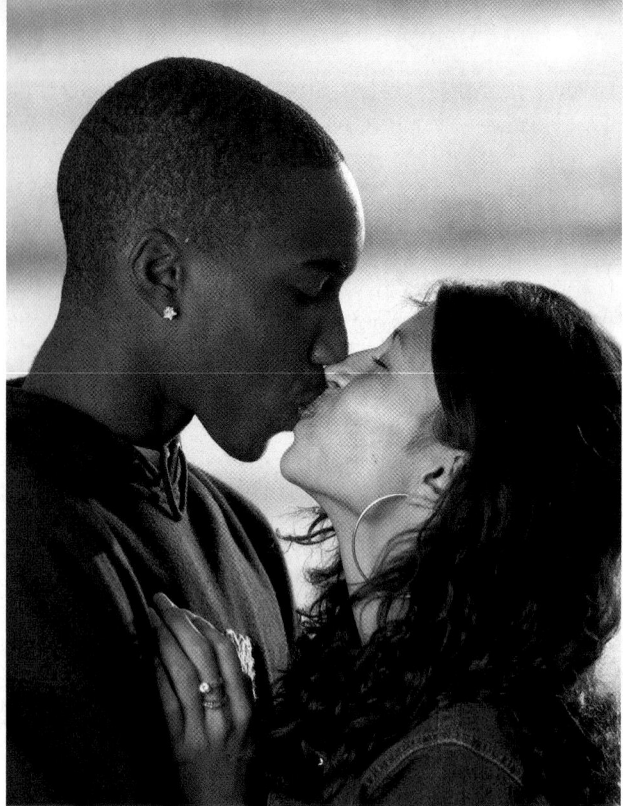

Human sexuality is not just a matter of bodies responding to each other. This couple's physical experiences together will be powerfully affected by their emotions, ideas, and values and by the quality of their relationship.

forms of physical stimulation carry emotional overtones. Kissing, caressing, and fondling express affection and caring. The emotional charge they give to a sexual interaction is at least as significant to sexual arousal as the purely physical stimulation achieved by touching.

## The Sexual Response Cycle

Noted sex researchers William Masters and Virginia Johnson were the first to describe in detail the human sexual response cycle. Men and women respond physiologically with a predictable set of reactions, regardless of the nature of the stimulation.

Two physiological mechanisms explain most genital and bodily reactions during sexual arousal and orgasm. These mechanisms are vasocongestion and myotonia. **Vasocongestion** is the engorgement of tissues that results when more blood flows into an organ than is flowing out. Thus, the penis becomes erect on the same principle that makes a garden hose become stiff when the water is turned on. **Myotonia** is increased muscular tension, which culminates in rhythmical muscular contractions during orgasm.

Four phases characterize the sexual response cycle:

1. In the *excitement phase,* the penis becomes erect as its tissues become engorged with blood. The testes expand and are pulled upward within the scrotum. In women, the clitoris and the labia are similarly engorged with blood, and the vaginal walls become moist with lubricating fluid.

2. The *plateau phase* is an extension of the excitement phase. Reactions become more marked. In men, the penis becomes harder, and the testes become larger. In women, the lower part of the vagina swells, as its upper end expands and vaginal lubrication increases.

3. In the *orgasmic phase,* or **orgasm,** rhythmic contractions occur along the man's penis, urethra, prostate gland, seminal vesicles, and muscles in the pelvic and anal regions. These involuntary muscular contractions lead to the ejaculation of **semen,** which consists of sperm cells from the testes and secretions from the prostate gland and seminal vesicles. In women, contractions occur in the lower part of the vagina and in the uterus, as well as in the pelvic region and the anus.

4. In the *resolution phase,* all the changes initiated during the excitement phase are reversed. Excess blood drains from tissues, the muscles in the region relax, and the genital structures return to their unstimulated state.

More general physical reactions accompany the genital changes in both men and women. Beginning with the excitement phase, nipples become erect, the woman's breasts begin to swell, and in both sexes the skin of the chest becomes flushed; these changes are more marked in women. The heart rate doubles by the plateau phase, and respiration becomes faster. During orgasm, breathing becomes irregular and the person may moan or cry out. A feeling of warmth leads to increased sweating during the resolution phase. Deep relaxation and a sense of well-being pervade the body and the mind.

Male orgasm is marked by the ejaculation of semen. After ejaculation, men enter a *refractory period,* during which they cannot be restimulated to orgasm. Women do not have a refractory period, and immediate restimulation to orgasm is possible.

## Sexual Problems

Both physical and psychological factors can interfere with sexual functioning. If you are in poor physical health or experiencing high levels of stress or anxiety, sexual functioning may be negatively affected. Difficulties may be caused by infection and other sexual health problems. Disturbances in sexual desire, performance, or satisfaction are referred to as **sexual dysfunctions.**

**Common Sexual Health Problems** Some problems with sexual functioning are due to treatable or preventable infections or other sexual health problems. Conditions that affect women include the following:

- *Vaginitis,* inflammation of the vagina, is caused by a variety of organisms: *Candida* (yeast infection), *Trichomonas* (trichomoniasis), and the overgrowth of a variety of bacteria (bacterial vaginosis).
- *Endometriosis* is the growth of endometrial tissue (tissue normally found lining the uterus) outside the

uterus. Endometriosis can cause serious problems if left untreated because the endometrial tissue can scar and partially or completely block the oviducts, causing infertility (difficulty conceiving) or sterility (the inability to conceive).

- *Pelvic inflammatory disease (PID)* is an infection of the uterus, oviducts, or ovaries caused when microorganisms spread to these areas from the vagina. Approximately 50–75% of PID cases are caused by sexually transmitted organisms associated with diseases such as gonorrhea and chlamydia. PID can cause scarring of the oviducts, resulting in infertility or sterility.

Sexual health problems that affect men include the following:

- *Prostatitis* is inflammation or infection of the prostate gland.
- *Testicular cancer* occurs most commonly in men in their twenties and thirties. A rare cancer, it has a very high cure rate if detected early.

**Sexual Dysfunctions** The term *sexual dysfunction* encompasses disturbances in sexual desire, performance, or satisfaction. A wide variety of physical conditions and drugs may interfere with sexual functioning; psychological causes and problems in intimate relationships can be important factors in some cases.

**COMMON SEXUAL DYSFUNCTIONS** Common sexual dysfunctions in men include erectile dysfunction (previously called impotence), the inability to have or maintain an erection sufficient for sexual intercourse; premature ejaculation, ejaculation before or just on penetration of the vagina or anus; and retarded ejaculation, the inability to ejaculate once an erection is achieved. Many men experience occasional difficulty achieving an erection or ejaculating because of excessive alcohol consumption, fatigue, or stress.

Two sexual dysfunctions in women are vaginismus, in which the woman experiences painful involuntary muscular spasms when sexual intercourse is attempted, and orgasmic dysfunction, the inability to experience orgasm. Vaginismus is a conditioned reflex probably related to fear of intercourse. Orgasmic dysfunction has been the subject of a great deal of discussion over the years, as people debated the nature of the female orgasm and what constitutes dysfunction in women. Many women experience orgasm but not during intercourse, or they experience orgasm during intercourse only if the clitoris is directly stimulated at the same time. In general, the inability to experience orgasm under certain circumstances is a problem only if the woman considers it so.

**TREATING SEXUAL DYSFUNCTION** Most forms of sexual dysfunction are treatable. The first step is to have a thorough physical examination to identify any underlying medical condition that may be responsible for the problem. Heart disease, diabetes, smoking, drug use, and medications can all inhibit sexual response.

If physical problems continue to interfere with sexual response, many treatments are available, particularly for erectile dysfunction. In 1998, Viagra (sildenafil citrate), the first-ever prescription pill for erectile dysfunction, was introduced; it quickly became the most successful new prescription drug in history. Since the introduction of Viagra, two other oral medications with actions similar to Viagra, Cialis (tadalafil) and Levitra (vardenafil), have been approved by the FDA. All three work by enhancing the effects of nitric oxide, a chemical that relaxes smooth muscles in the penis. This increases the amount of blood flow and allows a natural erection to occur in response to sexual stimulation. They are effective in about 70% of users, but there are potential side effects, including headaches, indigestion, facial flushing, and back pain.

Recent research found that there has been a more than 300% increase in Viagra use by men between the ages of 18 and 45 since 1998—possibly due to use of the drug for recreational rather than medical purposes. Research suggests that medication may cut the refractory period in men who do not have erectile dysfunction; younger men may also be using it to cope with performance anxiety or the effects of other drugs. Consumers should also note that as many as half of the Viagra pills sold on the Internet may be counterfeit.

If no physical problem is found, a sexual dysfunction may be psychosocial in origin. Psychosocial causes of dysfunction include troubled relationships, a lack of sexual skills, irrational attitudes and beliefs, anxiety, and psychosexual trauma, such as sexual abuse or rape. Many of these problems can be addressed by sex therapy methods that seek to modify the beliefs and behavior patterns that are interfering with satisfactory sexual relationships.

Women who seek treatment for orgasmic dysfunction often have not had the chance to learn through trial and error what types of stimulation will excite them and bring them to orgasm. Most sex therapists prefer to treat this problem with **masturbation** (genital self-stimulation).

### Terms

**vasocongestion** The accumulation of blood in tissues and organs.

**myotonia** Increased muscular tension.

**orgasm** The discharge of accumulated sexual tension with characteristic genital and bodily manifestations and a subjective sensation of intense pleasure.

**semen** Seminal fluid, consisting of sperm cells and secretions from the prostate gland and seminal vesicles.

**sexual dysfunction** A disturbance in sexual desire, performance, or satisfaction.

**masturbation** Self-stimulation for the purpose of sexual arousal and orgasm.

Vw

Mind/Body/Spirit

## Sexual Decision Making

Choosing to have sex can change a relationship as well as an individual's life. In making decisions about sexual activity, you owe it to yourself and your partner to think and talk honestly about your choices. Consider the following issues:

- *Your background, beliefs, and goals.* What are your religious, moral, and/or personal values regarding relationships and sex? What are your priorities at this time, and how will a sexual relationship fit into your goals and plans for the future? Are you physically, emotionally, and financially ready to accept the potential consequences of the choices you make? How will you feel if you act in ways that are not consistent with your values and goals?
- *Your relationship with your partner.* How do you feel about your partner and your relationship? Do you respect and trust each other? Do you feel comfortable talking about sexual issues, and have you discussed contraception, pregnancy, and safer sex? How do you think having sex will affect your relationship and how you feel about yourself and your partner? What does having sex mean to each of you?
- *Your reasons for having sex.* Are you feeling pressured to have sex? Are you afraid of losing your partner if you say no? Are you too embarrassed, shy, or insecure to say no or discuss waiting? Are you being honest with yourself and your partner about your reasons for moving into a sexual relationship?

Personal decisions about sex should always be respected. You have the right to make your own choices and to do only what you feel comfortable with. When you make choices about sex based on self-respect, along with physical, emotional, and spiritual considerations, you'll be more likely to feel good about your decisions—now and in the future—and to enhance your health and well-being.

Women are taught about their own anatomy and sexual responses and then are encouraged to experiment with masturbation until they experience orgasm.

## SEXUAL BEHAVIOR

Many behaviors stem from sexual impulses, and sexual expression takes a variety of forms. Probably the most basic aspect of sexuality is reproduction, the process of producing offspring. As important as reproduction is, the intention of creating a child accounts for only a small measure of sexual activity; most people have sex for other reasons as well.

Adult sexuality can include any of the sexual behaviors and practices described in this chapter. In mature love relationships, people ideally can integrate all the aspects of intimacy—physical, sexual, emotional—so that sexuality is a deeply meaningful part of how they express love (see the box "Sexual Decision Making").

### Sexual Orientation

As discussed in Chapter 4, sexual orientation is a consistent pattern of emotional and sexual attraction based on biological sex. It exists along a continuum that ranges from exclusive heterosexuality (attraction to people of the other sex) through bisexuality (attraction to people of both sexes) to exclusive homosexuality (attraction to people of one's own sex). The terms *straight* and *gay* are often used to refer to heterosexuals and homosexuals, respectively, and female homosexuals are also referred to as lesbians.

Sexual orientation involves feelings and self-concept, and individuals may or may not express their sexual orientation in their behavior. In national surveys, about 2–6% of men identify themselves as homosexuals and about 1.5% of women identify themselves as lesbians. Many theories have been proposed to account for the development of sexual orientation. Most scientists today agree that sexual orientation is most likely the result of the complex interaction of biological, psychological, and social factors, possibly different in the case of each individual.

### Varieties of Human Sexual Behavior

Most people express their sexuality in a variety of ways. Some sexual behaviors are aimed at self-stimulation only, such as masturbation, whereas other practices involve interaction with others in behaviors such as kissing and intercourse. Some people choose not to express their sexuality and practice celibacy instead.

**Celibacy** Continuous abstention from sexual activities, termed **celibacy**, can be a conscious and deliberate choice, or it can be necessitated by circumstances. Health considerations and religious and moral beliefs may lead some people to celibacy, particularly until marriage or until an acceptable partner appears. A disadvantage of the celibate life is that it may lack physical contact and affection.

Many people use the related term *abstinence* to refer to avoidance of just one sexual activity—intercourse. The use of abstinence to prevent pregnancy and sexually transmitted diseases is discussed in Chapters 6 and 13.

**Autoeroticism and Masturbation** The most common form of **autoeroticism** is **erotic fantasy**, creating imaginary experiences that range from fleeting thoughts to elaborate scenarios. Masturbation involves manually stimulating the genitals, rubbing them against objects (such as a pillow), or using stimulating devices such as vibrators. It may be used as a substitute for sexual intercourse or as part of sexual activity with a partner.

**Touching and Foreplay** Tactile stimulation, or touching, is integral to sexual experiences, whether in the form of massage, kissing, fondling, or holding. Our entire body surface is a sensory organ, and touching almost anywhere can enhance intimacy and sexual arousal. Touching can convey a variety of messages, including affection, comfort, and a desire for further sexual contact.

**Oral-Genital Stimulation** **Cunnilingus** (the stimulation of the female genitals with the lips and tongue) and **fellatio** (the stimulation of the penis with the mouth) are quite common practices. Oral sex may be practiced either as part of foreplay or as a sex act culminating in orgasm. Like all acts of sexual expression between two people, oral sex requires the cooperation and consent of both partners.

**Anal Intercourse** About 10% of heterosexuals and 50% of homosexual males regularly practice anal stimulation and penetration by the penis or a finger. Because the anus is composed of delicate tissues that tear easily under such pressure, anal intercourse is one of the riskiest of sexual behaviors associated with the transmission of HIV and the bacteria that cause gonorrhea and syphilis. The use of condoms is highly recommended for anyone engaging in anal sex. Special care and precaution should be exercised if anal sex is practiced.

**Sexual Intercourse** For most adults, most of the time, **sexual intercourse** is the ultimate sexual experience. Men and women engage in coitus—make love—to fulfill both sexual and psychological needs. The most common heterosexual practice is the man inserting his erect penis into the woman's dilated and lubricated vagina after sufficient arousal. Psychological factors and the quality of the relationship are more important to overall sexual satisfaction than sophisticated or exotic sexual techniques.

## Atypical and Problematic Sexual Behaviors

In American culture, many kinds of sexual behavior are accepted. However, some types of sexual expression are considered harmful; they may be against the law or classified as mental disorders, or both. Because sexual behavior occurs on a continuum, it is sometimes difficult to differentiate a behavior that is simply atypical from one that is harmful. When attempting to evaluate an unusual sexual behavior, experts consider the issues of consent between partners and whether physical or psychological harm is done to the individual or to others.

The use of force and coercion in sexual relationships is one of the most serious problems in human interactions. The most extreme manifestation of sexual coercion—forcing a person to submit to another's sexual desires—is rape, but sexual coercion occurs in many subtler forms, such as sexual harassment. Sexual coercion—including rape, the sexual abuse of children, and sexual harassment—is discussed in detail in Chapter 16.

## Commercial Sex

Conflicting feelings about sexuality are apparent in the attitudes of Americans toward commercial sex: prostitution and sexually oriented materials such as videos, magazines, and books. Our society condemns sexually explicit material and prostitution, but it also provides their customers.

**Pornography** Derived from the Greek word meaning "the writing of prostitutes," pornography is now often defined as obscene literature, art, or movies. A major problem in identifying pornographic material is that different people and communities have different opinions about what is obscene. Differing definitions of obscenity have led to many legal battles over potentially pornographic materials. Currently, the sale and rental of pornographic materials is restricted so that only adults can legally obtain them; materials depicting children in sexual contexts are illegal in any format or setting.

The appearance of thousands of sexually oriented Web sites has expanded the number of people with access to pornographic materials and has made enforcing pornography laws more difficult. People who might have hesitated to buy magazines or rent videos in person can now access sexually explicit material privately and anonymously. Of special concern is the increased availability of illegal materials, such as child pornography, that previously could be acquired only with great difficulty and at great legal risk.

**Prostitution** The exchange of sexual services for money is prostitution. Prostitutes may be men, women, or children, and the buyer of a prostitute's services is nearly always a man. Except in parts of Nevada, prostitution is illegal in the United States. Most customers are white, middle-class, middle-aged, and married. Although they

### Terms

**celibacy** Continuous abstention from sexual activity.

**autoeroticism** Behavior aimed at sexual self-stimulation.

**erotic fantasy** Sexually arousing thoughts and daydreams.

**cunnilingus** Oral stimulation of the female genitals.

**fellatio** Oral stimulation of the penis.

**sexual intercourse** Sexual relations involving genital union; also called *coitus,* and also known as making love.

Take Charge

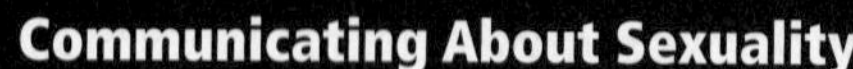

## Communicating About Sexuality

To talk with your partner about sexuality, follow the general suggestions for effective communication given in Chapter 4. Getting started may be the most difficult part. Some people feel more comfortable if they begin by talking about talking—that is, initiating a discussion about why people are so uncomfortable talking about sexuality. Talking about sexual histories—how partners first learned about sex or how family and cultural background influenced sexual values and attitudes—is another way to get started. Reading about sex can also be a good beginning: Partners can read an article or book and then discuss their reactions.

Be honest about what you feel and what you want from your partner. Cultural and personal obstacles to discussing sexual subjects can be difficult to overcome, but self-disclosure is important for successful relationships. Research indicates that when one partner openly discusses attitudes and feelings, the other partner is more likely to do the same. If your partner seems hesitant to open up, try asking open-ended or either/or questions: "Where do you like to be touched?" or "Would you like to talk about this now or wait until later?"

If something is bothering you about your sexual relationship, choose a good time to initiate a discussion with your partner. Be specific and direct but also tactful. Focus on what you actually observe, rather than on what you think the behavior means. "You didn't touch or hug me when your friends were around" is an observation. "You're ashamed of me around your friends" is an inference about your partner's feelings. Try focusing on a specific behavior that concerns you rather than on the person as a whole—your partner can change behaviors but not his or her entire personality. For example, you could say "I'd like you to take a few minutes away from studying to kiss me" instead of "You're so caught up in your work, you never have time for me."

If you are going to make a statement that your partner may interpret as criticism, try mixing it with something positive: "I love spending time with you, but I feel annoyed when you. . . ." Similarly, if your partner says something that upsets you, don't lash back. An aggressive response may make you feel better in the short run, but it will not help the communication process or the quality of the relationship.

If you want to say no to some sexual activity, say no unequivocally. Don't send mixed messages. If you are afraid of hurting your partner's feelings, offer an alternative if it's appropriate: "I am uncomfortable with that. How about . . . ?"

If you're in love, you may think that the sexual aspects of a relationship will work out magically without discussion. However, partners who never talk about sex deny themselves the opportunity to increase their closeness and improve their relationship.

come from a wide variety of backgrounds, prostitutes are usually motivated to join the profession because of money.

AIDS is a major concern for prostitutes and their customers. Many prostitutes are injecting drug users or are involved with men who are. The rate of HIV infection among prostitutes varies widely, but in some parts of the country it is as high as 25–50%.

## Responsible Sexual Behavior

Healthy sexuality is an important part of adult life. It can be a source of pleasurable experiences and emotions and an important part of intimate partnerships. But sexual behavior also carries many responsibilities, and you need to make choices about your sexuality that contribute to your well-being and that of your partner.

**Open, Honest Communication** Each partner needs to clearly indicate what sexual involvement means to him or her. Does it mean love, fun, a permanent commitment, or something else? The intentions of both partners should be clear. For strategies on how to talk about sexual issues with your partner, refer to the box "Communicating About Sexuality."

**Agreed-On Sexual Activities** No one should pressure or coerce a partner. Sexual behaviors should be consistent with the sexual values, preferences, and comfort level of both partners. Everyone has the right to refuse sexual activity at any time.

**Sexual Privacy** Intimate relationships involving sexual activity are based on trust, and that trust can be violated if partners reveal private information about the relationship to others. Sexual privacy also involves respecting other people—not engaging in activities in the presence of others that would make them uncomfortable.

**Using Contraception** If pregnancy is not desired, contraception should be used during sexual intercourse. Both partners need to take responsibility for protecting against unwanted pregnancy. Partners should discuss contraception before sexual involvement begins.

**Safer Sex** Both partners should be aware of and practice safer sex to guard against sexually transmitted diseases (STDs). The U.S. Surgeon General stated in his 2001 *Call to Action to Promote Sexual Health and Responsible Sexual Behavior* that the United States faces a significant challenge to the sexual health of its people due to the high levels of STDs. Many sexual behaviors carry the risk of STDs, including HIV infection. Partners should be honest about their health and any medical conditions and work out a plan for protection. Behaviors that carry no risk of HIV infection are those that don't involve the exchange of body fluids (blood, semen, and vaginal secretions). Anyone who is not in a mutually monogamous relationship with an uninfected partner and who wishes to have sex should always use a condom.

**Sober Sex** The use of alcohol or drugs in sexual situations increases the risk of unplanned, unprotected sexual activity. This is particularly true of young adults, many of whom engage in episodes of binge drinking during social events. Alcohol and drugs impair judgment and should not be used in association with sexual activity.

**Taking Responsibility for Consequences** Individuals should be aware of the physical and emotional consequences of their sexual behavior and accept responsibility for them. Consequences include pregnancy, STDs, and emotional changes in the relationship between partners.

## UNDERSTANDING FERTILITY

Conceiving a child is a highly complex process. Although many couples conceive readily, others can testify to the difficulties that can be encountered.

### Conception

The process of **conception** involves the **fertilization** of an ovum (egg) from a woman by a sperm from a man. Every month during a woman's fertile years, her body prepares itself for conception and pregnancy. In one of her **ovaries** an egg ripens and is released from its **follicle.** The egg, about the size of a pinpoint, travels through an **oviduct**, or **fallopian tube**, to the **uterus** in 3–4 days. The **endometrium,** or lining of the uterus, has already thickened for the implantation of a **fertilized egg,** or *zygote*. If the egg is not fertilized, it lasts about 24 hours and then disintegrates. It is expelled along with the uterine lining during menstruation.

Sperm cells are produced in the man's **testes** and ejaculated from his penis into the woman's vagina during sexual intercourse. Sperm cells are much smaller than eggs. The typical ejaculate contains millions of sperm, but only a few complete the journey through the uterus and up the fallopian tube to the egg. As sperm approach the egg, they release enzymes that soften this outer layer. Enzymes from hundreds of sperm must be released in order for the egg's outer layer to soften enough to allow one sperm cell to penetrate. The first sperm cell that bumps into a spot that is soft enough can swim into the egg cell. It then merges with the nucleus of the egg, and fertilization occurs. The egg then releases a chemical that makes it impenetrable by other sperm.

The ovum carries the hereditary characteristics of the mother and her ancestors; sperm cells carry the hereditary characteristics of the father and his ancestors. Each parent cell—egg or sperm—contains 23 chromosomes, each of

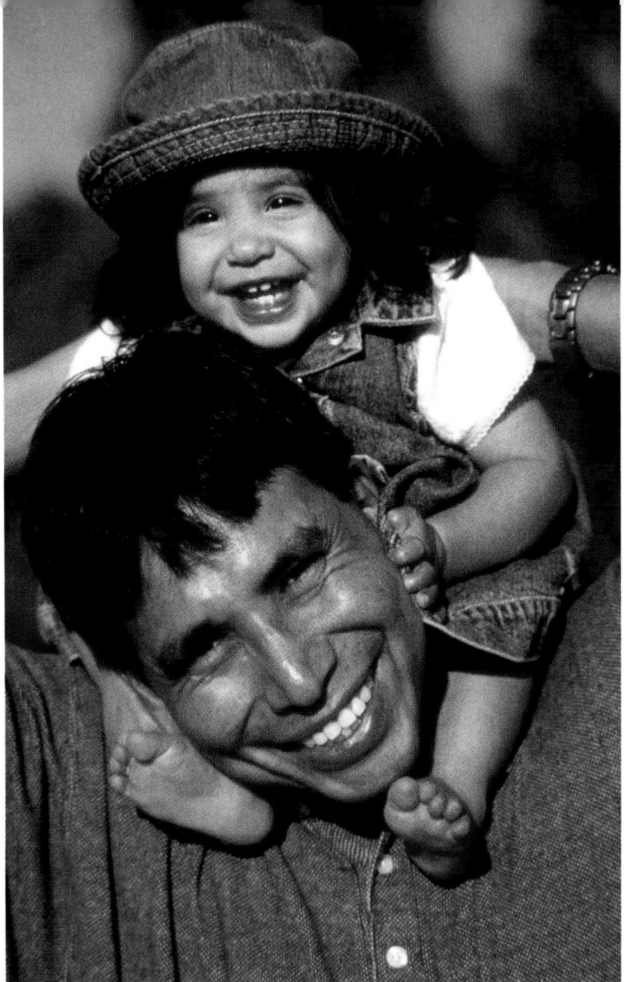

Having a child is one of the most important and rewarding experiences a person can undertake. Careful preparation can help maximize the benefits for both parents and children.

which contains genes, packages of chemical instructions for the developing baby. Genes provide the blueprint for a unique individual.

**Terms**

**conception** The fusion of ovum and sperm, resulting in a fertilized egg.

**fertilization** The initiation of biological reproduction: the union of the nucleus of an egg cell with the nucleus of a sperm cell.

**ovary** One of the two female reproductive organs that produce ova (eggs) and sex hormones.

**follicle** One of many saclike structures within the ovary in which eggs mature.

**oviduct (fallopian tube)** One of two passages through which eggs travel from the ovaries to the uterus; the site of fertilization.

**uterus** The hollow, thick-walled, muscular organ in which the fertilized egg develops; the womb.

**endometrium** The mucous membrane that forms the inner lining of the cavity of the uterus.

**fertilized egg** The egg after penetration by a sperm; a *zygote*.

**testis** One of two male reproductive organs; the testes are the site of sperm production.

The usual course of events is that one egg and one sperm unite to produce one fertilized egg and one baby. But if the ovaries release two (or more) eggs during ovulation and if both eggs are fertilized, twins will develop. These twins will be no more alike than siblings from different pregnancies, because each will have come from a different fertilized egg. Twins who develop this way are referred to as **fraternal twins;** they may be the same sex or different sexes. Twins can also develop from the division of a single fertilized egg into two cells that develop separately. Because these babies share all genetic material, they will be **identical twins.**

## Infertility

Although the main concern for many women and men, especially if they are young and single, is how *not* to get pregnant, the reverse is true for millions of couples who have difficulty conceiving. **Infertility** is usually defined as the inability to conceive after trying for a year or more. It affects about 6 million couples—10% of the reproductive-age population of the United States.

**Female Infertility** Female infertility usually results from one of two key causes—tubal blockage (40%) or failure to ovulate (40%). An additional 10% of cases of infertility are due to anatomical abnormalities, benign growths in the uterus, thyroid disease, and other uncommon conditions; the remaining 10% of cases are unexplained.

Blocked fallopian tubes are most commonly the result of *pelvic inflammatory disease (PID),* a serious complication of several sexually transmitted diseases. Most cases of PID are associated with untreated cases of chlamydia or gonorrhea. Tubal blockages can also be caused by prior surgery or by *endometriosis,* a condition in which endometrial (uterine) tissue grows outside of the uterus. This tissue responds to hormones and can cause pain, bleeding, scarring, and adhesions. Endometriosis is typically treated with hormonal therapy and surgery.

### Terms

VW

**fraternal twins** Twins who develop from separate fertilized eggs; not genetically identical.

**identical twins** Twins who develop from the division of a single zygote; genetically identical.

**infertility** The inability to conceive after trying for a year or more.

**cloning** Asexual reproduction in which offspring are genetically identical to one parent. DNA from the cell of one animal is transferred to an egg from which DNA has been removed; the egg is then placed in a surrogate and develops as though it were an embryo derived from two parents.

**trimester** One of the three 3-month periods of pregnancy.

**fetus** The developmental stage of a human from the 9th week after conception to the moment of birth.

Age impacts fertility; beginning at around age 30, a woman's fertility naturally begins to decline. Age is probably the main factor in ovulation failure. Exposure to toxic chemicals or radiation also appears to reduce fertility, as does cigarette smoking. Daughters born to women who were given diethylstilbestrol (DES) during pregnancy are at risk for a variety of problems with conception.

**Male Infertility** The leading causes of infertility among men are low sperm count, lack of sperm motility (the ability to move spontaneously), misshapen sperm, and blocked passageways between the testes and the urethra. Smoking may cause reduced sperm counts and abnormal sperm. The sons of mothers who took DES may have increased sperm abnormalities and fertility problems. Certain prescription and illegal drugs also affect the number of sperm. Large doses of marijuana, for example, cause lower sperm counts and suppress certain reproductive hormones. Other causes of sperm problems include injury to the testicles, infection (especially from mumps during adulthood), birth defects, subjecting the testes to high temperatures, and exposure to toxic environmental substances such as lead, radiation, or pollutants that mimic the effects of hormones.

**Treating Infertility** About 90% of infertile couples receive a physical diagnosis for their condition; for the remaining 10%, the cause of the infertility remains unexplained. Most cases of infertility are treated with conventional medical therapies: Surgery can repair oviducts, clear up endometriosis, and correct anatomical problems in both men and women. Fertility drugs can help women ovulate, although they carry the risk of causing multiple births. If these conventional treatments don't work, couples can turn to more advanced techniques.

**INTRAUTERINE INSEMINATION** Male infertility can sometimes be overcome by collecting and concentrating the man's sperm and introducing it by syringe into a woman's vagina or uterus, a procedure known as artificial (intrauterine) insemination. The sperm can be provided by the woman's partner or, if there are severe problems with his sperm or he carries a serious genetic disorder, by a donor.

**IVF, GIFT, AND ZIFT** Three related techniques for overcoming infertility involve removing mature eggs from a woman's ovary. In in vitro fertilization (IVF), the harvested eggs are mixed with sperm in a laboratory dish. If eggs are successfully fertilized, one or more of the resulting embryos are inserted into the woman's uterus. In gamete intrafallopian transfer (GIFT), eggs and sperm are surgically placed into the fallopian tubes prior to fertilization. In zygote intrafallopian transfer (ZIFT), eggs are fertilized outside the woman's body and surgically introduced into the oviducts after they begin to divide. Variations on these three techniques are also becoming available (see the box "Reproductive Technology").

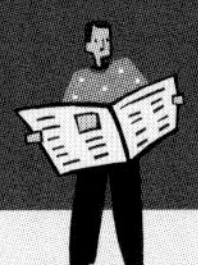

## In the News: Reproductive Technology

In the United States, more than 45,000 infants are born each year as a result of assisted reproductive technology (ART) techniques like IVF, GIFT, and ZIFT. Research into the areas of genetics and cloning promise even more breakthroughs for ART treatments. With these advances, however, come many medical, ethical, and legal questions. Below are a few of the most advanced techniques currently in use and under study.

*Use of donor eggs, donor sperm, and/or donor embryos* is fairly common in ART treatments. In some instances, this results in a child with a complex network of biological and legal parents. For example, in the case of IVF involving donor eggs and sperm and a surrogate mother, who are the legal parents of the child?

The use of donor eggs and embryos has also allowed women in their 50s to complete pregnancy and deliver a baby. The resulting offspring is no more genetically related to the woman than an adopted child would be. Use of ART in women of this age is controversial.

*Intracytoplasmic sperm injection (ICSI),* in which a single sperm is injected into a mature egg, was originally developed to overcome cases of severe male infertility; it is now used for a broader range of conditions. Concerns have been raised because some studies have linked ICSI to an increase in genetic defects in offspring. In addition, ICSI allows men who are infertile due to Y chromosome defects to have children, even though any sons they have will inherit the defect and also be infertile.

*Cryopreservation* of ovarian tissue and/or unfertilized eggs has been studied as a possible means of preserving fertility in women undergoing cancer therapy. In 2004, the first woman gave birth after having ovarian tissue removed and frozen prior to cancer chemotherapy and then reimplanted. This technique could potentially be used in women who choose to delay childbearing, and several controversial companies offer this technique to women in their 30s.

*Freezing embryos* is common in ART because multiple eggs are usually harvested and fertilized during IVF. If the initial IVF cycle is unsuccessful, the backup embryos can be used for additional attempts. Once ART treatment is completed, couples may choose to donate leftover embryos for use by another infertile couple or to have them destroyed. A more controversial potential use of extra embryos is for the creation of stem cell lines (see Chapter 14).

*Preimplantation genetic diagnosis,* in which embryos created through IVF undergo genetic analysis before implantation in the womb, was originally developed to help couples at risk for genetic diseases. It has now begun to be offered by some physicians for sex selection in couples who have no fertility problems. This is considered controversial because a particular gender isn't a disease that needs to be prevented, and there remains the difficult question of what becomes of the "wrong sex" embryos—freezing, donation, destruction, or use in research.

*Injection of the cytoplasm* (the material in a cell that surrounds the nucleus) from a younger woman's egg into an older woman's egg has begun to be used as a possible means of reducing genetic errors in the older woman's egg. These errors occur in so-called mitochondrial DNA, genetic material in the cytoplasm of the cell that is passed along unchanged to offspring.

*Nuclear transfer,* a technique related to cytoplasm injection, uses cloning technology—the transfer of the nucleus from an older woman's egg into an egg from a younger woman from which the nucleus has been removed. In cytoplasm injection and nuclear transfer, the offspring carry DNA from two women—nuclear DNA from one woman and mitochondrial DNA from a second woman—and so have three genetic "parents."

*What about cloning?* **Cloning** is different from any of the techniques discussed above because it is a form of asexual reproduction. A clone carries the genes of only one person, not two. However, as described above, the cloning technique of nuclear transfer could potentially be used in the treatment of infertility. Nuclear transfer could theoretically also be used to create a child that is the genetic offspring of two people of the same sex. In 2004, scientists announced that they had created a mouse from two unfertilized eggs.

**SURROGATE MOTHERHOOD** This controversial practice involves a contract between an infertile couple and a fertile woman who agrees to carry a fetus. The surrogate mother agrees to be artificially inseminated by the father's sperm or to undergo IVF with the couple's embryo, to carry the baby to term, and to give it to the couple at birth. Some people think that surrogate motherhood is essentially an arrangement to sell a baby, and they worry about the psychological consequences for children who learn that their mothers "sold" them. Experience has shown, too, that some surrogate mothers have a very difficult time giving up the baby.

Most infertility treatments are expensive and emotionally draining, and their success is uncertain. One measure you can take now to avoid infertility is to protect yourself against STDs and to treat promptly and completely any disease you do contract. Also, couples who are ready should consider trying to conceive prior to the woman's late 30s to decrease the probability of age-related infertility.

## PREGNANCY

Pregnancy is usually discussed in terms of **trimesters**—three periods of about 3 months (or 13 weeks) each. During the first trimester, the mother experiences a few physical changes and some fairly common symptoms. During the second trimester, often the most peaceful time of pregnancy, the mother gains weight, looks noticeably pregnant, and may experience a general sense of well-being if she is happy about having a child. The third trimester is the hardest for the mother because she must breathe, digest, excrete, and circulate blood for herself and the growing **fetus.**

## Pregnancy Tests

The earliest tests for pregnancy are chemical tests designed to detect the presence of **human chorionic gonadotropin (HCG)**, a hormone produced by the implanted fertilized egg. These tests may be performed as early as 2 weeks after fertilization. Home pregnancy tests can be very reliable, but the instructions must be followed carefully. If a home test done at the time of a missed menstrual period is negative, retesting after another week is recommended. In the first day or two following a missed period, the concentration of HCG may be too low to be detected by the test.

## Changes in the Woman's Body

Hormonal changes begin as soon as the egg is fertilized, and for the next 9 months the woman's body nourishes the fetus and adjusts to its growth. Let's take a closer look at the changes of early, middle, and late pregnancy.

**Early Signs and Symptoms** Early recognition of pregnancy is important, especially for women with physical problems and nutritional deficiencies. The following symptoms are not absolute indications of pregnancy, but they are reasons to visit a gynecologist:

- *A missed menstrual period.* If an egg has been fertilized and implanted in the uterine wall, the endometrium is retained to nourish the embryo.
- *Slight bleeding.* Slight bleeding may follow implantation of the fertilized egg. Because this happens about the time a period is expected, the bleeding is sometimes mistaken for menstrual flow.
- *Nausea.* About two-thirds of pregnant women feel nauseated, probably as a reaction to increased levels of progesterone and other hormones. Often called morning sickness, some women have it all day long. It frequently begins during the 3rd or 4th week and disappears by the 12th week. In some cases, it can last throughout a pregnancy.
- *Breast tenderness.* Some women experience breast tenderness, swelling, and tingling, usually described as different from the tenderness experienced before menstruation.
- *Increased urination.* Increased frequency of urination can occur soon after the missed period.
- *Sleepiness, fatigue, and emotional upset.* These symptoms result from hormonal changes.

### Terms

**human chorionic gonadotropin (HCG)** A hormone produced by the fertilized egg that can be detected in the urine or blood of the mother within a few weeks of conception.

**Braxton Hicks contractions** Uterine contractions that occur during the third trimester of pregnancy, preparing for labor.

The first reliable physical signs of pregnancy can be distinguished about 4 weeks after a woman misses her menstrual period. A softening of the uterus just above the cervix, called *Hegar's sign,* and other changes in the cervix and pelvis are apparent during a pelvic examination. The labia minora and the cervix may take on a purple color rather than their usual pink hue.

**Continuing Changes in the Woman's Body**
During the first 3 months, the uterus enlarges to about three times its nonpregnant size; by the 4th month, it is large enough to make the abdomen protrude. By the 7th or 8th month, the uterus pushes up into the rib cage, which makes breathing slightly more difficult. The breasts enlarge and are sensitive; by week 8, they may tingle or throb. The pigmented area around the nipple, the areola, darkens and broadens.

Early in pregnancy, the muscles and ligaments attached to bones begin to soften and stretch. The joints between the pelvic bones loosen and spread, making it easier to have a baby but harder to walk. The circulatory system becomes more efficient to accommodate the blood volume, which increases by 50%, and the heart pumps it more rapidly. The mother's lungs also become more efficient, and her rib cage widens to permit her to inhale up to 40% more air.

Women of normal weight gain an average of 18–25% of their initial weight: 20–28 pounds for a woman weighing 110; 23–32 pounds for a woman weighing 128. Women who begin pregnancy underweight are advised to gain more; obese women are advised to gain less. About 60% of weight gained relates directly to the baby and 40% accumulates over the mother's entire body as fluid and fat.

**Changes During the Later Stages of Pregnancy** By the end of the 6th month, the increased needs of the fetus place a burden on the mother's lungs, heart, and kidneys. Her back may ache from the pressure of the baby's weight and from having to throw her shoulders back to keep her balance while standing (Figure 5-4). Her body retains more water, perhaps up to 3 extra quarts of fluid. Her legs, hands, ankles, or feet may swell, and she may be bothered by leg cramps, heartburn, or constipation. Despite discomfort, both her digestion and her metabolism are working at top efficiency.

The uterus prepares for childbirth with preliminary contractions, called **Braxton Hicks contractions.** Unlike true labor contractions, these are usually short, irregular, and painless. The mother may only be aware that at times her abdomen is hard to the touch. These contractions become more frequent and intense as the delivery date approaches.

In the 9th month, the baby settles into the pelvic bones, usually head down, fitting snugly. This process, called *lightening,* allows the uterus to sink down about 2 inches, producing a visible change in the mother's profile. Pelvic pressure increases, and pressure on the diaphragm lightens. Breathing becomes easier; urination becomes more

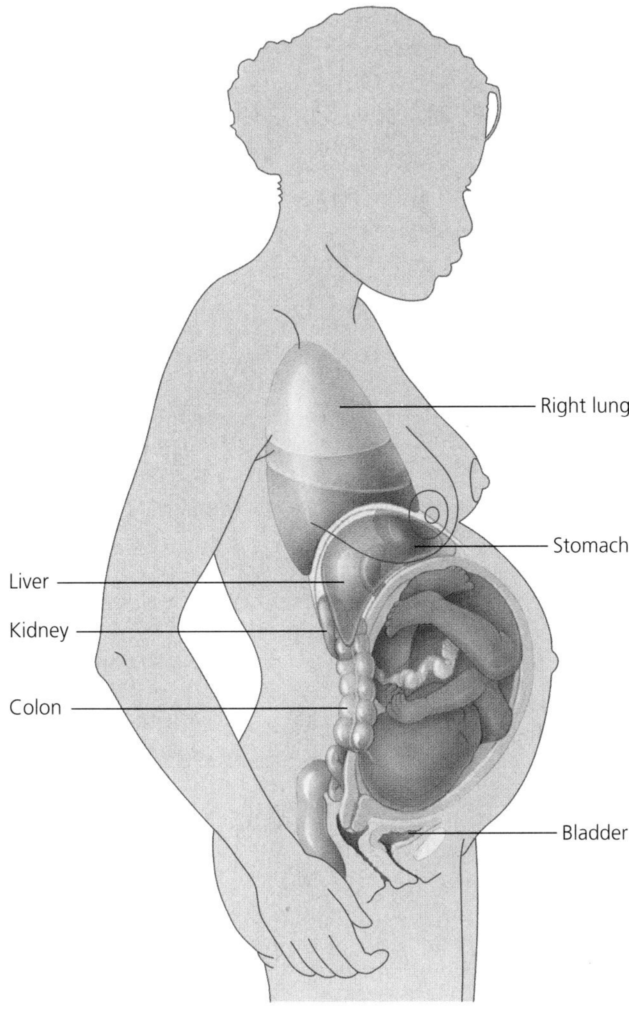


**Figure 5-4 The woman and fetus during the third trimester of pregnancy.** Pressure from the rapidly growing fetus on the mother's lungs, bladder, stomach, and other organs may cause shortness of breath, heartburn, and the need for frequent urination. The mother's uterus has expanded to 50–60 times its original size.

frequent. Sometimes, after a first pregnancy, the baby doesn't settle down into the pelvis until labor begins.

The third trimester is the time of greatest physical stress during the pregnancy. A woman may find that her physical abilities are limited by her size, but many also feel a great deal of happy excitement and anticipation. The fetus may already be looked upon as a member of the family, and both parents may begin talking to the fetus and interacting with it by patting the mother's belly. The upcoming birth will probably be a focus for both the woman and her partner (see the box "Pregnancy Tasks for Fathers").

## Fetal Development

Now that we've seen what happens to the mother's body during pregnancy, let's consider the development of the fetus (Figure 5-5).

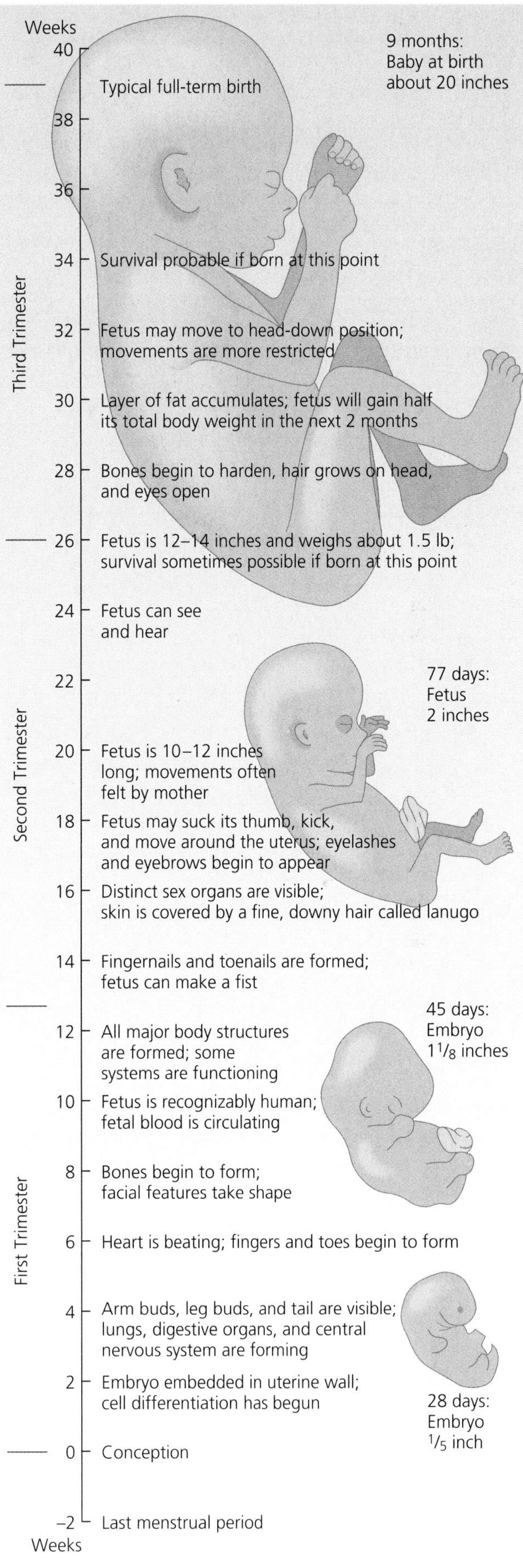


**Figure 5-5 A chronology of milestones in prenatal development.**

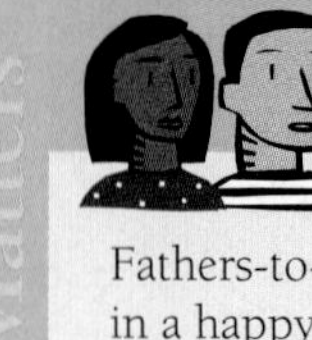

Gender Matters

## Pregnancy Tasks for Fathers

Fathers-to-be can play an important role in a happy and successful pregnancy.

### Before the Pregnancy

- *Consider your lifestyle and health habits.* A healthy lifestyle can help boost fertility and improve pregnancy outcome. Being too thin or too heavy may lower a man's sperm count, as may marijuana use. Men who smoke and drink have a lower concentration of sperm and a lower percentage of active sperm. Exposure to chemicals on the job may also play a role in poor pregnancy outcomes.
- *Check your budget, financial situation, and insurance status.* What is the paternal leave policy at your place of employment? Do you have health insurance, life insurance, disability insurance, and a will? Do you (and your partner or child) qualify for special benefits such as Medicaid? Can you make a budget and stick to it? Try putting away extra money every month now—both to practice living on a tighter budget and to actually save up for baby.
- *Get any necessary health checks and genetic counseling.* Testing for STDs may be recommended for some men; many STDs have no symptoms but can be potentially dangerous for the developing fetus, especially if the mother contracts the infection during her pregnancy. Genetic screening and counseling may be recommended for couples at risk for a specific inherited disease.

### During the Pregnancy

- *Help your partner stay healthy during the pregnancy.* If you smoke, quit; secondhand smoke is dangerous for the developing fetus. Support your partner by making other lifestyle changes and/or joining her in any changes she's making; for example, drink nonalcoholic beverages, take walks with her, get extra sleep.
- *Help around the home and with planning for the baby.* Help shop for necessary clothes and equipment, and help get your residence ready for a baby. Pregnancy is hard work, so providing extra help with household chores and errands can be an important element of support. (Due to the risk of infection by toxoplasmosis, one specific chore that should be avoided by pregnant women is handling cat litter; if you and your partner have a cat, emptying the litter box should be your job.)
- *Be involved.* Go to all the prenatal visits, birth preparation or education classes, hospital and nursery tours, and so on. Learn more about pregnancy, childbirth, and parenting by reading books, visiting Internet sites, and talking with others.

### After the Baby Arrives

- *Help meet your baby's needs.* If your job allows, take parental leave to help with the new baby. Support the new mother by helping with baby care (feeding, diaper changes), laundry, shopping, and other chores. Take turns or join the mother when the baby needs care or feeding during the night.
- *Support your partner, and reach out to others for help.* It is normal for a new mother to be tired and to experience mood changes, and some men also experience anxiety about their new role. Good communication between partners and help from supportive relatives and friends can help new parents adjust.

SOURCES: March of Dimes. 2004. *Just for Dad: Becoming a Dad* (http://www.modimes.org/pnhec/362_757.asp; retrieved September 8, 2004); Jensen, T. K., et al. 2004. Body mass index in relation to semen quality and reproductive hormones among 1,558 Danish men. *Fertility and Sterility* 82(4): 863–870; Martini, A. C., et al. 2004. Effects of alcohol and cigarette consumption on human seminal quality. *Fertility and Sterility* 82(2): 374–377.

**The First Trimester** About 30 hours after the egg is fertilized, the cell divides, and this process of cell division repeats many times. On about the fourth day after fertilization, the cluster, now about 32–128 cells and hollow, arrives in the uterus; this is a **blastocyst.** On about the sixth or seventh day, the blastocyst attaches to the uterine wall, usually along the upper curve; over the next few days, it becomes firmly implanted and begins to draw nourishment from the endometrium, the uterine lining.

The blastocyst becomes an **embryo** by about the end of the 2nd week after fertilization. The inner cells of the blastocyst separate into three layers. One layer becomes inner body parts, the digestive and respiratory systems; the middle layer becomes muscle, bone, blood, kidneys, and sex glands; and the third layer becomes the skin, hair, and nervous tissue. The outermost shell of cells becomes the **placenta, umbilical cord,** and **amniotic sac.** A network of blood vessels called chorionic villi eventually forms the placenta. The human placenta is a two-way exchange of nutrients and waste materials between the mother and the fetus. The placenta brings oxygen and nutrients to the fetus and transports waste products out. The placenta does not provide a perfect barrier between the fetal circulation and the maternal circulation, however. Some blood cells are exchanged and certain substances, such as alcohol, pass freely from the maternal circulation through the placenta to the fetus.

The period between weeks 2 and 9 is a time of rapid differentiation and change. All the major body structures are formed during this time, including the heart, brain, liver, lungs, and sex organs; the eyes, nose, ears, arms, and legs also appear. Some organs begin to function—the heart begins to beat, and the liver starts producing blood cells. Because body structures are forming, the developing organism is vulnerable to damage from environmental influences such as drugs and infections (discussed in detail in sections that follow).

By the end of the 2nd month, the brain sends out impulses that coordinate the functioning of other organs.

The embryo is now a fetus, and most further changes will be in the size and refinement of working body parts. In the 3rd month, the fetus begins to be quite active. By the end of the first trimester, the fetus is about 4 inches long and weighs 1 ounce.

**The Second Trimester** To grow during the second trimester, to about 14 inches and 1.5 pounds, the fetus must have large amounts of food, oxygen, and water, which come from the mother through the placenta. All body systems are operating, and the fetal heartbeat can be heard with a stethoscope. Fetal movements can be felt by the mother beginning in the 4th or 5th month. Against great odds, a fetus born prematurely at the end of the second trimester might survive.

**The Third Trimester** The fetus gains most of its birth weight during the last 3 months. Some of the weight is fatty tissue under the skin that insulates the fetus and supplies food. The fetus must obtain large amounts of calcium, iron, and nitrogen from the food the mother eats. Some 85% of the calcium and iron she consumes goes into the fetal bloodstream.

Although the fetus may live if it is born during the 7th month, it needs the fat layer acquired in the 8th month and time for the organs, especially the respiratory and digestive organs, to develop. It also needs the immunity supplied by the antibodies in the mother's blood during the final 3 months. The antibodies protect the fetus against many of the diseases to which she has acquired immunity. These immunities wear off within 6 months after birth, but breast milk can help the baby further resist infections because it also contains maternal antibodies.

**Diagnosing Fetal Abnormalities** Information about the health and sex of a fetus can be obtained prior to birth through prenatal testing.

**Ultrasonography** (also called *ultrasound*) uses high-frequency sound waves to create a **sonogram,** or visual image, of the fetus in the uterus. Sonograms show the position of the fetus, its size and gestational age, and the presence of certain anatomical problems. Sonograms can sometimes be used to determine the sex of the fetus. Sonograms are considered safe for a pregnant woman and the fetus, but the FDA advises against "keepsake" sonograms performed for no medical purpose.

**Amniocentesis** involves the removal of fluid from the uterus with a long, thin needle inserted through the abdominal wall. It is usually performed between 14 and 18 weeks into the pregnancy, although earlier amniocentesis is becoming available at some centers. A genetic analysis of the fetal cells in the fluid can reveal the presence of chromosomal disorders, such as Down syndrome, and some genetic diseases, including Tay-Sachs disease (see the box "Ethnicity and Genetic Diseases" on p. 104). The sex of the fetus can also be determined.

A newer alternative is **chorionic villus sampling (CVS),** which can be performed earlier in pregnancy than amniocentesis, between weeks 10 and 12. This procedure involves removal through the cervix (by catheter) or abdomen (by needle) of a tiny section of chorionic villi, which contain fetal cells that can be analyzed.

The **triple marker screen (TMS)** is a maternal blood test that can be used to help identify fetuses with neural tube defects, Down syndrome, and other anomalies. Blood is taken from the mother at 16–19 weeks of pregnancy and analyzed for three hormone levels—human chorionic gonadotropin (HCG), unconjugated estriol, and alpha-fetoprotein (AFP). The three hormone levels are compared to appropriate standards, and the results are used to estimate the probability that the fetus has particular anomalies.

A new first trimester screening test for Down syndrome combines ultrasound evaluation of the thickness of the back of the fetus's neck with maternal blood testing. This test can be done between the 10th and 14th week of pregnancy. If results indicate an increased risk of abnormality, further diagnostic studies such as amniocentesis can be done for confirmation.

## The Importance of Prenatal Care

Adequate prenatal care—a nutritious diet, exercise, adequate rest, avoidance of drugs, and regular medical evaluation—is essential to the lifelong health of both mother and baby.

### Terms

Vw

**blastocyst** A stage of development, days 6–14, when the cell cluster becomes the embryo and placenta.

**embryo** The stage of development between blastocyst and fetus; about weeks 2–8.

**placenta** The organ through which the fetus receives nourishment and empties waste via the mother's circulatory system; after birth, the placenta is expelled from the uterus.

**umbilical cord** The cord connecting the placenta and fetus, through which nutrients pass.

**amniotic sac** A membranous pouch enclosing and protecting the fetus, containing amniotic fluid.

**ultrasonography** The use of high-frequency sound waves to view the fetus in the uterus; also known as *ultrasound*.

**sonogram** The visual image of the fetus produced by ultrasonography.

**amniocentesis** A process in which amniotic fluid is removed and analyzed to detect possible birth defects.

**chorionic villus sampling (CVS)** Surgical removal of a tiny section of chorionic villi to be analyzed for genetic defects.

**triple marker screen (TMS)** Measurement of alpha-fetoprotein, estriol, and human chorionic gonadotropin to assess risk of fetal anomalies.

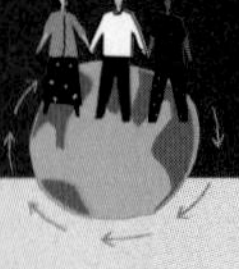

## Ethnicity and Genetic Diseases

Genes carry the chemical instructions that determine the development of hundreds of individual traits, including disease risks, in every human being. Many traits and conditions involve multiple genes and environmental influences. However, some diseases can be traced to a mutation in a single gene.

Children inherit one set of genes from each parent. If only one copy of an abnormal gene is necessary to produce a disease, then it is termed a *dominant* gene. Diseases that are carried by dominant genes seldom skip a generation: Anyone who carries the gene will probably get the disease. If two copies of an abnormal gene (one from each parent) are necessary for a disease to occur, then the gene is called *recessive*. Many common diseases caused by recessive genes occur disproportionately in certain ethnic groups. Prospective parents who come from the same ethnic group can be tested for any recessive diseases found in that group. If both are carriers, each of their children will have about a 25% chance of developing the disease.

Learning all you can about diseases that affect members of your ethnic group can be a lifesaver. Not only can you learn about the risk to your children, but you may also discover there are things you can do to manage the disease and reduce its impact.

- *Sickle-cell disease* affects about 1 out of every 500 African Americans and 1 out of every 1200 Latinos. In this disease, the red blood cells, which carry oxygen to the body's tissues, change shape; the normal doughnut-shaped cells become sickle-shaped. These altered cells carry less oxygen and clog small blood vessels.

People who inherit one gene for sickle-cell disease (about 1 in 12 African Americans) experience only mild symptoms; those with two genes become severely, often fatally, ill. Interestingly, people who inherit one sickle-cell gene are far more resistant to malaria than are those without the gene, leading geneticists to conclude that the sickle-cell trait might have developed in tropical regions as an adaptation to the widespread presence of malaria.

If you are at risk for sickle-cell disease, you can

1. Get genetic counseling to help determine your family's genetic pattern and the degree of risk to you and your potential offspring
2. Take particular care to reduce stress and respond to minor infections, because red blood cells become sickle-shaped during periods of stress on the body
3. Get regular checkups and appropriate treatment

- *Hemochromatosis* ("iron overload") affects about 1 in 250 Americans; most at risk are people of Northern European (especially Irish), Mediterranean, and Hispanic descent. In people with hemochromatosis, the body absorbs and stores up to ten times the normal amount of iron. Over time, iron deposits form in the joints, liver, heart, and pancreas. If untreated, hemochromatosis can cause organ failure and death.

Early symptoms are often vague, but early detection and treatment are necessary to prevent damage. If you have any family members with the disorder, get tested. Treatment involves reducing iron stores by removing blood from the body (a process also known as phlebotomy or "bloodletting").

- *Tay-Sachs disease,* another recessive disorder, occurs annually in approximately 1 out of every 1000 Jews of Eastern European ancestry. People with Tay-Sachs disease are unable to metabolize fat properly; as a result, the brain and other nerve tissues deteriorate. Affected children begin by showing weaknesses in their movements and eventually develop blindness and seizures. This disease is fatal, and death usually occurs by age 3 or 4.

If you are of Eastern European Jewish ancestry and are planning to have children, genetic counseling and blood testing will help you assess the chances that you and your mate will produce a child with Tay-Sachs disease.

- *Cystic fibrosis* occurs in 1 in every 2000 Caucasians per year; about 1 in 20 carries one copy of the cystic fibrosis gene. Because essential enzymes of the pancreas are deficient, nutrients are not properly absorbed. Thick mucus impairs functioning in the lungs and intestinal tracts of people with this disease. The disease is often fatal in early childhood, but medical treatments are increasingly effective in reducing symptoms and prolonging life. In some cases, symptoms do not appear until early adulthood.

If there is a history of cystic fibrosis in your family and you plan to have children, genetic tests and counseling can help in assessing the risk to your prospective offspring.

- *Thalassemia* is a blood disease found most often among Italians, Greeks, and, to a lesser extent, African Americans and Asians. When inherited from one parent, this form of anemia is mild; when two genes are present, the disease is severe and can cause fetal death. Children with this condition require repeated blood transfusions, eventually resulting in a damaging iron buildup. New medical interventions, such as genetic engineering, bone marrow transplants, and chemicals that bind with excess iron and remove it from the body, offer promise. Stem cell transplantation of cells obtained from the umbilical cord blood of an unaffected sibling or donor is already being used in some cases.

If you are at risk of carrying thalassemia, you can

1. Get regular checkups and monitor your health for symptoms
2. Learn symptom management
3. Get genetic counseling to assess the risk to your offspring

- *Lactose intolerance* is a less serious condition affecting about 30–50 million Americans, including a majority of Asian Americans, Native Americans, and African Americans. Although all people are dependent on milk in the early years, by about age 4 many lose the ability to absorb lactose, the chief nutrient in milk. This lactose intolerance results from an absence of lactase, an enzyme that permits the efficient digestion of milk. When lactose-intolerant people ingest more than 1 or 2 servings of milk or dairy products, they suffer from gas pains and diarrhea. Studies show that lactose intolerance is especially prevalent in cultures where milk is relatively unimportant after weaning, suggesting that evolutionary adaptation has played a role in its development.

If you suspect lactose intolerance, see your physician for a test. If you are lactose intolerant, use trial and error to determine how many servings of dairy products you can consume without symptoms. If you react to very small amounts of lactose, try lactose-reduced products or lactase drops or tablets.

Other health problems that have a hereditary component and that disproportionately affect certain ethnic groups include diabetes, osteoporosis, high blood pressure, alcoholism, and certain types of cancer. These links are discussed in later chapters.

**Regular Checkups** In the woman's first visit to her obstetrician, she will be asked for a detailed medical history of herself and her family. The physician or midwife will note any hereditary conditions that may assume increased significance during pregnancy. The tendency to develop gestational diabetes (diabetes during pregnancy only), for example, can be inherited; appropriate treatment during pregnancy reduces the risk of serious harm.

The woman is given a complete physical exam and is informed about appropriate diet. She returns for regular checkups throughout the pregnancy, during which her blood pressure and weight gain are measured, her urine is analyzed, and the size and position of the fetus are monitored. Regular prenatal visits also give the mother a chance to discuss her concerns and assure herself that everything is proceeding normally.

**Blood Tests** A blood sample is taken during the initial prenatal visit to determine blood type and detect possible anemia or Rh incompatibilities. The Rh factor is a blood protein. If an Rh-positive father and an Rh-negative mother conceive an Rh-positive baby, the baby's blood will be incompatible with the mother's. This condition is completely treatable with a serum called Rh-immune globulin. Blood may also be tested for evidence of hepatitis B, syphilis, rubella immunity, thyroid problems, and, with the mother's permission, HIV infection.

**Prenatal Nutrition** The saying that a pregnant woman needs to "eat for two" is true. A nutritious diet throughout pregnancy is essential for both the fetus and the mother. A woman needs to consume about 250–500 extra calories per day during pregnancy; and about 500 or more extra calories per day while breastfeeding. To ensure a balanced intake of key nutrients, pregnant women should follow the U.S. Department of Agriculture's Food Guide, which is described in detail in Chapter 9. It advocates a balance of servings from five key food groups: fruits; vegetables; grains; lean meat, poultry, fish, dry beans, eggs, and nuts; and milk, yogurt, and cheese. It is also important to consume an adequate amount of fluids—the equivalent of about 11 cups per day of liquid from beverages and foods.

Adequate intake of the B vitamin folic acid before conception and in the early weeks of pregnancy has been shown to decrease the risk of neural tube defects, including spina bifida. Any woman capable of becoming pregnant should consume at least 400 μg (0.4 mg) of folic acid daily from fortified foods and/or supplements, in addition to folate from a varied diet. For women who have already had a pregnancy involving a fetus with a neural tube defect, the CDC recommends consulting with a physician about taking a much larger amount of folic acid (4 mg). Folate is found naturally in leafy green vegetables, legumes, citrus fruits, and most berries.

Some physicians may prescribe vitamin and mineral supplements for women who are pregnant or trying to get pregnant. Supplements may be for a particular nutrient, such as folic acid or iron, or may be a multivitamin and mineral supplement. It is important not to supplement beyond a physician's advice or to take herbal dietary supplements without consulting a physician.

Food safety is another key issue because foodborne pathogens can be particularly dangerous during pregnancy. Pregnant women should wash their hands thoroughly before preparing or eating food and after handling raw meats or using the bathroom. All fruits and vegetables should be washed, and foods should be cooked thoroughly and leftovers reheated until steaming hot. One particularly dangerous bacterium is *Listeria monocytogenes*, which can cause miscarriage or birth defects; it is most often found in undercooked or ready-to-eat meat, poultry, or seafood; soft cheeses; and unpasteurized milk or juice.

One further recommendation relates to fish: Most types of fish are good choices for a healthy diet, but a few types can be contaminated with mercury or industrial pollutants. The FDA advises pregnancy women not to eat swordfish, shark, king mackerel, or tilefish; to limit albacore tuna consumption to 6 ounces per week; to limit overall fish consumption to 12 ounces per week; and to check with local health departments before consuming any game fish.

See Chapter 9 for more on healthy nutrition habits and food safety.

**Avoiding Drugs and Other Environmental Hazards** In addition to the food the mother eats, the drugs she takes and the chemicals she is exposed to affect the fetus. Everything the mother ingests may eventually reach the fetus in some proportion. Some drugs harm the fetus but not the mother because the fetus is in the process of developing and because the proper dose for the mother is a massive dose for the fetus.

During the first trimester, when the major body structures are rapidly forming, the fetus is extremely vulnerable to environmental factors such as viral infections, radiation, drugs, and other **teratogens,** any of which can cause **congenital malformations,** or birth defects. The most susceptible body parts are those growing most rapidly at the time of exposure. The rubella (German measles) virus, for example, can cause a congenital malformation of a delicate system such as the eyes or ears, leading to blindness or deafness, if exposure occurs during the first trimester, but it does no damage later in the pregnancy. Other drugs can cause damage throughout prenatal development.

### Terms

VW

**teratogen** An agent or influence that causes physical defects in a developing fetus.

**congenital malformation** A physical defect existing at the time of birth, either inherited or caused during gestation.

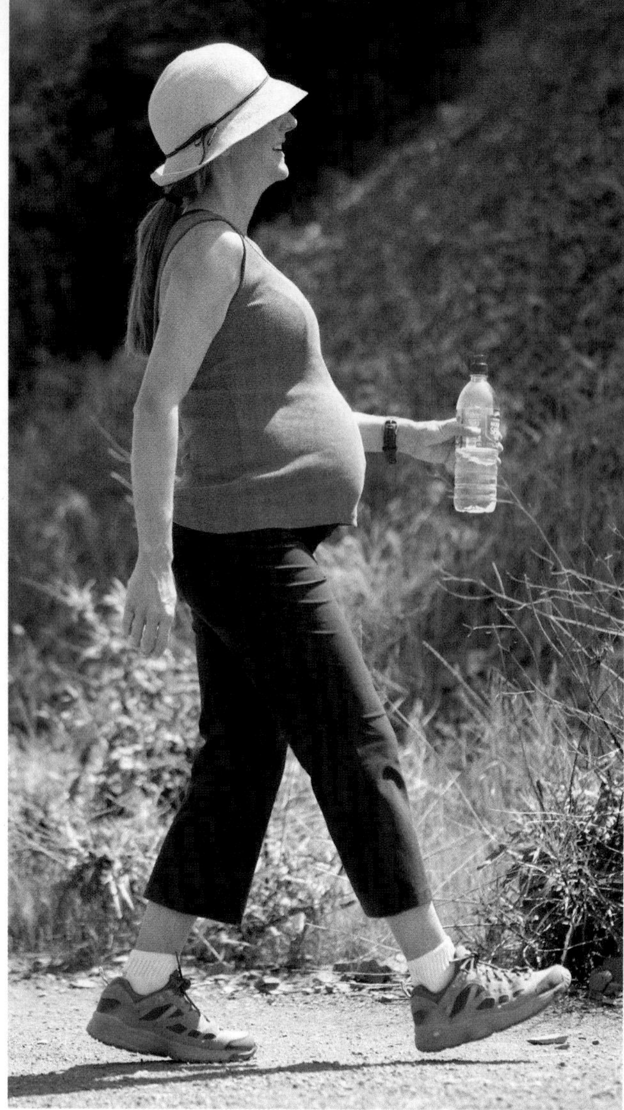

A woman's body changes drastically during pregnancy to accommodate and nourish the growing fetus. Prenatal exercise helps this woman stay healthy while her body works to sustain two lives.

Prenatal exposure to drugs can lead to serious problems. Cigarette smoking is associated with increased risk of miscarriage, low birth weight, chromosomal damage, and infant death. In high doses, caffeine also increases the risk of miscarriage. Getting drunk just one time during pregnancy may be enough to cause brain damage in a fetus. A high level of alcohol consumption during pregnancy is associated with miscarriages, stillbirths, and, in live babies, **fetal alcohol syndrome (FAS).** A baby born with FAS is likely to suffer from a small head and body size, unusual facial characteristics, congenital heart defects, joint problems, mental impairment, and abnormal behaviors patterns. During pregnancy, total abstinence from alcohol and other psychoactive drugs is recommended to help ensure the health of the fetus. Prescription and nonprescription drugs, including vitamins and other dietary supplements, can also harm the fetus and should be used only under medical supervision.

Infections, including those that are sexually transmitted, are another serious problem for the fetus if contracted either before or during birth. Rubella, syphilis, gonorrhea, hepatitis B, Group B streptococcus, herpes simplex, and HIV are among the most dangerous infections for the fetus. Treatment of the mother or immunization of the baby just after birth can help prevent problems from many infections. Women at risk for HIV infection should be tested before or during pregnancy because early treatment can dramatically reduce the chance that the virus will be passed to the fetus; some experts advocate universal HIV screening for pregnant women.

**Prenatal Activity and Exercise** Physical activity during pregnancy contributes to mental and physical wellness. Women can continue working at their jobs until late in their pregnancy, provided the work isn't so physically demanding that it jeopardizes their health. At the same time, pregnant women need more rest and sleep to maintain their own well-being and that of the fetus.

A moderate exercise program during pregnancy does not adversely affect pregnancy or birth; in fact, regular exercise appears to improve a woman's chance of an on-time delivery. The amniotic sac protects the fetus, and normal activities will not harm it. A woman who exercised before becoming pregnant can often continue her program, with appropriate modifications to maintain her comfort and safety. A pregnant woman who hasn't been exercising and wants to start should first consult a physician. Regular cardiorespiratory endurance exercise is recommended. Walking, swimming, and stationary cycling are all good choices; more strenuous activities that could result in a fall, such as skiing, skating, or horseback riding, are best delayed until after the birth. Recommendations for exercising safely during pregnancy include the following:

- Exercise regularly (at least three times a week) rather than intermittently.
- After 20 weeks of pregnancy, avoid exercise that requires lying on your back. Research indicates that this position restricts blood flow to the uterus. Also avoid prolonged periods of motionless standing.
- Modify the intensity of your exercise according to how you feel. Stop exercising if you feel fatigued, and don't exercise to exhaustion. You may find that non–weight-bearing exercises such as swimming and cycling are more comfortable than weight-bearing activities in the later months of pregnancy; they also minimize the risk of injury.
- Avoid any type of exercise that has the potential for even mild abdominal trauma, and take care when performing any activity in which balance is important or in which losing balance would be dangerous. Pregnancy shifts your center of gravity.
- Avoid heat stress, particularly during the first trimester, by drinking an adequate amount of fluid,

wearing appropriate clothing, and avoiding activity in hot and humid weather.

- If you experience any unusual symptoms, stop exercising and consult your physician. Warning signs include pain, vaginal bleeding, dizziness, rapid heartbeat, shortness of breath, and uterine contractions.
- Resume prepregnancy exercise routines gradually. Many of the changes of pregnancy persist for 4–6 weeks after delivery.

*Kegel exercises,* to strengthen the pelvic floor muscles, are also recommended for pregnant women. These exercises are performed by alternately contracting and releasing the muscles used to stop the flow of urine. Each contraction should be held for about 5 seconds. Kegel exercises should be done several times a day, for a total of about 50 repetitions daily.

**Preparing for Birth** Childbirth classes are almost a routine part of the prenatal experience for both mothers and fathers these days. These classes typically teach the details of the birth process as well as relaxation techniques to help deal with the discomfort of labor and delivery. The mother learns and practices a variety of techniques so she will be able to choose what works best for her during labor when the time comes. The father typically acts as a coach, supporting his partner emotionally and helping her with her breathing and relaxing. He remains with her throughout labor and delivery, even when a cesarean section is performed. It can be an important and fulfilling time for the parents to be together.

## Complications of Pregnancy and Pregnancy Loss

Pregnancy usually proceeds without major complications. Sometimes, however, complications may prevent full-term development of the fetus or affect the health of the infant at birth. As discussed earlier in the chapter, exposure to harmful substances, such as alcohol or drugs, can harm the fetus. Other complications are caused by physiological problems or genetic abnormalities.

**Ectopic Pregnancy** In an **ectopic pregnancy,** the fertilized egg implants and begins to develop outside of the uterus, usually in an oviduct. Ectopic pregnancies usually occur because the fallopian tube is blocked, most often as a result of pelvic inflammatory disease; smoking also increases a woman's risk for ectopic pregnancy. The embryo may spontaneously abort, or the embryo and placenta may continue to expand until they rupture the oviduct. Sharp pain on one side of the abdomen or in the lower back, usually in about the 7th or 8th week, may signal an ectopic pregnancy, and there may be irregular bleeding. If bleeding from a rupture is severe, surgical removal of the embryo and the oviduct may be necessary to save the mother's life, although microsurgery can sometimes be used to repair the damaged oviduct. If diagnosed early, before the oviduct ruptures, ectopic pregnancy can often be successfully treated without surgery with injections of methotrexate.

**Spontaneous Abortion** A **spontaneous abortion,** or **miscarriage,** is the termination of pregnancy before the 20th week. It is estimated that 10–40% of pregnancies end this way, some without the woman's awareness that she was even pregnant. Most miscarriages occur between the 6th and 8th weeks of pregnancy, and most—about 60%—are due to chromosomal abnormalities in the fetus. Certain occupations that involve exposure to chemicals may increase the likelihood of a spontaneous abortion.

**Preeclampsia** A disease unique to human pregnancy, **preeclampsia** is characterized by high blood pressure, leaking of protein into urine, and edema (fluid retention), which typically causes swelling of the hands and face. Symptoms may include sudden weight gain, severe headache, abdominal pain, blurred vision, and swelling. If preeclampsia is not treated, it can cause seizures, a condition called **eclampsia.** Other potential problems from preeclampsia include liver and kidney damage, internal bleeding, poor fetal growth, and fetal death. Changes in blood pressure and the presence of excess protein in the urine are usually noticed and tracked during routine prenatal examinations. Women with mild preeclampsia may be monitored and advised to rest in bed at home. Because more severe cases can be life-threatening for the woman and her fetus, patients may be hospitalized for close monitoring and treatment to prevent seizures. Preeclampsia affects about 7% of pregnant women.

**Low Birth Weight** A **low-birth-weight (LBW)** baby is one that weighs less than 5.5 pounds at birth. LBW babies may be premature (born before the 37th week of pregnancy) or full-term. Babies who are born

### Terms

VW

**fetal alcohol syndrome (FAS)** A combination of birth defects caused by excessive alcohol consumption by the mother during pregnancy.

**ectopic pregnancy** A pregnancy in which the embryo develops outside of the uterus, usually in the fallopian tube.

**spontaneous abortion (miscarriage)** Termination of pregnancy at less than 20 weeks' gestation when the uterine contents are expelled; causes include an abnormal uterus, insufficient hormones, and genetic or physical fetal defects.

**preeclampsia** A condition of pregnancy characterized by high blood pressure, edema, and protein in the urine.

**eclampsia** A severe, potentially life-threatening form of preeclampsia, characterized by convulsions and coma.

**low birth weight (LBW)** Weighing less than 5.5 pounds at birth, often the result of prematurity.

small even though they're full-term are referred to as small-for-date babies. Most LBW babies will grow normally, but some will experience problems. Although they are at greater risk than bigger babies for complications during infancy, small-for-date babies tend to have fewer problems than premature infants. The most fundamental problem of prematurity is that many of the infant's organs are not sufficiently developed. Even mild prematurity increases an infant's risk of dying in the first month or year of life. Premature infants are subject to respiratory problems and infections. They may have difficulty eating because they may be too small to suck a breast or bottle and their swallowing mechanism may be underdeveloped. As they get older, premature infants may have problems such as learning difficulties, behavior problems, poor hearing and vision, and physical awkwardness. Adequate prenatal care is the best means of preventing LBW.

**Infant Mortality** The U.S. rate of infant mortality, the death of a child of less than 1 year of age, is near its lowest point ever; however, it remains far higher than that of most of the developed world. Causes of infant death are congenital problems, infectious diseases, and injuries. In the United States, about 2800 infant deaths per year are due to **sudden infant death syndrome (SIDS),** in which an apparently healthy infant dies suddenly while sleeping. The number of SIDS deaths has decreased since 1992, when the "Back to Sleep" campaign was instituted to make people aware that putting babies to bed on their backs rather than on their stomachs significantly reduces the risk of SIDS. Other risk factors for SIDS include abnormalities in heart structure or rhythm or in brain receptors controlling breathing; exposing a fetus or infant to tobacco smoke, alcohol, or other drugs; and putting a baby to bed on a soft mattress or with fluffy bedding, pillows, or stuffed toys. Overbundling a baby or keeping a baby's room too warm also increases the risk of SIDS; because of this, SIDS deaths are more common in the colder months.

### Terms

VW

**sudden infant death syndrome (SIDS)** The sudden death of an apparently healthy infant during sleep.

**labor** The act or process of giving birth to a child, expelling it with the placenta from the mother's body by means of uterine contractions.

**contraction** Shortening of the muscles in the uterine wall, which causes effacement and dilation of the cervix and assists in expelling the fetus.

**transition** The last part of the first stage of labor, during which the cervix becomes fully dilated; characterized by intense and frequent contractions.

**Apgar score** A formalized system for assessing a newborn's need for medical assistance.

## CHILDBIRTH

By the end of the ninth month of pregnancy, most women are tired of being pregnant; both parents are eager to start a new phase of their lives. Most couples find the actual process of birth to be an exciting and positive experience.

### Choices in Childbirth

Many couples today can choose the type of practitioner and the environment they want for the birth of their child. A high-risk pregnancy is probably best handled by a specialist physician in a hospital with a nursery, but for low-risk births, many options are available.

Parents can choose to have their baby delivered by a physician (an obstetrician or family practitioner) or by a certified nurse-midwife. Most babies in the United States are delivered in hospitals or in freestanding alternative birth centers; only about 2% of women choose to have their babies at home. Many hospitals have introduced alternative birth centers in response to criticisms of traditional hospital routines. Alternative birth centers provide a comfortable, emotionally supportive environment in close proximity to up-to-date medical equipment. It's important for prospective parents to discuss all aspects of labor and delivery with their physician or midwife beforehand so they can learn what to expect and can state their preferences.

### Labor and Delivery

The birth process occurs in three stages (Figure 5-6). **Labor** begins when hormonal changes in both the mother and the baby cause strong, rhythmic uterine **contractions** to begin. These contractions exert pressure on the cervix and cause the lengthwise muscles of the uterus to pull on the circular muscles around the cervix, causing effacement (thinning) and dilation (opening) of the cervix. The contractions also pressure the baby to descend into the mother's pelvis, if it hasn't already. The entire process of labor and delivery usually takes between 2 and 36 hours, depending on the size of the baby, the baby's position in the uterus, the size of the mother's pelvis, the strength of the uterine contractions, the number of prior deliveries, and other factors. The length of labor is generally shorter for second and subsequent births.

**The First Stage of Labor** The first stage of labor averages 13 hours for a first birth, although there is a wide variation among women. It begins with cervical effacement and dilation and continues until the cervix is completely dilated (10 centimeters). Contractions usually last about 30 seconds and occur every 15–20 minutes at first, more often later. Early in the first stage, a small amount of bleeding may occur as a plug of slightly bloody mucus that blocked the opening of the cervix during pregnancy is expelled. In some women, the amniotic sac ruptures

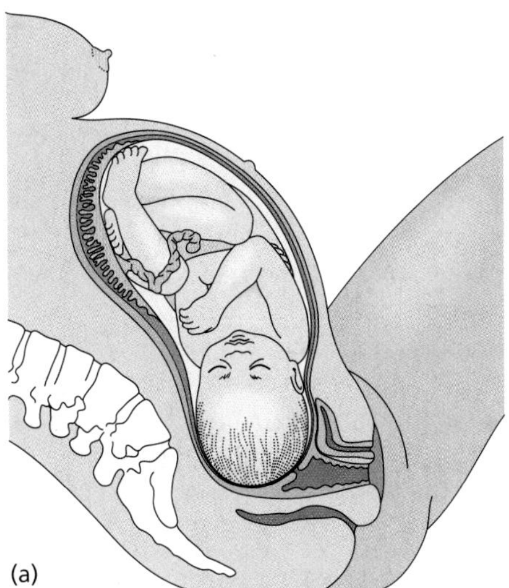


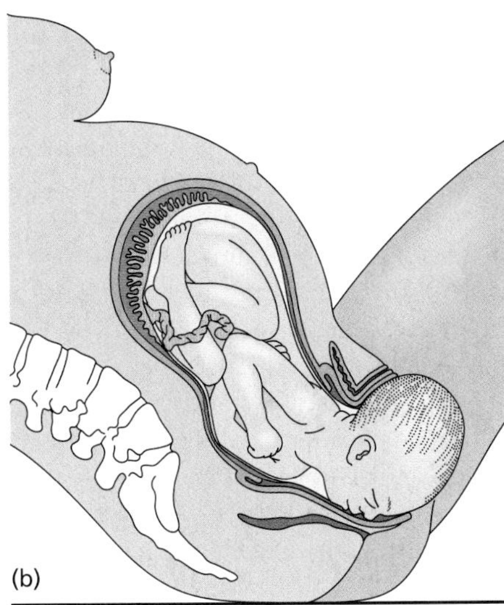


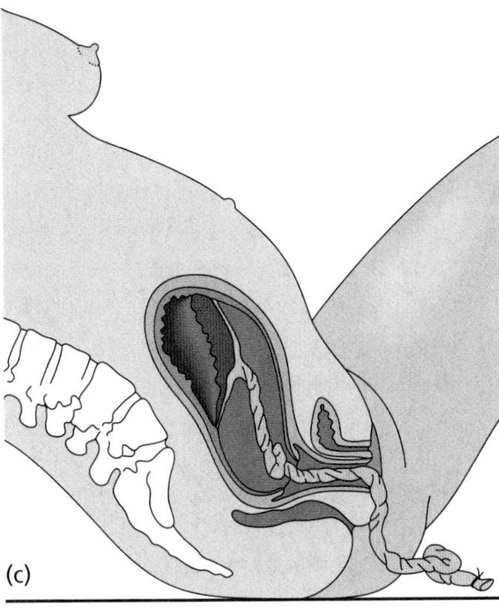


**Figure 5-6 Birth: labor and delivery.** (a) The first stage of labor; (b) the second stage of labor: delivery of the baby; (c) the third stage of labor: expulsion of the placenta.

and the fluid rushes out; this is sometimes referred to as the "water breaking."

The last part of the first stage of labor, called **transition,** is characterized by strong and frequent contractions, much more intense than in the early stages of labor. Contractions may last 60–90 seconds and occur every 1–3 minutes. During transition the cervix opens completely, to a diameter of about 10 centimeters. The head of the fetus usually measures 9–10 centimeters; thus once the cervix has dilated completely, the head can pass through. Many women report that transition, which normally lasts about 30–60 minutes, is the most difficult part of labor.

**The Second Stage of Labor** The second stage of labor begins with complete cervical dilation and ends with the delivery of the baby. The baby is slowly pushed down, through the bones of the pelvic ring, past the cervix, and into the vagina, which it stretches open. The mother bears down with the contractions to help push the baby down and out. Some women find this the most difficult part of labor; others find that the contractions and bearing down bring a sense of relief. The baby's back bends, the head turns to fit through the narrowest parts of the passageway, and the soft bones of the baby's skull move together and overlap as it is squeezed through the pelvis. When the top of the head appears at the vaginal opening, the baby is said to be crowning.

As the head of the baby emerges, the physician or midwife will remove any mucus from the mouth and nose, wipe the baby's face, and check to ensure that the umbilical cord is not around the neck. With a few more contractions, the baby's shoulders and body emerge. As the baby is squeezed through the pelvis, cervix, and vagina, the fluid in the lungs is forced out by the pressure on the baby's chest. Once this pressure is released as the baby emerges from the vagina, the chest expands and the lungs fill with air for the first time. The baby will still be connected to the mother via the umbilical cord, which is not cut until it stops pulsating. The baby will appear wet and often is covered with a milky substance. The baby's head may be oddly shaped at first, due to the molding of the soft plates of bone during birth, but it usually takes on a more rounded appearance within 24 hours.

**The Third Stage of Labor** In the third stage of labor, the uterus continues to contract until the placenta is expelled. This stage usually takes 5–20 minutes. If the placenta does not come out on its own, the physician or midwife may exert gentle pressure on the abdomen to help with its delivery. Breastfeeding soon after delivery helps control uterine bleeding because it stimulates the secretion of a hormone that makes the uterus contract; massaging the abdomen may also help.

In the meantime, the physical condition of the baby will be assessed with the **Apgar score,** a formalized system for assessing the baby's need for medical assistance during the first few minutes of life. Heart rate, respiration, color, reflexes, and muscle tone are individually rated with a score of 0–2, and a total score between 0 and 10 is given at 1 and 5 minutes after birth. A score of 7–10 at 5 minutes is considered normal. The baby is then usually wrapped securely in a blanket and returned to the mother, who may begin to nurse the baby right away.

**Pain Relief During Labor and Delivery** Women vary in how much pain they experience in childbirth. It is recommended that women and their partners learn about labor and what kinds of choices are available for pain relief. Childbirth preparation courses are a good place to start. Breathing and relaxation techniques such as Lamaze or Bradley have been used effectively.

The most commonly employed medical intervention for pain relief is the epidural. This procedure involves placing a thin plastic catheter between the vertebrae in the lower back. Medication that reduces the transmission of pain signals to the brain is given through this catheter. The amount of medication given is quite low and does not accumulate in the baby or interfere with the baby's transition after birth. The mother is awake and is an active participant in the birth. Women can also elect to have narcotics for pain relief during labor, but these medications usually provide less pain relief than the epidural and, if given shortly before the birth, can cause the baby to be less vigorous at birth.

**Cesarean Deliveries** About 26% of the babies born in the United States are delivered by **cesarean section,** in which the baby is removed through a surgical incision in the abdominal wall and uterus. Cesarean sections are necessary when a baby cannot be delivered vaginally—for example, if the baby's head is bigger than the mother's pelvic girdle or if the baby is in an unusual position. If the mother has a serious health condition such as high blood pressure, a cesarean may be safer for her than labor and a vaginal delivery. Other reasons for cesarean delivery include abnormal or difficult labor, fetal distress, and the presence of a dangerous infection like herpes that can be passed to the baby during delivery.

### Terms

Vw

**cesarean section** A surgical incision through the abdominal wall and uterus, performed to deliver a fetus.

**postpartum period** The period of about 3 months after delivering a baby.

**lactation** The production of milk.

**colostrum** A yellowish fluid secreted by the mammary glands around the time of childbirth until milk comes in, about the third day.

**postpartum depression** An emotional low that may be experienced by the mother following childbirth.

Repeat cesarean deliveries are also very common. About 85% of American women who have had one child by cesarean have subsequent children delivered the same way. Although the risk of complications from a vaginal delivery after a previous cesarean delivery is low, there is a small (1%) risk of serious complication to the mother and baby if the previous uterine scar opens during labor. For this reason, women and their doctors may choose to deliver by elective repeat caesarean.

A cesarean section is major surgery and carries some risk, but it is relatively safe. A regional anesthetic such as a spinal or epidural anesthetic may be used so the woman can remain conscious during the operation. The father may be present.

## The Postpartum Period

The **postpartum period,** a stage of about 3 months following childbirth, is a time of critical family adjustments. Parenthood—a job that goes on around the clock without relief—begins literally overnight, and the transition can cause considerable physical and emotional stress.

Currently, just over 60% of mothers breast feed their infants for some period, up from about 10% in 1970. **Lactation,** the production of milk, begins about 3 days after childbirth. Prior to that time (sometimes as early as the second trimester), **colostrum** is secreted by the nipples. Colostrum contains antibodies that help protect the newborn from infectious diseases and is also high in protein.

The American Academy of Pediatrics recommends breastfeeding exclusively for 6 months, in combination with solid food until the baby is 1 year of age, and then for as long after that as a mother and baby desire. Human milk is perfectly suited to the baby's nutritional needs and digestive capabilities, and it supplies the baby with antibodies. Breastfeeding decreases the incidence of infant ear infections, allergies, anemia, diarrhea, and bacterial meningitis; breastfed babies are less likely to be overweight when they reach preschool age. One study has even suggested that children who are breastfed do better in school and score higher on standardized tests. Breastfeeding is also beneficial to the mother: It stimulates contractions that help the uterus return to normal more rapidly, contributes to postpregnancy weight loss, and may reduce the risk of ovarian cancer, breast cancer, and postmenopausal hip fracture.

For some women, physical problems such as tenderness or infection of the nipples can make breastfeeding difficult. If a woman has an illness or requires drug treatment, she may have to bottle-feed her baby because drugs and infectious agents may show up in breast milk. Breastfeeding can be restrictive, making it especially difficult for working mothers. Employers rarely provide nursing breaks, so bottlefeeding or the use of a breast pump (to express milk for use while the mother is away from her infant) may be the only practical alternatives. Bottlefeeding makes it easier to tell how much milk an infant is taking in, and bottlefed infants tend to sleep longer. Bottlefeeding also allows the father or other caregiver to share in the nurturing process. Both breastfeeding and bottlefeeding can be part of loving, secure parent-child relationships.

Many women experience fluctuating emotions during the postpartum period as hormone levels change. The physical stress of labor, as well as dehydration, blood loss, and other physical factors, contributes to lowering the woman's stamina. About 50–80% of new mothers experience "baby blues," characterized by episodes of sadness, weeping, anxiety, headache, sleep disturbances, and irritability. A mother may feel lonely and anxious about caring for her infant. About 10% of new mothers experience **postpartum depression,** a more disabling syndrome characterized by despondency, mood swings, guilt, and occasional hostility. Rest, sharing feelings and concerns with others, and relying on supportive relatives and friends for assistance are usually helpful in dealing with mild cases of the baby blues or postpartum depression, which generally lasts only a few weeks. If the depression is serious, professional treatment may be needed.

Another feature of the postpartum period is the development of attachment—the strong emotional tie that grows between the baby and the adult who cares for the baby. Parents can foster secure attachment relationships in the early weeks and months by responding sensitively to the baby's true needs. A secure attachment relationship helps the child develop and function well socially, emotionally, and mentally.

For most people, the arrival of a child provides a deep sense of joy and accomplishment. However, adjusting to parenthood requires effort and energy. Talking with friends and relatives about their experiences during the first few weeks or months with a baby can help prepare new parents for the period when the baby's needs may require all the energy that both parents have to expend. But the pleasures of nurturing a new baby are substantial, and many parents look back on this time as one of the most significant and joyful of their lives.

**Tips for Today**

Wellness includes understanding and enjoying your own sexuality. This means understanding your sexual anatomy, physiology, and functioning; your sexual orientation; and the various ways of expressing your sexuality and of interacting sexually with others. Preparation for being a parent begins long before pregnancy; it includes healthy lifestyle choices in all the areas of wellness.

*Right now you can*

- Take a few moments to reflect on and articulate to yourself exactly what your beliefs are about sexual relationships at this point in your life. Consider your values, emotions, plans, and resources; also consider whether you are acting in accordance with your beliefs.
- If you are in a sexual relationship, ask yourself whether you are acting responsibly and in the best interest of yourself and your partner 100% of the time. For example, do you always respect each other's wishes and limits when it comes to sexual activity? Do you always avoid mixing sex and alcohol or drugs? If the answer to these or any similar questions is no, resolve to change that behavior.
- Take some time to think about whether *you* want to have children; try to cut through the cultural, societal, family, and personal expectations that may stand in the way of your making the decision you really want to make.
- Think of one thing your mother or father did as a parent that you particularly disliked; if you become a parent, how can you keep from repeating that behavior with your own children?
- Think of one thing your mother or father did as a parent that you particularly liked; if you become a parent, how can you make sure you do the same thing with your own children?

## SUMMARY

- The female external sex organs are called the vulva; the clitoris plays an important role in sexual arousal and orgasm. The vagina leads to the internal sex organs, including the uterus, oviducts, and ovaries.
- The male external sex organs are the penis and the scrotum; the glans of the penis is an important site of sexual arousal. Internal sexual structures include the testes, vasa deferentia, seminal vesicles, and prostate gland.
- The menstrual cycle consists of four phases: menses, the estrogenic phase, ovulation, and the progestational phase.
- The ovaries gradually cease to function as women approach age 50 and enter menopause. The pattern of male sexual responses changes with age, and testosterone production gradually decreases.
- The sexual response cycle has four stages: excitement, plateau, orgasm, and resolution.
- Physical and psychological problems can both interfere with sexual functioning. A treatment for sexual dysfunction first addresses any underlying medical conditions and then looks at psychosocial problems.
- Human sexual behaviors include celibacy, erotic fantasy, masturbation, touching, cunnilingus, fellatio, anal intercourse, and coitus.
- Responsible sexuality includes open, honest communication; agreed-on sexual activities; sexual privacy; using contraception; safer sex practices; sober sex; and taking responsibility for consequences.
- Fertilization is a complex process culminating when a sperm penetrates the membrane of the egg released

from the woman's ovary. Infertility affects about 10% of the reproductive-age population of the United States.

- During pregnancy, the uterus enlarges until it pushes up into the rib cage; the breasts enlarge and may secrete colostrum; the muscles and ligaments soften and stretch; and the circulatory system becomes more efficient.
- The fetal anatomy is almost completely formed in the first trimester and is refined in the second; during the third trimester, the fetus grows and gains most of its weight.
- Prenatal tests include ultrasound, amniocentesis, chorionic villus sampling, and triple marker screening.
- Important elements of prenatal care include regular check-ups; good nutrition; avoiding drugs, alcohol, tobacco, infections, and other harmful environmental agents; regular physical activity; and childbirth classes.
- Pregnancy usually proceeds without major complications. Problems that can occur include ectopic pregnancy, spontaneous abortion, preeclampsia, and low birth weight.
- The first stage of labor begins with contractions that exert pressure on the cervix, causing effacement and dilation. The second stage begins with complete cervical dilation and ends when the baby emerges. The third stage of labor is expulsion of the placenta.
- During the postpartum period, the mother's body begins to return to its prepregnancy state, and she begins to breast-feed. Both mother and father must adjust to their new roles as parents.

## Take Action

1. **Learn more:** Many reputable self-help books about sexual functioning are available in libraries and bookstores. If you're not satisfied with your level of knowledge and understanding, consider consulting some other sources.

2. **Listen to birth stories:** Interview your parents to find out what your birth was like. What were the cultural conditions like at the time, and what were their personal preferences? Find out as much as you can about hospital procedure, the use of anesthetics, length of hospital stay, and so on. Did your father have a role in your birth? If possible, also interview your grandparents or someone of their generation and someone who became a parent in the past few years. How were their experiences different from that of your parents'?

## For More Information

### Books

American College of Obstetricians and Gynecologists. 2005. *Your Pregnancy and Birth*, 4th ed. Washington, D.C.: ACOG. *An excellent guide to conception, pregnancy, and birth.*

Carlson, K. J., S. A. Eisenstat, and T. Ziporyn. 2004. *The New Harvard Guide to Women's Health*. Cambridge, Mass.: Belknap Press; Simon, H. B. 2004. *The Harvard Medical School Guide to Men's Health: Lessons from the Harvard Men's Health Studies*. New York: Free Press. *These books provide research-based information about a wide variety of health issues, including sexuality, contraception, and sexually transmitted diseases.*

Strong, B., et al. 2005. *Human Sexuality in Contemporary America*, 5th ed. New York: McGraw-Hill. *A comprehensive introduction to human sexuality.*

Tsiaras, A., and B. Werth. 2002. *From Conception to Birth: A Life Unfolds*. New York: Doubleday. *The story of prenatal development and birth, told in text and in stunning photographs and medical imaging.*

### Organizations, Hotlines, and Web Sites

*American College of Obstetricians and Gynecologists (ACOG).* Provides written materials relating to many aspects of preconception care, pregnancy, and childbirth.
202-638-5577
http://www.acog.org

*The American Society for Reproductive Medicine.* Provides up-to-date information on all aspects of infertility.
205-978-5000
http://www.asrm.org

*Center for Young Women's Health.* Includes information about topics such as menstruation, gynecological exams, eating disorders, body piercing, and sexual health.
http://www.youngwomenshealth.org

*Dr. Drew.* Provides answers to frequently asked questions about sexuality and relationships, geared toward young adults.
http://www.drDrew.com

*Generational Health.* Helps you create a family health tree online and provides information about detection and screening for any conditions that are common in your family history.
http://www.generationalhealth.com

*La Leche League International.* Provides advice and support for breastfeeding mothers.
800-LaLeche
http://www.lalecheleague.org

*Male Health Center.* A commercial site that provides a variety of information on male sexual health topics.
http://www.malehealthcenter.com

*The March of Dimes.* Provides public education materials on many pregnancy-related topics, including preconception care, genetic screening, diet and exercise, and the effects of smoking and drinking during pregnancy.
888-MODIMES; 914-428-7100
http://www.modimes.org

*National Institute of Child Health and Human Development.* Provides information about reproductive and genetic problems; sponsors the "Back to Sleep" campaign to fight SIDS.
800-505-CRIB (Back to Sleep hotline)
http://www.nichd.nih.gov

*New York University Sexual Disorders Screening*. Provides interactive online screening tests for common sexual disorders.
http://www.med.nyu.edu/psych/screens/disorder_male.html (men)
http://www.med.nyu.edu/psych/screens/disorder_women.html (women)

*Sexuality Information and Education Council of the United States (SIECUS)*. Provides information on many aspects of sexuality and has an extensive library and numerous publications.
http://www.siecus.org

The following sites include information, graphics, and video clips of fetal development:

*Nova/Odyssey of Life*
http://www.pbs.org/wgbh/nova/odyssey/clips

*Visible Embryo*
http://visembryo.com

See also the listings for Chapters 4, 6, and 13.

## Selected Bibliography


American Academy of Pediatrics Section on Breastfeeding. 2005. Breastfeeding and the use of human milk. *Pediatrics* 115(2): 496–506.

American Psychological Association. 2005. *Answers to Your Questions About Sexual Orientation and Homosexuality* (http://www.apa.org/publinfo/answers.html; retrieved February 22, 2005).

Centers for Disease Control and Prevention. 2004. Assisted reproductive technology surveillance, United States, 2001. *MMWR Surveillance Summaries* 53(SS01): 1–20.

Centers for Disease Control and Prevention. 2004. Use of vitamins containing folic acid among women of childbearing age—United States, 2004. *Morbidity and Mortality Weekly Report* 53(36): 847–850.

Cole, L. A., et al. 2004. Accuracy of home pregnancy tests at the time of missed menses. *American Journal of Obstetrics and Gynecology* 190(1): 100–105.

Currie, J., and M. Rich. 2004. Fit and well: Maintaining women's participation in pre- and postnatal exercise. *ACSM's Health and Fitness Journal*, July/August.

de la Chica, R. A., et al. 2005. Chromosomal instability in amniocytes from fetuses of mothers who smoke. *Journal of the American Medical Association* 293(10): 1212–1222.

Delate, T., V. Simmons, and B. Motheral. 2004. Patterns of use of sildenafil among commercially insured adults in the United States, 1998–2002. *International Journal of Impotence Research* 16: 313–318.

Ehrenberg, H. M., et al. 2004. The influence of obesity and diabetes on the risk of cesarean delivery. *American Journal of Obstetrics and Gynecology* 191(3): 969–974.

Fink, K., C. Carson, and R. DeVellis. 2002. Adult circumcision outcomes study: Effect on erectile function, penile sensitivity, sexual activity and satisfaction. *Journal of Urology* 167: 2113–2116.

Forsum, E. 2004. Energy requirements during pregnancy: Old questions and new findings. *American Journal of Clinical Nutrition* 79(6): 933–934.

Freeman, E. W. 2004. Luteal phase administration of agents for the treatment of premenstrual dysphoric disorder. *CNS Drugs* 18(7): 453–468.

Gades, N. M., et al. 2005. Association between smoking and erectile dysfunction: A population-based study. *American Journal of Epidemiology* 161(4): 346–351.

Grady-Weliky, T. A. 2003. Clinical practice. Premenstrual dysphoric disorder. *New England Journal of Medicine* 348(5): 433–438.

Hutcheson, J. C. 2004. Male neonatal circumcision: Indications, controversies and complications. *Urologic Clinics of North America* 31(3): 461–471.

Jernstrom, H., et al. 2004. Breast-feeding and the risk of breast cancer in BRCA1 and BRCA2 mutation carriers. *Journal of the National Cancer Institute* 96(14): 1094–1098.

Kalb, C. 2004. Brave new babies. *Newsweek*, 26 January.

Laumann, E. O., et al. 2005. Sexual problems among women and men aged 40–80 y: Prevalence and correlates identified in the Global Study of Sexual Attitudes and Behaviors. *International Journal of Impotence Research* 17(1): 39–57.

Landon, M.B., et al. 2004. Maternal and perinatal outcomes associated with a trial of labor after prior cesarean delivery. *New England Journal of Medicine* 351(25): 2581–2589.

Levine, R. J., et al. 2005. Urinary placental growth factor and risk of preeclampsia. *Journal of the American Medical Association* 293(1): 77–85.

Martindale, D. 2004. Mickey has two moms. *Scientific American*, July.

Mortensen, E. L., et al. 2002. The association between duration of breastfeeding and adult intelligence. *Journal of the American Medical Association* 287(18): 2365–2371.

National Center for Health Statistics. 2005. Explaining the 2001–2 infant mortality increase. *National Vital Statistics Reports* 53(12).

Nelson, C. P., et al. 2005. The increasing incidence of newborn circumcision: Data from the nationwide inpatient sample. *Journal of Urology* 173(3): 978–981.

Pills for erectile dysfunction: Now there are three. 2004. *Harvard Men's Health Watch*, April.

Rados, C. 2004. FDA cautions against ultrasound "keepsake" images. *FDA Consumer*, January/February.

Stoll, B. J., et al. 2004. Neurodevelopmental and growth impairment among extremely low-birth-weight infants with neonatal infection. *Journal of the American Medical Association* 292(19): 2357–2365.

Strong, B., et al. 2005. *Human Sexuality: Diversity in Contemporary America*, 5th ed. New York: McGraw-Hill.

U.S. Surgeon General. 2001. *The Surgeon General's Call to Action to Promote Sexual Health and Responsible Sexual Behavior* (http://www.surgeongeneral.gov/library/sexualhealth/call.htm; retrieved October 10, 2002).

Wang, L., et al. 2004. Stress and dysmenorrhoea: A population based prospective study. *Occupational and Environmental Medicine* 61(12): 1021–1026.

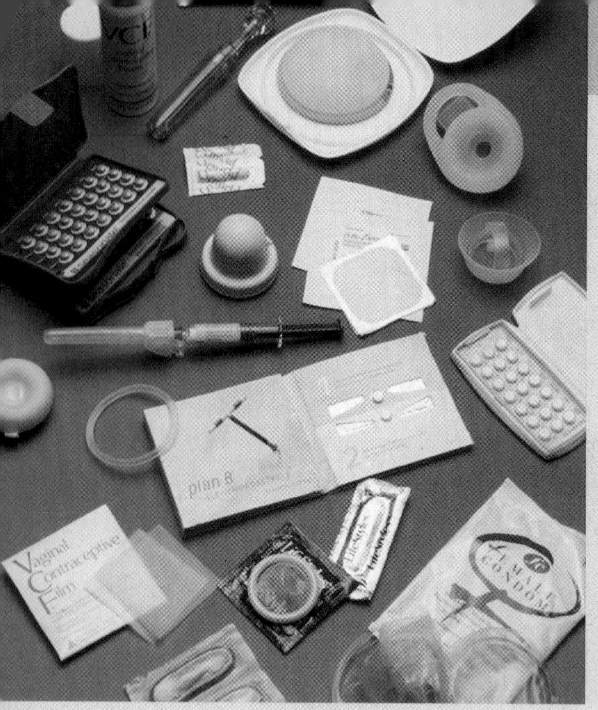


# 6

## Looking AHEAD

After reading this chapter, you should be able to

- Explain how contraceptives work and how to interpret information about a contraceptive method's effectiveness, risks, and benefits
- List the most popular contraceptives, and discuss their advantages, disadvantages, and effectiveness
- Choose a method of contraception based on the needs of the user and the safety and effectiveness of the method
- Describe the history, current legal status, and debate over abortion in the United States
- Describe the methods of abortion available in the United States

# Contraception and Abortion

In her lifetime, the ovaries of an average woman release over 400 eggs, one a month for about 35 years. Each egg is capable of developing into a human embryo if fertilized by one of the millions of sperm a man produces in every ejaculate. Furthermore, unlike most other mammals, humans are capable of sexual activity at any time of the month or year. These facts help explain why people have always had a compelling interest in controlling fertility and in preventing unwanted pregnancies.

Today, people have many options when it comes to making decisions about their sexual and **contraceptive** behavior. In addition to the primary purpose of preventing pregnancy, many types of contraception play an important role in protecting against **sexually transmitted diseases (STDs).** Being informed about the realities and risks and making responsible decisions about sexual and contraceptive behavior are crucial components of lifelong wellness. Among the most important choices of your life will be deciding what type of sexual involvement is best for you; equally critical is the commitment to always protect yourself against unwanted pregnancy and STDs.

## PRINCIPLES OF CONTRACEPTION

The underlying principle of contraception is to block the female's egg from uniting with the male's sperm (conception), thereby preventing pregnancy. A variety of effective approaches in preventing conception are based on different principles of birth control. *Barrier methods* work by physically blocking the sperm from reaching the egg. Diaphragms, condoms, and several other methods are based on this principle. *Hormonal methods*, such as oral contraceptives (birth control pills), alter the biochemistry of the woman's body, preventing ovulation (the release of the egg) and producing changes that make it more difficult for the sperm to reach the egg if ovulation does occur. So-called *natural methods* of contraception are based on the fact that egg and sperm have to be present at the same time if fertilization is to occur. Finally, *surgical methods*—female and male sterilization—more or less permanently prevent transport of the sperm or eggs to the site of conception.

All contraceptive methods have advantages and disadvantages that make them appropriate for some people but not for others or the best choice at one period of life but not at another. Factors that affect the choice of method include effectiveness, convenience, cost, reversibility, side effects and risks, and protection against STDs. Later in this chapter, we help you sort through these factors to decide on the method that's best for you.

Contraceptive effectiveness is partly determined by the reliability of the method itself—the failure rate if it were always used exactly as directed ("perfect use"). Effectiveness is also determined by characteristics of the user, including fertility of the individual, frequency of intercourse, and,

**Visit the *Core Concepts in Health* Online Learning Center (www.mhhe.com/inselbrief10e) for study aids and many additional resources.**

more important, how consistently and correctly the method is used. This "typical use" **contraceptive failure rate** is based on studies that directly measure the percentage of women experiencing an unintended pregnancy in the first year of contraceptive use. For example, the 8% failure rate of oral contraceptives means 8 out of 100 typical users will become pregnant in the first year. This failure rate is likely to be lower for women who are consistently careful in following instructions and higher for those who are frequently careless; the "perfect use" failure rate is 0.3%.

Another measure of effectiveness is the **continuation rate**—the percentage of people who continue to use the method after a specified period of time. This measure is important because many unintended pregnancies occur when a method is stopped and not immediately replaced with another. Thus, a contraceptive with a high continuation rate would be more effective at preventing pregnancy than one with a low continuation rate.

## REVERSIBLE CONTRACEPTION

Reversibility is an extremely important consideration for young adults when they choose a contraceptive method, because most people either plan to have children or at least want to keep their options open until they're older. In this section we discuss the reversible contraceptives, beginning with the hormonal methods, then moving to the barrier methods, and finally covering the natural methods.

### Oral Contraceptives: The Pill

During pregnancy, the corpus luteum secretes progesterone and estrogen in amounts high enough to suppress ovulation. **Oral contraceptives (OCs),** or birth control pills, prevent ovulation by mimicking the hormonal activity of the corpus luteum. The active ingredients in OCs are estrogen and progestins, laboratory-made compounds that are closely related to progesterone.

In addition to preventing ovulation, the birth control pill has other backup contraceptive effects. It inhibits the movement of sperm by thickening the cervical mucus, alters the rate of ovum transport by means of its hormonal effects on the oviducts, and may prevent implantation by changing the lining of the uterus, in the unlikely event that a fertilized ovum reaches that area.

The most common type of OC is the combination pill. Each 1-month packet contains 3 weeks of pills that combine varying types and amounts of estrogen and progestin. Most packets also include a 1-week supply of inactive pills to be taken following the hormone pills; others simply instruct the woman to take no pills at all for 1 week before starting the next cycle. During the week in which no hormones are taken, a light menstrual period occurs.

A newer option that became available in 2003 is the extended-cycle OC Seasonale. With Seasonale, a woman takes active pills for 84 consecutive days, followed by inactive pills for a week; this pattern reduces the number of menstrual periods from 13 per year to just 4 per year. However, spotting and slight bleeding are quite common, especially during the first months of use.

Another, much less common, type of OC is the minipill, a small dose of a synthetic progesterone taken every day of the month. Because the minipill contains no estrogen, it has fewer side effects and health risks, but it is associated with more irregular bleeding patterns.

A woman is usually advised to start the first cycle of pills with a menstrual period to increase effectiveness and eliminate the possibility of unsuspected pregnancy. She must take each month's pills completely and according to instructions. Taking a few pills just prior to having sexual intercourse will not provide effective contraception. A backup method is recommended during the first week and any subsequent cycle in which the woman forgets to take any pills.

**Advantages** The main advantage of the oral contraceptive is its high degree of effectiveness in preventing pregnancy. Nearly all unplanned pregnancies result because the pills were not taken as directed. The pill is relatively simple to use and does not require any interruptions that could hinder sexual spontaneity. Most women also enjoy the predictable regularity of periods, as well as the decrease in cramps and blood loss. For young women, the reversibility of the pill is especially important; **fertility**—the ability to reproduce—returns after the pill is discontinued (although not always immediately). Medical advantages include a decreased incidence of benign breast disease, iron-deficiency anemia, pelvic inflammatory disease (PID), ectopic pregnancy, colon and rectal cancer, endometrial cancer (of the lining of the uterus), and ovarian cancer.

**Disadvantages** Although oral contraceptives do lower the risk of PID, they do not protect against HIV infection or other STDs in the lower reproductive tract. OCs

**Terms**

**contraceptive** Any agent that can prevent conception; condoms, diaphragms, intrauterine devices, and oral contraceptives are examples.

**sexually transmitted disease (STD)** Any of several contagious diseases contracted through intimate sexual contact.

**contraceptive failure rate** The percentage of women using a particular contraceptive method who experience an unintended pregnancy in the first year of use.

**continuation rate** The percentage of women who continue to use a particular contraceptive after a specified period of time.

**oral contraceptive (OC)** Any of various hormone compounds (estrogen and progestins) in pill form that prevent conception by preventing ovulation.

**fertility** The ability to reproduce.

have been associated with increased cervical chlamydia. Regular condom use is recommended for an OC user, unless she is in a long-term, mutually monogamous relationship with an uninfected partner.

OCs can cause a variety of minor side effects, including morning nausea and swollen breasts during the first few months of use. Other side effects include depression, nervousness, changes in sex drive, dizziness, generalized headaches, migraine, bleeding between periods, and changes in vaginal discharge. Serious but uncommon side effects include blood clots, stroke, and heart attack, concentrated mostly in older women who smoke or have a history of circulatory disease. OC users may be slightly more prone to high blood pressure, blood clots in the legs and arms, and benign liver tumors. Most adverse effects of OCs disappear after pill use is discontinued, and studies show no long-term effect on mortality.

Birth control pills are not recommended for women with a history of blood clots, heart disease or stroke, any form of cancer or liver tumor, or impaired liver function. Women with certain other health conditions or behaviors, including migraines, high blood pressure, cigarette smoking, and sickle-cell disease, require close monitoring.

In trying to decide whether to use oral contraceptives, each woman needs to weigh the benefits against the risks with the help of a health care professional. A woman can take several steps to decrease her risk from OC use:

1. Request a low-dosage pill.
2. Stop smoking.
3. Follow the dosage carefully and consistently.
4. Be alert to preliminary danger signals, which can be remembered with the word ACHES:

   Abdominal pain (severe)

   Chest pain (severe), cough, shortness of breath or sharp pain on breathing in

   Headaches (severe), dizziness, weakness, or numbness, especially if one-sided

   Eye problems (vision loss or blurring) and/or speech problems

   Severe leg pain (calf or thigh)
5. Have regular checkups to monitor blood pressure, weight, and urine, and have an annual examination of the thyroid, breasts, abdomen, and pelvis.
6. Have regular **Pap tests** to check for early cervical changes. Because OC use may temporarily increase some women's susceptibility to the STDs chlamydia and gonorrhea, regular screening for those diseases is also recommended.

For most women, the known, directly associated risk of death from taking birth control pills is much lower than the risk of death from pregnancy (Table 6-1).

**Table 6-1 Contraceptive and Abortion Risks**

| | Risk of Death in Any Given Year |
|---|---|
| Oral contraceptives | |
| Nonsmoker | 1 in 66,700 |
| Age less than 35 | 1 in 200,000 |
| Age 35–44 | 1 in 28,600 |
| Heavy smoker (25 or more cigarettes/day) | 1 in 1,700 |
| Age less than 35 | 1 in 5,300 |
| Age 35–44 | 1 in 700 |
| IUDs | 1 in 10,000,000 |
| Barrier methods, spermicides | none |
| Fertility awareness methods, withdrawal | none |
| Sterilization | |
| Laparoscopic tubal ligation | 1 in 38,500 |
| Hysterectomy | 1 in 1,600 |
| Vasectomy | 1 in 1,000,000 |
| Legal abortion | |
| Before 9 weeks | 1 in 262,800 |
| 9–12 weeks | 1 in 100,100 |
| 13–15 weeks | 1 in 34,400 |
| After 15 weeks | 1 in 10,200 |
| Illegal abortion | 1 in 3,000 |
| Pregnancy and childbirth | 1 in 10,000 |

SOURCES: Hatcher, R. A., et al. 2004. *Contraceptive Technology*, 18th ed. New York: Ardent Media; Carlson, K. J., S. A. Eisenstat, and T. Ziporyn. 2004. *The New Harvard Guide to Women's Health*. Cambridge, Mass.: Harvard University Press.

**Effectiveness** If taken exactly as directed, the failure rate of OCs is extremely low (0.3%). However, among average users, lapses such as forgetting to take a pill do occur, and a typical first-year failure rate is 8%. The continuation rate for OCs is 68% after 1 year.

## Contraceptive Skin Patch

The thin, 1¾-inch square contraceptive skin patch (OrthoEvra) slowly releases an estrogen and a progestin into the bloodstream. The patch prevents pregnancy in the same way as combination OCs. Each patch is worn continuously for 1 week and is replaced on the same day of the week for 3 consecutive weeks. The fourth week is patch-free, allowing a woman to have her menstrual period.

The patch can be worn on the upper outer arm, abdomen, buttocks, or upper torso (excluding the breasts); it is designed to stick to skin even during bathing or swimming. If a patch should fall off for more than a day, users start a new 4-week cycle of patches and rely on a backup method of contraception for the first week. In studies of the device, the patch detached and had to be replaced in fewer than 3% of cases.

**Advantages** With both perfect and typical use, the patch is as effective as OCs in preventing pregnancy. Compliance seems to be higher with the patch than with OCs, probably because the patch requires weekly instead of daily action. Medical benefits are likely to be comparable to those of OCs.

**Disadvantages** With patch use, additional measures must be taken for protection against STDs. Minor side effects are similar to those of OCs, although breast discomfort may be more common in patch users. Some women also experience skin irritation around the patch. More serious complications and precautions are thought to be similar to those of OCs, including an increased risk of side effects among women who smoke.

**Effectiveness** With perfect use, the failure rate is very low (0.3%) in the first year of use. The typical failure rate is 8%. The product appears to be less effective when used by women weighing more than 198 pounds.

## Vaginal Contraceptive Ring

The NuvaRing is a vaginal ring that resembles the rim of a diaphragm and is molded with a mixture of progestin and estrogen. The 2-inch ring slowly releases hormones and maintains blood hormone levels comparable to those found with OC use; it prevents pregnancy in the same way as OCs. A woman inserts the ring anytime during the first 5 days of her menstrual period and leaves it in place for 3 weeks. During the fourth week, which is ring-free, her next menstrual period occurs. A new ring is then inserted. Backup contraception must be used for the first 7 days of the first ring use or if the ring has been removed for more than 3 hours during use.

**Advantages** The NuvaRing offers 1 month of protection with no daily or weekly action required. It does not require a fitting by a clinician, and exact placement in the vagina is not critical as it is with a diaphragm. Medical benefits are probably similar to those of OCs.

**Disadvantages** The NuvaRing gives no protection against STDs. Side effects are roughly comparable to those seen with OC use, except for a lower incidence of nausea and vomiting. Other side effects may include vaginal discharge, vaginitis, and vaginal irritation. Medical risks also are similar to those found with OC use.

**Effectiveness** As with the pill and patch, the perfect use failure rate is 0.3% and the typical use failure rate is 8%.

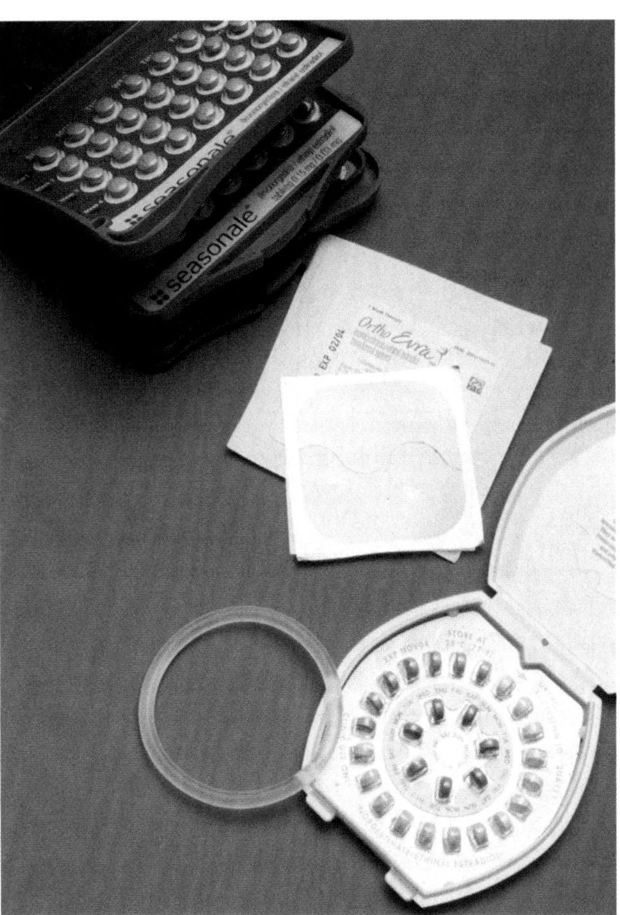


Reversible hormonal contraceptives are available in several forms. To maintain hormone levels in the blood, oral contraceptives are taken daily, the contraceptive patch is replaced weekly, and the vaginal ring is left in place for 3 weeks.

## Contraceptive Implants

Contraceptive implants are placed under the skin and deliver a small but steady dose of hormones over a period of several years. In 1990, the Norplant contraceptive implant became available in the United States. Norplant consists of six flexible, matchstick-size capsules that contain progestin, a synthetic progesterone. The capsules are placed under the skin, usually on the inside of a woman's upper arm in a fan-shaped configuration. The progestin in Norplant has several contraceptive effects: Hormonal shifts may inhibit ovulation and affect development of the uterine lining, thickening of cervical mucus inhibits the movement of sperm, and transport of the egg through the fallopian tubes may be slowed.

The use of Norplant by American women dropped substantially after its first few years of availability because

**Term**

**Pap test** A scraping of cells from the cervix for examination under a microscope to detect cancer.

of ongoing lawsuits and related complaints, and Norplant is no longer being distributed. Current users can leave the implants in place for the full 5 years, however. Other types of contraceptive implants may soon be available; these include a single capsule device, Implanon, and the two-capsule Norplant 2. Contraceptive implants are best suited for women who wish to have continuous and long-term protection against pregnancy.

**Advantages** Norplant implants are highly effective. After insertion of the implants, no further action is required for up to 5 years of protection; at the same time, contraceptive effects are quickly reversed upon removal. Because Norplant, unlike the combination pill, contains no estrogen, it carries a lower risk of certain side effects, such as blood clots and other cardiovascular complications. The thickened cervical mucus resulting from Norplant use has a protective effect against PID.

**Disadvantages** Like the pill, Norplant gives no protection against HIV infection and STDs in the lower reproductive tract. Although the implants are barely visible, their appearance may bother some women. The most common side effects of contraceptive implants are menstrual irregularities, including longer menstrual periods, spotting between periods, or having no bleeding at all. The menstrual cycle usually becomes more regular after 1 year of use. Less common side effects include headaches, weight gain, breast tenderness, nausea, acne, and mood swings. Cautions and more serious health concerns are similar to those associated with oral contraceptives but are less common.

**Effectiveness** Typical failure rates are very low (0.05%) in the first year, increasing slowly with each additional year of use. The cumulative failure rate of Norplant at the end of 5 years is about 1.9%.

## Injectable Contraceptives

The first injectable contraceptive approved for use in the United States was Depo-Provera, which uses long-acting progestins. Injected into the arm or buttocks, Depo-Provera is usually given every 12 weeks, although it actually provides effective contraception for a few weeks beyond that. As another progestin-only contraceptive, it prevents pregnancy in the same ways as Norplant.

Lunelle, an injectable containing both estrogen and progestin, was approved for use in the United States in 2000. Lunelle injections are given every month rather than every 3 months as with Depo-Provera. Lunelle prevents pregnancy in the same way as OCs. (Lunelle became unavailable in 2002 following a voluntary recall and manufacturing hold; for its current status, check with your health care provider.)

**Advantages** Injectable contraceptives are highly effective and require little action on the part of the user. Because the injections leave no trace and involve no ongoing supplies, injectables allow women almost total privacy in their decision to use contraception. Like Norplant, Depo-Provera has no estrogen-related side effects; it requires only periodic injections rather than the minor surgical procedures of implant insertion and removal. Lunelle, which does contain estrogen, has many of the same benefits as oral contraceptives and may be preferred by women who do not want to take a pill every day.

**Disadvantages** Injectable contraceptives provide no protection against HIV infection and STDs in the lower reproductive tract. A woman must visit a health care facility every month (Lunelle) or every 3 months (Depo-Provera) to receive the injections. The side effects of Depo-Provera are similar to those of Norplant; menstrual irregularities are the most common, and after 1 year of using Depo-Provera many women have no menstrual bleeding at all. Weight gain is a common side effect of both Depo-Provera and Lunelle. After discontinuing the use of Depo-Provera, women may experience temporary infertility for up to 12 months.

Reasons for not using Depo-Provera are similar to those for not using Norplant; contraindications for Lunelle are similar to those for OCs. Extended use of Depo-Provera is associated with decreased bone density, a risk factor for osteoporosis; women are advised to use Depo-Provera as a long-term contraceptive (longer than 2 years, for example) only if other methods are inadequate.

**Effectiveness** Perfect use failure rates are 0.3% with Depo-Provera and 0.5% for Lunelle. With typical use, failure rates increase to 3% for both types of injectables in the first year of use. The 1-year continuation rate for both Depo-Provera and Lunelle is about 56%.

## Emergency Contraception

Emergency contraception refers to postcoital methods—those used after unprotected sexual intercourse. An emergency contraceptive may be appropriate if a regularly used method has failed (for example, if a condom breaks) or if unprotected sex has occurred. Emergency contraceptives are designed only for emergency use and should not be relied on as a regular method.

The most frequently used emergency contraceptive is a two-dose regimen of certain oral contraceptives. Postcoital pills appear to work primarily by inhibiting or delaying ovulation and by altering the transport of sperm and/or eggs.

Two products specifically designed for emergency contraception have been approved by the FDA for use in the United States—Plan B and Preven. Plan B contains two progestin-only pills that may be taken together or in separate doses; efficacy and side effects (nausea, breast tenderness) are similar for the two regimens. The first dose should be taken as soon as possible within 120 hours after inadequately protected sex. If the doses are split, the second dose is usually taken 12 hours after the first and may be taken more than 120 hours after unprotected sex. If taken within 24 hours after intercourse, Plan B may prevent as many as 95% of expected pregnancies. Overall, Plan B reduces pregnancy risk by about 89%. (In 2004, the manufacturer of Preven stopped making the product, but existing stocks can still be used. The Preven kit contains two pills, both containing estrogen and progestin.)

Emergency contraceptive pills are available without a prescription in many European countries, and several U.S. states allow pharmacists to dispense emergency contraceptive packets directly, without a physician prescription (California, Washington, Alaska, New Mexico, Maine, and Hawaii, as of 2005). The FDA is considering Plan B as an over-the-counter (OTC) medication. Emergency contraceptives are available by prescription in all states, but not all physicians, hospitals, and/or pharmacies prescribe or provide emergency contraceptive pills, even in cases of sexual assault. For more information on availability, call the emergency contraception hotline (888-NOT-2-LATE).

Intrauterine devices, discussed in the next section, can also be used for emergency contraception if inserted within 5 days of unprotected intercourse. In addition, mifepristone, the "abortion pill," is being studied as another possible option.

## The Intrauterine Device (IUD)

The **intrauterine device (IUD)** is a small plastic device placed in the uterus as a contraceptive. Two IUDs are available in the United States: the Copper T-380A (also known as the ParaGard), which gives protection for up to 10 years, and the Levonorgestral IUD (Mirena), which releases small amounts of progestin and is effective for up to 5 years.

Researchers do not know exactly how IUDs prevent pregnancy. They may cause biochemical changes in the uterus and affect the movement of sperm and eggs; although less likely, they may also interfere with implantation of fertilized eggs. Mirena slowly releases very small amounts of hormones, which impedes fertilization or implantation.

An IUD must be inserted and removed by a trained professional. The device is threaded into a sterile inserter, which is introduced through the cervix; a plunger pushes the IUD into the uterus. The threads protruding from the cervix are trimmed so that only 1–1½ inches remain in the upper vagina.

**Advantages** Intrauterine devices are highly reliable and are simple and convenient to use, requiring no attention except for a periodic check of the string position. They do not require the woman to anticipate or interrupt sexual activity. Usually IUDs have only localized side effects, and in the absence of complications they are considered a fully reversible contraceptive.

**Disadvantages** Heavy menstrual flow and bleeding and spotting between periods may occur, although with Mirena menstrual periods tend to become shorter and lighter over time. Another side effect is pain, particularly uterine cramps and backache, which seem to occur most often in women who have never been pregnant. Spontaneous expulsion of the IUD happens to 5–6% of women within the first year, most commonly during the first months after insertion.

A serious but rare complication of IUD use is pelvic inflammatory disease (PID). Most pelvic infections among IUD users are relatively mild and can be treated successfully with antibiotics. However, early and adequate treatment is critical—a lingering infection can lead to tubal scarring and subsequent infertility.

Some physicians advise against the use of IUDs by young women who have never been pregnant because of the increased incidence of side effects in this group and the risk of infection with the possibility of subsequent infertility. Early IUD danger signals are abdominal pain, fever, chills, foul-smelling vaginal discharge, irregular menstrual periods, and other unusual vaginal bleeding. A change in string length should also be noted. An annual checkup is important for IUD users. IUDs offer no protection against STDs.

**Effectiveness** The typical failure rate of IUDs during the first year of use is 0.8% for the ParaGard and 0.1% for Mirena. Effectiveness can be increased by periodically checking to see that the device is in place and by using a backup method for the first few months after IUD insertion. The continuation rate of IUDs is about 80% after 1 year of use.

## Male Condoms

The **male condom** is a thin sheath designed to cover the penis during sexual intercourse. Most brands available in the United States are made of latex, although condoms made of polyurethane are also now available. Condoms

### Terms

**intrauterine device (IUD)** A plastic device inserted into the uterus as a contraceptive.

**male condom** A sheath, usually made of thin latex (synthetic rubber), that covers the penis during sexual intercourse; used for contraception and to prevent STDs.

Vw

prevent sperm from entering the vagina and provide protection against disease. Condom sales have increased dramatically in recent years, primarily because they are the only method that provides substantial protection against HIV infection as well as some protection against other STDs. At least one-third of all male condoms are bought by women. Women are more likely to contract an STD from an infected partner than men are. Women also face additional health risks from STDs, including cervical cancer, PID, ectopic pregnancy (which is potentially life-threatening), and infertility.

The man or his partner must put the condom on the penis before it is inserted into the vagina, because the small amounts of fluid that may be secreted unnoticed prior to **ejaculation** often contain sperm capable of causing pregnancy. The rolled-up condom is placed over the head of the erect penis and unrolled down to the base of the penis, leaving a half-inch space (without air) at the tip to collect semen (Figure 6-1). Some brands of condoms have a reservoir tip designed for this purpose. Uncircumcised men must first pull back the foreskin of the penis. Partners must be careful not to damage the condom with fingernails, rings, or other rough objects.

Prelubricated condoms are available containing the **spermicide** nonoxynol-9, the same agent found in many of the contraceptive creams that women use. However, there is no evidence that spermicidal condoms are more effective than condoms without spermicide, even though they cost more. Furthermore, these condoms have been associated with urinary tract infections in women and, if they cause tissue irritation, an increased risk of HIV transmission.

If desired, users can lubricate their own condoms with contraceptive foam, creams, or jelly. If vaginal irritation occurs with these products, water-based preparations such as K-Y Jelly can be used. Any products that contain mineral or vegetable oil—including baby oil, many lotions, regular Vaseline petroleum jelly, cooking oils (corn oil, Crisco, butter, and so on), and some vaginal lubricants and anti-fungal or anti-itch creams—should never be used with latex condoms; they can cause latex to begin to disintegrate within 60 seconds, thus greatly increasing the chance of condom breakage. (Polyurethane is not affected by oil-based products.)

**Advantages** Condoms are easy to purchase and are available without prescription or medical supervision (see the box "Buying and Using Over-the-Counter Contraceptives"). Simple to use, they provide for greater male participation in contraception (see the box "Men's Involvement in Contraception" on p. 122). Their effects are immediately and completely reversible. In addition to being free of medical side effects (other than occasional allergic reactions), latex condoms help protect against STDs. Condoms made of polyurethane are appropriate for people who are allergic to latex. However, they are more likely to slip or break than latex condoms, and therefore may give less protection against STDs and pregnancy. (Lambskin condoms permit the passage of HIV and other disease-causing organisms, so they can be used only for pregnancy prevention, not the prevention of STDs.) Except for abstinence, correct and consistent use of latex male condoms offers the most reliable available protection against the transmission of HIV.

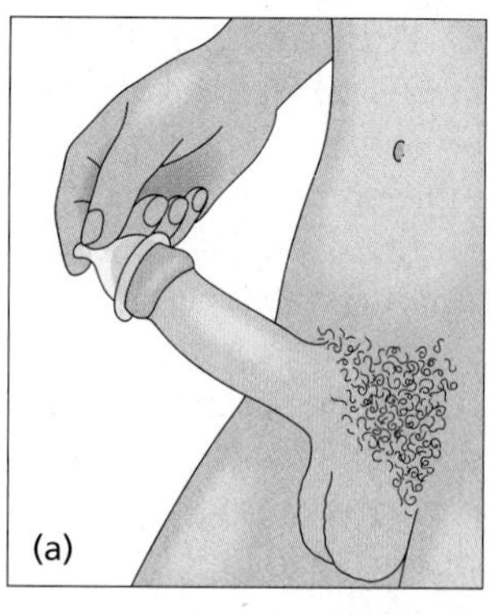

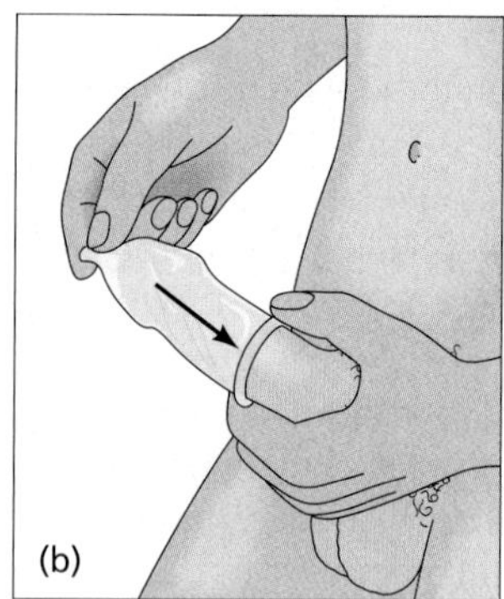

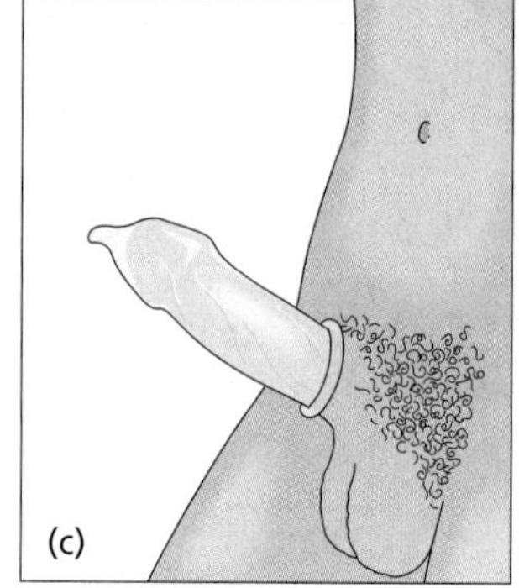

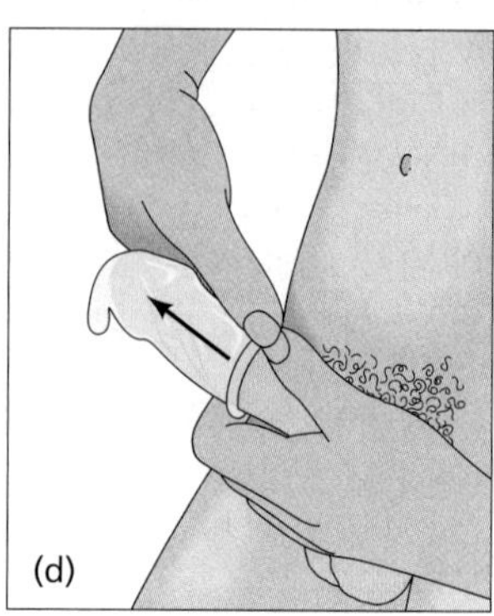


**Figure 6-1 Use of the male condom.** (a) Place the rolled-up condom over the head of the erect penis. Hold the top half-inch of the condom (with air squeezed out) to leave room for semen. (b) While holding the tip, unroll the condom onto the penis. Gently smooth out any air bubbles. (c) Unroll the condom down to the base of the penis. (d) To avoid spilling semen after ejaculation, hold the condom around the base of the penis as the penis is withdrawn. Remove the condom away from your partner, taking care not to spill any semen.

**Disadvantages** The two most common complaints about condoms are that they diminish sensation and interfere with spontaneity. Although some people find these drawbacks serious, others consider them only minor disadvantages.

**Effectiveness** First-year rates among typical users average about 15%. At least some pregnancies happen because the condom is carelessly removed after ejaculation.

## Terms

VW

**ejaculation** An abrupt discharge of semen from the penis after sexual stimulation.

**spermicide** A chemical agent that kills sperm.

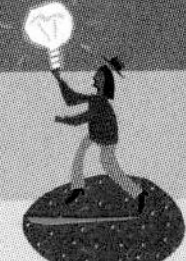

## Buying and Using Over-the-Counter Contraceptives



You can buy several types of contraceptives without a prescription. These have several advantages—they are readily accessible and relatively inexpensive, they are moderately effective at preventing pregnancy, and some offer some protection against HIV infection and other STDs. But like all methods, over-the-counter contraceptives work only if they are used correctly. The following guidelines can help you maximize the effectiveness of your method of choice.

### Male Condoms

- *Buy latex condoms.* If you're allergic to latex, use a polyurethane condom or wear a lambskin condom under a latex one. Lambskin condoms provide no STD protection; polyurethane condoms may provide less protection against pregnancy and STDs than latex condoms do, but more studies are needed.
- *Buy and use condoms while they are fresh.* Packages have an expiration date or a manufacturing date. Don't use a condom after the expiration date or more than 5 years after the manufacturing date (2 years if it contains spermicide).
- *Try different styles and sizes.* Male condoms come in a variety of textures, colors, shapes, lubricants, and sizes. Shop around until you find a brand that's right for you. Condom widths and lengths vary by about 10–20%. A condom that is too tight may be uncomfortable and more likely to break; one that is too loose may slip off.
- *Use "thinner" condoms with caution.* Condoms advertised as "thinner" are often no thinner than others, and those that really are the thinnest tend to break more easily.
- *Don't remove the condom from an individual sealed wrapper until you're ready to use it.* Open the packet carefully. Don't use a condom if it's gummy, dried out, or discolored. Keep extra condoms on hand.
- *Store condoms correctly.* Don't leave condoms in extreme heat or cold, and don't carry them in a pocket wallet.
- *Use only water-based lubricants.* Never use oil-based lubricants like Vaseline or hand lotion, as they may cause a latex condom to break. Avoid oil-based vaginal products.
- *Use male condoms correctly* (see Figure 6-1). Use a new condom every time you have intercourse. Misuse is by far the leading reason that condoms fail.
- *Use emergency contraceptive pills if a condom slips or breaks.*

### Female Condoms

- *Make sure your condom comes with the necessary supplies and information.* The Reality female condom comes individually wrapped. With your condom, you should receive a leaflet containing instructions and a small bottle of additional lubricant.
- *Buy and use female condoms while they are fresh.* Check the expiration dates on the condom packet and the lubricant bottle.
- *Buy several condoms.* Buy one or more for practice before using one during sex. Have a backup in case you have a problem with insertion or use.
- *Read the leaflet instructions carefully.* Practice inserting the condom and checking that it's in the proper position.
- *Use the female condom correctly.* Make sure the penis is inserted into the pouch and that the outer ring is not pushed into the vagina. Add lubricant around the outer ring if needed.
- *Use emergency contraception pills if a condom slips or breaks.*

### Contraceptive Sponges

- *Buy and use contraceptive sponges when they are fresh.* Check the expiration date on each package.
- *Read and follow the package instructions carefully.* Moisten the sponge with water and place high in the vagina.
- *Use each sponge only once.* The sponge may be left in place for up to 24 hours without the addition of spermicide for repeated intercourse.

### Spermicides

- *Try different types of spermicides.* You may find one type easier or more convenient to use. Foams come in aerosol cans and are similar to shaving cream in consistency. Foams are thicker than creams, which are thicker than jellies. Foams, creams, and jellies usually require applicators; spermicidal suppositories and films do not.
- *Read and follow the package directions carefully.* Cans of foam must be shaken before use. Jellies and creams are often inserted with an applicator just outside the entrance to the cervix. Suppositories and film must be placed with a finger.
- *Pay close attention to the timing of use.* Follow the package instructions for inserting the spermicide at the appropriate time before intercourse actually occurs. Spermicides have a fairly narrow window of effectiveness. Be sure to also allow the recommended amount of time for suppositories and films to dissolve.
- *Use an additional full dose for each additional act of intercourse.*
- *Leave the spermicide in place for 8 hours after the last act of intercourse.*
- *Consider using spermicides with another form of birth control.* These include a condom, diaphragm, or cervical cap. Combined use provides greater protection against pregnancy.

### Emergency Contraceptive Pills

Researchers estimate that 51,000 abortions were prevented by use of emergency contraception in 2000, and the FDA is considering changing the status of emergency contraceptive pills from prescription to over-the-counter. Several states allow women to obtain the pills from a pharmacist without a prescription. If emergency contraceptive pills become more widely available over the counter, it will be important for users to follow the instructions carefully.

Gender Matters

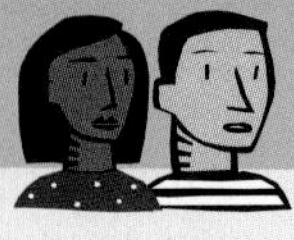

## Men's Involvement in Contraception

In past years, women have accepted the primary responsibility of contraception, along with related side effects and health risks, partly because of the wider spectrum of methods available to them and partly because women have greater personal investment in preventing pregnancy and childbearing. However, male participation is critical, in part because condom use is central to safer sex even when OCs or other female methods are being used. What can be done to increase men's involvement in contraception? Around the world, experts are trying diverse approaches:

- Develop programs and campaigns that stress the importance of information, counseling, and medical care relating to sexual and reproductive matters from adolescence on. Men are less likely than women to seek regular checkups, but regular care for men would benefit men in their own right and both men and women as individuals, couples, and families.
- Recruit and train male health workers, who can be important advocates and role models for healthful behaviors. Expand educational material and clinical programs that focus on male contraception and reproductive health.
- Focus on men as obstacles to women's contraceptive use and as an untapped group of potential users. Educate men about the ways in which stereotypical views of male or female sexuality can inhibit good reproductive health for both men and women. Stress the importance of shared responsibility.
- Develop educational and clinical programs specifically targeted at young men. Men in their early 20s are most likely to engage in risky sexual behaviors and to have adverse reproductive health outcomes. Surveys indicate that most men use a condom the first time they have intercourse, but condom use subsequently declines—and there is much greater reliance on female contraceptive methods.

What can individuals do? Men can increase their participation in contraception in the following ways:

- Initiate and support communication regarding contraception and STD protection.
- Buy and use condoms whenever appropriate.
- Help pay contraceptive costs.
- Be available for shared responsibility in the resolution of an unintended pregnancy, should one occur.

SOURCES: United Nations Population Fund. 2004. *The State of World Population Report 2004*. New York: UNFPA; Alan Guttmacher Institute. 2004. *In Their Own Right: Addressing the Sexual and Reproductive Health of American Men*. New York: Alan Guttmacher Institute; Armstrong, B. 2003. The young men's clinic: Addressing men's reproductive health and responsibilities. *Perspectives on Sexual and Reproductive Health* 35(5): 220–225.

Some may also occur because of breakage or slippage, which may happen 1–2 times in every 100 instances of use for latex condoms and up to 10 times in every 100 instances for polyurethane condoms. Breakage is more common among inexperienced users. Other contributing factors include poorly fitting condoms, insufficient lubrication, excessively vigorous sex, and improper storage (because heat destroys rubber, latex condoms should not be stored for long periods in a wallet or a car's glove compartment). To help ensure quality, condoms should not be used past their expiration date or more than 5 years past their date of manufacture (2 years for those with spermicide). It is important to note, however, that most condom failures are due to inconsistent or improper use, not problems with condom quality.

If a condom breaks or is carelessly removed, the risk of pregnancy can be reduced somewhat by the immediate use of a vaginal spermicide. Some clinicians also recommend keeping emergency contraceptive pills on hand.

## Female Condoms

A female condom is a latex or polyurethane pouch that a woman or her partner inserts into her vagina. The female condom currently available is a disposable device that comes in one size and consists of a soft, loose-fitting polyurethane sheath with two flexible rings. The ring at the closed end is inserted into the vagina and placed at the cervix much like a diaphragm. The ring at the open end remains outside the vagina. The walls of the condom protect the inside of the vagina.

The directions that accompany the condom should be followed closely. It can be inserted up to 8 hours before intercourse and should be used with the supplied lubricant or a spermicide to prevent penile irritation. As with male condoms, users need to take care not to tear the condom during insertion or removal. Following intercourse, the woman should remove the condom immediately, before standing up. By twisting and squeezing the outer ring, she can prevent the spilling of semen.

**Advantages** Female condoms can be inserted before sexual activity and are thus less disruptive than male condoms. Because the outer part of the condom covers the area around the vaginal opening as well as the base of the penis during intercourse, it offers potentially better protection against genital warts or herpes. The polyurethane pouch can be used by people who are allergic to latex. And because polyurethane is thin and pliable, there is little loss of sensation. When used correctly, the female condom should theoretically provide protection against HIV transmission and STDs comparable to that of the latex male condom. However, in research involving typical users, the female condom was less effective in preventing both pregnancy and STDs. With careful instruction and practice, effectiveness can be improved.

**Disadvantages** As with the traditional condom, interference with spontaneity is likely to be a common complaint. The outer ring, which hangs visibly outside the vagina, may be bothersome during foreplay. Female condoms, like male condoms, are made for one-time use. A single female condom costs about four times as much as a single male condom.

**Effectiveness** The typical first-year failure rate of the female condom is 21%.

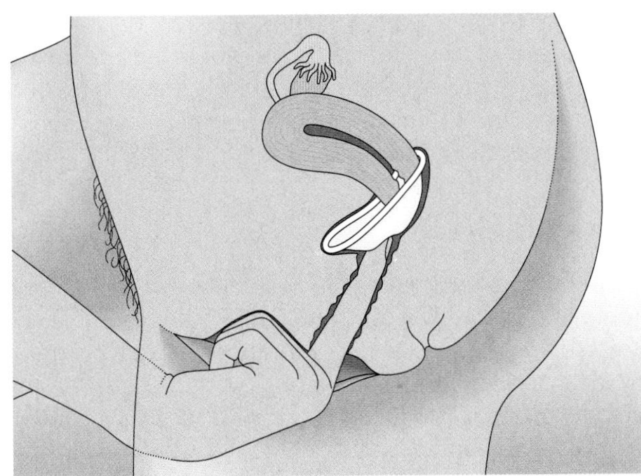

Figure 6-2 The diaphragm properly positioned.

## The Diaphragm with Spermicide

The **diaphragm** is a dome-shaped cup of thin rubber stretched over a collapsible metal ring. When correctly used with spermicidal cream or jelly, the diaphragm covers the cervix, blocking sperm from entering the uterus. A diaphragm can be obtained only by prescription. Because of individual anatomical differences, a diaphragm must be carefully fitted by a trained clinician to ensure both comfort and effectiveness. The fitting should be checked with each routine annual medical examination, as well as after childbirth, abortion, or a weight change of more than 10 pounds.

The woman spreads spermicidal jelly or cream on the diaphragm, squeezing it into a long narrow shape with the thumb and forefinger, inserting it into the vagina, and pushing it up along the back wall of the vagina as far as it will go. The cervix should be completely covered, and the front rim of the diaphragm should be tucked behind the pubic bone (Figure 6-2). If more than 6 hours elapse between the time of insertion and the time of intercourse, additional spermicide must be applied. The diaphragm must be left in place for at least 6 hours after the last act of coitus to give the spermicide enough time to kill all the sperm.

To remove the diaphragm, the woman simply hooks the front rim down from the pubic bone with one finger and pulls it out. She should wash it with mild soap and water, rinse it, pat it dry, and then examine it for holes or cracks. After inspecting the diaphragm, she should dust it with cornstarch (*not* talcum powder, which may damage it and irritate the vagina) and store it in its case.

**Advantages** A diaphragm can be inserted up to 6 hours before intercourse. Its use can be limited to times of sexual activity only, and it allows for immediate and total reversibility. The diaphragm is free of medical side effects (other than rare allergic reactions). When used along with spermicidal jelly or cream, it offers significant protection against gonorrhea and possibly chlamydia, STDs that are transmitted only by semen and for which the cervix is the sole site of entry. Diaphragm use can also protect the cervix from semen infected with the human papillomavirus, which has been implicated as an important factor in cellular changes in the cervix that can lead to cancer. However, the diaphragm is unlikely to protect against STDs that can be transmitted through vaginal or vulvar surfaces (in addition to the cervix), including HIV infection, genital herpes, and syphilis.

**Disadvantages** Diaphragms must always be used with a spermicide, so a woman must keep both of these somewhat bulky supplies with her whenever she anticipates sexual activity. Diaphragms require extra attention, since they must be cleaned and stored with care to preserve their effectiveness. Some women cannot wear a diaphragm because of their vaginal or uterine anatomy or because of frequent bladder infections. It has also been associated with a slightly increased risk of **toxic shock syndrome (TSS)**, an occasionally fatal bacterial infection. To diminish the risk of TSS, a woman should wash her hands carefully with soap and water before inserting or removing the diaphragm, should not use the diaphragm during menstruation or in the presence of an abnormal vaginal discharge, and should never leave the device in place for more than 24 hours.

### Terms

Vw

**diaphragm** A contraceptive device consisting of a flexible, dome-shaped cup that covers the cervix and prevents sperm from entering the uterus.

**toxic shock syndrome (TSS)** A bacterial disease usually associated with tampon use; can also occur in men; symptoms include weakness, cold and clammy hands, fever, nausea, and headache. TSS can progress to life-threatening complications, including very low blood pressure (shock) and kidney and liver failure.

**Effectiveness** Typical failure rates are 16% during the first year of use. The main causes of failure are incorrect insertion, inconsistent use, and inaccurate fitting. If a diaphragm slips during intercourse, a woman may choose to use emergency contraception.

## Lea's Shield

Lea's Shield, a one-size-fits-all diaphragm-like device, was approved by the FDA in 2002 and is now available by prescription. Made of silicone rubber, it can be used by people allergic to latex, and it is not damaged by petroleum-based products. The shield has a valve allowing the flow of air and fluids from the cervix as well as a loop that aids in insertion and removal. The device may be inserted at any time prior to intercourse, but should be left in place for 8 hours after last intercourse; it can be worn for up to 48 hours. Like the diaphragm, it must be used with spermicide. Studies completed thus far have reported advantages, disadvantages, and failure rates similar to those of the diaphragm.

## The Cervical Cap

The **cervical cap**, another barrier device, is a thimble-shaped rubber or plastic cup that fits snugly over the cervix and is held in place by suction. The cap comes in various sizes and must be fitted by a trained clinician. It is used in a manner similar to that of the diaphragm, with a small amount of spermicide being placed in the cup before each insertion.

**Advantages** Advantages of the cervical cap are similar to those associated with diaphragm use and include partial STD protection. It is an alternative for women who cannot use a diaphragm because of anatomical reasons or recurrent urinary tract infections. Because the cap fits tightly, it does not require a fresh dose of spermicide with repeated intercourse. It may be left in place for up to 48 hours (compared with 24 hours for the diaphragm).

**Disadvantages** Along with most of the disadvantages associated with the diaphragm, difficulty with insertion and removal is more common for cervical cap users. In addition, some studies have indicated that women who use the cap rather than the diaphragm initially have a higher rate of abnormal Pap test results. Because there may be a slightly increased risk of TSS with prolonged use, the cap should not be left in place for more than 48 hours.

**Effectiveness** Studies indicate that for women who have never had children, cervical cap failure rate is about 16%, similar to that of the diaphragm. For women who have given birth, the failure rate goes up to about 32%.

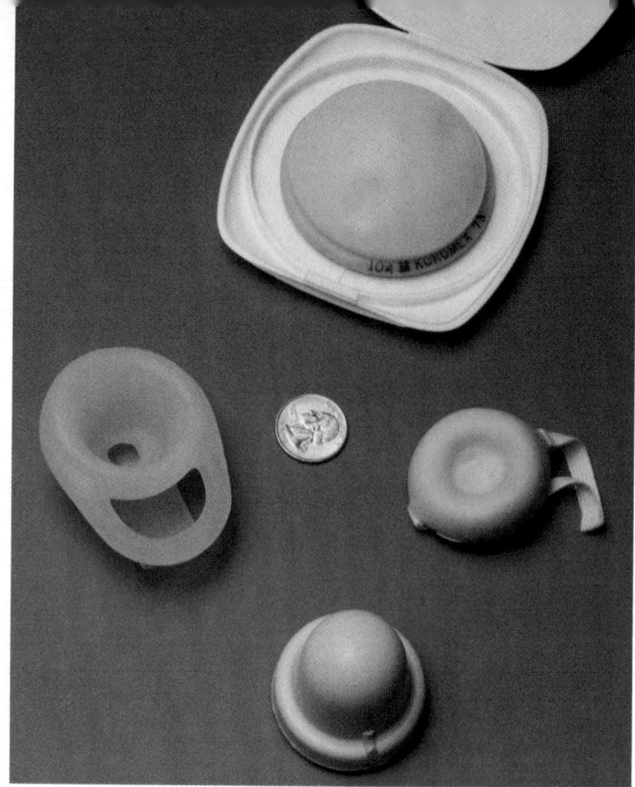

The diaphragm (top), Lea's Shield (left), and cervical cap (bottom) work by covering the mouth of the cervix, blocking sperm from entering the cervix; all require a prescription. The sponge (right), which is available without a prescription or fitting, acts as a barrier, a spermicide, and a seminal fluid absorbent.

## The Contraceptive Sponge

The **sponge** was sold in the United States between 1983 and 1995, at which time the original manufacturer decided to withdraw the contraceptive rather than bring its manufacturing plant up to FDA standards. The safety or effectiveness of the sponge itself was never in question, and FDA approval of the product was never rescinded. A new company bought the rights to the sponge and reintroduced it in Canada in 2003; the company expects to have it on the U.S. market in 2005.

The sponge is a round, absorbent device about 2 inches in diameter with a polyester loop on one side (for removal) and a concave dimple on the other side, which helps it fit snugly over the cervix. The sponge is made of polyurethane and is presaturated with the same spermicide that is used in contraceptive creams and foams. The spermicide is activated when moistened with a small amount of water just before insertion. The sponge, which can be used only once, acts as a barrier, as a spermicide, and as a seminal fluid absorbent.

**Advantages** The sponge offers advantages similar to those of the diaphragm and cervical cap, including partial protection against some STDs. In addition, sponges can be obtained without a prescription or professional fitting, and they may be safely left in place for 24 hours without the addition of spermicide for repeated intercourse.

**Disadvantages** Reported disadvantages include difficulty with removal and an unpleasant odor if left in place for more than 18 hours. Allergic reactions, such as irritation of the vagina, are more common with the sponge than with other spermicide products, probably because the overall dose contained in each sponge is significantly higher than that used with other methods. If irritation of the vaginal lining does occur, the risk of yeast infections and STDs (including HIV) may increase. Because the sponge has also been associated with toxic shock syndrome, the same precautions must be taken as described for diaphragm use.

**Effectiveness** The typical effectiveness of the sponge is slightly lower than that of the diaphragm (20% failure rate during the first year of use) for women who have never experienced childbirth. For women who have had a child, however, sponge effectiveness is significantly lower than diaphragm effectiveness.

## Vaginal Spermicides

Spermicidal compounds developed for use with a diaphragm have been adapted for use without a diaphragm by combining them with a bulky base. Foams, creams, and jellies must be placed deep in the vagina near the cervical entrance and must be inserted no more than 30 minutes before intercourse. The spermicidal suppository is small and easily inserted like a tampon; it is important to wait at least 15 minutes after insertion before having intercourse. The Vaginal Contraceptive Film (VCF)® is a paper-thin 2-inch square of film that contains spermicide. It is folded over one or two fingers and placed high in the vagina. After an hour, the effectiveness of spermicides is drastically reduced, and a new dose must be inserted. Another application is also required before each repeated act of coitus. If the woman wants to **douche,** she should wait for at least 6 hours after the last intercourse to make sure that there has been time for the spermicide to kill all the sperm; douching is not recommended, however, because it can irritate vaginal tissue and may increase the risk of various infections.

**Advantages** The use of vaginal spermicides is relatively simple and can be limited to times of sexual activity. They are readily available in most drugstores and do not require a prescription or a pelvic examination. Spermicides allow for complete and immediate reversibility, and the only medical side effects are occasional allergic reactions. Vaginal spermicides may provide limited protection against some STDs but should never be used instead of condoms for reliable protection.

**Disadvantages** When used alone, vaginal spermicides must be inserted shortly before intercourse, so their use may be seen as an annoying disruption. Spermicides can alter the balance of bacteria in the vagina and may increase the occurrence of yeast infections and urinary tract infections. This method does not protect against STDs, and overuse of spermicides can irritate vaginal tissues; if this occurs, the risk of HIV transmission may actually increase.

**Effectiveness** The typical failure rate is about 29% during the first year of use. Spermicide use is generally recommended only in combination with other barrier methods or as a backup to other contraceptives.

## Abstinence, Fertility Awareness, and Withdrawal

Millions of people throughout the world do not use any of the contraceptive methods we have described, either because of religious conviction or cultural prohibitions or because of poverty or lack of information and supplies. If they use any method at all, they are likely to use one of the following relatively "natural" methods of attempting to prevent conception.

**Abstinence** The decision not to engage in sexual intercourse for a chosen period of time, or **abstinence,** has been practiced throughout history for a variety of reasons. Until relatively recently, many people abstained because they had no other contraceptive measures. Today, few American women rely on periodic abstinence as a contraceptive method. For those who do, other methods may simply seem unsuitable. Concern about possible side effects, STDs, and unwanted pregnancy may be factors. For others, the most important reason for choosing abstinence is a moral one, based on cultural or religious beliefs or strongly held personal values. Individuals may feel that sexual intercourse is appropriate only for married couples or for people in serious, committed relationships. Abstinence may also be considered the wisest choice in terms of an individual's emotional needs. A period of abstinence may be useful as a time to focus energies on other aspects of interpersonal or personal growth.

Anyone can practice abstinence at any time, including people who are not yet sexually active, those who are

### Terms

V w

**cervical cap** A thimble-shaped cup that fits over the cervix, to be used with spermicide.

**sponge** A contraceptive device about 2 inches in diameter that fits over the cervix and acts as a barrier, spermicide, and seminal fluid absorbent.

**douche** To apply a stream of water or other solutions to a body part or cavity such as the vagina; not a contraceptive technique.

**abstinence** Avoidance of sexual intercourse; a method of contraception.

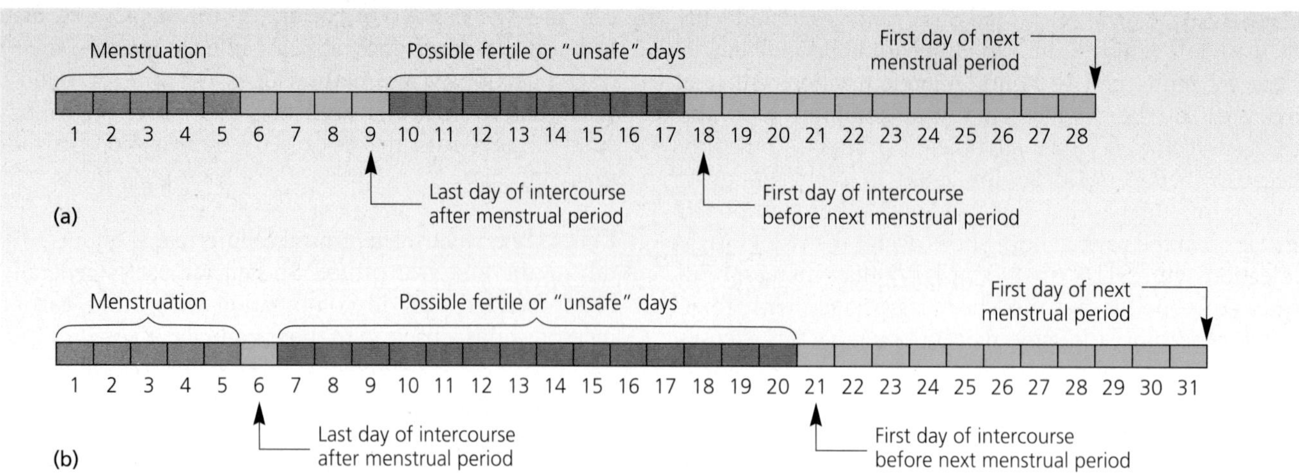


**Figure 6-3 The fertility awareness method of contraception.** This chart shows the safe and unsafe days for (a) a woman with a regular 28-day cycle and (b) a woman with an irregular cycle ranging from 25 to 31 days.

beginning a relationship with a new partner, and those who are not currently in a relationship. Couples may choose abstinence to allow time for their relationship to grow. A period of abstinence allows partners to get to know each other better and to develop trust and respect for each other. Many couples who do choose to abstain from sexual intercourse in the traditional sense turn to other mutually satisfying alternatives. When open communication between partners exists, many new avenues may be explored. These may include dancing, massage, hugging, kissing, petting, mutual masturbation, and oral-genital sex. Sexual feelings and intimacy may be expressed and satisfied through a wide range of activities.

**The Fertility Awareness Method** The basis for the **fertility awareness method (FAM)** is abstinence from coitus during the fertile phase of a woman's menstrual cycle. Ordinarily only one egg is released by the ovaries each month, and it lives about 24 hours unless it is fertilized. Sperm deposited in the vagina may be capable of fertilizing an egg for up to 6–7 days, so conception can theoretically occur only during 8 days of any cycle. Predicting which 8 days is difficult; several methods can be used.

The *calendar method* is based on the knowledge that the average woman releases an egg 14–16 days before her next period begins. Few women menstruate with complete regularity, so a record of the menstrual cycle must be kept for 12 months, during which time some other method of contraception must be used. The first day of each period is counted as day 1. To determine the first fertile, or "unsafe," day of the cycle, subtract 18 from the number of days in the shortest cycle (Figure 6-3). To determine the last unsafe day of the cycle, subtract 11 from the number of days in the longest cycle.

A variation of the calendar method known as the Standard Days Method (SDM) can be used by women with regular menstrual cycles between 26 and 32 days long. Couples must avoid unprotected intercourse on days 8 through 19 of the woman's cycle. Some women who use SDM use a string of color-coded beads known as CycleBeads™ to track their fertile ("unsafe") days.

The *temperature method* is based on the knowledge that a woman's body temperature drops slightly just before ovulation and rises slightly after ovulation. A woman using the temperature method records her basal (resting) body temperature (BBT) every morning before getting out of bed and before eating or drinking anything. Once the pattern is apparent (usually after about 3 months), the unsafe period for intercourse can be calculated as the interval from day 5 (day 1 is the first day of the period) until 3 days after the rise in BBT. To arrive at a shorter unsafe period, some women combine the calendar and temperature methods, calculating the first unsafe day from the shortest cycle of the calendar chart and the last unsafe day as the third day after a rise in BBT.

The *mucus method* (or Billings method) is based on changes in the cervical secretions throughout the menstrual cycle. During the estrogenic phase, cervical mucus increases and is clear and slippery. At the time of ovulation, some women can detect a slight change in the texture of the mucus and find that it is more likely to

## Terms

**fertility awareness method (FAM)** A method of preventing conception based on avoiding intercourse during the fertile phase of a woman's cycle.

**sterilization** Surgically altering the reproductive system to prevent pregnancy. Vasectomy is the procedure in males; tubal sterilization or hysterectomy is the procedure in females.

**Table 6-2 Contraceptive Methods and STD Protection**

| Method | Level of Protection |
|---|---|
| Hormonal methods | Do not protect against HIV or STDs in lower reproductive tract; increase risk of cervical chlamydia; provide some protection against PID. |
| IUD | Does not protect against STDs; associated with PID in first month after insertion. |
| Latex or polyurethane male condom | Best method for protection against STDs (if used correctly); does not protect against infections from lesions that are not covered by the condom. (Lambskin condoms do not protect against STDs.) |
| Female condom | Theoretically should reduce the risk of STDs, but research results are not yet available. |
| Diaphragm, sponge, or cervical cap | Protects against cervical infections and PID. Research results regarding HIV protection are contradictory, but diaphragms, sponges, and cervical caps are not as effective as male condoms and should not be relied on for protection. |
| Spermicide | Modestly reduces the risk of some vaginal and cervical STDs; does not reduce the risk of HIV, chlamydia, or gonorrhea. If vaginal irritation occurs, infection risk may increase. |
| FAM | Does not protect against STDs. |
| Sterilization | Does not protect against STDs. |
| Abstinence | Complete protection against STDs (as long as all activities that involve the exchange of body fluids are avoided). |

Abstinence or sex with a mutually monogamous, uninfected partner is the surest way to protect yourself against HIV and other STDs. Barring this, correct and consistent use of latex male condoms provides the best protection against STDs.

form an elastic thread when stretched between thumb and finger. After ovulation, these secretions become cloudy and sticky and decrease in quantity. Infertile, safe days are likely to occur during the relatively dry days just before and after menstruation. These additional clues have been found to be helpful by some couples who rely on the fertility awareness method.

FAM is not recommended for women who have very irregular cycles—about 15% of all menstruating women. Any woman for whom pregnancy would be a serious problem should not rely on FAM alone, because the failure rate is high—approximately 25% during the first year of use. FAM offers no protection against STDs.

**Withdrawal** In withdrawal, or coitus interruptus, the male removes his penis from the vagina just before he ejaculates. Withdrawal has a relatively high failure rate because the male has to overcome a powerful biological urge. In addition, because preejaculatory fluid may contain viable sperm, pregnancy can occur even if the man withdraws prior to ejaculation. Sexual pleasure is often affected because the man must remain in control and the sexual experience of both partners is interrupted.

Failure rates for typical use are about 27% in the first year. Men who are less experienced with sexual intercourse and withdrawal or who have difficulty in foretelling when ejaculation will occur have higher failure rates. Withdrawal does not protect against STDs.

### Combining Methods

Couples can choose to combine the preceding methods in a variety of ways, both to add STD protection and/or to increase contraceptive effectiveness. For example, condoms are strongly recommended along with OCs whenever there is a risk of STDs (Table 6-2). Foam may be added to condom use to increase protection against both STDs and pregnancy. For many couples, and especially for women, the added benefits far outweigh the extra effort and expense.

Table 6-3 summarizes the effectiveness of available contraceptive methods.

## PERMANENT CONTRACEPTION: STERILIZATION

**Sterilization** is permanent, and it is highly effective at preventing pregnancy. At present it is the most commonly used method both in the United States and in the world. It is especially popular among couples who have been married 10 or more years, as well as couples who have had all the children they intend to have. Sterilization provides no protection against STDs.

An important consideration in choosing sterilization is that, in most cases, it cannot be reversed and should be considered permanent. Some couples choosing male

**Table 6-3 Contraceptive Effectiveness**

| Method | Percentage of Women Experiencing an Unintended Pregnancy in the First Year of Use | |
|---|---|---|
| | Typical Use | Perfect Use |
| Mirena IUD | 0.1 | 0.1 |
| Male sterilization (vasectomy) | 0.15 | 0.1 |
| Female sterilization | 0.5 | 0.5 |
| ParaGard (Copper T-380A) | 0.8 | 0.6 |
| Lunelle injections | 3 | 0.05 |
| Depo-Provera injections | 3 | 0.3 |
| Oral contraceptives | 8 | 0.3 |
| OrthoEvra patch | 8 | 0.3 |
| NuvaRing | 8 | 0.3 |
| Male condom (latex or polyurethane) | 15 | 2 |
| Diaphragm with spermicide | 16 | 6 |
| Cervical cap with spermicide* | 16 | 9 |
| Sponge* | 16 | 9 |
| Female condom | 21 | 5 |
| Fertility awareness method | 25 | |
| Calendar alone | | 9 |
| Combination of FAM methods | | 2 |
| Withdrawal | 27 | 4 |
| Spermicides (alone) | 29 | 18 |
| Chance (no method) | 85 | 85 |

*For women who have given birth, the rates of unintended pregnancy increase to 32% for typical use and 26% for perfect use for the cervical cap and to 32% for typical use and 20% for perfect use for the sponge.

SOURCE: Hatcher, R. A., et al. 2004. *Contraceptive Technology,* 18th rev. ed. New York: Ardent Media. Reprinted by permission of Ardent Media, Inc.

sterilization store sperm as a way of extending the option of childbearing. Male sterilization may be preferable to female sterilization because the overall cost of a female procedure is about four times that of a male procedure, and women are much more likely than men to experience both minor and major complications following the operation. Furthermore, feelings of regret seem to be somewhat more prevalent in women than in men after sterilization.

## Male Sterilization: Vasectomy

The procedure for male sterilization, **vasectomy,** involves severing the vasa deferentia, two tiny ducts that transport sperm from the testes to the seminal vesicles. The testes continue to produce sperm, but the sperm are absorbed into the body. Because the testes contribute only about 10% of the total seminal fluid, the actual quantity of ejaculate is only slightly reduced. Hormone production from the testes continues with very little change, and secondary sex characteristics are not altered.

Vasectomy is ordinarily performed in a physician's office and takes about 30 minutes. A local anesthetic is injected into the skin of the scrotum near the vasa. Small incisions are made at the upper end of the scrotum where it joins the body, and the vas deferens on each side is exposed, severed, and tied off or sealed by electrocautery. A plastic clamp (Vasclip) the size of a grain of rice was approved by the FDA in 2003 and may become more popular as more physicians become trained and experienced in its use. Pain and swelling are usually slight; bleeding and infection occasionally develop but are usually easily treated. Fewer complications occur with an alternative procedure involving a midline puncture rather than incisions; this "no-scalpel" technique is used in about 30% of vasectomies performed in the United States.

Vasectomy is highly effective. In a small number of cases, a severed vas rejoins itself, so some physicians advise yearly examination of a semen sample. The overall failure rate for vasectomy is 0.15%. Although some surgeons report pregnancy rates of about 80% for partners of men who have their vasectomies reversed within 10 years of the original procedure, most studies report figures in the 50% range.

## Female Sterilization

The most common method of female sterilization involves severing, or in some manner blocking, the oviducts, thereby preventing the egg from reaching the uterus and the sperm from entering the fallopian tubes. Ovulation and menstruation continue, but the unfertilized eggs are released into the abdominal cavity and absorbed. Although progesterone levels in the blood may decline slightly, hormone production by the ovaries and secondary sex characteristics are generally not affected.

**Tubal sterilization** is most commonly performed by a method called **laparoscopy.** A laparoscope, a tube containing a small light, is inserted through a small abdominal incision, and the surgeon looks through it to locate the fallopian tubes. Instruments are passed either through the laparoscope or through a second small incision, and the two fallopian tubes are sealed off with ties or staples or by electrocautery. General anesthesia is usually used; the operation takes about 15 minutes. Tubal sterilization can also be performed shortly after a vaginal delivery, or in the case of cesarean section immediately after the uterine incision is repaired.

Although tubal sterilization is somewhat riskier than vasectomy, with a rate of minor complications of about 6–11%, it is the more common procedure (see the box "Contraceptive Use Among American Women" on p. 130). Potential problems include bowel injury, wound infection, and bleeding. Serious complications are rare, and the death rate is low. The failure rate for tubal sterilization is about 0.5%. When pregnancies do occur, an increased percentage of them are ectopic. Because reversibility rates are low and the procedure is costly, female sterilization should be considered permanent.

A new female sterilization device was approved by the FDA in 2002. The Essure System consists of tiny spring-like metallic implants that are inserted through the vagina, into the fallopian tubes, using a special catheter. Within several months, scar tissue forms over the implants, blocking the tubes. **Hysterectomy,** removal of the uterus, is the preferred method of sterilization for only a small number of women, usually those with preexisting menstrual problems.

## WHICH CONTRACEPTIVE METHOD IS RIGHT FOR YOU?

Each person must consider many variables in deciding which method is most acceptable and appropriate for her or him:

1. *Health risks.* Is there anything in your personal or family medical history that would affect your choice of method? For each method you consider, what are the potential health risks that apply to you? For example, IUDs are not recommended for young women without children because of an increased risk of pelvic infection and subsequent infertility. Hormonal methods should be used only after a clinical evaluation of your medical history. Other methods have only minor and local side effects. Talk with your physician about the potential health effects of different methods for you.

2. *The implications of an unplanned pregnancy.* How would an unplanned pregnancy affect you and your future? What are your feelings regarding the options—abortion, adoption, or raising a child? If effectiveness is of critical importance to you, carefully consider the ways the effectiveness of each method can be improved. Abstinence is 100% effective, if maintained. If used correctly, hormonal methods offer very good protection against pregnancy. Barrier methods can be combined with spermicides to improve their effectiveness.

3. *STD risk.* How likely are you to be exposed to any sexually transmitted diseases? Have you and your partner been screened for STDs recently? Have you openly and honestly discussed your past sexual behavior? Condom use is of critical importance whenever any risk of STDs is present. This is especially true when you are not in an exclusive, long-term relationship or when you are taking the pill, because cervical changes that occur during hormone use may increase vulnerability to certain diseases. Abstinence or activities that don't involve intercourse or any other exchange of body fluids can be a satisfactory alternative for some people.

4. *Convenience and comfort level.* How do your partner and you view each of the methods? Which would you most likely use consistently? The hormonal methods are generally ranked high in this category, unless there are negative side effects and health risks or forgetting to take pills is a problem for you. Some people think condom use disrupts spontaneity and lowers penile sensitivity. (Creative approaches to condom use and improved quality can decrease these concerns.) The diaphragm, cervical cap, contraceptive sponge, female condom, and spermicides can be inserted before intercourse begins but are still considered a significant inconvenience by some.

5. *Type of relationship.* How easy is it for you to talk with your partner about contraception (see the box "Talking with a Partner About Contraception" on p. 131)? How willing is he or she to be involved? Barrier methods require more motivation and sense of responsibility from *each* partner than hormonal methods do. When the method depends on the cooperation of one's partner, assertiveness is necessary, no matter how difficult. This is especially true in new relationships, when condom use is most important. When sexual activity is infrequent, a barrier method may make more sense than an IUD or one of the hormonal methods.

6. *Ease and cost of obtaining and maintaining each method.* If a physical exam and clinic follow-up are required, how readily accessible is this to you? Can you and your partner afford the associated expenses of the method? Investigate the costs of different methods. Find out if your insurance covers any of the costs.

7. *Religious or philosophical beliefs.* Are any of the methods unacceptable to you because of your personal beliefs? For some, abstinence and/or FAM may be the only permissible contraceptive methods.

### Terms

VW

**vasectomy** The surgical severing of the ducts that carry sperm to the ejaculatory duct.

**tubal sterilization** Severing or in some manner blocking the oviducts, preventing eggs from reaching the uterus.

**laparoscopy** Examining the internal organs by inserting a tube containing a small light through an abdominal incision.

**hysterectomy** Total or partial surgical removal of the uterus.

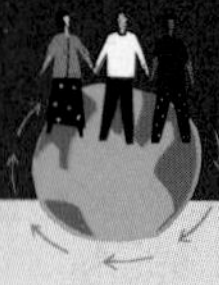

## Contraceptive Use Among American Women

About 62 million women in the United States are in their childbearing years (15–44) and thus face decisions about contraception. Overall, about 62% of American women use some form of contraception, and most of the remaining 38% are either sterile, pregnant or trying to become pregnant, or not sexually active. Only 7% of American women are fertile, sexually active, and not seeking pregnancy *and* not using contraceptives; this small group accounts for almost half of the 3 million unintended pregnancies that occur each year. The unintended pregnancies that occur among contraceptive users are usually the result of inconsistent or incorrect use of methods. For example, one-third of barrier method users report not using their method every time they have intercourse.

Oral contraceptives and female sterilization are the two most popular methods among American women (see figure). However, choice of contraceptive method and consistency of use vary with age, marital status, and other factors:

- *Age:* Sterilization is much more common among older women, particularly those who are over 35 years of age and/or who have had children. Older women are also much more likely to use reversible methods consistently—they are least likely to miss pills and most likely to use barrier methods during every act of intercourse. Young women between ages 15 and 17 who use OCs are more likely by far to miss pills than women in any other age group.
- *Marital status:* Women who are or were married have much higher rates of sterilization than women who have never been married. Those who have never been married have high rates of OC and condom usage.
- *Ethnicity:* Overall rates of contraceptive use and use of OCs are highest among white women. Female sterilization, implants, and injectables are more often used by African American women and Latinas, and IUD use is highest among Latinas. Condom use is highest among Asian American women and similar across other ethnic groups. Male sterilization is much more common among white men than among men of other ethnic groups.
- *Socioeconomic status and educational attainment:* Low socioeconomic status and low educational attainment are associated with high rates of female sterilization and low rates of pill and condom use. However, women who are poor or have low educational attainment and who do use OCs have higher rates of consistent use than women who are wealthier or have more education. About 20% of women age 15–44 lack adequate health insurance, increasing the cost and difficulty of obtaining contraceptives.

Some trends in contraceptive use may also reflect the differing priorities and experiences of women and men. For example, female sterilization is more expensive and carries greater health risks than male sterilization—yet it is more than twice as common. (Worldwide, female sterilization is more than four times as common as male sterilization.) This pattern may reflect culturally defined gender roles and the fact that women are more directly affected by unintended pregnancy. In surveys, women rate pregnancy prevention as the single most important factor when choosing a contraceptive method; in contrast, men rate STD prevention as equally important.

SOURCES: Alan Guttmacher Institute. 2005. *Facts in Brief: Contraceptive Use*. New York: Alan Guttmacher Institute; Alan Guttmacher Institute. 2004. *Issues in Brief: Preventing Unintended Pregnancy in the U.S.* (http://www.agi-usa.org/pubs/ib2004no3.html; retrieved August 23, 2004); National Center for Health Statistics. 2004. Use of contraception and use of family planning services in the United States: 1982–2002. *Advance Data from Vital and Health Statistics*, No. 350. Grady, W. R., D. H. Klepinger, and A. Nelson-Wally. 1999. Contraceptive characteristics: The perceptions and priorities of men and women. *Family Planning Perspectives* 31(4): 168–175.

Women not using contraception (38.1% of U.S. women)
Sterile for noncontraceptive reasons or with sterile male partner (3.1%)
Sexually active (7.4%)
Pregnant, post-partum, or seeking pregnancy (9.5%)
Not sexually active (18.1%)
Method reported by women using contraception (61.9% of U.S. women)
Female sterilization (16.7%)
Oral contraceptives (18.9%)
Condoms (11.1%)
Male sterilization (5.7%)
Withdrawal (2.5%)
3-month injectable (3.3%)
Fertility awareness method (0.9%)
Diaphragm (0.2%)
Implant, one-month injectable, or patch (0.8%)
IUDs (1.3%)
Other (0.6%)

**Contraceptive use among American women age 15–44 years.**

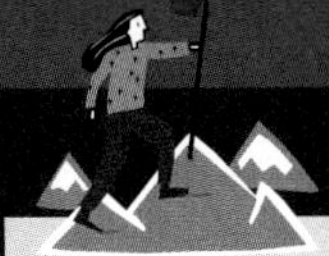

Take Charge

## Talking with a Partner About Contraception

Many people have a difficult time talking about contraception with a potential sex partner. How should you bring it up? And whose responsibility is it, anyway? Talking about the subject may be embarrassing at first, but imagine the possible consequences of *not* talking about it. An unintended pregnancy or a sexually transmitted disease could profoundly affect you for the rest of your life. Talking about contraception is one way of showing that you care about yourself, your partner, and your future.

Before you talk with your partner, explore your own thoughts and feelings. Find out the facts about different methods of contraception, and decide which one you think would be most appropriate for you. If you're nervous about having this discussion with your partner, it may help to practice with a friend.

Pick a good time to bring up the subject. Don't wait until you've started to have sex. A time when you're both feeling comfortable and relaxed will maximize your chances of having a good discussion. Tell your partner what you know about contraception and how you feel about using it, and talk about what steps you both need to take to get and use a method you can live with. Listen to what your partner has to say, and try to understand his or her point of view. You may need to have more than one discussion, and it may take some time for both of you to feel comfortable with the subject. *But don't have sex until this issue is resolved.*

If you want your partner to be involved but he or she isn't interested in talking about contraception, or if he or she leaves all the responsibility for it up to you, consider whether this is really a person you want to be sexually involved with. If you decide to go ahead with the involvement, you may want to enlist the support of a friend, family member, or health care worker to help you make and implement decisions about the essential issue of contraception.

Whatever your needs, circumstances, or beliefs, *do* make a choice about contraception. Not choosing anything is the one method known *not* to work. This is an area in which taking charge of your health has immediate and profound implications for your future.

## THE ABORTION ISSUE

In the United States today, few issues are as complex and emotion-filled as abortion. Although most public attention has focused on legal definitions and restrictions, the most difficult aspects of abortion actually take place at a much more personal level. Because the majority of women having abortions are young, many college students have had some type of direct exposure to these more personal experiences of abortion.

The word **abortion**, by strict definition, means the expulsion of an embryo or fetus from the uterus before it is sufficiently developed to survive. As commonly used, however, *abortion* refers only to those expulsions that are artificially induced by mechanical means or drugs, and *miscarriage* is generally used for a spontaneous abortion, one that occurs naturally with no causal intervention. In this chapter, *abortion* will mean a deliberately induced expulsion.

### The History of Abortion in the United States

For more than two centuries, abortion policy in the United States followed English common law, which made the practice a crime only when performed after "quickening" (fetal movement that begins at about 20 weeks). Opposition to abortion gained minimal attention until the mid-1800s, when newspaper advertisements for abortion preparations became common and concern grew that women were using abortion as a means of birth control (and perhaps to cover up extramarital activity). There was much discussion about the corruption of morality among women in the United States, and by the 1900s abortion was illegal in every state. These antiabortion laws stayed in effect until the 1960s, when courts began to invalidate them on the grounds of constitutional vagueness and violation of the right to privacy (see the box "Timeline of Selected Key Abortion Decisions and Legislation" on p. 132).

### Current Legal Status

In 1973, the U.S. Supreme Court made abortion legal in the landmark case of *Roe v. Wade*. To replace the restrictions most states still imposed at that time, the justices divided pregnancy into three parts, or trimesters, giving a pregnant woman less choice about abortion as she advances toward full term. In the first trimester, the abortion decision must be left to the judgment of the pregnant woman and her physician. During the second trimester, similar rights remain but a state may regulate factors that protect the health of the woman, such as type of facility where an abortion may be performed. In the third trimester, when the fetus is viable (capable of survival

**Term**

**abortion** The expulsion or removal of an embryo or fetus from the uterus.

VW

In the News

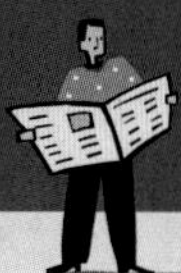

## Timeline of Selected Key Abortion Decisions and Legislation

WW

**1700s to mid-1800s** Abortion is generally legal throughout the United States.

**Mid-1800s to mid-1900s** Abortion becomes illegal in all 50 states, with certain exceptions that vary by state (for example, to save the life of the mother). The federal Comstock Act of 1873 makes it illegal to distribute or possess information about, or devices or medications for, contraception or abortion.

**1965** *Griswold v. Connecticut:* The Supreme Court overturns a law prohibiting use of contraceptives by married couples, stating that it violates the right of marital privacy guaranteed in the Bill of Rights.

**1967–1973** Some states rewrite their abortion laws, including four states that repeal abortion bans.

**1972** *Eisenstadt v. Baird:* The Supreme Court overturns a law banning distribution of contraceptives to unmarried adults, stating that the ban violates the equal protection clause of the constitution.

**1973** *Roe v. Wade:* The Supreme Court strikes down a Texas law banning abortion and rules that abortion is encompassed within the constitutional right to privacy. The court divides pregnancy into three trimesters and states that during the first trimester, decisions about abortion should be left up to the woman and her physician. After the first trimester, states may regulate abortion in ways related to maternal health; once the fetus is viable, states may regulate or ban abortion except when abortion is necessary to preserve the life or health of the mother.

**1976** *Planned Parenthood of Central Missouri v. Danforth:* The Supreme Court rules against a statute that requires married women to obtain their spouse's approval before having an abortion and requires minors to obtain written parental consent.

**1980** *Harris v. McRae:* The Supreme Court upholds restrictions on Medicaid funding for abortions except as needed to protect the life of the mother or in other special circumstances.

**1986** *Thornburgh v. American College of Obstetricians and Gynecologists:* The Supreme Court strikes down a law requiring any woman seeking an abortion to receive a state-scripted lecture from her physician about potential risks and possible alternatives.

**1989** *Webster v. Reproductive Health Services:* The Supreme Court upholds a state law prohibiting the use of public facilities for abortions that are not medically necessary and requiring physicians to do viability testing on fetuses of more than 20 weeks' gestation.

**1991** *Rust v. Sullivan:* The Supreme Court rules that clinics receiving federal Title X (family planning) funding can be prohibited from counseling, referring, or providing information about abortions.

**1992** *Planned Parenthood of Southeastern Pennsylvania v. Casey:* The Supreme Court upholds the *Roe* decision but allows states to restrict abortion access as long as the restrictions do not impose an undue burden on women seeking abortions. It upholds a provision requiring minors to obtain consent from one parent or a judge (judicial bypass) to obtain an abortion.

**1994** Congress passes the Freedom of Access to Clinics Act, making it a crime to injure, intimidate, or interfere through threats, force, or physical obstruction with a woman's right to obtain reproductive health services, including abortion.

**2000** The FDA approves mifepristone (RU-486), the abortion pill.

**2000** *Stenberg v. Carhart:* The Supreme Court finds a law banning partial-birth abortion unconstitutional because it lacks an exception for the health of the mother and imposes an undue burden on women seeking abortions.

**2003** Congress passes and President Bush signs the Partial Birth Abortion Ban Act with no exception to the ban in cases of risk to a woman's health.

**2004** The Partial Birth Abortion Ban Act is declared unconstitutional by federal judges in San Francisco, New York, and Lincoln, Nebraska; the decisions are expected to be appealed to the Supreme Court.

SOURCES: Cornell University Legal Information Institute. 2004. *U.S. Supreme Court Decisions* (http://supct.law.cornell.edu/supct/; retrieved November 15, 2004); CBS News. 2004. *Abortion Timeline* (http://www.cbsnews.com/htdocs/abortion/timeline.html; retrieved November 15, 2004); National Public Radio. 2003. *History of the Abortion Debate: Timeline of Significant Supreme Court Decisions* (http://www.npr.org/news/specials/roevwade/timeline.html; retrieved November 15, 2004).

outside of the uterus), a state may regulate and even bar all abortions except those considered necessary to preserve the mother's life or health.

Today, abortion remains legal throughout the United States, but rulings by the Supreme Court in 1989 *(Webster v. Reproductive Health Services)* and 1992 *(Planned Parenthood of Southeastern Pennsylvania v. Casey)* allow states to regulate abortion throughout pregnancy as long as an "undue burden" is not imposed on women seeking the procedure. As a result, states have passed a variety of laws, including bans on the use of public funding, employees, and facilities for abortion services; mandatory counseling and waiting periods; insurance prohibitions; and requirements for parental consent for minors. In addition to state abortion restrictions, the U.S. Congress has barred the use of federal Medicaid funds to pay for abortions, except when a woman's life is in danger or in cases of rape or incest. Concerns have been raised that a two-tiered system has been created—one for women with means and another for those without.

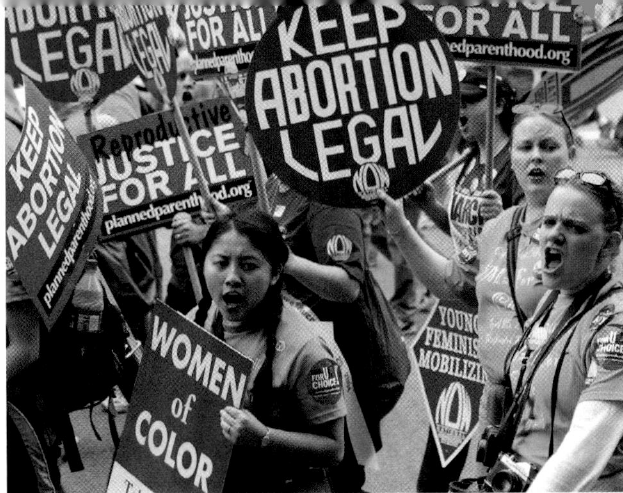

KEEP ABORTION LEGAL
KEEP ABORTION LEGAL
WOMEN of COLOR
Pro-choice groups believe that the decision to end or continue a pregnancy is a personal matter that should be left up to the individual.

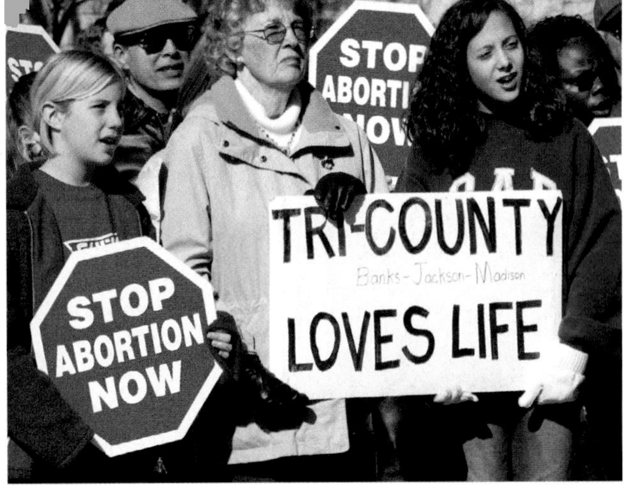

STOP ABORTION NOW
TRI-COUNTY
Banks-Jackson-Madison
LOVES LIFE
Pro-life groups oppose abortion on the basis of their belief that life begins at the moment of conception.

## Moral Considerations

Along with the legal debates are ongoing arguments between pro-life and pro-choice groups regarding the ethics of abortion. Central to the pro-life position is the belief that the fertilized egg must be valued as a human being from the moment of conception and that abortion at any time is equivalent to murder. This group holds that any woman who has sexual intercourse knows that pregnancy is a possibility, and should she willingly have intercourse and get pregnant, she is morally obligated to carry the pregnancy through. Pro-life followers encourage adoption for women who feel they are unable to raise the child and point out how many couples are seeking babies for adoption. Pro-life individuals do not consider the availability of legal abortion as essential to women's well-being but view it instead as having an overall destructive effect on our traditional morals and values.

In contrast, the pro-choice viewpoint holds that distinctions must be made between the stages of fetal development and that preserving the fetus early in pregnancy (or *gestation*) is not always the ultimate moral concern. Members of this group maintain that women must have the freedom to decide whether and when to have children; they argue that pregnancy can result from contraceptive failure or other factors out of a woman's control. When pregnancy does occur, pro-choice individuals believe that the most moral decision possible must be determined according to each situation and that, in some cases, greater injustice would result if abortion were not an option. If legal abortions were not available, pro-choice supporters say, "back-alley shops" and do-it-yourself techniques, with their many health risks, as well as the births of unplanned children, would again grow in number. Others argue that discrimination in health care would result, since wealthy women could travel for a legal abortion elsewhere.

Some people strongly identify exclusively with either the pro-life or the pro-choice stance, but many have moral beliefs that are blurred, less defined, and in some cases a mixture of the two. Although the most vocal groups in the abortion debate tend to paint a black-and-white picture, the majority of Americans view abortion as a complex issue without any easy answers.

## Public Opinion

In general, U.S. public opinion on abortion seems to change depending on the specific situation. Many individuals approve of legal abortion as an option when destructive health or welfare consequences could result from continuing pregnancy, but they do not advocate abortion as a simple way out of an inconvenient situation. Overall, most adults in the United States continue to approve of legal abortion and are opposed to overturning the basic right to abortion established in *Roe v. Wade* (Figure 6-4). But the amount of public support varies considerably depending on the circumstances surrounding the abortion request. For example, more Americans are in favor of legal abortion in a situation in which the woman's life is endangered (85%) than in cases where the baby is physically impaired (56%) or the woman or family cannot afford to raise the child (35%). Similarly, more people are in favor of allowing legal abortion in the first 3 months of pregnancy (66%) than in the second 3 months (25%).

## Personal Considerations

For the pregnant woman who is considering abortion, the usual legal and moral arguments may sound meaningless as she attempts to weigh the many short- and long-term ramifications for all lives directly concerned. If she chooses abortion, can she accept that decision in terms of her own religious and moral beliefs? What are her long-range feelings likely to be regarding this decision? What are her partner's feelings regarding abortion, and how will she deal with his response?

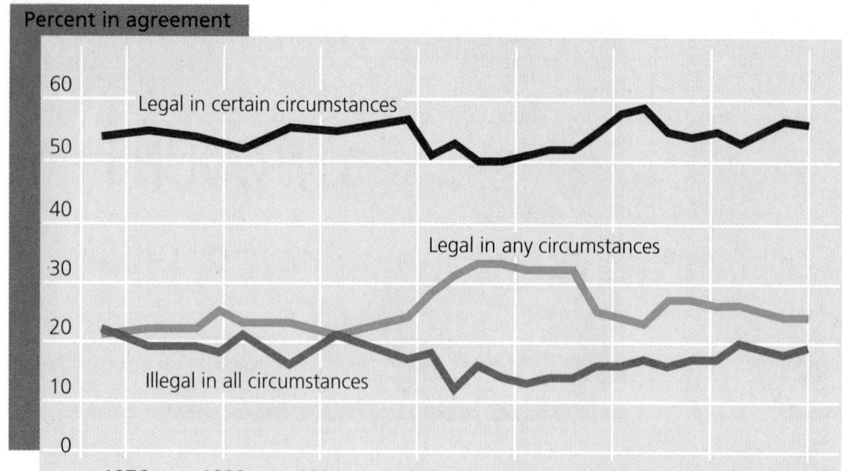


VITAL STATISTICS

**Figure 6-4 Public opinion about abortion.** The graph represents responses to this question: Do you think abortions should be legal under any circumstances, legal only under certain circumstances, or illegal in all circumstances? SOURCE: Gallup Organization. 2004. *Gallup Poll Tuesday Briefing: Abortion* (http://www.gallup.com/content/print.aspx?ci=1574; retrieved September 7, 2004).

For the woman who decides against abortion and chooses instead to continue the pregnancy, there are other questions. If she decides to raise the child herself, will she have the resources to do it well? Is a supportive, lasting relationship with her partner likely? If not, how does she feel about being a single parent?

If the pregnant woman considers adoption, she will have to try to predict what her emotional responses will be throughout the full-term pregnancy and the adoption process. What are her long-range feelings likely to be? What type of adoption would be most appropriate? (The box "The Adoption Option" on p. 136 addresses some of these questions.)

## Current Trends

With the increased accessibility to legalized abortion following the mid-1970s, the rate of late abortions dropped steadily, until fewer than 2% of all abortions were performed at more than 20 weeks and fewer than 12% at more than 12 weeks by the 1990s (Figure 6-5). The overall abortion *rate* rose during most of the 1970s, leveled off around 1980, and decreased in the 1990s (Figure 6-6). As much as 43% of the decline in abortion between 1994 and 2000 may be attributable to the use of emergency contraception (see Chapter 6). Possible future influences on the number, rate, and timing of abortions in the United States include legal decisions, more widespread availability of emergency contraceptives, and the increasing use of medical abortion.

Since the 1989 *Webster* and 1992 *Casey* decisions, many states have imposed additional restrictions on abortion. In 2004, 29 states required mandatory counseling, in 26 states followed by a waiting period; 34 states required parental consent or notification for minors; more than half of the states banned certain abortion procedures; and 35 states severely restricted the use of public funds for abortion. Research into the effects of these restrictions has been mixed. Parental consent and notification laws may result in minors traveling out of state to obtain abortions.

Adding to the legal restrictions is the growing scarcity of physicians willing to provide abortion services. Currently, 87% of all U.S. counties, 96% of nonmetropolitan counties, and about 57% of metropolitan areas have no abortion providers. It is unclear whether the approval of mifepristone for medical abortion will significantly affect

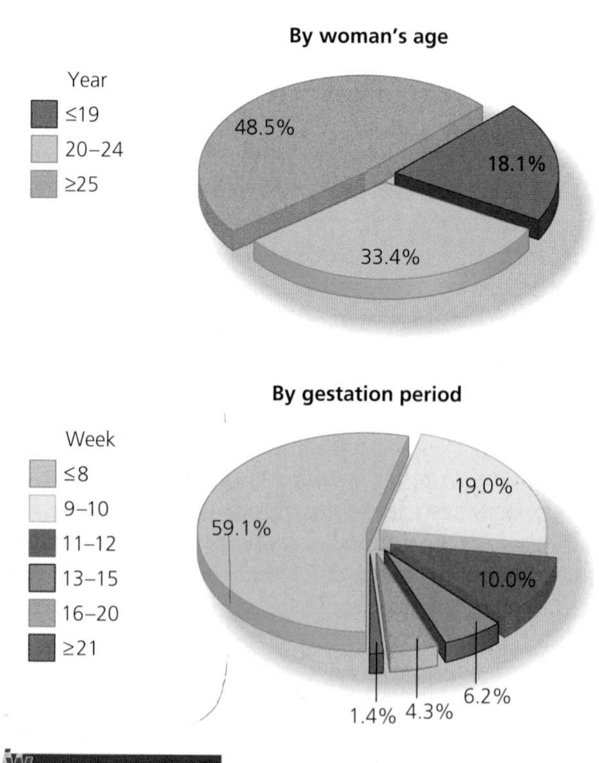


VITAL STATISTICS

**Figure 6-5 Distribution of abortions by the woman's age and by the weeks of gestation.** SOURCE: Centers for Disease Control and Prevention. 2004. Abortion surveillance—United States, 2001. *Morbidity and Mortality Weekly Report Surveillance Summaries* 53 (SS-9).

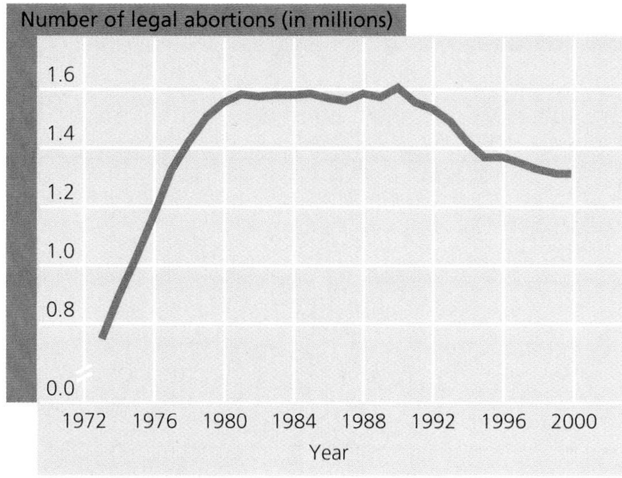


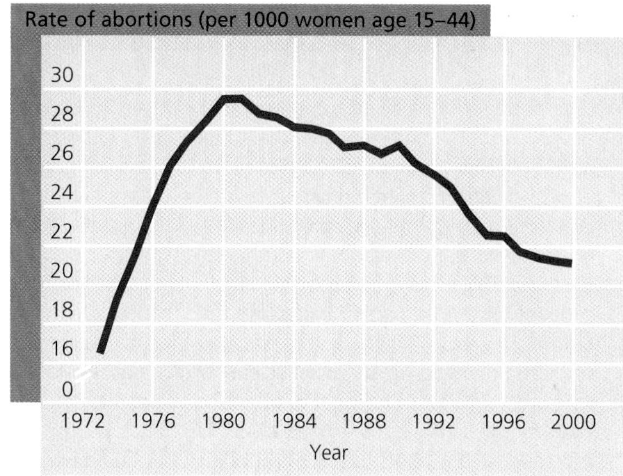


VW VITAL STATISTICS

**Figure 6-6 Number and rate of abortions in the United States.** SOURCE: Finer, L. B., and S. K. Henshaw. 2003. Abortion incidence and services in the United States in 2000. *Perspectives on Sexual and Reproductive Health* 35(1): 6–15.

these numbers. The diminishing number of providers is due in part to increased anti-abortion protests and violence, including arson, bombings, and the murders of several physicians and clinic workers. Women living in areas that have restrictive laws and few abortion providers may continue to obtain abortions, but they are likely to face significant increases in expense and time delays.

Unless accompanied by a greater effort at preventing unwanted pregnancy, legal changes alone will probably not dramatically reduce the number of abortions. At current rates, about 40% of American women will have had at least one abortion by the time they are 45 years old. Based on national research, the typical American woman having an abortion is age 20–30, has a previous birth, has never been married, is poor, lives in a metropolitan area, and is Christian.

## Methods of Abortion

Abortion methods can be divided into two categories: surgical and medical. Surgical abortion is by far the most common, accounting for about 98% of all abortions performed in the United States. Medical abortion, in which medications are used to induce abortion, may become more common following the approval in 2000 of mifepristone (Mifeprex).

**Suction curettage** (also called *vacuum aspiration*) is the most common method for abortions performed from the 6th to the 12th week of pregnancy. It is used in about 90% of all abortions performed in the United States. In this procedure, the cervix is dilated and a suction curette, a specially designed hollow tube, is then inserted into the uterus. The curette is attached to the rubber tubing of an electric pump, and suction is applied to the uterus, and the uterine lining is scraped with a metal curette to remove any remaining tissue. The entire procedure takes only 5–10 minutes and has a low risk of complications.

Because suction curettage is believed to be safer and more effective when performed at least 6 or 7 weeks after the last menstrual period, women seeking abortion early in pregnancy are sometimes told to wait several weeks. A relatively new option for women at the very earliest stages of pregnancy is a surgical procedure called **manual vacuum aspiration (MVA).** In MVA, the cervix is dilated, and a plastic tube attached to a handheld syringe is inserted through the cervix. The uterus is emptied with gentle suction provided by the syringe.

Medical abortion, ending a pregnancy with medications rather than surgery, is an option for women who are in the early phase of pregnancy. A combination of drugs is given that causes the embryo and products of conception to be passed out through the vagina, as in a natural miscarriage. The drug mifepristone, also called RU-486 or the "abortion pill," is approved for use under medical supervision up to 49 days following the last menstrual period. A woman takes a dose of mifepristone and follows it up two days later with a second drug, misoprostol, which induces contractions. Abortion can take anywhere from a few hours to several weeks; about 75% of abortions occur within 24 hours. Two weeks after taking mifepristone, a woman must return to her health care

### Terms

VW

**suction curettage** Removal of the embryo or fetus by means of suction; also called *vacuum aspiration.*

**manual vacuum aspiration (MVA)** The vacuum aspiration of uterine contents shortly after a missed period using a handheld syringe.

In Focus

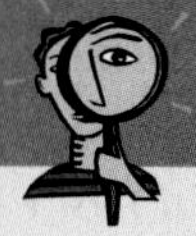

## The Adoption Option

One of the options available to a woman facing an unplanned pregnancy is adoption. Between 1952 and 1972, nearly 9% of unmarried pregnant women gave their children up for adoption; currently, however, only about 2% of women choose to place a child for adoption. This decline is probably due to a variety of factors, including increased rates of contraceptive use and an easing of the social stigma of single parenthood. The drop in adoption rates in the 1970s probably reflected an increase in the abortion rate following the 1973 legalization of abortion; however, since 1990 adoption rates have remained steady, while the abortion rate has declined, indicating that women are not choosing abortion over adoption.

If you are pregnant and considering adoption, make sure you explore all possibilities before you make a final choice. The decision to go through an unwanted pregnancy and then give the baby to another family is difficult and takes tremendous love, maturity, and courage. Adoption is permanent: The adoptive parents will raise your child and have legal authority for his or her welfare. Think about your life now and in the future as you weigh alternatives. There are many people who can help you consider your options, including your partner, friends, family members, or a professional counselor at a crisis pregnancy center, a family planning clinic, or a family services, social services, or adoption agency. A counselor should always treat you with respect and be willing to discuss all your options with you—keeping the baby, having an abortion, or arranging an adoption. If you aren't comfortable with a particular counselor, find a different one.

There are two types of adoptions, confidential and open. In confidential adoption, the birth parents and the adoptive parents never know each other. Adoptive parents will be given any information, such as medical information, that they would need to help take care of the child. A later meeting between the child and birth parents is possible in confidential adoption, however, if the birth parents leave information with the agency or lawyer who handled the adoption and/or in a national adoption registry.

In an open adoption, the birth parents and adoptive parents know something about each other. There are different levels of openness, ranging from reading a brief description of prospective adoptive parents to meeting them and sharing full information. Birth parents may also be able to arrange to stay in touch with the family over the years, by visiting, calling, or writing. Some women feel that an open adoption enables them to keep in touch with a baby they will always love; others feel that this would be too difficult and decide against contact with the adoptive family.

In all states, you can work with a licensed child-placing (adoption) agency. In most, you can also work directly with an adopting couple or their attorney; this is called a private or independent adoption. Prospective adoptive parents can be located through personal ads, a physician, adoptive parent support groups, national matching services, and family members and friends.

You will also need to consider the reaction and rights of the birth father. A woman can choose to have an abortion without the consent or knowledge of the father, but once the baby is born, the father has certain rights. These rights vary from state to state, but, at a minimum, most states require that the birth father be notified of the adoption.

As with abortion, there are emotional and physical risks associated with pregnancy, childbirth, and adoption. Throughout the adoption process, make sure that you have the help you need and that you carefully consider all your options. Deciding how to handle an unplanned pregnancy is important, and you have the power to make your own decisions.

SOURCES: National Adoption Information Clearinghouse. 2000. *Are You Pregnant and Thinking About Adoption?* (http://naic.acf.hhs.gov/pubs/f_pregna.cfm; retrieved November 16, 2004); National Adoption Information Clearinghouse. 2000. *Placing Children for Adoption* (http://naic.acf.hhs.gov/pubs/s_place.cfm; retrieved November 16, 2004).

provider for a follow-up visit. The two-drug regimen has a rate of completed abortion of about 92–95%; the success rate is highest in early pregnancy.

Only about 1 in 10 abortions is performed after the 12th week of pregnancy. The method most commonly used for abortion from 13 to 24 weeks of pregnancy is **dilation and evacuation (D & E).** The cervix is opened using dilators, which gradually expand the cervix overnight. The next day, the uterus is emptied using surgical instruments and the aspirating machine. *Partial birth abortion* is a nonmedical term for a particular type of D & E. In this procedure, the fetal limbs and body are delivered first and then the skull is collapsed to allow it to pass more easily through the cervix. This procedure is performed only rarely, but it can be useful in the presence of particular fetal anomalies such as severe hydrocephalus (a condition in which fluid collects around the brain, causing brain damage and an enlarged head). Chemically induced labor is another infrequently used method of late abortion.

### Term

VW **dilation and evacuation (D & E)** The method of abortion most commonly used between 13 and 24 weeks of pregnancy. Following dilation of the cervix, both vacuum aspiration and curettage instruments are used as needed.

## Complications of Abortion

Along with questions regarding the actual procedure of abortion, many people have concerns about possible aftereffects. More information is gradually being gathered on this important subject.

**Possible Physical Effects** The incidence of immediate problems following an abortion (infection, bleeding, trauma to the cervix or uterus, and incomplete abortion requiring repeat curettage) varies widely. The potential for problems is significantly reduced by a woman's good health, early timing of the abortion, use of the suction method, performance by a well-trained clinician, and the availability and use of prompt follow-up care.

Studies on long-term complications—subsequent infertility, spontaneous second abortions, premature delivery, and babies of low birth weight—have not revealed any major risks with the most common abortion methods. A few studies have reported that women who have abortions have an increased risk of breast cancer. However, a well-designed study of 1.5 million Danish women found no connection between a woman's abortion history and her risk of breast cancer. A 2003 workshop convened by the National Cancer Institute and a 2004 analysis published in the journal *Lancet* also concluded that having an abortion or miscarriage does not increase a woman's subsequent risk of breast cancer.

Problems related to infection can be minimized through preabortion testing and treatment for gonorrhea, chlamydia, and other infections. Postabortion danger signs are fever above 100°F; abdominal pain or swelling, cramping, or backache; abdominal tenderness (to pressure); prolonged or heavy bleeding; foul-smelling vaginal discharge; vomiting or fainting; and delay in resuming menstrual periods (6 weeks or more).

Some cramping and bleeding are an expected part of ending a pregnancy. In rare cases, life-threatening bleeding, infections, or other problems can occur following a miscarriage, surgical abortion, or medical abortion. Prompt medical attention should be sought if heavy bleeding, severe abdominal pain, or fever occurs.

**Possible Psychological Effects** After an exhaustive review completed in 1988, the then surgeon general, C. Everett Koop, concluded that the available evidence failed to demonstrate either a negative or a positive long-term impact of abortion on mental health. More recent research has resulted in the same general conclusion. Psychological responses vary and depend on the individual woman's psychological makeup, family background, current personal and social relationships, cultural attitudes, and many other factors. A woman who has specific goals with a somewhat structured life pattern may be able to incorporate her decision to have an abortion as the unequivocally best and acceptable course more easily than a woman who feels uncertain about her future.

Although many women experience great relief after an abortion and virtually no negative feelings, some go through a period of ambivalence. Along with relief, they often feel a mixture of other responses, such as guilt, regret, loss, sadness, and/or anger. For a woman who does experience psychological or emotional effects after an abortion, talking with a close friend or family member can be very helpful. Supportive people can help her feel positive about herself and her decision. In a few cases, unresolved emotions may persist, and a woman should seek professional counseling.

**Tips for Today**

Your decisions about contraception and abortion are among the most important you will make in your life. They affect your physical and emotional health, your relationship and family choices, and your career and life plans. You may never have to face an unintended pregnancy, but you should know what choices you would have—abortion, adoption, parenthood—as well as where you stand on the issue.

*Right now you can*

- Visualize the life you hope to have in 5 years, 10 years, and 15 years. Does it include a relationship, a family, children? Are you doing anything right now—such as taking a chance on an unintended pregnancy—that could prevent you from realizing your dreams?
- If you are sexually active or considering becoming so, make an appointment with a physician or health care practitioner to discuss which contraceptive method is right for you.
- Take some time to examine your feelings about becoming a parent unexpectedly. Consider your views on the morality of abortion. Refer to the boxes in this chapter for some thoughtful ideas about the subject.

## SUMMARY

- The choice of contraceptive method depends on effectiveness, convenience, cost, reversibility, side effects and risk factors, and protection against STDs.
- Hormonal methods may include a combination of estrogen and progestins or progesterone alone. Hormones may be delivered via pills, patch, vaginal ring, implants, or injections. They prevent ovulation, inhibit the movement of sperm, and affect the uterine lining so that implantation is prevented.
- The most commonly used emergency contraceptives are two-dose regimens of OCs.
- IUDs may cause biochemical changes in the uterus, affect movement of sperm and eggs, or interfere with the implantation of the egg in the uterus.
- Male condoms are simple to use, immediately reversible, and provide STD protection; female condoms are available but are more difficult to use.
- The diaphragm, Lea's Shield, cervical cap, and contraceptive sponge cover the cervix and block sperm from entering; all are used with or contain spermicide.
- Vaginal spermicides come in the form of foams, creams, jellies, suppositories, and film.

- So-called natural methods include abstinence, withdrawal, and fertility awareness method (FAM).
- Vasectomy—male sterilization—involves severing the vasa deferentia. Female sterilization involves severing or blocking the oviducts.
- Issues to be considered in choosing a contraceptive include the individual health risks of each method, the implications of an unplanned pregnancy, STD risk, convenience and comfort level, type of relationship, the cost and ease of obtaining and maintaining each method, and religious or philosophical beliefs.
- The 1973 *Roe v. Wade* Supreme Court case devised new standards to govern abortion decisions; based on the trimesters of pregnancy, it limited a woman's choices as her pregnancy advanced.
- Although the Supreme Court continued to uphold its 1973 decision, it gave states further power to regulate abortion in *Webster v. Reproductive Health Services* and *Planned Parenthood of Southeastern Pennsylvania v. Casey.*
- The controversy between pro-life and pro-choice viewpoints focuses on the issue of when life begins. Overall public opinion in the United States supports legal abortion in at least some circumstances and opposes overturning *Roe v. Wade.*
- Methods of abortion include suction curettage, manual vacuum aspiration, dilation and evacuation, and medical abortion using mifepristone.
- Physical complications following abortion can be minimized by overall good patient health, early timing, use of the suction method, a well-trained physician, and follow-up care. Psychological aftereffects of abortion vary with the individual.

## Take Action

1. **Visit a health care provider:** Make an appointment with a physician or other health care provider to review the health risks of different contraceptive methods as they apply to you. For each method, determine whether any risk factors associated with its use apply to you or your partner.

2. **Visit a drugstore:** Visit a local drugstore and make a list of the contraceptives sold there, along with their prices. Next, investigate the costs of prescription contraceptive methods by contacting your physician, medical clinic, and/or pharmacy. Estimate the annual cost of regular use for each method, and rank the methods from most to least expensive.

3. **Conduct an opinion survey:** Survey your classmates about their position on the abortion issue. How many people consider themselves pro-choice and how many pro-life? How strong are their opinions? What, if anything, might cause them to change their minds? Do opinions seem to depend on age, gender, or any other factor?

## For More Information

### Books

Harris, M. M., ed. 2004. *Abortion: An Eternal Social and Moral Issue.* Farmington Hills, Mich.: Thomson Gale. *A brief reference outlining legal, political, and ethical issues.*

Hatcher, R. A., et al. 2004. *A Pocket Guide to Managing Contraception, 2004–2005.* Tiger, Ga.: Bridging the Gap Foundation. *An easy-to-use, reliable source of contraceptive information.*

Hatcher, R. A., et al. 2005. *Safely Sexual,* 2nd ed. New York: Ardent Media. *Realistic recommendations on the prevention of unplanned pregnancy, as well as HIV infection and other STDs.*

National Abortion and Reproductive Rights Action League Foundation. 2005. *Who Decides? A State-by-State Review of Abortion and Reproductive Rights.* Washington, D.C.: NARAL Foundation. *An in-depth annual review of the legal status of reproductive rights in the United States.*

Tone, A. 2001. *Devices and Desires: Men, Women, and the Commercialization of Contraception in the United States.* New York: Hill and Wang. *An engaging history of contraception in America.*

### WW Organizations, Hotlines, and Web Sites

*Abortion Law Homepage.* Includes an overview of the background and state of U.S abortion law, including the text of major legal decisions.
http://hometown.aol.com/abtrbng

*The Alan Guttmacher Institute.* A nonprofit institute for reproductive health research, policy analysis, and public education.
http://www.agi-usa.org

*Association of Reproductive Health Professionals.* Offers educational materials about contraception and other reproductive health issues; the Web site includes an interactive questionnaire to help people choose contraceptive methods.
http://www.arhp.org

*Emergency Contraception Web Site and Hotline.* Provides extensive information about emergency contraception.
888-NOT-2-LATE
http://www.not-2-late.com

*It's Your Sex Life.* Provides information about sexuality, relationships, contraceptives, and STDs; geared toward teenagers and young adults.
http://www.itsyoursexlife.com

*National Abortion and Reproductive Rights Action League.* Provides information on the politics of the pro-choice movement.
202-973-3000
http://www.naral.org

*National Adoption Information Clearinghouse.* Provides resources on all aspects of adoption.
888-251-0075
http://naic.acf.hhs.gov

*National Right to Life Committee.* Provides information on alternatives to abortion and the politics of the pro-life movement.
202-626-8800
http://www.nrlc.org

*Planned Parenthood Federation of America.* Provides information on family planning, contraception, and abortion and provides counseling services.
800-230-PLAN
http://www.plannedparenthood.org

*Reproductive Health Online (Reproline).* Presents information on contraceptive methods currently available and those under study for future use.
http://www.reproline.jhu.edu

*U.S. Food and Drug Administration: Mifepristone.* Provides information on the testing, labeling, and use of mifepristone.
http://www.fda.gov/cder/drug/infopage/mifepristone

See also the listings for Chapters 5 and 13.

## Selected Bibliography


Ashok, P. W., et al. 2005. Patient preference in a randomized study comparing medical and surgical abortion at 10–13 weeks gestation. *Contraception* 71(2): 143–8.

Beral, V., et al. 2004. Breast cancer and abortion: Collaborative reanalysis of data from 53 epidemiological studies, including 83,000 women with breast cancer from 16 countries. *Lancet* 363(9414): 1007–1016.

Berenson, A. B., et al. 2004. Effects of hormonal contraception on bone mineral density after 24 months of use. *Obstetrics and Gynecology* 103(5 Pt 1): 899–906.

Broen, A. N., et al. 2004. Psychological impact on women of miscarriage versus induced abortion: A 2-year follow-up study. *Psychosomatic Medicine* 66: 265–271.

Burkman, R., et al. 2004. Safety concerns and health benefits associated with oral contraception. *American Journal of Obstetrics and Gynecology* 190(4 Suppl): 5–22.

Burkman, R. T., 2004. The transdermal contraceptive system. *American Journal of Obstetrics and Gynecology* 190(4 Suppl): 49–53.

Centers for Disease Control and Prevention. 2004. Abortion surveillance—United States, 2001. *Morbidity and Mortality Weekly Report* 53(SS–9).

Chen, A., et al. 2004. Mifepristone-induced early abortion and outcome of subsequent wanted pregnancy. *American Journal of Epidemiology* 160(2): 110–117.

Espey, E., et al. 2005. Abortion education in medical schools: a national survey. *American Journal of Obstetrics and Gynecology* 192(2): 640–3.

Food and Drug Administration. 2004. *Medication Guide: Mifeprex* (http://www.fda.gov/cder/drug/infopage/mifepristone/medicationguide.htm; retrieved November 15, 2004).

Grimes, D. A. 2005. Risks of mifepristone abortion in context. *Contraception* 71(3): 161.

Harper, C. C., et al. 2004. Tolerability of levonorgestrel emergency contraception in adolescents. *American Journal of Obstetrics and Gynecology* 191(4): 1158–1163.

Hatcher, R. A., et al. 2004. *Contraceptive Technology,* 18th ed. New York: Ardent Media.

Henshaw, S. K., and L. B. Finer. 2003. The accessibility of abortion services in the United States, 2001. *Perspectives on Sexual Reproductive Health* 35(1): 16–24.

International Medical Advisory Panel. 2004. IMAP statement on emergency contraception. *International Planned Parenthood Federation Medical Bulletin* 38(1): 1–3.

Johansson, E. D., and R. Sitruk-Ware. 2004. New delivery systems in contraception: Vaginal rings. *American Journal of Obstetrics and Gynecology* 190(4 Suppl): 54–59.

Jones, R. K., J. E. Darroch, and S. K. Henshaw. 2002. Contraceptive use among U.S. women having abortions in 2000–2001. *Perspectives on Sexual and Reproductive Health* 34(6): 294–303.

Jones, R. K., J. E. Darroch, and S. K. Henshaw. 2002. Patterns in the socioeconomic characteristics of women obtaining abortions in 2000–2001. *Perspectives on Sexual and Reproductive Health* 34(5): 226–235.

Kero, A., and A. Lalos. 2004. Reactions and reflections in men, 4 and 12 months post-abortion. *Journal of Psychosomatic Obstetrics and Gynaecology* 25(2): 135–143.

Litt, I. F. 2005. Placing emergency contraception in the hands of women. *Journal of the American Medical Association* 293(1): 98–99.

National Abortion and Reproductive Rights Action League. 2004. *Who Decides: A State-by-State Review of Abortion and Reproductive Rights* (http://www.naral.org; retrieved November 16, 2004).

National Cancer Institute. 2003. *Cancer Facts: Abortion, Miscarriage, and Breast Cancer Risk* (http://cis.nci.nih.gov/fact/3_75.htm; retrieved November 16, 2004).

Pruitt, S. L., and P. D. Mullen. 2005. Contraception or abortion? Inaccurate descriptions of emergency contraception in newspaper articles, 1992–2002. *Contraception* 71(1): 14–21.

Raine, T. R., et al. 2005. Direct access to emergency contraception through pharmacies and effect on unintended pregnancy and STIs. *Journal of the American Medical Association* 293(1): 54–62.

Rorbye, D., M. Norgaard, and L. Nilas. 2005. Medical versus surgical abortion: Comparing satisfaction and potential confounders in a partly randomized study. *Human Reproduction* 20(3): 834–838.

Scholes, D., et al. 2005. Change in bone mineral density among adolescent women using and discontinuing depot medroxyprogesterone acetate contraception. *Archives of Pediatrics and Adolescent Medicine* 159(2): 139–44.

Shafii, T., et al. 2004. Is condom use habit forming? Condom use at sexual debut and subsequent condom use. *Sexually Transmitted Diseases* 31(6): 366–372.

Trussell, J., et al. 2004. The role of emergency contraception. *American Journal of Obstetrics and Gynecology* 190(4 Suppl): 30–38.

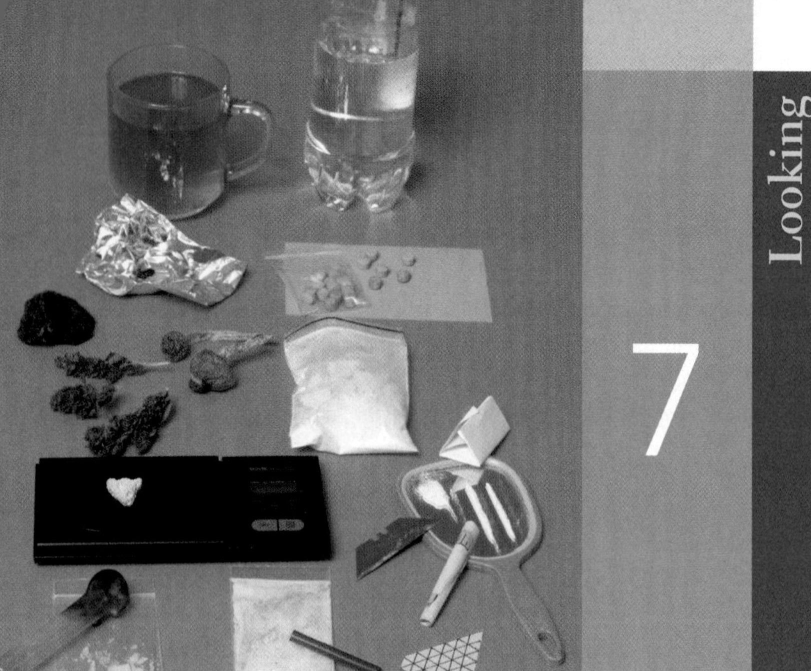

7

## Looking AHEAD

After reading this chapter, you should be able to

- Define and discuss the concepts of addictive behavior, substance abuse, and substance dependence
- Explain factors contributing to drug use and dependence
- List the major categories of psychoactive drugs and describe their effects, methods of use, and potential for abuse and dependence
- Discuss social issues related to psychoactive drug use and its prevention and treatment
- Evaluate the role of drugs and other addictive behaviors in your life and identify your risk factors for abuse or dependence

# The Use and Abuse of Psychoactive Drugs

The use of **drugs** for both medical and social purposes is widespread in American society (Table 7-1). Many people believe that every problem, no matter how large or small, has or should have a chemical solution. For fatigue, many turn to caffeine; for insomnia, sleeping pills; for anxiety or boredom, alcohol or other recreational drugs. Advertisements, social pressures, and the human desire for quick solutions to life's difficult problems all contribute to the prevailing attitude that drugs can ease all pain. Unfortunately, using drugs can—and often does—have serious consequences.

The most serious consequences are abuse and addiction. The drugs most often associated with abuse are **psychoactive drugs**—those that alter a person's experiences or consciousness. In the short term, psychoactive drugs can cause **intoxication**, a state in which sometimes unpredictable physical and emotional changes occur. A person who is intoxicated may experience potentially serious changes in physical functioning, and his or her emotions and judgment may be affected in ways that lead to uncharacteristic and unsafe behavior. In the long term, recurrent drug use can have profound physical, emotional, and social effects.

## ADDICTIVE BEHAVIOR

Although addiction is most often associated with drug use, many experts now extend the concept of addiction to other areas. **Addictive behaviors** are habits that have gotten out of control, with resulting negative effects on a person's health. Looking at the nature of addiction and a range of addictive behaviors can help us understand similar behaviors when they involve drugs.

### Terms

VW

**drug** Any chemical other than food intended to affect the structure or function of the body.

**psychoactive drug** A drug that can alter a person's consciousness or experience.

**intoxication** The state of being mentally affected by a chemical (literally, a state of being poisoned).

**addictive behavior** Any habit that has gotten out of control, resulting in a negative effect on one's health.

VITAL STATISTICS

**Table 7-1 Nonmedical Drug Use Among Americans**

| | Percentage Using Substance in the Past 30 Days | |
|---|---|---|
| | College Students (age 18–22) | All Americans (age 12 and older) |
| Any illicit drug | 21.4 | 8.2 |
| Tobacco (all forms) | 36.4 | 29.8 |
| Cigarettes | 31.4 | 25.4 |
| Smokeless tobacco | 3.8 | 3.3 |
| Cigars | 10.5 | 5.4 |
| Pipe tobacco | 0.9 | 0.7 |
| Alcohol | 64.9 | 50.1 |
| Binge alcohol use | 43.5 | 22.6 |
| Marijuana/hashish | 18.4 | 6.2 |
| Cocaine | 2.1 | 1.0 |
| Crack | 0.0 | 0.3 |
| Heroin | 0.0 | 0.1 |
| Hallucinogens | 1.8 | 0.4 |
| LSD | 0.4 | 0.1 |
| Ecstasy | 0.6 | 0.2 |
| Inhalants | 0.6 | 0.2 |
| Psychotherapeutics* | 5.8 | 2.7 |
| Pain relievers | 4.4 | 2.0 |
| Tranquilizers | 1.3 | 0.8 |
| Stimulants | 1.3 | 0.5 |
| Methamphetamine | 0.1 | 0.3 |
| Sedatives | 0.1 | 0.1 |

*Nonmedical use of prescription-type pain relievers, tranquilizers, stimulants, or sedatives.

SOURCE: Office of Applied Studies, Substance Abuse and Mental Health Services Administration. 2004. *National Survey on Drug Use and Health* (http://oas.samhsa.gov/nhsda.htm; retrieved December 6, 2004).

## What Is Addiction?

The word *addiction* tends to be a highly charged one for most people. We may jokingly say we're addicted to fudge swirl ice cream or our morning jog, but most of us think of true addiction as a habitual and uncontrollable behavior, usually involving the use of a drug. Some people think of addiction as a moral flaw or a personal weakness. Others think addictions arise from certain personality traits, genetic factors, or socioeconomic influences. Views on the causes of addictions have an impact on our attitudes toward people with addictive disorders, as well as on the approaches to treatment.

Historically, the term *addiction* was applied only when the habitual use of a drug produced chemical changes in the user's body. One such change is physical tolerance, in which the body adapts to a drug so that the initial dose no longer produces the original emotional or psychological effects. This process, caused by chemical changes, means the user has to take larger and larger doses of the drug to achieve the same high. The concept of addiction as a disease process, one based in brain chemistry, rather than a moral failing, has led to many advances in the understanding and treatment of drug addiction.

Some scientists think that other behaviors may share some of the chemistry of drug addiction. Activities like gambling, eating, exercising, and sex trigger the release of brain chemicals that cause a pleasurable rush in much the same way that psychoactive drugs do. The brain's own chemicals thus become the "drug" that can cause addiction. These theorists suggest that drug addiction and addiction to other pleasurable behaviors have a common mechanism in the brain. In this view, addiction is partly the result of our own natural wiring.

However, and very important, the view that addiction is based in our brain chemistry does *not* imply that an individual bears no responsibility for his or her addictive behavior. Many experts believe that it is inaccurate and counterproductive to think of all bad habits and excessive behaviors as diseases. They point to other factors, especially lifestyle and personality traits, that play key roles in the development of addictive behaviors.

## Characteristics of Addictive Behavior

It is often difficult to distinguish between a healthy habit and one that has become an addiction. Experts have identified some general characteristics typically associated with addictive behaviors:

- *Reinforcement.* Addictive behaviors are physically and/or psychologically reinforcing. Some aspect of the behavior produces pleasurable physical and/or emotional states or relieves negative ones.
- *Compulsion or craving.* The individual feels a strong compulsion—a compelling need—to engage in the behavior, often accompanied by obsessive planning for the next opportunity to perform it.
- *Loss of control.* The individual loses control over the behavior and cannot block the impulse to engage in it. He or she may deny that the behavior is problematic or may have tried but failed to control it.
- *Escalation.* Addiction often involves a pattern of escalation, in which more and more of a particular substance or activity is required to produce its desired effects. This escalation typically means that a person must give an increasing amount of his or her time, attention, and resources to the behavior.
- *Negative consequences.* The behavior continues despite serious negative consequences, such as problems with academic or job performance, personal relationships, and health; legal or financial troubles are also typical.

## The Development of Addiction

There is no single cause of addiction. Instead, characteristics of an individual person, of the environment in which the person lives, and of the substance or behavior he or she abuses combine in an addictive behavior.

We all engage in activities that are potentially addictive. Some of these activities can be part of a wellness lifestyle if they are done appropriately and in moderation, but if a behavior starts to be excessive, it may become an addiction. An addiction often starts when a person does something he or she thinks will bring pleasure or help avoid pain. The activity may be drinking a beer, going on the Internet, playing the lottery, or going shopping. If it works, and the behavior does bring pleasure or alleviates pain, the person is likely to repeat it. He or she becomes increasingly dependent on the behavior, and tolerance may develop—that is, the person needs more of the behavior to feel the same effect. Eventually, the behavior becomes a central focus of the person's life, and there is a deterioration in other areas, such as school performance or relationships. The behavior no longer brings pleasure, but it is necessary to avoid the pain of going without it.

Many common behaviors are potentially addictive, but most people who engage in them do not develop problems. The reason, again, lies in the combination of factors that are involved in the development of addiction, including personality, lifestyle, heredity, the social and physical environment, and the nature of the substance or behavior in question. For a behavior to become an addiction, these diverse factors must come together in a certain way. For example, nicotine, the psychoactive drug in tobacco, has a very high potential for physical addiction; but a person who doesn't choose to try cigarettes, perhaps because of family influence or a tendency to develop asthma, will never develop nicotine addiction.

## Characteristics of People with Addictions

The causes and course of an addiction are extremely varied, but people with addictions do seem to share some characteristics. Many use the substance or activity as a substitute for other, healthier, coping strategies. People vary in their ability to manage their lives, and those who have the most trouble dealing with stress and painful emotions may be more susceptible to addiction.

Some people may have a genetic predisposition to addiction to a particular substance; such predispositions may involve variations in brain chemistry. People with addictive disorders usually have a distinct preference for a particular addictive behavior. They also often have problems with impulse control and self-regulation and tend to be risk takers.

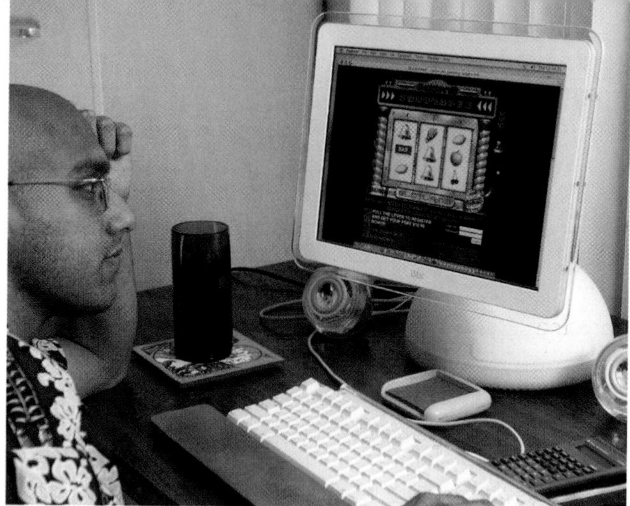

Most people who gamble do so casually and occasionally, but for a few the habit spins out of control and becomes the central focus of their life. The availability of gambling on the Internet makes it even more difficult for pathological gamblers to control their compulsion.

## Examples of Addictive Behaviors

The use and abuse of psychoactive drugs is explored in detail later in the chapter. In this section, we examine some behaviors that are not related to drugs and that can become addictive for some people.

**Compulsive or Pathological Gambling** Many people gamble casually by putting a dollar in the office football pool or buying a lottery ticket. But some become compulsive gamblers, unable to resist or control the urge to gamble, even in the face of financial and personal ruin. Most compulsive gamblers say they are seeking excitement even more than money. Increasingly larger bets are necessary to produce the desired level of excitement. A series of losses can lead to a perceived need to keep placing bets to win back the money. When financial resources become strained, the person may lie or steal to pay off debts. The consequences of compulsive gambling are not just financial; the suicide rate of compulsive gamblers is 20 times higher than that of the general population.

Compulsive gamblers may gamble to relieve negative feelings and become restless and irritable when they are unable to gamble. Compulsive gambling may begin or flare up in times of stress. The earlier a person starts to gamble, the more likely he or she is to become a pathological gambler. Gambling is often linked to other risky behaviors, and many compulsive gamblers also have drug and alcohol abuse problems.

The American Psychiatric Association (APA) recognizes pathological gambling as a mental disorder and lists ten characteristic behaviors, including preoccupation with gambling, unsuccessful efforts to cut back or quit, using gambling to escape problems, and lying to family members to conceal the extent of involvement with gambling. Compulsive gambling shares many of these behaviors with other addictions, including drug use. About

1.1 million teens and 1.9 million adults in the United States may be compulsive gamblers. These numbers may increase due to the spread of legalized gambling, both on the Internet and on American Indian tribal reservations.

In a recent survey of more than 10,000 students from more than 100 colleges, 42% of students reported having gambled at least once in the past year, and about 3% reported gambling at least once a week. Rates were significantly higher among men than women. Other characteristics associated with gambling among college students included more time watching TV, more time using a computer nonacademically, less time studying, lower grades, participation in intercollegiate athletics, and alcohol use and binge drinking.

**Compulsive Spending or Shopping** Nearly everyone splurges at the mall or goes into debt once in a while. But a compulsive spender repeatedly gives in to the impulse to buy much more than he or she needs or can afford. For the compulsive shopper, spending may serve to relieve painful feelings such as depression or anxiety, or it may produce positive emotions such as excitement or happiness. Compulsive spenders usually buy luxury items rather than daily necessities. Men tend to buy cars, exercise equipment, and sporting gear; women tend to buy clothes, jewelry, and perfume. Some experts link compulsive shopping with neglect or abuse during childhood; it also seems to be associated with eating disorders, depression, and bipolar disorder. Some compulsive shoppers are helped by antidepressant medications.

Compulsive shoppers are usually significantly distressed by their behavior and its social, personal, and financial consequences. Characteristics of out-of-control spending include shopping in order to "feel better," using money or time that had been set aside for other purposes, hiding spending from others, and spending so much that the shopper goes into debt or engages in illegal activities such as shoplifting or writing bad checks.

**Internet Addiction** Some recent research has indicated that surfing the World Wide Web can also be addictive. In order to spend more time online, Internet addicts skip important social, school, or recreational activities, thereby damaging personal relationships and jeopardizing academic and job performance. Despite the negative consequences they are experiencing, they don't feel able to stop. The Internet addicts identified in one study averaged 38 online hours per week. Internet addicts may feel uncomfortable or be moody when they are not online. They may be preoccupied with getting back online and may stay there longer than they intend. As with other addictive behaviors, online addicts may be using their behavior to alleviate stress or avoid painful emotions.

Activities by Internet addicts may take many forms, some of which, such as e-mail and chat rooms, are specific to the online format. However, widespread access to the Internet may expose many more people to other potentially addictive behaviors, including gambling, shopping, and sex. There are thousands of online gambling sites and millions of online stores that allow people to gamble or shop from their homes at all times of the day or night; in addition, sites featuring online auctions or stock trading offer activities that are very similar to gambling. It remains to be seen whether increasing access to the Internet among Americans will lead to more problems with many types of addictive behaviors.

Other behaviors that can become addictive include eating, watching TV, and working. Any substance or activity that becomes the focus of a person's life at the expense of other needs and interests can be damaging to health.

We turn now to the substances most commonly associated with addiction: psychoactive drugs.

## DRUG USE, ABUSE, AND DEPENDENCE

Drugs are chemicals other than food that are intended to affect the structure or function of the body. They include prescription medicines such as antibiotics and antidepressants; nonprescription, or over-the-counter (OTC), substances such as alcohol, tobacco, and caffeine products; and illegal substances such as LSD and heroin.

### Drug Abuse and Dependence

The APA's *Diagnostic and Statistical Manual of Mental Disorders* is the authoritative reference for defining all sorts of behavioral disorders, including those related to drugs. The APA has chosen not to use the term *addiction,* in part because it is so broad and has so many connotations. Instead, the APA refers to two forms of substance (drug) disorders: substance abuse and substance dependence. Both are maladaptive patterns of substance use that lead to significant impairment or distress. Although the APA's definitions are more precise and more directly related to drug use, they clearly encompass the general characteristics of addictive behavior described in the last section.

**Drug Abuse** As defined by the APA, **substance abuse** involves one or more of the following:

- Recurrent drug use, resulting in a failure to fulfill major responsibilities at work, school, or home

**Term**

**substance abuse** A maladaptive pattern of use of any substance that persists despite adverse social, psychological, or medical consequences. The pattern may be intermittent, with or without tolerance and physical dependence.

Vw

- Recurrent drug use in situations in which it is physically hazardous, such as before or while driving a car
- Recurrent drug-related legal problems
- Continued drug use despite persistent social or interpersonal problems caused or exacerbated by the effects of the drug

The pattern of use may be constant or intermittent, and **physical dependence** may or may not be present. For example, a person who smokes marijuana once a week and cuts classes because he or she is high is abusing marijuana, even though he or she is not physically dependent.

**Drug Dependence** **Substance dependence** is a more complex disorder and is what many people associate with the idea of addiction. The seven specific criteria the APA uses to diagnose substance dependence are listed below. The first two are associated with physical dependence; the final five are associated with compulsive use. To be considered dependent, an individual must experience a cluster of three or more of these seven symptoms during a 12-month period.

1. *Developing tolerance to the substance.* When a person requires increased amounts of a substance to achieve the desired effect or notices a markedly diminished effect with continued use of the same amount, he or she has developed **tolerance.** For example, heavy heroin users may need to take ten times the amount they took at the beginning in order to achieve the desired effect.
2. *Experiencing withdrawal.* In an individual who has maintained prolonged, heavy use of a substance, a drop in its concentration within the body can result in unpleasant physical and cognitive **withdrawal** symptoms. For example, nausea, vomiting, and tremors are common withdrawal symptoms for alcohol, opioids, and sedatives.
3. *Taking the substance in larger amounts or over a longer period than was originally intended.*
4. *Expressing a persistent desire to cut down or regulate substance use.* This desire is often accompanied by many unsuccessful efforts to reduce or discontinue use of the substance.
5. *Spending a great deal of time obtaining the substance, using the substance, or recovering from its effects.*
6. *Giving up or reducing important social, school, work, or recreational activities because of substance use.* A dependent person may withdraw from family activities and hobbies in order to use the substance in private or to spend more time with substance-using friends.
7. *Continuing to use the substance in spite of recognizing that it is contributing to a psychological or physical problem.*

If a drug-dependent person experiences either tolerance or withdrawal, he or she is considered physically dependent. However, not everyone who experiences tolerance or withdrawal is drug dependent and dependence can occur without a physical component, based solely on compulsive use.

## Who Uses Drugs?

The use and abuse of drugs occur at all income and education levels, among all ethnic groups, and at all ages. One reason for our society's concern with the casual or recreational use of illegal drugs is that it is not really possible to know when drug use will lead to abuse or dependence. Some casual users develop substance-related problems; others do not. Some psychoactive drugs are more likely than others to lead to dependence (Table 7-2). People who begin to use drugs at very young ages have a greater risk for dependence and serious health consequences.

Although we can't accurately predict which drug users will become drug abusers, researchers have identified

**Table 7-2 Psychoactive Drugs and Their Potential for Producing Dependence**

| | Potential for Dependence | |
|---|---|---|
| **Drug** | **Physical** | **Psychological** |
| Nicotine | Very high | Very high |
| Heroin | Very high | Very high |
| Methamphetamine smoked ("ice") | Very high | Very high |
| Crack cocaine | Possible | Very high |
| Alcohol | High | High |
| Methaqualone | High | High |
| Barbiturates | High | Moderate |
| Amphetamine | Possible | High |
| Cocaine | Possible | High |
| Diazepam (Valium) | Low | High |
| PCP | Unknown | High |
| Chloral hydrate ("mickey") | Moderate | Moderate |
| Codeine | Moderate | Moderate |
| Marijuana/ hashish | Unknown | Moderate |
| Inhalants | Unknown | Moderate |
| Steroids | Possible | Possible |
| LSD | None | Unknown |
| MDMA (ecstasy) | Unknown | Unknown |

SOURCES: National Clearinghouse for Alcohol and Drug Information. 2002. *Drugs of Abuse* (http://www.health.org/govpubs/rpo926; retrieved December 8, 2004); Beers, M. H., and R. Berkow, eds. 1999. *Merck Manual of Diagnosis and Therapy,* 17th ed. Rahway, N.J.: Merck; Food and Drug Administration. 1995. Nicotine in cigarettes and smokeless tobacco products is a drug and these products are nicotine delivery devices under the Federal Food, Drug, and Cosmetic Act. *Federal Register* 60(155): 41454–41459.

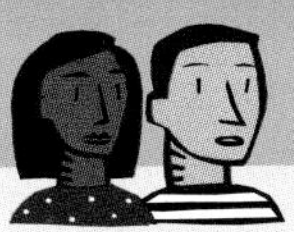

## Gender Differences in Drug Use and Abuse

Men are more likely than women to use, abuse, and be dependent on illicit drugs. Rates of use are similar in males and females age 12–17, but among those 18 and older, more men than women use drugs and have problems associated with drug use (see table). Men account for about 80% of arrests for drug abuse violations, 70% of admissions for treatment, and 65% of drug-related deaths.

There are also gender differences in why and how young people use drugs. Young males tend to use alcohol or drugs for sensation seeking or to enhance their social status, factors tied to culturally based gender roles. Young women tend to use drugs to improve mood, increase confidence, and reduce inhibitions. Boys are likelier to receive offers to use drugs in public settings, whereas girls are likelier to receive offers in a private place such as a friend's residence.

Despite overall lower rates of drug use, females may have unique biological vulnerabilities to certain drugs, and they may move more quickly from use to abuse. Major life transitions, including the physical and emotional changes associated with puberty, increase the risk of drug use and abuse for girls more so than for boys. Certain other drug abuse risk factors are also more common in female adolescents, including depression, low self-esteem, eating disorders, and a history of physical or sexual abuse.

Adolescent boys and girls share some protective factors relating to drug abuse, including positive family relationships and extracurricular activities; religious involvement is protective for both boys and girls but may be more protective for girls. Among older men and women, marriage, children, and employment are associated with lower rates of drug abuse and dependence. Rates of drug abuse and dependence among married adults are less than half of those among unmarried adults; similar patterns are seen when comparing adults who live with children versus those who do not live with children and adults who are employed versus those who are unemployed.

**National Survey Results: Percent Reporting in Past Year**

| | Males | Females |
|---|---|---|
| Illicit drug use* | 17.2 | 12.4 |
| Age 12–17 | 21.7 | 21.9 |
| Age 18–25 | 38.6 | 30.5 |
| Age 26 and older | 12.6 | 8.1 |
| Drove under influence of illicit drug | 6.6 | 2.8 |
| Illicit drug abuse or dependence | 3.7 | 2.1 |
| Treatment for drug dependence | 1.0 | 0.5 |

*Illicit drugs include marijuana/hashish, cocaine, heroin, hallucinogens, inhalants, and prescription-type psychotherapeutics used nonmedically.

SOURCES: Office of Applied Studies, Substance Abuse and Mental Health Services Administration. 2004. *The NSDUH Report: Gender Differences in Substance Dependence and Abuse,* October 29; Office of National Drug Control Policy. 2004. *Women and Drugs* (http://whitehousedrugpolicy.gov/drugfact/women/index.html; retrieved December 7, 2004); National Center on Addiction and Substance Abuse at Columbia University. 2003. *The Formative Years: Pathways to Substance Abuse Among Girls and Young Women Ages 8–22.* New York: National Center on Addiction and Substance Abuse.

some characteristics that place young people at higher-than-average risk for *trying* illicit drugs. Being male is one risk factor: Although gender differences in drug use are gradually narrowing, males are still about twice as likely as females to abuse illicit drugs (see the box "Gender Differences in Drug Use and Abuse"). An adolescent who has a poor self-image; lacks self-control; uses tobacco; has an eating disorder; is aggressive, impulsive, or moody; or suffers from attention-deficit/hyperactivity disorder (ADHD) may be at increased risk for trying drugs. A thrill-seeking or risk-taking personality is another factor. People who drive too fast or who don't wear safety belts may have this personality type, which is characterized by a sense of invincibility.

Belonging to a peer group or family that accepts or rewards drug use is a significant risk factor for trying illicit drugs. Chaotic home environments, dysfunctional families, lack of supervision, and parental abuse also increase risk. Young people who live in disadvantaged areas are more likely to be offered drugs at a young age, increasing their risk of drug use. However, drug use rates among middle-class youths with college-educated parents tend

### Terms

VW

**physical dependence** The result of physiological adaptation that occurs in response to the frequent presence of a drug; typically associated with tolerance and withdrawal.

**substance dependence** A cluster of cognitive, behavioral, and physiological symptoms that occur in an individual who continues to use a substance despite suffering significant substance-related problems, leading to significant impairment or distress; also known as *addiction*.

**tolerance** Lower sensitivity to a drug so that a given dose no longer exerts the usual effect and larger doses are needed.

**withdrawal** Physical and psychological symptoms that follow the interrupted use of a drug on which a user is physically dependent; symptoms may be mild or life-threatening.

Mind/Body/Spirit

## Spirituality and Drug Abuse

The use of alcohol and other drugs is intertwined with spirituality and religion. Some religions use drugs in the quest for spiritual transcendence: American Indian, Polynesian, African, and other indigenous religions have used psychoactive drugs such as peyote, khat, alcohol, and hashish for expanding consciousness and developing personal spirituality. For other religions, the use of psychoactive drugs is seen as a threat to spirituality. In Islam, for example, the consumption of alcohol and certain other drugs is strictly forbidden. Although there are diverse religious viewpoints on drug use, many religions infer some link between psychoactive drugs and spirituality.

In studies of American teens and adults, spiritual or religious involvement is generally associated with a lower risk of trying psychoactive drugs and, for those who do use drugs, a lower risk of heavy use and dependence. The mechanism for this protective effect is unclear; possibilities include the adoption of a strict code of behavior or set of principles that forbids drug use, the presence of a social support system for abstinence or moderation, and the promotion of a large, complex set of values that includes avoidance of drug use. The relationship between religious faith and avoidance of drug use appears to be even stronger in teens than in adults. Overall, people who spend time regularly engaging in spiritual practices such as prayer and transcendental meditation have lower rates of drug abuse.

People with current substance-abuse problems tend to have lower rates of religious affiliation and involvement and lower levels of spiritual wellness, characterized by a lack of a sense of meaning in life. One of the hallmarks of drug dependence is spending increasing amounts of time and energy obtaining and using drugs; such a pattern of behavior inevitably reduces the resources an individual puts toward developing physical, emotional, and spiritual wellness.

What about those seeking to break their dependence on drugs? Among people in treatment for substance abuse, higher levels of religious faith and spirituality may contribute to the recovery process. A study of people recovering from alcohol or other drug abuse found that spirituality and religiosity were associated with increased coping skills, greater optimism about life, greater resilience to stress, and greater perceived social support. If, for a particular individual, there is a spiritual aspect to his or her substance-abuse problem, then it is likely that spirituality may also play a role in recovery.

More research is needed to clarify the relationships among spirituality, religion, drug use, and recovery. One of the difficulties in conducting research in this area is the difficulty in defining and measuring spirituality and religious involvement. Spirituality is a complex part of human nature, involving behavior, belief, and experience. And although behaviors such as the spiritual practices of prayer or meditation can be measured, it is more difficult to determine what such practices mean to an individual and her or his overall sense of self.

SOURCES: Substance Abuse and Mental Health Network. 2004. Religious beliefs and substance use among youths. *NSDUH Report*, January; Plante, T. G., and D. A. Pardini. 2000. Religious denomination affiliation and psychological health: Results from a substance abuse population. Presented at the American Psychological Association Annual Convention, August 7; Miller, L., M. Davies, and S. Greenwald. 2000. Religiosity and substance use and abuse among adolescents in the national comorbidity survey. *Journal of the American Academy of Child and Adolescent Psychiatry* 39(9): 1190–1197; Miller, W. R. 1998. Researching the spiritual dimensions of alcohol and other drug problems. *Addiction* 93(7): 979–990.

to catch up with, and in some cases outstrip, those of other groups by the time students reach the twelfth grade.

What about people who *don't* use drugs? Not surprisingly, people who perceive drug use as risky and who disapprove of it are less likely to use drugs than those who believe otherwise. Drug use is also less common among people who have positive self-esteem and self-concept and who are assertive, independent thinkers who are not controlled by peer pressure. Self-control, social competence, optimism, academic achievement, and regular church attendance are also linked to lower rates of drug use (see the box "Spirituality and Drug Abuse"). Home environments are also influential: Coming from a strong family, one that has a clear policy on drug use, is another characteristic of people who don't use drugs.

## Why Do People Use Drugs?

Young people, especially those from middle-class backgrounds, are frequently drawn to drugs by the allure of the exciting and illegal. They may be curious, rebellious, or vulnerable to peer pressure. They may want to appear to be daring and to be part of the group. Young people may want to imitate adult models in their lives or in the movies. Most people who have taken illicit drugs have done so on an experimental basis, typically trying the drug one or more times but not continuing. The main factors in the initial choice of a drug are whether it is available and whether other people around are already using it.

Although some people use drugs because they want to alter their mood or are seeking a spiritual experience, others are motivated by a desire to escape boredom, anxiety, depression, feelings of worthlessness, or other distressing symptoms of psychological problems. They use drugs as a way to cope with the difficulties they are experiencing in life. The common practice in our society of seeking a drug solution to every problem is a factor in the widespread reliance on both illicit and prescription drugs.

For people living in poverty in the inner cities, many of these reasons for using drugs are magnified. The problems are more devastating, the need for escape more compelling. Furthermore, the buying and selling of drugs provide access to an unofficial, alternative economy that may seem like an opportunity for success.

### Risk Factors for Dependence

Why do some people use psychoactive drugs without becoming dependent, whereas others aren't as lucky? The answer seems to be a combination of physical, psychological, and social factors. Some people may be born with certain characteristics of brain chemistry or metabolism that make them more vulnerable to drug dependence. Psychological risk factors for drug dependence include difficulty in controlling impulses and a strong need for excitement, stimulation, and immediate gratification. Feelings of rejection, hostility, aggression, anxiety, or depression are also associated with drug dependence. People may turn to drugs to blot out their emotional pain. People with mental illnesses have a very high risk of substance dependence.

### Other Risks of Drug Use

Dependence is not the only serious potential consequence of drug use.

**Intoxication** People who are under the influence of drugs—intoxicated—may act in uncharacteristic and unsafe ways because both their physical and mental functioning are impaired. They are more likely to be injured from a variety of causes, including falls, drowning, and automobile crashes; to engage in unsafe sex, increasing their risk for sexually transmitted diseases and unintended pregnancy; and to be involved in incidents of aggression and violence, including sexual assault.

**Unintended Side Effects** Psychoactive drugs have many effects beyond the alteration of consciousness. These effects range from nausea and constipation to paranoia, depression, and heart failure. Some drugs also carry the risk of potentially fatal overdose.

**Unknown Drug Constituents** There is no quality control in the illegal drug market, so the composition, dosage, and toxicity of street drugs is highly variable. Studies of samples indicate that many street drugs don't contain their promised primary ingredient; in some cases, a drug may be present in unsafe dosages or mixed with other drugs to boost the effects. Careless manufacturing practices can result in the presence of toxic contaminants.

**Risks Associated with Injection Drug Use** Many injection drug users (IDUs) share or reuse needles, syringes, and other injection equipment, which can easily become contaminated with the user's blood. Small amounts of blood can carry enough human immunodeficiency virus (HIV) and hepatitis C virus (HCV) to be infectious. Unsterile injection practices can cause skin and other infections.

The surest way to prevent diseases related to injection drug use is never to inject drugs. Syringe exchange programs (SEPs)—in which IDUs can turn in a used syringe and get back a new one free—have been advocated to help slow the spread of HIV and reduce the rates and cost of other health problems associated with injection drug use. Getting people off drugs is clearly the best solution, but there are far more IDUs (an estimated 1.5 million in the United States) than treatment facilities can currently handle.

**Legal Consequences** Many psychoactive drugs are illegal, so using them can result in large fines and/or imprisonment. The FBI reports nearly 1.7 million drug-related arrests each year. Possession of marijuana, heroin, or cocaine are the most commonly reported violations.

## HOW DRUGS AFFECT THE BODY

The psychoactive drugs discussed in this chapter have complex and variable effects, many of which can be traced to changes in brain chemistry. However, the same drug may affect different people differently or the same person in different ways under different circumstances. Beyond a fairly predictable general change in brain chemistry, the effects of a drug may vary depending on three general categories of factors: drug factors, user factors, and social factors.

### Changes in Brain Chemistry

Psychoactive drugs produce most of their key effects by acting on brain chemistry in a characteristic fashion. Each psychoactive drug acts on one or more neurotransmitters, either increasing or decreasing their concentration and actions. Cocaine, for example, affects dopamine, a neurotransmitter thought to play a key role in the process of reinforcement—the brain's way of telling itself "That's good; do the same thing again." Heroin, nicotine, alcohol, and amphetamines also affect dopamine levels through their effects on the brain.

The duration of a drug's effect depends on many factors and may range from 5 minutes (crack cocaine) to 12 or more hours (LSD). As drugs circulate through the body, they are metabolized by the liver and eventually excreted by the kidneys in urine. Small amounts may also be eliminated in other ways, including in sweat, in breast milk, and via the lungs.

## Drug Factors

When different drugs or dosages produce different effects, the differences are usually caused by one or more of five different drug factors:

1. The **pharmacological properties** of a drug are its overall effects on a person's body chemistry, behavior, and psychology. The pharmacological properties also include the amount of a drug required to exert various effects, the time course of these effects, and other characteristics, such as a drug's chemical composition.

2. The **dose-response function** is the relationship between the amount of drug taken and the type and intensity of the resulting effect. Many psychological effects of drugs reach a plateau in the dose-response function, so that increasing the dose does not increase the effect any further. However, all drugs have more than one effect, and the dose-response functions usually are different for different effects. This means that increasing the dose of any drug may begin to result in additional effects, which are likely to be increasingly unpleasant or dangerous at high doses.

3. The **time-action function** is the relationship between the time elapsed since a drug was taken and the intensity of its effect. The effects of a drug are greatest when concentrations of the drug in body tissues are changing fastest, especially if they are increasing.

4. The person's *drug use history* may influence the effects of a drug. A given amount of alcohol, for example, will generally affect a habitual drinker less than an occasional drinker. Tolerance to some drugs, such as LSD, builds rapidly. To experience the same effect, a user has to abstain from the drug for a period of time before that dosage will again exert its original effects.

5. The *method of use (or route of administration)* has a direct effect on how strong a response a drug produces. Methods of use include ingestion, inhalation, injection, and absorption through the skin or tissue linings. Drugs are usually injected in one of three ways: intravenously (IV, or mainlining), intramuscularly (IM), or subcutaneously (SC, or skin popping). If a drug is taken by a method that allows the drug to enter the bloodstream and reach the brain rapidly, the effects are usually stronger and the potential for dependence greater than when the method involves slower absorption. For example, injecting a drug intravenously produces stronger effects than swallowing the same drug. Inhaling a drug, such as when tobacco or crack cocaine is smoked, produces very rapid effects on the brain.

## User Factors

The second category of factors that determine how a person will respond to a particular drug involves certain physical and psychological characteristics. Body mass is one variable. The effects of a certain dose of a drug on a 100-pound person will be twice as great as on a 200-pound person. Other variables include general health and genetic factors. For example, some people have an inherited ability to rapidly metabolize a cough suppressant called dextromethorphan, which also has psychoactive properties. These people must take a higher-than-normal dose to get a given cough-suppressant effect.

If a person's biochemical state is already altered by another drug, this too can make a difference. Some drugs intensify the effects of other drugs, as is the case with alcohol and sedatives. Some drugs block the effects of other drugs, such as when a tranquilizer is used to relieve anxiety caused by cocaine. Interactions between drugs, including many prescription and OTC medications, can be unpredictable and dangerous.

One physical condition that requires special precautions is pregnancy. It can be risky for a woman to use any drugs at all during pregnancy, including alcohol and common OTC preparations like cough medicine. The risks are greatest during the first trimester, when the fetus's body is rapidly forming and even small biochemical alterations in the mother can have a devastating effect on fetal development. Even later, the fetus is more susceptible than the mother to the adverse effects of any drugs she takes. The fetus may even become physically dependent on a drug being taken by the mother and suffer withdrawal symptoms after birth.

Sometimes a person's response to a drug is strongly influenced by the user's expectations about how he or she will react (the psychological *set*). With large doses, the drug's chemical properties do seem to have the strongest effect on the user's response. But with small doses, psychological (and social) factors are often more important. When people strongly believe that a given drug will affect them a certain way, they are likely to experience those effects regardless of the drug's pharmacological properties. In one study, regular users of marijuana reported a moderate level of intoxication **(high)** after using a cigarette that smelled and tasted like marijuana but contained no THC, the active ingredient in marijuana. This is an example of the **placebo effect**—when a person receives an inert substance yet responds as if it were an active drug. In other studies, subjects who smoked low doses of real marijuana that they believed to be a placebo experienced no effects from the drug. Clearly, the user's expectations had a greater effect on the smokers than the drug itself.

## Social Factors

The *setting* is the physical and social environment surrounding the drug use. If a person uses marijuana at home with trusted friends and pleasant music, the effects are likely to be different from the effects if the same dose is taken in an austere experimental laboratory with an impassive research technician. Similarly, the dose of alcohol that produces mild euphoria and stimulation at a noisy, active cocktail party might induce sleepiness and slight depression when taken at home while alone.

## REPRESENTATIVE PSYCHOACTIVE DRUGS

What are the major psychoactive drugs, and how do they produce their effects? We discuss six different representative groups in this chapter: (1) opioids, (2) central nervous system depressants, (3) central nervous system stimulants, (4) marijuana and other cannabis products, (5) hallucinogens, and (6) inhalants (Figure 7-1).

### Opioids

Also called *narcotics,* **opioids** are natural or synthetic (laboratory-made) drugs that relieve pain, cause drowsiness, and induce **euphoria.** Especially in small doses, opioids have beneficial medical uses, including pain relief. Opium, morphine, heroin, methadone, codeine, hydrocodone, oxycodone, meperidine, and fentanyl are examples of drugs in this category. Opioids tend to reduce anxiety and produce lethargy, apathy, and an inability to concentrate. Opioid users become less active and less responsive to frustration, hunger, and sexual stimulation. These effects are more pronounced in novice users; with repeated use, many effects diminish.

Opioids are typically injected or absorbed into the body from the stomach, intestines, nasal membranes (from snorting or sniffing), or lungs (from smoking). Effects depend on the method of administration. If brain levels of the drug change rapidly, more immediate effects will result. Although the euphoria associated with opioids is an important factor in their abuse, many people experience a feeling of uneasiness when they first use these drugs. Users also often feel nauseated and vomit, and they may have other unpleasant sensations. Even so, the abuse of opioids often results in dependence. Tolerance can develop rapidly and be pronounced. Withdrawal symptoms include cramps, chills, sweating, nausea, tremors, irritability, and feelings of panic.

Users who sniff or smoke heroin avoid the special disease risks of injection drug use, including HIV infection, but dependence can readily result from sniffing and smoking heroin. In addition, the potentially high but variable purity of street heroin poses a risk of unintentional overdose. Symptoms of overdose include respiratory depression, coma, and constriction of the pupils; death can result.

Problems with abuse have recently been reported for oxycodone and hydrocodone, narcotics found in prescription pain relievers including OxyContin and Vicodin. When taken as prescribed in tablet form, these drugs treat moderate to severe chronic pain and do not typically lead to abuse. However, like other opioids, use of prescription painkillers can lead to abuse and dependence. Oxycodone and hydrocodone can be abused orally; the long-acting form of oxycodone is also sometimes crushed and snorted or dissolved and injected, providing a powerful heroin-like high. When taken in large doses or combined with other drugs, oxycodone and hydrocodone can cause fatal respiratory depression.

### Central Nervous System Depressants

Central nervous system **depressants,** also known as **sedative-hypnotics,** slow down the overall activity of the **central nervous system (CNS).** The result can range from mild **sedation** to death. CNS depressants include alcohol (discussed in Chapter 8), barbiturates, and other sedatives.

**Types** The various types of barbiturates (downers or downs) are similar in chemical composition and action, but they differ in how quickly and how long they act. Antianxiety agents, also called sedatives or **tranquilizers,** include the benzodiazepines such as Xanax, Valium, Librium, clonazepam (Klonopin), and flunitrazepam (Rohypnol). Other CNS depressants include methaqualone (Quaalude), ethchlorvynol (Placidyl), chloral hydrate ("mickey"), and gamma hydroxy butyrate (GHB, or "liquid ecstasy").

**Effects** CNS depressants reduce anxiety and cause mood changes, impaired muscular coordination, slurring of speech, and drowsiness or sleep. Mental functioning is also affected, but the degree varies from person to person and also depends on the kind of task the person is trying to do. Most people become drowsy with small doses, although a few become more active.

#### Terms

**pharmacological properties** The overall effects of a drug on a person's behavior, psychology, and chemistry.

**dose-response function** The relationship between the amount of a drug taken and the intensity or type of the resulting effect.

**time-action function** The relationship between the time elapsed since a drug was taken and the intensity of its effect.

**high** The subjectively pleasing effects of a drug, usually felt quite soon after the drug is taken.

**placebo effect** A response to an inert or innocuous medication given in place of an active drug.

**opioid** Any of several natural or synthetic drugs that relieve pain and cause drowsiness and/or euphoria; examples are opium, morphine, and heroin; also called *narcotic.*

**euphoria** An exaggerated feeling of well-being.

**depressant, or sedative-hypnotic** A drug that decreases nervous or muscular activity, causing drowsiness or sleep.

**central nervous system (CNS)** The brain and spinal cord.

**sedation** The induction of a calm, relaxed, often sleepy state.

**tranquilizer** A CNS depressant that reduces tension and anxiety.

| Category | Representative drugs | Street names | Appearance | Methods of use | Short-term effects |
|---|---|---|---|---|---|
| **Opioids** | Heroin | Dope, H, junk, brown sugar, smack | White/dark brown powder; dark tar or coal-like substance | Injected, smoked, snorted | Relief of anxiety and pain; euphoria; lethargy, apathy, drowsiness, confusion, inability to concentrate; nausea, constipation, respiratory depression |
| | Opium | Big O, black stuff, hop | Dark brown or black chunks | Swallowed, smoked | |
| | Morphine | M, Miss Emma, monkey, white stuff | White crystals, liquid solution | Injected, swallowed, smoked | |
| | Oxycodone, codeine, hydrocodone | Oxy, O.C., killer, Captain Cody, schoolboy, vike | Tablets, powder made from crushing tablets | Swallowed, injected, snorted | |
| **Central nervous system depressants** | Barbiturates | Barbs, reds, red birds, yellows, yellow jackets | Colored capsules | Swallowed, injected | Reduced anxiety, mood changes, lowered inhibitions, impaired muscle coordination, reduced pulse rate, drowsiness, loss of consciousness, respiratory depression |
| | Benzodiazepines (e.g., Valium, Xanax, Rohypnol) | Candy, downers, tranks, roofies, forget-me pill | Tablets | Swallowed, injected | |
| | Methaqualone | Ludes, quad, quay | Tablets | Injected, swallowed | |
| | Gamma hydroxy butyrate (GHB) | G, Georgia home boy, grievous bodily harm | Clear liquid, white powder | Swallowed | |
| **Central nervous system stimulants** | Amphetamine, methamphet-amine | Bennies, speed, black beauties, uppers, chalk, crank, crystal, ice, meth | Tablets, capsules, white powder, white crystals | Injected, swallowed, smoked, snorted | Increased heart rate, blood pressure, metabolism; increased mental alertness and energy; nervousness, insomnia, impulsive behavior; reduced appetite |
| | Cocaine, crack cocaine | Blow, C, candy, coke, flake, rock, toot | White powder, beige pellets or rocks | Injected, smoked, snorted | |
| | Ritalin | JIF, MPH, R-ball, Skippy | Tablets | Injected, swallowed, snorted | |
| **Marijuana and other cannabis products** | Marijuana | Dope, grass, joints, Mary Jane, reefer, skunk, weed | Dried leaves and stems | Smoked, swallowed | Euphoria, slowed thinking and reaction time, confusion, anxiety, impaired balance and coordination, increased heart rate |
| | Hashish | Hash, hemp, boom, gangster | Dark, resin-like compound formed into rocks or blocks | Smoked, swallowed | |
| **Hallucinogens** | LSD | Acid, boomers, blotter, yellow sunshines | Blotter paper, liquid, gelatin tabs, pills | Swallowed, absorbed through mouth tissues | Altered states of perception and feeling; nausea; increased heart rate, blood pressure; delirium; impaired motor function; numbness, weakness |
| | Mescaline (peyote) | Buttons, cactus, mesc | Brown buttons, liquid | Swallowed, smoked | |
| | Psilocybin | Shrooms, magic mushrooms | Dried mushrooms | Swallowed | |
| | Ketamine | K, special K, cat valium, vitamin K | Clear liquid, white or beige powder | Injected, snorted, smoked | |
| | PCP | Angel dust, hog, love boat, peace pill | White to brown powder, tablets | Injected, swallowed, smoked, snorted | |
| | MDMA (ecstasy) | X, peace, clarity, Adam | Tablets | Swallowed | |
| **Inhalants** | Solvents, aerosols, nitrites, anesthetics | Laughing gas, poppers, snappers, whippets | Household products, sprays, glues, paint thinner, petroleum products | Inhaled through nose or mouth | Stimulation, loss of inhibition, slurred speech, loss of motor coordination, loss of consciousness |

**Figure 7-1 Commonly abused drugs and their effects** SOURCES: National Institute on Drug Abuse. 2004. *Commonly Abused Drugs* (http://www.drugabuse.gov/DrugPages/DrugsofAbuse.html; retrieved December 9, 2004); U.S. Drug Enforcement Agency. 2004. *Photo Library* (http://www.usdoj.gov:80/dea/photo_library.html; retrieved December 9, 2004); U.S. Drug Enforcement Agency. 2004. *Drug Briefs and Backgrounds* (http://www.usdoj.gov:80/dea/concern/concern.htm; retrieved December 9, 2004).

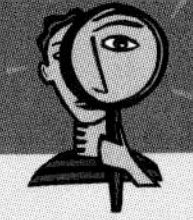

## Club Drugs

Club drugs include a variety of very different drugs that are part of the popular dance culture of clubs and raves—all-night dance parties held in fields or abandoned buildings. Some people refer to club drugs as soft drugs because they see them as recreational—more for the casual, weekend user—rather than as addictive. But club drugs have many potential negative effects and are particularly potent and unpredictable when mixed with alcohol. Substitute drugs are often sold in place of club drugs, putting users at risk for taking dangerous combinations of unknown drugs.

***MDMA*** *(ecstasy, E, X, XTC, Adam, hug drug, lover's speed):* Taken in pill form, MDMA (methylenedioxymethamphetamine) is a stimulant with mildly hallucinogenic and amphetamine-like effects. Users may experience euphoria, increased energy, and a heightened sense of belonging. In club settings, using MDMA can produce dangerously high body temperature and potentially fatal dehydration; some users experience confusion, depression, anxiety, paranoia, muscle tension, involuntary teeth clenching, blurred vision, nausea, and seizures. Even low doses can affect concentration, judgment, and driving ability. Tolerance can develop, leading users to take the drug more frequently (on a daily basis), to use higher doses, or to combine MDMA with other drugs, including Prozac, to enhance the drug's effects. In addition to MDMA, many ecstasy tablets include other drugs such as methamphetamine, ephedrine, or cocaine. At high doses or mixed with other drugs, MDMA is extremely dangerous; most deaths linked to MDMA have occurred as a result of multidrug toxicity or traumatic injuries.

Animal studies have found that moderate to high doses of MDMA are toxic to nerve cells producing serotonin and may cause long-lasting damage; human studies are ongoing. MDMA users perform worse than nonusers on complex cognitive tasks of memory, attention, and general intelligence. Long-term effects may include physical symptoms and psychological problems such as confusion or paranoia. Pregnant women who use MDMA are at increased risk for having a baby with congenital malformations and long-term impairment in memory and other cognitive functions.

***LSD*** *(acid, boomers, yellow sunshines, red dragon):* A popular and potent hallucinogen, LSD (lysergic acid diethylamide) is sold in tablets or capsules, in liquid form, or on small squares of paper called blotters. LSD increases heart rate and body temperature and may cause nausea, tremors, sweating, numbness, and weakness. (See pp. 155–156 for more on LSD.)

***Ketamine*** *(special K, vitamin K, K, cat valium, jet):* A veterinary anesthetic that can be taken in powdered or liquid form, ketamine may cause hallucinations and impaired attention and memory. At higher doses, ketamine can cause delirium, amnesia, high blood pressure, and potentially fatal respiratory problems. Tolerance to ketamine develops rapidly.

***GHB*** *(Georgia home boy, G, grievous bodily harm, liquid ecstasy):* GHB (gamma hydroxybutyrate) can be produced in clear liquid, white powder, tablet, and capsule form; it is often made in basement chemistry labs, where toxic substances may unintentionally be added or produced. GHB is a CNS depressant that in large doses or when taken in combination with alcohol or other depressants can cause sedation, loss of consciousness, respiratory arrest, and death. GHB may cause prolonged and potentially life-threatening withdrawal symptoms.

***Rohypnol*** *(roofies, roche, forget-me pill):* Taken in tablet form, Rohypnol (flunitrazepam) is a sedative that is ten times more potent than Valium. Its effects, which are magnified by alcohol, include reduced blood pressure, dizziness, confusion, gastrointestinal disturbances, and loss of consciousness. Users of Rohypnol may develop physical and psychological dependence on the drug.

An additional problem associated with GHB, Rohypnol, and several other club drugs is their potential use as "date rape drugs." Because they can be added to beverages surreptitiously, these drugs may be unknowingly consumed by intended rape victims. In addition to depressant effects, some drugs also cause *anterograde amnesia,* the loss of memory of things occurring while under the influence of the drug. Because of concern about GHB, Rohypnol, and other similarly abused drugs, Congress passed the "Drug-Induced Rape Prevention and Punishment Act," which increased federal penalties for use of any controlled substance to aid in sexual assault.

**From Use to Abuse** People are usually introduced to CNS depressants either through a medical prescription or through drug-using peers. The use of Rohypnol and GHB is often associated with dance clubs and raves (see the box "Club Drugs"). Most CNS depressants, including alcohol, can lead to classical physical dependence. Tolerance, sometimes for up to 15 times the usual dose, can develop with repeated use. Tranquilizers have been shown to produce physical dependence even at ordinary prescribed doses. Withdrawal symptoms can be more severe than those accompanying opioid dependence. They may begin as anxiety, shaking, and weakness but may turn into convulsions and possibly cardiovascular collapse and death.

While intoxicated, people on depressants cannot function very well. They are mentally confused and are frequently obstinate, irritable, and abusive. Even prescription use of benzodiazepines increases the risk of automobile crashes. After long-term use, depressants like alcohol can lead to generally poor health and brain damage, with impaired ability to reason and make judgments.

Too much depression of the central nervous system slows respiration and may stop it entirely. CNS depressants are particularly dangerous in combination with another depressant, such as alcohol. Rohypnol is ten times more potent than Valium and can be fatal if combined with alcohol. GHB is often produced clandestinely, resulting in widely varying degrees of purity.

## Central Nervous System Stimulants

CNS **stimulants** speed up the activity of the nervous or muscular system. Under their influence, the heart rate accelerates, blood pressure rises, blood vessels constrict, the pupils of the eyes and the bronchial tubes dilate, and gastric and adrenal secretions increase. There is greater muscular tension and sometimes an increase in motor activity. Small doses usually make people feel more awake and alert, less fatigued and bored. The most common CNS stimulants are cocaine, amphetamines, nicotine (discussed in Chapter 8), ephedrine, and caffeine.

**Cocaine** Usually derived from the leaves of coca shrubs that grow high in the Andes Mountains in South America, cocaine—also known as "coke" or "snow"—is a potent CNS stimulant. Cocaine is usually snorted and absorbed through the nasal mucosa or injected intravenously, providing rapid increases of the drug's concentration in the blood and therefore fast, intense effects. Another method of use involves processing cocaine with baking soda and water, yielding the ready-to-smoke form of cocaine known as crack. Crack is typically available as small beads or pellets smokable in glass pipes.

**EFFECTS** The effects of cocaine are usually intense but short-lived. The euphoria lasts from 5 to 20 minutes and ends abruptly, to be replaced by irritability, anxiety, or slight depression. When cocaine is absorbed via the lungs, it reaches the brain in about 10 seconds, and the effects are particularly intense. The effects from IV injections occur almost as quickly—in about 20 seconds. Since the mucous membranes in the nose briefly slow absorption, the onset of effects from snorting takes 2–3 minutes. Heavy users may inject cocaine intravenously every 10–20 minutes to maintain the effects.

The larger the cocaine dose and the more rapidly it is absorbed into the bloodstream, the greater the immediate—and sometimes lethal—effects. Sudden death from cocaine is most commonly the result of excessive CNS stimulation that causes convulsions and respiratory collapse, irregular heartbeat, extremely high blood pressure, blood clots, and possibly heart attack or stroke. Although rare, fatalities can occur in healthy young people. Chronic cocaine use produces inflammation of the nasal mucosa, which can lead to persistent bleeding and ulceration of the septum between the nostrils. The use of cocaine may also cause paranoia and/or aggressiveness.

**COCAINE USE DURING PREGNANCY** A woman who uses cocaine during pregnancy is at higher risk for miscarriage, premature labor, and stillbirth. She is more likely to deliver a low-birth-weight baby who has a small head circumference. Her infant may be at increased risk for defects of the genitourinary tract, cardiovascular system, central nervous system, and extremities. It is difficult to pinpoint the effects of cocaine because many women who use cocaine also use tobacco and/or alcohol. Infants whose mothers use cocaine may also be born intoxicated; cocaine also passes into breast milk and can intoxicate a breastfeeding infant.

In the long term, prenatal cocaine exposure may cause subtle changes in the brain that affect specific cognitive and motor skills. Behavioral problems—disorganization, poor social skills, and hyperactivity—have also been reported. Although fetal cocaine exposure is an important issue, the type and magnitude of effects produced by nicotine are similar, and there are nearly 20 times more infants exposed to cigarettes than to cocaine.

**Amphetamines** Amphetamines (uppers) are a group of potent synthetic stimulants. Some common drugs in this family are amphetamine (Benzedrine), dextroamphetamine (Dexedrine), and methamphetamine (Methedrine). Popular names for these drugs include speed, crank, chalk, ice, crystal, and meth.

**EFFECTS** Small doses of amphetamines usually make people feel more alert and wide-awake and less fatigued or bored. Amphetamines generally increase motor activity but do not measurably alter a normal, rested person's ability to perform tasks calling for challenging motor skills or complex thinking. When amphetamines do improve performance, it is primarily by counteracting fatigue and boredom. Amphetamines in small doses also increase heart rate and blood pressure and change sleep patterns.

Amphetamines are sometimes used to curb appetite, but after a few weeks the user develops tolerance and higher doses are necessary. When people stop taking the drug, their appetite usually returns, and they gain back the weight they lost unless they have made permanent changes in eating behavior.

**FROM USE TO ABUSE** Much amphetamine abuse begins as an attempt to cope with a temporary situation. A student cramming for an exam or an exhausted long-haul truck driver can go a little longer by taking amphetamines, but the results can be disastrous. The likelihood of making bad judgments significantly increases. The stimulating effects may also wear off suddenly, and the user may precipitously feel exhausted or fall asleep ("crash").

### Terms

VW

**stimulant** A drug that increases nervous or muscular activity.

**state dependence** A situation in which information learned in a drug-induced state is difficult to recall when the effect of the drug wears off.

Another problem is **state dependence,** the phenomenon whereby information learned in a certain drug-induced state is difficult to recall when the person is not in that same physiological state. Test performance may deteriorate when students use drugs to study and then take tests in their normal, nondrug state.

**DEPENDENCE** Repeated use of amphetamines, even in moderate doses, often leads to tolerance and the need for increasingly larger doses. Long-term use of amphetamines at high doses can cause paranoia, hallucinations, delusions, and incoherence. Methamphetamine users have signs of brain damage similar to those seen in Parkinson's disease patients that appear to persist even after drug use ceases, causing impaired memory and motor coordination. Withdrawal symptoms may include muscle aches and tremors, along with profound fatigue, deep depression, despair, and apathy. Chronic high-dose amphetamine use is often associated with pronounced psychological cravings and obsessive drug-seeking behavior.

Women who use amphetamines during pregnancy risk premature birth, stillbirth, low birth weight, and early infant death. Babies born to amphetamine-using mothers have a higher incidence of cleft palate, cleft lip, and deformed limbs. They may also experience symptoms of withdrawal from amphetamines.

**Ritalin** A stimulant with amphetamine-like effects, Ritalin (methylphenidate) is used to treat attention-deficit/hyperactivity disorder. When taken orally at prescribed levels, it has little potential for abuse. When injected or snorted, however, dependence and tolerance can rapidly result. In a 2003 survey, 4.7% of college students reported having used Ritalin in the previous year.

**Caffeine** Caffeine is probably the most popular psychoactive drug and also one of the most ancient. It is found in coffee, tea, cocoa, soft drinks, headache remedies, and OTC preparations like NōDōz. In ordinary doses, caffeine produces greater alertness and a sense of well-being. It also decreases feelings of fatigue or boredom, and using caffeine may enable a person to keep at physically exhausting or repetitive tasks longer. Such use is usually followed, however, by a sudden letdown. Caffeine does not noticeably influence a person's ability to perform complex intellectual tasks unless fatigue or boredom have already affected normal performance.

Caffeine mildly stimulates the heart and respiratory system, increases muscular tremor, and enhances gastric secretion. Higher doses may cause nervousness, anxiety, irritability, headache, disturbed sleep, and gastric irritation or peptic ulcers. In people with high blood pressure, caffeine can cause blood pressure to rise even further above normal; in people with type 2 diabetes, caffeine may cause glucose and insulin levels to rise after meals. Some people, especially children, are quite vulnerable to the adverse effects of caffeine. They become wired: hyperactive and overly sensitive to any stimulation in their environment. In rare instances, the disturbance is so severe that there is misperception of their surroundings—a toxic psychosis.

Drinks containing caffeine are rarely harmful for most individuals, but some tolerance develops, and withdrawal symptoms of irritability, headaches, and even mild depression do occur. Thus, although we don't usually think of caffeine as a dependence-producing drug, for some people it is. People can usually avoid problems by simply decreasing their daily intake of caffeine (Figure 7-2).

Milligrams of caffeine
Coffee
Brewed (8 oz.), 135
Instant (8 oz.), 95
Espresso (2 oz.), 90
Cappuccino (2 oz.), 90
Decaffeinated (8 oz.), 5
Tea
Snapple (16 oz.), 48
Black, bag or leaf (8 oz.), 40
Green, bag or leaf (8 oz.), 30
Instant, hot or iced (8 oz.), 25
Herbal, 0
Soft drinks (12 oz)
Mountain Dew, 55
Coca-Cola, 45
Pepsi-Cola, 37
7-Up, Sprite, 0
Desserts/dairy products
Coffee ice cream (1 cup), 50
Dannon coffee yogurt (8 oz.), 45
Dark chocolate (1 oz.), 20
Cocoa or hot chocolate (8 oz.), 6
Milk chocolate (1 oz.), 6
Dannon cappuccino yogurt (8 oz.), 0
Over-the-counter medications (1 tablet)
Vivarin, 200
NōDōz, 100
Excedrin, 65
Anacin, 32
Midol, 32
Yog
0
25
50
75
100
125
150
175
200


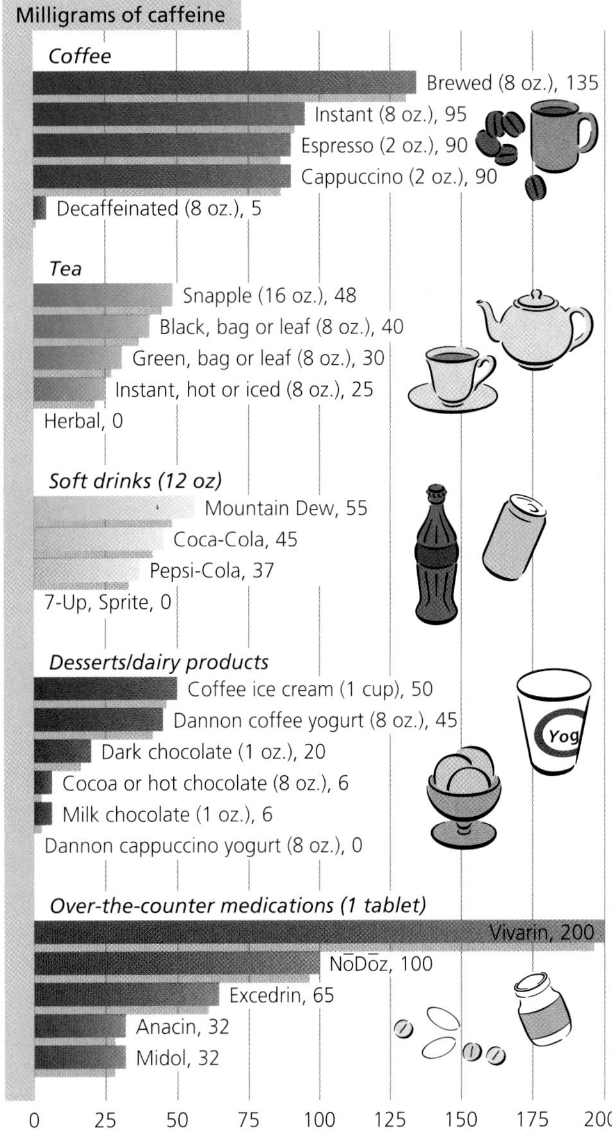

**Figure 7-2 Common sources of caffeine.** The caffeine content of products varies with the brand and preparation method; the values shown here are averages. Among Americans, the average daily intake is about 230 milligrams. SOURCES: Become a bean counter. 2000. *Prevention,* July; International Food Information Council. 1998. *Everything You Need to Know About Caffeine* (http://ific.org/publications/brochures/caffeinebroch.cfm; retrieved December 8, 2004); Caffeine content of foods and drugs. 1996. *Nutrition Action Healthletter,* December.

## Marijuana and Other Cannabis Products

Marijuana is the most widely used illegal drug in the United States (cocaine is second). More than 40% of Americans—more than 90 million—have tried marijuana at least once; among 21–25-year-olds, more than 50% have tried marijuana.

Marijuana is a crude preparation of various parts of the Indian hemp plant *Cannabis sativa,* which grows in most parts of the world. THC (tetrahydrocannabinol) is the main active ingredient in marijuana. Based on THC content, the potency of marijuana preparations varies widely. Marijuana plants that grow wild often have less than 1% THC in their leaves, whereas when selected strains are cultivated by separation of male and female plants (*sinsemilla*), the bud leaves from the flowering tops may contain 7–8% THC. Hashish, a potent preparation made from the thick resin that exudes from the leaves, may contain up to 14% THC. Marijuana is usually smoked, but it can also be ingested.

**Short-Term Effects** The effects of a low dose of marijuana are strongly influenced both by the user's expectations and by past experiences. At low doses, marijuana users typically experience euphoria, a heightening of subjective sensory experiences, a slowing down of the perception of passing time, and a relaxed, laid-back attitude. These pleasant effects are the reason this drug is so widely used. With moderate doses, these effects become stronger, and the user can also expect to have impaired memory function, disturbed thought patterns, lapses of attention, and feelings of **depersonalization,** in which the mind seems to be separated from the body.

The effects of marijuana in higher doses are determined mostly by the drug itself rather than by the user's expectations and setting. Very high doses produce feelings of depersonalization, as well as marked sensory distortion and changes in body image (such as a feeling that the body is very light). Inexperienced users sometimes think these sensations mean they are going crazy and become anxious or even panicky. Such reactions resemble a bad trip on LSD, but they happen much less often, are less severe, and do not last as long.

### Terms

VW

**depersonalization** A state in which a person loses the sense of his or her reality or perceives his or her body as unreal.

**hallucinogen** Any of several drugs that alter perception, feelings, or thoughts; examples are LSD, mescaline, and PCP.

**synesthesia** A condition in which a stimulus evokes not only the sensation appropriate to it but also another sensation of a different character, such as when a color evokes a specific smell.

**altered states of consciousness** Profound changes in mood, thinking, and perception.

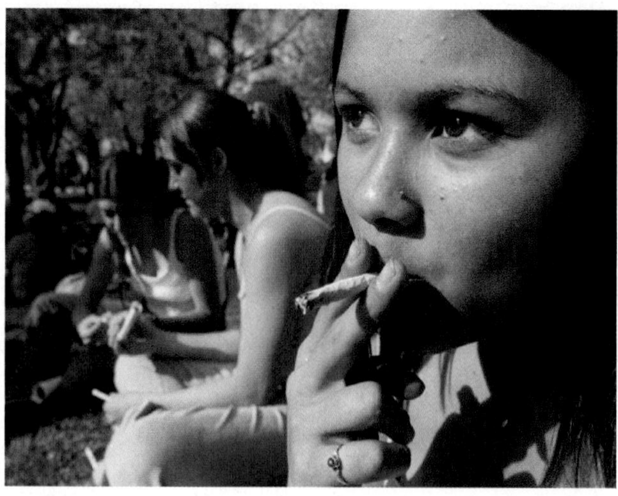

Marijuana is the most widely used illegal drug in the United States. At low doses, marijuana users typically experience euphoria and a relaxed attitude. Further research is needed to determine its precise physiological and psychological effects, particularly for chronic use.

Physiologically, marijuana increases heart rate and dilates certain blood vessels in the eyes, which creates the characteristic bloodshot eyes. The user may also feel less inclined toward physical exertion and may feel particularly hungry or thirsty (see the box "Medical Marijuana").

**Long-Term Effects** The most probable long-term effect of smoking marijuana is respiratory damage, including impaired lung function, chronic bronchial irritation, and precancerous changes in the lungs. People who smoke marijuana may be at increased risk for emphysema and cancer of the head and neck; among people with chronic conditions like cancer and AIDS, marijuana use is associated with increased risk of fatal lung infections. Heavy users who are frequently intoxicated experience subtle impairments of attention and memory that may or may not be reversible following long-term abstinence. Long-term use may also decrease testosterone levels and sperm counts and increase sperm abnormalities.

Heavy marijuana use during pregnancy may cause impaired fetal growth and development and low birth weight. Marijuana may act synergistically with alcohol to increase the damaging effects of alcohol on the fetus. THC rapidly enters breast milk and may impair an infant's early motor development.

Regular users of marijuana can develop tolerance; some develop dependence, and researchers estimate that 1.5% of Americans meet the APA criteria for marijuana dependence. Withdrawal symptoms may occur in the majority of dependent or heavy users; common symptoms include anger or aggression, irritability, nervousness or restlessness, sleep difficulties, and decreased appetite or weight loss. Withdrawal symptoms begin about 1–2 days after cessation of marijuana use and typically last 1–2 weeks. As with all drugs that relieve "bad"

In the News

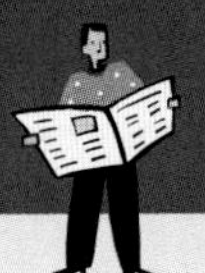

## Medical Marijuana

The question of whether marijuana has any medical uses has been hotly debated. Cannabis preparations were once medically prescribed for a variety of illnesses, but most such uses are no longer supported by research. A legal, prescription form of THC called dronabinol has been available in a capsule for some patients since 1985. However, many patients argue that oral THC is not as effective as smoked marijuana; the chemicals are absorbed more rapidly when marijuana is smoked and compounds in marijuana other than THC may contribute to its effects. Part of the difficulty in making a case for or against medical marijuana based on current research is that most patient testimonials are based on smoked marijuana, whereas most published research utilized THC in pill form.

A 1999 government-commissioned report from the Institute of Medicine (IOM) concluded that substances in marijuana have potential therapeutic value for pain relief, for control of nausea and vomiting in chemotherapy patients, and for stimulating appetite in people with AIDS-related wasting. Although effective drugs already exist for these conditions, marijuana may be suitable for patients who do not respond to other therapies. The report said that short-term use of marijuana could be considered for patients with debilitating symptoms.

The IOM report recommended further studies and the development of alternative methods of drug delivery—inhalers, patches, or under-the-tongue sprays, for example—that would safely deliver set doses of specific compounds in marijuana. As described in the chapter, smoking marijuana can cause respiratory damage and impair lung function; it may also increase cancer risk. Beyond the risks from smoking, the IOM report found that the range of problems associated with marijuana is not out of line with problems associated with other medications available in the United States.

A number of states have passed laws legalizing marijuana for medical uses; these laws are intended to shield users from laws against possessing marijuana and to protect physicians who recommend its use. However, purchasing, prescribing, or possessing marijuana is a federal crime. Under federal drug laws, marijuana is classified as a schedule I drug, defined as being potentially addictive, having no medical uses, and being unsafe for use under medical supervision (heroin and LSD are also schedule I drugs; cocaine is a schedule II drug because it has accepted medical uses). Opponents of allowing medical use of marijuana fear that making the drug more available would expand nonmedical use among the general population.

Several cases relating to medical marijuana have been heard by the U.S. Supreme Court. In 2003, the Court upheld the right of physicians to discuss marijuana with patients for medical purposes; however, an earlier ruling found that a so-called cannabis cooperative that was distributing marijuana to patients was not exempt from federal drug laws. And in June 2005, the Court ruled that patients using homegrown marijuana on the advice of a physician for personal, noncommercial use are still subject to federal drug law and can be prosecuted—even if they live in a state that allows such use. The debate over medical marijuana is likely to continue.

SOURCES: Reefer Rx: Marijuana as medicine. 2004. *Harvard Health Letter,* September; U.S. Department of Justice. 2004. *Supreme Court Briefs: No. 03-1454: Ashcroft v. Raich* (http://www.usdoj.gov/osg/briefs/2004/3mer/2mer/toc3index.html; retrieved December 7, 2004); Institute of Medicine. 1999. *Marijuana and Medicine: Assessing the Science Base.* Washington, D.C.: National Academy Press.

feelings and produce "good" feelings, marijuana can become the focus of the user's life, to the exclusion of other activities. Drug uses appear to be related, and the chronic marijuana user is more likely to be a heavy user of tobacco, alcohol, and other dangerous drugs.

## Hallucinogens

**Hallucinogens** are a group of drugs whose predominant pharmacological effect is to alter the user's perceptions, feelings, and thoughts. Hallucinogens include LSD (lysergic acid diethylamide), mescaline, psilocybin, STP (4-methyl-2,5-dimethoxyamphetamine), DMT (dimethyltryptamine), MDMA (3,4-methylene-dioxymethamphetamine), ketamine, and PCP (phencyclidine). These drugs are most commonly ingested or smoked.

**LSD** LSD is one of the most powerful psychoactive drugs. Tiny doses will produce noticeable effects in most people, such as an altered sense of time, visual disturbances, an improved sense of hearing, mood changes, and distortions in how people perceive their bodies. Dilation of the pupils and slight dizziness, weakness, and nausea may also occur. With larger doses, users may experience a phenomenon known as **synesthesia,** feelings of depersonalization, and other changes in the perceived relationship between the self and external reality.

Many hallucinogens induce tolerance so quickly that after only one or two doses their effects decrease substantially. The user must then stop taking the drug for several days before his or her system can be receptive to it again. These drugs cause little drug-seeking behavior and no physical dependence or withdrawal symptoms.

The immediate effects of low doses of hallucinogens are largely determined by expectations and setting. Many effects are hard to describe because they involve subjective and unusual dimensions of awareness—the **altered states of consciousness** for which these drugs are famous. For this reason, hallucinogens have acquired a certain aura not associated with other drugs. People have taken LSD in search of a religious or mystical experience or in the hope of exploring new worlds.

A severe panic reaction, which can be terrifying in the extreme, can result from taking any dose of LSD. It is impossible to predict when a panic reaction will occur. Even after the drug's chemical effects have worn off, spontaneous flashbacks and other psychological disturbances can occur. **Flashbacks** are perceptual distortions and bizarre thoughts that occur after the drug has been entirely eliminated from the body.

**Other Hallucinogens** Most other hallucinogens have the same general effects as LSD, but there are some variations. For example, MDMA has both hallucinogenic and amphetamine-like properties. Tolerance to MDMA develops quickly, and high doses can cause anxiety, delusions, and paranoia. (See p. 151 for more on MDMA.)

PCP, also known as "angel dust," "hog," and "peace pill," reduces and distorts sensory input, especially **proprioception,** the sensation of body position and movement; it creates a state of sensory deprivation. Because it can be easily made, PCP is often available illegally and is sometimes used as an inexpensive replacement for other psychoactive drugs. The effects of ketamine are similar to those of PCP—confusion, agitation, aggression, and lack of coordination—but they tend to be less predictable. Tolerance to either drug can develop rapidly.

Mescaline, derived from the peyote cactus, is the ceremonial drug of the Native American Church. It causes effects similar to LSD, including altered perception and feeling; increased body temperature, heart rate, and blood pressure; weakness and trembling; and sleeplessness. Obtaining mescaline is expensive, so most street mescaline is diluted LSD or a mixture of other drugs. Hallucinogenic effects can be obtained from certain mushrooms (*Psilocybe mexicana*, or "magic mushrooms"), certain morning glory seeds, nutmeg, jimsonweed, and other botanical products, but unpleasant side effects, such as dizziness, have limited the popularity of these products.

## Inhalants

Inhaling certain chemicals can produce effects ranging from heightened pleasure to delirium and death. Inhalants fall into several major groups: (1) volatile solvents, which are found in products such as paint thinner, glue, and gasoline; (2) aerosols, which are sprays that contain propellants and solvents; (3) nitrites, such as butyl nitrite and amyl nitrite; and (4) anesthetics, which include nitrous oxide, or laughing gas.

### Terms

VW

**flashback** A perceptual distortion or bizarre thought that recurs after the chemical effects of a drug have worn off.

**proprioception** The sensation of body position and movement, from muscles, joints, and skin.

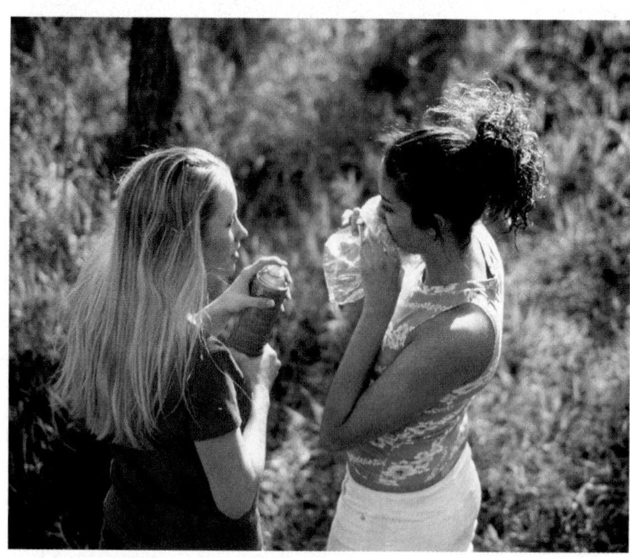

Inhalant use is difficult to monitor and control because inhalants are found in many inexpensive and legal products. Low doses of inhalants may cause a user to feel slightly stimulated; higher concentrations can cause a loss of consciousness, heart failure, and death.

Inhalant use is difficult to control because inhalants are easy to obtain. They are present in a variety of seemingly harmless products, from dessert-topping sprays to underarm deodorants, that are both inexpensive and legal. Using the drugs also requires no illegal or suspicious paraphernalia. Inhalant users get high by sniffing, snorting, "bagging" (inhaling fumes from a plastic bag), or "huffing" (placing an inhalant-soaked rag in the mouth).

Although different in makeup, nearly all inhalants produce effects similar to those of anesthetics, which slow down body functions. Low doses may cause users to feel slightly stimulated; at higher doses, users may feel less inhibited and less in control. Sniffing high concentrations of the chemicals in solvents or aerosol sprays can cause a loss of consciousness, heart failure, and death. High concentrations of any inhalant can also cause death from suffocation by displacing the oxygen in the lungs and central nervous system. Deliberately inhaling from a bag or in a closed area greatly increases the chances of suffocation. Other possible effects of the excessive or long-term use of inhalants include damage to the nervous system (impaired perception, reasoning, memory, and muscular coordination); hearing loss; increased risk of cancer; and damage to the liver, kidneys, and bone marrow.

## DRUG USE: THE DECADES AHEAD

Drug research will undoubtedly provide new information, new treatments, and new chemical combinations in the decades ahead. Mounting public concern has led to great debate and a wide range of opinions about what should be done. Efforts to combat the problem include

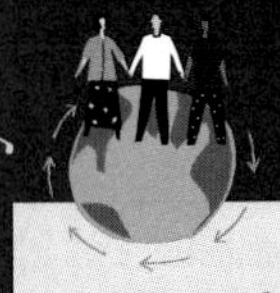

## Drug Use and Ethnicity: Risk Factors and Protective Factors

Surveys of the U.S. population find a variety of trends in drug use and abuse among ethnic groups (see table). In general, rates of drug use and abuse are highest among people who identify themselves as American Indians or Alaska Natives or as being of two races; rates are lowest among Asian Americans. In addition to the general trends shown in the table, there are also trends relating to age and to specific drugs. For example, African American teens have relatively low rates of drug use; rates climb among older blacks. Hallucinogen use is relatively prevalent among whites and Latinos, while inhalant use is more common among Native Hawaiians and other Pacific Islander Americans.

However, as is true for many areas of health, ethnic trends are influenced by a complex interplay of other factors, including educational and employment status and parental education and socioeconomic status. High income, high education, and full-time employment are associated with lower rates of drug use and abuse in adults and their children. People living in communities with high rates of poverty, crime, and unemployment have higher than average rates of drug use, and specific drugs may also be more available—and their abuse more common—in certain areas.

Strong cultural identity is associated with reduced risk of drug use and abuse among all groups. Other protective factors include the following:

- *Parental and community disapproval of drug and alcohol use:* Parents of African American and Asian American children tend to have more restrictive drug and alcohol use norms than white parents, and black parents tend to monitor their children's activities and friendships more closely than white parents.
- *Close family ties:* Asian American teens are the likeliest to come from intact homes. Black teens, although least likely to come from intact homes, often come from single-parent households with close extended family ties.
- *Focus on schooling and education:* Teens from families who value education and where parents help with homework and limit weeknight time with friends have lower rates of drug use.

**National Survey Results**

| | Lifetime Drug Use | Past Year Drug Use | Past Month Drug Use | Past Year Abuse or Dependence |
|---|---|---|---|---|
| Whites | 49.2 | 14.9 | 8.3 | 2.8 |
| African Americans | 44.6 | 15.4 | 8.7 | 3.1 |
| Latinos | 37.0 | 14.7 | 8.0 | 3.4 |
| Asian Americans | 25.6 | 7.1 | 3.8 | 1.5 |
| American Indians and Alaska Natives | 62.4 | 18.9 | 12.1 | 4.8 |
| Native Hawaiians and Pacific Islander Americans | 51.0 | 18.5 | 11.1 | 5.6 |
| Two or more races | 60.1 | 20.1 | 12.0 | 5.0 |

SOURCES: Office of Applied Studies, Substance Abuse and Mental Health Services Administration. 2004. *National Survey on Drug Use and Health* (http://oas.samhsa.gov/nhsda.htm; retrieved December 6, 2004); Johnston, L. D., et al. 2003. *Monitoring the Future: National Survey Results on Drug Use, 1975–2003: Volume I, Secondary School Students* (NIH Publication No. 04-5507). Bethesda, Md.: National Institute on Drug Abuse; National Center on Addiction and Substance Abuse at Columbia University. 2003. *The Formative Years: Pathways to Substance Abuse Among Girls and Young Women Ages 8–22.* New York: National Center on Addiction and Substance Abuse.

workplace drug testing, tougher law enforcement and prosecution, and treatment and education.

## Drugs, Society, and Families

The economic cost of drug use is staggering. Each year, Americans spend over $50 billion on illegal drugs, with an additional $100 billion going to cover enforcement, prevention, treatment, lost wages, and drug-related injuries and crime. But the costs are more than just financial; they are also paid in human pain and suffering.

The criminal justice system is inundated with people accused of crimes related to drug possession, sale, or use. More than 2 million arrests are made each year for drug and alcohol violations, and over 100,000 people are in jail for violating drug laws. Many assaults and murders are committed when people try to acquire or protect drug territories, settle disputes about drugs, or steal from dealers. Violence and the use of guns are more common in neighborhoods where drug trafficking is prevalent. Addicts commit more robberies and burglaries than criminals not on drugs. People under the influence of drugs, especially alcohol, are more likely to commit violent crimes like rape and murder than people who do not use drugs. Although often associated with poor inner-city areas and ethnic minorities, drug-related problems affect all groups and every area of the country (see the box "Drug Use and Ethnicity: Risk and Protective Factors").

Drug use is also a health care issue for society. In the United States, illegal drug use leads to more than 500,000 emergency room admissions and nearly 20,000 deaths annually. Although it is in the best interest of society to treat addicts who want help, there is not nearly enough space in treatment facilities to help the estimated 5 million Americans in need of immediate treatment. Drug addicts who want to quit, especially those among the urban poor, often have to wait a year or more for acceptance into a residential care or other treatment program.

Drug abuse also takes a toll on individuals and families. Children born to women who use drugs such as alcohol, tobacco, or cocaine may have long-term health problems. Drug use in families can become a vicious cycle. Observing adults around them using drugs, children assume it is an acceptable way to deal with problems. Problems such as abuse, neglect, lack of opportunity, and unemployment become contributing factors to drug use and serve to perpetuate the cycle.

## Legalizing Drugs

Pointing out that many of the social problems associated with drugs are related to prohibition rather than to the effects of the drugs themselves, some people have argued for various forms of drug legalization or decriminalization. Proposals range from making drugs such as marijuana and heroin available by prescription to allowing licensed dealers to sell some of these drugs to adults. Proponents argue that crimes by drug users are usually committed to buy drugs that cost relatively more than alcohol and tobacco because they are produced illegally and that making some currently illicit drugs legal—but putting controls on them similar to those used for alcohol, tobacco, and prescription drugs—could eliminate many of the problems related to drug use.

Opponents of drug legalization argue that allowing easier access to drugs would expose many more people to possible abuse and dependence. Drugs would be cheaper and easier to obtain, and drug use would be more socially acceptable. Legalizing drugs could cause an increase in drug use among children and teenagers. Opponents point out that alcohol and tobacco are major causes of disease and death in our society and that they should not be used as models for other practices.

## Drug Testing

It has been estimated that as many as 10% of workers use psychoactive drugs on the job. For some occupations, such as air traffic controllers, truck drivers, and train engineers, drug use can create significant hazards, sometimes involving hundreds of people. Some people believe that the dangers are so great that all workers should be tested and that anyone found with traces of drugs in the blood or urine should be either fired or treated. Others insist that this would violate people's right to privacy and to freedom from unreasonable search, guaranteed by the Fourth Amendment. Opponents point out that most jobs do not involve hazards, so employees who take drugs are not any more dangerous than employees who do not.

Despite the expense, many employers now test their employees, and the U.S. armed forces test military personnel regularly. People in jobs involving transportation—truck drivers, bus drivers, train engineers, airline pilots—are required by federal law to be tested regularly to ensure public safety. The primary criterion leading most companies to use drug testing is the company's liability if an employee under the influence of a drug makes a mistake that could potentially harm others. If a person tests positive for drugs, the employer may provide drug counseling or treatment, suspend the employee until he or she tests negative, or fire the individual.

## Treatment for Drug Dependence

A variety of programs is available to help people break their drug habits, but there is no single best method of treatment. The relapse rate is high for all types of treatment but is similar to the rate of relapse seen in people being treated for diabetes, high blood pressure, and asthma. Being treated is better than not being treated. To be successful, treatment must deal with the reasons behind people's drug abuse and help them develop behaviors, attitudes, and a social support system that will help them remain drug-free.

**Medication-Assisted Treatment** Medications are increasingly being used in addiction treatment—to reduce the craving for the abused drug or to block or oppose its effects. Perhaps the best-known medication for drug abuse is methadone, a synthetic drug used as a substitute for heroin. Use of methadone prevents withdrawal reactions and reduces the craving for heroin; it enables dependent people to function normally in social and vocational activities, although they remain dependent on methadone. The narcotic buprenorphine, approved for treatment of opioid addiction, also reduces cravings.

Medication therapy is relatively simple and inexpensive and is therefore popular. However, the relapse rate is high. Combining drug therapy with psychological and social services improves success rates, underscoring the importance of psychological factors in dependence.

**Treatment Centers** Treatment centers offer a variety of short-term and long-term services, including hospitalization, detoxification, counseling, and other mental health services. The therapeutic community is a specific type of center, a residential program run in a completely drug-free atmosphere. Administered by ex-addicts, these programs use confrontation, strict discipline, and unrelenting peer pressure to attempt to resocialize the addict with a different set of values. Halfway houses, transitional settings between a 24-hour-a-day program and independent living, can be an important phase of treatment.

**Self-Help Groups and Peer Counseling** Groups such as Alcoholics Anonymous (AA) and Narcotics Anonymous (NA) have helped many people. People treated in drug substitution programs or substance-abuse treatment centers are often urged or required to join a self-help group as part of their recovery. These groups follow a 12-step program. Group members' first step is to acknowledge that they have a problem over which they

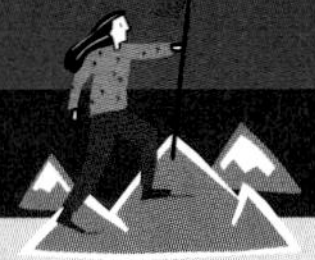

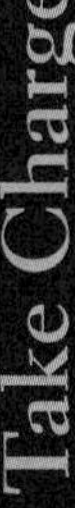

Take Charge

## If Someone You Know Has a Drug Problem . . .

If you notice changes in behavior and mood in someone you know, they may signal a growing dependence on drugs. Signs that a person's life is beginning to focus on drugs include the following:

- Sudden withdrawal or emotional distance
- Rebellious or unusually irritable behavior
- A loss of interest in usual activities or hobbies
- A decline in school performance
- A sudden change in the chosen group of friends
- Changes in sleeping or eating habits
- Frequent borrowing of money or stealing
- Secretive behavior about personal possessions, such as a backpack or the contents of a drawer
- Deterioration of physical appearance

If you believe a family member or friend has a drug problem, obtain information about resources for drug treatment available on your campus or in your community. Communicate your concern, provide him or her with information about treatment options, and offer your support during treatment. If the person continues to deny having a problem, you may want to talk with an experienced counselor about setting up an intervention—a formal, structured confrontation designed to end denial by having family, friends, and other caring individuals present their concerns to the drug user. Participants in an intervention would indicate the ways in which the individual is hurting others as well as himself or herself. If your friend or family member agrees to treatment, encourage him or her to attend a support group such as Narcotics Anonymous or Alcoholics Anonymous. And finally, examine your relationship with the abuser for signs of codependency. If necessary, get help for yourself; friends and family of drug users can often benefit from counseling.

have no control. Peer support is a critical ingredient of these programs, and members usually meet at least once a week. Each member is paired with a sponsor to call on for advice and support if the temptation to relapse becomes overwhelming. Chapters of AA and NA meet on some college campuses; community-based chapters are listed in the phone book and in local newspapers.

Many colleges also have peer counseling programs, in which students are trained to help other students who have drug problems. A peer counselor's role may be as limited as referring a student to a professional with expertise in substance dependence for an evaluation or as involved as helping arrange a leave of absence from school for participation in a drug-treatment program. Most peer counseling programs are founded on principles of strict confidentiality. Peer counselors may also be able to help students who are concerned about a classmate or loved one with an apparent drug problem (see the box "If Someone You Know Has a Drug Problem . . .").

**Harm Reduction Strategies** Recognizing that many attempts at treatment are at first unsuccessful and that a drug-free society may be an unobtainable goal, some experts advocate the use of harm reduction strategies. The goal of harm reduction is to minimize the negative effects of drug use and abuse; a common example is the use of designated drivers to reduce alcohol-related motor vehicle crashes. In terms of illicit drugs, drug substitution programs such as methadone maintenance are one form of harm reduction; although participants remain drug dependent, the negative individual and social consequences of their drug use is reduced. Syringe exchange programs, designed to reduce transmission of HIV and hepatitis C, are another harm reduction approach. Some experts have also suggested free testing of street drugs for purity and potency to help users avoid unintentional toxicity or overdose. Harm reduction strategies are controversial, in part because they measure success not in terms of overall levels of drug use and dependence but rather in terms of the harm caused by drug use in terms of illness, death, and crime.

**Codependency** Many treatment programs also offer counseling for those who are close to drug abusers. Drug abuse takes a toll on friends and family members, and counseling can help people work through painful feelings of guilt and powerlessness. **Codependency,** in which a person close to the drug abuser is controlled by the abuser's behavior, sometimes develops. Codependent people may come to believe that love, approval, and security are contingent on their taking care of the abuser. People can become codependent naturally because they want to help when someone they love becomes dependent on a drug. They may assume that their good intentions will persuade the drug user to stop.

Codependent people often engage in behaviors that remove or soften the effects of the drug use on the user—so-called *enabling* behaviors. However, the habit of enabling can inhibit a drug-dependent person's recovery because the person never has to experience the consequences of his or her behavior.

### Term

**codependency** A relationship in which a non–substance-abusing partner or family member is controlled by the abuser's behavior; codependent people frequently engage in enabling behaviors.

VW

Have you ever been an enabler in a relationship? You may have, if you've ever done any of the following:

- Given someone one more chance to stop abusing drugs, then another, and another . . .
- Made excuses or lied for someone to his or her friends, teachers, or employer
- Joined someone in drug use and blamed others for your behavior
- Loaned money to someone to continue drug use
- Stayed up late waiting for or gone out searching for someone who uses drugs
- Felt embarrassed or angry about the actions of someone who uses drugs
- Ignored the drug use because the person got defensive when you brought it up
- Not confronted a friend or relative who was obviously intoxicated or high on a drug

If you come from a codependent family or see yourself developing codependency relationships or engaging in enabling behaviors, consider acting now to make changes in your patterns of interaction.

## Preventing Drug Abuse

Obviously, the best solution to drug abuse is prevention. Government attempts at controlling the drug problem tend to focus on stopping the production, importation, and distribution of illegal drugs. Creative effort also has to be put into stopping the demand for drugs. Indirect approaches to prevention involve building young people's self-esteem, improving their academic skills, and increasing their recreational opportunities. Direct approaches involve giving information about the adverse effects of drugs and teaching tactics that help students resist peer pressure to use drugs in various situations.

Prevention efforts need to focus on the different motivations individuals have for using and abusing specific drugs at different ages. For example, adolescents in junior or senior high school are often more responsive to peer counselors. Many young adults tend to be influenced by efforts that focus on health education. For all ages, it is important to provide nondrug alternatives that speak to the individual's or group's specific reasons for using drugs, such as recreational facilities, counseling, greater opportunities for leisure activities, and places to socialize. Reminding young people that most people, no matter what age, are *not* users of illegal drugs, do *not* smoke cigarettes, and do *not* get drunk frequently is a critical part of preventing substance abuse.

## The Role of Drugs in Your Life

Whatever your experience has been up to now, it's likely that you will encounter drugs at some point in your life. To make sure you'll have the inner resources to resist peer pressure and make your own decision, cultivate a variety of activities you enjoy doing, realize that you are entitled to have your own opinion, and don't neglect your self-esteem.

**Issues to Consider** Before you try a psychoactive drug, consider the following questions:

- *What are the risks involved?* Many drugs carry an immediate risk of injury or death. Most involve the longer-term risk of abuse and dependence.
- *Is using the drug compatible with your goals?* Consider how drug use will affect your education and career objectives, your relationships, your future happiness, and the happiness of those who love you.
- *What are your ethical beliefs about drug use?* Consider whether using a drug would cause you to go against your personal ethics, religious beliefs, social values, or family responsibilities.
- *What are the financial costs?* Many drugs are expensive, especially if you become dependent on them.
- *Are you trying to solve a deeper problem?* Drugs will not make emotional pain go away; in the long run, they will only make it worse. If you are feeling depressed or anxious, seek help from a mental health professional instead of self-medicating with drugs.

Like all aspects of health-related behavior, making responsible decisions about drug use depends on information, knowledge, and insight into yourself. Many choices are possible; making the ones that are right for you is what counts.

**What to Do Instead of Drugs** If you have used or considered using drugs, think carefully about your reasons for doing so. Consider trying healthier strategies for dealing with difficult emotions and peer pressure. For ideas, look over the following list of reasons for drug use and suggested alternative activities:

- *Bored?* Go for a walk or a run; stimulate your senses at a museum or a movie; challenge your mind with a new game or book; introduce yourself to someone new.
- *Stressed?* Practice relaxation or visualization; try to slow down and open your senses to the natural world; get some exercise.
- *Shy or lonely?* Talk to a counselor; enroll in a shyness clinic; learn and practice communication techniques.
- *Feeling low on self-esteem?* Focus on the areas in which you are competent; give yourself credit for the things you do well. A program of regular exercise can also enhance self-esteem.
- *Depressed or anxious?* Talk to a friend, parent, or counselor.
- *Apathetic or lethargic?* Force yourself to get up and get some exercise to energize yourself; assume

responsibility for someone or something outside yourself; volunteer.

- *Searching for meaning?* Try yoga or meditation; explore spiritual experiences through religious groups, church, prayer, or reading.
- *Afraid to say no?* Take a course in assertiveness training; get support from others who don't want to use drugs; remind yourself that you have the right and the responsibility to make your own decisions.
- *Still feeling peer pressure?* Begin to look for new friends or roommates. Take a class or join an organization that attracts other health-conscious people.

**Tips for Today**

The essence of wellness is taking charge of your life. Dependence on drugs or compulsive activities is the very opposite of wellness, because it involves relinquishing control over your life to chemical substances or forces outside yourself. The best treatment for dependence is prevention—not starting in the first place—but it's never too late to regain control of your life.

*Right now you can*

- Go outside and sit on a park bench, or walk around outside at half your normal pace, opening all your senses to the beauty of nature. If you can't get to a beautiful place, close your eyes and visualize one. See if you can experience a "natural high."
- Substitute some bottled water for your caffeinated soda, and make your next cup of coffee half decaf.
- Consider whether someone you love has a drug problem; if so, consider how you can best help that person face and solve the problem.
- Plan to get enough sleep this week, so you won't feel the need for stimulants to be awake and alert.
- Examine what you've been doing lately to see if you are truly making your own decisions—or if some substance or out-of-control behavior has you in its power; if so, start thinking about how to regain control.

## SUMMARY

- Addictive behaviors are reinforcing. Addicts experience a strong compulsion for the behavior and a loss of control over it; an escalating pattern of abuse with serious negative consequences may result.
- The sources or causes of addiction include heredity, personality, lifestyle, and environmental factors. People may use an addictive behavior as a means of alleviating stress or painful emotions.
- Many common behaviors are potentially addictive, including gambling, shopping, Internet use, eating, and working.
- Drug abuse is a maladaptive pattern of drug use that persists despite adverse social, psychological, or medical consequences.
- Drug dependence involves taking a drug compulsively, which includes neglecting constructive activities because of it and continuing to use it despite experiencing adverse effects resulting from its use. Tolerance and withdrawal symptoms are often present.
- The effect of a drug depends on the properties of the drug and how it's used (drug factors), the physical and psychological characteristics of the user (user factors), and the physical and social environment surrounding the drug use (social factors).
- Opioids relieve pain, cause drowsiness, and induce euphoria; they reduce anxiety and produce lethargy, apathy, and an inability to concentrate.
- CNS depressants slow down the overall activity of the nerves; they reduce anxiety and cause mood changes, impaired muscular coordination, slurring of speech, and drowsiness or sleep.
- CNS stimulants speed up the activity of the nerves, causing acceleration of the heart rate, a rise in blood pressure, dilation of the pupils and bronchial tubes, and an increase in gastric and adrenal secretions.
- Marijuana usually causes euphoria and a relaxed attitude at low doses; very high doses produce feelings of depersonalization and sensory distortion.
- Hallucinogens alter perception, feelings, and thought and may cause an altered sense of time, visual disturbances, and mood changes.
- Inhalants are present in a variety of harmless products. Their use can lead to loss of consciousness, heart failure, suffocation, and death.
- Economic and social costs of drug abuse include the financial costs of law enforcement, treatment, and health care and the social costs of crime, violence, and family problems.
- Approaches to treatment include medication, treatment centers, self-help groups, and peer counseling; many programs also offer counseling to family members.

## Take Action

1. **Research local addiction services:** Find out what types of services are available on your campus or in your community to handle drug dependence and other addictive behaviors. If there are none, what services are needed? Locate the school official and public health agency responsible for your campus and community, and ask why these needs aren't being met.

## Changing Your Drug Habits

Behavior Change Strategy

This behavior change strategy focuses on one of the most commonly used drugs—caffeine. If you are concerned about your use of a different drug or another type of addictive behavior, you can devise your own plan based on this one and on the steps outlined in Chapter 1.

Because caffeine supports certain behaviors that are characteristic of our culture, such as sedentary, stressful work, you may find yourself relying on coffee (or tea, chocolate, or cola) to get through a busy schedule. Such habits often begin in college. Fortunately, it's easier to break a habit before it becomes entrenched as a lifelong dependency.

When you are studying for exams, the forced physical inactivity and the need to concentrate even when fatigued may lead you to overuse caffeine. But caffeine doesn't help unless you are already sleepy. And it does not relieve any underlying condition (you are just more tired when it wears off). How can you change this pattern?

### Self-Monitoring

Keep a log of how much caffeine you eat or drink. Use a measuring cup to measure coffee or tea. Using Figure 7-2, convert the amounts you eat or drink into an estimate expressed in milligrams of caffeine. Be sure to include all forms, such as chocolate bars and OTC medications, as well as caffeine candy, colas, cocoa or hot chocolate, chocolate cake, tea, and coffee.

### Self-Assessment

At the end of the week, add up your daily totals and divide by 7 to get your daily average in milligrams. How much is too much? At more than 250 mg per day, you may well be experiencing some adverse symptoms. If you are experiencing at least five of the following symptoms, you may want to cut down: restlessness, nervousness, excitement, insomnia, flushed face, excessive sweating, gastrointestinal problems, muscle twitching, rambling thoughts and speech, irregular heartbeat, periods of inexhaustibility, and excessive pacing or movement.

### Set Limits

Can you restrict your caffeine intake to a daily total, and stick to this contract? If so, set a cutoff point, such as one cup of coffee. Pegging it to a specific time of day can be helpful, because then you won't confront a decision at any other point (and possibly fail). If you find you cannot stick to your limit, you may want to cut out caffeine altogether; abstinence can be easier than moderation for some people. If you experience caffeine withdrawal symptoms (headache, fatigue), you may want to cut your intake more gradually.

### Find Other Ways to Keep Up Your Energy

If you are fatigued, it makes sense to get enough sleep or exercise more, rather than drowning the problem in coffee or tea. Different people need different amounts of sleep; you may also need more sleep at different times, such as during a personal crisis or an illness. Also, exercise raises your metabolic rate for hours afterward—a handy fact to exploit when you want to feel more awake and want to avoid an irritable caffeine jag. And if you've been compounding your fatigue by not eating properly, try filling up on complex carbohydrates such as whole-grain bread or crackers instead of candy bars.

**Tips on Cutting Out Caffeine** Here are some more ways to decrease your consumption of caffeine:

- Keep some noncaffeinated drinks on hand, such as decaffeinated coffee, herbal teas, mineral water, bouillon, or hot water.
- Alternate between hot and very cold liquids.
- Fill your coffee cup only halfway.
- Avoid the office or school lunchroom or cafeteria and the chocolate sections of the grocery store. (Often people drink coffee or tea and eat chocolate simply because they're available.)
- Read labels of over-the-counter medications to check for hidden sources of caffeine.

2. **Survey attitudes:** Survey three older adults and three young students about their attitudes toward legalizing marijuana. Are there any differences? If so, what accounts for these differences? What kinds of reasons do they give for their positions?

3. **Analyze media portrayals:** Look at a current movie or television program, paying special attention to how drug use is portrayed. What messages are being conveyed? If possible, compare a recent movie with one made 10–20 years ago. Has the presentation of drug use changed? If so, how?

## For More Information

### Books

Booth, M. 2004. *Cannabis: A History*. New York: Thomas Dunne Books. *Provides historical information and covers current issues about marijuana from a variety of perspectives.*

Julien, R. M. 2004. *A Primer of Drug Action*, 10th ed. New York: Worth. *A guide to the actions, uses, and side effects of psychoactive drugs.*

Ray, O. S., and C. Ksir. 2006. *Drugs, Society, and Human Behavior*, 11th ed. New York: McGraw-Hill. *Examines drugs and behavior from the behavioral, pharmacological, historical, social, legal, and clinical perspectives.*

Roleff, T. L., and H. Cothran. 2004. *Drug Abuse: Opposing Viewpoints*. San Diego: Greenhaven Press. *Explores key issues relating to drug use and abuse.*

### Organizations, Hotlines, and Web Sites

*Center for On-Line Addiction*. Contains information about Internet and cybersex addiction.
http://netaddiction.com

*ClubDrugs.Org*. Provides information on drugs commonly classified as "club drugs."
http://www.clubdrugs.org

*Do It Now Foundation.* Provides youth-oriented information about drugs.
http://www.doitnow.org

*Drug Enforcement Administration: Drugs of Abuse.* Provides basic facts about major drugs of abuse, including penalties for drug trafficking.
http://www.dea.gov/concern/concern.htm

*Gamblers Anonymous.* Includes questions to help diagnose gambling problems and resources for getting help.
http://www.gamblersanonymous.org

*Higher Eduction Center for Alcohol and Other Drug Prevention.* Gives information about alcohol and drug abuse on campus and links to related sites.
http://www.edc.org/hec

*Indiana Prevention Resource Center.* A clearinghouse of information and links on substance-abuse topics, including specific psychoactive drugs and issues such as drug testing and drug legalization.
http://www.drugs.indiana.edu

*Narcotics Anonymous (NA).* Similar to Alcoholics Anonymous, NA sponsors 12-step meetings and provides other support services for drug abusers.
818-773-9999
http://www.na.org

There are also 12-step programs that focus on specific drugs:
Cocaine Anonymous
http://www.ca.org
Marijuana Anonymous
http://www.marijuana-anonymous.org

*National Center on Addiction and Substance Abuse (CASA) at Columbia University.* Provides information about the costs of substance abuse to individuals and society.
http://www.casacolumbia.org

*National Clearinghouse for Alcohol and Drug Information.* Provides statistics, information, and publications on substance abuse, including resources for people who want to help friends and family members overcome substance-abuse problems.
http://www.health.org

*National Drug Information, Treatment, and Referral Hotlines.* Sponsored by the SAMHSA Center for Substance Abuse Treatment, these hotlines provide information on drug abuse and on HIV infection as it relates to substance abuse; referrals to support groups and treatment programs are available.
800-662-HELP
800-729-6686 (Spanish)
800-487-4889 (TDD for hearing impaired)

*National Institute on Drug Abuse.* Develops and supports research on drug-abuse prevention programs; fact sheets on drugs of abuse are available on the Web site or via recorded phone messages, fax, or mail.
http://www.drugabuse.gov

See also the listings for Chapter 8.

## Selected Bibliography


American Psychiatric Association. 2001. *Diagnostic and Statistical Manual of Mental Disorders,* Fourth Edition, Text Revision. *(DSM-IV).* Washington, D.C.: American Psychiatric Association.

Budney, A. J., et al. 2004. Review of the validity and significance of cannabis withdrawal syndrome. *American Journal of Psychiatry* 161(11): 1967–1977.

Compton, W. M., et al. 2004. Prevalence of marijuana use disorder in the United States. *Journal of the American Medical Association* 291(17): 2114–2121.

Delaney-Black, V., et al. 2004. Prenatal cocaine: Quantity of exposure and gender moderation. *Journal of Developmental and Behavioral Pediatrics* 25(4): 254–263.

Engwall, D., R. Hunter, and M. Steinberg. 2004. Gambling and other risk behaviors on university campuses. *Journal of American College Health* 52(6): 245–255.

Herning, R. I., et al. 2005. Cerebrovascular perfusion in marijuana users during a month of monitored abstinence. *Neurology* 64(3): 488–493.

Hurd, Y. L., et al. 2005. Marijuana impairs growth in mid-gestation fetuses. *Neurotoxicology and Teratology* 27(2): 221–229.

Johnston, L. D., et al. 2004. *Monitoring the Future: National Survey Results on Drug Use, 1975–2003. Volume II: College Students and Adults Ages 19–45* (NIH Publication No. 04-5508). Bethesda, Md.: National Institute on Drug Abuse.

Juliano, L. M., and R. R. Griffiths. 2004. A critical review of caffeine withdrawal: Empirical validation of symptoms and signs, incidence, severity, and associated features. *Psychopharmacology* 176(1): 1–29.

Kish, S. J., et al. 2000. Striatal serotonin is depleted in brain of a human MDMA (ecstasy) user. *Neurology* 55(2): 294–296.

LaBrie, R. A., et al. 2003. Correlates of college student gambling in the United States. *Journal of American College Health* 52(2): 53–62.

McBride, B. F., et al. 2004. Electrocardiographic and hemodynamic effects of a multicomponent dietary supplement containing ephedra and caffeine. *Journal of the American Medical Association* 291(4): 216–221.

National Institute on Drug Abuse. 2004. *Inhalant Abuse: What Are the Medical Consequences of Inhalant Abuse?* (http://www.drugabuse.gov/ResearchReports/Inhalants/Inhalants4.html; retrieved December 6, 2004).

Parrott, A. C. 2005. Chronic tolerance to recreational MDMA (3,4-methylenedioxymethamphetamine) or ecstasy. *Journal of Psychopharmacology* 19(1): 71–83.

Ramaekers, J. G., et al. 2004. Dose-related risk of motor vehicle crashes after cannabis use. *Drug and Alcohol Dependence* 73(2): 109–119.

Savoca, M. R., et al. 2005. Association of ambulatory blood pressure and dietary caffeine in adolescents. *American Journal of Hypertension* 18(1): 116–120.

Singer, L. T., et al. 2004. Cognitive outcomes of preschool children with prenatal cocaine exposure. *Journal of the American Medical Association* 291(20): 2448–2456.

Solowij, N., et al. 2002. Cognitive functioning of long-term heavy cannabis users seeking treatment. *Journal of the American Medical Association* 287(9): 1123–1131.

Strote, J., J. E. Lee, and H. Wechsler. 2002. Increased MDMA use among college students: Results of a national survey. *Journal of Adolescent Health* 30: 64–72.

Substance Abuse and Mental Health Services Administration. 2005. Nonmedical oxycodone users: A comparison with heroin users. *The NSDUH Report,* January.

U.S. Drug Enforcement Agency. 2002. *DEA Drug Briefs: OxyContin* (http://www.dea.gov/concern/oxycodone.html; retrieved November 12, 2002).

Wareing, M., et al. 2005. Visuo-spatial working memory deficits in current and former users of MDMA ('ecstasy'). *Human Psychopharmacology* 20(2): 115–23.

World Health Organization. 2004. *Facts and Figures: Management of Substance Abuse* (http://www.who.int/substance_abuse/facts/en; retrieved September 15, 2004).

Zakzanis, K. K., and D. A. Young. 2001. Memory impairment in abstinent MDMA ("ecstasy") users: A longitudinal investigation. *Neurology* 56: 966–969.

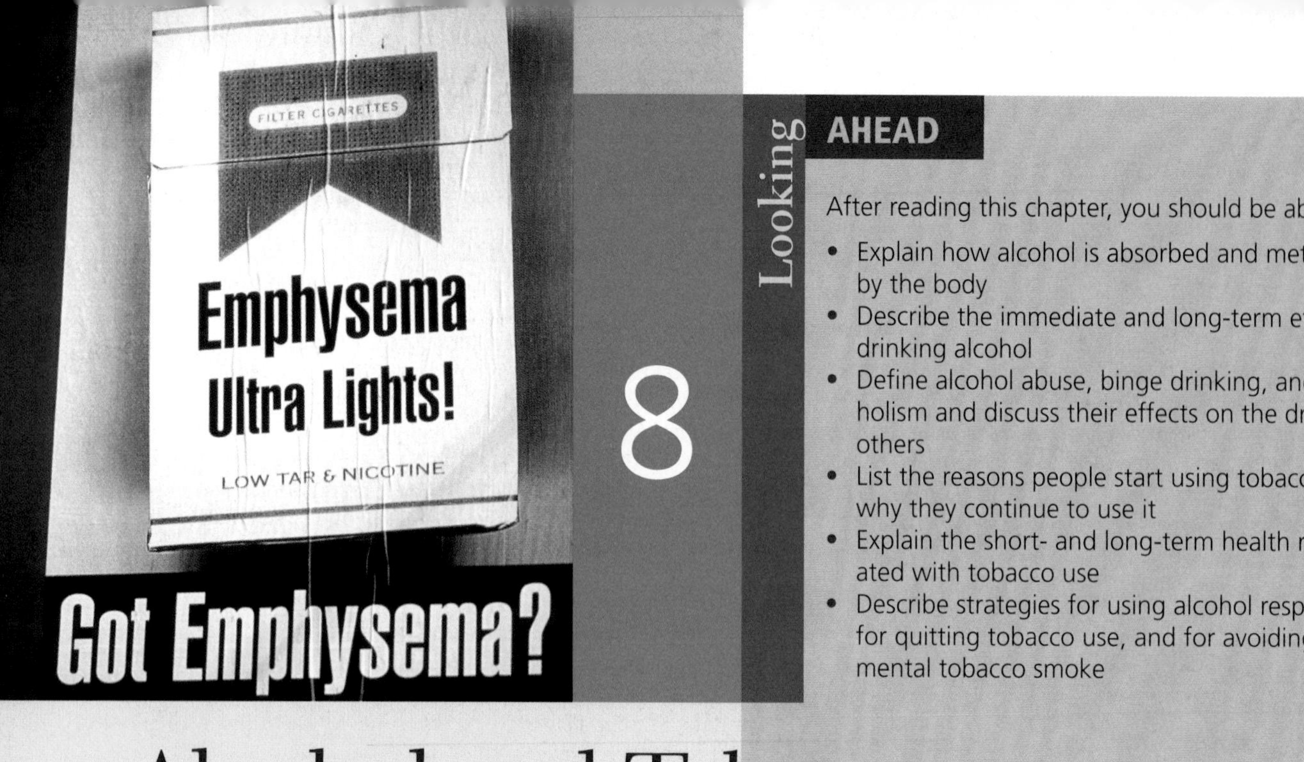


## Looking AHEAD

After reading this chapter, you should be able to

- Explain how alcohol is absorbed and metabolized by the body
- Describe the immediate and long-term effects of drinking alcohol
- Define alcohol abuse, binge drinking, and alcoholism and discuss their effects on the drinker and others
- List the reasons people start using tobacco and why they continue to use it
- Explain the short- and long-term health risks associated with tobacco use
- Describe strategies for using alcohol responsibly, for quitting tobacco use, and for avoiding environmental tobacco smoke

# 8 Alcohol and Tobacco

When we hear about the dangers of drugs, most of us think of illicit drugs such as marijuana, heroin, and ecstasy. Stories of violence and deaths related to the sale and use of illegal drugs often appear in the news. Less attention is given to the drugs that are actually responsible for the most injuries and deaths in the United States—**alcohol** and **tobacco.** Indeed, alcohol and tobacco are seldom even thought of as drugs. The truth is that both alcohol and **nicotine** (the psychoactive drug in tobacco) are powerful drugs that can have a devastating impact on wellness. Each year, alcohol use is responsible for about 85,000 deaths, and tobacco use, 435,000; smoking is the leading preventable cause of death in this country.

Many people think of alcohol the way it's portrayed in advertisements, on television, and in movies—as part of a good time, an integral ingredient of celebrations. However, like other drugs, alcohol can impair functioning in the short term and cause devastating damage in the long term. About half of American adults abstain from alcohol use or drink fewer than 12 drinks per year. About 22% are light or occasional drinkers, and about 29% are risky drinkers, meaning they occasionally or regularly drink excessively. Through automobile crashes and other injuries, alcohol is the leading cause of death among people age 15 to 24.

Although the proportion of cigarette smokers among Americans has dropped over the last four decades, tobacco use remains widespread, and nearly 1 in 4 adults smoke. Male and female smokers lose an average of 13.2 and 14.5 years of life, respectively. Nonsmokers subjected to the smoke of others also suffer. Exposure to **environmental tobacco smoke (ETS)** causes more than 60,000 deaths annually, and smoking by pregnant women is responsible for up to 10% of all infant deaths in this country.

Avoiding tobacco and using alcohol wisely, if at all, are important parts of a healthy lifestyle. This chapter explores the reasons people use alcohol and tobacco, how these drugs affect health, and how people can make healthy and responsible choices about the role of alcohol and tobacco in their lives.

## THE NATURE OF ALCOHOL

How does alcohol affect people? Does it affect some people differently than others? Can some people handle alcohol? Is it possible to drink a safe amount of alcohol? Many misconceptions about the effects of alcohol can be cleared up by taking a closer look at the chemistry of alcohol and how it is absorbed and metabolized by the body.

### The Chemistry of Alcohol

Ethyl alcohol is the psychoactive ingredient in all alcoholic beverages. Beer, a mild intoxicant brewed from a

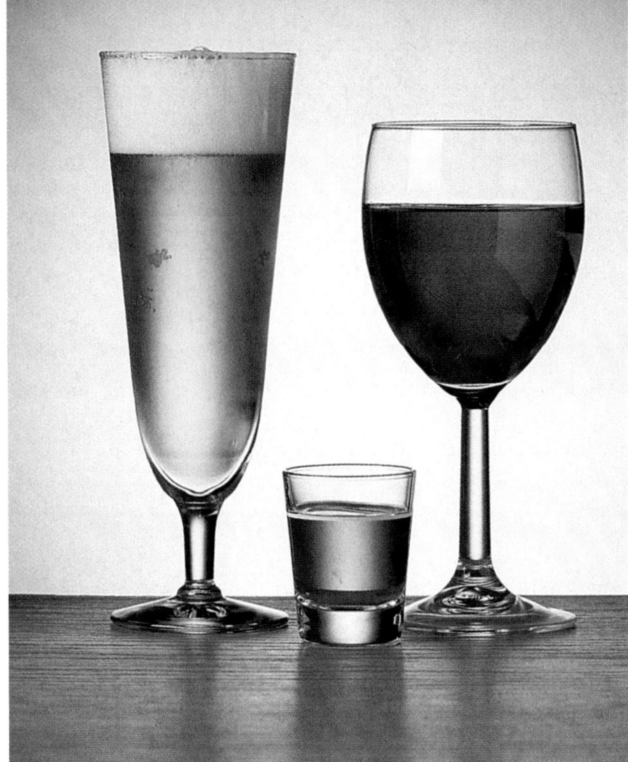

Ethyl alcohol is the common psychoactive drug found in all alcoholic beverages. One drink—a 12-ounce beer, a 1.5-ounce cocktail, or a 5-ounce glass of wine—contains about 0.5–0.6 ounce of ethyl alcohol.

mixture of grains, usually contains 3–6% alcohol by volume. Ales and malt liquors are 6–8% alcohol by volume. Wines are made by *fermenting* the juices of grapes or other fruits. The concentration of alcohol in table wines is about 9–14%. *Fortified wines,* so named because alcohol has been added to them, contain about 20% alcohol; these include sherry, port, and Madeira. Stronger alcoholic beverages, called *hard liquors,* are made by *distilling* brewed or fermented grains or other products. These beverages, including gin, whiskey, brandy, rum, tequila, vodka, and liqueurs, usually contain 35–50% alcohol.

The concentration of alcohol in a beverage is indicated by the **proof value,** which is two times the percentage concentration. For example, if a beverage is 100 proof, it contains 50% alcohol. Two ounces of 100-proof whiskey contain 1 ounce of pure alcohol. The proof value of hard liquors can usually be found on the bottle labels. When alcohol consumption is discussed, "one drink" refers to a 12-ounce bottle of beer, a 5-ounce glass of table wine, or a cocktail with 1.5 ounces of 80-proof liquor. Each of these different drinks contains approximately the same amount of alcohol: 0.5–0.6 ounce.

Alcohol provides 7 calories per gram, and the alcohol in one drink (14–17 grams) supplies about 100–120 calories. Most alcoholic beverages also contain some carbohydrate, so, for example, one beer provides about 150 total calories. The "light" in light beer refers to calories; a light beer typically has close to the same alcohol content as a regular beer and about two-thirds the calories. People who choose to drink alcohol should remember to count the calories in alcoholic beverages toward their total daily calorie intake to avoid unintentional weight gain.

## Absorption

When a person ingests alcohol, about 20% is rapidly absorbed from the stomach into the bloodstream. About 75% is absorbed through the upper part of the small intestine. Any remaining alcohol enters the bloodstream further along the gastrointestinal tract. Once in the bloodstream, alcohol produces feelings of intoxication. The rate of absorption is affected by a variety of factors. For example, the carbonation in a beverage like champagne increases the rate of alcohol absorption. Food in the stomach slows the rate of absorption, as does the drinking of highly concentrated alcoholic beverages such as hard liquor. But remember: *All* alcohol a person consumes is eventually absorbed.

## Metabolism and Excretion

Alcohol is quickly transported throughout the body by the blood. Because alcohol easily moves through most biological membranes, it is rapidly distributed throughout most body tissues. The main site of alcohol **metabolism** is the liver, though a small amount of alcohol is metabolized in the stomach. (See the box "Metabolizing Alcohol: Our Bodies Work Differently" on p. 166 for more information.) About 2–10% of ingested alcohol is not metabolized in the liver or other tissues but is excreted unchanged by the lungs, kidneys, and sweat glands. Excreted alcohol causes the telltale smell on a drinker's breath and is the basis of breath and urine analyses for alcohol levels.

### Terms

VW

**alcohol** The intoxicating ingredient in fermented liquors; a colorless, pungent liquid.

**tobacco** The leaves of cultivated tobacco plants prepared for smoking, chewing, or use as snuff.

**nicotine** A poisonous, addictive substance found in tobacco and responsible for many of the effects of tobacco.

**environmental tobacco smoke (ETS)** Smoke that enters the atmosphere from the burning end of a cigarette, cigar, or pipe, as well as smoke that is exhaled by smokers; also called *secondhand smoke.*

**proof value** Two times the percentage of alcohol by volume; a beverage that is 50% alcohol by volume is 100 proof.

**metabolism** The chemical transformation of food and other substances in the body into energy and wastes.

Dimensions of Diversity

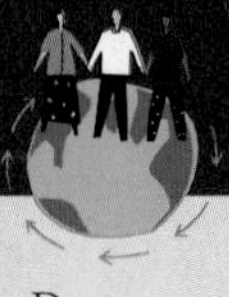

## Metabolizing Alcohol: Our Bodies Work Differently

Do you notice that you react differently to alcohol than some of your friends do? If so, you may be noticing genetic differences in alcohol metabolism that are associated with ethnicity. Alcohol is metabolized mainly in the liver, where it is broken down by an enzyme called alcohol dehydrogenase, producing a by-product called acetaldehyde (see the figure). Acetaldehyde is responsible for many of the unpleasant effects of alcohol abuse. Another enzyme, acetaldehyde dehydrogenase, breaks this product down further.

Some people, including many of Asian descent or of certain Jewish population groups, have genes that cause them to produce somewhat different forms of the two enzymes that metabolize alcohol. The result is high concentrations of acetaldehyde in the brain and other tissues, producing a host of unpleasant symptoms. When people with these enzymes drink alcohol, they experience a physiological reaction referred to as *flushing syndrome.* Their skin feels hot, their heart and respiration rates increase, and they may get a headache, vomit, or break out in hives. Drinking makes some people so uncomfortable that it's unlikely they could ever become addicted to alcohol.

The body's response to acetaldehyde is the basis for treating alcohol abuse with the drug disulfiram (Antabuse), which inhibits the action of acetaldehyde dehydrogenase. When a person taking disulfiram ingests alcohol, acetaldehyde levels increase rapidly, and he or she develops an intense flushing reaction along with weakness, nausea, vomiting, and other disagreeable symptoms.

How people behave in relation to alcohol is influenced in complex ways by many factors, including social and cultural ones. But in this case at least, individual choices and behavior are strongly influenced by a specific genetic characteristic.

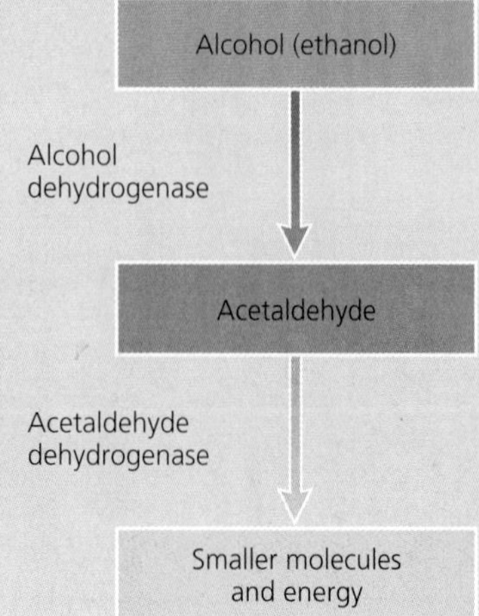


## Alcohol Intake and Blood Alcohol Concentration

**Blood alcohol concentration (BAC),** a measure of intoxication, is determined by the amount of alcohol consumed in a given amount of time and by individual factors:

- *Body weight:* In most cases, a smaller person develops a higher BAC than a larger person after drinking the same amount of alcohol. A smaller person has less overall body tissue into which alcohol can be distributed.
- *Percent body fat:* A person with a higher percentage of body fat will usually develop a higher BAC than a more muscular person of the same weight. Alcohol does not concentrate as much in fatty tissue as in muscle and most other tissues, in part because fat has fewer blood vessels.
- *Sex:* Women metabolize less alcohol in the stomach than men do because the stomach enzyme that breaks down alcohol before it enters the bloodstream is four times more active in men than in women. This means that more unmetabolized alcohol is released into the bloodstream in women. Because women are also generally smaller than men and have a higher percentage of body fat, women will have a higher BAC than men after consuming the same amount of alcohol. Hormonal fluctuations may also affect the rate of alcohol metabolism, making a woman more susceptible to high BACs at certain times during her menstrual cycle (usually just prior to the onset of menstruation).

BAC also depends on the balance between the rate of alcohol absorption and the rate of alcohol metabolism. A man who weighs 150 pounds and has normal liver function metabolizes about 0.3 ounce of alcohol per hour, the equivalent of about half a 12-ounce bottle of beer or a 5-ounce glass of wine. The rate of alcohol metabolism varies among individuals and is largely determined by genetic factors and drinking behavior. Contrary to popular myths, this metabolic rate *cannot* be influenced by exercise, breathing deeply, eating, drinking coffee, or taking other drugs. The rate of alcohol metabolism is the same whether a person is asleep or awake.

If a person absorbs slightly less alcohol each hour than he or she can metabolize in an hour, the BAC remains low. People can drink large amounts of alcohol this way over a long period of time without becoming noticeably intoxicated; however, they do run the risk of significant long-term health hazards (described later in the chapter). If a person is absorbing alcohol more quickly than it can be metabolized, the BAC will steadily increase, and he or she will become more and more drunk (Table 8-1). How fast you drink makes a big difference in how high your BAC will be. Consuming several drinks over a period of 2 or 3 hours is likely to cause intoxication, followed on the next day by a hangover; chugging the same amount of alcohol in an hour or less could be lethal.

**Table 8-1 The Effects of Alcohol**

| BAC (%) | Common Behavioral Effects | Hours Required to Metabolize Alcohol |
|---|---|---|
| 0.00–0.05 | Slight change in feelings, usually relaxation and euphoria. Decreased alertness. | 2–3 |
| 0.05–0.10 | Emotional instability, with exaggerated feelings and behavior. Reduced social inhibitions. Impairment of reaction time and fine motor coordination. Increasingly impaired during driving. Legally drunk at 0.08%. | 3–6 |
| 0.10–0.15 | Unsteadiness in standing and walking. Loss of peripheral vision. Driving is extremely dangerous. | 6–10 |
| 0.15–0.30 | Staggering gait. Slurred speech. Pain and other sensory perceptions greatly impaired. | 10–24 |
| More than 0.30 | Stupor or unconsciousness. Anesthesia. Death possible at 0.35% and above. Can result from rapid or binge drinking with few earlier effects. | More than 24 |

## ALCOHOL AND HEALTH

The effects of alcohol consumption on health depend on the individual, the circumstances, and the amount of alcohol consumed.

### The Immediate Effects of Alcohol

BAC is a primary factor determining the effects of alcohol (see Table 8-1). At low concentrations, alcohol tends to make people feel relaxed and jovial, but at higher concentrations people are more likely to feel angry, sedated, or sleepy. Alcohol is a CNS depressant, and its effects vary because body systems are affected to different degrees at different BACs. At any given BAC, the effects of alcohol are more pronounced when the BAC is rapidly increasing than when it is slowly increasing, steady, or decreasing. The effects of alcohol are more pronounced if a person drinks on an empty stomach, because alcohol is absorbed more quickly and the BAC rises more quickly.

**Low Concentrations of Alcohol** The effects of alcohol can first be felt at a BAC of about 0.03–0.05%. These effects may include light-headedness, relaxation, and a release of inhibitions. Most drinkers experience mild euphoria and become more sociable. When people drink in social settings, alcohol often seems to act as a stimulant, enhancing conviviality or assertiveness. This apparent stimulation occurs because alcohol depresses inhibitory centers in the brain.

**Higher Concentrations of Alcohol** At higher concentrations, the pleasant effects tend to be replaced by more negative ones: interference with motor coordination, verbal performance, and intellectual functions. The drinker often becomes irritable and may be easily angered or given to crying. When the BAC reaches 0.1%, most sensory and motor functioning is reduced, and many people become sleepy. Vision, smell, taste, and hearing become less acute. At 0.2%, most drinkers are completely unable to function, either physically or psychologically, because of the pronounced depression of the central nervous system, muscles, and other body systems. Coma usually occurs at a BAC of 0.35%, and any higher level can be fatal.

Alcohol causes flushing and sweating, which lower body temperature. Alcohol use also disturbs normal sleep patterns.

**Alcohol Hangover** Despite all the jokes about hangovers, anyone who has experienced a severe hangover knows they are no laughing matter. The symptoms include headache, shakiness, nausea, diarrhea, fatigue, and impaired mental functioning. During a hangover, heart rate and blood pressure increase, making some individuals more vulnerable to heart attacks. Brain wave measurement shows diffuse slowing of brain waves for up to 16 hours after BAC drops to zero. Studies of pilots, drivers, and skiers all indicate that coordination and cognition are impaired in a person with a hangover, increasing the risk of injury.

The best treatment for hangover is prevention. Nearly all men can expect a hangover if they drink more than 5 or 6 drinks; for women, the number is 3 or 4. Drinking less, drinking more slowly, and consuming nonalcoholic liquids decrease the risk of hangover. If you do get a

**Term**

**blood alcohol concentration (BAC)** The amount of alcohol in the blood in terms of weight per unit volume; used as a measurement of intoxication.

VW

Take Charge

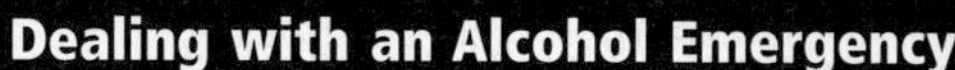

## Dealing with an Alcohol Emergency

Remember: Being very drunk is potentially life-threatening. Helping a drunken friend could save a life.

- Be firm but calm. Don't engage the person in an argument or discuss her drinking behavior while she is intoxicated.
- Get the person out of harm's way—don't let her drive or wander outside. Don't let her drink any more alcohol.
- If the person is unconscious, don't assume she is just "sleeping it off." Place her on her side with her knees up. This position will help prevent choking if the person should vomit.
- Stay with the person—you need to be ready to help if she vomits or stops breathing.
- Don't try to give the person anything to eat or drink, including coffee or other drugs. Don't give cold showers or try to make her walk around. None of these things help anyone to sober up, and they can be dangerous.

Call 911 immediately in any of the following instances:

- You can't wake the person even with shouting or shaking.
- The person is taking fewer than 8 breaths per minute or her breathing seems shallow or irregular.
- You think the person took other drugs in addition to alcohol.
- The person has had an injury, especially a blow to the head.
- The person drank a large amount of alcohol within a short period of time and then became unconscious. Death caused by alcohol poisoning most often occurs when the blood alcohol level rises very quickly due to rapid ingestion of alcohol.

If you aren't sure what to do, call 911. You may save a life.

hangover, remember that your ability to drive is definitely impaired, even after your BAC has returned to zero.

**Alcohol Poisoning** Drinking large amounts of alcohol over a short period of time can rapidly raise the BAC into the lethal range. A common scenario for alcohol poisoning is that inexperienced drinkers try to outdo each other by consuming glass after glass of alcohol as rapidly as possible. Death from alcohol poisoning may be caused either by central nervous system and respiratory depression or by inhaling fluid or vomit into the lungs. The amount of alcohol it takes to make a person unconscious is dangerously close to a fatal dose. Special care should be taken to ensure the safety of anyone who has been drinking heavily, especially if the person becomes unconscious (see the box "Dealing with an Alcohol Emergency"). Children are at high risk from unintentional alcohol poisoning.

**Using Alcohol with Other Drugs** Alcohol-drug combinations are the number-one cause of drug-related deaths in this country. Using alcohol while taking any other drug that can cause CNS depression increases the effects of both drugs, potentially leading to coma, respiratory depression, and death. Examples of common drugs that can result in oversedation when combined with alcohol include barbiturates, Valium-like drugs, narcotics such as codeine, and OTC antihistamines such as Benadryl. For people who consume three or more drinks per day, use of OTC pain relievers like aspirin, ibuprofen, or acetaminophen increases the risk of stomach bleeding or liver damage. Some antibiotics and diabetes medications can also interact dangerously with alcohol. Many illegal drugs are especially dangerous when combined with alcohol. Life-threatening overdoses occur at much lower doses when heroin and other narcotics are combined with alcohol.

The safest strategy is to not combine alcohol with any other drug—prescription, over-the-counter, or illegal. If in doubt, ask your pharmacist or physician before using any drug in combination with alcohol, or just don't do it.

**Alcohol-Related Injuries and Violence** The combination of impaired judgment, weakened sensory perception, reduced inhibitions, impaired motor coordination, and, often, increased aggressiveness and hostility that characterizes alcohol intoxication can be dangerous or even deadly. Through homicide, suicide, automobile crashes, and other incidents, alcohol kills over 75,000 Americans each year. Alcohol use contributes to over 50% of all murders, assaults, and rapes, and alcohol is frequently found in the bloodstream of both perpetrators and victims. Nearly 80% of people who attempt suicide have been drinking, and about half of all successful suicides are alcoholics. Alcohol use more than triples the chances of fatal injuries during leisure activities such as swimming and boating, and more than half of all fatal falls and serious burns happen to people who have been drinking. Being drunk is clearly hazardous to your health.

**Alcohol and Sexual Decision Making** Alcohol seriously affects a person's ability to make wise decisions about sex. Heavy drinkers are more likely to engage in unplanned sexual activity; to have unprotected sex; to have multiple sex partners; and to engage in other forms of high-risk sexual behavior. Rates of sexually transmitted diseases and unwanted pregnancy are higher among people who drink heavily than among people who drink moderately or not at all.

Women who binge-drink are at increased risk for rape and other forms of nonconsensual sex. The laws regarding sexual consent are clear: A person who is very drunk or passed out cannot consent to sex. If you have sex with a person who is drunk or unconscious, you are committing sexual assault. Claiming that you were drunk at the time won't absolve you of your legal and moral responsibility for this serious crime.

## Drinking and Driving

Every year, more than 800,000 people are injured in alcohol-related automobile crashes—an average of *1 person every 40 seconds*. About 40% of the more than 44,000 crash fatalities in 2003 were alcohol-related. Even low doses of alcohol increase the risk of automobile crashes, but as the dose increases, the risk goes up at a spectacular rate (Figure 8-1). Still, in surveys, more than one in four of U.S. drivers admit to having used alcohol or another drug within 2 hours before driving a vehicle.

In addition to an increased risk of injury and death, driving while intoxicated can have serious legal consequences. Drunk driving is against the law. In 2005, the legal limit for BAC was 0.08% in all states and the District of Columbia. Under current zero-tolerance laws in many states, drivers under age 21 who have consumed *any* alcohol may have their licenses suspended. There are stiff penalties for drunk driving, including fines, loss of license, confiscation of vehicle, and jail time.

People who drink and drive are unable to drive safely because their judgment is impaired, their reaction time is slower, and their coordination is reduced. The number of drinks it takes the average person to reach various BACs is shown in Figure 8-2. However, any amount of alcohol impairs your ability to drive safely, and fatigue augments alcohol's effects. If you are out of your home and drinking, find an alternative means of transportation or follow the practice of having a *designated driver*, an individual who refrains from drinking in order to provide safe transportation home for others in the group.

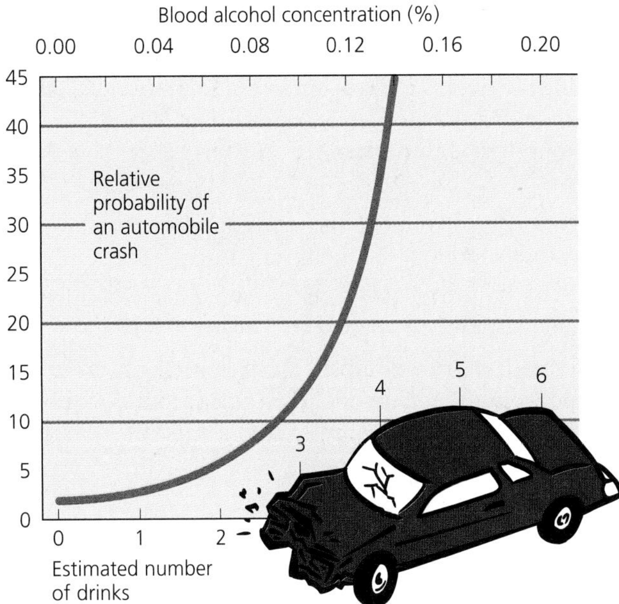


**Figure 8-1 The dose-response relationship between BAC and automobile crashes.**

It's more difficult to protect yourself against someone else who drinks and drives. Learn to be alert to the erratic driving that signals an impaired driver. Warning signs include wide, abrupt, and illegal turns; straddling the center line or lane marker; driving on the shoulder; weaving, swerving, or nearly striking an object or another vehicle; following too closely; erratic speed; driving with headlights off at night; and driving with the window down in very cold weather. If you see any of these signs, try the following strategies:

- If the driver is ahead of you, maintain a safe following distance. Don't try to pass.

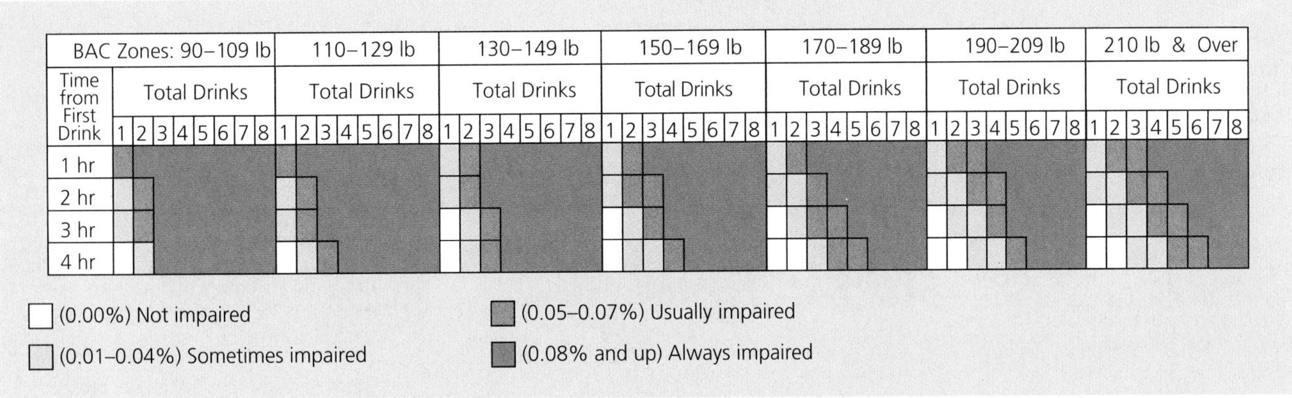


**Figure 8-2 Approximate blood alcohol concentration and body weight.** This chart illustrates the BAC an average person of a given weight would reach after drinking the specified number of drinks in the time shown. The legal limit for BAC is 0.08%; for drivers under 21 years of age, many states have zero-tolerance laws that set BAC limits of 0.01% or 0.02%.

- If the driver is behind you, turn right at the nearest intersection, and let the driver pass.
- If the driver is approaching your car, move to the shoulder and stop. Avoid a head-on collision by sounding your horn or flashing your lights.
- When approaching an intersection, slow down and stay alert for vehicles that don't appear to be slowing in preparation for stopping at a stop sign or red light.
- Make sure your safety belt is fastened and children are in approved safety seats.
- Report suspected impaired drivers to the nearest police station by phone. Give a description of the vehicle, license number, location, and direction the vehicle is headed.

## The Effects of Chronic Use

Because alcohol is distributed throughout most of the body, it can affect many different organs and tissues (Figure 8-3).

**The Digestive System** Even in relatively small amounts, alcohol can alter the normal functioning of the liver. Within just a few days of heavy alcohol consumption, fat begins to accumulate in liver cells, resulting in the development of "fatty liver." If drinking continues, inflammation of the liver can occur, resulting in alcoholic hepatitis. With continued alcohol use, however, liver cells are progressively damaged and then permanently destroyed. The destroyed cells are replaced by fibrous scar tissue, a condition known as **cirrhosis.** Alcohol-precipitated cirrhosis is the twelfth leading cause of death in the United States.

Alcohol can inflame the pancreas, causing nausea, vomiting, abnormal digestion, and severe pain. Unlike cirrhosis, which usually occurs after years of fairly heavy alcohol use, pancreatitis can occur after just one or two severe binge-drinking episodes. Acute pancreatitis is often fatal and can also develop into a chronic condition. Overuse of alcohol is also a common cause of bleeding in the gastrointestinal tract.

**The Cardiovascular System** The effects of alcohol on the cardiovascular system depend on the amount of alcohol consumed. Moderate doses of alcohol—less than one drink a day for women and two drinks a day for men—may reduce the risk of heart disease and heart attack in some

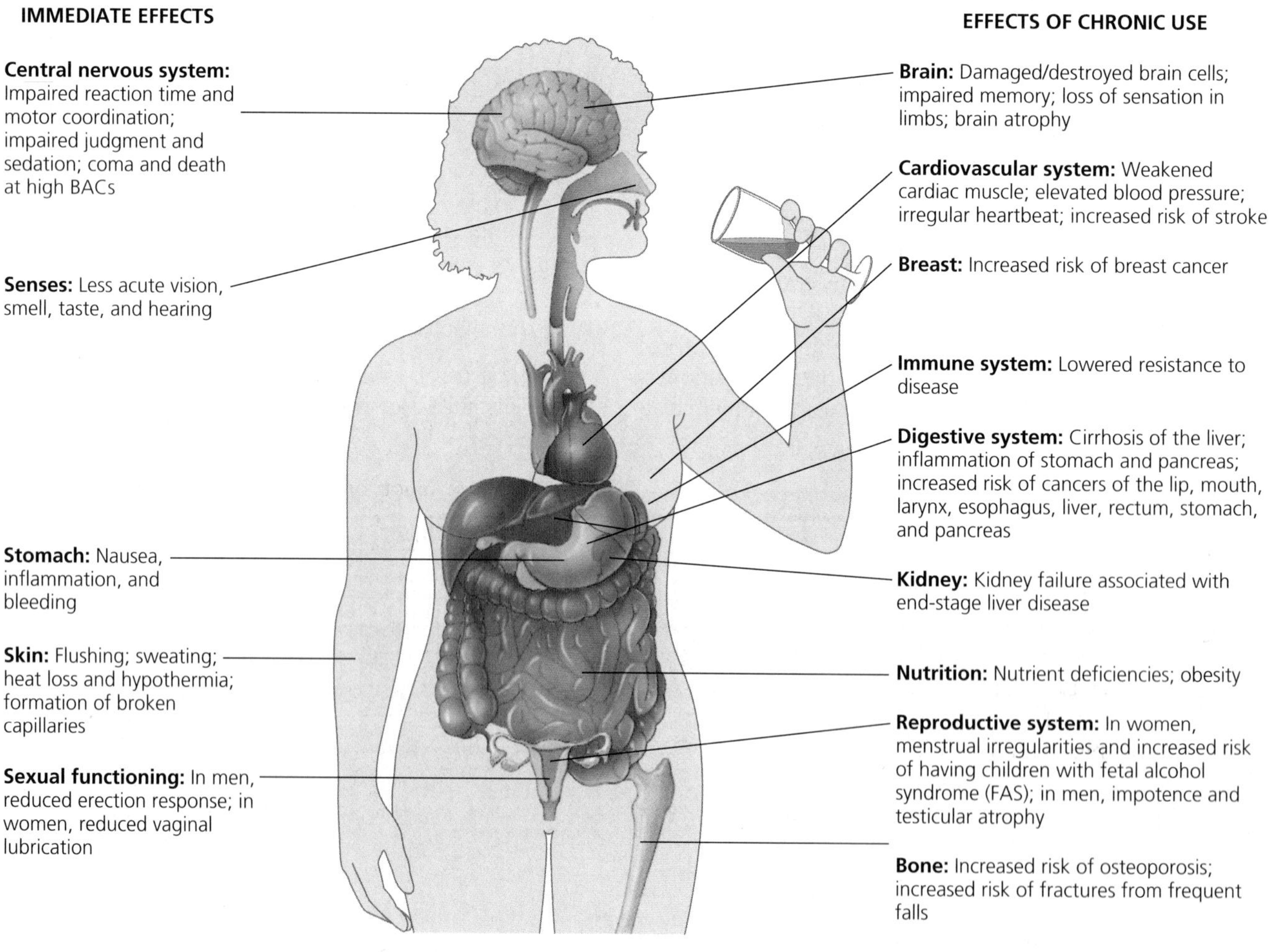

**Figure 8-3 The immediate and long-term effects of alcohol use.**

people. However, higher doses of alcohol have harmful effects on the cardiovascular system. In some people, more than two drinks a day will elevate blood pressure, making stroke and heart attack more likely. Some alcoholics show a weakening of the heart muscle, a condition known as **cardiac myopathy.** Binge drinking can cause "holiday heart," a syndrome characterized by serious abnormal heart rhythms, which usually appear within 24 hours of a binge episode.

**Cancer** Alcoholics have a cancer rate about ten times higher than that of the general population. They are particularly vulnerable to cancers of the throat, larynx, esophagus, upper stomach, liver, and pancreas. Drinking three or more alcoholic beverages per day doubles a woman's risk of developing breast cancer. Some studies have linked even moderate drinking to increased risk for cancers of the breast, mouth, throat, and esophagus. The U.S. Department of Health and Human Services classifies alcoholic beverages as known human carcinogens.

**Brain Damage** Heavy social drinkers and alcoholics show evidence of brain damage. Men who have 100 or more drinks per month and women who have 80 or more drinks per month experience impairment of memory, processing speed, attention, and balance. Brain shrinkage has also been found among heavy drinkers; slight reduction in brain volume has been seen even in moderate drinkers, although it is unclear whether this indicates the death of nerve cells.

**Mortality** As an ancient proverb states, "Those who worship Bacchus [the god of wine] die young." Excessive alcohol consumption is a factor in six of the ten leading causes of death for Americans. Average life expectancy among alcoholics is about 58 years; heavy drinkers may die in their 20s or 30s. About half the deaths caused by alcohol are due to chronic conditions such as cirrhosis and cancer; the other half are due to acute conditions or events such as car crashes, falls, and suicide.

## The Effects of Alcohol Use During Pregnancy

Alcohol ingested during pregnancy is harmful to the developing fetus. The damage depends on the stage of pregnancy and the amount of alcohol consumed. Alcohol use in early pregnancy can cause a miscarriage. Getting drunk just one time during the final 3 months of pregnancy, when brain cells are developing rapidly, can cause fetal brain damage. Moderate to heavy alcohol use can cause a collection of birth defects known as **fetal alcohol syndrome (FAS).** Children with FAS have a characteristic mixture of deformities that include a small head, abnormal facial structure, heart defects, and other physical abnormalities; most are mentally impaired, and their physical and mental growth is slower than normal.

FAS is a permanent, incurable condition that causes lifelong disability; it is by far the most common preventable cause of mental retardation in the Western world. Full-blown FAS occurs in 1 or 2 out of every 1000 live births in the United States. Many more babies are born with **alcohol-related neurodevelopmental disorder (ARND).** Children with ARND appear physically normal but often have significant learning and behavioral disorders.

No one is sure exactly how much alcohol use is required to cause FAS, but no amount of alcohol during pregnancy is considered safe. The adverse effects of alcohol are especially pronounced when women drink early in pregnancy. For this reason, women who are trying to conceive or who are sexually active without using effective contraception should abstain from alcohol in order to avoid inadvertently harming their fetus even before they know they are pregnant. Experts agree that the safest course of action is complete abstinence from alcohol during pregnancy.

Any alcohol consumed by a nursing mother quickly enters the breast milk. What impact this has on the child or on the mother's milk production is a matter of controversy. However, many physicians advise nursing mothers to abstain from drinking alcohol because of the belief that any amount may have negative effects on the baby's brain development.

## Possible Health Benefits of Alcohol

Numerous studies have shown that, on average, light to moderate drinkers live longer than either abstainers or heavy drinkers. But although moderate alcohol consumption may provide some health benefits for a given individual, for many people the dangers of alcohol are much greater than the potential benefits. A recent large-scale study found that the risks and benefits of drinking alcohol vary considerably with the age of the drinker. If you are 35 or younger, your odds of dying *increase* in direct proportion to the amount of alcohol you drink. Among people under age 35, even light drinkers have slightly higher mortality rates than nondrinkers. In other words, young adults who drink *any* amount of alcohol are more likely to die than nondrinkers of the same age. Alcohol consumption

### Terms

VW

**cirrhosis** A disease in which the liver is severely damaged by alcohol, other toxins, or infection.

**cardiac myopathy** Weakening of the heart muscle through disease.

**fetal alcohol syndrome (FAS)** A characteristic group of birth defects caused by excessive alcohol consumption by the mother, including facial deformities, heart defects, and physical and mental impairments.

**alcohol-related neurodevelopmental disorder (ARND)** Cognitive and behavioral problems seen in people whose mothers drank alcohol during pregnancy.

appears to confer health benefits primarily to older individuals, with the greatest benefits seen in people age 65 and older. Moderate drinking may also benefit people who currently have or are at high risk for certain diseases such as coronary heart disease or diabetes.

Moderate drinking is not without risk, however. It increases the risk of dying from unintentional injuries, violence, and certain types of cancer. In women, even moderate drinking may increase the risk of breast cancer. There is also a risk that moderate drinking will not stay moderate. People who avoid alcohol because they or family members have had problems with dependence in the past should not start drinking for their health. People with conditions such as depression that are worsened by alcohol use should probably avoid even moderate drinking. Nor should drinkers use this information as an excuse to overindulge; any health benefits of alcohol are negated by heavy use. In addition, there are many situations in which consuming any amount of alcohol is unwise, including during pregnancy, while taking medication that may interact with alcohol, and when driving or engaging in another activity that requires attention, skill, or coordination.

The bottom line is that limited, regular consumption of alcohol may be beneficial for some adults, but there is a narrow window of benefit, and excessive drinking causes serious health problems. If you drink alcoholic beverages, you should do it in moderation, with meals, at times when consumption does not put you or others at risk. Moderate drinking means no more than one drink a day for women and two drinks a day for men.

## ALCOHOL ABUSE AND DEPENDENCE

Abuse of and dependence on alcohol affect more than just the drinker. Friends, family members, coworkers, strangers that drinkers encounter on the road, and society as a whole pay the physical, emotional, and financial costs of the misuse of alcohol.

### Alcohol Abuse

As explained in Chapter 7, the APA's *Diagnostic and Statistical Manual of Mental Disorders* makes a distinction between substance abuse and substance dependence. **Alcohol abuse** is recurrent alcohol use that has negative consequences, such as drinking in dangerous situations (before driving, for instance), or drinking patterns that result in academic, professional, interpersonal, or legal difficulties. **Alcohol dependence,** or **alcoholism,** involves more extensive problems with alcohol use, usually involving physical tolerance and withdrawal. Alcoholism is discussed in greater detail later in the chapter.

Other authorities use different definitions to describe problems associated with drinking. The important point is that one does not have to be an alcoholic to have problems with alcohol. The person who drinks only once a month, perhaps after an exam, but then drives while intoxicated is an alcohol abuser.

How can you tell if you are beginning to abuse alcohol or if someone you know is doing so? Look for the following warning signs:

- Drinking alone or secretively
- Using alcohol deliberately and repeatedly to perform or get through difficult situations
- Feeling uncomfortable on certain occasions when alcohol is not available
- Escalating alcohol consumption beyond an already established drinking pattern
- Consuming alcohol heavily in risky situations, such as before driving
- Getting drunk regularly or more frequently than in the past
- Drinking in the morning or at other unusual times

### Binge Drinking

As a group, college students spend more money on alcohol than on textbooks and all nonalcoholic beverages combined. A common form of alcohol abuse on college campuses is **binge drinking.** In surveys of students on over 100 college campuses, 44% reported binge drinking, defined as having five drinks in a row for men or four in a row for women on at least one occasion in the 2 weeks prior to the survey. Some 23% of all students were found to be frequent binge drinkers, defined as having at least three binges during the 2-week period. Students living at fraternity houses had the highest rate of binge drinking, up to 80%. Men were more likely to binge than women, and white students had higher rates of binge drinking than students of other ethnicities. Nineteen percent of students (about 1 in 5) abstained from alcohol.

Binge drinking has a profound effect on students' lives. Frequent binge drinkers were found to be three to seven times more likely than non–binge drinkers to engage in unplanned or unprotected sex, to drive after drinking, and to get hurt or injured (see Table 8-2). Binge drinkers were also more likely to miss classes, get behind in schoolwork, and argue with friends. The more frequent the binges, the more problems the students encountered. Despite their experiences, fewer than 1% of the binge drinkers identified themselves as problem drinkers.

Binge drinking kills dozens of American college students each year. Some die from acute alcohol poisoning. The typical scenario involves a hazing ritual, a competition, or a bet that involves drinking a large amount of alcohol very quickly. This kind of fast, heavy drinking can result in unconsciousness and death very quickly, before anyone realizes that something is seriously wrong. Many other students die from alcohol-related injuries, including those from motor vehicle crashes.

VITAL STATISTICS

**Table 8-2 The Effects of Binge Drinking on College Students**

| Alcohol-Related Problem | Percentage of Students Experiencing Problems: Non–Binge Drinkers | Percentage of Students Experiencing Problems: Frequent Binge Drinkers |
|---|---|---|
| Drove after drinking alcohol | 18 | 58 |
| Did something they regretted | 17 | 62 |
| Argued with friends | 10 | 43 |
| Engaged in unplanned sex | 9 | 41 |
| Missed a class | 9 | 60 |
| Got behind in schoolwork | 9 | 42 |
| Had unprotected sex | 4 | 21 |
| Got hurt or injured | 4 | 28 |
| Got into trouble with police | 2 | 14 |
| Had five or more of these problems since school year began | 4 | 48 |

SOURCE: Wechsler, H., and B. Wuethrich. 2002. *Dying to Drink: Confronting Binge Drinking on College Campuses.* Emmaus, Pa.: Rodale.

Binge drinking also affects nonbingeing students. At schools with high rates of binge drinking, the nonbingers were up to twice as likely to report being bothered by the alcohol-related behaviors of others than were students at schools with lower rates of binge drinking. These problems included having sleep or studying disrupted; having to take care of a drunken student; being insulted or humiliated; experiencing unwanted sexual advances; and being pushed, hit, or assaulted (see the box "College Binge Drinking").

## Alcoholism

As mentioned earlier, alcoholism, or alcohol dependence, is usually characterized by tolerance to alcohol and withdrawal symptoms. Everyone who drinks—even nonalcoholics—develops tolerance after repeated alcohol use. As described in Chapter 7, *tolerance* means that a drinker needs more alcohol to achieve intoxication or the desired effect, that the effects of continued use of the same amount of alcohol are diminished, or that the drinker can function adequately at doses or a BAC that would produce significant impairment in a casual user. Heavy users of alcohol may need to consume about 50% more than they originally needed in order to experience the same degree of intoxication.

Withdrawal occurs when someone who has been using alcohol heavily for several days or more suddenly stops drinking or markedly reduces intake. Symptoms of withdrawal include trembling and nervousness and sometimes even hallucinations and seizures.

**Patterns and Prevalence** Alcoholism occurs among people of all ethnic groups and at all socioeconomic levels. There are different patterns of alcohol dependence, including these four common ones: (1) Regular daily intake of large amounts, (2) Regular heavy drinking limited to weekends, (3) Long periods of sobriety interspersed with binges of daily heavy drinking lasting for weeks or months, (4) Heavy drinking limited to periods of stress. Once established, alcoholism often exhibits a pattern of exacerbations and remissions. Alcoholism is not hopeless, however; many alcoholics do achieve permanent abstinence.

According to the National Survey on Drug Use and Health, about 16.1 million Americans are heavy drinkers and 54 million are binge drinkers. Studies suggest that the lifetime risk of alcoholism in the United States is about 10% for men and about 3% for women.

**Health Effects** Tolerance and withdrawal can have a serious impact on health. Symptoms of withdrawal include trembling hands (shakes or jitters), a rapid pulse and accelerated breathing rate, insomnia, nightmares, anxiety, and gastrointestinal upset. These symptoms usually begin 5–10 hours after alcohol intake is decreased and improve after 4–5 days; occasionally anxiety, insomnia, and other symptoms persist for 6 months or more.

More severe withdrawal symptoms occur in about 5% of alcoholics. These include seizures (sometimes called rum fits), confusion, and hallucinations. Still less common is **DTs (delirium tremens),** a medical emergency characterized by severe disorientation, confusion, epileptic-like seizures, and vivid hallucinations, often of vermin. The mortality rate from DTs can be as high as 15%.

Alcoholics face all the health risks associated with intoxication and chronic drinking described earlier in the chapter. Some of the damage is compounded by nutritional

### Terms

**alcohol abuse** The use of alcohol to a degree that causes physical damage, impairs functioning, or results in behavior harmful to others.

**alcohol dependence** A pathological use of alcohol or impairment in functioning due to alcohol; characterized by tolerance and withdrawal symptoms; alcoholism.

**alcoholism** A chronic psychological disorder characterized by excessive and compulsive drinking.

**binge drinking** Periodically drinking alcohol to the point of severe intoxication.

**DTs (delirium tremens)** A state of confusion brought on by the reduction of alcohol intake in an alcohol-dependent person; other symptoms are sweating, trembling, anxiety, hallucinations, and seizures.

In the News

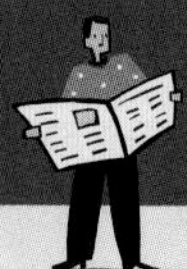

## College Binge Drinking

An estimated 1700 college students age 18–24 die from alcohol-related injuries and alcohol overdoses each year. To many people, heavy drinking is considered a normal and integral part of college life. But research has shown that the pattern of excessive binge drinking common on many of today's college campuses has had a devastating impact on far too many students, as well as on their families and communities.

What are some of the facts about college drinking? A recent survey of 14,000 students at U.S. 4-year colleges found that 31% of college students meet the medical criteria for a diagnosis of alcohol abuse and 6% for a diagnosis of alcohol dependence. Alcohol use and abuse are linked to many serious problems on campus; the annual toll includes the following:

- A total of 500,000 students between 18 and 24 are unintentionally injured in alcohol-related incidents (motor vehicle crashes, fights, falls, and so on).
- More than 600,000 students are assaulted by another student who has been drinking.
- More than 70,000 students are victims of alcohol-related sexual assault, including date rape. Nearly 75% of female rape victims were raped while intoxicated.
- Hundreds of thousands of students engage in unsafe sex while intoxicated, resulting in dramatically increased risk for STDs and unwanted pregnancy.
- As many as 2.1 million students drive while under the influence of alcohol.
- About 1.2–1.5% of college students attempt suicide because of drinking or drug use.

Heavy alcohol use detracts from the college experience of drinkers and nondrinkers alike. The National Advisory Council Task Force on Alcohol Abuse and Alcoholism calls for an overhaul of the campus drinking culture. Unfortunately, drinking to excess has been a college tradition for decades. Changing long-entrenched campus drinking habits will require effort on the part of students, college administrators, parents, and communities alike. According to the Task Force, changes must occur on three levels:

1. Ultimately, *individual students* must take responsibility for their own behavior. Students who enter college as nonbingers should be supported, and treatment should be readily available to problem drinkers. Groups at special risk for increasing or established problem drinking behavior include first-year students, Greek organization members, and athletes.

2. The *student body as a whole* must work to discourage alcohol abuse. This effort might include promoting alcohol-free activities for students, reducing the availability of alcohol, and avoiding the social and commercial promotion of alcohol on campus. Fraternities and sororities must be involved in these changes, as the most serious binge drinking tends to occur among their members. The Greek system must substitute genuine camaraderie for alcohol-saturated events.

3. *Colleges and surrounding communities* must cooperate to discourage excessive drinking. Laws that prohibit excessive and underage drinking must be fairly enforced. Students who commit crimes while under the influence must receive appropriate punishment, including restitution to any victims. College administrators must find other funding sources to replace the financial support that currently flows in from the alcohol industry in exchange for advertising and promotion of their products on college campuses.

SOURCES: Hingson, R., et al. 2005. Magnitude of alcohol-related mortality and morbidity among U.S. college students ages 18–24. *Annual Review of Public Health* 26: 259–279; Mohler-Kuo, M., et al. 2004. Correlates of rape while intoxicated in a national sample of college women. *Journal of Studies on Alcohol* 65(1): 37–45; Wechsler, H., and B. Wuethrich. 2002. *Dying to Drink: Confronting Binge Drinking on College Campuses.* Emmaus, Pa.: Rodale; National Institute on Alcohol Abuse and Alcoholism. 2002. *A Call to Action: Changing the Culture of Drinking at U.S. Colleges* (http://www.collegedrinkingprevention.gov/Reports/TaskForce/TaskForce_TOC.aspx; retrieved October 10, 2002).

deficiencies that often accompany alcoholism. A mental problem associated with alcohol use is profound memory gaps (blackouts).

**Social and Psychological Effects** Alcohol use causes more serious social and psychological problems than all other forms of drug abuse combined. For every person who is an alcoholic, another three or four people are directly affected.

Alcoholics frequently suffer from mental disorders in addition to alcohol dependence. Alcoholics are much more likely than nonalcoholics to suffer from clinical depression, panic disorder, schizophrenia, and antisocial personality disorders. People with anxiety or panic attacks may try to use alcohol to lessen their anxiety, even though alcohol often makes these disorders worse.

An estimated 3 million Americans age 14–17 show signs of potential alcohol dependence. These numbers are far greater than those associated with cocaine, heroin, or marijuana use. The social and psychological consequences of excessive drinking in young people are more difficult to measure than the risks to physical health. One consequence is that excessive drinking interferes with learning the interpersonal and job-related skills required for adult life. Perhaps most important is that people who were excessive drinkers in college are more likely to have social, occupational, and health problems 20 years later. Despite media attention on cocaine and other drugs, alcohol abuse remains our society's number-one drug-abuse problem.

**Causes of Alcoholism** The precise causes of alcoholism are unknown, but many factors are probably involved. Some studies suggest that as much as 50–60% of a person's risk for alcoholism is determined by genetic factors. But not all children of alcoholics become alcoholic, and it is clear that other factors are involved. A person's risk of developing alcoholism may be increased by certain personality disorders, having grown up in a violent or otherwise troubled household, and imitating the alcohol abuse of peers and other role models. People who begin drinking excessively in their teens are especially prone to binge drinking and alcoholism later in life. Certain social factors have also been linked with alcoholism, including urbanization, disappearance of the extended family, a general loosening of kinship ties, increased mobility, and changing values.

**Treatment** Some alcoholics recover without professional help. How often this occurs is unknown, but possibly as many as one third stop drinking on their own or reduce their drinking enough to eliminate problems. Often these spontaneous recoveries are linked to an alcohol-related crisis, such as a health problem or the threat of being fired. Most alcoholics, however, require a treatment program of some kind in order to stop drinking. Many different kinds of programs exist. No single treatment works for everyone, so a person may have to try different programs before finding the right one. Over 1 million Americans enter treatment for alcoholism every year.

One of the oldest and best-known recovery programs is Alcoholics Anonymous (AA). AA consists of self-help groups that meet several times each week in most communities and follow a 12-step program. Important steps for people in these programs include recognizing that they are "powerless over alcohol" and must seek help from a "higher power" in order to regain control of their lives. By verbalizing these steps, the alcoholic directly addresses the denial that is often prominent in alcoholism and other addictions. Many AA members have a sponsor of their choosing who is available by phone 24 hours a day for individual support and crisis intervention.

Alcoholics Anonymous is generally recognized as an effective mutual help program, but not everyone responds to its style and message, and other recovery approaches are available. Some, like Rational Recovery and Women for Sobriety, deliberately avoid any emphasis on higher spiritual powers. A more controversial approach to problem drinking is offered by the group Moderation Management, which encourages people to manage their drinking behavior by limiting intake or abstaining.

Al-Anon is a companion program to AA that consists of groups for families and friends of alcoholics. In Al-Anon, spouses and others explore how they enabled the alcoholic to drink by denying, rationalizing, or covering up his or her drinking and how they can change this codependent behavior.

Other types of programs include inpatient hospital rehabilitation, employee assistance programs, and school-based programs. There are also some pharmacological treatments for alcoholism:

- *Disulfiram* (Antabuse) inhibits the metabolic breakdown of acetaldehyde and causes patients to flush and feel ill when they drink, thus theoretically inhibiting impulse drinking.
- *Naltrexone* reduces the craving for alcohol and decreases the pleasant, reinforcing effects of alcohol without making the user ill.
- *Acamprosate* (Campral), approved by the FDA in 2004, helps people maintain alcohol abstinence after they have stopped drinking. It is unclear precisely how it works, but it appears to act on the brain pathways related to alcohol abuse.

In people who abuse alcohol and have significant depression or anxiety, the use of antidepressant or antianxiety medication can improve both mental health and drinking behavior. Drug therapy is usually combined with psychosocial treatment.

## Gender and Ethnic Differences

Alcohol abusers come from all socioeconomic levels and cultural groups, but there are notable differences in patterns of drinking between men and women and among different ethnic groups (Table 8-3).

VITAL STATISTICS

**Table 8-3 Prevalence of Alcohol Abuse and Dependence**

| | Past Year Prevalence (Percentage) | |
|---|---|---|
| | Alcohol Abuse | Alcohol Dependence |
| **Gender** | | |
| Men | 6.9 | 5.4 |
| Women | 2.6 | 2.3 |
| **Ethnicity** | | |
| White | 5.1 | 3.8 |
| African American | 3.3 | 3.6 |
| American Indians and Alaska Natives | 5.8 | 6.4 |
| Asian Americans and Pacific Islander Americans | 2.1 | 2.4 |
| Latinos | 4.0 | 4.0 |
| **Total population** | **4.7** | **3.8** |

SOURCE: Grant, B., et al. 2004. The 12-month prevalence and trends in DSM-IV alcohol abuse and dependence: United States, 1991–1992 and 2001–2002. *Drug and Alcohol Dependence* 74(3): 223–234.

Take Charge

## Drinking Behavior and Responsibility

### Examine Your Attitudes and Behavior

Think about how you really feel about drinking: Is it of little consequence to you or perhaps even an intrusion into your college experience? Or is alcohol the key ingredient for any and all fun activities? How do you perceive nondrinkers at a party where others are drinking?

Also consider the sources of your ideas about alcohol. How was alcohol used in your family when you were growing up? How is it used—or how do you think it's used—by students at your school? And how is alcohol use portrayed in advertisements you're exposed to? Try examining some alcohol ads to determine what messages they convey, what audiences they target, and what effect they may have on you and your attitudes about drinking.

Finally, carefully examine your drinking behavior. If you drink alcohol, what are your reasons for doing so? Is your drinking behavior moderate and responsible? Or do you frequently overindulge and suffer negative consequences? Try tracking your alcohol use in your health journal for a week or two to help evaluate your drinking behavior.

### Drink Moderately and Responsibly

- *Drink slowly and space your drinks.* Sip your drinks, and alternate them with nonalcoholic choices. Don't drink alcoholic beverages to quench your thirst, and avoid drinks made with carbonated mixers.
- *Eat before and while drinking.* Don't drink on an empty stomach. Food in your stomach will slow the rate at which alcohol is absorbed and thus often lower the peak BAC.
- *Know your limits and your drinks.* Learn how different BACs affect you and how to keep your BAC and behavior under control.
- *Be aware of the setting.* In dangerous situations, such as driving or operating complicated machinery, abstinence is the only appropriate choice.
- *Use designated drivers.* Arrange carpools to and from parties or events where alcohol will be served. Rotate the responsibility for acting as a designated driver.
- *Learn to enjoy activities without alcohol.* If you can't have fun without drinking, you may have a problem with alcohol.

### Encourage Responsible Drinking in Others

- *Encourage responsible attitudes.* Learn to express disapproval about someone who has drunk too much. Don't treat the choice to abstain as strange. The majority of American adults drink moderately or not at all.
- *Be a responsible host.* Serve only enough alcohol for each guest to have a moderate number of drinks, and serve lots of nonalcoholic choices. Always serve food along with alcohol, and stop serving alcohol an hour or more before people will leave. Insist that a guest who drinks too much take a taxi, ride with someone else, or stay overnight rather than drive.
- *Hold drinkers fully responsible for their behavior.* Pardoning unacceptable behavior fosters the attitude that the behavior is due to the drug rather than the person.
- *Take community action.* Find out about prevention programs on your campus or in your community. Consider joining an action group such as Students Against Destructive Decisions (SADD) or Mothers Against Drunk Driving (MADD); visit www.sadd.org and www.madd.org.

**Men** Men account for the majority of alcohol-related deaths and injuries in the United States; many of these result from acute conditions related to intoxication, such as motor vehicle crashes, falls, drowning, suicide, and homicide. Traditional or stereotypic gender roles and ideas regarding masculinity and drinking behavior may promote excessive alcohol consumption among men (see the box "Drinking Behavior and Responsibility"). Among white American men, excessive drinking often begins in the teens or twenties and progresses gradually through the thirties until the individual is clearly identifiable as an alcoholic by the time he is in his late thirties or early forties. Other men remain controlled drinkers until later in life, sometimes becoming alcoholic in association with retirement, the inevitable losses of aging, boredom, illness, or psychological disorders.

**Women** Women tend to become alcoholic at a later age and with fewer years of heavy drinking. It is not unusual for women in their forties or fifties to become alcoholic after years of controlled drinking. Women alcoholics develop cirrhosis and other medical complications more often than men. Women alcoholics may have more medical problems because they are less likely to seek early treatment. In addition, there may be an inherently greater biological risk for women who drink.

**African Americans** Although as a group African Americans use less alcohol than most other groups (including whites), they face disproportionately high levels of alcohol-related birth defects, cirrhosis, cancer, hypertension, and other medical problems. In addition, blacks are more likely than members of other ethnic groups to be victims of alcohol-related homicides, criminal assaults, and injuries. AA groups of predominantly African Americans have been shown to provide effective treatment, perhaps because essential elements of AA—sharing common experiences, mutual acceptance of one another as human beings, and trusting a higher power—are already a part of African American culture.

**Latinos** Drinking patterns among Latinos vary significantly, depending on their specific cultural background and how long they and their families have lived in the United States. Drunk driving and cirrhosis are the most common causes of alcohol-related death and injury among Hispanic men. Hispanic women are more likely to abstain from alcohol than white or black women, but those who do drink are at special risk for problems. Treating the entire family as a unit is an important part of treatment because family pride, solidarity, and support are important aspects of Latino culture. Some Hispanics do better during treatment if treatment efforts are integrated with the techniques of *curanderos* (folk healers) and *espiritistas* (spiritists).

**Asian Americans** Asian Americans have lower-than-average rates of alcohol abuse, although acculturation may weaken the generally strong Asian community sanctions against alcohol use. For many Asian Americans, though, the genetically based physiological aversion to alcohol remains a deterrent to abuse. For those needing treatment, ethnic agencies, health care professionals, and ministers seem to be the most effective sources.

**American Indians and Alaska Natives** Alcohol abuse is one of the most widespread and severe health problems among American Indians and Alaska Natives, especially for adolescents and young adults. The rate of alcoholism among American Indians is twice that of the general population, and the death rate from alcohol-related causes is about eight times higher. Treatment may be more effective if it reflects tribal values. Some healers have incorporated aspects of American Indian religions into the therapeutic process, using traditional sweat houses, prayers, and dances.

### Helping Someone with an Alcohol Problem

Helping a friend or relative with an alcohol problem requires skill and tact. One of the first steps is making sure you are not an enabler or codependent, perhaps unknowingly allowing someone to continue excessively using alcohol. Enabling takes many forms. One of the most common is making excuses or covering up for the alcohol abuser—for example, saying "he has the flu" when it is really a hangover. Whenever you find yourself minimizing or lying about someone's drinking behavior, a warning bell should sound. Another important step is open, honest labeling—"I think you have a problem with alcohol." Such explicit statements usually elicit emotional rebuttals and may endanger a relationship. In the long run, however, you are not helping your friends by allowing them to deny their problems with alcohol or other drugs. Even when problems are acknowledged, there is usually reluctance to get help. Your best role might be to obtain information about the available resources and persistently encourage their use.

## WHY PEOPLE USE TOBACCO

Roughly 70 million Americans, including nearly 4 million adolescents, use tobacco. Each day more than 2000 teenagers become regular smokers, and at least one-third of them will die prematurely because of tobacco. Most smokers understand the risks of tobacco use: More than 80% of adult smokers believe tobacco will shorten their life and would like to quit. Each year roughly 40% of smokers quit for at least a day, but 9 out of 10 of them are smoking again within a year.

### Nicotine Addiction

The primary reason people continue to use tobacco despite the health risks is that they have become addicted to a powerful psychoactive drug: nicotine. Many researchers consider nicotine to be the most physically addictive of all the psychoactive drugs. Neurological studies indicate that nicotine acts on the brain in much the same way as cocaine and heroin. Nicotine reaches the brain via the bloodstream seconds after it is inhaled or, in the case of spit tobacco, absorbed through membranes of the mouth or nose. It triggers the release of powerful chemical messengers in the brain, including epinephrine, norepinephrine, and dopamine. But unlike street drugs, most of which are used to achieve a high, nicotine's primary attraction seems to lie in its ability to modulate everyday emotions.

At low doses, nicotine acts as a stimulant: It increases heart rate and blood pressure and, in adults, can enhance alertness, concentration, rapid information processing, memory, and learning. People type faster on nicotine, for instance. In some circumstances, nicotine acts as a mild sedative. Most commonly, nicotine relieves symptoms such as anxiety, irritability, and mild depression in tobacco users who are experiencing withdrawal. Tobacco users are able to fine-tune nicotine's effects and regulate their moods by increasing or decreasing their intake of the drug.

All tobacco products contain nicotine, and the use of any of them can lead to addiction. Nicotine addiction fulfills the criteria for substance dependence described in Chapter 7, including loss of control, tolerance, and withdrawal.

**Loss of Control** Three out of four smokers want to quit but find they cannot. People who quit smoking have a relapse rate similar to rates for alcoholics and heroin addicts. Regular tobacco users live according to a rigid cycle

Mind/Body/Spirit

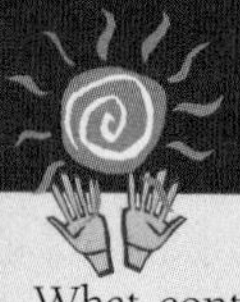

## Tobacco Use and Religion: Global Views

What contributions can the world's religions make to efforts to limit tobacco use? This was the question behind a meeting attended by representatives of the major religions of the world at the headquarters of the World Health Organization (WHO).

### Tobacco Use as a Violation of Religious Principles

A primary thread among all the religions is a condemnation of tobacco use for its damaging effects on the body. Most religions regard the human body as the dwelling place of the spirit; as such, it deserves care and respect.

The Baha'i faith, for example, strongly discourages smoking as unclean and unhealthy. For Hindus, smoking goes against one of the primary spiritual practices, the care of the body. The Roman Catholic Church endorses the age-old adage "a sound mind in a sound body." For Muslims, one of the five essential principles on which religious law is based is the protection of the integrity of the individual. In Judaism, people are urged to "choose life" and to choose whatever strengthens the capacity to live. Buddhists believe that the body doesn't belong to the person at all—even suicide is considered murder—and one must do nothing to harm it.

A second common thread is the notion that dependence and addiction run counter to ideas of freedom, choice, and human dignity. Buddhism teaches a path of freedom—a way of life without dependence on anything. Hindus regard tobacco use as a *vyasana,* a dependence that is not necessary for the preservation of health. Protestant churches caution that any form of dependence is contrary to the notion of Christian freedom.

A third argument against tobacco use is the immorality of imposing secondhand smoke on nonsmokers, which is seen as inflicting harm on others. In Hinduism, harming others is sinful. In the Jewish tradition, those who force nonsmokers to breathe smoke jeopardize the lives of others, and to do so is to jeopardize the whole universe.

### The Role of Individual Responsibility

Most religions focus on the role of individual responsibility in overcoming dependence on tobacco. In Buddhism, for example, people must assume responsibility for their habits; they practice introspection to understand the cause of problems within themselves and the effects of their actions on others. The principles of Islam are based on notions of responsibility and protection; a fundamental message is that you are responsible for your body and for your health.

### Religion and Tobacco Control

Common threads again emerged in discussions of how the problem of tobacco use should be approached. The Islamic view is that the campaign to control tobacco use must be based on awareness, responsibility, and justice. Developing awareness means providing information on the global problem. Fostering responsibility means helping people understand what they need to do to attain well-being. Emphasizing social and human justice means helping the farmers and societies that depend on tobacco cultivation to find alternative crops.

According to the representative from the Geneva Interreligious Platform (a project involving Hindus, Buddhists, Jews, Christians, Muslims, and Baha'is), the best approach is prevention. Here, the rights of nonsmokers clearly prevail over the freedom of smokers. In support of this position, the common religious exhortation not to do unto others what you would not have them do unto you can be invoked. Further, adequate information should be provided to counter the deceptive images projected by tobacco industry advertising, especially where minors are concerned. Protection of the weak and denunciation of dishonesty are underlying values of all religious traditions.

Religious traditions can best assist adult smokers by reminding them of two principles: one, the value of liberation from any form of slavery, and two, respect for life out of deference to the source of all life, which religions call by different names—God, ultimate reality, and so on—but which is the supreme value of any religious commitment.

SOURCE: World Health Organization Tobacco Free Initiative. 1999. *Meeting Report: Meeting on Tobacco and Religion* (3 May 1999). Geneva: World Health Organization.

of need and gratification. On average, they can go no more than 40 minutes between doses of nicotine; otherwise, they begin feeling edgy and irritable and have trouble concentrating. If ignored, nicotine cravings build until getting a cigarette or some spit tobacco becomes a paramount concern, crowding out other thoughts. Tobacco users become adept, therefore, at keeping a steady amount of nicotine circulating in the blood and going to the brain. They may plan their daily schedule around opportunities to satisfy their nicotine cravings; this loss of control and personal freedom can affect all the dimensions of wellness (see the box "Tobacco Use and Religion: Global Views").

**Tolerance and Withdrawal** Using tobacco builds up tolerance. Where one cigarette may make a beginning smoker nauseated and dizzy, a long-term smoker may have to chain-smoke a pack or more to experience the same effects. For most regular tobacco users, sudden abstinence from nicotine produces predictable withdrawal symptoms, which come on several hours after the last dose of nicotine. These can include severe cravings, insomnia, confusion, tremors, difficulty concentrating, fatigue, muscle pains, headache, nausea, irritability, anger, and depression. Although most of these symptoms of physical dependence pass in 2 or 3 days, many ex-smokers report intermittent, intense urges to smoke for years after quitting.

Compared with older smokers, adolescents become heavy smokers and develop dependence after fewer cigarettes. Nicotine addiction can start within a few days of smoking and after just a few cigarettes. Over half of teenagers who try cigarettes progress to daily use, and about half of those who ever smoke daily progress to nicotine dependence. In polls, about 75% of smoking teens state they wish they had never started.

## Social and Psychological Factors

Social and psychological forces combine with physiological addiction to maintain the tobacco habit. Many people, for example, have established habits of smoking while doing something else—while talking, working, drinking, and so on. The spit tobacco habit is also associated with certain situations—studying, drinking coffee, or playing sports. It is difficult for these people to break their habits because the activities they associate with tobacco use continue to trigger their urge.

## Why Start in the First Place?

A junior high school girl takes up smoking in an attempt to appear older. A high school boy uses spit tobacco in the bullpen, emulating the major league ball players he admires. An overweight first-year college student turns to cigarettes, hoping they will curb her appetite. Smoking rates among American youth rose steadily through the 1990s but have begun to decline.

Children and teenagers constitute 90% of all new smokers in this country: Every day, an estimated 2000 adolescents become regular cigarette smokers, while hundreds of others take up snuff or chewing tobacco. The average age for starting smokers is 13; for spit tobacco users, 10. Meanwhile, children—especially girls—are beginning to experiment with tobacco at ever-younger ages. The earlier people begin smoking, the more likely they are to become heavy smokers—and to die of tobacco-related disease.

**Rationalizing the Dangers** Making the decision to smoke requires minimizing or denying both the health risks of tobacco use and the tremendous pain, disability, emotional trauma, family stress, and financial expense involved in tobacco-related diseases such as cancer and emphysema. A sense of invincibility, characteristic of many adolescents and young adults, also contributes to the decision to use tobacco. Young people may persuade themselves they are too intelligent, too lucky, or too healthy to be vulnerable to tobacco's dangers (see the box "Building Motivation to Quit Smoking").

**Listening to Advertising** Advertising is a powerful influence. The tobacco industry spends more than $12 billion each year on advertising that links tobacco products with desirable traits such as confidence, popularity, sexual attractiveness, and slenderness. The tobacco industry has perfected techniques that target young people. Young smokers are the ones most likely to purchase the most familiar brands. Thus, the most heavily advertised cigarettes—Marlboro, Camel, and Newport—are the choice of 90% of teen smokers. Only a third of adult smokers, who prefer less expensive generic cigarettes, choose these brands.

Young people are not the only group targeted. Certain brands are designed to appeal primarily to men, women, or particular ethnic groups. For example, Virginia Slims tries to appeal to women by associating the brand with confidence and sexual attractiveness. Magazines that are targeted at African American audiences receive proportionately more revenues from cigarette advertising than do other consumer magazines. Billboards advertising tobacco products are placed in black communities four or five times more often than in primarily white communities.

**Emulating Smoking Onscreen** In the top-grossing films in 2002–2003, smoking was portrayed in more than 73% of the films, including 82% of PG-13 films; smoking was often shown positively as a means to relieve tension or as something to do while socializing. Negative consequences resulting from tobacco use were depicted for only 3% of the major characters who used tobacco. By showing smoking in an unrealistically positive light, films may be acting as advertisement.

Studies of adolescents have consistently found a strong association between seeing tobacco use in films and trying cigarettes. Some groups equate seeing a favorite actor smoke on-screen with now-banned celebrity television advertisements for cigarettes. They suggest an automatic R rating for any film that shows tobacco use, equating smoking with violence, strong language, sexuality, and nudity in determining a film's rating. The debate over the prevalence and effects of smoking is likely to continue.

## Who Uses Tobacco?

Currently, about 25% of men and 20% of women smoke cigarettes (Table 8-4). Rates of smoking vary, based on gender, age, ethnicity, and education level. Adults with less than a twelfth-grade education are three times as likely to smoke cigarettes as those with a college degree. The reverse is true for cigars: Cigar smoking is most common among the affluent and those with high educational attainment.

Although all states ban the sale of tobacco to anyone under 18 years of age, at least 500 million packs of cigarettes and 26 million containers of chewing tobacco are consumed by minors each year. About 15% of middle school students use some form of tobacco. Among high school students, about 28% smoke cigarettes at least occasionally and 15% smoke cigars. An estimated 8%,

Take Charge

## Building Motivation to Quit Smoking

A common misconception among smokers is that a few cigarettes a day aren't enough to cause harm. Perhaps this is why a recent survey showed that among college students who smoke, 75% smoke 10 or fewer cigarettes a day. These smokers are ignoring the very real health risks of even one cigarette. The U.S. Public Health Service suggests a "5 R's" strategy to enhance motivation to quit. If you are a smoker or are trying to help one, think about these areas of concern and see if they help develop a desire and readiness to make a real attempt at quitting.

*Relevance:* Think about the personal relevance of quitting tobacco use. What would the effects be on your family and friends? How would your daily life improve? What is the most important way that quitting would change your life?

*Risks:* There are immediate risks, such as shortness of breath, infertility, and impotence, and long-term risks, including cancer, heart disease, and respiratory problems. Remember, smoking is harmful both to you and to anyone exposed to your smoke.

*Rewards:* The list of the rewards of quitting is almost endless, including improving immediate and long-term health, saving money, and feeling better about yourself. You can also stop worrying about quitting and set a good example for others.

*Roadblocks:* What are the potential obstacles to quitting? Are you worried about withdrawal symptoms, weight gain, or lack of support? How can these barriers be overcome?

*Repetition:* Revisit your reasons for quitting and strengthen your resolve until you are ready to prepare a plan. Most people make several attempts to quit before they succeed. Relapsing once does not mean that you will never succeed.

If someone you care about uses tobacco, you can try the following strategies to help them quit.

1. **Ask** about tobacco use. How many cigarettes does your girlfriend smoke each day? How long has your roommate been dipping snuff?
2. **Advise** tobacco users to stop. Express your concern over the tobacco user's habit. "When we're close, the smell of smoke on your hair and breath bothers me. I've noticed you cough a lot and your voice is raspy. I'm worried about your health. You should stop."
3. **Assess** the tobacco user's willingness to quit. "Next week would be a good time to try to quit. Would you be willing to give it a try?"
4. **Assist** the tobacco user who is willing to stop. To coincide with your partner's quit date, take him away for a romantic weekend far from the places he associates with smoking. Offer to be an exercise partner. Call once a day to offer support and help. Bring gifts of low-calorie snacks or projects that occupy the hands. If the quitter lapses, be encouraging. A lapse doesn't have to become a relapse.
5. **Arrange** follow-up. Maintaining abstinence is an ongoing process. Celebrate milestones of 1 week, 1 month, 1 year without tobacco. Note how much better your friend's or partner's car, room, and person smell, how much healthier he or she is, and how much you appreciate not having to breathe tobacco smoke.

SOURCES: Rigotti, N. A., J. E. Lee, and H. Wechsler. 2000. U.S. college students' use of tobacco products. *Journal of the American Medical Association* 284(6): 699–705; Fiore, M. C., et al. 2000. *Treating Tobacco Use and Dependence*. Clinical Practice Guidelines. Rockville, Md.: U.S. Department of Health and Human Services.

including 11% of white male students, use spit tobacco. Male college athletes and professional baseball players report even higher rates of spit tobacco use.

## HEALTH HAZARDS

Tobacco adversely affects nearly every part of the body, including the brain, stomach, mouth, and reproductive organs.

### Tobacco Smoke: A Toxic Mix

Tobacco smoke contains hundreds of damaging chemical substances, including acetone (nail polish remover), ammonia, hexamine (lighter fluid), and toluene (industrial solvent). Smoke from a typical unfiltered cigarette contains about 5 billion particles per cubic millimeter—50,000 times as many as are found in an equal volume of smoggy urban air. These particles, when condensed, form the brown, sticky mass called **cigarette tar.**

**Carcinogens and Poisons** At least 43 chemicals in tobacco smoke are linked to the development of cancer. Other substances in tobacco cause health problems because they damage the lining of the respiratory tract or decrease the lungs' ability to fight off infection. Tobacco also contains poisonous substances, including arsenic and hydrogen cyanide. In addition to being an addictive psychoactive drug, nicotine is also a poison and can be fatal in high doses. Many cases of nicotine poisoning occur each year in toddlers and infants who pick up and eat cigarette butts they find at home or on the playground. Cigarette smoke contains carbon monoxide, the deadly gas in automobile exhaust, in concentrations 400 times greater than is considered safe in industrial workplaces. Carbon monoxide displaces oxygen in red blood cells, depleting the body's supply of life-giving oxygen for extra work.

VITAL STATISTICS

**Table 8-4 Who Smokes?**

| | Percentage of Smokers | | |
|---|---|---|---|
| | Men | Women | Total |
| **Ethnic group (age ≥ 18)** | | | |
| White | 26 | 22 | 24 |
| Black | 27 | 19 | 22 |
| Asian | 19 | 7 | 13 |
| American Indian/ Alaska Native | 40 | 41 | 41 |
| Latino | 23 | 11 | 17 |
| **Education (age ≥ 25)** | | | |
| ≤8 years | 25 | 13 | 20 |
| 9–11 years | 39 | 31 | 34 |
| 12 years (no diploma) | 32 | 30 | 31 |
| GED diploma | 48 | 38 | 42 |
| 12 years (diploma) | 30 | 22 | 26 |
| Associate degree | 24 | 20 | 22 |
| Undergraduate degree | 14 | 11 | 12 |
| Graduate degree | 8 | 6 | 7 |
| **Total** | 25 | 20 | 22 |

SOURCE: Centers for Disease Control and Prevention. 2004. Cigarette smoking among adults—United States, 2002. *Morbidity and Mortality Weekly Report* 53(20): 427–431.

**Additives** Tobacco manufacturers use additives to manipulate the taste and effect of cigarettes and other tobacco products. Many of the nearly 600 chemicals used in manufacturing cigarettes are approved as safe when used as food additives, but some form cancer-causing agents when they are heated or burned. Examples of additives include flavoring agents that mask the harsh, bitter taste of tobacco, and ammonia, which boosts the amount of nicotine delivered by cigarettes. Chemicals from cocoa and licorice also act as bronchodilators; like menthol, they open the lung's airways and make it easier for nicotine to enter the bloodstream. Other additives make sidestream smoke (the uninhaled smoke from a burning cigarette) less obvious and objectionable, presumably to reduce social pressures from nonsmokers.

**"Light" and Low-Tar Cigarettes** Some smokers switch to low-tar, low-nicotine, or filtered cigarettes because they believe them to be healthier alternatives. But there is no such thing as a safe cigarette, and smoking behavior is a more important factor in tar and nicotine intake than the type of cigarette smoked. Smokers who switch to a low-nicotine brand often compensate by smoking more cigarettes, inhaling more deeply, taking larger or more frequent puffs, or blocking ventilation holes with lips or fingers to offset the effects of filters. Studies have found that people who smoke "light" cigarettes inhale up to eight times as much tar and nicotine as printed on the label. Use of "light" and low-tar cigarettes does not reduce the risk of smoking-related illnesses, and they provide *no* benefit to smokers' health.

**Menthol Cigarettes** Concerns have also been raised about menthol cigarettes. About 70% of African American smokers smoke these cigarettes, as compared to 22% of whites. Studies have found that blacks absorb more nicotine than other groups and metabolize it more slowly; they also have lower rates of successful quitting. The anesthetizing effect of menthol, which may allow smokers to inhale more deeply and hold smoke in their lungs for a longer period, may be partly responsible for these differences.

## The Immediate Effects of Smoking

The beginning smoker often has symptoms of mild nicotine poisoning: dizziness; faintness; rapid pulse; cold, clammy skin; and sometimes nausea, vomiting, and diarrhea. The effects of nicotine on smokers vary, depending greatly on the size of the nicotine dose and how much tolerance previous smoking has built up. Nicotine can either excite or tranquilize the nervous system, depending on dosage.

Nicotine has many other immediate effects (Figure 8-4). It stimulates the part of the brain called the **cerebral cortex.** It also stimulates the adrenal glands to discharge adrenaline. And it inhibits the formation of urine; constricts the blood vessels, especially in the skin; accelerates the heart rate; and elevates blood pressure. Higher blood pressure, faster heart rate, and constricted blood vessels require the heart to pump more blood. Smoking depresses hunger contractions and dulls the taste buds; smokers who quit often notice that food tastes much better. Smoking is not useful for weight loss, however. (Smoking for decades may lessen or prevent age-associated weight gain for some smokers, but for people under 30, smoking is not associated with weight loss.)

## The Long-Term Effects of Smoking

Smoking is linked to many deadly and disabling diseases. The total amount of tobacco smoke inhaled is a key factor contributing to disease: People who smoke more cigarettes per day, inhale deeply, puff frequently, smoke cigarettes down to the butts, or begin smoking at an early age run a greater risk of disease than do those who smoke more moderately or who do not smoke at all.

**Terms**

**cigarette tar** A brown, sticky mass created when the chemical particles in tobacco smoke condense.

**cerebral cortex** The outer layer of the brain, which controls complex behavior and mental activity.

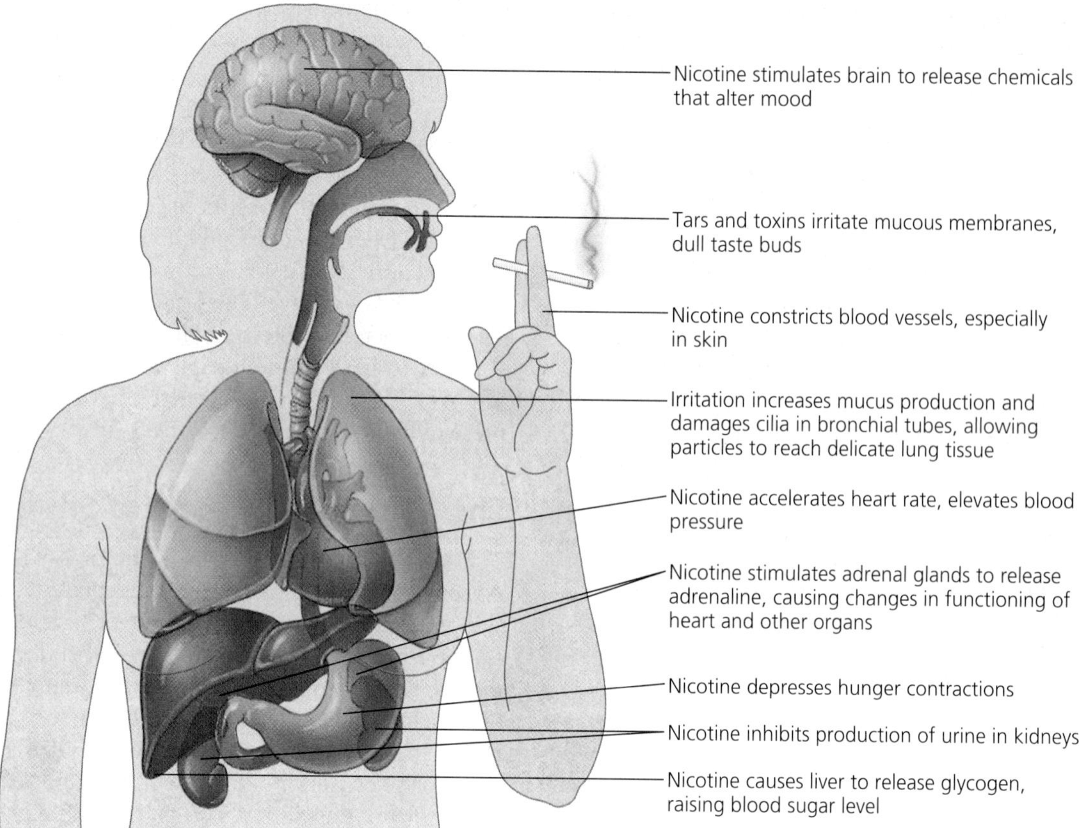


**Figure 8-4 The short-term effects of smoking a cigarette.**

**Cardiovascular Disease** Although lung cancer tends to receive the most publicity, one form of cardiovascular disease, **coronary heart disease (CHD)**, is actually the most widespread single cause of death for cigarette smokers. CHD often results from atherosclerosis, a condition in which fatty deposits called plaques form on the inner walls of heart arteries, causing them to narrow and stiffen. Smoking and exposure to environmental tobacco smoke (ETS) permanently accelerate the rate of plaque accumulation in the coronary arteries—50% for smokers, 25% for ex-smokers, and 20% for people regularly exposed to ETS. If the plaque completely blocks the flow of blood to a portion of the heart, a heart attack occurs. CHD can also interfere with the heart's electrical activity, resulting in disturbances of the normal heartbeat rhythm.

Smokers have a death rate from CHD that is 70% higher than that of nonsmokers. The risks of CHD decrease rapidly when a person stops smoking; this is particularly true for younger smokers, whose coronary arteries have not yet been extensively damaged. Cigarette smoking has also been linked to other cardiovascular diseases, including the following:

- *Stroke,* a sudden interference with the circulation of blood in a part of the brain, resulting in the destruction of brain cells
- *Aortic aneurysm,* a bulge in the aorta caused by a weakening in its walls
- *Pulmonary heart disease,* a disorder of the right side of the heart, caused by changes in the blood vessels of the lungs

**Lung Cancer and Other Cancers** Cigarette smoking is the primary cause of lung cancer. Benzo(a)pyrene, a chemical found in tobacco smoke, causes genetic mutations in lung cells. Those who smoke two or more packs of cigarettes a day have lung cancer death rates 12–25 times greater than those of nonsmokers. The dramatic rise in lung cancer rates among women in the past 40 years clearly parallels the increase of smoking in this group; lung cancer now exceeds breast cancer as the leading cause of cancer deaths among women. The risk of developing lung cancer increases with the number of cigarettes smoked each day, the number of years of smoking, and the age at which the person started smoking.

Evidence suggests that after 1 year without smoking, the risk of lung cancer decreases substantially. After 10 years, the risk of lung cancer among ex-smokers is 50% of that of continuing smokers. The sooner one quits, the better: If smoking is stopped before cancer has started, lung tissue tends to repair itself, even if cellular changes that can lead to cancer are already present.

Research has also linked smoking to cancers of the trachea, mouth, esophagus, larynx, pancreas, bladder, kidney, breast, cervix, stomach, liver, colon, and skin.

**Chronic Obstructive Lung Disease** The lungs of a smoker are constantly exposed to dangerous chemicals and irritants, and they must work harder to function adequately. The stresses placed on the lungs by smoking can permanently damage lung function and lead to *chronic obstructive lung disease (COLD)*, also known as chronic obstructive pulmonary disease. COLD is the fourth leading cause of death in the United States. This progressive and disabling disorder consists of several different but related diseases; emphysema and chronic bronchitis are two of the most common.

EMPHYSEMA Smoking is the primary cause of **emphysema,** a particularly disabling condition in which the walls of the air sacs in the lungs lose their elasticity and are gradually destroyed. The lungs' ability to obtain oxygen and remove carbon dioxide is impaired. A person with emphysema is breathless, is constantly gasping for air, and has the feeling of drowning. The heart must pump harder and may become enlarged. People with emphysema often die from a damaged heart. There is no known way to reverse this disease. In its advanced stage, the victim is bedridden and severely disabled.

CHRONIC BRONCHITIS Persistent, recurrent inflammation of the bronchial tubes characterizes **chronic bronchitis.** When the cell lining of the bronchial tubes is irritated, it secretes excess mucus. Bronchial congestion is followed by a chronic cough, which makes breathing more and more difficult. If smokers have chronic bronchitis, they face a greater risk of lung cancer, no matter how old they are or how many (or few) cigarettes they smoke. Chronic bronchitis seems to be a shortcut to lung cancer.

**Other Respiratory Damage** Even when the smoker shows no signs of lung impairment or disease, cigarette smoking damages the respiratory system. Normally the cells lining the bronchial tubes secrete mucus, a sticky fluid that collects particles of soot, dust, and other substances in inhaled air. Mucus is carried up to the mouth by the continuous motion of the cilia, hairlike structures that protrude from the inner surface of the bronchial tubes. If the cilia are destroyed or impaired, or if the pollution of inhaled air is more than the system can remove, the protection provided by cilia is lost.

Cigarette smoke first slows and then stops the action of the cilia. Eventually it destroys them, leaving delicate membranes exposed to injury from substances inhaled in cigarette smoke or from polluted air. This interference with the functioning of the respiratory system often leads rapidly to the conditions known as smoker's throat and smoker's cough, as well as to shortness of breath. Other respiratory effects of smoking include a worsening of allergy and asthma symptoms and an increase in the smoker's susceptibility to colds.

**Other Concerns** Smokers are more likely to develop peptic ulcers and to die from them; they have higher rates of heartburn. Smoking reduces fertility in both men and women and is linked to pregnancy complications; men who smoke are twice as likely as nonsmokers to experience impotence and have a higher proportion of defective sperm (see the box "Gender and Tobacco Use" on p. 184). Smoking dulls the senses of taste and smell and increases the risk of hearing loss and blindness; it causes premature skin wrinkling and baldness, tooth decay and stains, gum disease, and a persistent tobacco odor in clothes and hair. Smokers have higher rates of motor vehicle crashes, fire-related injuries, and back pain.

Smoking is also expensive: The average per-pack price of cigarettes is about $4, meaning a pack-a-day habit costs nearly $1500 each year for cigarettes alone. Other costs, including higher insurance premiums, bring the annual total up to $3000. One study estimated that the total cost for a 24-year-old—including cigarettes, lost earnings, insurance costs, and harm done by environmental tobacco smoke—is nearly $40 per pack.

**Cumulative Effects** The cumulative effects of tobacco use fall into two general categories. The first category is reduced life expectancy. A male who takes up smoking before age 15 and continues to smoke is only half as likely to live to age 75 as a male who never smokes. If he inhales deeply, he risks losing a minute of life for every minute of smoking. Females who have similar smoking habits also have a reduced life expectancy. Smoking reduces their life expectancy by more than 10 years.

The second category involves quality of life. A national health survey begun in 1964 shows that smokers spend one-third more time away from their jobs because of illness than nonsmokers. Both men and women smokers show a greater rate of acute and chronic disease than people who have never smoked. Smokers become disabled at

### Terms

VW

**coronary heart disease (CHD)** Cardiovascular disease caused by hardening of the arteries that supply oxygen to the heart muscle; also called *coronary artery disease.*

**emphysema** A disease characterized by a loss of lung tissue elasticity and breakup of the air sacs, impairing the lungs' ability to obtain oxygen and remove carbon dioxide.

**chronic bronchitis** Recurrent, persistent inflammation of the bronchial tubes.

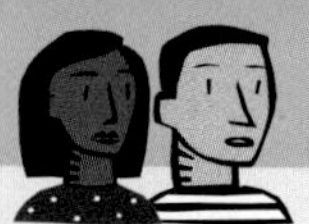

Gender Matters

## Gender and Tobacco Use

American men are currently more likely than women to smoke, but women younger than age 23 are becoming smokers at a faster rate than any other population segment. As the rate of smoking among women approaches that of men, so do rates of tobacco-related illness and death. Lung cancer, emphysema, and cardiovascular diseases sicken and kill both men and women who smoke, and more American women now die each year from lung cancer than from breast cancer.

Although overall risks of tobacco-related illness are similar for women and men, sex appears to make a difference in some diseases. Women, for example, are more at risk for smoking-related blood clots and strokes than are men, and the risk is even greater for women using oral contraceptives. Among men and women with the same smoking history, the odds for developing three major types of cancer, including lung cancer, is 1.2–1.7 times higher in women than in men. One possible explanation for this difference is that women are more likely to use low-tar cigarettes and thus engage in compensatory behaviors such as deep inhalation, which is linked to increased respiratory damage. Women may also have a greater biological vulnerability to lung cancer.

For both men and women, tobacco use is associated with increased incidence of sex-specific health problems. Men who smoke increase their risk of erectile dysfunction and infertility due to reduced sperm density and motility. Women who smoke have higher rates of osteoporosis (a bone-thinning disease that can lead to fractures), thyroid-related diseases, and depression.

Women who smoke also have risks associated with reproduction and the reproductive organs. Smoking is associated with greater menstrual bleeding, greater duration of painful menstrual cramps, and more variability in menstrual cycle length. Smokers have a more difficult time becoming pregnant, and they reach menopause on average a year or two earlier than nonsmokers. When women smokers become pregnant, they face increased chances of miscarriage or placental disorders that lead to bleeding and premature delivery; rates of ectopic pregnancy, preeclampsia, and stillbirth are also higher among women who smoke. Smoking is a risk factor for cervical cancer.

When women decide to try to stop smoking, they are more likely than men to join a support group. Overall, though, women are less successful than men in quitting. Women report more severe withdrawal symptoms when they stop smoking and are more likely than men to report cravings in response to social and behavioral cues associated with smoking. For men, relapse to smoking is often associated with work or social pressure; women are more likely to relapse when sad or depressed or concerned about weight gain. Women and men also respond differently to medications: Nicotine replacement therapy appears to work better for men, whereas the non-nicotine medication bupropion appears to work better for women.

younger ages than nonsmokers and have more years of unhealthy life in addition to a shorter life span.

## Other Forms of Tobacco Use

Many smokers have switched from cigarettes to other forms of tobacco, such as spit (smokeless) tobacco, cigars and pipes, clove cigarettes, and bidis. However, each of these alternatives is far from safe.

**Spit (Smokeless) Tobacco** More than 5 million adults and about 6% of all high school students are current spit tobacco users. Spit tobacco comes in two major forms: snuff and chewing tobacco (chew). In snuff, the tobacco leaf is processed into a coarse, moist powder and mixed with flavorings. Snuff is usually sold in small tins. Users place a "pinch," "dip," or "quid" between the lower lip or cheek and gum and suck on it. In chewing tobacco, the tobacco leaf may be shredded ("leaf"), pressed into bricks or cakes ("plugs"), or dried and twisted into rope-like strands ("twists"). Users place a wad of tobacco in their mouth and then chew or suck it to release the nicotine. All types of smokeless tobacco cause an increase in saliva production, and the resulting tobacco juice is spit out or swallowed.

The nicotine in spit tobacco—along with flavorings and additives—is absorbed through the gums and lining of the mouth. Holding an average-size dip in the mouth for 30 minutes delivers about the same amount of nicotine as two or three cigarettes. Because of its nicotine content, spit tobacco is highly addictive. Some users keep it in their mouth even while sleeping.

Although not as dangerous as smoking cigarettes, the use of spit tobacco carries many health risks. Changes can occur in the mouth after only a few weeks of use: Gums and lips become dried and irritated and may bleed. White or red patches may appear inside the mouth; this condition, known as *leukoplakia,* can lead to oral cancer (see below). About 25% of regular spit tobacco users have *gingivitis* (inflammation) and recession of the gums and bone loss around the teeth, especially where the tobacco is usually placed. The senses of taste and smell are usually dulled. In addition, other people find the presence of wads of tobacco in the mouth, stained teeth, bad breath, and behaviors such as frequent spitting to be unpleasant.

One of the most serious effects of spit tobacco is an increased risk of oral cancer—cancers of the lip, tongue, cheek, throat, gums, roof and floor of the mouth, and larynx. Spit tobacco contains at least 28 chemicals known to cause cancer, and long-term snuff use may increase the risk of oral cancer by as much as 50 times. Surgery to treat oral cancer is often disfiguring and may involve removing parts of the face, tongue, cheek, or lip.

Dipping and chewing tobacco produce blood levels of nicotine similar to those in cigarette smokers. High blood levels of nicotine have dangerous effects on the cardiovascular system, including elevation of blood pressure, heart rate, and blood levels of certain fats. Other chemicals in spit tobacco are believed to pose risks to developing fetuses.

**Cigars and Pipes** The popularity of cigars is highest among white males age 18–44 with higher-than-average income and education, but women are also smoking cigars in record numbers. Cigar use is also growing among young people: In the latest government surveys, 12% of high school students reported having smoked at least one cigar in the previous month. An estimated 2% of Americans, mostly males who also smoke cigarettes, are pipe smokers.

Cigars are made from rolled whole tobacco leaves; pipe tobacco is made from shredded leaves and often flavored. Users absorb nicotine through the gums and lining of the mouth. Cigars contain more tobacco than cigarettes and so contain more nicotine and produce more tar when smoked. Large cigars may contain as much tobacco as a whole pack of cigarettes and take 1–2 hours to smoke.

The smoke from cigars contains many of the same toxins and carcinogens as the smoke from cigarettes, some in much higher quantities. The health risks of cigars depend on the number of cigars smoked and whether the smoker inhales. Because most cigar and pipe users do not inhale, they have a lower risk of cancer and cardiovascular and respiratory diseases than cigarette smokers. However, their risks are substantially higher than those of nonsmokers.

Nicotine addiction is another concern. Most adults who smoke cigars do so only occasionally, and there is little evidence that use of cigars by adults leads to addiction. The recent rise in cigar use among teens has raised concerns, however, because nicotine addiction almost always develops in the teen or young adult years.

**Clove Cigarettes and Bidis** Clove cigarettes, also called "kreteks" or "chicartas," are made of tobacco mixed with chopped cloves; they are imported primarily from Indonesia and Pakistan. Clove cigarettes contain almost twice as much tar, nicotine, and carbon monoxide as conventional cigarettes and so have all the same health hazards. Some chemical constituents of cloves may also be dangerous. For example, eugenol, an anesthetic compound found in cloves, may impair the respiratory system's ability to detect and defend against foreign particles. There have been a number of serious respiratory injuries and deaths from the use of clove cigarettes.

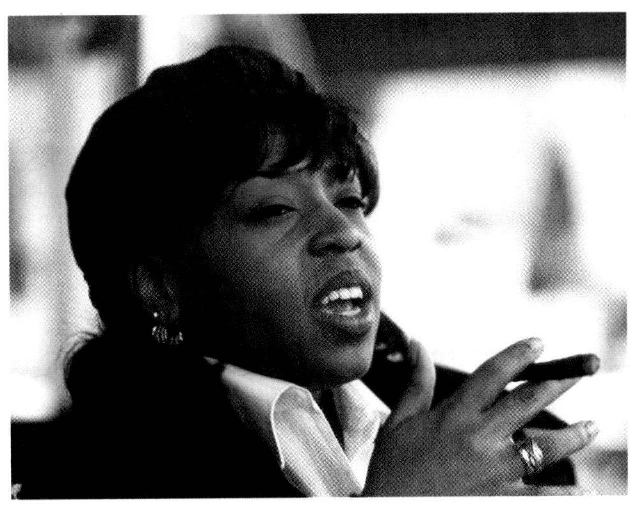

Cigars contain more tobacco than cigarettes and so produce more tar when smoked. Cigar smokers face an increased risk of cancer even if they don't inhale the smoke.

Bidis, or "beadies," are small cigarettes imported from India that contain species of tobacco different from those used by U.S. cigarette manufacturers. The tobacco in bidis is hand-rolled in Indian ebony leaves (tendu) and then often flavored; clove, mint, chocolate, and fruit varieties are available. Bidis contain up to four times more nicotine than and twice as much tar as U.S. cigarettes.

## THE EFFECTS OF SMOKING ON THE NONSMOKER

In a watershed decision in 1993, the U.S. Environmental Protection Agency (EPA) designated **environmental tobacco smoke (ETS)** a Class A carcinogen—an agent known to cause cancer in humans. In 2000, the Department of Health and Human Services' National Toxicology Program classified ETS as a "known human carcinogen." These designations put ETS in the same category as notorious cancer-causing agents like asbestos. Every year, ETS causes thousands of deaths from lung cancer and heart disease and is responsible for hundreds of thousands of respiratory infections in young children.

### Environmental Tobacco Smoke

Environmental tobacco smoke, or *secondhand smoke,* consists of mainstream smoke and sidestream smoke.

**Term**

**environmental tobacco smoke (ETS)** Smoke that enters the atmosphere from the burning end of a cigarette, cigar, or pipe, as well as smoke that is exhaled by smokers; also called *secondhand smoke.*

VW

Smoke exhaled by smokers is referred to as **mainstream smoke. Sidestream smoke** enters the atmosphere from the burning end of a cigarette, cigar, or pipe. Undiluted sidestream smoke, because it is not filtered through either a cigarette filter or a smoker's lungs, has significantly higher concentrations of the toxic and carcinogenic compounds found in mainstream smoke. For example, compared to mainstream smoke, sidestream smoke has (1) twice as much tar and nicotine; (2) three times as much benzo(a)pyrene, a carcinogen; (3) almost three times as much carbon monoxide, which displaces oxygen from red blood cells; and (4) three times as much ammonia.

Nearly 85% of the smoke in a room where someone is smoking comes from sidestream smoke. Of course, sidestream smoke is diffused through the air, so nonsmokers don't inhale the same concentrations of toxic chemicals that the smoker does. Still, the concentrations can be high. In rooms where people are smoking, levels of carbon monoxide, for instance, can exceed those permitted by Federal Air Quality Standards for outside air.

The secondhand smoke from a cigar can be even more dangerous than that from cigarettes. The EPA has found that the output of carcinogenic particles from a cigar exceeds that of three cigarettes, and cigar smoke contains up to 30 times more carbon monoxide.

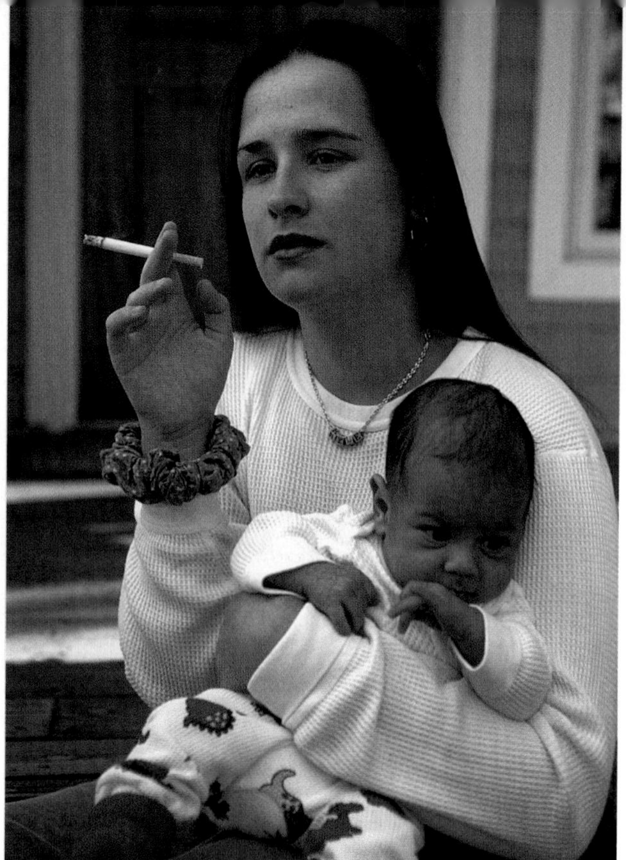

It is estimated that 19 million American infants and children are regularly exposed to environmental tobacco smoke. ETS can cause SIDS, trigger respiratory infections, cause or aggravate asthma, contribute to middle-ear infections, and impair development.

**ETS Effects** Studies show that up to 25% of nonsmokers subjected to ETS develop coughs, 30% develop headaches and nasal discomfort, and 70% suffer from eye irritation. Other symptoms range from breathlessness to sinus problems. People with allergies tend to suffer the most. The odor of tobacco smoke clings to skin and clothes—another unpleasant effect of ETS.

But ETS causes more than just annoyance and discomfort; it causes 3000 lung cancer deaths annually. People who live, work, or socialize among smokers face a 24–50% increase in lung cancer risk. ETS is also responsible for about 60,000 deaths from cardiovascular disease each year. Scientists have been able to measure changes that contribute to lung tissue damage and potential tumor promotion in the bloodstreams of healthy young test subjects who spend just 3 hours in a smoke-filled room. After just 30 minutes of exposure to ETS, the endothelial function in the coronary arteries of healthy nonsmokers is reduced to the same level as that of smokers. And nonsmokers can still be affected by the harmful effects of ETS hours after they have left a smoky environment. Carbon monoxide, for example, lingers in the bloodstream 5 hours later.

**Infants, Children, and ETS** ETS causes up to 18,600 cases of low birth weight each year and also significantly increases the risk for sudden infant death syndrome. Children under 5 whose primary caregiver smokes 10 or more cigarettes per day have measurable blood levels of nicotine and tobacco carcinogens. Chemicals in tobacco smoke also show up in breast milk, and breastfeeding may pass more chemicals to the infant of a smoking mother than direct exposure to ETS.

ETS triggers up to 300,000 cases of bronchitis, pneumonia, and other respiratory infections in infants and toddlers each year, resulting in up to 15,000 hospitalizations. ETS is a risk factor for asthma in children who have not previously displayed symptoms of the disease, and it aggravates the symptoms of the 200,000 to 1 million children who already have asthma. ETS is also linked to reduced lung function and fluid buildup in the middle ear, a contributing factor in middle-ear infections. Children and teens exposed to ETS score lower on tests of reading and reasoning. Later in life, people exposed to ETS as children are at increased risk for lung cancer, emphysema, and chronic bronchitis.

Why are infants and children so vulnerable? Because they breathe faster than adults, they inhale more air—and more of the pollutants in the air. Because they also weigh less, they inhale three times more pollutants per unit of body weight than adults do. And because their young lungs are still growing, this intake can impair optimal development. The problem is widespread: About 19 million American children are exposed to ETS.

**Avoiding ETS** Given the health risks of exposure to ETS, try these strategies to keep the air around you safe:

- *Speak up tactfully.* Smokers may not know the dangers they are causing or may not know it bothers you.
- *Display reminders.* Put up signs asking smokers to refrain in your home, work area, and car.
- *Don't allow smoking in your home or room.* Get rid of ashtrays and ask smokers to light up outside.
- *Open a window.* If you cannot avoid being in a room with a smoker, at least try to provide some ventilation.
- *Sit in the nonsmoking section in restaurants and other public areas.* Complain to the manager if none exists.
- *Fight for a smoke-free work environment.* Join with your coworkers to either eliminate all smoking indoors or confine it to certain areas.
- *Discuss quitting strategies.* Social pressure is a major factor in many former smokers' decisions to quit. Help the smokers in your life by sharing quitting strategies with them.

### Smoking and Pregnancy

Smoking almost doubles a pregnant woman's chance of having a miscarriage, and it significantly increases her risk of ectopic pregnancy. Maternal smoking causes an estimated 4600 infant deaths in the United States each year, primarily due to premature delivery and smoking-related problems with the placenta. Maternal smoking is a major factor in low birth weight, which puts newborns at high risk for infections and other serious problems. If a nonsmoking mother is regularly exposed to ETS, her infant is also at greater risk for low birth weight. Recent studies have also shown that babies whose mothers smoked during pregnancy had higher rates of colic, clubfoot, cleft lip and palate, and impaired lung function; they may also have genetic damage.

Babies born to mothers who smoke more than two packs a day perform poorly on developmental tests in the first hours after birth, compared to babies of nonsmoking mothers. Later in life, obesity, hyperactivity, short attention span, and lower scores on spelling and reading tests all occur more frequently in children whose mothers smoked during pregnancy than in those born to nonsmoking mothers. Prenatal tobacco exposure has also been associated with behavioral problems in children, including immaturity, emotional instability, physical aggression, and hyperactivity. Males born to smoking mothers have higher rates of adolescent and adult criminal activity, suggesting that maternal smoking may cause brain damage that increases the risk of criminal behavior.

### The Cost of Tobacco Use to Society

The health care costs associated with smoking exceed $75 billion per year. If the cost of lost productivity from sickness, disability, and premature death is included, the total is closer to $157 billion. This works out to $7.18 per pack of cigarettes, far more than the average $0.84 per pack tax collected by states to offset tobacco-related medical costs.

In order to recoup public health care expenditures, 43 state attorneys general filed suit against tobacco companies. In March 1997, Liggett Group settled its part of the suit by agreeing to turn over internal documents and to pay a portion of its profits to cover tobacco-related medical expenses and anti-smoking campaigns. In November 1998, an agreement was reached that settled 39 state lawsuits and applied to seven states that never filed suit. (Four states—Florida, Minnesota, Mississippi, and Texas—settled their suits separately for a total of $40 billion.) The 1998 Master Settlement Agreement (MSA) requires the tobacco companies to pay states $206 billion over 25 years; it also limits or bans certain types of advertising, promotions, and lobbying. In exchange, the tobacco industry settled the state lawsuits and is protected from future suits by states, counties, towns, and other public entities. Tobacco companies passed the costs of the settlement on to smokers. Although the bulk of the money states receive from the MSA is intended for tobacco control, many states are using most or all of the funds for other purposes.

## WHAT CAN BE DONE?

Every hour, 60 Americans die from preventable smoking-related diseases. Today there are more avenues than ever before for individual and group action against this major public health threat.

### Action at Many Levels

In recent years, thousands of local anti-smoking ordinances have been passed to restrict or ban smoking in schools, restaurants, stores, and workplaces. Many private employers, fearing worker's compensation claims based on exposure to workplace smoke, have banned smoking on the job. State legislatures have also passed many tough anti-tobacco laws. California has one of the most aggressive—and successful—programs, combining taxes on cigarettes, graphic advertisements, and bans on smoking in bars and restaurants. In the past decade, per-capita cigarette consumption fell by 50% in California, and lung cancer cases and heart disease deaths both declined.

**Terms**

**mainstream smoke** Smoke that is inhaled by a smoker and then exhaled into the atmosphere.

**sidestream smoke** Smoke that comes from the burning end of a cigarette, cigar, or pipe.

Vw

At the federal level, smoking has been banned on virtually all domestic airplane flights. The World Health Organization has taken the lead in international anti-tobacco efforts through sponsorship of World No-Tobacco Day and the Framework Convention on Tobacco Control (FCTC), an international treaty designed to improve tobacco control efforts worldwide. FCTC entered into force in February 2005; the United States signed the treaty in 2004 but it has not yet been ratified and written into U.S. law.

With their immensely profitable industry shrinking, tobacco companies have redirected marketing efforts toward minorities, the poor, and young women, populations among whom smoking rates are still high. Another controversial practice is that of pushing the export of cigarettes to developing nations. The need to exercise public pressure to keep the tobacco companies in check will persist.

### What You Can Do

When a smoker violates a no-smoking designation, complain. If your favorite restaurant or shop doesn't have a nonsmoking policy, ask the manager to adopt one. If you see children buying tobacco, report this illegal activity to the facility manager or the police. Learn more about addiction and tobacco cessation so you can better support the tobacco users you know. Vote for candidates who support anti-tobacco measures; contact local, state, and national representatives to express your views.

Cancel your subscriptions to magazines that carry tobacco advertising; send a letter to the publisher explaining your decision. Voice your opinion about other positive representations of tobacco use. (A recent study found that more than two-thirds of children's animated feature films have featured tobacco or alcohol use with no clear message that such practices were unhealthy.) Volunteer with the American Lung Association, the American Cancer Society, or the American Heart Association.

These are just some of the many ways in which individuals can help support tobacco prevention and stop-smoking efforts. Nonsmokers not only have the right to breathe clean air but also have the right to take action to help solve one of society's most serious public health threats.

## HOW A TOBACCO USER CAN QUIT

Since 1964, over 50% of all adults who have ever smoked have quit. Giving up tobacco is a long-term, intricate process. Tobacco users move through predictable stages—from being uninterested in stopping, to thinking about change, to making a concerted effort to stop, to finally maintaining abstinence. But most attempt to quit several times before they finally succeed. Relapse is a normal part of the process.

### The Benefits of Quitting

Giving up tobacco provides immediate health benefits to men and women of all ages (Table 8-5). The younger

**Table 8-5 Benefits of Quitting Smoking**

**Within 20 minutes of your last cigarette:**
- You stop polluting the air
- Blood pressure drops to normal
- Pulse rate drops to normal
- Temperature of hands and feet increases to normal

**8 hours:**
- Carbon monoxide level in blood drops to normal
- Oxygen level in blood increases to normal

**24 hours:**
- Chance of heart attack decreases

**48 hours:**
- Nerve endings start regrowing
- Ability to smell and taste is enhanced

**2–3 months:**
- Circulation improves
- Walking becomes easier
- Lung function increases up to 30%

**1–9 months:**
- Coughing, sinus congestion, fatigue, and shortness of breath all decrease

**1 year:**
- Heart disease death rate is half that of a smoker

**5 years:**
- Stroke risk drops nearly to the risk for nonsmokers

**10 years:**
- Lung cancer death rate drops to 50% of that of continuing smokers
- Incidence of other cancers (mouth, throat, larynx, esophagus, bladder, kidney, and pancreas) decreases
- Risk of ulcer decreases

**15 years:**
- Risk of lung cancer is about 25% of that of continuing smokers
- Risks of heart disease and death are close to those for nonsmokers

SOURCES: American Lung Association. 2002. *Benefits of Quitting* (http://www.lungusa.org/tobacco/quit_ben.html; retrieved November 25, 2002); American Cancer Society. 2000. *Quitting Smoking* (http://www.cancer.org/tobacco/quitting.html; retrieved July 10, 2000).

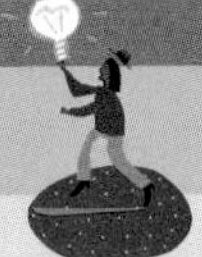

## Smoking Cessation Products

Critical Consumer

### Nicotine Replacement Therapy

As the name suggests, nicotine replacement therapy involves supplying the tobacco user with nicotine from a source other than standard tobacco products. This allows a user to overcome the psychological and behavioral aspects of a tobacco habit without simultaneously having to endure the physical symptoms of withdrawal. Although still harmful, nicotine replacement provides a cleaner form of nicotine. It avoids the thousands of poisons and tars that are found in burning tobacco and delivers a lower dose of nicotine than most smokers receive. After a few weeks or months of use, the reforming tobacco user begins to taper off use of the replacement, alleviating withdrawal symptoms.

There are several types of nicotine replacements, each with advantages and disadvantages. None of them are safe to use if the smoker plans to continue using tobacco; nicotine is a powerful stimulant, and an overdose can cause serious health complications. Studies have shown that combining nicotine replacement therapy with behavioral counseling can double the number of smokers who quit.

*Nicotine patches* can be purchased in varying strengths without a prescription. The patches release a controlled and steady supply of nicotine through the skin for 16 or 24 hours, depending on the type selected. Smokers often begin by using a full-strength patch and then switch to a weaker one to decrease the nicotine dosage. The most common side effects of the patch are skin irritation and redness, which can often be cleared up by switching to another brand.

Another nonprescription option is *nicotine gum.* When chewed, the gum releases nicotine that is absorbed through the mucous membranes of the mouth. Most users chew one or two pieces per hour. An advantage of the gum versus the patch is that it allows the user to control the nicotine doses, so that the smoker can chew more during a craving. Long-term dependence seems to be a problem for some gum users. Research has shown that 15–20% of gum users who successfully quit smoking continued using the gum for a year or longer, despite the recommended 6-month limit on use.

A new over-the-counter nicotine replacement product, the *nicotine lozenge* Commit, was approved by the FDA in 2002. The lozenge comes in two strengths and is designed to be taken for 12 weeks. Side effects may include nausea and heartburn.

*Nicotine nasal spray* and *nicotine inhalers* are available only by prescription. The nasal spray immediately relieves withdrawal symptoms by delivering nicotine to the bloodstream through the nose. The most common side effects are nasal irritation and sinus problems. Inhalers are plastic rods with a nicotine plug. When the smoker puffs on the rod, the plug produces a nicotine vapor that goes to the mouth instead of the lungs. A benefit of the inhaler is that it mimics hand and mouth actions of smoking.

### Non-Nicotine Medications

One of the most exciting developments in smoking cessation has been the use of bupropion (Zyban), a prescription antidepressant that affects neurotransmitters related to nicotine cravings. In one study of quitting success, 36% of nicotine patch users quit for at least the month, 49% of bupropion users quit, and 58% of users of both the patch and bupropion quit. Another study found that quitters who use bupropion tend to gain less weight than quitters who do not; an especially significant difference was seen among women. Bupropion has also been shown to be successful in helping even the most hardened smokers quit. If bupropion is not effective, there are two other drugs that may be prescribed, clonidine and nortriptyline; however, neither has been approved by the FDA specifically for nicotine dependence.

people are when they stop smoking, the more pronounced the health improvements. And these improvements gradually but invariably increase as the period of nonsmoking lengthens. It's never too late to quit, though. According to a U.S. Surgeon General's report, people who quit smoking, regardless of age, live longer than people who continue to smoke.

## Options for Quitting

Most tobacco users—76% in a recent survey—want to quit, and half of those who want to quit will make an attempt this year. What are their options? No single method works for everyone, but each does work for some people some of the time. Choosing to quit requires developing a strategy for success. Some people quit cold turkey, whereas others taper off slowly. There are over-the-counter and prescription products that help many people (see the box "Smoking Cessation Products" for more on these options). Behavioral factors that have been shown to increase the chances of a smoker's permanent smoking cessation are support from others and regular exercise. Support can come from friends and family and/or formal group programs sponsored by organizations such as the American Cancer Society, the American Lung Association, and the Seventh-Day Adventist Church or by your college health center or community hospital.

Free telephone quitlines are emerging as a popular and effective strategy to help stop smoking. Quitlines are staffed by trained counselors who help each caller plan a personal quitting strategy, usually including a combination of nicotine replacement therapy, changes in daily habits, and emotional support. In 2004, the Department of Health and Human Services established a national toll-free number, 1-800-QUITNOW (1-800-784-8669), to serve as a single access point for smokers seeking information and assistance in quitting.

Most smokers in the process of quitting experience both physical and psychological effects of nicotine withdrawal, and exercise can help with both. For many smokers, their tobacco use is associated with certain times and places—following a meal, for example. Resolving to walk after dinner instead of lighting up provides a distraction from cravings and eliminates the cues that trigger a desire to smoke. In addition, many people worry about weight gain associated with quitting. Although most ex-smokers do gain a few pounds, at least temporarily, incorporating exercise into a new tobacco-free routine lays the foundation for healthy weight management. The health risks of adding a few pounds are far outweighed by the risks of continued smoking; it's estimated that a smoker would have to gain 75–100 pounds to equal the health risks of smoking a pack a day.

As with any significant change in health-related behavior, giving up tobacco requires planning, sustained effort, and support. It is an ongoing process, not a one-time event. The Behavior Change Strategy describes the steps that successful quitters follow.

**Tips for Today**

Alcohol and tobacco cause far more injuries and deaths in the United States than any other drug. To achieve wellness, it's important to avoid tobacco use and ETS exposure and to use alcohol in moderation, if at all. If tobacco or alcohol use is a problem for you or someone you care about, there are many things you can do to improve the situation.

*Right now you can*

- Ask your roommates or friends if they know that binge drinking can be fatal; if they don't know, give them the facts about it; also share with them the information in this chapter about how to deal with an alcohol emergency.
- If you drink, plan ahead for the next party you attend, figuring out how you can limit yourself to one or two drinks.
- If you smoke, think about the next time you'll want a cigarette, such as while talking on the phone this afternoon or relaxing after dinner tonight. Visualize yourself enjoying this activity without a cigarette in your hand. Imagine yourself as a healthier, more robust person. See if you get pleasure or satisfaction from thinking of yourself as a nonsmoker, an ex-smoker, or someone liberated from dependence on cigarettes.
- If you use tobacco, go outside for a short walk or a stretch to limber up. Breathe deeply. Tell a friend you've just decided to quit.
- Resolve to talk to someone you know who uses tobacco, offering support and assistance if the person is interested in quitting.

## SUMMARY


- After being absorbed into the bloodstream in the stomach and small intestine, alcohol is transported throughout the body. If people drink more alcohol each hour than the body can metabolize, blood alcohol concentration (BAC) increases.
- Alcohol is a CNS depressant. At low doses, it tends to make people feel relaxed. At higher doses, alcohol interferes with motor and mental functioning; at very high doses, alcohol poisoning, coma, and death can occur.
- Alcohol use increases the risk of injury and violence; drinking before driving is particularly dangerous.
- Continued alcohol use has negative effects on the digestive and cardiovascular systems and increases cancer risk and overall mortality.
- Pregnant women who drink risk giving birth to children with a cluster of birth defects known as fetal alcohol syndrome (FAS). Even occasional drinking during pregnancy can cause brain injury in the fetus.
- Alcohol abuse involves drinking in dangerous situations or drinking to a degree that causes academic, professional, interpersonal, or legal difficulties.
- Alcohol dependence, or alcoholism, is characterized by more extensive problems with alcohol, usually involving tolerance and withdrawal.
- Binge drinking is a common form of alcohol abuse on college campuses that has negative effects on both drinking and nondrinking students.
- Physical consequences of alcoholism include the direct effects of tolerance and withdrawal, as well as all the problems associated with chronic drinking. Treatment approaches include mutual support groups like AA and pharmacological treatments.
- Smoking is the largest preventable cause of ill health and death in the United States. Regular tobacco use causes physical dependence on nicotine, characterized by loss of control, tolerance, and withdrawal.
- People who begin smoking are usually imitating others or responding to seductive advertising. Smoking is associated with low education level and the use of other drugs.
- Tobacco smoke is made up of hundreds of different chemicals, including some that are carcinogenic or poisonous or that damage the respiratory system.
- Nicotine acts on the nervous system as a stimulant or a depressant. It can cause blood pressure and heart rate to increase, straining the heart.
- Smoking causes cardiovascular disease, lung and other cancers, respiratory damage, and many other disorders. Tobacco use leads to lower life expectancy and to a diminished quality of life.
- The use of spit tobacco leads to nicotine addiction and is linked to oral cancers. Cigars, pipes, clove cigarettes, and bidis are not safe alternatives to cigarettes.

## Kicking the Tobacco Habit

You can look forward to a longer and healthier life if you join the 47 million Americans who have quit using tobacco. The steps for quitting described below are discussed in terms of the most popular tobacco product in the United States—cigarettes—but they can be adapted for all forms of tobacco.

### Gather Information

Collect personal smoking information in a detailed journal about your smoking behavior. Write down the time you smoke each cigarette of the day, the situation you are in, how you feel, where you smoke, and how strong your craving for the cigarette is, plus any other information that seems relevant. Part of the job is to identify patterns of smoking that are connected with routine situations (for example, the coffee break smoke, the after-dinner cigarette, the tension-reduction cigarette). Use this information to discover the behavior patterns involved in your smoking habit.

### Make the Decision to Quit

Choose a date in the near future when you expect to be relatively stress-free and can give quitting the energy and attention it will require. Don't choose a date right before or during finals week, for instance. Consider making quitting a gift: Choose your birthday as your quit date, for example, or make quitting a Father's Day or Mother's Day present. You might also want to coordinate your quit date with a buddy—a fellow tobacco user who wants to quit or a nonsmoker who wants to give up another bad habit or begin an exercise program. Tell your friends and family when you plan to quit. Ask them to offer encouragement and help hold you to your goal.

Decide what approach to quitting will work best for you. Will you go cold turkey, or will you taper off? Will you use nicotine patches or gum? Will you join a support group or enlist the help of a buddy? Prepare a contract for quitting, as discussed in Chapter 1. Set firm dates and rewards, and sign the contract. Post it in a prominent place.

### Prepare to Quit

One of the most important things you can do to prepare to quit is to develop and practice nonsmoking relaxation techniques. Many smokers find that they use cigarettes to help them unwind in tense situations or to relax at other times. If this is true for you, you'll need to find and develop effective substitutes. It takes time to become proficient at relaxation techniques, so begin practicing before your quit date. Refer to the detailed discussion of relaxation techniques in Chapter 2.

Other things you can do to help prepare for quitting include the following:

- Make an appointment to see your physician. Ask about OTC and prescription aids for tobacco cessation and whether one or more might be appropriate for you.
- Make a dentist's appointment to have your teeth cleaned the day after your target quit date.
- Start an easy exercise program, if you're not exercising regularly already.
- Buy some sugarless gum. Stock your kitchen with low-calorie snacks.
- Clean out your car, and air out your house. Send your clothes out for dry cleaning.
- Throw away all your cigarette-related paraphernalia (ashtrays, lighters, etc.).
- The night before your quit day, get rid of all your cigarettes. Have fun with this—get your friends or family to help you tear them up.
- Make your last few days of smoking inconvenient: Smoke only outdoors and when alone. Don't do anything else while you smoke.

### Quitting

Your first few days without cigarettes will probably be the most difficult. It's hard to give up such a strongly ingrained habit, but remember that millions of Americans have done it—and you can, too. Plan and rehearse the steps you will take when you experience a powerful craving. Avoid or control situations that you know from your journal are powerfully associated with your smoking. If your hands feel empty without a cigarette, try holding or fiddling with a small object such as a paper clip or pencil.

Social support can also be a big help. Arrange with a buddy to help you with your weak moments, and call him or her whenever you feel overwhelmed by an urge to smoke. Tell people you've just quit. You may discover many inspiring former smokers who can encourage you and reassure you that it's possible to quit and lead a happier, healthier life. Find a formal support group to join if you think it will help.

### Maintaining Nonsmoking

The lingering smoking urges that remain once you've quit should be carefully tracked and controlled because they can cause relapses if left unattended. Keep track of these urges in your journal to help you deal with them. If certain situations still trigger the urge for a cigarette, change something about the situation to break past associations. If stress or boredom causes strong smoking urges, use a relaxation technique, take a brisk walk, have a stick of gum, or substitute some other activity for smoking.

Don't set yourself up for a relapse. If you allow yourself to get overwhelmed at school or work or to gain weight, it will be easier to convince yourself that now isn't the right time to quit. This *is* the right time. Continue to practice time-management and relaxation techniques. Exercise regularly, eat sensibly, and get enough sleep. These habits will not only ensure your success at remaining tobacco-free but also serve you well in stressful times throughout your life. In fact, former smokers who have quit for at least 3 months report reduced stress levels, probably because quitting smoking lowers overall arousal.

Watch out for patterns of thinking that can make nonsmoking more difficult. Focus on the positive aspects of not smoking, and give yourself lots of praise—you deserve it. Stick with the schedule of rewards you developed for your contract.

Keep track of the emerging benefits that come from having quit. Items that might appear on your list include improved stamina, an increased sense of pride at having kicked a strong addiction, a sharper sense of taste and smell, no more smoker's cough, and so on. Keep track of the money you're saving by not smoking, and spend it on things you really enjoy. And if you do lapse, be gentle with yourself. Lapses are a normal part of quitting. Forgive yourself, and pick up where you left off.

- Environmental tobacco smoke (ETS) contains high concentrations of toxic chemicals and can cause lung cancer and heart disease. Children whose parents smoke are especially susceptible to respiratory diseases.
- Smoking during pregnancy increases the risk of miscarriage, stillbirth, congenital abnormalities, premature birth, and low birth weight. SIDS, behavior problems, and long-term impairments in development are also risks.
- Giving up smoking is a difficult and long-term process. Although most ex-smokers quit on their own, some smokers benefit from stop-smoking programs, OTC and prescription medications, and support groups.

## Take Action

1. **Interview peers:** Interview some of your fellow students about their drinking habits. How much do they drink, and how often? Are they more likely to drink on certain days or in certain circumstances? Are there any habits that seem to be common to most students? How do your own drinking habits compare to those of people you interviewed?

2. **Identify alcohol ads and points of sale in your community:** Look around your neighborhood and note the types of alcohol advertisements you find. How many are there, and what groups are being targeted—for example, young people, college students, or people of a particular ethnic group? Also identify where alcohol is sold: In what types of stores, and in how many locations? Is there a cluster of bars in a particular location? If you notice patterns that suggest marketing or sales targeted at particular groups, consider bringing your findings to the attention of community leaders.

3. **Interview successful quitters:** Interview one or two former tobacco users about their experiences with tobacco and the methods they used to quit. Why did they start smoking or using tobacco, how old were they when they started, and how long did their habit continue? What made them decide to quit? How did they quit? What could a current tobacco user learn from their experience of quitting?

## For More Information

### Books

Carr, A. 2005. *The Easy Way to Stop Smoking*. New York: Sterling. *A helpful guide to quitting.*

Gilman, S. L., ed. 2004. *Smoke: A Global History of Smoking*. London: Reaktion Books. *A look at smoking and its effects, including history and issues related to culture, art, and gender.*

Kinney, J., and G. Leaton. 2006. *Loosening the Grip: A Handbook of Alcohol Information*, 8th ed. New York: McGraw-Hill. *A fascinating book about alcohol, including information on physical effects, abuse, alcoholism, and cultural aspects of alcohol use.*

Wechsler, H., and B. Wuethrich. 2003. *Dying to Drink: Confronting Binge Drinking on College Campuses*. Emmaus, Pa.: Rodale. *An in-depth review of the problem of binge drinking that lays out solutions for students, schools, parents, and communities; written by the lead researcher of the College Alcohol Study.*

Zailckas, K. 2005. *Smashed: Story of a Drunken Girlhood*. New York: Viking. *A 24-year-old writes about her own experiences of drinking through high school and college; also includes information from surveys and research into the effects of alcohol use.*

### Organizations, Hotlines, and Web Sites

*Al-Anon Family Group Headquarters.* Provides information and referrals to local Al-Anon and Alateen groups. The Web site includes a self-quiz to determine if you are affected by someone's drinking.
888-4AL-ANON
http://www.al-anon.alateen.org

*Alcoholics Anonymous (AA) World Services.* Provides general information on AA, literature on alcoholism, and information about AA meetings and related 12-step organizations.
212-870-3400
http://www.alcoholics-anonymous.org

*Alcohol Treatment Referral Hotline.* Provides referrals to local intervention and treatment providers.
800-ALCOHOL

*American Cancer Society (ACS).* Sponsor of the annual Great American Smokeout; provides information on the dangers of tobacco, as well as tools for prevention and cessation for both smokers and users of spit tobacco.
800-ACS-2345
http://www.cancer.org

*American Lung Association.* Provides information on lung diseases, tobacco control, and environmental health.
800-LUNG-USA; 212-315-8700
http://www.lungusa.org

*CDC's Tobacco Information and Prevention Source (TIPS).* Provides research results, educational materials, and tips on how to quit smoking.
800-CDC-1311
http://www.cdc.gov/tobacco

*The College Alcohol Study. Harvard School of Public Health.* Provides information about and results from the recent studies of binge drinking on college campuses.
http://www.hsph.harvard.edu/cas

*College Drinking Prevention: Students.* Includes information about alcohol, including myths about alcohol use and an interactive look at how alcohol affects the body.
http://www.collegedrinkingprevention.gov/students

*HadEnough.Org.* Provides information and a self-quiz on binge drinking among college students.
http://www.hadenough.org

*National Association for Children of Alcoholics (NACoA).* Provides information and support for children of alcoholics.
888-554-COAS
http://www.nacoa.net

*National Clearinghouse for Alcohol and Drug Information/ Prevention Online.* Provides statistics and information on alcohol abuse, including resources for people who want to help friends and family members overcome alcohol-abuse problems.

800-729-6686

http://www.health.org

*National Institute on Alcohol Abuse and Alcoholism (NIAAA).* Provides booklets and other publications on a variety of alcohol-related topics, including fetal alcohol syndrome, alcoholism treatment, and alcohol use and minorities.

http://www.drugabuse.gov

*Quitnet.* Provides interactive tools and questionnaires, support groups, a library, news on tobacco issues, and quitting programs for both smokers and spit tobacco users.

http://www.quitnet.com

*Smokefree.Gov.* Provides step-by-step strategies for quitting as well as expert support via telephone or instant messaging.

http://www.smokefree.gov

1-800-QUITNOW

http://www.cancer.gov (additional information)

*World Health Organization Tobacco Free Initiative.* Promotes the goal of a tobacco-free world.

http://www.who.int/tobacco/en

See also the listings for Chapter 9.

## Selected Bibliography


Anthonisen, N. R., et al. 2005. The effects of a smoking cessation intervention on 14.5-year mortality: A randomized clinical trial. *Annals of Internal Medicine* 142(4): 233–239.

Campaign for Tobacco-Free Kids. 2004. *State Cigarette Excise Tax Rates and Rankings* (http://tobaccofreekids.org/research/factsheets/pdf/0097.pdf; retrieved December 19, 2004).

Centers for Disease Control and Prevention. 2004. Alcohol-attributable deaths and years of potential life lost, United States, 2001. *Morbidity and Mortality Weekly Report* 53(37): 866–870.

Centers for Disease Control and Prevention. 2004. Smoking during pregnancy—United States, 1990–2002. *Morbidity and Mortality Weekly Report* 53(39): 911–915.

Dawson, D. A., et al. 2005. Recovery from DSM-IV alcohol dependence: United States, 2001–2002. *Addiction* 100(3): 281–292.

de la Chica, R. A., et al. 2005. Chromosomal instability in amniocytes from fetuses of mothers who smoke. *Journal of the American Medical Association* 293(10): 1212–1222.

Distefan, J. M., J. P. Pierce, and E. A. Gilpin. 2004. Do favorite movie stars influence adolescent smoking initiation? *American Journal of Public Health* 94(7): 1239–1244.

Doll, R., et al. 2004. Mortality in relation to smoking: 50 years' observations on male British doctors. *British Medical Journal* 328(7455): 1519.

Gades, N. M., et al. 2005. Association between smoking and erectile dysfunction: a population-based study. *American Journal of Epidemiology* 161(4): 346–351.

Giovino, G. A., et al. 2004. Epidemiology of menthol cigarette use. *Nicotine & Tobacco Research* 6(Suppl 1): S67–S81.

Grant, B., et al. 2004. The 12-month prevalence and trends in DSM-IV alcohol abuse and dependence: United States, 1991–1992 and 2001–2002. *Drug and Alcohol Dependence* 74(3): 223–234.

Hanaoka, T., et al. 2005. Active and passive smoking and breast cancer risk in middle-aged Japanese women. *International Journal of Cancer* 114(2): 317–322.

Harvard College Alcohol Study. 2005. *Binge Drinking on Campus Lower in States with Fewer Adult Binge Drinkers and Stronger Alcohol Control Laws* (http://www.hsph.harvard.edu/cas/Documents/state/state_pr.html; retrieved March 14, 2005).

Henschke, C. I., and O. S. Miettinen. 2004. Women's susceptibility to tobacco carcinogens. *Lung Cancer* 43(1): 1–5.

Hingson, R., et al. 2005. Magnitude of alcohol-related mortality and morbidity among U.S. college students ages 18–24. *Annual Review of Public Health* 26: 259–279.

Jacobson, S. W., et al. 2004. Maternal age, alcohol abuse history, and quality of parenting as moderators of the effects of prenatal alcohol exposure on 7.5-year intellectual function. *Alcoholism: Clinical and Experimental Research* 28(11): 1732–1745.

McCarty, C. A., et al. 2004. Continuity of binge and harmful drinking from late adolescence to early adulthood. *Pediatrics* 114(3): 714–719.

Meyerhoff, D. J., et al. 2004. Effects of heavy drinking, binge drinking, and family history of alcoholism on regional brain metabolites. *Alcoholism: Clinical and Experimental Research* 28(4): 650–651.

Monti, P. M., et al. 2005. Adolescence: Booze, brains, and behavior. *Alcohol: Clinical and Experimental Research* 29(2): 207–220.

Mukamal, K. J., et al. 2005. Alcohol and risk for ischemic stroke in men: The role of drinking patterns and usual beverage. *Annals of Internal Medicine* 142(1): 11–19.

National Cancer Institute. 2004. *The Truth About "Light" Cigarettes: Questions and Answers* (http://cis.nci.nih.gov/fact/3_74.htm; retrieved September 3, 2004).

National Institute on Alcohol Abuse and Alcoholism. 2005. *2001–2002 Survey Finds That Many Recover from Alcoholism; Researchers Identify Factors Associated with Abstinent and Non-Abstinent Recovery* (http://www.niaaa.nih.gov/press/2005/Recovery.htm; retrieved March 14, 2005).

National Institute on Alcohol Abuse and Alcoholism. 2004. *Alcohol—An Important Women's Health Issue.* Alcohol Alert No. 62. Bethesda, Md.: National Institute on Alcohol Abuse and Alcoholism.

Nelson, T. F., et al. 2005. The state sets the rate: The relationship of college binge drinking to state binge drinking rates and selected state alcohol control policies. *American Journal of Public Health* 95(3): 441–446.

Office of Applied Studies, Substance Abuse and Mental Health Services Administration. 2004. *National Survey on Drug Use and Health* (http://oas.samhsa.gov/nhsda.htm; retrieved December 6, 2004).

Pletcher, M. J., et al. 2005. Alcohol consumption, binge drinking, and early coronary calcification: Findings from the coronary artery risk development in young adults (CARDIA) study. *American Journal of Epidemiology* 161(5): 423–433.

Shiffman, S., M. E. Di Marino, and J. L. Pillitteri. 2005. The effectiveness of nicotine patch and nicotine lozenge in very heavy smokers. *Journal of Substance Abuse Treatment* 28(1): 49–55.

Slutske, W. S. 2005. Alcohol use disorders among US college students and their non-college-attending peers. *Archives of General Psychiatry* 62(3): 321–327.

Vineis, P., et al. 2005. Environmental tobacco smoke and risk of respiratory cancer and chronic obstructive pulmonary disease in former smokers and never smokers in the EPIC prospective study. *British Medical Journal* 330(7486): 277.

Weitzman, E. R. 2004. Poor mental health, depression, and associations with alcohol consumption, harm and abuse in a national sample of young adults in college. *Journal of Nervous and Mental Disease* 192(4): 269–277.

Yolton, K., et al. 2005. Exposure to environmental tobacco smoke and cognitive abilities among U.S. children and adolescents. *Environmental Health Perspectives* 113(1): 98–103.

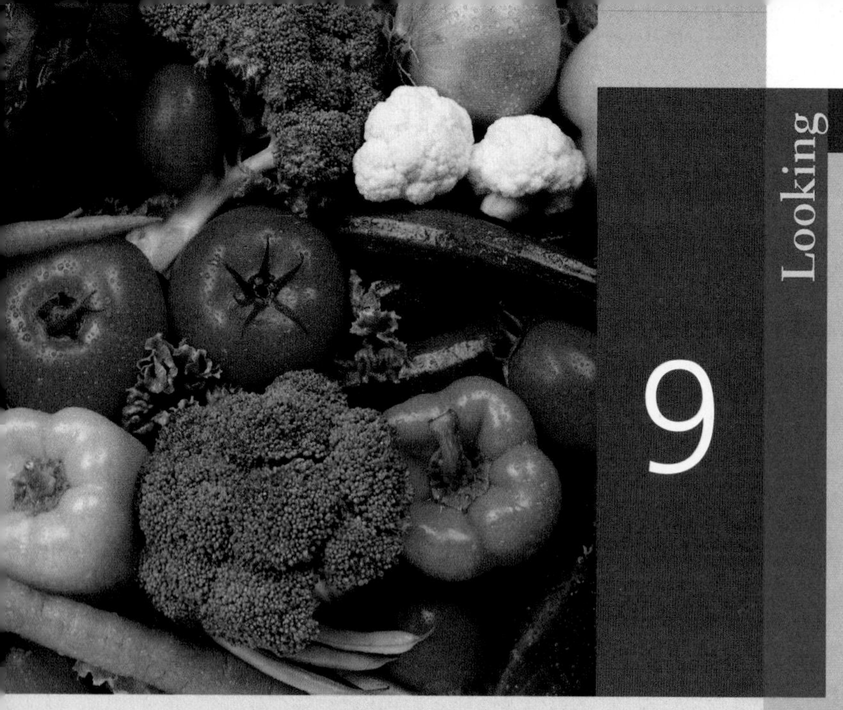

# 9

## Looking AHEAD

After reading this chapter, you should be able to

- List the essential nutrients, and describe the functions they perform in the body
- Describe the guidelines that have been developed to help people choose a healthy diet, avoid nutritional deficiencies, and reduce their risk of diet-related chronic diseases
- Discuss nutritional guidelines for vegetarians and for special population groups
- Explain how to use food labels and other consumer tools to make informed choices about foods
- Put together a personal nutrition plan based on affordable foods that you enjoy and that will promote wellness, today as well as in the future

# Nutrition Basics

In your lifetime, you'll spend about 6 years eating—about 70,000 meals and 60 tons of food. What you choose to eat can have profound effects on your health and well-being. Of particular concern is the connection between lifetime nutritional habits and the risk of major chronic diseases, including heart disease, cancer, stroke, and diabetes. Choosing foods that provide adequate amounts of the nutrients you need while limiting the substances linked to disease should be an important part of your daily life. The food choices you make will significantly influence your health—both now and in the future.

This chapter provides the basic principles of **nutrition.** It introduces the six classes of essential nutrients, explaining their roles in the functioning of the body. It also provides different sets of guidelines that you can use to design a healthy diet plan. Finally, it offers practical tools and advice to help you apply the guidelines to your own life. Diet is an area of your life in which you have almost total control. Using your knowledge and understanding of nutrition to create a healthy diet plan is a significant step toward wellness.

## NUTRITIONAL REQUIREMENTS: COMPONENTS OF A HEALTHY DIET

When you think about your diet, you probably do so in terms of the foods you like to eat—a turkey sandwich and a glass of milk or black beans and rice. What's important for your health, though, are the nutrients contained in those foods. Your body requires proteins, fats, carbohydrates, vitamins, minerals, and water—about 45 **essential nutrients.** The word *essential* in this context means that you must get these substances from food because your body is unable to manufacture them at all, or at least not fast enough to meet your physiological needs. Your body obtains these nutrients through the process of **digestion,** in which the foods you eat are broken down into compounds your gastrointestinal tract can absorb and your body can use (Figure 9-1).

The energy in foods is expressed as **kilocalories.** One kilocalorie represents the amount of heat it takes to raise the temperature of 1 liter of water 1°C. A person needs about 2000 kilocalories per day to meet his or her energy needs. In common usage, people usually refer to kilocalories as *calories,* which is technically a much smaller energy unit: (1 kilocalorie contains 1000 calories). We use the familiar word *calorie* in this chapter to stand for the larger energy unit; you'll also find the word *calorie* on food labels.

Of the six classes of essential nutrients, three supply energy:

- Fat = 9 calories per gram
- Protein = 4 calories per gram
- Carbohydrate = 4 calories per gram

(Alcohol, although it is not an essential nutrient, also supplies energy, providing 7 calories per gram.) The high caloric content of fat is one reason experts often advise

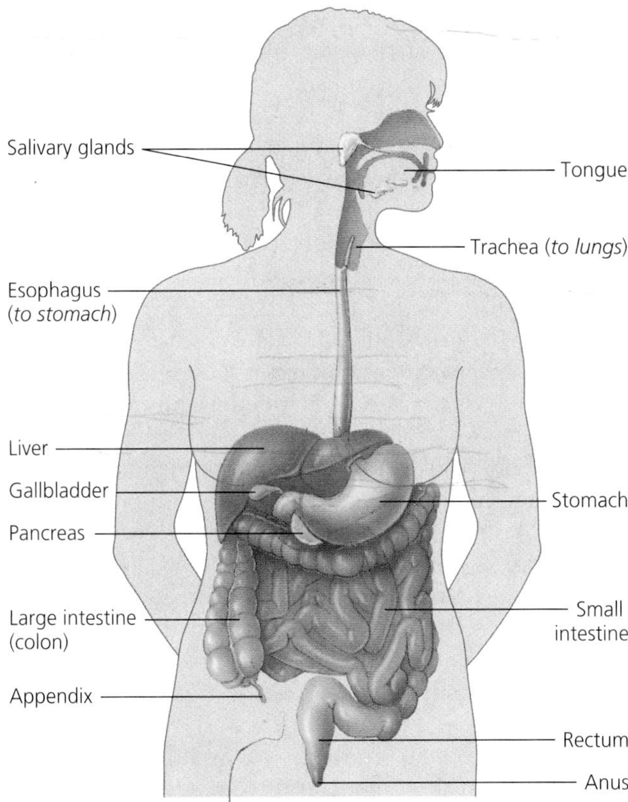


**Figure 9-1 The digestive system.** Food is partially broken down by being chewed and mixed with saliva in the mouth. After traveling to the stomach via the esophagus, food is broken down further by stomach acids. As food moves through the digestive tract, it is mixed by muscular contractions and broken down by chemicals. Most absorption of nutrients occurs in the small intestine, aided by secretions from the pancreas, gallbladder, and intestinal lining. The large intestine reabsorbs excess water; the remaining solid wastes are collected in the rectum and excreted through the anus.

against high fat consumption; most of us do not need the extra calories to meet energy needs. Regardless of their source, calories consumed in excess of energy needs are converted to fat and stored in the body.

But just meeting energy needs is not enough; our bodies require adequate amounts of all the essential nutrients to grow and function properly.

## Proteins—The Basis of Body Structure

**Proteins** form important parts of the body's main structural components: muscles and bones. Proteins also form important parts of blood, enzymes, some hormones, and cell membranes. As mentioned above, proteins can provide energy (4 calories per gram) for the body.

**Amino Acids** The building blocks of proteins are called **amino acids.** Twenty common amino acids are found in food; nine of these are essential: histidine, isoleucine, leucine, lysine, methionine, phenylalanine, threonine, tryptophan, and valine. The other eleven amino acids can be produced by the body, given the presence of the needed components supplied by foods.

**Complete and Incomplete Proteins** Individual protein sources are considered *complete* if they supply all the essential amino acids in adequate amounts and *incomplete* if they do not. Meat, fish, poultry, eggs, milk, cheese, and soy provide complete proteins. Incomplete proteins, which come from other plant sources such as **legumes** and nuts, are good sources of most essential amino acids but are usually low in one or two.

Certain combinations of vegetable proteins, such as wheat and peanuts in a peanut butter sandwich, allow each vegetable protein to make up for the amino acids missing in the other protein. The combination yields a complete protein. Many traditional food pairings, such as beans and rice or corn and beans, emerged as dietary staples because they are complementary proteins. Proteins consumed throughout the course of the day can complement each other to form a pool of amino acids the body can draw from to produce the necessary proteins. About two-thirds of the protein in the American diet comes from animal sources (red meat and milk); therefore, the American diet is rich in essential amino acids.

**Recommended Protein Intake** Adequate daily intake of protein for adults is 0.8 gram per kilogram (0.36 gram per pound) of body weight, corresponding to 50 grams of protein per day for someone who weighs 140 pounds and 65 grams of protein for someone who weighs 180 pounds. This amount of protein is easily obtained from popular foods: 3 ounces of lean meat, poultry, or fish or ½ cup of tofu contains about 20–25 grams of protein; 1 cup of dry beans (legumes such as pinto and kidney beans), 15–20 grams; 1 cup of milk or yogurt or 1½ ounces of cheese, 8–12 grams; and

### Terms

V W

**nutrition** The science of food and how the body uses it in health and disease.

**essential nutrients** Substances the body must get from foods because it cannot manufacture them at all or fast enough to meet its needs. These nutrients include proteins, fats, carbohydrates, vitamins, minerals, and water.

**digestion** The process of breaking down foods in the gastrointestinal tract into compounds the body can absorb.

**kilocalorie** A measure of energy content in food; 1 kilocalorie represents the amount of heat needed to raise the temperature of 1 liter of water 1°C; commonly referred to as *calorie.*

**protein** An essential nutrient; a compound made of amino acids that contain carbon, hydrogen, oxygen, and nitrogen.

**amino acids** The building blocks of proteins.

**legumes** Vegetables such as peas and beans that are high in fiber and are also important sources of protein.

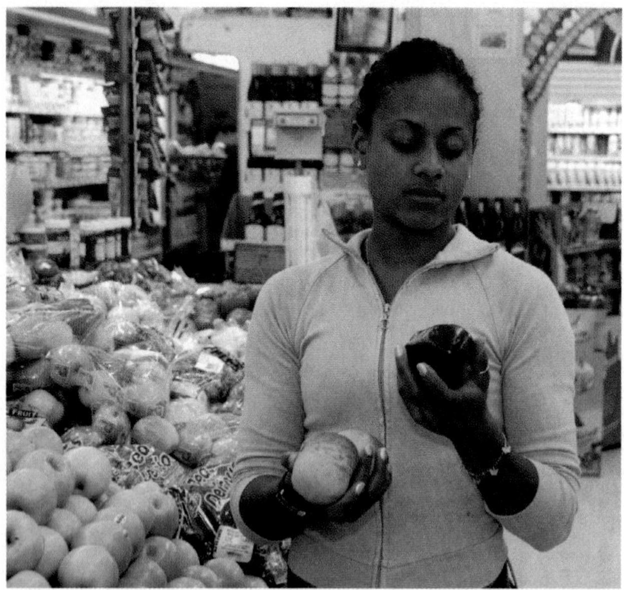

Our bodies require adequate amounts of all essential nutrients—water, proteins, carbohydrates, fats, vitamins, and minerals—in order to grow and function properly. Choosing foods to satisfy these nutritional requirements is an important part of a healthy lifestyle.

cereals, grains, nuts, and vegetables, about 2–4 grams of protein per serving.

Most Americans meet or exceed the protein intake needed for adequate nutrition. Protein consumed beyond what the body needs is synthesized into fat for energy storage or burned for energy requirements. Consuming somewhat above daily needs is not harmful, but it can contribute fat to the diet because protein-rich foods are often fat-rich as well. A very high protein intake can also strain the kidneys. A fairly broad range of protein intakes is associated with good health, and the Food and Nutrition Board recommends that the amount of protein adults eat should fall within the range of 10–35% of total daily calorie intake. The average American diet includes about 15–16% of total daily calories as protein.

## Fats—Essential in Small Amounts

Fats, also known as *lipids,* are the most concentrated source of energy, at 9 calories per gram. The fats stored in your body represent usable energy, they help insulate your body, and they support and cushion your organs. Fats in the diet help your body absorb fat-soluble vitamins, as well as add important flavor and texture to foods. Fats are the major fuel for the body during rest and light activity. Two fats, linoleic acid and alpha-linolenic acid, are essential components of the diet.

**Types and Sources of Fats** Most of the fats in food are in the form of triglycerides, which are composed of a glycerol molecule (an alcohol) plus three fatty acids. A fatty acid is made up of a chain of carbon atoms with oxygen attached at one end and hydrogen atoms attached along the length of the chain. Fatty acids differ in the length of their carbon atom chains and in their degree of saturation (the number of hydrogens attached to the chain). If every available bond from each carbon atom in a fatty acid chain is attached to a hydrogen atom, the fatty acid is said to be **saturated.** If not all the available bonds are taken up by hydrogens, the carbon atoms in the chain will form double bonds with each other. Such fatty acids are called *unsaturated fats*. If there is only one double bond, the fatty acid is called **monounsaturated.** If there are two or more double bonds, the fatty acid is called **polyunsaturated.** The essential fatty acids, linoleic and alpha-linolenic acids, are both polyunsaturated. The different types of fatty acids have different characteristics and different effects on your health.

Food fats are usually composed of both saturated and unsaturated fatty acids; the dominant type of fatty acid determines the fat's characteristics. Food fats containing large amounts of saturated fatty acids are usually solid at room temperature; they are generally found naturally in animal products. The leading sources of saturated fat in the American diet are red meats (hamburger, steak, roasts), whole milk, cheese, hot dogs, and lunch meats. Food fats containing large amounts of unsaturated fatty acids are usually from plant sources and are liquid at room temperature. Olive, canola, safflower, and peanut oils contain mostly monounsaturated fatty acids. Soybean, corn, and cottonseed oils contain mostly polyunsaturated fatty acids.

There are notable exceptions to these generalizations. When unsaturated vegetable oils undergo the process of **hydrogenation,** a mixture of saturated and unsaturated fatty acids is produced. Hydrogenation turns many of the double bonds in unsaturated fatty acids into single bonds, increasing the degree of saturation and producing a more solid fat from a liquid oil. Hydrogenation also changes some unsaturated fatty acids to **trans fatty acids,** unsaturated fatty acids with an atypical shape that affects their behavior in the body. Food manufacturers use hydrogenation to increase the stability of an oil so it can be reused for deep frying, to improve the texture and extend the shelf life of certain foods, and to transform a liquid oil into margarine or vegetable shortening.

Leading sources of trans fats in the American diet are deep-fried fast foods such as french fries and fried chicken (typically fried in vegetable shortening rather than oil); baked and snack foods such as pot pies, cakes, cookies, pastries, doughnuts, and chips; and stick margarine. In general, the more solid a hydrogenated oil is, the more saturated and trans fats it contains; for example, stick margarines typically contain more saturated and trans fats than do tub or squeeze margarines. Small amounts of trans fatty acids are found naturally in meat and milk.

Hydrogenated vegetable oils are not the only plant fats that contain saturated fats. Palm and coconut oils, although derived from plants, are also highly saturated. However, fish oils, derived from an animal source, are rich in polyunsaturated fats.

**Fats and Health** Different types of fats have very different effects on health. Many studies have examined the effects of dietary fat intake on blood **cholesterol** levels and the risk of heart disease. Saturated and trans fatty acids raise blood levels of **low-density lipoprotein (LDL),** or "bad" cholesterol, thereby increasing a person's risk of heart disease. Unsaturated fatty acids lower LDL. Monounsaturated fatty acids, such as those found in olive and canola oils, may also increase levels of **high-density lipoproteins (HDL),** or "good" cholesterol, providing even greater benefits for heart health. In large amounts, trans fatty acids may lower HDL. Thus, to reduce the risk of heart disease, it is important to choose unsaturated fats instead of saturated and trans fats. (See Chapter 12 for more on cholesterol and a heart-healthy diet.)

Most Americans consume more saturated fat than trans fat (12% versus 2–4% of total daily calories). However, health experts are particularly concerned about trans fats because of their double negative effect on heart health—they both raise LDL and lower HDL—and because there is less public awareness of trans fats. The saturated fat content of prepared foods has been listed on nutrition labels since 1994. By January 2006, food labels will also include trans fat content. Until that time consumers can check for the presence of trans fats by examining the ingredient list of a food: If a food contains partially hydrogenated oil or vegetable shortening, it contains trans fat.

Although saturated and trans fats pose health hazards, other fats can be beneficial. When used in place of saturated fats, monounsaturated fatty acids, as found in avocados, most nuts, and olive, canola, peanut, and safflower oils, improve cholesterol levels and may help protect against some cancers. **Omega-3 fatty acids,** a form of polyunsaturated fat found primarily in fish, may be even more healthful. Omega-3s and the compounds the body makes from them have a number of heart-healthy effects; and nutritionists recommend that Americans increase the proportion of omega-3s in their diet by eating fish two or more times a week. Salmon, tuna, trout, mackerel, herring, sardines, and anchovies are all good sources of omega-3s; lesser amounts are found in plant sources, including dark-green leafy vegetables; walnuts; flaxseeds; and canola, walnut, and flaxseed oils.

Most of the polyunsaturated fats currently consumed by Americans are omega-6s, primarily from corn oil and soybean oil. Foods rich in omega-6s are important because they contain the essential nutrient linoleic acid. However, some nutritionists recommend that people reduce the proportion of omega-6s they consume in favor of omega-3s. To make this adjustment, use canola oil rather than corn oil in cooking, and check for corn, soybean, or cottonseed oil in products such as mayonnaise, margarine, and salad dressing.

In addition to its effects on heart disease risk, dietary fat can affect health in other ways. Diets high in fatty red meat are associated with an increased risk of certain forms of cancer, especially colon cancer. A high-fat diet can also make weight management more difficult. Because fat is a concentrated source of calories (9 calories per gram versus 4 calories per gram for protein and carbohydrate), a high-fat diet is often a high-calorie diet that can lead to weight gain. In addition, there is some evidence that calories from fat are more easily converted to body fat than calories from protein or carbohydrate.

Although more research is needed on the precise effects of different types and amounts of fat on overall health, a great deal of evidence points to the fact that most people benefit from keeping their overall fat intake at recommended levels and choosing unsaturated fats instead of saturated and trans fats. The types of fatty acids and their effects on health are summarized in Figure 9-2.

**Recommended Fat Intake** To meet the body's demand for essential fats, adult men need about 17 grams per day of linoleic acid and 1.6 grams per day of alpha-linolenic acid; adult women need 12 grams of linoleic acid and 1.1 grams of alpha-linolenic acid. Only 3–4 teaspoons

### Terms

**saturated fat** A fat with no carbon-carbon double bonds; usually solid at room temperature.

**monounsaturated fat** A fat with one carbon-carbon double bond; liquid at room temperature.

**polyunsaturated fat** A fat containing two or more carbon-carbon double bonds; liquid at room temperature.

**hydrogenation** A process by which hydrogens are added to unsaturated fats, increasing the degree of saturation and turning liquid oils into solid fats. Hydrogenation produces a mixture of saturated fatty acids and standard and trans forms of unsaturated fatty acids.

**trans fatty acid** A type of unsaturated fatty acid produced during the process of hydrogenation; trans fats have an atypical shape that affects their chemical activity.

**cholesterol** A waxy substance found in the blood and cells and needed for synthesis of cell membranes, vitamin D, and hormones.

**low-density lipoprotein (LDL)** Blood fat that transports cholesterol to organs and tissues; excess amounts result in the accumulation of deposits on artery walls.

**high-density lipoprotein (HDL)** Blood fat that helps transport cholesterol out of the arteries, thereby protecting against heart disease.

**omega-3 fatty acids** Polyunsaturated fatty acids commonly found in fish oils that are beneficial to cardiovascular health; the endmost double bond occurs three carbons from the end of the fatty acid chain.

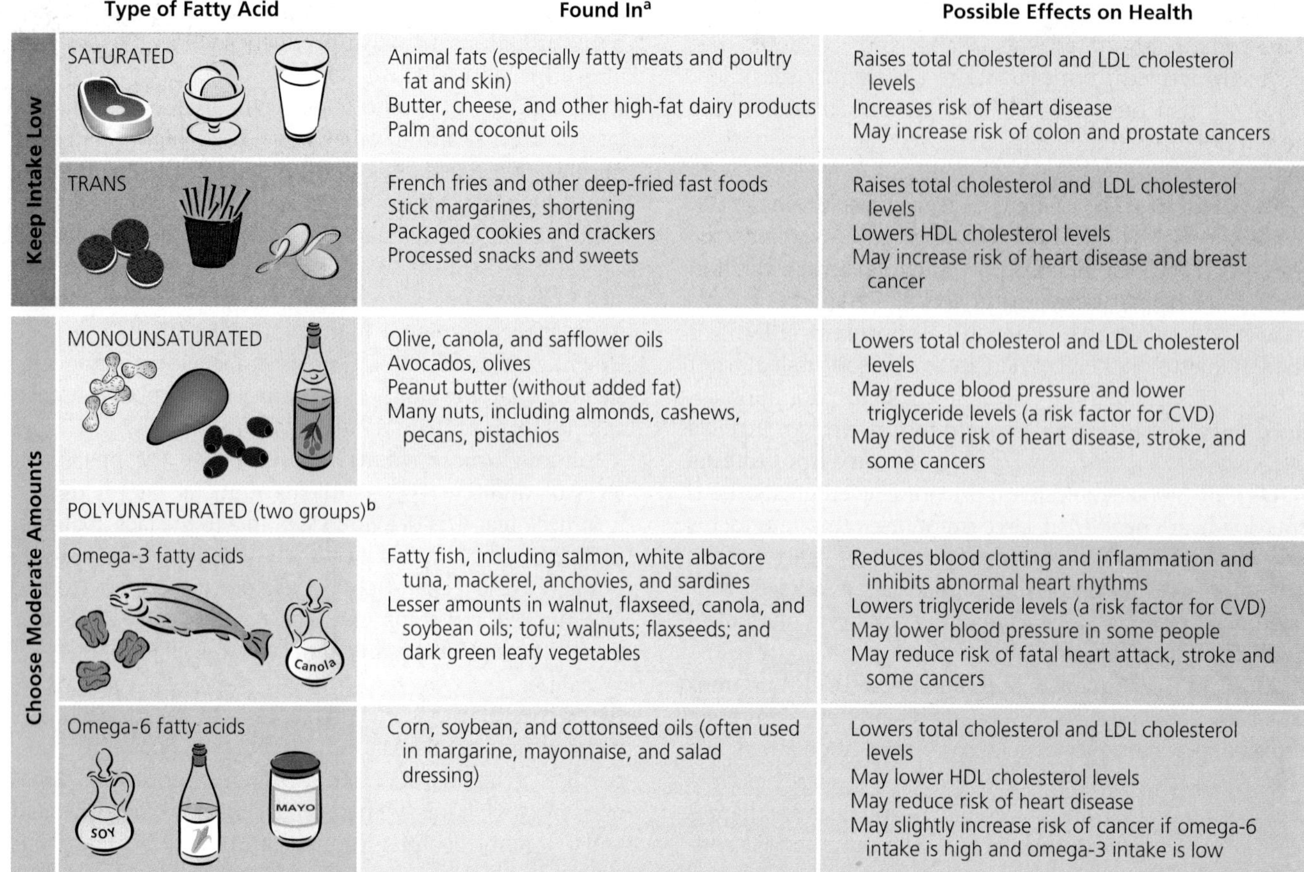

| | Type of Fatty Acid | Found In[a] | Possible Effects on Health |
|---|---|---|---|
| Keep Intake Low | SATURATED | Animal fats (especially fatty meats and poultry fat and skin)<br>Butter, cheese, and other high-fat dairy products<br>Palm and coconut oils | Raises total cholesterol and LDL cholesterol levels<br>Increases risk of heart disease<br>May increase risk of colon and prostate cancers |
| | TRANS | French fries and other deep-fried fast foods<br>Stick margarines, shortening<br>Packaged cookies and crackers<br>Processed snacks and sweets | Raises total cholesterol and LDL cholesterol levels<br>Lowers HDL cholesterol levels<br>May increase risk of heart disease and breast cancer |
| Choose Moderate Amounts | MONOUNSATURATED | Olive, canola, and safflower oils<br>Avocados, olives<br>Peanut butter (without added fat)<br>Many nuts, including almonds, cashews, pecans, pistachios | Lowers total cholesterol and LDL cholesterol levels<br>May reduce blood pressure and lower triglyceride levels (a risk factor for CVD)<br>May reduce risk of heart disease, stroke, and some cancers |
| | POLYUNSATURATED (two groups)[b] | | |
| | Omega-3 fatty acids | Fatty fish, including salmon, white albacore tuna, mackerel, anchovies, and sardines<br>Lesser amounts in walnut, flaxseed, canola, and soybean oils; tofu; walnuts; flaxseeds; and dark green leafy vegetables | Reduces blood clotting and inflammation and inhibits abnormal heart rhythms<br>Lowers triglyceride levels (a risk factor for CVD)<br>May lower blood pressure in some people<br>May reduce risk of fatal heart attack, stroke and some cancers |
| | Omega-6 fatty acids | Corn, soybean, and cottonseed oils (often used in margarine, mayonnaise, and salad dressing) | Lowers total cholesterol and LDL cholesterol levels<br>May lower HDL cholesterol levels<br>May reduce risk of heart disease<br>May slightly increase risk of cancer if omega-6 intake is high and omega-3 intake is low |



[a] Food fats contain a combination of types of fatty acids in various proportions; for example, canola oil is composed mainly of monounsaturated fatty acids (62%) but also contains polyunsaturated (32%) and saturated (6%) fatty acids. Food fats are categorized here according to their predominant fatty acid.

[b] The essential fatty acids are polyunsaturated: Linoleic acid is an omega-6 fatty acid and alpha-linolenic acid is an omega-3 fatty acid.

**Figure 9-2 Types of fatty acids and their possible effects on health.** The health effects of dietary fats are still being investigated. In general, nutritionists recommend that we consume a diet moderate in fat overall and that we choose unsaturated fats instead of saturated and trans fats. Monounsaturated fats and omega-3 polyunsaturated fats may be particularly good choices for promoting health. Eating lots of fat of any type can provide excess calories because all types of fats are rich sources of energy (9 calories per gram).

(15–20 grams) of vegetable oil per day incorporated into your diet will supply the essential fats. Most Americans consume sufficient amounts of the essential fats; limiting unhealthy fats is a much greater health concern.

Limits for total fat, saturated fat, and trans fat intake have been set by a number of government and research organizations. In 2002, the Food and Nutrition Board of the Institute of Medicine released recommendations for the balance of energy sources in a healthful diet. These new recommendations, called Acceptable Macronutrient Distribution Ranges (AMDRs), are based on ensuring adequate intake of essential nutrients while also reducing the risk of chronic diseases such as heart disease and cancer. As with protein, a range of levels of fat consumption is associated with good health; the AMDR for total fat is 20–35% of total calories. Although more difficult for consumers to monitor, AMDRs have also been set for omega-6 fatty acids (5–10%) and omega-3 fatty acids (0.6–1.2%) as part of total fats intake. Because any amount of saturated and trans fats increases the risk of heart disease, the Food and Nutrition Board recommends that saturated fat and trans fat intake be kept as low as possible; most fat in a healthy diet should be unsaturated.

For advice on setting individual intake goals, see the box "Setting Intake Goals for Protein, Fat, and Carbohydrate." To determine how close you are to meeting your personal intake goals for fat, keep a running total over the course of the day. For prepared foods, food labels list the number of grams of fat, protein, and carbohydrate; the breakdown for popular fast-food items can be found in the Appendix. Nutrition information is also available in many grocery stores, in inexpensive published nutrition guides, and online. For most Americans, meeting recommendations for fat intake means lowering intake of saturated and trans fats and maintaining total fat intake within the healthy range. You can still eat high-fat foods, but it makes good sense to limit the size of your portions and to balance your intake with low-fat foods.

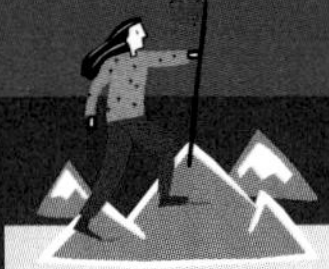

Take Charge

## Setting Intake Goals for Protein, Fat, and Carbohydrate

Goals have been established by the Food and Nutrition Board to help ensure adequate intake of the essential amino acids, fatty acids, and carbohydrate. The daily goals for adequate intake for adults are as follow:

| | Men | Women |
|---|---|---|
| Protein | 56 grams | 46 grams |
| Fat: Linoleic acid | 17 grams | 12 grams |
| Alpha-linolenic acid | 1.6 grams | 1.1 grams |
| Carbohydrate | 130 grams | 130 grams |

Protein intake goals can be calculated more specifically by multiplying your body weight in kilograms by 0.8 or your body weight in pounds by 0.36. (Refer to the Nutrition Resources section at the end of the chapter for information for specific age groups and life stages.)

To meet your daily energy needs, you need to consume more than the minimally adequate amounts of the energy-providing nutrients listed above, which alone supply only about 800–900 calories. The Food and Nutrition Board provides additional guidance in the form of Acceptable Macronutrient Distribution Ranges (AMDRs). The ranges can help you balance your intake of the energy-providing nutrients in ways that ensure adequate intake while reducing the risk of chronic disease. The AMDRs for protein, total fat, and carbohydrate are as follow:

| | |
|---|---|
| Protein | 10–35% of total daily calories |
| Total fat | 20–35% of total daily calories |
| Carbohydrate | 45–65% of total daily calories |

To set individual goals, begin by estimating your total daily energy (calorie) needs; if your weight is stable, your current energy intake is the number of calories you need to maintain your weight at your current activity level. Next, select percentage goals for protein, fat, and carbohydrate. You can allocate your total daily calories among the three classes of macronutrients to suit your preferences; just make sure that the three percentages you select total 100% and that you meet the minimum intake goals listed. Two samples reflecting different total energy intake and nutrient intake goals are shown in the table below.

To translate your own percentage goals into daily intake goals expressed in calories and grams, multiply the appropriate percentages by total calorie intake and then divide the results by the corresponding calories per gram. For example, a fat limit of 35% applied to a 2200-calorie diet would be calculated as follows: 0.35 × 2200 = 770 calories of total fat; 770 ÷ 9 calories per gram = 86 grams of total fat. (Remember that, fat has 9 calories per gram and that protein and carbohydrate have 4 calories per gram.)

**Two Sample Macronutrient Distributions**

| | | Sample 1 | | Sample 2 | |
|---|---|---|---|---|---|
| Nutrient | AMDR | Individual Goals | Amounts for a 1600-Calorie Diet | Individual Goals | Amounts for a 2800-Calorie Diet |
| Protein | 10–35% | 15% | 240 calories = 60 grams | 30% | 840 calories = 210 grams |
| Fat | 20–35% | 30% | 480 calories = 53 grams | 25% | 700 calories = 78 grams |
| Carbohydrate | 45–65% | 55% | 880 calories = 220 grams | 45% | 1260 calories = 315 grams |

SOURCE: Food and Nutrition Board, Institute of Medicine, National Academies. 2002. *Dietary Reference Intakes: Applications in Dietary Planning,* Washington, D.C.: National Academies Press. © 2003 by the National Academy of Sciences. Reprinted with permission from the National Academies Press, Washington, D.C.

## Carbohydrates—An Ideal Source of Energy

**Carbohydrates** are needed in the diet primarily to supply energy for body cells. Some cells, such as those found in the brain and other parts of the nervous system and in blood, use only carbohydrates for fuel. During high-intensity exercise, muscles also use primarily carbohydrates for fuel.

**Simple and Complex Carbohydrates** Carbohydrates are classified into two groups: simple and complex. Simple carbohydrates contain only one or two sugar units in each molecule; they include sucrose (table sugar), fructose (fruit sugar, honey), maltose (malt sugar), and lactose (milk sugar). Simple carbohydrates provide much of the sweetness in foods and are found naturally in fruits and milk and are added to soft drinks, fruit drinks, candy, and sweet desserts. There is no evidence that any type of simple sugar is more nutritious than others.

**Term**

**carbohydrate** An essential nutrient; sugars, starches, and dietary fiber are all carbohydrates.

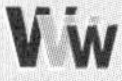

Complex carbohydrates consist of chains of many sugar molecules; they include starches and most types of dietary fiber. Starches are found in a variety of plants, especially grains (wheat, rye, rice, oats, barley, millet), legumes (dry beans, peas, and lentils), and tubers (potatoes and yams). Most other vegetables contain a mixture of starches and simple carbohydrates. Fiber, discussed in the next section, is found in grains, fruits, and vegetables.

During digestion, your body breaks down starches and double sugars into single sugar molecules, such as **glucose,** for absorption. Once glucose is in the bloodstream, the pancreas releases the hormone insulin, which allows cells to take up glucose and use it for energy. The liver and muscles also take up glucose to provide carbohydrate storage in the form of **glycogen.** Some people have problems controlling blood glucose levels, a disorder called diabetes mellitus (see Chapter 10).

**Refined Carbohydrates Versus Whole Grains** Complex carbohydrates can be further divided between refined, or processed, carbohydrates and unrefined carbohydrates, or whole grains. Before they are processed, all grains are **whole grains,** consisting of an inner layer, germ; a middle layer, the endosperm; and an outer layer, bran. During processing, the germ and bran are often removed, leaving just the starchy endosperm. The refinement of whole grains transforms whole-wheat flour to white flour, brown rice to white rice, and so on.

Refined carbohydrates usually retain all the calories of their unrefined counterparts, but they tend to be much lower in fiber, vitamins, minerals, and other beneficial compounds. Unrefined carbohydrates tend to take longer to chew and digest than refined ones; they also enter the bloodstream more slowly. This slower digestive pace tends to make people feel full sooner and for a longer period. Also, a slower rise in blood glucose levels following consumption of complex carbohydrates may help in the management of diabetes. Whole grains are also high in dietary fiber and so have all the benefits of fiber. Consumption of whole grains has been linked to a reduced risk of heart disease, diabetes, high blood pressure, stroke, and certain forms of cancer. For all these reasons, whole grains are recommended over those that have been refined. See the box "Choosing More Whole-Grain Foods" for tips on increasing your intake of whole grains.

**Glycemic Index and Glycemic Response** Insulin and glucose levels rise and fall following a meal or snack containing any type of carbohydrate. Some foods cause a quick and dramatic rise in glucose and insulin levels; others have a slower, more moderate effect. A food that has a strong effect on blood glucose levels is said to have a high **glycemic index.** Some studies have found that consuming a meal containing high glycemic index foods may increase appetite, and that over the long term, diets rich in these foods may increase risk of diabetes and heart disease for some people. High glycemic index foods do not, as some popular diets claim, directly cause weight gain beyond the calories they contain.

Attempting to base food choices on glycemic index can be a difficult task, however. Although unrefined complex carbohydrates and high-fiber foods generally tend to have a low glycemic index, patterns are less clear for other types of foods and do not follow a easy distinction such as that of simple versus complex carbohydrates. For example, some fruits with fairly high levels of simple carbohydrates have only a moderate effect on blood glucose levels, whereas white rice, potatoes, and white bread, which are rich in complex carbohydrates, have a high glycemic index. The body's response to carbohydrates also depends on many other factors, such as how foods are combined and prepared and the fitness status of the individual.

This complexity is one reason major health organizations have not issued specific guidelines for glycemic index. For people with particular health concerns, glycemic index may be an important consideration; however, it should not be the sole criterion for food choices. For example, ice cream has a lower glycemic index than brown rice or carrots—but that doesn't make it a healthier choice overall. Remember that most unrefined grains, fruits, vegetables, and legumes are rich in nutrients, have a relatively low energy density, and have low-to-moderate glycemic index. Choose a variety of vegetables daily, and avoid heavy consumption of white potatoes. Limit foods that are high in added sugars but provide few other nutrients. Some studies have singled out regular soda, with its large dose of rapidly absorbable sugar, as specifically linked to increased diabetes risk.

**Recommended Carbohydrate Intake** On average, Americans consume 200–300 grams of carbohydrate per day, well above the 130 grams needed to meet the body's requirement for essential carbohydrate. A range of intakes is associated with good health, and experts recommend that adults consume 45–65% of total daily calories as carbohydrate, about 225–325 grams of carbohydrate for someone consuming 2000 calories per day. The focus should be on consuming a variety of foods rich in complex carbohydrates, especially whole grains.

Although the Food and Nutrition Board set an AMDR for added sugars of 25% or less of total daily calories, many health experts recommend an even lower intake. World Health Organization guidelines suggest a limit of 10% of total daily calories from added sugars; limits set by the USDA in 2005 are even lower, with a maximum of about 8 teaspoons (32 grams) suggested for someone consuming 2000 calories per day. Foods high in added sugar are generally high in calories and low in nutrients and fiber, thus providing empty calories. To reduce your intake of added sugars, limit soft drinks, candy, sweet

Take Charge

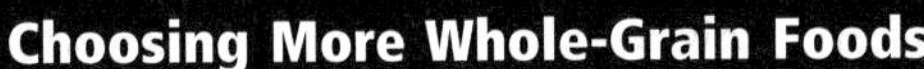

## Choosing More Whole-Grain Foods

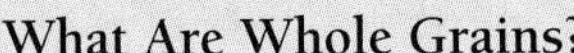

### What Are Whole Grains?

The first step in increasing your intake of whole grains is to correctly identify them. The following are whole grains:

| | |
|---|---|
| whole wheat | whole-grain corn |
| whole rye | popcorn |
| whole oats | brown rice |
| oatmeal | whole-grain barley |

More unusual choices include bulgur (cracked wheat), millet, kasha (roasted buckwheat kernels), quinoa, wheat and rye berries, amaranth, wild rice, graham flour, whole-grain kamut, whole-grain spelt, and whole-grain triticale.

Wheat flour, unbleached flour, enriched flour, and degerminated corn meal are not whole grains. Wheat germ and wheat bran are also not whole grains, but they are the constituents of wheat typically left out when wheat is processed and so are healthier choices than regular wheat flour, which typically contains just the endosperm.

### Reading Food Packages to Find Whole Grains

To find packaged foods rich in whole grains, read the list of ingredients and check for special health claims related to whole grains. The *first* item on the list of ingredients should be one of the whole grains listed above. In addition, the FDA allows manufacturers to include special health claims for foods that contain 51% or more whole-grain ingredients. Such products may contain a statement such as the following on their packaging: "Rich in whole grain," "Made with 100% whole grain," or "Diets rich in whole-grain foods may help reduce the risk of heart disease and certain cancers." However, many whole-grain products will not carry such claims.

### Incorporating Whole Grains into Your Daily Diet

- *Bread:* Look for sandwich breads, bagels, English muffins, buns, and pita breads with a whole grain listed as the first ingredient.
- *Breakfast cereals:* Check the ingredient list for whole grains. Whole-grain choices include oatmeal, muesli, shredded wheat, and some types of raisin bran, bran flakes, wheat flakes, toasted oats, and granola.
- *Rice:* Choose brown rice or rice blends that include brown rice.
- *Pasta:* Look for whole-wheat, whole-grain kamut, or whole-grain spelt pasta.
- *Tortillas:* Choose whole-wheat or whole-corn tortillas.
- *Crackers and snacks:* Some varieties of crackers are made from whole grains, including some flatbreads or crispbreads, woven wheat crackers, and rye crackers. Other whole-grain snack possibilities include popcorn, popcorn cakes, brown rice cakes, whole-corn tortilla chips, and whole-wheat fig cookies. Be sure to check food labels for fat content, as many popular snacks are high in fat.
- *Mixed-grain dishes:* Combine whole grains with other foods to create healthy mixed dishes such as tabouli; soups made with hulled barley or wheat berries; and pilafs, casseroles, and salads made with brown rice, whole-wheat couscous, kasha, millet, wheat bulgur, or quinoa.

If your grocery store doesn't carry all of these items, try your local health food store.

desserts, and sweetened fruit drinks. The simple carbohydrates in your diet should come mainly from fruits, which are excellent sources of vitamins and minerals, and from low-fat or fat-free milk and other dairy products, which are high in protein and calcium.

## Fiber—A Closer Look

*Fiber* is the term given to nondigestible carbohydrates provided by plants. Instead of being digested, like starch, fiber passes through the intestinal tract and provides bulk for feces in the large intestine, which in turn facilitates elimination. In the large intestine, some types of fiber are broken down by bacteria into acids and gases, which explains why consuming too much fiber can lead to intestinal gas. Because humans cannot digest fiber, it is not a source of carbohydrate in the diet; however, the consumption of fiber is necessary for good health.

**Types of Fiber** The Food and Nutrition Board has defined two types of fiber: dietary fiber and functional fiber. **Dietary fiber** refers to the nondigestible carbohydrates (and the noncarbohydrate substance lignin) that are present

### Terms

**glucose** A simple sugar that is the body's basic fuel.

**glycogen** An animal starch stored in the liver and muscles.

**whole grain** The entire edible portion of a grain such as wheat, rice, or oats, consisting of the germ, endosperm, and bran. During milling or processing, parts of the grain are removed, often leaving just the endosperm.

**glycemic index** A measure of how the ingestion of a particular food affects blood glucose levels.

**dietary fiber** Nondigestible carbohydrates and lignin that are intact in plants.

naturally in plants such as grains, legumes, and vegetables. **Functional fiber** refers to nondigestible carbohydrates that have been either isolated from natural sources or synthesized in a lab and then added to a food product or dietary supplement. **Total fiber** is the sum of dietary and functional fiber.

Fibers have different properties that lead to different physiological effects in the body. For example, viscous fibers such as those found in oat bran or legumes can delay stomach emptying, slow the movement of glucose into the blood after eating, and reduce absorption of cholesterol. Other types of fiber, such as those found in wheat bran or psyllium seed, increase fecal bulk and help prevent constipation, hemorrhoids, and **diverticulitis.** A diet high in fiber can help reduce the risk of type 2 diabetes and heart disease as well as improve gastrointestinal health. Some studies have linked high-fiber diets with reduced risk of colon and rectal cancer; other studies have suggested that other characteristics of diets rich in fruits, vegetables, and whole grains may be responsible for this reduction in risk.

**Sources of Fiber** All plant foods contain some dietary fiber. Fruits, legumes, oats (especially oat bran), and barley all contain the viscous types of fiber that help lower blood glucose and cholesterol levels. Wheat (especially wheat bran), other grains and cereals, and vegetables are good sources of cellulose and other fibers that help prevent constipation. Psyllium, which is often added to cereals or used in fiber supplements and laxatives, improves intestinal health and also helps control glucose and cholesterol levels. The processing of packaged foods can remove fiber, so it is important to rely on fresh fruits and vegetables and foods made from whole grains as your main sources of fiber.

**Recommended Fiber Intake** To reduce the risk of chronic disease and maintain intestinal health, the Food and Nutrition Board recommends a daily fiber intake of 38 grams for adult men and 25 grams for adult women. Americans currently consume about half this amount. Fiber should come from foods, not supplements, which should be used only under medical supervision. To increase the amount of fiber in your daily diet to recommended levels, try the following strategies:

- Choose whole-grain foods instead of those made from processed grains. Select high-fiber breakfast cereals (those with 5 or more grams of fiber per serving).
- Eat whole, unpeeled fruits rather than drinking fruit juice. Top cereals, yogurt, and desserts with berries, unpeeled apple slices, or other fruit.
- Include legumes in soups and salads. Combine raw vegetables with pasta, rice, or beans in salads.
- Substitute bean dip for cheese-based or sour cream–based dips or spreads. Use raw vegetables rather than chips for dipping.

## Vitamins—Organic Micronutrients

**Vitamins** are organic (carbon-containing) substances required in small amounts to regulate various processes within living cells (Table 9-1). Humans need 13 vitamins; 4 are fat-soluble (A, D, E, and K), and 9 are water-soluble (C, and the 8 B-complex vitamins: thiamin, riboflavin, niacin, vitamin B-6, folate, vitamin B-12, biotin, and pantothenic acid).

**Functions of Vitamins** Many vitamins help chemical reactions take place. They provide no energy to the body directly but help unleash the energy stored in carbohydrates, proteins, and fats. Vitamins are critical in the production of red blood cells and the maintenance of the nervous, skeletal, and immune systems. Some vitamins act as **antioxidants,** which help preserve healthy cells in the body. Key vitamin antioxidants include vitamin E, vitamin C, and the vitamin A precursor beta-carotene. (Antioxidants are described later in the chapter.)

**Sources of Vitamins** The human body does not manufacture most of the vitamins it requires and must obtain them from foods. Vitamins are abundant in fruits, vegetables, and grains. In addition, many processed foods, such as flour and breakfast cereals, contain added vitamins. A few vitamins are made in certain parts of the body: The skin makes vitamin D when it is exposed to sunlight, and intestinal bacteria make vitamin K.

**Vitamin Deficiencies and Excesses** If your diet lacks sufficient amounts of a particular vitamin, characteristic symptoms of deficiency develop (see Table 9-1.) For example, vitamin A deficiency can cause blindness, and vitamin B-6 deficiency can cause seizures. Vitamin deficiency diseases are most often seen in developing countries; they are relatively rare in the United States

### Terms

Ww

**functional fiber** Nondigestible carbohydrates either isolated from natural sources or synthesized; these may be added to foods and dietary supplements.

**total fiber** The total amount of dietary fiber and functional fiber in the diet.

**diverticulitis** A digestive disorder in which abnormal pouches form in the walls of the intestine and become inflamed.

**vitamins** Carbon-containing substances needed in small amounts to help promote and regulate chemical reactions and processes in the body.

**antioxidant** A substance that can lessen the breakdown of food or body constituents by free radicals; actions include binding oxygen, donating electrons to free radicals, and repairing damage to molecules.

## Table 9-1 Facts About Vitamins

| Vitamin | Important Dietary Sources | Major Functions | Signs of Prolonged Deficiency | Toxic Effects of Megadoses |
|---|---|---|---|---|
| **Fat-Soluble** | | | | |
| Vitamin A | Liver, milk, butter, cheese, and fortified margarine; carrots, spinach, and other orange and deep-green vegetables and fruits | Maintenance of vision, skin, linings of the nose, mouth, digestive and urinary tracts, immune function | Night blindness; dry, scaling skin; increased susceptibility to infection; loss of appetite; anemia; kidney stones | Liver damage, miscarriage and birth defects, headache, vomiting and diarrhea, vertigo, double vision, bone abnormalities |
| Vitamin D | Fortified milk and margarine, fish oils, butter, egg yolks (sunlight on skin also produces vitamin D) | Development and maintenance of bones and teeth, promotion of calcium absorption | Rickets (bone deformities) in children; bone softening, loss, and fractures in adults | Kidney damage, calcium deposits in soft tissues, depression, death |
| Vitamin E | Vegetable oils, whole grains, nuts and seeds, green leafy vegetables, asparagus, peaches | Protection and maintenance of cellular membranes | Red blood cell breakage and anemia, weakness, neurological problems, muscle cramps | Relatively nontoxic, but may cause excess bleeding or formation of blood clots |
| Vitamin K | Green leafy vegetables; smaller amounts widespread in other foods | Production of factors essential for blood clotting and bone metabolism | Hemorrhaging | None reported |
| **Water-Soluble** | | | | |
| Biotin | Cereals, yeast, egg yolks, soy flour, liver; widespread in foods | Synthesis of fat, glycogen, and amino acids | Rash, nausea, vomiting, weight loss, depression, fatigue, hair loss | None reported |
| Folate | Green leafy vegetables, yeast, oranges, whole grains, legumes, liver | Amino acid metabolism, synthesis of RNA and DNA, new cell synthesis | Anemia, weakness, fatigue, irritability, shortness of breath, swollen tongue | Masking of vitamin B-12 deficiency |
| Niacin | Eggs, poultry, fish, milk, whole grains, nuts, enriched breads and cereals, meats, legumes | Conversion of carbohydrates, fats, and protein into usable forms of energy | Pellagra (symptoms include diarrhea, dermatitis, inflammation of mucous membranes, dementia) | Flushing of the skin, nausea, vomiting, diarrhea, liver dysfunction, glucose intolerance |
| Pantothenic acid | Animal foods, whole grains, broccoli, potatoes; widespread in foods | Metabolism of fats, carbohydrates, and proteins | Fatigue, numbness and tingling of hands and feet, gastrointestinal disturbances | None reported |
| Riboflavin | Dairy products, enriched breads and cereals, lean meats, poultry, fish, green vegetables | Energy metabolism; maintenance of skin, mucous membranes, and nervous system structures | Cracks at corners of mouth, sore throat, skin rash, hypersensitivity to light, purple tongue | None reported |
| Thiamin | Whole-grain and enriched breads and cereals, organ meats, lean pork, nuts, legumes | Conversion of carbohydrates into usable forms of energy, maintenance of appetite and nervous system function | Beriberi (symptoms include muscle wasting, mental confusion, anorexia, enlarged heart, nerve changes) | None reported |
| Vitamin B-6 | Eggs, poultry, fish, whole grains, nuts, soybeans, liver, kidney, pork | Metabolism of amino acids and glycogen | Anemia, convulsions, cracks at corners of mouth, dermatitis, nausea, confusion | Neurological abnormalities and damage |
| Vitamin B-12 | Meat, fish, poultry, fortified cereals | Synthesis of blood cells; other metabolic reactions | Anemia, fatigue, nervous system damage, sore tongue | None reported |
| Vitamin C | Peppers, broccoli, spinach, brussels sprouts, citrus fruits, strawberries, tomatoes, potatoes, cabbage, other fruits and vegetables | Maintenance and repair of connective tissue, bones, teeth, and cartilage; promotion of healing; aid in iron absorption | Scurvy, anemia, reduced resistance to infection, loosened teeth, joint pain, poor wound healing, hair loss, poor iron absorption | Urinary stones in some people, acid stomach from ingesting supplements in pill form, nausea, diarrhea, headache, fatigue |

SOURCES: Food and Nutrition Board, Institute of Medicine, National Academies. 2001. *Dietary Reference Intakes Tables* (http://www.iom.edu/file.asp?id=21372; retrieved December 21, 2004). The complete Dietary Reference Intake reports are available from the National Academy Press (http://www.nap.edu); Shils, M. E., et al., eds. 1998. *Modern Nutrition in Health and Disease,* 9th ed. Baltimore: Williams & Wilkins.

because vitamins are readily available from our food supply. However, intakes below recommended levels can have adverse effects on health even if they are not low enough to cause a deficiency disease. For example, low intake of folate and vitamins B-6 and B-12 has been linked to increased heart disease risk.

Extra vitamins in the diet can also be harmful, especially when taken as supplements. High doses of vitamin A are toxic and increase the risk of birth defects, for example. Even when vitamins are not taken in excess, relying on supplements for an adequate intake of vitamins can be a problem. There are many substances in foods other than vitamins and minerals, and some of these compounds may have important health effects. Later in the chapter we discuss specific recommendations for vitamin intake and when a vitamin supplement is advisable. For now, keep in mind that it's best to obtain most of your vitamins from foods rather than supplements.

## Minerals—Inorganic Micronutrients

**Minerals** are inorganic (non–carbon-containing) elements you need in relatively small amounts to help regulate body functions, aid in the growth and maintenance of body tissues, and help release energy (Table 9-2). There are about 17 essential minerals. The major minerals, those that the body needs in amounts exceeding 100 milligrams per day, include calcium, phosphorus, magnesium, sodium, potassium, and chloride. The essential trace minerals, those that you need in minute amounts, include copper, fluoride, iodide, iron, selenium, and zinc.

Characteristic symptoms develop if an essential mineral is consumed in a quantity too small or too large for good health. The minerals commonly lacking in the American diet are iron, calcium, potassium, and magnesium. Focus on good food choices for these (see Table 9-2). Lean meats are rich in iron, whereas low-fat or fat-free dairy products are excellent choices for calcium. Potassium is found in leafy green vegetables, white and sweet potatoes, bananas, and other fruits and vegetables. Plant foods such as whole grains and leafy vegetables are good sources of magnesium. Iron-deficiency **anemia** is a problem in many age groups, and researchers fear poor calcium intakes are sowing the seeds for future **osteoporosis,** especially in women. See Chapter 14 for more information on osteoporosis; the box "Eating for Healthy Bones" has tips for building and maintaining bone density.

### Terms

VW

**minerals** Inorganic compounds needed in relatively small amounts for regulation, growth, and maintenance of body tissues and functions.

**anemia** A deficiency in the oxygen-carrying material in the red blood cells.

**osteoporosis** A condition in which the bones become extremely thin and brittle and break easily.

**free radical** An electron-seeking compound that can react with fats, proteins, and DNA, damaging cell membranes and mutating genes in its search for electrons; produced through chemical reactions in the body and by exposure to environmental factors such as sunlight and tobacco smoke.

## Water—Vital but Often Ignored

Water is the major component in both foods and the human body: You are composed of about 50–60% water. Your need for other nutrients, in terms of weight, is much less than your need for water. You can live up to 50 days without food, but only a few days without water. Water is distributed all over the body, among lean and other tissues and in blood and other body fluids. Water is used in the digestion and absorption of food and is the medium in which most of the chemical reactions take place within the body. Some water-based fluids, like blood, transport substances around the body, whereas other fluids serve as lubricants or cushions. Water also helps regulate body temperature.

Water is contained in almost all foods, particularly in liquids, fruits, and vegetables. The foods and fluids you consume provide 80–90% of your daily water intake; the remainder is generated through metabolism. You lose water each day in urine, feces, and sweat and through evaporation from your lungs.

Most people can maintain a healthy water balance by consuming beverages at meals and drinking fluids in response to thirst. Water and other beverages typically make up about 80% of your fluid intake; the remainder comes from foods, especially fruits and vegetables. In 2004, the Food and Nutrition Board set levels of adequate water intake to maintain hydration; all fluids, including those containing caffeine, can count toward your total daily fluid intake. Under these guidelines, men need to consume about 3.7 total liters of water, with 3.0 liters (about 13 cups) coming from beverages; women need 2.7 total liters, with 2.2 liters (about 9 cups) coming from beverages (see Table 1 in the Nutrition Resources section at the end of the chapter). If you exercise vigorously or live in a hot climate, you need to consume additional fluids to maintain a balance between water consumed and water lost.

## Other Substances in Food

Many substances in food are not essential nutrients but may influence health.

**Antioxidants** When the body uses oxygen or breaks down certain fats or proteins as a normal part of metabolism, it gives rise to substances called **free radicals.** Environmental factors such as cigarette smoke, exhaust

## Table 9-2 Facts About Selected Minerals

| Mineral | Important Dietary Sources | Major Functions | Signs of Prolonged Deficiency | Toxic Effects of Megadoses |
|---|---|---|---|---|
| Calcium | Milk and milk products, tofu, fortified orange juice and bread, green leafy vegetables, bones in fish | Formation of bones and teeth, control of nerve impulses, muscle contraction, blood clotting | Stunted growth in children, bone mineral loss in adults; urinary stones | Kidney stones, calcium deposits in soft tissues, inhibition of mineral absorption, constipation |
| Fluoride | Fluoridated water, tea, marine fish eaten with bones | Maintenance of tooth and bone structure | Higher frequency of tooth decay | Increased bone density, mottling of teeth, impaired kidney function |
| Iodine | Iodized salt, seafood, processed foods | Essential part of thyroid hormones, regulation of body metabolism | Goiter (enlarged thyroid), cretinism (birth defect) | Depression of thyroid activity, hyperthyroidism in susceptible people |
| Iron | Meat and poultry, fortified grain products, dark green vegetables, dried fruit | Component of hemoglobin, myoglobin, and enzymes | Iron-deficiency anemia, weakness, impaired immune function, gastrointestinal distress | Nausea, diarrhea, liver and kidney damage, joint pains, sterility, disruption of cardiac function, death |
| Magnesium | Widespread in foods and water (except soft water); especially found in grains, legumes, nuts, seeds, green vegetables, milk | Transmission of nerve impulses, energy transfer, activation of many enzymes | Neurological disturbances, cardiovascular problems, kidney disorders, nausea, growth failure in children | Nausea, vomiting, diarrhea, central nervous system depression, coma; death in people with impaired kidney function |
| Phosphorus | Present in nearly all foods, especially milk, cereal, peas, eggs, meat | Bone growth and maintenance, energy transfer in cells | Impaired growth, weakness, kidney disorders, cardiorespiratory and nervous system dysfunction | Drop in blood calcium levels, calcium deposits in soft tissues, bone loss |
| Potassium | Meats, milk, fruits, vegetables, grains, legumes | Nerve function and body water balance | Muscular weakness, nausea, drowsiness, paralysis, confusion, disruption of cardiac rhythm | Cardiac arrest |
| Selenium | Seafood, meat, eggs, whole grains | Defense against oxidative stress, regulation of thyroid hormone action | Muscle pain and weakness, heart disorders | Hair and nail loss, nausea and vomiting, weakness, irritability |
| Sodium | Salt, soy sauce, salted foods, tomato juice | Body water balance, acid-base balance, nerve function | Muscle weakness, loss of appetite, nausea, vomiting; deficiency is rarely seen | Edema, hypertension in sensitive people |
| Zinc | Whole grains, meat, eggs, liver, seafood (especially oysters) | Synthesis of proteins, RNA, and DNA; wound healing; immune response; ability to taste | Growth failure, loss of appetite, impaired taste acuity, skin rash, impaired immune function, poor wound healing | Vomiting, impaired immune function, decline in blood HDL levels, impaired copper absorption |

SOURCES: Food and Nutrition Board, Institute of Medicine, National Academies. 2001. *Dietary Reference Intakes Tables* (http://www.iom.edu/file.asp?id=21372; retrieved December 21, 2004). The complete Dietary Reference Intake reports are available from the National Academy Press (http://www.nap.edu); Shils, M. E., et al., eds. 1998. *Modern Nutrition in Health and Disease,* 9th ed. Baltimore: Williams & Wilkins.

fumes, radiation, excessive sunlight, certain drugs, and stress can increase free radical production. A free radical is a chemically unstable molecule that will react with fats, proteins, and DNA, damaging cell membranes and mutating genes. Because of this, free radicals have been implicated in aging, cancer, cardiovascular disease, and other degenerative diseases like arthritis.

Antioxidants found in foods can help protect the body from damage by free radicals in several ways. Some dietary antioxidants prevent or reduce the formation of free radicals; others remove free radicals from the body by reacting with them directly by donating electrons. Antioxidants can also repair some types of free radical damage after it occurs. Some antioxidants, such as vitamin C, vitamin E, and selenium, are also essential nutrients; others, such as carotenoids, found in yellow, orange, and deep-green vegetables, are not. Obtaining a regular intake of these nutrients is vital for the health of the body. Many fruits and vegetables are rich in antioxidants.

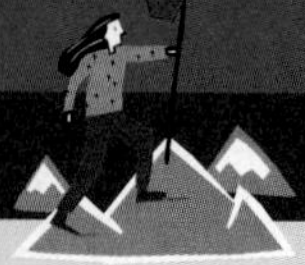
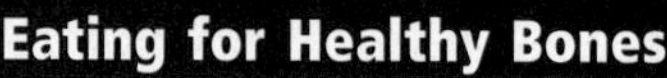

Take Charge

## Eating for Healthy Bones

Osteoporosis is a condition in which bones become dangerously thin and fragile over time. An estimated 10 million Americans over age 50 have osteoporosis, and another 34 million are at risk. Most bone mass is built by age 18, and after bone density peaks between the ages of 25 and 35, bone mass is slowly lost over time. To prevent osteoporosis, the best strategy is to build as much bone as possible during your young years and then do everything you can to maintain it as you age. Up to 50% of bone loss is determined by controllable lifestyle factors, especially diet and exercise habits. Key nutrients include the following:

***Calcium*** Consuming an adequate amount of calcium is important throughout life to build and maintain bone mass. Americans average 600–800 mg of calcium per day, only about half of what is recommended. Milk, yogurt, and calcium-fortified orange juice, bread, and cereals are all good sources. Nutritionists suggest that you obtain calcium from foods first and then take supplements only if needed to make up the difference.

***Vitamin D*** Vitamin D is necessary for bones to absorb calcium; a daily intake of 5 µg is recommended for adults age 19–50. Vitamin D can be obtained from foods and is manufactured by the skin when it is exposed to sunlight. Candidates for vitamin D supplements include people who don't eat many foods rich in vitamin D; those who have dark skin or who don't expose their face, arms, and hands to the sun (without sunscreen) for 5–15 minutes a few times each week; and people who live north of an imaginary line roughly between Boston and the Oregon–California border (the sun is weaker in northern latitudes).

***Vitamin K*** Vitamin K promotes the synthesis of proteins that help keep bones strong. Broccoli and leafy green vegetables are rich in vitamin K.

***Other Nutrients*** Other nutrients that may play an important role in bone health include vitamin C, magnesium, potassium, manganese, zinc, copper, and boron. On the flip side, there are several dietary substances that may have a *negative* effect on bone health, especially if consumed in excess: alcohol, caffeine, sodium, retinol (a form of vitamin A), and soda. Protein can help build bone if calcium intake is adequate, but if calcium intake is low, protein may cause calcium loss from bone.

Finally, it is important to combine a healthy diet with regular exercise. Weight-bearing aerobic activities, if performed regularly, help build and maintain bone mass throughout life. Strength training improves bone density, muscle mass, strength, and balance, protecting against both bone loss and falls, a major cause of fractures. See Chapter 10 for tips on creating a complete, personalized exercise program.

**Phytochemicals** Antioxidants fall into the broader category of **phytochemicals,** substances found in plant foods that may help prevent chronic disease. Researchers have just begun to identify and study all the different compounds found in foods, and many preliminary findings are promising. For example, certain substances found in soy foods may help lower cholesterol levels. Sulforaphane, a compound isolated from broccoli and other **cruciferous vegetables,** may render some carcinogenic compounds harmless. Allyl sulfides, a group of chemicals found in garlic and onions, appear to boost the activity of cancer-fighting immune cells.

If you want to increase your intake of phytochemicals, it is best to obtain them by eating a variety of fruits, vegetables, and grains rather than relying on supplements. Like many vitamins and minerals, isolated phytochemicals may be harmful if taken in high doses. In addition, it is likely that their health benefits are the result of chemical substances working in combination. See Chapter 12 for more on the role of phytochemicals in disease prevention.

## NUTRITIONAL GUIDELINES: PLANNING YOUR DIET

Various tools have been created by scientific and government groups to help people design healthy diets. The **Dietary Reference Intakes (DRIs)** are standards for nutrient intake designed to prevent nutritional deficiencies and reduce the risk of chronic disease. **Dietary Guidelines for Americans** have been established to promote health and reduce the risk for major chronic diseases through diet and physical activity. Further guidance symbolized by **MyPyramid** provides daily food intake patterns that meet the DRIs and are consistent with the Dietary Guidelines for Americans.

### Dietary Reference Intakes (DRIs)

How much vitamin C, iron, calcium, and other nutrients do you need to stay healthy? The Food and Nutrition Board establishes dietary standards, or recommended intake levels, for Americans of all ages. The current set of standards, called Dietary Reference Intakes (DRIs), is relatively new, having been introduced in 1997. An earlier set of standards, called the **Recommended Dietary Allowances (RDAs),** focused on preventing nutritional deficiency diseases such as anemia. The DRIs have a broader focus because of research that looked not just at the prevention of nutrient deficiencies but also at the role of nutrients in promoting optimal health and preventing chronic diseases such as cancer, osteoporosis, and heart disease.

The DRIs include standards for both recommended intakes and maximum safe intakes. The recommended intake of each nutrient is expressed as either a *Recommended*

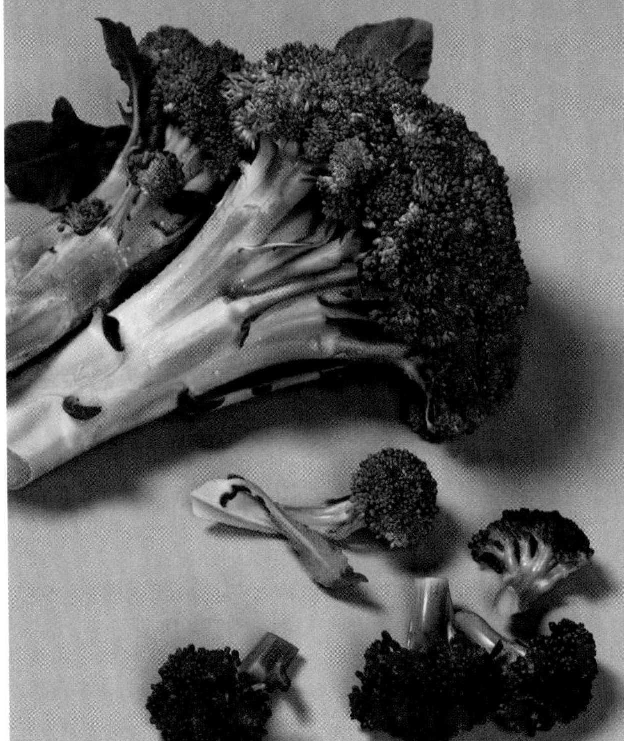

Cruciferous vegetables are rich in phytochemicals and essential vitamins and minerals. Most Americans can obtain adequate amounts of essential nutrients as well as other beneficial compounds by consuming a healthy, varied diet that favors nutrient-dense foods.

*Dietary Allowance (RDA)* or *Adequate Intake (AI)*. An AI is set when there is not enough information available to set an RDA value; regardless of the type of standard used, however, the DRI represents the best available estimate of intake for optimal health. The *Tolerable Upper Intake Level (UL)* sets the maximum daily intake that is unlikely to cause health problems in a healthy person. (However, there is no established benefit from consuming nutrients at levels above the RDA or AI). The DRIs can be found in the Nutrition Resources section at the end of the chapter.

**Should You Take Supplements?** The aim of the DRIs is to guide you in meeting your nutritional needs primarily with food, rather than with vitamin and mineral supplements. Supplements lack potentially beneficial phytochemicals and fibers that are found only in whole foods. Most Americans can obtain most of the vitamins and minerals they need to prevent deficiencies by consuming a varied, nutritionally balanced diet.

The question of whether to take supplements is a serious one. Some vitamins and minerals are dangerous when ingested in excess, as shown in Tables 9-1 and 9-2. Large doses of particular nutrients can also cause health problems by affecting the absorption of other vitamins and minerals. For these reasons, think carefully about whether to take supplements; consider consulting a physician or registered dietitian.

In setting the DRIs, the Food and Nutrition Board recommended supplements of particular nutrients for the following groups:

- Women who are capable of becoming pregnant should obtain 400 μg per day of folic acid (the synthetic form of the vitamin folate) from fortified foods and/or supplements in addition to folate from a varied diet. Research indicates that this level of folate intake will reduce the risk of neural tube defects. Since 1998, enriched breads, flours, cornmeals, rice, noodles, and other grain products have been fortified with small amounts of folic acid. Folate is found naturally in leafy green vegetables, legumes, oranges and orange juice, and strawberries.
- People over age 50 should consume foods fortified with vitamin B-12, B-12 supplements, or a combination of the two in order to meet the majority of the RDA of 2.4 μg of B-12 daily. Up to 30% of people over 50 may have problems absorbing protein-bound B-12 in foods. Vitamin B-12 in supplements and fortified foods is more readily absorbed and can help prevent a deficiency.

Because of the oxidative stress caused by smoking, the Food and Nutrition Board also recommends that smokers consume 35 mg *more* vitamin C per day than the RDA set for their age and sex (for adults, recommended daily vitamin C intakes for nonsmokers are 90 mg for men and 75 mg for women). However, supplements are not usually needed because this extra vitamin C can easily be obtained from foods. For example, one cup of orange juice has about 100 mg of vitamin C.

Supplements may also be recommended in other cases. Women with heavy menstrual flows may need extra

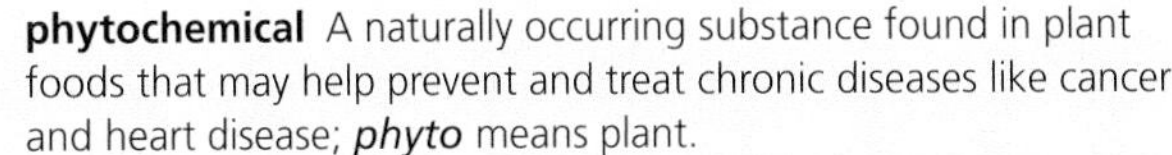

## Terms

**phytochemical** A naturally occurring substance found in plant foods that may help prevent and treat chronic diseases like cancer and heart disease; ***phyto*** means plant.

**cruciferous vegetables** Vegetables of the cabbage family, including cabbage, broccoli, brussels sprouts, kale, and cauliflower; the flower petals of these plants form the shape of a cross, hence the name.

**Dietary Reference Intakes (DRIs)** An umbrella term for four types of nutrient standards: Adequate Intake (AI), Estimated Average Requirement (EAR), and Recommended Dietary Allowance (RDA) set levels of intake considered adequate to prevent nutrient deficiencies and reduce the risk of chronic disease; Tolerable Upper Intake Level (UL) sets the maximum daily intake that is unlikely to cause health problems.

**Dietary Guidelines for Americans** General principles of good nutrition intended to help prevent certain diet-related diseases.

**MyPyramid** A food-group plan that provides practical advice to ensure a balanced intake of the essential nutrients.

**Recommended Dietary Allowances (RDAs)** Amounts of certain nutrients considered adequate to prevent deficiencies in most healthy people; will eventually be replaced by the broader Dietary Reference Intakes (DRIs).

Vw

iron to compensate for the monthly loss. The elderly, people with dark skin, and people exposed to little sunlight may need extra vitamin D from vitamin D–fortified foods and/or supplements that contain vitamin D. Some vegetarians may need supplemental calcium, iron, zinc, and vitamin B-12, depending on their food choices. Newborns need a single dose of vitamin K, which must be administered under the direction of a physician. People who consume few calories, who have certain diseases, or who take certain medications may need specific vitamin and mineral supplements; such supplement decisions must be made by a physician because some vitamins and minerals counteract the actions of certain medications.

In deciding whether to take a vitamin and mineral supplement, consider whether you already regularly consume a fortified breakfast cereal. Many breakfast cereals contain almost as many nutrients as a multivitamin pill. If you do decide to take a supplement, choose a balanced formulation that contains 50–100% of the Daily Value (see below) for vitamins and minerals. Avoid supplements containing large doses of particular nutrients.

**Daily Values** Because the DRIs are far too cumbersome to use as a basis for food labels, the U.S. Food and Drug Administration uses another set of dietary standards, the **Daily Values.** The Daily Values are based on several different sets of guidelines and represent appropriate intake levels for a 2000-calorie diet. The percent Daily Value shown on a food label shows how well that food contributes to your recommended daily intake. Food labels are described in detail later in the chapter.

## Dietary Guidelines for Americans

To provide general guidance for choosing a healthy diet, the U.S. Department of Agriculture (USDA) and the U.S. Department of Health and Human Services (DHHS) have jointly issued Dietary Guidelines for Americans, most recently in 2005. These guidelines are intended for healthy children age 2 and older and adults of all ages. Key recommendations include the following:

- Consume a variety of nutrient-dense foods within and among the basic food groups, while staying within energy needs.
- Control calorie intake to manage body weight.
- Be physically active every day.
- Increase daily intake of foods from certain groups: fruits and vegetables, whole grains, and fat-free or low-fat milk and milk products.

### Term

VW **Daily Values** A simplified version of the RDAs used on food labels; also included are values for nutrients with no RDA per se.

- Choose fats wisely for good health, limiting intake of saturated and trans fats.
- Choose carbohydrates wisely for good health, limiting intake of added sugars.
- Choose and prepare foods with little salt, and consume potassium-rich foods.
- If you drink alcoholic beverages, do so in moderation.
- Keep foods safe to eat.

Following these guidelines promotes health and reduces risk for chronic diseases, including heart disease, cancer, diabetes, stroke, osteoporosis, and obesity. What follows is a brief summary of the guidelines.

### Adequate Nutrients within Calorie Needs

Many people consume more calories than they need while failing to meet recommended intakes for all nutrients. Most people need to choose meals and snacks that are high in nutrients but low to moderate in calories. The USDA's MyPyramid food plan, described in detail in the next section, translates nutrient recommendations into food choices. (Another plan, the DASH plan, also reflects the recommendations in the Dietary Guidelines; for more on this plan, visit the Web site for the Dietary Guidelines at www.healthierus.gov/dietaryguidelines.) You can obtain all the nutrients and other substances you need by choosing the recommended number of daily servings from basic food groups and following the advice about selecting nutrient-dense foods within the groups. Following these plans would mean that many Americans would have to make some general dietary changes:

- Eat more dark green vegetables, orange vegetables, legumes, fruits, whole grains, and low-fat and fat-free milk and milk products.
- Eat less refined grains, saturated fat, trans fat, cholesterol, added sugars, and calories.

For maximum nutrition, it is important to consume foods from all the food groups daily and to consume a variety of nutrient-dense foods within the groups. Nutrient-dense foods are those that provide substantial amounts of vitamins and minerals and relatively few calories. Americans currently consume many foods and beverages that are low in nutrient density, making it difficult or impossible to meet nutrient needs without overconsuming calories (see the box "America's Poor Eating Habits"). Selecting nutrient-dense foods—low-fat forms of foods in each group and those free of added sugars—allows you to meet your nutrient needs without overconsuming calories and unhealthy food components such as saturated and trans fats.

**Weight Management** Overweight and obesity are a major public health problem in the United States. Calorie intake and physical activity (see next section) work together

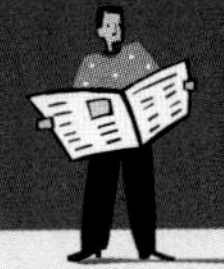

## America's Poor Eating Habits

The typical American diet has changed significantly in recent decades—and not for the better. The top ten sources of calories in the American diet, which together account for more than 30% total energy intake, do not reflect healthy eating habits (see table). Americans now consume too many calories, often in the form of added sugars and fats, but too few vitamins and minerals, in part because intake of fruits, vegetables, and milk products is relatively low.

Consumption of regular sodas and sweetened fruit drinks has nearly doubled since 1970, and Americans consume an average of 152 pounds of added sugars each year. Milk consumption has dropped 40% since 1970 as children and young adults have switched to sodas, which now account for nearly 10% of daily calories for those age 12–19. Americans now eat out much more than in the past—more than 40% of Americans eat out at least once on a typical day—and foods eaten outside the home tend to be higher in calories and lower in nutrients than foods prepared at home.

### Individual Choice

Individual choice is certainly a key component in recent dietary shifts. Low prices and convenience are valued by American consumers, and there has been a rapid increase in the availability of affordable, convenient, and tasty foods. Many foods with these characteristics do not have a healthy nutritional profile; they tend to be energy-dense and nutrient-poor. American consumers know they should make better choices—but they frequently fail to do so.

### Environmental Influences

While acknowledging the role of personal responsibility, some experts also point to environmental factors. Convenience foods are now widely available for purchase, and in many urban neighborhoods in particular, it is easier to buy fast food than fruits and vegetables. In part because sugar is inexpensive, many foods high in added sugars are inexpensive. (Federal subsidies for corn make high-fructose corn syrup, which is found in a wide variety of processed foods, very inexpensive.)

The food industry spends over $30 billion a year on advertising, special promotions, and supermarket slotting fees, with $10 billion of this directed at children. McDonald's alone spends over $1 billion each year on ads, compared to just $1 million spent by the National Cancer Institute for its "5 to 9 a Day" fruits and vegetables campaign.

Many ads target children under age 10, who researchers have found cannot distinguish between advertising and informational programming. (A study of Australian children ages 9–10 found that more than half believed that Ronald McDonald "knows best" when it comes to what children should eat.) Most ads during children's programming feature large portions of sweetened breakfast cereals, fruit-flavored drinks, and fast food. Teen programming features three times as many ads for soft drinks as for milk, a ratio that mirrors consumption patterns.

And young people can now consume fast food at school: About 30% of public high schools offer some type of brand-name fast food, and food ads are featured in television programming shown in schools. (Some school districts have raised money by accepting marketing deals with brand-name soda and fast-food companies.)

### What Can Be Done?

Several different strategies have been proposed to promote personal responsibility and combat negative environmental forces:

- Change the price structure of food. Add small taxes on soft drinks, fast food, and other nutrient-poor foods to subsidize (and lower) the costs of healthy foods and to fund campaigns to promote healthy diet and activity habits.
- Prominently print or post basic nutrition information for meals ordered in restaurants and for convenience and fast foods. For example, the calorie, sugar, and fat content of sodas and popcorn could be printed on the cups in which they are served at schools, restaurants, and movie theaters.
- Restrict food advertising aimed at children, and ban commercials for unhealthy foods on school television programs.
- Require that all meals sold on school grounds meet federal nutrition recommendations; ban paid marketing agreements between schools and fast-food and soft-drink companies.
- Increase public awareness of factors that promote unhealthy food choices, including low cost, accessibility, convenience, and taste (added sugars and fats).

If you're concerned about your own eating habits and those of people in your community, speak with your consumer dollars. Make it a priority to purchase healthy foods when they are offered. In addition, be aware of outside influences on your food choices. This chapter—and the resources listed at the end of the chapter—provide many suggestions for choosing delicious, convenient, and healthy foods.

### Top Ten Sources of Calories in the American Diet

| Food | Percent of Total Calories |
|---|---|
| Regular soft drinks | 7.1 |
| Cake, sweet rolls, doughnuts, pastries | 3.6 |
| Hamburgers, cheeseburgers, meatloaf | 3.1 |
| Pizza | 3.1 |
| Potato chips, corn chips, popcorn | 2.9 |
| Rice | 2.7 |
| Rolls, buns, English muffins, bagels | 2.7 |
| Cheese or cheese spread | 2.6 |
| Beer | 2.6 |
| French fries, fried potatoes | 2.2 |

SOURCES: Block, G. 2004. Foods contributing to energy intake in the US: Data from NHANES III and NHANES 1999–2000. *Journal of Food Composition and Analysis* 17(2004): 439–447; Brownell, K. D. 2004. *Food Fight.* New York: McGraw-Hill; Liebman, B. 2002. The changing American diet. *Nutrition Action HealthLetter,* December; Nestle, M., and M. F. Jacobson. 2000. Halting the obesity epidemic: A public health policy approach. *Public Health Reports* 115: 12–24.

to influence body weight. Most Americans need to reduce the amount of calories they consume, increase their level of physical activity, and make wiser food choices. Many adults gain weight slowly over time, but even small changes in behavior can help avoid weight gain.

Evaluate your body weight in terms of body mass index (BMI), a measure of relative body weight that also takes height into account (see Chapter 11 for instructions on how to determine your BMI). If your current weight is healthy, aim to avoid weight gain. Do so by increasing physical activity and making small cuts in calorie intake. Choose nutrient-dense foods and sensible portion sizes. Avoiding weight gain is easier than losing weight: For example, for most adults, a reduction of 50 to 100 calories per day may prevent gradual weight gain, whereas a reduction of 500 calories or more per day may be needed initially for weight loss.

Monitoring weight regularly helps people know if they need to adjust their food intake or physical activity to maintain a healthy weight. Those who need to lose weight should aim for slow, steady weight loss by decreasing calorie intake, maintaining adequate nutrient intake, and increasing physical activity. In terms of macronutrient intake, use the AMDR ranges described earlier in the chapter for dietary planning; within these healthy ranges, total calorie intake is what counts for weight management rather than specific percentages of particular macronutrients.

**Physical Activity** Regular physical activity improves fitness, helps manage weight, promotes psychological well-being, and reduces risk of heart disease, high blood pressure, cancer, and diabetes. Become active if you are inactive, and maintain or increase physical activity if you are already active. The amount of daily physical activity recommended for you depends on your current health status and goals.

- To reduce the risk of chronic disease, aim to accumulate at least 30 minutes (adults) or 60 minutes (children) of moderate physical activity—the equivalent of brisk walking at a pace of 3–4 miles per hour—beyond your usual activity at work, home, and school. Greater health benefits can be obtained by engaging in more vigorous activity or activity of longer duration.
- To help manage body weight and prevent gradual, unhealthy weight gain, engage in 60 minutes of moderately to vigorously intense activity on most days of the week.
- To sustain weight loss in adulthood, engage daily in at least 60–90 minutes of moderate physical activity.

You can do the activity all at once or spread it out over several 10-minute or longer bouts during the day; choose activities you enjoy and can do regularly. You can boost fitness by engaging in exercises specifically designed for the health-related fitness components: cardiorespiratory endurance exercises, stretching exercises for flexibility, and resistance training for muscular strength and endurance. See Chapter 10 for advice on increasing daily physical activity and creating a complete fitness program.

**Food Groups to Encourage** Many Americans do not consume the recommended amounts of fruits, vegetables, whole grains, and low-fat or fat-free milk products—all of which have health benefits.

**FRUITS AND VEGETABLES** Fruits and vegetables are important sources of dietary fiber, vitamins, and minerals. For a 2000-calorie diet, about 4½ cups or the equivalent (9 servings) of fruits and vegetables each day is recommended. Eat a variety of fruits—fresh, frozen, canned, or dried—rather than fruit juice for most of your fruit choices. For vegetables, choose a variety of colors and kinds. Eat more of the following types of vegetables:

- Dark green vegetables, such as broccoli, kale, and other dark leafy greens
- Orange vegetables, such as carrots, sweet potatoes, pumpkin, and winter squash
- Legumes, such as pinto beans, kidney beans, black beans, garbanzo beans, split peas, and lentils

Other fruits and vegetables that are important sources of nutrients of concern include tomatoes and tomato products, red sweet peppers, cabbage and other cruciferous vegetables, bananas, citrus fruits, berries, and melons. See the discussion of MyPyramid for more advice on choosing fruits and vegetables.

**WHOLE GRAINS** Whole grains provide more fiber and nutrients than refined grains, and intake of whole grains reduces the risk of chronic disease and helps with weight maintenance. For a 2000-calorie diet, 6 ounce-equivalents (6 servings) of grains each day are recommended; at least half of these servings should be whole grains. (One ounce is about 1 slice of bread, 1 cup of cereal flakes, or ½ cup of cooked pasta or rice.) The remaining grain servings should be from enriched or whole-grain products. Refer back to p. 201 for information on identifying whole-grain products.

**LOW-FAT AND FAT-FREE MILK AND MILK PRODUCTS** Regular consumption of milk and milk products can reduce the risk of low bone mass throughout life. Choosing low-fat and fat-free dairy products helps to control calorie intake and reduce intake of saturated fat and cholesterol. For adults, the equivalent of 3 daily cups of fat-free or low-fat milk or milk products is recommended; 1½ ounces of cheese is the equivalent of 1 cup of milk. Yogurt and lactose-free milk are options for people who are lactose intolerant, as is use of the enzyme lactase prior to the consumption of milk products. For individuals who avoid all milk products, nondairy calcium sources include fortified cereals and beverages, tofu prepared with calcium sulfate, green leafy vegetables, soybeans, and certain fish and seafood.

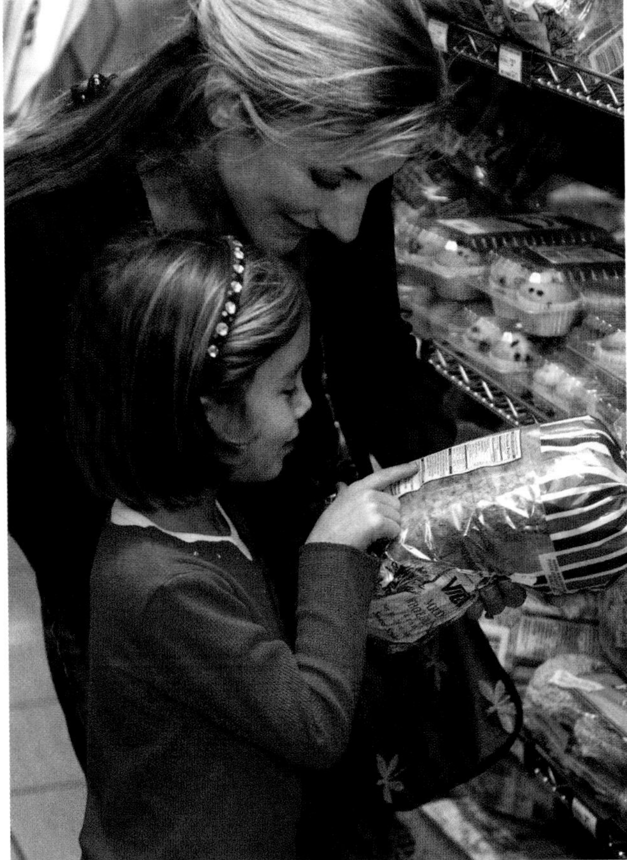

Whole grains provide more nutrients and fiber than refined grains, and they may help reduce the risk of chronic disease. Half of your daily grain servings should come from whole grains. To check if a food contains whole grains, read the ingredient list on a food label.

**Fats** A diet low in saturated fat, trans fat, and cholesterol helps keep blood cholesterol low and reduces the risk for heart disease. A diet containing omega-3 fats from fish also reduces the risk for heart disease. Goals for fat intake for most adults are as follows:

Total fat: 20–35% of total daily calories

Saturated fat: Less than 10% of total daily calories

Trans fat: As little as possible

Cholesterol: Less than 300 mg per day

Most fats in the diet should come from sources of unsaturated fats, such as fish, nuts, and vegetable oils. Refer to the box "Reducing the Saturated and Trans Fats in Your Diet" for specific suggestions.

Cholesterol is found only in animal foods. If you need to reduce your cholesterol intake, limit your intake of foods that are particularly high in cholesterol, including egg yolks, dairy fats, certain shellfish, and liver and other organ meats; watch your serving sizes of animal foods. Food labels list the fat and cholesterol content of foods.

Two servings per week of fish rich in heart-healthy omega-3 fatty acids are also recommended for people at high risk for heart disease. However, for certain groups, intake limits are set for varieties of fish that may contain mercury; see p. 213 for more information. Fish rich in omega-3 fatty acids include salmon, mackerel, and trout.

**Carbohydrates** Fruits, vegetables, whole grains, and fat-free or low-fat milk can provide the recommended amount of carbohydrate. Choose foods rich in fiber often—for example, choose whole fruits instead of juices and whole grains instead of refined grains. Legumes are another good source of fiber.

People who consume foods and beverages high in added sugars tend to consume more calories but smaller amounts of vitamins and minerals than those who limit their intake of added sugars. A food is likely high in sugar if one of the following appears first or second in the list of ingredients or if several are listed: sugar (any type, including beet, brown, invert, raw, and cane), corn syrup or sweetener, fruit juice concentrate, honey, malt syrup, molasses, syrup, cane juice, or dextrose, fructose, glucose, lactose, maltose, or sucrose.

To reduce added sugar consumption, cut back on soft drinks, candies, sweet desserts (cakes, cookies, pies), fruit drinks, and other foods high in added sugars. Drink water rather than sweetened drinks, and don't let sodas and other sweets crowd out more nutritious foods, such as low-fat milk. Regular soda is the leading source of both added sugars and calories in the American diet, but it provides little in the way of nutrients except sugar. The 10 teaspoons of sugar in a 12-ounce soda can exceed the recommended daily limit for added sugars for someone consuming 2000 calories per day; for more on added sugar limits, see the discussion of MyPyramid.

Keep your teeth and gums healthy by limiting consumption of sweet or starchy foods between meals and brushing and flossing regularly; drinking fluoridated water also reduces the risk of dental caries.

**Sodium and Potassium** Many people can reduce their chance of developing high blood pressure or lower already elevated blood pressure by consuming less salt; reducing blood pressure lowers the risk for stroke, heart disease, and kidney disease. Salt is made up of the minerals sodium and chloride, and although both of these minerals are essential for normal body function, we need only small amounts (1500 mg per day for adults). Most Americans consume much more salt than they need. The goal is to reduce sodium intake to less than 2300 mg per day, the equivalent of about 1 teaspoon of salt. Certain groups, including people with hypertension, African Americans, and older adults, benefit from an even lower sodium intake (no more than 1500 mg per day).

Salt is found mainly in processed and prepared foods; smaller amounts may also be added during cooking or at the table. To lower your intake of salt, choose fresh or plain frozen meat, poultry, seafood, and vegetables most often; these are lower in salt than processed forms are.

Take Charge

## Reducing the Saturated and Trans Fats in Your Diet

Your overall goal is to limit total fat intake to no more than 35% of total calories. Within that limit, favor unsaturated fats from vegetable oils, nuts, and fish over saturated and trans fats from animal products and foods made with hydrogenated vegetable oils or shortening. Saturated and trans fat intake should be kept as low as possible within a nutritionally adequate diet.

- Be moderate in your consumption of foods high in fat, including fast food, commercially prepared baked goods and desserts, deep-fried foods, meat, poultry, nuts and seeds, and regular dairy products.
- When you do eat high-fat foods, limit your portion sizes, and balance your intake with foods low in fat.
- Choose lean cuts of meat, and trim any visible fat from meat before and after cooking. Remove skin from poultry before or after cooking.
- Drink fat-free or low-fat milk instead of whole milk, and use lower-fat varieties in puddings, soups, and baked products. Substitute plain low-fat yogurt, blender-whipped low-fat cottage cheese, or buttermilk for sour cream.
- Use vegetable oil instead of butter or margarine. Use tub or squeeze margarine instead of stick margarine. Look for margarines that are free of trans fats. Minimize intake of coconut or palm oil.
- Season vegetables, seafood, and meats with herbs and spices rather than with creamy sauces, butter, or margarine.
- Try lemon juice on salad, or use a yogurt-based salad dressing instead of mayonnaise or sour cream dressings.
- Steam, boil, bake, or microwave vegetables, or stir-fry them in a small amount of vegetable oil.
- Roast, bake, or broil meat, poultry, or fish so that fat drains away as the food cooks.
- Use a nonstick pan for cooking so that added fat will be unnecessary; use a vegetable spray for frying. Kitchen stores sell non-aerosol spray bottles to use with regular cooking oils.
- Chill broths from meat or poultry until the fat becomes solid. Spoon off the fat before using the broth.
- Substitute egg whites for whole eggs when baking; limit the number of egg yolks when scrambling eggs.
- Choose fruits as desserts most often.
- Eat a low-fat vegetarian main dish at least once a week.

Check and compare the sodium content in processed foods, including frozen dinners, cheeses, soups, salad dressings, sauces, and canned mixed dishes. Add less salt during cooking and at the table, and limit your use of high-sodium condiments like soy sauce, ketchup, mustard, pickles, and olives. Use lemon juice, herbs, and spices instead of salt to enhance the flavor of foods.

Along with lowering salt intake, increasing potassium intake helps lower blood pressure. Fruits, vegetables, and most milk products are available in forms that contain no salt, and many of these are sources of potassium. Potassium-rich foods include leafy green vegetables, sweet and white potatoes, winter squash, soybeans, tomato sauce, bananas, peaches, apricots, cantaloupes, and orange juice.

**Alcoholic Beverages** Alcoholic beverages supply calories but few nutrients. Drinking in moderation is defined as no more than one drink per day for women and no more than two drinks per day for men. People who should not drink at all include individuals who cannot restrict their drinking to moderate levels; women who are pregnant or breastfeeding or who may become pregnant; children and adolescents; people with specific health conditions; individuals who plan to drive or operate machinery or engage in any activity that requires attention, skill, or coordination; and individuals taking prescription or over-the-counter medications that can interact with alcohol. If you choose to drink alcoholic beverages, do so sensibly, moderately, and with meals. Never drink in situations where it may put you or others at risk.

**Food Safety** Safe foods are those that pose little risk from harmful bacteria, viruses, parasites, toxins, or chemical or physical contaminants. Foodborne diseases affect more about 76 million Americans each year, resulting in more than 5000 deaths. Actions by consumers can reduce the occurrence of foodborne illness significantly (see the box "Food Safety"). It is especially important to be careful with perishable foods such as poultry, meats, eggs, shellfish, milk products, and fresh fruits and vegetables.

## USDA's MyPyramid

Many Americans are familiar with the USDA Food Guide Pyramid, the food guidance system that was first released in 1992. Since the initial release of the Pyramid, scientists have updated both nutrient recommendations (the DRIs) and the Dietary Guidelines for Americans. So, as the 2005 Dietary Guidelines revision was being prepared, the USDA reassessed its overall food guidance system and released MyPyramid in April 2005 (Figure 9-3, p. 214).

A variety of experts have proposed other food-group plans. Some of these address perceived shortcomings in the USDA plans, and some adapt the basic 1992 Pyramid to special populations. The USDA Center for Nutrition Policy and Promotion (www.usda.gov/cnpp) has more on

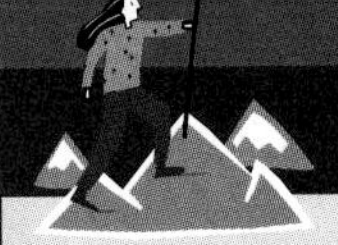

## Food Safety

- Don't buy food in containers that leak, bulge, or are severely dented. Refrigerated foods should be cold, and frozen foods should be solid.
- Refrigerate perishable items as soon as possible after purchase. Use or freeze fresh meats within 3–5 days and fresh poultry, fish, and ground meat within 1–2 days.
- Store raw meat, poultry, fish, and shellfish in containers in the refrigerator so that the juices don't drip onto other foods. Keep these items away from other foods, surfaces, utensils, or serving dishes to prevent cross-contamination.
- Thaw frozen food in the refrigerator or in the microwave oven, not on the kitchen counter. Cook foods immediately after thawing.
- Thoroughly wash your hands with warm soapy water for 20 seconds before and after handling food, especially raw meat, fish, shellfish, poultry, or eggs.
- Make sure counters, cutting boards, dishes, utensils, and other equipment are thoroughly cleaned before and after use using hot soapy water. Wash dishcloths and kitchen towels frequently.
- If possible, use separate cutting boards for meat, poultry, and seafood and for foods that will be eaten raw, such as fruits and vegetables. Replace cutting boards once they become worn or develop hard-to-clean grooves.
- Thoroughly rinse and scrub fruits and vegetables with a brush, if possible, or peel off the skin.
- Cook foods thoroughly, especially beef, poultry, fish, pork, and eggs. Use a food thermometer to ensure that foods are cooked to a safe temperature. Hamburgers should be cooked to 160°F. Turn or stir microwaved food to make sure it is heated evenly throughout. When eating out, order hamburger cooked "well-done" and make sure foods are served piping hot.
- Refrigerate foods within 2 hours of purchase or preparation, and within 1 hour if the air temperature is above 90°F. Refrigerate foods at or below 40°F and freeze at or below 0°F. Use refrigerated leftovers within 3–4 days.
- Don't eat raw animal products, including raw eggs in homemade hollandaise sauce or eggnog. Use only pasteurized milk and juice, and look for pasteurized eggs, which are now available in some states.
- Cook eggs until they're firm, and fully cook foods containing eggs. Store eggs in the coldest part of the refrigerator, not in the door, and use them within 3–5 weeks.
- Avoid raw sprouts. Even sprouts grown under clean conditions in the home can be risky because bacteria may be present in the seeds. Cook sprouts before eating them.
- According to the USDA, "When in doubt, throw it out." Even if a food looks and smells fine, it may not be safe. If you aren't sure that a food has been prepared, served, and stored safely, don't eat it.

### Special Populations

Additional precautions are recommended for people at particularly high risk for foodborne illness—pregnant women, young children, older persons, and people with weakened immune systems or certain chronic illnesses. If you are a member of one of these groups, don't eat or drink any of the following products: unpasteurized juices; raw sprouts; raw (unpasteurized) milk and products made from unpasteurized milk; raw or undercooked meat, poultry, eggs, fish, and shellfish; and soft cheeses such as feta, Brie, Camembert, or blue-veined varieties. Avoid ready-to-eat foods such as hot dogs, luncheon meats, and cold cuts unless they are reheated until they are steaming hot.

### Guidelines for Fish Consumption

Overall, fish and shellfish are healthy sources of essential nutrients. However, mercury contamination that can occur particularly in predatory fish (large fish that eat smaller fish) is a concern because mercury can cause brain damage in fetuses and young children. To reduce exposure to the harmful effects of mercury, the FDA and the Environmental Protection Agency (EPA) issued the following guidelines for women who are or who may become pregnant and nursing mothers:

- Do not eat shark, swordfish, king mackerel, or tilefish.
- Eat up to 12 ounces a week of a variety of fish and shellfish that is lower in mercury, such as shrimp, canned light tuna, salmon, pollock, and catfish. Limit consumption of albacore tuna to 6 ounces per week.
- Check advisories about the safety of recreationally caught fish; if no information is available, limit consumption to 6 ounces per week.

The same FDA/EPA guidelines apply to children, although they should consume smaller servings.

Some experts have also expressed concern about the presence of toxins such as PCBs in farmed fish, especially farmed salmon. Consumers may wish to limit themselves to 8 ounces of farmed salmon per month. Fish should be labeled with its country of origin and state whether it is wild or farmed; most canned salmon is wild.

### Mad Cow Disease

A potential new threat from food is bovine spongiform encephalopathy (BSE), or "mad cow disease," a fatal degenerative disease caused by an abnormal protein that forms deposits in the brain. A variant form of the human version of this disease, known as Creutzfeldt-Jacob disease (CJD), is believed to be caused by eating beef contaminated with central nervous system tissue from BSE-infected cows. In December 2003, the first BSE-infected cow was identified in the United States; no meat or organs from this animal had made it into the food supply. Although the USDA states that the risk to human health from BSE is extremely low, additional steps are being taken to prevent the BSE protein from entering the food supply; visit the USDA Web site for more information (www.usda.gov/bse).

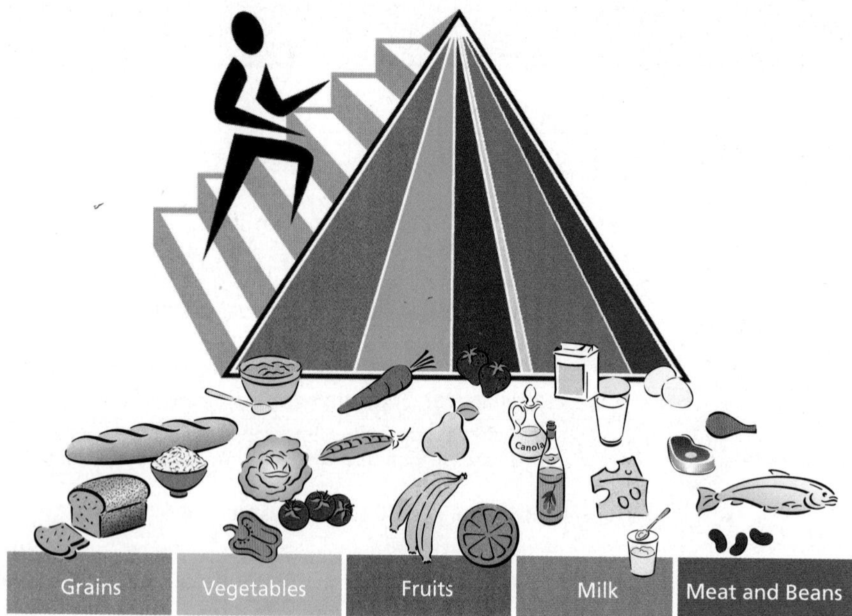


**Figure 9-3 USDA's MyPyramid.** The USDA food guidance system, called MyPyramid, can be personalized based on an individual's sex, age, and activity level; visit MyPyramid.gov to obtain a food plan appropriate for you. MyPyramid contains five main food groups plus oils (yellow band). Key consumer messages include the following:

- Grains: Make half your grains whole
- Vegetables: Vary your veggies
- Fruits: Focus on fruits
- Milk: Get your calcium-rich foods
- Meat and Beans: Go lean with protein

SOURCE: U.S. Department of Agriculture. 2005. *MyPyramid* (http://mypyramid.gov; retrieved April 20, 2005).

alternative food plans for special populations such as young children, older adults, and people choosing particular ethnic diets.

**Key Messages of MyPyramid** The new MyPyramid symbol (see Figure 9-3) has been developed to remind consumers to make healthy food choices and to be active every day. Key messages include the following:

- *Personalization* is represented by the person on the steps and the MyPyramid.gov site, which includes individualized recommendations, interactive assessments of food intake and physical activity, and tips for success.
- *Daily physical activity,* represented by the person climbing the steps, is important for maintaining a healthy weight and reducing the risk of chronic disease.
- *Moderation* of food intake is represented by the narrowing of each food group from bottom to top.
- *Proportionality* is represented by the different widths of the food group bands.
- *Variety* is represented by the color bands; foods from all groups are needed daily for good health.
- *Gradual improvement* is a good strategy; people can benefit from making small changes each day.

The MyPyramid chart in Figure 9-4 shows the food intake patterns recommended for different levels of calorie intake; Table 9-3 (p. 216) provides guidance for determining an appropriate calorie intake for weight maintenance. Use the table to identify an energy intake that is about right for you; then refer to the appropriate column in Figure 9-4. A personalized version of MyPyramid recommendations can also be obtained by visiting MyPyramid.gov. Each food group is described briefly below. Past experiences have shown that many Americans have trouble identifying serving sizes, so recommended daily intakes from each group are now given in terms of cups and ounces; see the box "Judging Portion Sizes" (p. 216) for additional advice.

**Grains** Foods from this group are usually low in fat and rich in complex carbohydrates, dietary fiber (if grains are unrefined), and many vitamins and minerals, including thiamin, riboflavin, iron, niacin, folic acid (if enriched or fortified), and zinc. Someone eating 2000 calories a day should include 6 ounce-equivalents each day, with half of those servings from whole grains such as whole-grain bread, whole-wheat pasta, high-fiber cereal, and brown rice. The following count as 1 ounce-equivalent:

- 1 slice of bread
- 1 small (2½-inch diameter) muffin
- 1 cup ready-to-eat cereal flakes
- ½ cup cooked cereal, rice, grains, or pasta
- 1 6-inch tortilla

Choose foods that are typically made with little fat or sugar (bread, rice, pasta) over those that are high in fat and sugar (croissants, chips, cookies, doughnuts).

**Vegetables** Vegetables contain carbohydrates, dietary fiber, vitamin A, vitamin C, folate, potassium, and other nutrients. They are also naturally low in fat. In a 2000-calorie diet, 2½ cups (5 servings) of vegetables should be included daily. Each of the following counts as 1 serving (½ cup or equivalent) of vegetables:

- ½ cup raw or cooked vegetables
- 1 cup raw leafy salad greens
- ½ cup vegetable juice

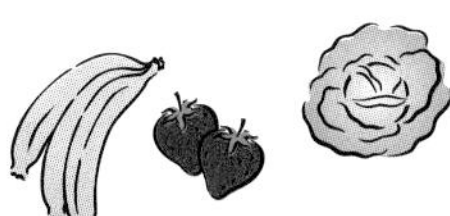 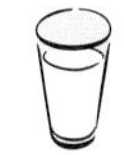 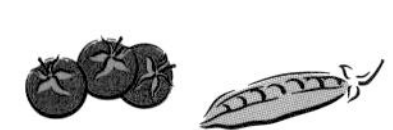 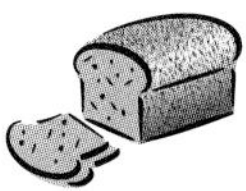 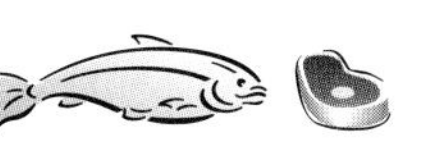 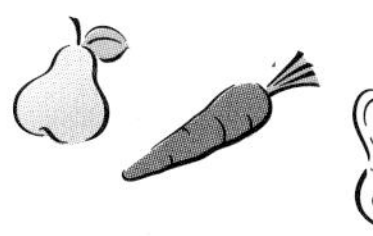 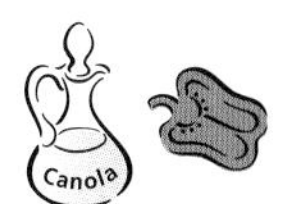

**Daily Amount of Food from Each Group**

Food group amounts shown in cups (c) or ounce-equivalents (oz-eq), with number of daily servings (srv) shown in parentheses; vegetable subgroup amounts are per week

| Calorie level | 1600 | 1800 | 2000 | 2200 | 2400 | 2600 | 2800 | 3000 |
|---|---|---|---|---|---|---|---|---|
| **Grains** | 5 oz-eq | 6 oz-eq | 6 oz-eq | 7 oz-eq | 8 oz-eq | 9 oz-eq | 10 oz-eq | 10 oz-eq |
| Whole grains | 3 oz-eq | 3 oz-eq | 3 oz-eq | 3.5 oz-eq | 4 oz-eq | 4.5 oz-eq | 5 oz-eq | 5 oz-eq |
| Other grains | 2 oz-eq | 3 oz-eq | 3 oz-eq | 3.5 oz-eq | 4 oz-eq | 4.5 oz-eq | 5 oz-eq | 5 oz-eq |
| **Vegetables** | 2 c (4 srv) | 2.5 c (5 srv) | 2.5 c (5 srv) | 3c (6 srv) | 3 c (6 srv) | 3.5 c (7 srv) | 3.5 c (7 srv) | 4 c (8 srv) |
| Dark green | 2 c/wk | 3 c/wk | 3 c/wk | 3 c/wk | 3 c/wk | 3 c/wk | 3 c/wk | 3 c/wk |
| Orange | 1.5 c/wk | 2 c/wk | 2 c/wk | 2 c/wk | 2 c/wk | 2.5 c/wk | 2.5 c/wk | 2.5 c/wk |
| Legumes | 2.5 c/wk | 3 c/wk | 3 c/wk | 3 c/wk | 3 c/wk | 3.5 c/wk | 3.5 c/wk | 3.5 c/wk |
| Starchy | 2.5 c/wk | 3 c/wk | 3 c/wk | 6 c/wk | 6 c/wk | 7 c/wk | 7 c/wk | 9 c/wk |
| Other | 5.5 c/wk | 6.5 c/wk | 6.5 c/wk | 7 c/wk | 7 c/wk | 8.5 c/wk | 8.5 c/wk | 10 c/wk |
| **Fruits** | 1.5 c (3 srv) | 1.5 c (3 srv) | 2 c (4 srv) | 2 c (4 srv) | 2 c (4 srv) | 2 c (4 srv) | 2.5 c (5 srv) | 2.5 c (5 srv) |
| **Milk** | 3 c | 3 c | 3 c | 3 c | 3 c | 3 c | 3 c | 3 c |
| **Lean meat and beans** | 5 oz-eq | 5 oz-eq | 5.5 oz-eq | 6 oz-eq | 6.5 oz-eq | 6.5 oz-eq | 7 oz-eq | 7 oz-eq |
| **Oils** | 5 tsp | 5 tsp | 6 tsp | 6 tsp | 7 tsp | 8 tsp | 8 tsp | 10 tsp |

The discretionary calorie allowances shown below are the calories remaining at each level after nutrient-dense foods in each food group are selected. Those trying to lose weight may choose not to use discretionary calories. For those wanting to maintain weight, discretionary calories may be used to increase the amount of food from each food group; to consume foods that are not in the lowest fat form or that contain added sugars; to add oil, fat, or sugars to foods; or to consume alcohol. The amounts below show how discretionary calories may be divided between solid fats and added sugars.

| Discretionary calories | 132 | 195 | 267 | 290 | 362 | 410 | 426 | 512 |
|---|---|---|---|---|---|---|---|---|
| **Solid fats** | 11 g | 15 g | 18 g | 19 g | 22 g | 24 g | 24 g | 29 g |
| **Added sugars** | 12 g (3 tsp) | 20 g (5 tsp) | 32 g (8 tsp) | 38 g (9 tsp) | 48 g (12 tsp) | 56 g (14 tsp) | 60 g (15 tsp) | 72 g (18 tsp) |

**Figure 9-4 MyPyramid food intake patterns.** To determine an appropriate amount of food from each group, find the column with your approximate daily energy intake. That column lists the daily recommended intake from each food group. Visit MyPyramid.gov for a personalized intake plan and for intakes for other calorie levels. SOURCE: U.S. Department of Health and Human Services and U.S. Department of Agriculture. *Dietary Guidelines for Americans,* 2005 (http://www.health.gov/dietaryguidelines; retrieved January 20, 2005).

Because vegetables vary in the nutrients they provide, it is important to consume a variety of types of vegetables to obtain maximum nutrition. Many Americans consume only a few different types of vegetables, with white potatoes (baked or served as french fries) being the most popular. To help boost variety, MyPyramid recommends servings from five different subgroups within the vegetables group; try to consume vegetables from several subgroups each day. (For clarity, Figure 9-4 shows servings from the subgroups in terms of weekly consumption.)

- Dark green vegetables like spinach, chard, collards, bok choy, broccoli, kale, romaine, and turnip and mustard greens
- Orange and deep yellow vegetables like carrots, winter squash, sweet potatoes, and pumpkin

Take Charge

## Judging Portion Sizes

Studies have shown that most people underestimate the size of their food portions, in many cases by as much as 50%. If you need to retrain your eye, try using measuring cups and spoons and an inexpensive kitchen scale when you eat at home. With a little practice, you'll learn the difference between 3 and 8 ounces of chicken or meat, and what a half-cup of rice really looks like. For quick estimates, use the following equivalents:

- 1 teaspoon of margarine = the tip of your thumb
- 1 ounce of cheese = your thumb, four dice stacked together, or an ice cube
- 3 ounces of chicken or meat = a deck of cards or an audiocassette tape
- 1 cup of pasta = a small fist or a tennis ball
- ½ cup of rice or cooked vegetables = an ice cream scoop or one-third of a can of soda
- 2 tablespoons of peanut butter = a ping-pong ball or large marshmallow
- 1 medium potato = a computer mouse
- 1–2-ounce muffin or roll = plum or large egg
- 2-ounce bagel = hockey puck or yo-yo
- 1 medium fruit (apple or orange) = baseball
- ¼ cup nuts = golf ball
- Small cookie or cracker = poker chip

**Table 9-3 MyPyramid Daily Calorie Intake Levels**

| Age (years) | Sedentary[a] | Moderately Active[b] | Active[c] |
|---|---|---|---|
| **Child** | | | |
| 2–3 | 1000 | 1000–1400 | 1000–1400 |
| **Female** | | | |
| 4–8 | 1200–1400 | 1400–1600 | 1400–1800 |
| 9–13 | 1400–1600 | 1600–2000 | 1800–2200 |
| 14–18 | 1800 | 2000 | 2400 |
| 19–30 | 1800–2000 | 2000–2200 | 2400 |
| 31–50 | 1800 | 2000 | 2200 |
| 51+ | 1600 | 1800 | 2000–2200 |
| **Male** | | | |
| 4–8 | 1200–1400 | 1400–1600 | 1600–2000 |
| 9–13 | 1600–2000 | 1800–2200 | 2000–2600 |
| 14–18 | 2000–2400 | 2400–2800 | 2800–3200 |
| 19–30 | 2400–2600 | 2600–2800 | 3000 |
| 31–50 | 2200–2400 | 2400–2600 | 2800–3000 |
| 51+ | 2000–2200 | 2200–2400 | 2400–2800 |

[a]A lifestyle that includes only the light physical activity associated with typical day-to-day life.
[b]A lifestyle that includes physical activity equivalent to walking about 1.5 to 3 miles per day at 3 to 4 miles per hour (30–60 minutes a day of moderate physical activity), in addition to the light physical activity associated with typical day-to-day life.
[c]A lifestyle that includes physical activity equivalent to walking more than 3 miles per day at 3 to 4 miles per hour (60 or more minutes a day of moderate physical activity), in addition to the light physical activity associated with typical day-to-day life.

SOURCE: U.S. Department of Agriculture. 2005. *MyPyramid Food Intake Pattern Calorie Levels* (http://mypyramid.gov/professionals; retrieved April 20, 2005).

- Legumes like pinto beans, kidney beans, black beans, lentils, chickpeas, and tofu; legumes can be counted as servings of vegetables *or* as alternatives to meat
- Starchy vegetables like corn, green peas, and white potatoes
- Other vegetables; tomatoes, bell peppers (red, orange, yellow, or green), green beans, and cruciferous vegetables like cauliflower are good choices

**Fruits** Fruits are rich in carbohydrates, dietary fiber, and many vitamins, especially vitamin C. For someone eating a 2000-calorie diet, 2 cups (4 servings) of fruits are recommended daily. The following each count as 1 serving (½ cup or equivalent) of fruit:

- ½ cup fresh canned or frozen fruit
- ½ cup fruit juice (100% juice)
- 1 small whole fruit
- ¼ cup dried fruit

Good choices from this group are citrus fruits and juices, melons, pears, apples, bananas, and berries. Choose whole fruits often—they are higher in fiber and often lower in calories than fruit juices. Fruit *juices* typically contain more nutrients and less added sugar than fruit *drinks*. For canned fruits, choose those packed in 100% fruit juice or water rather than in syrup.

**Milk** This group includes all milk and milk products, such as yogurt, cheeses (except cream cheese), and dairy desserts, as well as lactose-free and lactose-reduced products. Foods from this group are high in protein, carbohydrate, calcium, riboflavin, and vitamin D (if fortified).

Those consuming 2000 calories per day should include 3 cups of milk or the equivalent daily. Each of the following counts as the equivalent of 1 cup:

- 1 cup milk or yogurt
- ½ cup ricotta cheese
- 1½ ounces natural cheese
- 2 ounces processed cheese

Cottage cheese is lower in calcium than most other cheeses; ½ is equivalent to ¼ cup milk. Ice cream is also lower in calcium and higher in sugar and fat than many other dairy products; one scoop counts as ⅓ cup milk. To limit calories and saturated fat in your diet, it is best to choose servings of low-fat and fat-free items from this group.

**Meat and Beans** This group includes meat, poultry, fish, dry beans and peas, eggs, nuts, and seeds. These foods provide protein, niacin, iron, vitamin B-6, zinc, and thiamin; the animal foods in the group also provide vitamin B-12. For someone consuming a 2000-calorie diet, 5½ ounce-equivalents is recommended. The following each count as equivalent to 1 ounce:

- 1 ounce cooked lean meat, poultry, or fish
- ¼ cup cooked dry beans (legumes) or tofu
- 1 egg
- 1 tablespoon peanut butter
- ½ ounce nuts or seeds

One egg at breakfast, ½ cup of pinto beans at lunch, and a 3-ounce (cooked weight) hamburger at dinner would add up to the equivalent of 6 ounces of lean meat for the day. To limit your intake of saturated fat, choose lean cuts of meat and skinless poultry, and watch your serving sizes carefully. Choose at least one serving of plant proteins, such as black beans, lentils, or tofu, every day.

**Oils and Trans-Free Soft Fats** The Oils group represents the oils that are added to foods during processing, cooking, or at the table; oils and soft margarines include vegetables oils and soft vegetable oil table spreads that have no trans fats. These are major sources of vitamin E and unsaturated fatty acids, including the essential fatty acids. For a 2000-calorie diet, 6 teaspoons per day are recommended. One teaspoon is the equivalent of the following:

- 1 teaspoon vegetable oil or soft margarine
- 1 tablespoon salad dressing or light mayonnaise

Foods that are mostly oils include nuts, olives, avocados, and some fish. The following portions include about 1 teaspoon of oil: 8 large olives, ⅙ medium avocado, ½ tablespoon peanut butter, and ⅓ ounce roasted nuts. Food labels can help consumers identify the type and amount of fat in various foods.

**Discretionary Calories, Solid Fats, and Added Sugars** The suggested intakes from the basic food groups in MyPyramid assume that nutrient-dense forms are selected from each group; nutrient-dense forms are those that are fat-free or low-fat and that contain no added sugars. If this pattern is followed, then a small amount of additional calories can be consumed—the *discretionary calorie allowance.* Figure 9-4 shows the discretionary calorie allowance at each calorie level in MyPyramid.

People who are trying to lose weight may choose not to use discretionary calories. For those wanting to maintain weight, discretionary calories may be used to increase the amount of food from a food group; to consume foods that are not in the lowest fat form or that contain added sugars; to add oil, fat, or sugars to foods; or to consume alcohol. The amounts shown in Figure 9-4 show how discretionary calories may be divided between solid fats and added sugars. The values for additional fat target no more than 30% of total calories from fat and less than 10% of calories from saturated fat. Examples of discretionary solid fat calories include choosing higher-fat meats such as sausages, chicken with skin, or whole milk instead of fat-free milk, and topping foods with butter. For example, a cup of whole milk has 60 calories more than a cup of fat-free milk; these 60 calories would be counted as discretionary calories.

The suggested amounts of added sugars may be helpful limits for including some sweetened foods or beverages in the daily diet without exceeding energy needs or underconsuming other nutrients. For example, on a 2000-calorie diet, MyPyramid lists 32 grams (8 teaspoons) for discretionary intake of added sugars. In the American diet, added sugars are often found in sweetened beverages (regular soda, sweetened teas, fruit drinks), dairy products (ice cream, some yogurts), and grain products (bakery goods). For example, a 20-ounce regular soda has 260 calories from added sugars that would be counted as discretionary calories. The current American diet includes higher-than-recommended levels of sugar intake.

## The Vegetarian Alternative

Some people choose a diet with one essential difference from the diets we've already described—foods of animal origin (meat, poultry, fish, eggs, milk) are eliminated or restricted. Many do so for health reasons; vegetarian diets tend to be lower in saturated fat, cholesterol, and animal protein and higher in complex carbohydrates, dietary fiber, folate, vitamins C and E, carotenoids, and phytochemicals. Some people adopt a vegetarian diet out of concern for the environment, for financial considerations, or for reasons related to ethics or religion.

**Types of Vegetarian Diets** There are various vegetarian styles; the wider the variety of the diet eaten, the

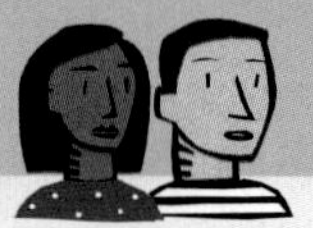

### How Different Are the Nutritional Needs of Women and Men?

When it comes to nutrition, men and women have a lot in common. Both sexes need the same essential nutrients, and the Dietary Guidelines for Americans apply equally to both. But beyond the basics, men and women need different amounts of essential nutrients and have different nutritional concerns.

Women tend to be smaller and weigh less than men, and thus have lower energy requirements and need to consume fewer calories than men to maintain a healthy weight. For most nutrients, women need the same or slightly lower amounts than men. But because women consume fewer calories, they may have more difficulty getting adequate amounts of all essential nutrients and need to focus on nutrient-dense foods.

Two nutrients of special concern to women are calcium and iron. Low calcium intake may be linked to the development of osteoporosis in later life. The *Healthy People 2010* report sets a goal of increasing from 40% to 75% the proportion of women age 20–49 who meet the dietary recommendation for calcium. Fat-free and low-fat dairy products and fortified cereal, bread, and orange juice are good choices for calcium-rich foods.

Menstruating women also have higher iron needs than other groups, and low iron intake can lead to iron-deficiency anemia. Lean red meat, green leafy vegetables, and fortified breakfast cereals are good sources of iron. As discussed earlier, all women capable of becoming pregnant should consume adequate folic acid from fortified foods and/or supplements.

Men are seldom thought of as having nutritional deficiencies because they generally have high-calorie diets. However, many men have a diet that does not follow recommended food intake patterns and includes more red meat and fewer fruits, vegetables, and whole grains than recommended. This dietary pattern is linked to heart disease and some types of cancer. A high intake of calories can lead to weight gain over time if a man's activity level decreases as he ages. To reduce chronic disease risk, men should focus on increasing their consumption of fruits, vegetables, and whole grains to obtain vitamins, minerals, fiber, and phytochemicals.

The "Eat 5 to 9 a Day for Better Health" program created by the National Cancer Institute and U.S. Department of Health and Human Services to promote increased intake of fruits and vegetables has been adapted to create the "Shoot for 9 for Better Health" message for men; for strategies and guidelines for consuming more fruits and vegetables, visit http://5aday.gov/9aday.

easier it is to meet nutritional needs. **Vegans** eat only plant foods. **Lacto-vegetarians** eat plant foods and dairy products. **Lacto-ovo-vegetarians** eat plant foods, dairy products, and eggs. According to recent polls, over 5 million American adults never eat meat, poultry, or fish and fall into one of these three groups. Others can be categorized as **partial vegetarians, semivegetarians,** or **pescovegetarians;** these individuals eat plant foods, dairy products, eggs, and usually a small selection of poultry, fish, and other seafood.

**A Food Plan for Vegetarians** MyPyramid can be adapted for use by vegetarians with only a few key modifications. For the meat and beans group, vegetarians can focus on the nonmeat choices of dry beans (legumes), nuts, seeds, eggs, and soy foods like tofu (soybean curd) and tempeh (a cultured soy product). Vegans and other vegetarians who do not consume any dairy products must find other rich sources of calcium (see below). Fruits, vegetables, and whole grains are healthy choices for people following all types of vegetarian diets.

A healthy vegetarian diet emphasizes a wide variety of plant foods. Although plant proteins are generally of lower quality than animal proteins, choosing a variety of plant foods will supply all of the essential amino acids. Choosing minimally processed and unrefined foods will maximize nutrient value and provide ample dietary fiber. Daily consumption of a variety of plant foods in amounts that meet total energy needs can provide all needed nutrients, although special care (and supplements) may be needed to obtain adequate amounts of vitamin B-12, vitamin D, calcium, iron, and zinc.

### Terms

VW

**vegan** A vegetarian who eats no animal products at all.

**lacto-vegetarian** A vegetarian who includes milk and cheese products in the diet.

**lacto-ovo-vegetarian** A vegetarian who eats no meat, poultry, or fish but does eat eggs and milk products.

**partial vegetarian, semivegetarian,** or **pescovegetarian** A vegetarian who includes eggs, dairy products, and/or small amounts of poultry and seafood in the diet.

## Dietary Challenges for Special Population Groups

The Dietary Guidelines for Americans and MyPyramid provide a basis that everyone can use to create a healthy diet. However, some population groups face special dietary challenges (see the box "How Different Are the Nutritional Needs of Women and Men?").

**College Students** Foods that are convenient for college students are not always the healthiest choices. It is easy for students who eat in buffet-style dining halls or food courts to overeat, and the foods offered are not

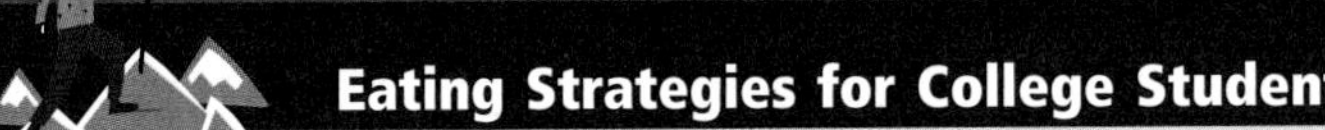

## Eating Strategies for College Students

Take Charge

### General Guidelines

- Eat slowly, and enjoy your food. Set aside a separate time to eat, and don't eat while you study.
- Eat a colorful, varied diet. The more colorful your diet is, the more varied and rich in fruits and vegetables it will be. Many Americans eat few fruits and vegetables, despite the fact that these foods are typically inexpensive, delicious, rich in nutrients, and low in fat and calories.
- Eat breakfast. You'll have more energy in the morning and be less likely to grab an unhealthy snack later on.
- Choose healthy snacks—fruits, vegetables, grains, and cereals—as often as you can.
- Drink water more often than soft drinks or other sweetened beverages. Rent a mini-refrigerator for your dorm room and stock up on healthy beverages.
- Pay attention to portion sizes.
- Combine physical activity with healthy eating. You'll feel better and have a much lower risk of many chronic diseases. Even a little exercise is better than none.

### Eating in the Dining Hall

- Choose a meal plan that includes breakfast, and don't skip it.
- Accept that dining hall food is not going to taste the same as home cooking. Find healthy dishes that you like.
- If menus are posted or distributed, decide what you want to eat before you get in line, and stick to your choices. Consider what you plan to do and eat for the rest of the day before making your choices.
- Ask for large servings of vegetables and small servings of meat and other high-fat main dishes. Build your meals around grains and vegetables.
- Try whole grains like brown rice, whole-wheat bread, and whole-grain cereals.
- Choose leaner poultry, fish, or bean dishes rather than high-fat meats and fried entrees.
- Ask that gravies and sauces be served on the side; limit your intake.
- Choose broth-based or vegetable soups rather than cream soups.
- At the salad bar, load up on leafy greens, beans, and fresh vegetables. Avoid mayonnaise-coated salads, bacon, croutons, and high-fat dressings. Put dressing on the side, and dip your fork into it rather than pouring it over the salad.
- Drink nonfat milk, water, mineral water, or 100% fruit juice rather than heavily sweetened fruit drinks, whole milk, or soft drinks.
- Choose fruit for dessert rather than pastries, cookies, or cakes.
- Do some research about the foods and preparation methods used in your dining hall or cafeteria. Discuss any suggestions you have with your food-service manager.

### Eating in Fast-Food Restaurants

- Most fast-food chains can provide a brochure with a nutritional breakdown of the foods on the menu. Ask for it. (See also the information in the appendix.)
- Order small single burgers with no cheese instead of double burgers with many toppings. If possible, ask for them broiled instead of fried.
- Ask for items to be prepared without mayonnaise, tartar sauce, sour cream, or other high-fat sauces. Ketchup, mustard, and fat-free mayonnaise or sour cream are better choices and are available at many fast-food restaurants.
- Choose whole-grain buns or bread for burgers and sandwiches.
- Choose chicken items made from chicken breast, not processed chicken.
- Order vegetable pizzas without extra cheese.
- If you order french fries or onion rings, get the smallest size, and/or share them with a friend.

### Eating on the Run

Are you chronically short of time? The following healthy and filling items can be packed for a quick snack or meal: fresh or dried fruit, fruit juices, raw fresh vegetables like carrots, plain bagels, bread sticks, whole-wheat fig bars, low-fat cheese sticks or cubes, low-fat crackers or granola bars, nonfat or low-fat yogurt, snack-size cereal boxes, pretzels, rice or corn cakes, plain popcorn, soup (if you have access to a microwave), or water.

necessarily high in essential nutrients and low in fat. The same is true of meals at fast-food restaurants, another convenient source of quick and inexpensive meals for busy students. Although no food is entirely bad, consuming a wide variety of foods is critical for a healthy diet. See the box "Eating Strategies for College Students" for tips on making healthy eating convenient and affordable.

**Older Adults** Nutrient needs do not change much as people age; but because older adults tend to become less active, they require fewer calories to maintain body weight. At the same time, the absorption of nutrients tends to be lower in older adults because of age-related changes in the digestive tract. Thus, they must consume nutrient-dense foods in order to meet their nutritional requirements. As discussed earlier, foods fortified with vitamin B-12 and/or B-12 supplements are recommended for people over age 50. Because constipation is a common problem, consuming foods high in fiber and getting adequate fluids are important goals.

**Athletes** Key dietary concerns for athletes are meeting their increased energy requirements and drinking enough fluids during practice and throughout the day to remain fully hydrated. Endurance athletes may also benefit from increasing the amount of carbohydrate in the diet to 60–70% of total daily calories; this increase should come in the form of complex, rather than simple, carbohydrates. Athletes for whom maintaining low body weight and body fat is important—such as skaters, gymnasts, and wrestlers—should consume adequate nutrients and avoid falling into unhealthy patterns of eating.

**People with Special Health Concerns** Many Americans have special health concerns that affect their dietary needs. For example, women who are pregnant or breastfeeding require extra calories, vitamins, and minerals (see Chapter 8). People with diabetes benefit from a well-balanced diet that is low in simple sugars, high in complex carbohydrates, and relatively rich in monounsaturated fats. People with high blood pressure need to control their weight and limit their sodium consumption. If you have a health problem or concern that may require a special diet, discuss your situation with a physician or registered dietitian.

## A PERSONAL PLAN: MAKING INFORMED CHOICES ABOUT FOOD

Now that you understand the basis of good nutrition and a healthy diet, you can put together a diet that works for you. Focus on the likely causes of any health problems in your life, and make specific dietary changes to address them. You may also have some specific areas of concern, such as interpreting food labels and dietary supplement labels, avoiding foodborne illnesses and environmental contaminants, and understanding food additives. We turn to these and other topics next.

### Reading Food Labels

Consumers can get help from food labels in applying the principles of the Dietary Guidelines for Americans. Since 1994, all processed foods regulated by either the FDA or the USDA have included standardized nutrition information on their labels. Every food label shows serving sizes and the amount of fat, saturated fat, cholesterol, sodium, total carbohydrate, dietary fiber, sugars, and protein in each serving. To make intelligent choices about food, learn to read and *understand* food labels (see the box "Using Food Labels").

### Reading Dietary Supplement Labels

Dietary supplements include vitamins, minerals, amino acids, herbs, glandular extracts, enzymes, and other compounds. Although dietary supplements are often thought to be safe and "natural," they contain powerful, bioactive chemicals that have the potential for harm. About one-quarter of all pharmaceutical drugs are derived from botanical sources, and even essential vitamins and minerals can have toxic effects if consumed in excess.

In the United States, supplements are not legally considered drugs and are not regulated the way drugs are. Before they are approved by the FDA and put on the market, drugs undergo clinical studies to determine safety, effectiveness, side effects and risks, possible interactions with other substances, and appropriate dosages. The FDA does not authorize or test dietary supplements, and supplements are not required to demonstrate either safety or effectiveness prior to marketing. Although dosage guidelines exist for some of the compounds in dietary supplements, dosages for many are not well established.

Although many ingredients in dietary supplements have been used for centuries in Eastern or European herbal medicine, some have been found to be dangerous or to interact with prescription or over-the-counter drugs in dangerous ways. Garlic supplements, for example, can cause bleeding if taken with anticoagulant ("blood thinning") medications. Even products that are generally considered safe can have side effects—St. John's wort, for example, increases the skin's sensitivity to sunlight and may decrease the effectiveness of oral contraceptives, drugs used to treat HIV infection, and other medications.

There are also key differences in how drugs and supplements are manufactured. FDA-approved medications are standardized for potency, and quality control and proof of purity are required. Dietary supplement manufacture is not as closely regulated, and there is no guarantee that a product even contains a given ingredient, let alone in the appropriate amount. The potency of herbal supplements tends to vary widely due to differences in growing and harvesting conditions, preparation methods, and storage. In addition, herbs can be contaminated or misidentified at any stage from harvest to packaging.

With increased consumer knowledge and demand, it is likely that both the research base and the manufacturing standards for supplements will improve. (The FDA proposed manufacturing standards in 2003.) To provide consumers with more reliable and consistent information about supplements, the FDA requires supplements to have labels similar to those found on foods (see the box "Using Dietary Supplement Labels").

Finally, it is important to remember that dietary supplements are no substitute for a healthy diet. Supplements do not provide all the known—or yet-to-be-discovered—benefits of whole foods. Supplements should also not be used as a replacement for medical treatment for serious illnesses.

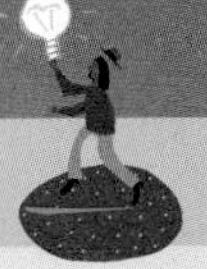



## Using Food Labels



Food labels are designed to help consumers make food choices based on the nutrients that are most important to good health. In addition to listing nutrient content by weight, the label puts the information in the context of a daily diet of 2000 calories that includes no more than 65 grams of fat (approximately 30% of total calories). For example, if a serving of a particular product has 13 grams of fat, the label will show that the serving represents 20% of the daily fat allowance. If your daily diet contains fewer or more than 2000 calories, you need to adjust these calculations accordingly.

Food labels contain uniform serving sizes. This means that if you look at different brands of salad dressing, for example, you can compare calories and fat content based on the serving amount. (Food label serving sizes may be larger or smaller than MyPyramid serving size equivalents, however.) Regulations also require that foods meet strict definitions if their packaging includes the terms *light, low-fat,* or *high-fiber* (see the sample label). Claims such as "good source of dietary fiber" or "low in saturated fat" on packages are signals that those products can wisely be included in your diet. Overall, the food label is an important tool to help you choose a diet that conforms to MyPyramid and the Dietary Guidelines.

### Selected Nutrient Content Claims and What They Mean

***Healthy*** A food that is low in fat, is low in saturated fat, has no more than 360–480 mg of sodium and 60 mg of cholesterol, *and* provides 10% or more of the Daily Value for vitamin A, vitamin C, protein, calcium, iron, or dietary fiber per serving.

***Light or lite*** One-third fewer calories or 50% less fat than a similar product.

***Reduced or fewer*** At least 25% less of a nutrient than a similar product; can be applied to fat ("reduced fat"), saturated fat, cholesterol, sodium, and calories.

***Extra or added*** 10% or more of the Daily Value per serving when compared to what a similar product has.

***Good source*** 10–19% of the Daily Value for a particular nutrient per serving.

***High, rich in, or excellent source of*** 20% or more of the Daily Value for a particular nutrient per serving.

***Low calorie*** 40 calories or less per serving.

***High fiber*** 5 g or more of fiber per serving.

***Good source of fiber*** 2.5–4.9 g of fiber per serving.

***Fat-free*** Less than 0.5 g of fat per serving.

***Low-fat*** 3 g of fat or less per serving.

***Saturated fat-free*** Less than 0.5 g of saturated fat and 0.5 g of trans fatty acids per serving.

***Low saturated fat*** 1 g or less of saturated fat per serving and no more than 15% of total calories.

***Cholesterol-free*** Less than 2 mg of cholesterol and 2 g or less of saturated fat per serving.

***Low cholesterol*** 20 mg or less of cholesterol and 2 g or less of saturated fat per serving.

***Low sodium*** 140 mg or less of sodium per serving.

***Very low sodium*** 35 mg or less of sodium per serving.

***Lean*** Cooked seafood, meat, or poultry with less than 10 g of fat, 4.5 g or less of saturated fat, and less than 95 mg of cholesterol per serving.

***Extra lean*** Cooked seafood, meat, or poultry with less than 5 g of fat, 2 g of saturated fat, and 95 mg of cholesterol per serving.

NOTE: As of April 2005, the FDA had not yet defined nutrient claims relating to carbohydrate, so foods labeled low- or reduced-carbohydrate do not conform to any approved standard.

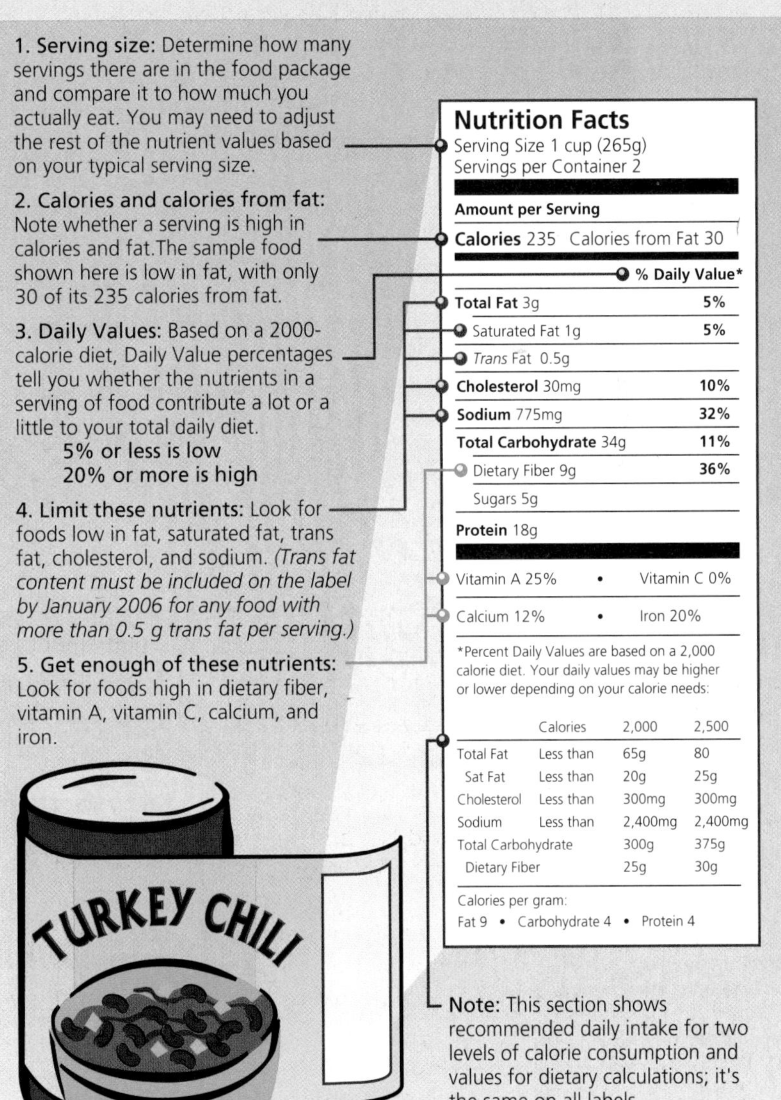

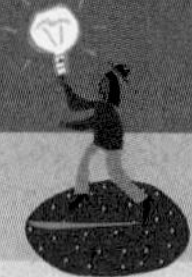

## Using Dietary Supplement Labels



Since 1999, specific types of information have been required on the labels of dietary supplements. In addition to basic information about the product, labels include a "Supplement Facts" panel, modeled after the "Nutrition Facts" panel used on food labels (see the label below). Under the Dietary Supplement Health and Education Act (DSHEA) and food labeling laws, supplement labels can make three types of health-related claims.

- *Nutrient-content claims,* such as "high in calcium," "excellent source of vitamin C," or "high potency." The claims "high in" and "excellent source of" mean the same as they do on food labels. A "high potency" single-ingredient supplement must contain 100% of its Daily Value; a "high potency" multi-ingredient product must contain 100% or more of the Daily Value of at least two-thirds of the nutrients present for which Daily Values have been established.
- *Health claims,* if they have been authorized by the FDA or another authoritative scientific body. The association between adequate calcium intake and lower risk of osteoporosis is an example of an approved health claim. Since 2003, the FDA has also allowed so-called *qualified* health claims for situations in which there is emerging but as yet inconclusive evidence for a particular claim. Such claims must include qualifying language such as "scientific evidence suggests but does not prove" the claim.
- *Structure-function claims,* such as "antioxidants maintain cellular integrity" or "this product enhances energy levels." Because these claims are not reviewed by the FDA, they must carry a disclaimer (see the sample label).

### Tips for Choosing and Using Dietary Supplements

- Check with your physician before taking a supplement. Many are not meant for children, elderly people, women who are pregnant or breast-feeding, people with chronic illnesses, or people taking prescription or OTC medications.
- Choose brands made by nationally known food and drug manufacturers or house brands from large retail chains. Due to their size and visibility, such sources are likely to have high manufacturing standards.
- Look for the USP-DSVP mark on the label, indicating that the product meets minimum safety and purity standards developed under the Dietary Supplement Verification Program (DSVP) by the United States Pharmacopeia (USP). The USP-DSVP mark means that the product (1) contains the ingredients stated on the label, (2) has the declared amount and strength of ingredients, (3) will dissolve effectively, (4) has been screened for harmful contaminants, and (5) has been manufactured using safe, sanitary, and well-controlled procedures. The National Nutritional Foods Association (NNFA) has a self-regulatory testing program for its members; other, smaller associations and labs, including ConsumerLab.Com, also test and rate dietary supplements.
- Follow the cautions, instructions for use, and dosage given on the label.
- If you experience side effects, discontinue use of the product and contact your physician. Report any serious reactions to the FDA's MedWatch monitoring program (800-FDA-1088; http://www.fda.gov/medwatch).

### For More Information About Dietary Supplements

ConsumerLab.Com: http://www.consumerlab.com

Food and Drug Administration: http://vm.cfsan.fda.gov/~dms/supplmnt.html

National Institutes of Health, Office of Dietary Supplements: http://dietary-supplements.info.nih.gov

National Nutritional Foods Association: http://www.nnfa.org

U.S. Department of Agriculture: http://www.nal.usda.gov/fnic/etext/000015.html

U.S. Pharmacopeia: http://www.usp.org/dietarysupplements

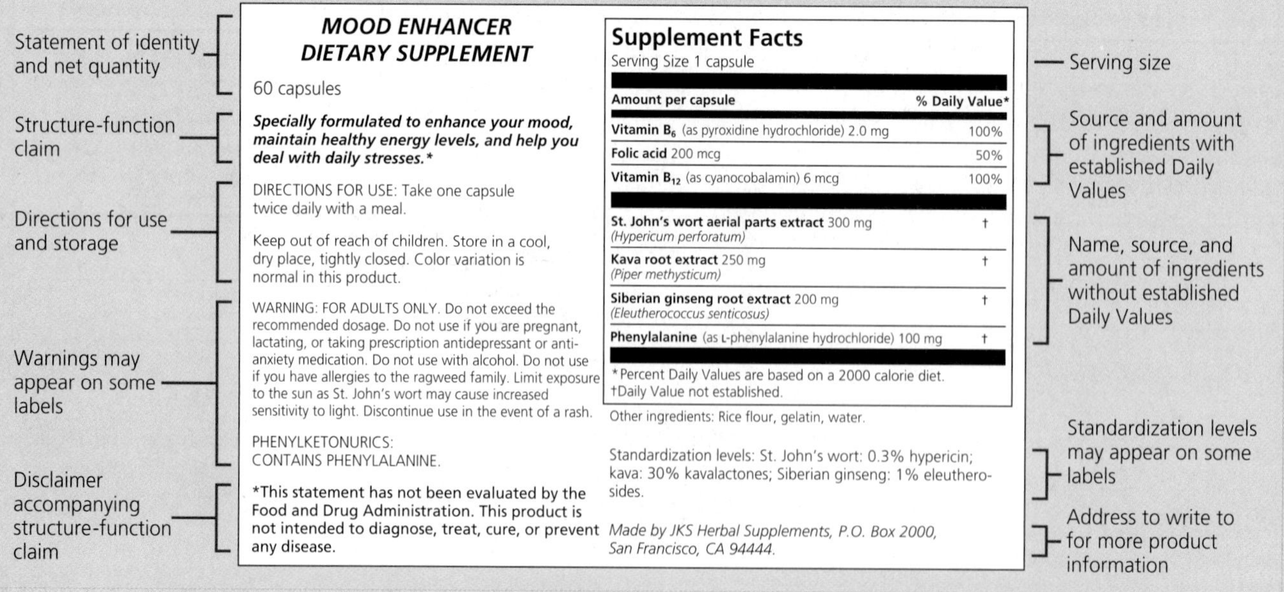

## Organic Foods

Some people who are concerned about pesticides and other environmental contaminants choose to buy foods that are **organic.** In December 2000, the USDA enacted a new national standard for organic foods to replace the older system of local, state, and private standards. To be certified as organic, foods must meet strict production, processing, handling, and labeling criteria. Organic crops must meet limits on pesticide residues; for meat, milk, eggs, and other animal products to be certified organic, animals must be given organic feed and access to the outdoors and may not be given antibiotics or growth hormones. The use of genetic engineering, ionizing radiation, and sewage sludge is prohibited (see below for more on irradiated and genetically modified foods). Products can be labeled "100% organic" if they contain all organic ingredients and "organic" if they contain at least 95% organic ingredients; all such products may carry the USDA organic seal. A product with at least 70% organic ingredients can be labeled "made with organic ingredients" but cannot use the USDA seal.

USDA ORGANIC

Organic foods are not necessarily chemical-free, however. They may be contaminated with pesticides used on neighboring lands or on foods transported in the same train or truck. However, they do tend to have lower levels of pesticide residues than conventionally grown crops. There are strict pesticide limits for all foods—organic and conventional—and the debate about the potential health effects of long-term exposure to small amounts of pesticide residues is ongoing.

## Additives in Food

Today, some 2800 substances are intentionally added to foods for one or more of the following reasons: (1) to maintain or improve nutritional quality, (2) to maintain freshness, (3) to help in processing or preparation, or (4) to alter taste or appearance. Additives make up less than 1% of our food. The most widely used are sugar, salt, and corn syrup; these three plus citric acid, baking soda, vegetable colors, mustard, and pepper account for 98% by weight of all food additives used in the United States.

Some additives, such as sulfites or monosodium glutamate (MSG), may be of concern for certain people, either because they are consumed in large quantities or because they cause some type of reaction. To protect yourself, eat a variety of foods in moderation. If you are sensitive to an additive, check food labels when you shop, and ask questions when you eat out.

## Food Irradiation

**Food irradiation** is the treatment of foods with gamma rays, X rays, or high-voltage electrons to kill potentially harmful pathogens, including bacteria, parasites, insects, and fungi that cause foodborne illness. It also reduces spoilage and extends shelf life.

Even though irradiation has been generally endorsed by agencies such as the World Health Organization, the Centers for Disease Control and Prevention, and the American Medical Association, few irradiated foods are currently on the market due to consumer resistance and skepticism. Studies haven't conclusively identified any harmful effects of food irradiation, and the newer methods of irradiation involving electricity and X rays do not require the use of any radioactive materials. Some irradiated foods may taste slightly different, just as pasteurized milk tastes slightly different than unpasteurized milk.

Studies indicate that when consumers are given information about the process of irradiation and the benefits of irradiated foods, most want to purchase them. All primary irradiated foods (meat, vegetables, and so on) are labeled with the flowerlike radura symbol and a brief information label. It is important to remember that although irradiation kills most pathogens, proper handling of irradiated foods is still critical for preventing foodborne illness.

## Genetically Modified Foods

Genetic engineering involves altering the characteristics of a plant, animal, or microorganism by adding, rearranging, or replacing genes in its DNA; the result is a **genetically modified (GM) organism.** New DNA may come from related species or from entirely different types of organisms. Many GM crops are already grown in the United States: About 75% of the current U.S. soybean crop has been genetically modified to be resistant to an herbicide used to kill weeds, and about 34% of the U.S. corn crop carries genes for herbicide resistance or pest resistance. Products made with GM organisms include juice, soda, nuts, tuna, frozen pizza, spaghetti sauce, canola oil, chips, salad dressings, and soup.

The potential benefits of GM foods cited by supporters include improved yields overall and in difficult growing conditions, increased disease resistance, improved nutritional content, lower prices, and less pesticide use. Critics of biotechnology argue that unexpected effects may occur: Gene manipulation could elevate levels of naturally

### Terms

**organic** A designation applied to foods grown and produced according to strict guidelines limiting the use of pesticides, non-organic ingredients, hormones, antibiotics, irradiation, genetic engineering, and other practices.

**food irradiation** The treatment of foods with gamma rays, X rays, or high-voltage electrons to kill potentially harmful pathogens and increase shelf life.

**genetically modified (GM) organism** A plant, animal, or microorganism in which genes have been added, rearranged, or replaced through genetic engineering.

Vw

occurring toxins or allergens, permanently change the gene pool and reduce biodiversity, and produce pesticide-resistant insects through the transfer of genes. Experience has shown that GM products are difficult to keep separate from non-GM products; animal escapes, cross-pollination, and contamination during processing are just a few ways GM organisms could potentially appear unexpectedly in the food supply or the environment.

According to the National Academy of Sciences, there is currently no proof that the GM food already on the market is unsafe. However, experts have recommended regulatory changes and further study of key issues, particularly the environmental effects of the escape of GM animals. Labeling has been another major concern, with surveys indicating that most Americans want to know if their food contains GM ingredients. Under current rules, the FDA requires special labeling only when a food's composition is changed significantly or when a known allergen such as a peanut gene is introduced into a food. The only foods guaranteed not to contain GM ingredients are those certified as organic.

## Food Allergies and Food Intolerances

For some people, consuming a particular food causes symptoms such as itchiness, swollen lips, or abdominal pain. Adverse reactions like these may be due to a food allergy or a food intolerance, and symptoms may range from annoying to life-threatening.

**Food Allergies** A true **food allergy** is a reaction of the body's immune system to a food or food ingredient. This immune reaction can occur within minutes of ingesting the food, resulting in symptoms that affect the skin (hives), gastrointestinal tract (cramps or diarrhea), respiratory tract (asthma), or mouth (swelling of the lips or tongue). The most severe response is a systemic reaction called anaphylaxis, which involves a potentially life-threatening drop in blood pressure.

Food allergies affect only about 2% of the adult population and about 4–6% of infants. Although numerous food allergens have been identified, just a few foods account for more than 90% of the food allergies in the United States: cow's milk, eggs, peanuts, tree nuts (walnuts, cashews, and so on), soy, wheat, fish, and shellfish. Individuals with food allergies, especially those prone to anaphylaxis, must diligently avoid trigger foods.

### Terms

VW

**food allergy** An adverse reaction to a food or food ingredient in which the immune system perceives a particular substance (allergen) as foreign and acts to destroy it.

**food intolerance** An adverse reaction to a food or food ingredient that doesn't involve the immune system; intolerances are often due to a problem with metabolism.

**Food Intolerances** Many people who believe they have food allergies may actually suffer from a much more common source of adverse food reactions, a **food intolerance.** In the case of a food intolerance, the problem usually lies with metabolism rather than with the immune system. Lactose intolerance, for example, occurs in people who are deficient in the enzyme lactase, which is needed to digest milk sugar (lactose). A more serious condition is intolerance of gluten, a protein component of some grains; in affected individuals, consumption of gluten damages the lining of the small intestine. Many people with food intolerances can consume small amounts of the food that affects them, and through trial and error, they can adjust their intake of the trigger food to an appropriate level.

If you suspect that you have a food allergy or intolerance, a good first step is to keep a food diary. Note everything you eat or drink, any symptoms you develop, and how long after eating the symptoms appear. Then make an appointment with your physician to go over your diary and determine if any additional tests are needed.

### Tips for Today

Eating is one of life's great pleasures. There are many ways to satisfy your nutrient needs, so you can create a healthy diet that takes into account your personal preferences and favorite foods. If your current eating habits are not as healthy as they could be, you can choose equally delicious foods that offer both short-term and long-term health benefits. Opportunities to improve your diet present themselves every day, and small changes add up.

*Right now you can*

- Substitute a healthy snack—an apple, a banana, or popcorn—for a bag of chips or cookies.
- Drink a glass of water, and put a bottle of water in your backpack for tomorrow.
- Plan to make healthy selections when you go to dinner, such as grilled or steamed vegetables instead of french fries or salmon instead of steak.
- Study the fast-food charts in the appendix and plan to order a healthy selection the next time you eat at your favorite fast-food restaurant.

## SUMMARY

- To function at its best, the human body requires about 45 essential nutrients in specific proportions. People get the nutrients needed to fuel their bodies and maintain tissues and organ systems from foods.
- Proteins, made up of amino acids, form muscles and bones and help make up blood, enzymes, hormones, and cell membranes. Foods from animal sources

Behavior Change Strategy

## Improving Your Diet by Choosing Healthy Beverages

After reading this chapter and completing the dietary assessment in Wellness Worksheet 9 in the Study Guide, you can probably identify several changes you could make to improve your diet. Here, we focus on choosing healthy beverages to increase intake of nutrients and decrease intake of empty calories from added sugars and fat. However, this model of dietary change can be applied to any modification you'd like to make to your diet. An additional plan for improving diet can be found in the Behavior Change Strategy in Chapter 12.

### Gather Data and Establish a Baseline

Begin by tracking your beverage consumption in your health journal. Write down the types and amounts of beverages you drink, including water. Also note where you were at the time and whether you obtained the beverage there or brought it with you. At the same time, investigate your options. Find out what other beverages you can easily obtain over the course of your daily routine. For example, what drinks are available in the dining hall where you eat lunch or at the food court where you often grab snacks? How many drinking fountains do you walk by over the course of the day? This information will help you put together a successful plan for change.

### Analyze Your Data and Set Goals

Evaluate your beverage consumption by dividing your typical daily consumption between healthy and less healthy choices. Use the following guide as a basis, and add other beverages to the lists as needed.

*Choose less often:*

- Regular soda
- Sweetened bottled iced tea
- Fruit beverages made with little fruit juice (usually labeled fruit drinks, punches, beverages, blends, or ades)
- Whole milk

*Choose more often:*

- Water—plain, mineral, and sparkling
- Low-fat or fat-free milk
- Fruit juice (100% juice)
- Unsweetened herbal tea

How many beverages do you consume daily from each category? What would be a healthy and realistic goal for change? For example, if your beverage consumption is currently evenly divided between the "choose more often" and "choose less often" categories (four from each list), you might set a final goal for your behavior change program of increasing your healthy choices by two (to six from the "more often" list and two from the "less often" list).

### Develop a Plan for Change

Once you've set your goal, you need to develop strategies that will help you choose healthy beverages more often. Consider the following possibilities:

- Keep healthy beverages on hand; if you live in a student dorm, rent a small refrigerator or keep bottled water, juice, fat-free milk, and other healthy choices in the dorm's kitchen refrigerator.
- Plan ahead, and put a bottle of water or 100% juice in your backpack every day.
- Check food labels on beverages for serving sizes, calories, and nutrients; comparison shop to find the healthiest choices, and watch your serving sizes. Use this information to make your "choose more often" list longer and more specific.
- If you eat out frequently, examine all the beverages available at the places you typically eat your meals. You'll probably find that healthy choices are available; if not, bring along your own drink or find somewhere else to eat.
- For a snack, try water and a piece of fruit rather than a heavily sweetened beverage.
- Create healthy beverages that appeal to you; for example, try adding slices of citrus fruit to water or mixing 100% fruit juice with sparkling water.

You may also need to make some changes in your routine to decrease the likelihood that you'll make unhealthy choices. For example, you might discover from your health journal that you always buy a soda after class when you pass a particular vending machine. If this is the case, try another route that allows you to avoid the machine. And try to guard against impulse buying by carrying water or a healthy snack with you every day.

To complete your plan, try some of the other behavior change strategies described in Chapter 1: Develop and sign a contract, set up a system of rewards, involve other people in your program, and develop strategies for challenging situations. Once your plan is complete, take action. Keep track of your progress in your health journal by continuing to monitor and evaluate your beverage consumption.

provide complete proteins; plants provide incomplete proteins.

- Fats, a concentrated source of energy, also help insulate the body and cushion the organs. Dietary fat intake should be 20–35% of total daily calories. Unsaturated fats should be favored over saturated and trans fats.
- Carbohydrates supply energy to the brain and other parts of the nervous system as well as to red blood cells. The body needs about 130 grams of carbohydrates a day, but much more is recommended.
- Fiber includes nondigestible carbohydrates provided mainly by plants. Adequate intake of fiber (38 grams per day for men and 25 grams per day for women) can help people manage diabetes and high cholesterol levels and improve intestinal health.
- The 13 vitamins needed in the diet are organic substances that promote specific chemical and cell processes within living tissue. Deficiencies or excesses can cause serious illnesses and even death.
- The approximately 17 minerals needed in the diet are inorganic substances that regulate body functions, aid in the growth and maintenance of body tissues, and help in the release of energy from foods.
- Water is used to digest and absorb food, transport substances around the body, lubricate joints and organs, and regulate body temperature.

- Foods contain other substances such as phytochemicals, which may not be essential nutrients but which reduce chronic disease risk.
- Dietary Reference Intakes (DRIs) are recommended intakes for essential nutrients that meet the needs of healthy people.
- The Dietary Guidelines for Americans address the prevention of diet-related diseases such as CVD, cancer, and diabetes. The guidelines advise us to consume a variety of foods while staying within calorie needs; manage body weight through calorie control and regular physical activity; eat more fruits, vegetables, whole grains, and reduced-fat dairy products; choose fats and carbohydrates wisely; eat less salt and more potassium; be moderate with alcohol intake, and handle foods safely.
- Choosing foods from each group in MyPyramid every day helps ensure the appropriate amounts of necessary nutrients.
- A vegetarian diet can meet human nutritional needs.
- Other dietary issues of concern include food and supplement labels, organic foods, food irradiation, and food allergies and intolerances.

## Take Action

1. **Examine ingredients and nutrient content:** Read the list of ingredients on three or four canned or packaged foods that you enjoy eating. If any ingredients are unfamiliar to you, find out what they are and why they have been used. A nutrition textbook from the library may be a helpful resource. Also examine and compare nutrient content using the food label. Are you surprised by the energy or nutrient content of any of the foods you examine?

2. **Investigate nutritional and dietary guidelines:** What guidelines are used to prepare the food served in your school? Are they consistent with what you've learned in this chapter? If not, try to find out more about the guidelines that have been used and why they were chosen.

3. **Prepare a flavorful low-fat vegetarian and/or ethnic meal.** Use the suggestions in the chapter, and check your local library for appropriate cookbooks. How do the foods included in the meal and the preparation methods differ from what you're used to?

4. **Keep a journal:** A nutrition journal is useful for evaluating and improving your diet. The very act of recording everything you eat may improve your dietary habits—you'll find yourself thinking before you eat and avoiding some unhealthy choices so that you don't have to record them in your journal. Keeping a journal boosts your awareness of your food choices and your portion sizes, and it reinforces your commitment to improving your diet.

5. **Volunteer in your community:** There are many opportunities for improving the nutritional status of members of your community. Consider volunteering at a food bank or a kitchen at a homeless shelter. Or find a community garden program for school children or low-income families—working in a vegetable garden increases your own connection to the food you eat and improves your community.

## For More Information

### Books

Duyff, R. L. 2002. *ADA Complete Food and Nutrition Guide,* 2nd ed. Chicago, Ill.: The American Dietetic Association. *An excellent review of current nutrition information.*

Insel, P., R. E. Turner, and D. Ross. 2004. *Nutrition,* 2nd ed. Sudbury, Mass.: Jones & Bartlett. *An introductory nutrition textbook.*

Katz, D., and M. Gonzalez. 2003. *The Way to Eat.* Chicago, Ill.: American Dietetic Association. *Guide to a lifetime of eating well and promoting good health, weight control, and enjoyment of food.*

Melina, V., and B. Davis. 2003. *The New Becoming Vegetarian: The Essential Guide to a Healthy Vegetarian Diet.* Summertown, Tn.: Healthy Living Publications. *Provides information on the health benefits of vegetarian diets and how to plan healthy meals.*

Selkowitz, A. 2000. *The College Student's Guide to Eating Well on Campus.* Bethesda, Md.: Tulip Hill Press. *Provides practical advice for students, including how to make healthy choices when eating in a dorm or restaurant and how to stock a first pantry.*

Wardlaw, G. M., and A. M. Smith. 2006. *Contemporary Nutrition.* New York: McGraw-Hill. *A review of major concepts in nutrition.*

### Newsletters

*Environmental Nutrition* (800-829-5384; http://www.environmentalnutrition.com)

*Nutrition Action Health Letter* (202-332-9110; http://www.cspinet.org)

*Tufts University Health & Nutrition Letter* (800-274-7581; http://www.healthletter.tufts.edu)

### WW Organizations, Hotlines, and Web Sites

*American Dietetic Association.* Provides a wide variety of nutrition-related educational materials.
800-877-1600
http://www.eatright.org

*American Heart Association: Delicious Decisions.* Provides basic information about nutrition, tips for shopping and eating out, and heart-healthy recipes.
http://www.deliciousdecisions.org

*FDA Center for Food Safety and Applied Nutrition.* Offers information about topics such as food labeling, food additives, dietary supplements, and foodborne illness.
http://vm.cfsan.fda.gov

*Food Safety Hotlines.* Provide information on safe purchase, handling, cooking, and storage of food.
888-SAFEFOOD (FDA)
800-535-4555 (USDA)

*Gateways to Government Nutrition Information.* Provide access to government resources relating to food safety and nutrition.
http://www.foodsafety.gov
http://www.nutrition.gov

*Harvard School of Public Health Nutrition Source.* Provides recent key research findings, including advice on interpreting news on nutrition; an overview of the Healthy Eating Pyramid, an alternative to the basic USDA pyramid; and suggestions for building a healthy diet.
http://www.hsph.harvard.edu/nutritionsource

*MyPyramid.gov.* Provides personalized dietary plans and interactive food and activity tracking tools.
http://mypyramid.gov

*National Academies' Food and Nutrition Board.* Provides information about the Dietary Reference Intakes and related guidelines.
http://www.iom.edu/board.asp?id=3788

*National Cancer Institute: Eat 5 to 9 a Day for Better Health.* Provides tips and recipes to help consumers increase their intake of fruits and vegetables.
http://5aday.nci.nih.gov

*Tufts University Nutrition Navigator.* Provides descriptions and ratings for many nutrition-related Web pages.
http://navigator.tufts.edu

*USDA Center for Nutrition Policy and Promotion.* Includes information on the Dietary Guidelines and MyPyramid.
http://www.usda.gov/cnpp

*USDA Food and Nutrition Information Center.* Provides a variety of materials and extensive links relating to the Dietary Guidelines, food labels, MyPyramid, and many other topics.
http://www.nal.usda.gov/fnic

*Vegetarian Resource Group.* Information and links for vegetarians and people interested in learning more about vegetarian diets.
http://www.vrg.org

You can obtain nutrient breakdowns of individual food items from the following sites:

*Nutrition Analysis Tool, University of Illinois, Urbana/Champaign*
http://www.nat.uiuc.edu

*USDA Nutrient Data Laboratory*
http://www.nal.usda.gov/fnic/foodcomp

See also the resources listed in the dietary supplements box on p. 222 and in the For More Information sections in Chapters 10–12 and 14.

## Selected Bibliography


Aldana, S. G., et al. 2005. Effects of an intensive diet and physical activity modification program on the health risks of adults. *Journal of the American Dietetic Association* 105(3): 371–381.

Block, G. 2004. Foods contributing to energy intake in the US: Data from NHANES III and NHANES 1999–2000. *Journal of Food Composition and Analysis* 17(2004): 439–447.

Clifton, P. M., J. B. Keogh, and M. Noakes. 2004. Trans fatty acids in adipose tissue and the food supply are associated with myocardial infarction. *Journal of Nutrition* 134: 874–879.

Cotton, P. A., et al. 2004. Dietary sources of nutrients among U.S. adults, 1994 to 1996. *Journal of the American Dietetic Association* 104: 921–930.

Ervin, R. B., et al. 2004. Dietary intake of selected minerals for the United States population: 1999–2000. *Advance Data from Vital and Health Statistics* No. 341.

Food and Drug Administration. 2004. *Backgrounder for the 2004 FDA/EPA Consumer Advisory: What You Need to Know About Mercury in Fish and Shellfish* (http://www.fda.gov/oc/opacom/hottopics/mercury/backgrounder.html; retrieved April 27, 2004).

Food and Drug Administration. 2004. *Commonly Asked Questions About BSE in Products Regulated by FDA's Center for Food Safety and Applied Nutrition* (http://www.cfsan.fda.gov/~comm/bsefaq.html; retrieved April 28, 2004).

Food and Drug Administration. 2004. *Fact Sheet: Carbohydrates* (http://www.fda.gov/oc/initiatives/obesity/factsheet.html; retrieved April 28, 2004).

Food and Nutrition Board, Institute of Medicine. 2002. *Dietary Reference Intakes for Energy, Carbohydrate, Fiber, Fat, Fatty Acids, Cholesterol, Protein, and Amino Acids.* Washington, D.C.: National Academy Press.

Food and Nutrition Board, Institute of Medicine. 2004. *Dietary Reference Intakes for Water, Potassium, Sodium, Chloride, and Sulfate.* Washington, D.C.: National Academy Press.

Hanley, D. A., and K. S. Davison. 2005. Vitamin D insufficiency in North America. *Journal of Nutrition* 135(2): 332–337.

He, K., et al. 2004. Accumulated evidence on fish consumption and coronary heart disease mortality: A meta-analysis of cohort studies. *Circulation* 109: 2705–2711.

Hites, R. A., et al. 2004. Global assessment of organic contaminants in farmed salmon. *Science* 303(5655): 225–229.

Houston, D. K., et al. 2005. Dairy, fruit, and vegetable intakes and functional limitations and disability in a biracial cohort. *American Journal of Clinical Nutrition* 81(2): 515–522.

Joint WHO/FAO Expert Consultation. 2003. *Diet, Nutrition, and the Prevention of Chronic Diseases.* Geneva:World Health Organization.

Kranz, S., et al. 2005. Adverse effect of high added sugar consumption on dietary intake in American preschoolers. *Journal of Pediatrics* 46(1): 105–111.

Liu, S., et al. 2003. Is intake of breakfast cereals related to total and cause-specific mortality in men? *American Journal of Clinical Nutrition* 77(3): 594–599.

Ma, Y., et al. 2005. Association between dietary carbohydrates and body weight. *American Journal of Epidemiology* 161(4): 359–367.

National Center for Health Statistics. 2003. Dietary intake of ten key nutrients for public health, United States: 1999–2000. *Advance Data from Vital and Health Statistics* No. 334.

Opotowsky, A. R., et al. 2004. Serum vitamin A concentration and the risk of hip fracture among women 50 to 74 years old in the United States. *American Journal of Medicine* 117(3): 169–174.

Pereira, M. A., et al. 2004. Dietary fiber and risk of coronary heart disease: A pooled analysis of cohort studies. *Archives of Internal Medicine* 164(4): 370–376.

U.S. Department of Agriculture, Center for Nutrition Policy and Promotion. 2005. *MyPyramid* (http://www.mypyramid.gov; retrieved April 20, 2005).

U.S. Department of Agriculture, Center for Nutrition Policy and Promotion. 2004. *The Food Guide Pyramid Update* (http://www.cnpp.usda.gov/pyramid-update; retrieved January 5, 2005).

U.S. Department of Health and Human Services and U.S. Department of Agriculture. 2005. *Dietary Guidelines for Americans, 2005* (http://www.health.gov/dietary guidelines; retrieved January 20, 2005).

U.S. Department of Health and Human Services and U.S. Department of Agriculture. 2005. *Finding Your Way to a Healthier You: Based on the Dietary Guidelines for Americans.* Home and Garden Bulletin No. 232-CP.

# Nutrition Resources

## Table 1 Dietary Reference Intakes (DRIs): Recommended Levels for Individual Intake

| Life Stage | Group | Biotin (μg/day) | Choline (mg/day)[a] | Folate (μg/day)[b] | Niacin (mg/day)[c] | Pantothenic Acid (mg/day) | Riboflavin (mg/day) | Thiamin (mg/day) | Vitamin A (μg/day)[d] | Vitamin B-6 (mg/day) | Vitamin B-12 (μg/day) | Vitamin C (mg/day)[e] | Vitamin D (μg/day)[f] | Vitamin E (mg/day)[g] |
|---|---|---|---|---|---|---|---|---|---|---|---|---|---|---|
| Infants | 0–6 months | 5 | 125 | 65 | 2 | 1.7 | 0.3 | 0.2 | 400 | 0.1 | 0.4 | 40 | 5 | 4 |
| | 7–12 months | 6 | 150 | 80 | 4 | 1.8 | 0.4 | 0.3 | 500 | 0.3 | 0.5 | 50 | 5 | 5 |
| Children | 1–3 years | 8 | 200 | **150** | **6** | 2 | **0.5** | **0.5** | **300** | **0.5** | **0.9** | **15** | 5 | **6** |
| | 4–8 years | 12 | 250 | **200** | **8** | 3 | **0.6** | **0.6** | **400** | **0.6** | **1.2** | **25** | 5 | **7** |
| Males | 9–13 years | 20 | 375 | **300** | **12** | 4 | **0.9** | **0.9** | **600** | **1.0** | **1.8** | **45** | 5 | **11** |
| | 14–18 years | 25 | 550 | **400** | **16** | 5 | **1.3** | **1.2** | **900** | **1.3** | **2.4** | **75** | 5 | **15** |
| | 19–30 years | 30 | 550 | **400** | **16** | 5 | **1.3** | **1.2** | **900** | **1.3** | **2.4** | **90** | 5 | **15** |
| | 31–50 years | 30 | 550 | **400** | **16** | 5 | **1.3** | **1.2** | **900** | **1.3** | **2.4** | **90** | 5 | **15** |
| | 51–70 years | 30 | 550 | **400** | **16** | 5 | **1.3** | **1.2** | **900** | **1.7** | **2.4**[h] | **90** | 10 | **15** |
| | >70 years | 30 | 550 | **400** | **16** | 5 | **1.3** | **1.2** | **900** | **1.7** | **2.4**[h] | **90** | 15 | **15** |
| Females | 9–13 years | 20 | 375 | **300** | **12** | 4 | **0.9** | **0.9** | **600** | **1.0** | **1.8** | **45** | 5 | **11** |
| | 14–18 years | 25 | 400 | **400**[i] | **14** | 5 | **1.0** | **1.0** | **700** | **1.2** | **2.4** | **65** | 5 | **15** |
| | 19–30 years | 30 | 425 | **400**[i] | **14** | 5 | **1.1** | **1.1** | **700** | **1.3** | **2.4** | **75** | 5 | **15** |
| | 31–50 years | 30 | 425 | **400**[i] | **14** | 5 | **1.1** | **1.1** | **700** | **1.3** | **2.4** | **75** | 5 | **15** |
| | 51–70 years | 30 | 425 | **400**[i] | **14** | 5 | **1.1** | **1.1** | **700** | **1.5** | **2.4**[h] | **75** | 10 | **15** |
| | >70 years | 30 | 425 | **400** | **14** | 5 | **1.1** | **1.1** | **700** | **1.5** | **2.4**[h] | **75** | 15 | **15** |
| Pregnancy | ≤18 years | 30 | 450 | **600**[j] | **18** | 6 | **1.4** | **1.4** | **750** | **1.9** | **2.6** | **80** | 5 | **15** |
| | 19–30 years | 30 | 450 | **600**[j] | **18** | 6 | **1.4** | **1.4** | **770** | **1.9** | **2.6** | **85** | 5 | **15** |
| | 31–50 years | 30 | 450 | **600**[j] | **18** | 6 | **1.4** | **1.4** | **770** | **1.9** | **2.6** | **85** | 5 | **15** |
| Lactation | ≤18 years | 35 | 550 | **500** | **17** | 7 | **1.6** | **1.4** | **1200** | **2.0** | **2.8** | **115** | 5 | **19** |
| | 19–30 years | 35 | 550 | **500** | **17** | 7 | **1.6** | **1.4** | **1300** | **2.0** | **2.8** | **120** | 5 | **19** |
| | 31–50 years | 35 | 550 | **500** | **17** | 7 | **1.6** | **1.4** | **1300** | **2.0** | **2.8** | **120** | 5 | **19** |
| *Tolerable Upper Intake Levels for Adults (19–70)* | | | *3500* | *1000*[k] | *35*[k] | | | | *3000* | *100* | | *2000* | *50* | *1000*[k] |

NOTE: The table includes values for the type of DRI standard—Adequate Intake (AI) or Recommended Dietary Allowance (RDA)—that has been established for that particular nutrient and life stage; RDAs are shown in **bold type.** The final row of the table shows the Tolerable Upper Intake Levels (ULs) for adults; refer to the full DRI report for information on other ages and life stages. A UL is the maximum level of daily nutrient intake that is likely to pose no risk of adverse effects. There is insufficient data to set ULs for all nutrients, but this does not mean that there is no potential for adverse effects; source of intake should be from food only to prevent high levels of intake of nutrients without established ULs. In healthy individuals, there is no established benefit from nutrient intakes above the RDA or AI.

[a]Although AIs have been set for choline, there are few data to assess whether a dietary supply of choline is needed at all stages of the life cycle, and it may be that the choline requirement can be met by endogenous synthesis at some of these stages.

[b]As dietary folate equivalents (DFE): 1 DFE = 1 μg food folate = 0.6 μg folate from fortified food or as a supplement consumed with food = 0.5 μg of a supplement taken on an empty stomach.

[c]As niacin equivalents (NE): 1 mg niacin = 60 mg tryptophan.

## Table 1 Dietary Reference Intakes (DRIs): Recommended Levels for Individual Intake (*continued*)

| Life Stage | Group | Vitamin K (μg/day) | Calcium (mg/day) | Chromium (μg/day) | Copper (μg/day) | Fluoride (mg/day) | Iodine (μg/day) | Iron (mg/day)[l] | Magnesium (mg/day) | Manganese (mg/day) | Molybdenum (μg/day) | Phosphorus (mg/day) | Selenium (μg/day) | Zinc (mg/day)[m] |
|---|---|---|---|---|---|---|---|---|---|---|---|---|---|---|
| Infants | 0–6 months | 2.0 | 210 | 0.2 | 200 | 0.01 | 110 | 0.27 | 30 | 0.003 | 2 | 100 | 15 | 2 |
| | 7–12 months | 2.5 | 270 | 5.5 | 220 | 0.5 | 130 | 11 | 75 | 0.6 | 3 | 275 | 20 | 3 |
| Children | 1–3 years | 30 | 500 | 11 | 340 | 0.7 | 90 | 7 | 80 | 1.2 | 17 | 460 | 20 | 3 |
| | 4–8 years | 55 | 800 | 15 | 440 | 1 | 90 | 10 | 130 | 1.5 | 22 | 500 | 30 | 5 |
| Males | 9–13 years | 60 | 1300 | 25 | 700 | 2 | 120 | 8 | 240 | 1.9 | 34 | 1250 | 40 | 8 |
| | 14–18 years | 75 | 1300 | 35 | 890 | 3 | 150 | 11 | 410 | 2.2 | 43 | 1250 | 55 | 11 |
| | 19–30 years | 120 | 1000 | 35 | 900 | 4 | 150 | 8 | 400 | 2.3 | 45 | 700 | 55 | 11 |
| | 31–50 years | 120 | 1000 | 35 | 900 | 4 | 150 | 8 | 420 | 2.3 | 45 | 700 | 55 | 11 |
| | 51–70 years | 120 | 1200 | 30 | 900 | 4 | 150 | 8 | 420 | 2.3 | 45 | 700 | 55 | 11 |
| | >70 years | 120 | 1200 | 30 | 900 | 4 | 150 | 8 | 420 | 2.3 | 45 | 700 | 55 | 11 |
| Females | 9–13 years | 60 | 1300 | 21 | 700 | 2 | 120 | 8 | 240 | 1.6 | 34 | 1250 | 40 | 8 |
| | 14–18 years | 75 | 1300 | 24 | 890 | 3 | 150 | 15 | 360 | 1.6 | 43 | 1250 | 55 | 9 |
| | 19–30 years | 90 | 1000 | 25 | 900 | 3 | 150 | 18 | 310 | 1.8 | 45 | 700 | 55 | 8 |
| | 31–50 years | 90 | 1000 | 25 | 900 | 3 | 150 | 18 | 320 | 1.8 | 45 | 700 | 55 | 8 |
| | 51–70 years | 90 | 1200 | 20 | 900 | 3 | 150 | 8 | 320 | 1.8 | 45 | 700 | 55 | 8 |
| | >70 years | 90 | 1200 | 20 | 900 | 3 | 150 | 8 | 320 | 1.8 | 45 | 700 | 55 | 8 |
| Pregnancy | ≤18 years | 75 | 1300 | 29 | 1000 | 3 | 220 | 27 | 400 | 2.0 | 50 | 1250 | 60 | 13 |
| | 19–30 years | 90 | 1000 | 30 | 1000 | 3 | 220 | 27 | 350 | 2.0 | 50 | 700 | 60 | 11 |
| | 31–50 years | 90 | 1000 | 30 | 1000 | 3 | 220 | 27 | 360 | 2.0 | 50 | 700 | 60 | 11 |
| Lactation | ≤18 years | 75 | 1300 | 44 | 1300 | 3 | 290 | 10 | 360 | 2.6 | 50 | 1250 | 70 | 14 |
| | 19–30 years | 90 | 1000 | 45 | 1300 | 3 | 290 | 9 | 310 | 2.6 | 50 | 700 | 70 | 12 |
| | 31–50 years | 90 | 1000 | 45 | 1300 | 3 | 290 | 9 | 320 | 2.6 | 50 | 700 | 70 | 12 |
| *Tolerable Upper Intake Levels for Adults (19–70)* | | | *2500* | | *10,000* | *10* | *1100* | *45* | *350*[k] | *11* | *2000* | *4000* | *400* | *40* |

[d]As retinol activity equivalents (RAEs): 1 RAE = 1 μg retinol, 12 μg β-carotene, or 24 μg α-carotene or β-cryptoxanthin. Preformed vitamin A (retinol) is abundant in animal-derived foods; provitamin A carotenoids are abundant in some dark yellow, orange, red, and deep-green fruits and vegetables. For preformed vitamin A and for provitamin A carotenoids in supplements, 1RE = 1 RAE; for provitamin A carotenoids in foods, divide the REs by 2 to obtain RAEs. The UL applies only to preformed vitamin A.

[e]Individuals who smoke require an additional 35 mg/day of vitamin C over that needed by nonsmokers; nonsmokers regularly exposed to tobacco smoke should ensure they meet the RDA for vitamin C.

[f]As cholecalciferol: 1 μg cholecalciferol = 40 IU vitamin D. DRI values are based on the absence of adequate exposure to sunlight.

[g]As α-tocopherol. Includes naturally occurring RRR-α-tocopherol and the 2R-stereoisomeric forms from supplements; does not include the 2S-stereoisomeric forms from supplements.

[h]Because 10–30% of older people may malabsorb food-bound B-12, those over age 50 should meet their RDA mainly with supplements or foods fortified with B-12.

[i]In view of evidence linking folate intake with neural tube defects in the fetus. It is recommended that all women capable of becoming pregnant consume 400 μg from supplements or fortified foods in addition to consuming folate from a varied diet.

[j]It is assumed that women will continue consuming 400 μg from supplements or fortified food until their pregnancy is confirmed and they enter prenatal care, which ordinarily occurs after the end of the periconceptional period—the critical time for formation of the neural tube.

[k]The UL applies only to intake from supplements, fortified foods, and/or pharmacological agents and not to intake from foods.

[l]Because the absorption of iron from plant foods is low compared to that from animal foods, the RDA for strict vegetarians is approximately 1.8 times higher than the values established for omnivores (14 mg/day for adult male vegetarians; 33 mg/day for premenopausal female vegetarians). Oral contraceptives (OCs) reduce menstrual blood losses, so women taking them need less daily iron; the RDA for premenopausal women taking OCs is 10.9 mg/day. For more on iron requirements for other special situations, refer to *Dietary Reference Intakes for Vitamin A, Vitamin K, Arsenic, Boron, Chromium, Copper, Iodine, Iron, Manganese, Molybdenum, Nickel, Silicon, Vanadium, and Zinc* (visit http://www.nap.edu for the complete report).

[m]Zinc absorption is lower for those consuming vegetarian diets so the zinc requirement for vegetarians is approximately twofold greater than for those consuming a nonvegetarian diet.

**Table 1 Dietary Reference Intakes (DRIs): Recommended Levels for Individual Intake (*continued*)**

| | | | | | Carbohydrate | | Total Fiber | Total Fat | Linoleic Acid | | Alpha-linolenic Acid | | Protein[n] | | |
|---|---|---|---|---|---|---|---|---|---|---|---|---|---|---|---|
| Life Stage | Group | Potassium (g/day) | Sodium (g/day) | Chloride (g/day) | RDA/AI (g/day) | AMDR[o] (%) | RDA/AI (g/day) | AMDR[o] (%) | RDA/AI (g/day) | AMDR[o] (%) | RDA/AI (g/day) | AMDR[o] (%) | RDA/AI (g/day) | AMDR[o] (%) | Water[p] (L/day) |
| Infants | 0–6 months | 0.4 | 0.12 | 0.18 | 60 | ND[q] | ND | [r] | 4.4 | ND[q] | 0.5 | ND[q] | 9.1 | ND[q] | 0.7 |
| | 7–12 months | 0.7 | 0.37 | 0.57 | 95 | ND[q] | ND | [r] | 4.6 | ND[q] | 0.5 | ND[q] | **13.5** | ND[q] | 0.8 |
| Children | 1–3 years | 3.0 | 1.0 | 1.5 | **130** | 45–65 | 19 | 30–40 | 7 | 5–10 | 0.7 | 0.6–1.2 | **13** | 5–20 | 1.3 |
| | 4–8 years | 3.8 | 1.2 | 1.9 | **130** | 45–65 | 25 | 25–35 | 10 | 5–10 | 0.9 | 0.6–1.2 | **19** | 10–30 | 1.7 |
| Males | 9–13 years | 4.5 | 1.5 | 2.3 | **130** | 45-65 | 31 | 25–35 | 12 | 5–10 | 1.2 | 0.6–1.2 | **34** | 10–30 | 2.4 |
| | 14–18 years | 4.7 | 1.5 | 2.3 | **130** | 45–65 | 38 | 25–35 | 16 | 5–10 | 1.6 | 0.6–1.2 | **52** | 10–30 | 3.3 |
| | 19–30 years | 4.7 | 1.5 | 2.3 | **130** | 45–65 | 38 | 20–35 | 17 | 5–10 | 1.6 | 0.6–1.2 | **56** | 10–35 | 3.7 |
| | 31–50 years | 4.7 | 1.5 | 2.3 | **130** | 45–65 | 38 | 20–35 | 17 | 5–10 | 1.6 | 0.6–1.2 | **56** | 10–35 | 3.7 |
| | 51–70 years | 4.7 | 1.3 | 2.0 | **130** | 45–65 | 30 | 20–35 | 14 | 5–10 | 1.6 | 0.6–1.2 | **56** | 10–35 | 3.7 |
| | >70 years | 4.7 | 1.2 | 1.8 | **130** | 45–65 | 30 | 20–35 | 14 | 5–10 | 1.6 | 0.6–1.2 | **56** | 10-35 | 3.7 |
| Females | 9–13 years | 4.5 | 1.5 | 2.3 | **130** | 45–65 | 26 | 25–35 | 10 | 5–10 | 1.0 | 0.6–1.2 | **34** | 10–30 | 2.1 |
| | 14–18 years | 4.7 | 1.5 | 2.3 | **130** | 45–65 | 26 | 25–35 | 11 | 5–10 | 1.1 | 0.6–1.2 | **46** | 10–30 | 2.3 |
| | 19–30 years | 4.7 | 1.5 | 2.3 | **130** | 45–65 | 25 | 20–35 | 12 | 5–10 | 1.1 | 0.6–1.2 | **46** | 10–35 | 2.7 |
| | 31–50 years | 4.7 | 1.5 | 2.3 | **130** | 45–65 | 25 | 20–35 | 12 | 5–10 | 1.1 | 0.6–1.2 | **46** | 10–35 | 2.7 |
| | 51–70 years | 4.7 | 1.3 | 2.0 | **130** | 45–65 | 21 | 20–35 | 11 | 5–10 | 1.1 | 0.6–1.2 | **46** | 10–35 | 2.7 |
| | >70 years | 4.7 | 1.2 | 1.8 | **130** | 45–65 | 21 | 20–35 | 11 | 5–10 | 1.1 | 0.6–1.2 | **46** | 10–35 | 2.7 |
| Pregnancy | ≤18 years | 4.7 | 1.5 | 2.3 | **175** | 45–65 | 28 | 20–35 | 13 | 5–10 | 1.4 | 0.6–1.2 | **71** | 10–35 | 3.0 |
| | 19–30 years | 4.7 | 1.5 | 2.3 | **175** | 45–65 | 28 | 20–35 | 13 | 5–10 | 1.4 | 0.6–1.2 | **71** | 10–35 | 3.0 |
| | 31–50 years | 4.7 | 1.5 | 2.3 | **175** | 45–65 | 28 | 20–35 | 13 | 5–10 | 1.4 | 0.6–1.2 | **71** | 10–35 | 3.0 |
| Lactation | ≤18 years | 5.1 | 1.5 | 2.3 | **210** | 45–65 | 29 | 20–35 | 13 | 5–10 | 1.3 | 0.6–1.2 | **71** | 10–35 | 3.8 |
| | 19–30 years | 5.1 | 1.5 | 2.3 | **210** | 45–65 | 29 | 20–35 | 13 | 5–10 | 1.3 | 0.6–1.2 | **71** | 10–35 | 3.8 |
| | 31–50 years | 5.1 | 1.5 | 2.3 | **210** | 45–65 | 29 | 20–35 | 13 | 5–10 | 1.3 | 0.6–1.2 | **71** | 10-35 | 3.8 |
| ***Tolerable Upper Intake Level for Adults (19–70)*** | | | 2.3 | 3.6 | | | | | | | | | | | |

[n]Daily protein recommendations are based on body weight for reference body weights. To calculate for a specific body weight, use the following values: 1.5 g/kg for infants, 1.1 g/kg for 1–3 years, 0.95 g/kg for 4–13 years, 0.85 g/kg for 14–18 years, 0.8 g/kg for adults, and 1.1 g/kg for pregnant (using prepregnancy weight) and lactating women.

[o]Acceptable Macronutrient Distribution Range (AMDR), expressed as a percent of total daily calories, is the range of intake for a particular energy source that is associated with reduced risk of chronic disease while providing intakes of essential nutrients. If an individual consumes in excess of the AMDR, there is a potential for increasing the risk of chronic diseases and/or insufficient intakes of essential nutrients.

[p]Total water intake from fluids and food.

[q]Not determinable due to lack of data of adverse effects in this age group and concern with regard to lack of ability to handle excess amounts. Source of intake should be from food only to prevent high levels of intake.

[r]For infants, Adequate Intake of total fat is 31 grams/day (0–6 months) and 30 grams per day (7–12 months) from breast milk and, for infants 7–12 months, complementary food and beverages.

SOURCE: Food and Nutrition Board, Institute of Medicine, National Academies. 2004. *Dietary Reference Intakes Tables* (http://www.iom.edu/file.asp?id=21372; retrieved December 21, 2004). The complete Dietary Reference Intake reports are available from the National Academy Press (http://www.nap.edu).

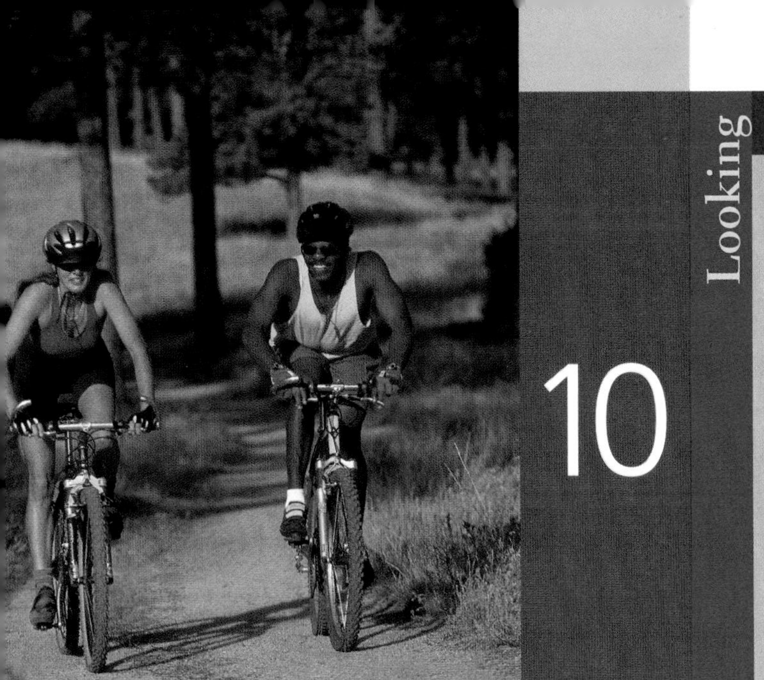

# 10

## Looking AHEAD

After reading this chapter, you should be able to

- Define physical fitness, and list the health-related components of fitness
- Explain the wellness benefits of physical activity and exercise
- Describe how to develop each of the health-related components of fitness
- Discuss how to choose appropriate exercise equipment, how to eat and drink for exercise, how to assess fitness, and how to prevent and manage injuries
- Put together a personalized exercise program that you enjoy and that will enable you to achieve your fitness goals

# Exercise for Health and Fitness

Your body is a wonderful moving machine. Your bones, joints, and ligaments provide a support system for movement; your muscles perform the motions of work and play; your heart and lungs nourish your cells as you move through your daily life. But your body is made to work best when it is physically active. It readily adapts to practically any level of activity and exercise: The more you ask of your body—your muscles, bones, heart, lungs—the stronger and more fit it becomes. The opposite is also true. Left unchallenged, bones lose their density, joints stiffen, muscles become weak, and cellular energy systems begin to degenerate. To be truly healthy, human beings must be active.

The benefits of physical activity are both physical and mental, immediate and far-reaching. Being physically fit makes it easier to do everyday tasks, such as lifting; it provides reserve strength for emergencies; and it helps people to look and feel good. Over the long term, physically fit individuals are less likely to develop heart disease, cancer, high blood pressure, diabetes, and many other degenerative diseases.

Unfortunately, modern life for most Americans provides few built-in occasions for vigorous activity. Technological advances have made our lives increasingly sedentary: We drive cars, ride escalators, watch television, and push papers around at school and work. According to *Healthy People 2010*, levels of physical activity remain low for all populations of Americans. In 1996, the U.S. Surgeon General published *Physical Activity and Health*, a report designed to reverse these trends and get Americans moving. The report's conclusions include the following:

- People of all ages, both male and female, benefit from regular physical activity.
- People can obtain significant health benefits by including a moderate amount of physical activity on most, if not all, days of the week.
- Additional health benefits can be gained through greater amounts of physical activity. People who can maintain a regular regimen of more vigorous or longer-duration activity are likely to obtain even greater benefits.
- Physical activity reduces the risk of premature mortality, improves psychological health, and is important for the health of muscle, bones, and joints.

Are you one of the 55% of Americans who are not regularly active? Or one of the 25% who are not active at all? This chapter will give you the basic information you need to put together a physical fitness program that will add fun and joy to life, and provide the foundation for a lifetime of fitness.

**Visit the Core Concepts in Health Online Learning Center (www.mhhe.com/inselbrief10e) for study aids and many additional resources.**

## WHAT IS PHYSICAL FITNESS?

**Physical fitness** is a set of physical attributes that allows the body to respond or adapt to the demands and stress of physical effort—that is, to perform moderate-to-vigorous levels of physical activity without becoming overly tired. Physical fitness has many components, some related to general health and others related more specifically to particular sports or activities. The five components of fitness most important for health are cardiorespiratory endurance, muscular strength, muscular endurance, flexibility, and body composition (proportion of fat to fat-free mass).

### Cardiorespiratory Endurance

**Cardiorespiratory endurance** is the ability to perform prolonged, large-muscle, dynamic exercise at moderate-to-high levels of intensity. When levels of cardiorespiratory fitness are low, the heart has to work very hard during normal daily activities and may not be able to work hard enough to sustain high-intensity physical activity in an emergency. As cardiorespiratory fitness improves, the heart begins to function more efficiently. It doesn't have to work as hard at rest or during low levels of exercise. The heart pumps more blood per heartbeat, resting heart rate slows down, blood volume increases, blood supply to the tissues improves, the body is better able to cool itself, and resting blood pressure decreases. A healthy heart can better withstand the strains of everyday life, the stress of occasional emergencies, and the wear and tear of time.

Cardiorespiratory endurance is considered a critically important component of health-related fitness because the functioning of the heart and lungs is so essential to overall wellness. A person simply cannot live very long or very well without a healthy heart. Low levels of cardiorespiratory fitness are linked with heart disease, the leading cause of death in the United States. Cardiorespiratory endurance is developed by activities that involve continuous rhythmic movements of large-muscle groups like those in the legs—for example, walking and cycling.

### Terms

**physical fitness** A set of physical attributes that allows the body to respond or adapt to the demands and stress of physical effort.

**cardiorespiratory endurance** The ability of the body to perform prolonged, large-muscle, dynamic exercise at moderate-to-high levels of intensity.

**muscular strength** The amount of force a muscle can produce with a single maximum effort.

**muscular endurance** The ability of a muscle or group of muscles to remain contracted or to contract repeatedly for a long period of time.

**flexibility** The range of motion in a joint or group of joints; flexibility is related to muscle length.

**body composition** The proportion of fat and fat-free mass (muscle, bone, and water) in the body.

### Muscular Strength

**Muscular strength** is the amount of force a muscle can produce with a single maximum effort. Strong, powerful muscles are important for the smooth and easy performance of everyday activities, such as carrying groceries, lifting boxes, and climbing stairs, as well as for emergency situations. They help keep the skeleton in proper alignment, preventing back and leg pain and providing the support necessary for good posture. Muscular strength has obvious importance in recreational activities. Strong people can hit a tennis ball harder, kick a soccer ball farther, and ride a bicycle uphill more easily.

Muscle tissue is an important element of overall body composition. Greater muscle mass makes possible a higher rate of metabolism and faster energy use, which help to maintain a healthy body weight. Strength training helps maintain muscle mass, function, and balance in older people, which greatly enhances their quality of life and prevents life-threatening injuries. Strength training has also been shown to benefit cardiovascular health. Muscular strength can be developed by training with weights or by using the weight of the body for resistance during calisthenic exercises such as push-ups and sit-ups.

### Muscular Endurance

**Muscular endurance** is the ability to resist fatigue and sustain a given level of muscle tension—that is, to hold a muscle contraction for a long period of time or to contract a muscle over and over again. Muscular endurance is important for good posture and for injury prevention. It helps people cope with the physical demands of everyday life and enhances performance in sports and work. Like muscular strength, muscular endurance is developed by stressing the muscles with a greater load (weight) than they are used to. The degree to which strength or endurance develops depends on the type and amount of stress that is applied.

### Flexibility

**Flexibility** is the ability to move the joints through their full range of motion. Although range of motion is not a significant factor in everyday activities for most people, inactivity causes the joints to become stiffer with age. Stiffness often causes older people to assume unnatural body postures, and it can lead to back, shoulder, or neck pain. Stretching exercises can help ensure a normal range of motion and pain-free joints.

## Body Composition

**Body composition** refers to the proportion of fat and fat-free mass (muscle, bone, and water) in the body. Healthy body composition involves a high proportion of fat-free mass and an acceptably low level of body fat. A person with excessive body fat is more likely to experience a variety of health problems, including heart disease, high blood pressure, stroke, joint problems, diabetes, gallbladder disease, cancer, and back pain. The best way to lose fat is through a lifestyle that includes a sensible diet and exercise. The best way to add muscle mass is through resistance training such as weight training. (Body composition is discussed in more detail in Chapter 11.)

# THE BENEFITS OF EXERCISE

As mentioned above, the human body is very adaptable. The greater the demands made on it, the more it adjusts to meet the demands—it becomes fit. Over time, immediate, short-term adjustments translate into long-term changes and improvements (Figure 10-1). For example, when breathing and heart rate increase during exercise, the heart gradually develops the ability to pump more blood with each beat. Then, during exercise, it doesn't have to beat as fast to meet the body's demand for oxygen.

Exercise is one of the most important things you can do to improve your level of wellness. Regular exercise increases energy levels, improves emotional and psychological

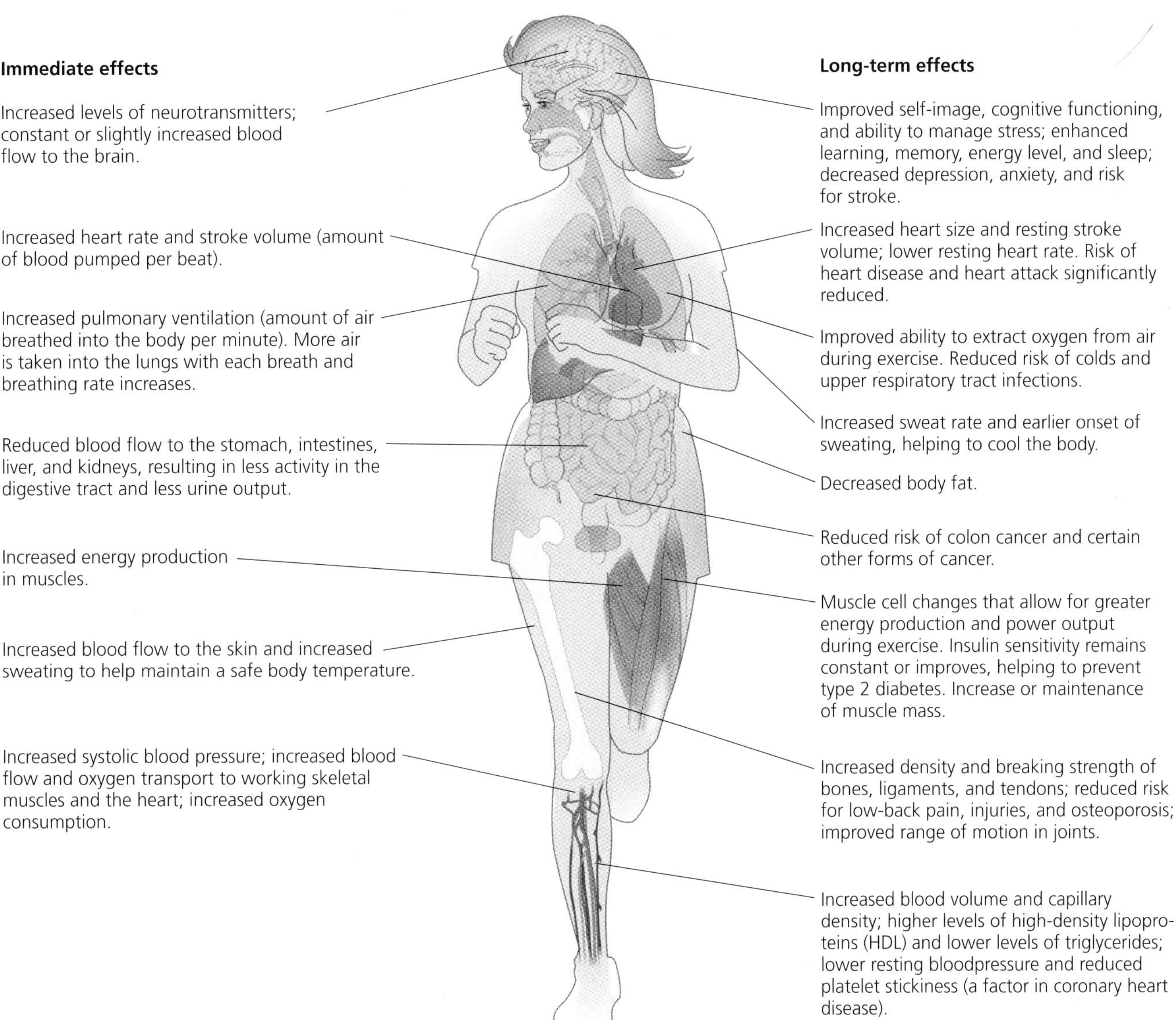


**Figure 10-1 Immediate and long-term effects of regular exercise.** When exercise is performed regularly, short-term changes in the body develop into more permanent adaptations; these long-term effects include improved ability to exercise, reduced risk of many chronic diseases, improved psychological and emotional well-being, and increased life expectancy.

well-being, and boosts the immune system. It prevents heart disease, some types of cancer, stroke, high blood pressure, insulin resistance, type 2 diabetes, obesity, and osteoporosis. At any age, people who exercise are less likely to die from all causes than are their sedentary peers. Worldwide, it is estimated that physical inactivity causes 1.9 million deaths per year.

## Improved Cardiorespiratory Functioning

Every time you take a breath, some of the oxygen in the air you take into your lungs is picked up by red blood cells and transported to your heart. From there, this oxygenated blood is pumped by the heart throughout the body to organs and tissues that use it. During exercise, the cardiorespiratory system (heart, lungs, and circulatory system) must work harder to meet the body's increased demand for oxygen. Regular endurance exercise improves the functioning of the heart and the ability of the cardiorespiratory system to carry oxygen to body tissues. It also reduces the risk of cardiovascular disease.

## More Efficient Metabolism

Endurance exercise improves metabolism, the process by which food is converted to energy and tissue is built. A physically fit person is better able to generate energy, to use carbohydrates and fats for energy, and to regulate hormones. Physical training may also protect the body's cells from damage from free radicals, which are produced during normal metabolism (see Chapter 9), and from inflammation caused by high blood pressure or cholesterol, nicotine, and overeating.

## Improved Body Composition

Exercise can improve body composition in several ways. Endurance exercise significantly increases daily calorie expenditure; it can also slightly raise *metabolic rate,* the rate at which the body burns calories, for several hours after an exercise session. Strength training increases muscle mass, thereby tipping the body composition ratio toward fat-free mass and away from fat. It can also help with losing fat because metabolic rate is directly proportional to fat-free mass: The more muscle mass, the higher the metabolic rate.

## Disease Prevention and Management

Regular physical activity lowers your risk of many chronic, disabling diseases. It can also help people with those diseases improve their health.

**Cardiovascular Disease** A sedentary lifestyle is one of the six major risk factors for **cardiovascular disease (CVD)** (see Chapter 12). People who are sedentary have CVD death rates significantly higher than those of fit individuals. Physical inactivity increases the risk of CVD by 50–240%. There is a dose-response relationship between exercise and CVD: The benefit of physical activity occurs at moderate levels of activity and increases with increasing levels of activity. Endurance exercise and strength training improve blood fat levels by increasing levels of high-density lipoproteins and decreasing levels of low-density lipoproteins and triglycerides. Exercise also reduces blood pressure and enhances the function of cells lining the arteries; it reduces the risk of heart disease, heart attack, and stroke.

**Cancer** Some studies have shown a relationship between increased physical activity and a reduction in a person's risk of all types of cancer, but these findings are not conclusive. There is strong evidence that exercise reduces the risk of colon cancer, and promising data that it reduces the risk of cancer of the breast and reproductive organs in women and cancer of the prostate in men.

**Osteoporosis** A special benefit of exercise, especially for women, is protection against osteoporosis, a disease that results in loss of bone density and poor bone strength. Weight-bearing exercise, which includes almost everything except swimming, helps build bone during the teens and twenties. Older people with denser bones can better endure the bone loss that occurs with aging. Strength training and impact exercises such as jumping rope can increase bone density throughout life. With stronger bones and muscles and better balance, fit people are less likely to experience debilitating falls and bone fractures.

**Type 2 Diabetes** People with diabetes are prone to heart disease, blindness, and severe problems of the nervous and circulatory systems. Exercise actually prevents the development of type 2 diabetes, the most common form. Exercise burns excess sugar and makes cells more sensitive to insulin; it also helps keep body fat at healthy levels. (Obesity is a key risk factor for type 2 diabetes.) For people who have diabetes, physical activity is an important part of treatment (see Chapter 11).

## Improved Psychological and Emotional Wellness

The joy of a well-hit cross-court backhand, the euphoria of a walk through the park, or the rush of a downhill schuss through deep powder snow provides pleasure that transcends health benefits alone. People who are physically active experience many social, psychological, and emotional benefits. They experience less stress and are buffered against the dangerous physical effects of stress. They are less likely to experience sleep problems, anxiety, or depression. They have enhanced learning and memory and improved self-image. Exercise also offers an arena for harmonious interaction with other people, as well as

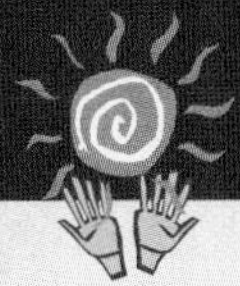

Mind/Body/Spirit

## Exercise and the Mind

If you've ever gone for a long, brisk walk after a hard day's work, you know how refreshing exercise can be. Exercise can improve mood, stimulate creativity, clarify thinking, relieve anxiety, and provide an outlet for anger or aggression. But why does exercise make you feel good? Does it simply take your mind off your problems? Or does it cause a physical reaction that affects your mental state?

Current research indicates that exercise triggers many physical changes in the body that can alter mood. Scientists are now trying to explain how and why exercise affects the mind. One theory has to do with the physical structure of the brain. The area of the brain responsible for the movement of muscles is near the area responsible for thought and emotion. As muscles work vigorously, the resulting stimulation in the muscle center of the brain may also stimulate the thought and emotion center, producing improvements in mood and cognitive functions.

Other researchers suggest that exercise stimulates the release of brain chemicals that affect mood. Exercise increases levels of **endorphins**, brain chemicals that can suppress fatigue, decrease pain, and produce euphoria. Levels of a chemical called anandamide are increased in people who exercise at a moderate intensity for an extended period. Anandamide produces effects similar to those of THC, the psychoactive chemical found in marijuana. The "runner's high" often experienced after running several miles may be due to the action of endorphins or anandamide.

A third area of research focuses on changes in brain activity during and after exercise. One change is an increase in alpha brain wave activity. Alpha waves indicate a highly relaxed state; meditation also induces alpha wave activity. A second change is an alteration in the levels of **neurotransmitters**, brain chemicals that increase alertness and reduce stress.

Higher levels of neurotransmitters such as serotonin may explain how exercise improves mild to moderate cases of depression. Researchers have found that exercise can be as effective as psychotherapy in treating depression, and even more effective when used in conjunction with other therapies. In addition to boosting neurotransmitter activity, exercise provides a distraction from stressful stimuli, enhances self-esteem, and may provide an opportunity for positive social interactions. Regular exercise also improves self-esteem and body image.

Although most people don't associate exercise with mental skills, physical activity has been shown to have positive effects on cognitive functioning in both the short term and the long term. Exercise improves alertness and memory and can help you perform cognitive tasks at your peak level. Exercise may also help boost creativity. In a study of college students, those who ran regularly or took aerobic dance classes scored significantly higher on standard psychological tests of creativity than sedentary students. Over the long term, exercise can slow and possibly even reverse certain age-related declines in cognitive performance, including slowed reaction time and loss of shortterm memory and nonverbal reasoning skills.

The message from this research is that exercise is a critical factor in developing *all* the dimensions of wellness, not just physical health. Even moderate exercise like walking briskly a few times per week can significantly improve your well-being. A lifetime of physical activity can leave you with a healthier body and a sharper, happier, more creative mind.

opportunities to strive and excel. See the box "Exercise and the Mind" for more information.

## Improved Immune Function

Exercise can have either positive or negative effects on the immune system, the physiological processes that protect us from disease. Moderate endurance exercise boosts immune function, whereas excessive training depresses it. Physically fit people get fewer colds and upper respiratory tract infections than people who are not fit.

## Prevention of Injuries and Low-Back Pain

Increased muscle strength provides protection against injury because it helps people maintain good posture and appropriate body mechanics when carrying out everyday activities such as walking, lifting, and carrying. Good muscle endurance in the abdomen, hips, lower back, and legs support the back in proper alignment and help prevent low-back pain.

## Improved Wellness over the Life Span

Although people differ in the maximum levels of fitness they can achieve through exercise, the wellness benefits of exercise are available to everyone (see the box "Exercise for People with Disabilities and Other Special Health Concerns" on p. 236). Exercising regularly may be the single most important thing you can do now to improve the quality of your life in the future. All the benefits of exercise continue to accrue but gain new importance as the resilience of youth begins to wane. Simply stated, exercising can help you live a longer and healthier life.

### Terms

VW

**cardiovascular disease (CVD)** A collective term for diseases of the heart and blood vessels.

**endorphins** Brain chemicals that seem to be involved in modulating pain and producing euphoria.

**neurotransmitters** Brain chemicals that transmit nerve impulses.

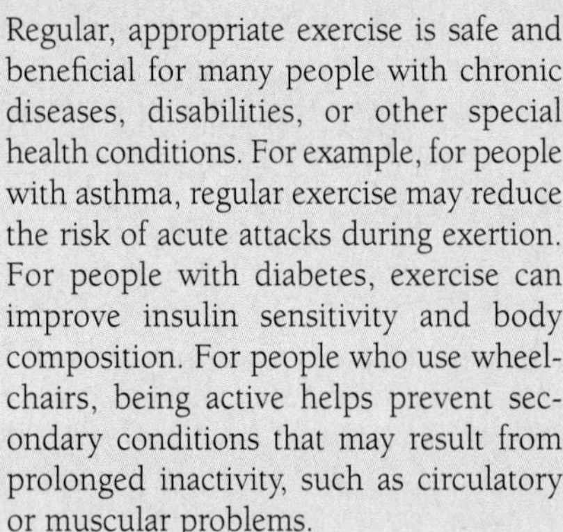

## Exercise for People with Disabilities and Other Special Health Concerns

Regular, appropriate exercise is safe and beneficial for many people with chronic diseases, disabilities, or other special health conditions. For example, for people with asthma, regular exercise may reduce the risk of acute attacks during exertion. For people with diabetes, exercise can improve insulin sensitivity and body composition. For people who use wheelchairs, being active helps prevent secondary conditions that may result from prolonged inactivity, such as circulatory or muscular problems.

For everyone, activity provides an emotional boost that helps support a positive attitude as well as opportunities to make new friends, increase self-confidence, and gain a sense of accomplishment. For many people with special health concerns, the risks associated with *not* exercising are far greater than those associated with a moderate program of regular exercise.

If you have a special health concern and have hesitated becoming more active, one helpful strategy is to take a class or join an exercise group specifically designed for your condition. Many health centers and support groups sponsor specially tailored activity programs. For example, health clubs may have modified aerobics classes, special weight training machines, and classes involving mild exercise in warm water; popular sports and recreational activities include adapted golf, swimming, and skiing, and wheelchair tennis, hockey, and basketball. Such a class or group activity can provide you with both expert advice and exercise partners who share your concerns and goals. If you prefer to exercise at home, exercise videos are available for people with a variety of conditions.

The fitness recommendations for the general population presented in this chapter can serve as general guidelines for any exercise program. However, for people with special health concerns, certain precautions and monitoring may be required. *Anyone with special health concerns should consult a physician before beginning an exercise program.* Guidelines and cautions for some common conditions are described below:

### Asthma

- Carry medication during workouts and avoid exercising alone. Use your inhaler before exercise, if recommended by your physician.
- Exercise regularly, and warm up and cool down slowly to reduce the risk of acute attacks.
- When starting a fitness program, choose self-paced endurance activities, especially those involving interval training (short bouts of exercise followed by a rest period).
- When possible, avoid circumstances that may trigger an asthma attack, including cold, dry air or pollen or dust. Drink water to keep your airways moist, and in cold weather, cover your mouth with a mask or scarf to warm and humidify the air you breathe. Swimming is a good activity choice for people with asthma.

### Diabetes

- Don't exercise alone; wear a bracelet identifying yourself as having diabetes.
- If you are taking insulin or another medication, you may need to adjust the timing and amount of each dose as you learn to balance your energy intake and output and your medication dosage.
- To prevent abnormally rapid absorption of injected insulin, inject it over a muscle that won't be exercised and wait at least an hour before exercising.
- Check blood sugar levels before, during, and after exercise, and adjust your diet or insulin dosage if needed. Avoid exercise if your blood sugar level is above 250 mg/dl, and ingest carbohydrates prior to exercise if your blood sugar level is below 100 mg/dl. Have high-carbohydrate foods available during a workout.
- Don't lift heavy weights. Check your skin regularly for blisters and abrasions, especially on your feet.

### Obesity

- For maximum benefit and minimum risk, begin with low- to moderate-intensity activities and increase intensity slowly as your fitness improves.
- To lose weight or maintain lost weight, exercise moderately 60 minutes or more every day; you can exercise all at once or divide your total activity time into sessions of 10 or more minutes.
- Choose non- or low-weight-bearing activities like swimming, water exercises, cycling, or walking.
- Stay alert for symptoms of heat-related problems during exercise.
- Try to include as much lifestyle physical activity in your daily routine as possible.
- Include strength training in your program to build or maintain muscle mass.

### Heart Disease and Hypertension

- Warm-up and cool-down sessions should be gradual and last at least 10 minutes.
- Exercise at a moderate rather than a high intensity; monitor your heart rate during exercise, and stop if you experience dizziness or chest pain.
- Increase exercise frequency, intensity, and time very gradually.
- Don't hold your breath when exercising as this can cause sudden, steep increases in blood pressure.
- Discuss the effects of your medication with your physician; for example, certain drugs for hypertension affect heart rate. If your physician has prescribed it, carry nitroglycerine with you during exercise.

### Arthritis

- Begin an exercise program as early as possible in the course of the disease.
- Warm up thoroughly before each workout to loosen stiff muscles and lower the risk of injury.
- Avoid high-impact activities that may damage arthritic joints; consider swimming or water aerobics.
- In strength training, pay special attention to muscles that support and protect affected joints; add weight very gradually.
- Perform flexibility exercises regularly.

### Osteoporosis

- If possible, choose low-impact weight-bearing activities to help safely maintain bone density.
- To prevent fractures, avoid any activity or movement that stresses the back or carries a risk of falling.
- Weight train to improve strength and balance and reduce the risk of falls and fractures, but avoid lifting heavy weights.

No matter what your level of ability or disability, you can make physical activity an integral part of your life.

# DESIGNING YOUR EXERCISE PROGRAM

The best exercise program has two primary characteristics: It promotes your health, and it's fun for you to do. Exercise does not have to be a chore. On the contrary, it can provide some of the most pleasurable moments of your day, once you make it a habit.

## Physical Activity and Exercise for Health and Fitness

*Physical activity* can be defined as any body movement carried out by skeletal muscles and requiring energy. Different types of physical activity can be arranged on a continuum based on the amount of energy they require. Quick, easy movements such as standing up or walking down a hallway require little energy or effort; more intense, sustained activities such as cycling 5 miles or running in a race require considerably more.

The term *exercise* is commonly used to refer to a subset of physical activity—planned, structured, repetitive movement of the body designed specifically to improve or maintain physical fitness. To develop fitness, a person must perform a sufficient amount of physical activity to stress the body and cause long-term physiological changes.

**Lifestyle Physical Activity for Health Promotion** The Surgeon General's report and joint guidelines from the CDC and the American College of Sports Medicine (ACSM) recommend that all Americans include a moderate amount of physical activity on most, preferably all, days of the week. The report suggests a goal of expending 150 calories per day, or about 1000 calories per week, in physical activity. Because energy expenditure is a function of both intensity and duration of activity, the same amount of benefit can be obtained in longer sessions of moderate-intensity activities as in shorter sessions of more strenuous activities. Thus, 15 minutes of running is equivalent to 30 minutes of brisk walking (Figure 10-2).

In this lifestyle approach to physical activity, the daily total of activity can be accumulated in multiple short bouts—for example, two 10-minute bicycle rides to and from class and a brisk 15-minute walk to the post office. Everyday tasks at school, work, and home can be structured to contribute to the daily activity total (see the box "Becoming More Active" on p. 238). The Surgeon General's report also recommends that people perform resistance training (exercising against an opposing force such as a weight) at least twice a week to build and maintain strength.

By increasing lifestyle physical activity in accordance with the guidelines given in the Surgeon General's report, people can expect to significantly improve their health and well-being. Such a program may not, however, increase physical fitness. A program of 30 minutes of lifestyle activity per day may also not be enough activity for some people to achieve and maintain a healthy body weight.

|  | |
|---|---|
| Washing and waxing a car for 45–60 minutes | ***Less Vigorous, More Time*** |
| Washing windows or floors for 45–60 minutes | |
| Playing volleyball for 45 minutes | |
| Playing touch football for 30–45 minutes | |
| Gardening for 30–45 minutes | |
| Wheeling self in wheelchair for 30–40 minutes | |
| Walking 1 3/4 miles in 35 minutes (20 min/mile) | |
| Basketball (shooting baskets) for 30 minutes | |
| Bicycling 5 miles in 30 minutes | |
| Dancing fast (social) for 30 minutes | |
| Pushing a stroller 1 1/2 miles in 30 minutes | |
| Raking leaves for 30 minutes | |
| Walking 2 miles in 30 minutes (15 min/mile) | |
| Water aerobics for 30 minutes | |
| Swimming laps for 20 minutes | |
| Wheelchair basketball for 20 minutes | |
| Basketball (playing a game) for 15–20 minutes | |
| Bicycling 4 miles in 15 minutes | |
| Jumping rope for 15 minutes | |
| Running 1 1/2 miles in 15 minutes (10 min/mile) | |
| Shoveling snow for 15 minutes | |
| Stairwalking for 15 minutes | ***More Vigorous, Less Time*** |

**Figure 10-2 Examples of moderate amounts of physical activity.** A moderate amount of physical activity is roughly equivalent to physical activity that uses approximately 150 calories of energy per day, or 1000 calories per week. Some activities can be performed at various intensities; the suggested durations correspond to expected intensity of effort. SOURCE: U.S. Department of Health and Human Services. 1996. *Physical Activity and Health. A Report of the Surgeon General: At-a-Glance.* Washington, D.C.: U.S. Department of Health and Human Services.

**Lifestyle Physical Activity for Health Promotion and Weight Management** Since the publication of the physical activity guidelines from the Surgeon General and the CDC/ACSM, other organizations have released physical activity recommendations that focus on specific health concerns. Because more than half of all U.S. adults are overweight, guidelines that focus on weight management such as those in the 2005 Dietary Guidelines for Americans are of particular interest. These guidelines recognize that for people who need to prevent weight gain, to lose weight, or to maintain weight loss, 30 minutes per day of physical activity may not be enough—and so they recommend 60–90 or more minutes per day of physical activity.

**Exercise Programs to Develop Physical Fitness** The Surgeon General's report also summarized the benefits of more formal exercise programs. It concluded that people can obtain even greater health benefits by increasing the duration and intensity of activity. Thus, a person who engages in a structured, formal exercise program

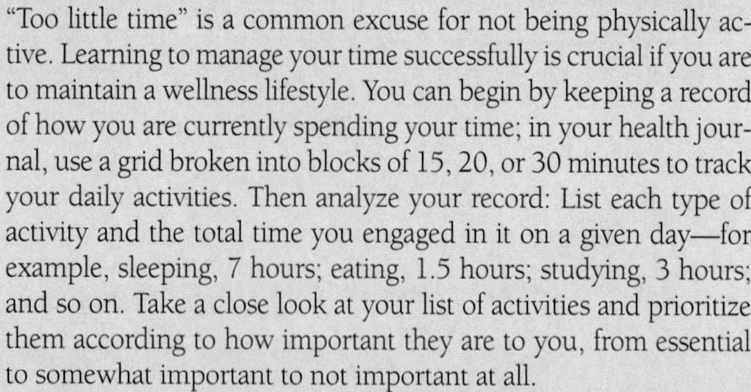

Take Charge

## Becoming More Active

"Too little time" is a common excuse for not being physically active. Learning to manage your time successfully is crucial if you are to maintain a wellness lifestyle. You can begin by keeping a record of how you are currently spending your time; in your health journal, use a grid broken into blocks of 15, 20, or 30 minutes to track your daily activities. Then analyze your record: List each type of activity and the total time you engaged in it on a given day—for example, sleeping, 7 hours; eating, 1.5 hours; studying, 3 hours; and so on. Take a close look at your list of activities and prioritize them according to how important they are to you, from essential to somewhat important to not important at all.

Based on the priorities you set, make changes in your daily schedule by subtracting time from some activities in order to make time for physical activity. Look particularly carefully at your leisure time activities and your methods of transportation; these are areas where it is easy to build in physical activity. Make changes using a system of tradeoffs. For example, you may decide to watch 10 fewer minutes of television in the morning in order to change your 5-minute drive to class into a 15-minute walk.

The following are just a few ways to become more active:

- Take the stairs instead of the elevator or escalator.
- Walk to the mailbox, post office, store, bank, or library whenever possible.
- Park your car a mile or even just a few blocks from your destination, and walk briskly.
- Do at least one chore every day that requires physical activity: wash the windows or your car, clean your room or house, mow the lawn, rake the leaves.
- Take study or work breaks to avoid sitting for more than 30 minutes at a time. Get up and walk around the library, your office, or your home or dorm; go up and down a flight of stairs.
- Stretch when you stand in line or watch TV.
- When you take public transportation, get off one stop down the line and walk to your destination.
- Go dancing instead of to a movie.
- Walk to visit a neighbor or friend rather than calling him or her on the phone. Go for a walk while you chat.
- Put your remote controls in storage; when you want to change TV or radio stations, get up and do it by hand.
- Take the dog for a walk (or an extra walk) every day.
- Play actively with children or go for a walk pushing a stroller.
- If weather or neighborhood safety rule out walking outside, look for alternate locations—an indoor track, enclosed shopping mall, or even a long hallway. Look for locations near or on the way between your campus, workplace, or residence.
- Being busy isn't the same thing as being active. Seize every opportunity to get up and walk around. Move more and sit less.

designed to measurably improve physical fitness will obtain even greater improvements in quality of life and greater reductions in disease and mortality risk.

### How Much Physical Activity Is Enough?

Some experts believe that people get most of the health benefits of a formal exercise program simply by becoming more active over the course of the day. Others think that the lifestyle approach sets too low an activity goal; they argue that people should exercise long and intensely enough to improve the body's capacity for exercise—that is, to improve physical fitness. There is probably truth in both positions.

Most experts agree that some physical activity is better than none but that more—as long as it does not result in injury or become obsessive—is probably better than some.

**Term**

Vw **cardiorespiratory endurance (aerobic) exercise** Rhythmical, large-muscle exercise for a prolonged period of time; partially dependent on the ability of the cardiovascular system to deliver oxygen to tissues.

Regular physical activity, regardless of intensity, makes you healthier and can help protect you against many chronic diseases. However, exercising at low intensities does little to improve physical fitness. Although you get many of the health benefits of exercise by simply being more active, you obtain even more benefits when you are physically fit.

A physical activity pyramid to guide you in meeting goals for physical activity is shown in Figure 10-3. If you are sedentary, start at the bottom of the pyramid and gradually increase the amount of moderate-intensity physical activity in your daily life. You don't have to exercise vigorously, but you should experience a moderate increase in your heart and breathing rates. If weight management is a concern for you, begin by achieving the goal of 30 minutes per day and then look to raise your activity level further, to 60 minutes per day or more.

For even greater benefits, move up to the next two levels of the pyramid, which illustrate parts of a formal exercise program. The American College of Sports Medicine has established guidelines for creating an exercise program that includes **cardiorespiratory endurance (aerobic) exercise,** strength training, and flexibility training (Table 10-1). Such a program will develop all the health-related components of physical fitness.

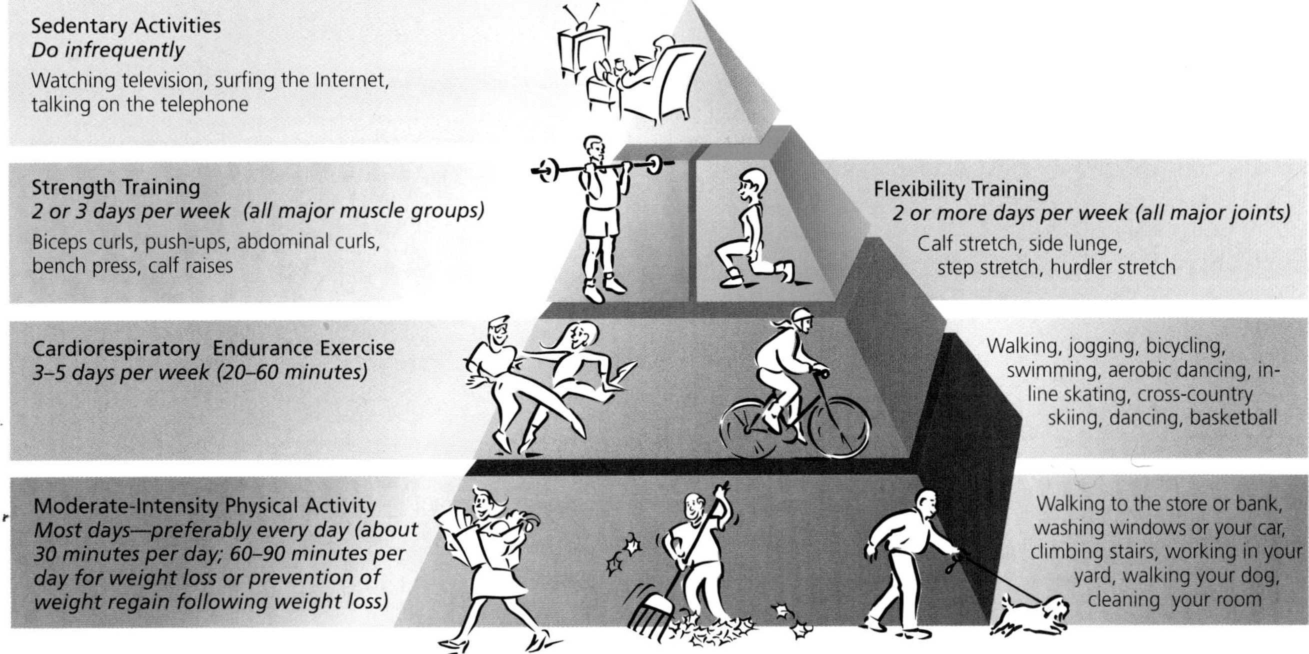


**Figure 10-3 Physical activity pyramid.** This physical activity pyramid is designed to help people become more active. If you are currently sedentary, begin at the bottom of the pyramid and gradually increase the amount of moderate-intensity physical activity in your life. Then begin a formal exercise program that includes cardiorespiratory endurance exercise, flexibility training, and strength training to help you develop all the health-related components of fitness.

## Table 10-1 Exercise Recommendations for Fitness Development in Healthy Adults

| | |
|---|---|
| **Exercise to Develop and Maintain Cardiorespiratory Endurance and Body Composition** | |
| Frequency of training | 3–5 days per week. |
| Intensity of training | 55/65–90% of maximum heart rate or 40/50–85% of maximum oxygen uptake reserve. The lower intensity values (55–64% of maximum heart rate and 40–49% of maximum oxygen uptake reserve) are most applicable to individuals who are quite unfit. For average individuals, intensities of 75–85% of maximum heart rate are appropriate; see p. 242 for instructions for determining target heart rate. |
| Time (duration) of training | 20–60 total minutes of continuous or intermittent (in sessions lasting 10 or more minutes) aerobic activity. Duration is dependent on the intensity of activity; thus, lower-intensity activity should be conducted over a longer period of time (30 minutes or more). Lower- to moderate-intensity activity of longer duration is recommended for the nonathletic adult. |
| Type (mode) of activity | Any activity that uses large-muscle groups, can be maintained continuously, and is rhythmical and aerobic in nature; for example, walking-hiking, running-jogging, cycling-bicycling, cross-country skiing, aerobic dance and other forms of group exercise, rope skipping, rowing, stair climbing, swimming, skating, and endurance game activities. |
| **Exercise to Develop and Maintain Muscular Strength and Endurance, Flexibility, and Body Composition** | |
| Resistance training | One set of 8–10 exercises that condition the major muscle groups should be performed 2 or 3 days per week. Most people should complete 8–12 repetitions of each exercise; for older and more frail people (approximately 50–60 years of age and above), 10–15 repetitions with a lighter weight may be more appropriate. Multiple-set regimens may provide greater benefits if time allows. |
| Flexibility training | Stretches for the major muscle groups should be performed a minimum of 2 or 3 days per week; at least four repetitions, held for 10–30 seconds, should be completed. |

SOURCE: American College of Sports Medicine. 1998. ACSM position stand. The recommended quantity and quality of exercise for developing and maintaining cardiorespiratory and muscular fitness and flexibility in healthy adults. *Medicine and Science in Sports and Exercise* 30(6): 975–991.

| | Lifestyle physical activity 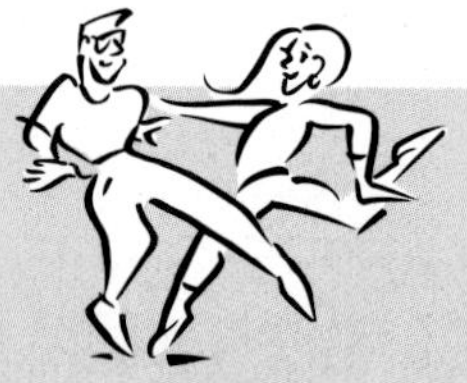 | Moderate exercise program 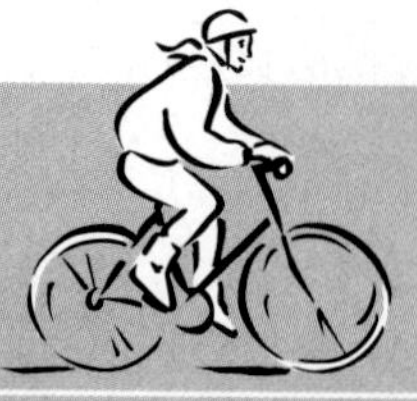 | Vigorous exercise program 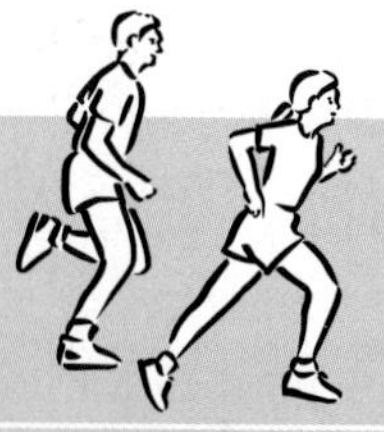 |
|---|---|---|---|
| **Description** | Moderate physical activity—an amount of activity that uses about 150 calories per day | Cardiorespiratory endurance exercise (20–60 minutes, 3–5 days per week); strength training and stretching exercises (2–3 days per week) | Cardiorespiratory endurance exercise (20–60 minutes, 3–5 days per week); interval training; strength training (3–4 days per week); and stretching exercises (3–5 days per week) |
| **Sample activities or program** | *One of the following:*<br>• Walking to and from work, 15 minutes each way<br>• Cycling to and from class, 10 minutes each way<br>• Yardwork for 30 minutes<br>• Dancing (fast) for 30 minutes<br>• Playing basketball for 20 minutes | • Jogging for 30 minutes, 3 days per week<br>• Weight training, 1 set of 8 exercises, 2 days per week<br>• Stretching exercises, 3 days per week | • Running for 45 minutes, 3 days per week<br>• Intervals: running 400 m at high effort 4 sets, 2 days per week<br>• Weight training, 3 sets of 10 exercises, 3 days per week<br>• Stretching exercises, 5 days per week |
| **Health and fitness benefits** | Better blood cholesterol levels, reduced body fat, better control of blood pressure, improved metabolic health, and enhanced glucose metabolism; improved quality of life; reduced risk of some chronic diseases<br><br>Greater amounts of activity can help prevent weight gain and promote weight loss | All the benefits of lifestyle physical activity, plus improved physical fitness (increased cardiorespiratory endurance, muscular strength and endurance, and flexibility) and even greater improvements in health and quality of life and reductions in chronic disease risk | All the benefits of lifestyle physical activity and a moderate exercise program, with greater increases in fitness and somewhat greater reductions in chronic disease risk<br><br>Participating in a vigorous exercise program may increase risk of injury and overtraining |

**Figure 10-4 Benefits of different amounts of physical activity and exercise.**

For a summary of the health and fitness benefits of different levels of physical activity, refer to Figure 10-4.

## First Steps

Are you thinking about starting a formal exercise program? A little planning can help make it a success.

**Medical Clearance** Previously inactive men over 40 and women over 50 should get a medical examination before beginning an exercise program. Diabetes, asthma, heart disease, and extreme obesity are conditions that may call for a modified program. If you have an increased risk of heart disease because of smoking, high blood pressure, or obesity, have a physical checkup, including an **electrocardiogram (ECG or EKG)**, before beginning an exercise program. This checkup will help ensure that your program will be a benefit to your health, rather than a potential hazard. The Canadian Society for Exercise Physiology has developed questionnaires to help evaluate exercise safety; visit their Web site to complete an appropriate questionnaire (www.csep.ca/forms.asp).

**Basic Principles of Physical Training** To put together an effective exercise program, a person should first understand the basic principles of physical training.

- *Specificity:* To develop a particular fitness component, you must perform exercises that are specifically designed for that component. For example, walking develops cardiorespiratory endurance, not flexibility. Specificity also applies to different parts of the body and to different sports and activities.
- *Progressive overload:* When the amount of exercise, called overload, is slowly and progressively increased, the body adapts by improving its functioning. Overload is determined by four dimensions, represented by the acronym FITT:

Frequency—how often

Intensity—how hard

Time—how long

Type—mode of activity

Later in the chapter, these dimensions of overload are described individually as they apply to each of the health-related components of fitness.

- *Reversibility:* The body adjusts to lower levels of physical activity in the same way it adjusts to higher levels. Consistency of activity is important.
- *Individual differences:* There are limits on the potential for fitness improvements and large individual differences in our ability to improve fitness and perform and learn sports skills. But physical training improves fitness and wellness regardless of heredity.

**Selecting Activities** If you have been inactive, you should begin slowly by gradually increasing the amount of moderate physical activity in your life (the bottom of the activity pyramid). Once your body has adjusted to your new level of activity, you will be ready to choose additional activities for your exercise program.

Consider your choices carefully. First, be sure the activities you choose contribute to your overall wellness. Choose activities that make sense for you. Are you competitive? If so, try racquetball, basketball, or squash. Do you prefer to exercise alone? Then consider cross-country skiing or road running. Have you been sedentary? A walking program may be a good place to start. Don't forget to consider issues of cost, time, and accessibility.

If you think you may have trouble sticking with an exercise program, find a structured activity that you can do with a buddy or a group. If you don't have any favorite sports or activities, try something new. Take a physical education class, join a health club, or sign up for jazz dancing. You're sure to find an activity that's both enjoyable and good for you.

## Cardiorespiratory Endurance Exercises

Exercises that condition your heart and lungs should have a central role in your fitness program. The best exercises for developing cardiorespiratory endurance stress a large portion of the body's muscle mass for a prolonged period of time. These include walking, jogging, running, swimming, bicycling, and aerobic dancing. Many popular sports and recreational activities, such as racquetball, tennis, basketball, and soccer, are also good if the skill level and intensity of the game are sufficient to provide a vigorous workout.

**Frequency** The optimal workout schedule for endurance training is 3–5 days per week. Beginners should start with 3 and work up to 5 days. Training more than 5 days a week can lead to injury.

**Intensity** Intensity is the crucial factor in attaining a significant training effect—that is, in increasing the body's cardiorespiratory capacity. A primary purpose of endurance training is to increase **maximal oxygen consumption ($VO_{2max}$)**. $VO_{2max}$ represents the maximum ability of the cells to use oxygen and is considered the best measure of cardiorespiratory capacity. Intensity of training is the crucial factor in improving $VO_{2max}$.

One of the easiest ways to determine exactly how intensely you should work involves measuring your heart rate. It is not necessary or desirable to exercise at your maximum heart rate—the fastest heart rate possible before exhaustion sets in—in order to improve your cardiorespiratory capacity. Beneficial effects occur at lower heart rates with a much lower risk of injury. **Target heart rate range** is the range of rates at which you should exercise to obtain cardiorespiratory benefits. To find out how you can determine the intensity at which you should exercise, refer to the box "Determining Your Target Heart Rate Range" on page 242.

**Time (Duration)** A total time of 20–60 minutes is recommended; exercise can take place in a single session or in multiple bouts lasting 10 or more minutes. The total duration of exercise depends on its intensity. To improve cardiorespiratory endurance during a low- to moderate-intensity activity such as walking or slow swimming, you should exercise for 45–60 minutes. For high-intensity exercise performed at the top of your target heart rate zone, a duration of 20 minutes is sufficient. It is usually best to start off with less vigorous activities and only gradually increase intensity.

**The Warm-Up and Cool-Down** It is always important to warm up before you exercise and to cool down afterward. Warming up enhances your performance and decreases your chances of injury. A warm-up session should include low-intensity movements similar to those in the activity that will follow. Examples of low-intensity movements are hitting forehands and backhands before a tennis game and running a 12-minute mile before progressing to an 8-minute one. Some people like to include stretching exercises in their warm-up. Experts recommend that you stretch *after* the active part of your warm-up, when your body temperature has been elevated. Studies have found that stretching prior to exercise can temporarily decrease muscle strength and power, so if a high-performance workout is your goal, it is best to stretch after a workout.

Cooling down after exercise is important to restore the body's circulation to its normal resting condition. When you are at rest, a relatively small percentage of your total blood volume is directed to muscles, but during exercise, as much as 85% of the heart's output is directed to them.

### Terms

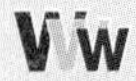

**electrocardiogram (ECG or EKG)** A recording of the changes in electrical activity of the heart.

**maximal oxygen consumption ($VO_{2max}$)** The body's maximum ability to transport and use oxygen.

**target heart rate range** The range of heart rates at which exercise yields cardiorespiratory benefits.

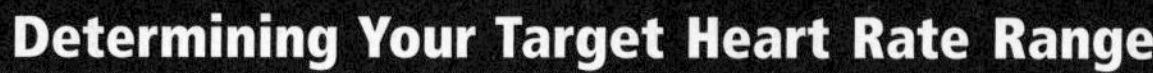

## Determining Your Target Heart Rate Range

Take Charge

Your target heart rate is the range of rates at which you should exercise to experience cardiorespiratory benefits. Your target heart rate range is based on your maximum heart rate, which can be estimated from your age. (If you are a serious athlete or face possible cardiovascular risks from exercise, you may want to have your maximum heart rate determined more accurately through a treadmill test in a physician's office, hospital, or sports medicine laboratory.) Your target heart rate is a range; the lower value corresponds to moderate-intensity exercise, while the higher value is associated with high-intensity activities. Target heart rate ranges are shown in the accompanying table.

You can monitor the intensity of your workouts by measuring your pulse either at your wrist or at one of your carotid arteries, located on either side of your Adam's apple. Your pulse rate drops rapidly after exercise, so begin counting immediately after you have finished exercising. You will obtain the most accurate results by counting beats for 10 seconds and then multiplying by 6 to get your heart rate in beats per minute (bpm). The 10-second counts corresponding to each target heart rate range are also shown in the table at right.

| Age (years) | Target Heart Rate Range (bpm)* | 10-Second Count (beats)* |
|---|---|---|
| 20–24 | 127–180 | 21–30 |
| 25–29 | 124–176 | 20–29 |
| 30–34 | 121–171 | 20–28 |
| 35–39 | 118–167 | 19–27 |
| 40–44 | 114–162 | 19–27 |
| 45–49 | 111–158 | 18–26 |
| 50–54 | 108–153 | 18–25 |
| 55–59 | 105–149 | 17–24 |
| 60–64 | 101–144 | 16–24 |
| 65+ | 97–140 | 16–23 |

*Target heart rates lower than those shown here are appropriate for individuals who are quite unfit. Ranges are based on the following formula: Target heart rate = 0.65 to 0.90 of maximum heart rate, assuming maximum heart rate = 220 − age.

During recovery from exercise, it is important to continue exercising at a low level to provide a smooth transition to the resting state.

## Developing Muscular Strength and Endurance

Any program designed to promote health should include exercises that develop muscular strength and endurance. A lean, healthy-looking body is certainly one of the goals and one of the benefits of an overall fitness program (see the box "Gender Differences in Muscular Strength").

**Types of Strength Training Exercises** Muscular strength and endurance can be developed in many ways, from weight training to calisthenics. Common exercises such as sit-ups, push-ups, pull-ups, and wall-sitting (leaning against a wall in a seated position and supporting yourself with your leg muscles) maintain the muscular strength of most people if they practice them several times a week. To condition and tone your whole body, choose exercises that work the major muscles of the shoulders, chest, back, arms, abdomen, and legs.

To increase muscular strength and endurance, you must do **resistance exercise**—exercises in which your muscles must exert force against a significant amount of resistance. Resistance can be provided by weights, exercise machines, or your own body weight. **Isometric (static) exercises** involve applying force without

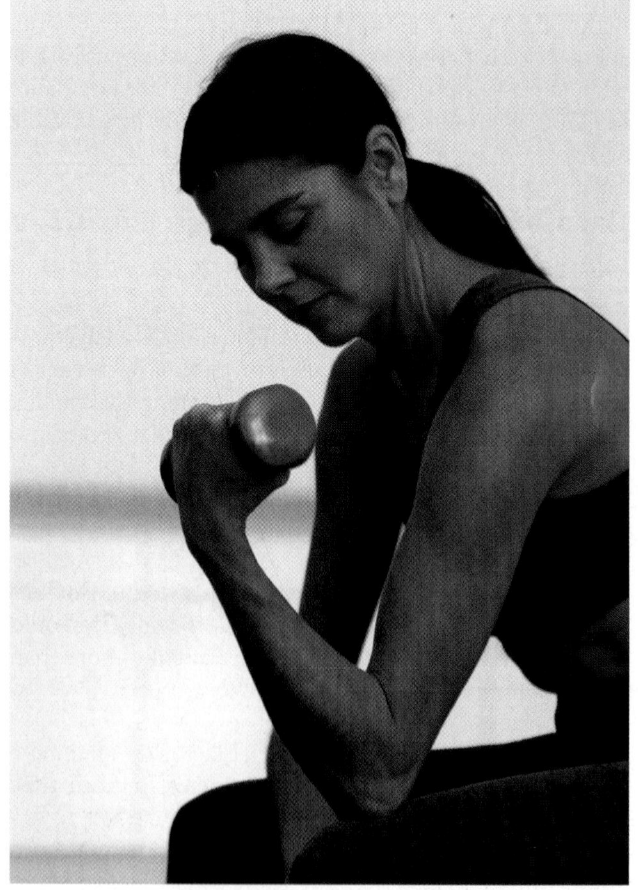

Building muscular strength is a key component of a fitness program. Weight training is just one way to increase strength, improve muscle tone, and enhance the overall appearance of the body.

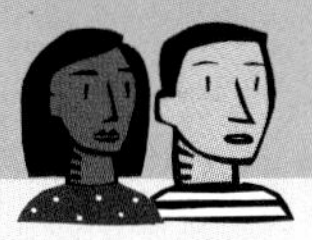

## Gender Differences in Muscular Strength

Men are generally stronger than women because they typically have larger bodies overall and a larger proportion of their total body mass is made up of muscle. But when strength is expressed per unit of muscle tissue, men are only 1–2% stronger than women in the upper body and about equal to women in the lower body. Individual muscle cells are larger in men, but the functioning of the cells is the same in both sexes.

Two factors that help explain these disparities between the sexes are testosterone levels and the speed of nervous control of muscle. Testosterone promotes the growth of muscle tissue in both males and females, but testosterone levels are about 6–10 times higher in men than in women, so men develop larger muscles. Also, because the male nervous system can activate muscles faster, men tend to have more power.

Some women are concerned that they will develop large muscles from strength training. Because of hormonal differences, most women do not develop big muscles unless they train intensely over many years or take steroids. Women do gain muscle and improve body composition through strength training, but they don't develop bulky muscles or gain significant amounts of weight. A study of average women who weight trained 2–3 days per week for 8 weeks found that the women gained about 1.75 pounds of muscle and lost about 3.5 pounds of fat.

Losing muscle over time is a much greater health concern for women than small gains in muscle weight in response to strength training, especially as any gains in muscle weight are typically more than balanced with loss of fat weight. Both men and women lose muscle mass and power as they age, but because men start out with more muscle when they are young and don't lose power as quickly as women, older women tend to have greater impairment of muscle function than older men. This may partially explain the higher incidence of life-threatening falls in older women.

The bottom line is that both men and women can increase strength through strength training. Women may not be able to lift as much weight as men, but pound for pound of muscle, they have nearly the same capacity to gain strength as men. The lifetime wellness benefits of strength training are available to everyone. Strength training is particularly beneficial for women because it helps prevent bone and muscle loss with aging and maintains fat-free weight during weight management programs.

SOURCES: Fahey, T. D. 2007. *Weight Training for Men and Women,* 6th ed. New York: McGraw-Hill; IDEA. 2001. *Fitness Tip—Why Women Need Weight Training* (http://www.ideafit.com/ftwomen.htm; retrieved October 22, 2002); Krivickas, L. S., et al. 2001. Age and gender-related differences in maximum shortening velocity of skeletal muscle fibers. *American Journal of Physical Medicine & Rehabilitation* 80: 447–455.

movement, such as when you contract your abdominal muscles. This static type of exercise is valuable for toning and strengthening muscles. Isometrics can be practiced anywhere and do not require any equipment. For maximum strength gains, hold an isometric contraction maximally for 6 seconds; do five to ten repetitions. Don't hold your breath—that can restrict blood flow to your heart and brain. Within a few weeks, you will notice the effect of this exercise. Isometrics are particularly useful when recovering from an injury.

**Isotonic (dynamic) exercises** involve applying force with movement, as, for example, in weight training exercises such as the bench press. These are the most popular type of exercises for increasing muscle strength and seem to be most valuable for developing strength that can be transferred to other forms of physical activity. They include exercises using barbells, dumbbells, weight machines, and the body's own weight, as in push-ups or sit-ups.

**Choosing Equipment** Weight machines are preferred by many people because they are safe, convenient, and easy to use. You just set the resistance (usually by placing a pin in the weight stack), sit down at the machine, and start working. Machines make it easy to isolate and work specific muscles. Free weights require more care, balance, and coordination to use, but they strengthen your body in ways that are more adaptable to real life. For free weights, you need to use a spotter, someone who stands by to assist in case you lose control over a weight.

**Choosing Exercises** A complete weight training program works all the major muscle groups: neck, upper back, shoulders, arms, chest, abdomen, lower back, thighs, buttocks, and calves. Different exercises work different muscles, so it usually takes about eight to ten exercises to get a complete workout for general fitness—for example, bench presses to develop the chest, shoulders, and upper arms; pull-ups to work the biceps and upper back; squats to develop the legs and buttocks; toe raises to work the calves; and so on. Refer to the Online Learning Center for a sample recommended program for strength training using either free weights, weight

### Terms

VW

**resistance exercise** Exercise that forces muscles to contract against increased resistance; also called *strength training.*

**isometric (static) exercise** The application of force without movement.

**isotonic (dynamic) exercise** The application of force with movement.

machines, or no weight equipment. A sample workout card for monitoring your progress and video clips of selected exercises are also included.

**Frequency** For general fitness, the American College of Sports Medicine recommends a frequency of 2 or 3 days per week. Allow your muscles a day of rest between workouts to avoid soreness and injury. If you enjoy weight training and would like to train more often, try working different muscle groups on alternate days.

**Intensity and Time** The amount of weight (resistance) you lift in weight training exercises is equivalent to intensity in cardiorespiratory endurance training; the number of repetitions of each exercise is equivalent to duration. In order to improve fitness, you must do enough repetitions of each exercise to temporarily fatigue your muscles. The number of repetitions needed to cause fatigue depends on the amount of resistance: the heavier the weight, the fewer repetitions to reach fatigue. In general, a heavy weight and a low number of repetitions (1–5) build strength, whereas a light weight and a high number of repetitions (20–25) build endurance. For a general fitness program to build both strength and endurance, try to do 8–12 repetitions of each exercise; a few exercises, such as abdominal crunches and calf raises, may require more.

To start, choose a weight that you can move easily through 8–12 repetitions. As you progress, add weight when you can do more than 12 repetitions of an exercise. If adding weight means you can do only 7 or 8 repetitions before your muscles fatigue, stay with that weight until you can again complete 12 repetitions. If you can do only 4–6 repetitions after adding weight, or if you can't maintain good form, you've added too much and should take some off.

For developing strength and endurance for general fitness, a single set (group) of each exercise is sufficient, provided you use enough resistance (weight) to fatigue your muscles. Doing more than one set of each exercise may increase strength development, and most serious weight trainers do at least three sets of each exercise. If you do perform more than one set of an exercise, rest long enough between sets to allow your muscles to recover.

As with cardiorespiratory endurance exercise, you should warm up before every weight training session and cool down afterward.

**A Caution About Supplements** No nutritional supplement or drug will change a weak, untrained person into a strong, fit person. Those changes require regular training that stresses the body and causes physiological adaptations. Supplements or drugs that promise quick, large gains in strength usually don't work and are often either dangerous or expensive, or both (see the box "Drugs and Supplements for Improved Athletic Performance"). The long-term effects of many supplements have not been studied, and over-the-counter supplements are not carefully regulated. Use your critical thinking skills to evaluate claims made about supplements, and stay with the proven method of a steady, progressive fitness program to build strength.

## Flexibility Exercises

Flexibility, or stretching, exercises are important for maintaining the normal range of motion in the major joints of the body. Some exercises, such as running, can actually decrease flexibility because they require only a partial range of motion. Like a good weight training program, a good stretching program includes exercises for all the major muscle groups and joints of the body: neck, shoulders, back, hips, thighs, hamstrings, and calves. Refer to the Online Learning Center for a sample recommended program for flexibility training.

**Proper Stretching Technique** Stretching should be performed statically. "Bouncing" (known as ballistic stretching) is dangerous and counterproductive. Stretching can be either active or passive. In active stretching, a muscle is stretched by a contraction of opposing muscles. In passive stretching, an outside force or resistance provided by yourself, a partner, gravity, or a weight helps your joints move through their range of motion. You can achieve a greater range of motion and a more intense stretch using passive stretching, but there is a greater risk of injury. The safest and most convenient technique may be active static stretching with a passive assist. For example, you might do a seated stretch of your calf muscles both by contracting the muscles on the top of your shin and by grabbing your feet and pulling them toward you.

**Frequency** Do stretching exercises a minimum of 2 or 3 days per week. You can set apart a special time for these exercises or do them after cardiorespiratory endurance exercise or strength training. You may develop more flexibility if you do them after exercise, during your cool-down, because your muscles are warmer then and can be stretched farther.

**Intensity and Time** For each exercise, stretch to the point of tightness in the muscle, and hold the position for 10–30 seconds. Rest for 30–60 seconds, and then repeat, trying to stretch a bit farther. Relax and breathe easily as you stretch. You should feel a pleasant, mild stretch as you let the muscles relax; stretching should not be painful. Do at least four repetitions of each exercise. A complete flexibility workout usually takes about 20–30 minutes.

Increase your intensity gradually over time. Improved flexibility takes many months to develop. There

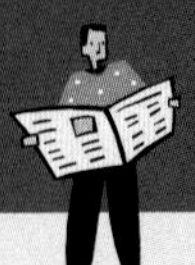

In the News

## Drugs and Supplements for Improved Athletic Performance

WW

The 2004 Olympic Games in Athens made headlines not just for athletic achievements but also for the record number of athletes testing positive for performance-enhancing drugs. Some athletes were banned from competition before or during the games; others had medals taken away after they failed postcompetition drug tests. The Olympic Movement Anti-Doping Code calls for the elimination of the use of performance-enhancing drugs in sports in order to both ensure respect for sports ethics and protect the health of athletes. In the wake of the BALCO legal case, which focused attention on use of steroids and other compounds by Olympic and professional athletes, the U.S. Congress and additional sports organizations began to consider stricter regulations regarding performance-enhancing drugs.

Drugs intended to enhance athletic performance are used not only by elite Olympic and professional athletes but also by active individuals of all fitness levels. About 2–6% of high school and college students report having used anabolic steroids, and over-the-counter dietary supplements are much more popular. Many such substances are ineffective and expensive, and many are also dangerous. A few of the most widely used compounds are described below.

***Anabolic Steroids*** These synthetic derivatives of testosterone are taken to increase strength, power, speed, endurance, muscle size, and aggressiveness. **Anabolic steroids** have dangerous side effects, including disruption of the body's hormone system, liver disease, acne, breast development and testicular shrinkage in males, masculinization in women and children, and increased risk of heart disease and cancer. Steroid users who inject the drugs face the same health risks as other injection drug users, including increased risk of HIV infection.

***Adrenal Androgens*** This group of drugs, which includes dehydroepiandrosterone (DHEA) and androstenedione, are typically taken to stimulate muscle growth and aid in weight control. The few studies of these agents done on humans show that they are of very little value in improving athletic performance, and they have side effects similar to those of anabolic steroids, especially when taken in high doses. In January 2005, androstenedione was reclassified and is no longer available without a prescription.

***Ephedra and Other Stimulants*** These drugs may be taken to increase training intensity, to suppress hunger, to reduce fatigue, and to promote weight loss. They raise heart rate and blood pressure and, at high doses, may increase the risk of heart attack, stroke, and heat-related illness. Several stimulants, including ephedra and phenylpropanolamine, were recently banned by the FDA.

***Erythropoietin (EPO)*** A naturally occurring hormone that boosts the concentration of red blood cells, EPO is typically used by endurance athletes to improve their performance. EPO can cause blood clots and death.

***Creatine Monohydrate*** Use of creatine supplements may improve performance in short-term, high-intensity, repetitive exercise and decrease the risk of injury. These supplements may increase water retention in muscles, giving the feeling of increased muscularity without an actual increase in muscle size. The long-term effects of creatine use, especially among young people, are not well established.

***Protein, Amino Acid, and Polypeptide Supplements*** Little research supports the use of such supplements, even in athletes on extemely heavy training regimens. The protein requirements of athletes are not much higher than those of sedentary individuals, and most people take in more than enough protein in their diets. By substituting supplements for food sources of protein, people may risk deficiencies in other key nutrients typically found in such foods, including iron and B vitamins.

***Chromium Picolinate*** Sold over the counter, chromium picolinate is a more easily digested form of the trace mineral chromium. Although often marketed as a means to build muscle and reduce fat, most studies have found no positive effects. Long-term use of high dosages may have serious health consequences.

are large individual differences in joint flexibility. Don't feel you have to compete with others during stretching workouts.

## Training in Specific Skills

The final component in your fitness program is learning the skills required for the sports or activities in which you choose to participate. The first step in learning a new skill is getting help. Sports like tennis, golf, sailing, and skiing require mastery of basic movements and techniques, so instruction from a qualified teacher can save you hours of frustration and increase your enjoyment of the sport. Skill is also important in conditioning activities such as jogging, swimming, and cycling. Even if you learned a sport as a child, additional instruction now can help you refine your technique.

## Putting It All Together

Now that you know the basic components of a fitness program, you can put them all together in a program that works for you. Refer to Figure 10-5 for a summary of the FITT principle for the health-related fitness components.

### Term

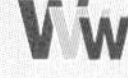

**anabolic steroids** Synthetic male hormones used to increase muscle size and strength.

| | Cardiorespiratory Endurance Training | Strength Training | Flexibility Training |
|---|---|---|---|
| **F**requency | 3–5 days per week | 2–3 days per week | 2–3 days per week, or more |
| **I**ntensity | 55/65–90% of maximum heart rate | Sufficient resistance to fatigue muscles | Stretch to the point of tension |
| **T**ime | 20–60 minutes in sessions lasting 10 minutes or more | 8–12 repetitions of each exercise, 1 or more sets | 4 repetitions of each exercise, held for 10–30 seconds |
| **T**ype | Continuous rhythmic activities using large muscle groups | Resistance exercises for all major muscle groups | Stretching exercises for all major joints |

**Figure 10-5 A summary of the FITT principle for the health-related components of fitness**

## GETTING STARTED AND STAYING ON TRACK

Once you have a program that fulfills your basic fitness needs and suits your personal tastes, adhering to a few basic principles will help you improve at the fastest rate, have more fun, and minimize the risk of injury.

### Selecting Instructors, Equipment, and Facilities

One of the best places to get help is an exercise class, where an expert instructor can help you learn the basics and answer your questions. A qualified personal trainer can also get you started on an exercise program or a new form of training. Make sure that your instructor or trainer has proper qualifications, such as a college degree in exercise physiology or physical education and certification by the American College of Sports Medicine (ACSM), National Strength and Conditioning Association (NSCA), or another professional organization.

Many Web sites provide fitness programs, including ongoing support and feedback via e-mail. Many of these sites charge a fee, so it is important to review the sites, decide which ones seem most appropriate, and if possible go through a free trial period before subscribing. Also remember to consider the reliability of the information at fitness Web sites, especially those that also advertise or sell products.

Try to purchase the best equipment you can afford. Good equipment will enhance your enjoyment and decrease your risk of injury. Appropriate safety equipment, such as pads and helmets for in-line skating, is particularly important. Before you invest in a new piece of equipment, investigate it. Is it worth the money? Does it produce the results its proponents claim for it? Is it safe? Does it fit properly, and is it in good working order? Does it provide a genuine workout? Will you really use it? Before you buy an expensive piece of equipment, try it out at a local gym to make sure that you'll use it regularly. Footwear is a key piece of equipment for almost any activity; see the box "Choosing Exercise Footwear" for shopping strategies.

If you are thinking of becoming a member of a health club or fitness center, be sure to choose one that has the right programs and equipment available at the times you will use them. Ask for a free trial workout, a 1-day pass, or an inexpensive 1- to 2-week trial membership before committing to a long-term contract. Be wary of promotional gimmicks and high-pressure sales tactics. Also make sure the facility is certified; look for the displayed names American College of Sports Medicine (ACSM); National Strength and Conditioning Association (NSCA); American Council on Exercise (ACE); Aerobics and Fitness Association of America (AFAA); or International Health, Racquet, and Sportsclub Association (IHRSA). These trade associations have established standards to help protect consumer health, safety, and rights.

### Eating and Drinking for Exercise

Most people do not need to change their eating habits when they begin a fitness program. In almost every case, a well-balanced diet contains all the energy and nutrients needed to sustain an exercise program. A balanced diet is also the key to improving your body composition when you begin to exercise more. One of the promises of a fitness program is a decrease in body fat and an increase in muscular body mass. The best way to control body fat is to follow a diet containing adequate but not excessive calories and to be physically active.

One of the most important principles to follow when exercising is to drink enough water. Sweating during exercise depletes the body's water supply and can lead to dehydration if fluids are not replaced. Serious dehydration

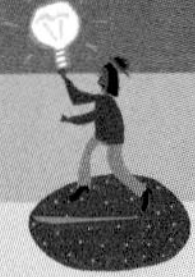

Critical Consumer

## Choosing Exercise Footwear

V W

When choosing athletic shoes, first consider the activity you've chosen for your exercise program. Shoes appropriate for different activities have very different characteristics. For example, running shoes typically have highly cushioned midsoles, rubber outsoles with elevated heels, and a great deal of flexibility in the forefoot. The heels of walking shoes tend to be lower, less padded, and more beveled than those designed for running. For aerobic dance, shoes must be flexible in the forefoot and have straight, nonflared heels to allow for safe and easy lateral movements. Court shoes also provide substantial support for lateral movements; they typically have outsoles made from white rubber that will not damage court surfaces.

Also consider the location and intensity of your workouts. If you plan to walk or run on trails, you should choose shoes with water-resistant, highly durable uppers and more outsole traction. If you work out intensely or have a relatively high body weight, you'll need thick, firm midsoles to avoid bottoming-out the cushioning system of your shoes.

Foot type is another important consideration. If your feet tend to roll inward excessively, you may need shoes with additional stability features on the inner side of the shoe to counteract this movement. If your feet tend to roll outward excessively, you may need highly flexible and cushioned shoes that promote foot motion. For aerobic dancers with feet that tend to roll inward or outward, mid-cut to high-cut shoes may be more appropriate than low-cut aerobic shoes or cross-trainers (shoes designed to be worn for several different activities). Compared with men, women have narrower feet overall and narrower heels relative to the forefoot. Most women will get a better fit if they choose shoes that are specifically designed for women's feet rather than those that are downsized versions of men's shoes.

For successful shoe shopping, keep the following strategies in mind:

- Shop at an athletic shoe or specialty store that has personnel trained to fit athletic shoes and a large selection of styles and sizes.
- Shop late in the day or, ideally, following a workout. Your foot size increases over the course of the day and as a result of exercise.
- Wear socks like those you plan to wear during exercise. If you have an old pair of athletic shoes, bring them with you. The wear pattern on your old shoes can help you select a pair with extra support or cushioning in the places you need it the most.
- Ask for help. Trained salespeople know which shoes are designed for your foot type and your level of activity. They can also help fit your shoes properly.
- Don't insist on buying shoes in what you consider to be your typical shoe size. Sizes vary from shoe to shoe. In addition, foot sizes change over time, and many people have one foot that is larger or wider than the other. Try several sizes in several widths, if necessary. Don't buy shoes that are too small.
- Try on both shoes, and wear them around for 10 or more minutes. Try walking on a noncarpeted surface. Approximate the movements of your activity: walk, jog, run, jump, and so on.
- Check the fit and style carefully:

  Is the toe box roomy enough? There should be at least one thumb's width of space from the longest toe to the end of the toe box.

  Do the shoes have enough cushioning? Do your feet feel supported when you bounce up and down?

  Do your heels fit snugly into the shoe? Do they stay put when you walk, or do they rise up?

  Are the arches of your feet right on top of the shoes' arch supports?

  Do the shoes feel stable when you twist and turn on the balls of your feet?

  Do you feel any pressure points?

- If the shoes are not comfortable in the store, don't buy them. Don't expect athletic shoes to stretch over time in order to fit your feet properly.
- Replace athletic shoes about every 3 months or 300–500 miles of jogging or walking.

can cause reduced blood volume, accelerated heart rate, elevated body temperature, muscle cramps, heat stroke, and other serious problems.

During heavy or prolonged exercise or exercise in hot weather, thirst alone isn't a good indication of how much fluid you need to drink. As a rule of thumb, drink at least 2 cups (16 ounces) of fluid 2 hours before exercise and then drink enough during exercise to match fluid loss in sweat—at least 1 cup of fluid every 20–30 minutes of exercise. To determine if you're drinking the right amount of fluid, weigh yourself before and after an exercise session: Any weight loss is due to fluid loss that needs to be replaced. Any weight gain is due to overconsumption of fluid.

Bring a bottle of water when you exercise so you can replace your fluids when they're depleted. For exercise sessions lasting less than 60–90 minutes, cool water is an excellent fluid replacement. For longer workouts, a sports drink that contains water and small amounts of electrolytes (sodium, potassium, and magnesium) and simple carbohydrates ("sugar," usually in the form of sucrose or glucose) is recommended.

## Managing Your Fitness Program

How can you tell when you're in shape? When do you stop improving and start maintaining? How can you stay motivated? If your program is going to become an integral part of your life, and if the principles behind it are going to serve you well in the years ahead, these are very important questions.

**Consistency: The Key to Physical Improvement** It is important to be able to recognize when you have achieved the level of fitness that is appropriate for you. Your body gets into shape by adapting to increasing levels of physical stress. If you don't push yourself by increasing the intensity of your workout—by adding weight or running a little faster or a little longer—no change will occur in your body. But if you subject your body to overly severe stress, it will break down and become distressed, or injured. Your body needs time to adapt to increasingly higher levels of stress. If you feel extremely sore and tired the day after exercising, then you have worked too hard.

Consistency is the key to getting into shape without injury. The best way to ensure consistency is to keep a training journal in which you record the details of your workouts: how far you ran, how much weight you lifted, how many laps you swam, and so on. This record will help you evaluate your progress and plan your workout sessions intelligently. Don't increase your exercise volume by more than 5–10% per week.

**Assessing Your Fitness** When are you "in shape"? It depends. One person may be out of shape running a mile in 5 minutes; another may be in shape running a mile in 12 minutes. As mentioned earlier, your ultimate level of fitness depends on your goals, your program, and your natural ability. The important thing is to set goals that make sense for you. If you are interested in finding out exactly how fit you are before you begin a program, the best approach is to get an assessment from a modern sports medicine laboratory.

**Preventing and Managing Athletic Injuries** It is important to learn how to deal with injuries so they don't derail your fitness program (Table 10-2). Some injuries require medical attention. Consult a physician for head and eye injuries, possible ligament injuries, broken bones, and internal disorders such as chest pain, fainting, and intolerance to heat. Also seek medical attention for

**Table 10-2 Care of Common Exercise Injuries and Discomforts**

| Injury | Symptoms | Treatment |
|---|---|---|
| Blister | Accumulation of fluid in one spot under the skin | Don't pop or drain it unless it interferes too much with your daily activities. If it does pop, clean the area with antiseptic and cover with a bandage. Do not remove the skin covering the blister. |
| Bruise (contusion) | Pain, swelling, and discoloration | R-I-C-E: rest, ice, compression, elevation. |
| Joint sprain | Pain, tenderness, swelling, discoloration, and loss of function | R-I-C-E; apply heat when the swelling has disappeared. Stretch and strengthen the affected area. |
| Muscle cramp | Painful, spasmodic muscle contractions | Gently stretch for 15–30 seconds at a time, and/or massage the cramped area. Drink fluids. |
| Muscle soreness or stiffness | Pain and tenderness in the affected muscle | Stretch the affected muscle gently; exercise at a low intensity; apply heat. |
| Muscle strain | Pain, tenderness, swelling, and loss of strength in the affected muscle | R-I-C-E; apply heat when swelling has disappeared. Stretch and strengthen the affected area. |
| Shin splints | Pain and tenderness on the front of the lower leg; sometimes also pain in the calf muscle | Rest; apply ice to the affected area several times a day and before exercise; wrap with tape for support. Stretch and strengthen muscles in the lower legs. Purchase good-quality footwear, and run on soft surfaces. |
| Side stitch | Pain on the side of the abdomen | Stretch the arm on the affected side as high as possible; if that doesn't help, try bending forward while tightening the abdominal muscles. |

SOURCE: Fahey, T. D., P. M. Insel, and W. T. Roth. 2005. *Fit and Well: Core Concepts and Labs in Physical Fitness and Wellness*, 6th ed. New York: McGraw-Hill.

apparently minor injuries that do not get better within a reasonable amount of time.

For minor cuts and scrapes, stop the bleeding and clean the wound with soap and water. Treat soft tissue injuries (muscles and joints) with the R-I-C-E principle:

**Rest:** Stop using the injured area as soon as you experience pain, protect it from further injury, and avoid any activity that causes pain.

**Ice:** Apply ice to the injured area to reduce swelling and alleviate pain. Apply ice immediately for 10–20 minutes, and repeat every few hours until the swelling disappears. Let the injured part return to normal temperature between icings, and do not apply ice to one area for more than 20 minutes (10 minutes if you are using a cold gel pack).

**Compression:** Wrap the injured area with an elastic or compression bandage between icings. If the area starts throbbing or begins to change color, the bandage may be wrapped too tightly. Do not sleep with the wrap on.

**Elevation:** Raise the injured area above heart level to decrease the blood supply and reduce swelling.

After about 36–48 hours, apply heat if the swelling has completely disappeared to help relieve pain, relax muscles, and reduce stiffness. Immerse the affected area in warm water or apply warm compresses, a hot water bottle, or a heating pad.

To prevent injuries in the future, follow a few basic guidelines:

1. Stay in condition; haphazard exercise programs invite injury.
2. Warm up thoroughly before exercise.
3. Use proper body mechanics when lifting objects or executing sports skills.
4. Don't exercise when you're ill or overtrained (experiencing extreme fatigue due to overexercising).
5. Use the proper equipment.
6. Don't return to your normal exercise program until athletic injuries have healed.

You can minimize the risk of injury by following safety guidelines, using proper technique and equipment, respecting signals from your body that something may be wrong, and treating any injuries that occur. Warm up, cool down, and drink plenty of fluids. Use special caution in extreme heat or humidity (over 80°F and/or 60% humidity): Exercise slowly, rest frequently in the shade, wear clothing that "breathes," and drink plenty of fluids; slow down or stop if you begin to feel uncomfortable. During hot weather, it's best to exercise in the early morning or evening, when temperatures are lowest.

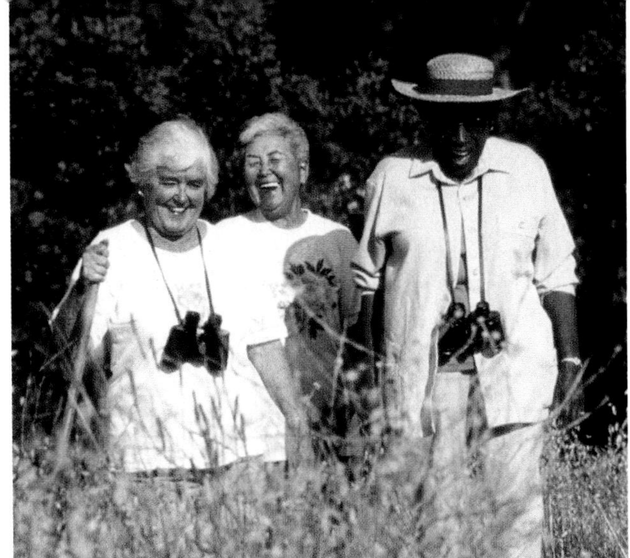

It makes sense to choose activities that will add enjoyment to your life for years to come. In this group of older people, we can see the rewards of a lifetime of fitness and smart exercise habits.

**Staying with Your Program** Once you have attained your desired level of fitness, you can maintain it by exercising regularly at a consistent intensity, three to five times a week. In general, if you exercise at the same intensity over a long period, your fitness will level out and can be maintained easily.

Adapt your program to changes in environment or schedule. If you walk in the summer, dress appropriately and walk in the winter as well. If you can't go out because of darkness or an unsafe neighborhood, walk in a local shopping mall or on campus or join a gym and walk on a treadmill. Changes in your job or family situation can also affect your exercise program. Remember that physical activity is important for your energy level, self-esteem, and well-being. You owe it to yourself to include physical activity in your day. Try to exercise before going to work or to do some physical activity during your lunch hour—even if it's only a short walk or a few trips up and down the stairs.

What if you run out of steam? Although good health is an important *reason* to exercise, it's a poor *motivator* for consistent adherence to an exercise program. It's a good idea to have a meaningful goal, anything from fitting into the same-size jeans you used to wear to successfully skiing down a more advanced slope. Signing a contract, exercising with a friend, and giving yourself frequent rewards are additional strategies.

Varying your program is another key strategy. Some people alternate two or more activities—swimming and jogging, for example—to improve a particular component of fitness. The practice, called **cross-training,** can

**Term**

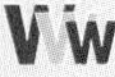

**cross-training** Participating in two or more activities to develop a particular component of fitness.

help prevent boredom and overuse injuries. Try new activities, especially ones that you will be able to do for the rest of your life. Get maps of the recreational or wilderness areas near you, and go exploring. Fill a canteen, pack a good lunch, and take along a wildflower or bird book. Every step you take will bring you closer to your ultimate goal—fitness and wellness that last a lifetime.

**Tips for Today**

Physical activity and exercise offer benefits in nearly every area of wellness, helping you generate energy, manage stress, control your weight, improve your mood, and, of course, become physically stronger and healthier. Building a program of regular exercise into your life is well worth the effort, even if it seems complicated or difficult at first. Even a low-to-moderate level of activity provides valuable health benefits. The important thing is to get moving: When in doubt, exercise!

*Right now you can*

- Get up and stretch.
- Go outside and take a brisk walk.
- Look at your calendar for the rest of the week and write in some physical activity—such as walking, running, biking, skating, swimming, hiking, or playing Frisbee—on as many days as you can; schedule the activity for a specific time, and stick to it.
- If you don't yet use the gym or fitness facility on your campus, go there now and begin planning how to use it.
- Call a friend and invite him or her to start a regular exercise program with you.

## SUMMARY

- The five components of physical fitness most important to health are cardiorespiratory endurance, muscular strength, muscular endurance, flexibility, and body composition.
- Exercise improves the functioning of the heart and the ability of the cardiorespiratory system to carry oxygen to the body's tissues. It also increases the efficiency of the body's metabolism and improves body composition.
- Exercise lowers the risk of cardiovascular disease, cancer, osteoporosis, and diabetes. It improves immune function and psychological health and helps prevent injuries and low-back pain.
- Everyone should accumulate at least 30–60 minutes per day of moderate endurance-type physical activity. Additional health and fitness benefits can be achieved through longer or more vigorous activity.
- Cardiorespiratory endurance exercises stress a large portion of the body's muscle mass. Endurance exercise should be performed 3–5 days per week for a total of 20–60 minutes per day. Intensity can be evaluated by measuring the heart rate.
- Warming up before exercising and cooling down afterward improve your performance and decrease your chances of injury.
- Exercises that develop muscular strength and endurance involve exerting force against a significant resistance. A strength training program for general fitness typically involves one set of 8–12 repetitions of 8–10 exercises, 2 or 3 days per week.
- A good stretching program includes exercises for all the major muscle groups and joints of the body. Do a series of active, static stretches (possibly with a passive assist) 2 or more days per week. Hold each stretch for 10–30 seconds; do at least four repetitions. Stretch when muscles are warm.
- Instructors, equipment, and facilities should be chosen carefully to enhance enjoyment and prevent injuries.
- A well-balanced diet contains all the energy and nutrients needed to sustain a fitness program. When exercising, remember to drink enough fluids.
- Rest, ice, compression, and elevation (R-I-C-E) are treatments for muscle and joint injuries.

## Take Action

1. **Investigate campus resources:** Go to your school's physical education office and ask for a comprehensive listing of all the exercise and fitness facilities available on your campus. Visit the facilities you haven't yet seen, and investigate the activities that take place there. If there are sports or activities you'd like to try, consider doing so.

2. **Investigate community resources:** Investigate the fitness clubs in your community. How do they compare with one another? How do they measure up in terms of the guidelines provided in this chapter?

3. **Count your steps:** One way to monitor physical activity is to purchase and wear a pedometer to count your daily steps. To begin, wear the pedometer for a week and determine your typical level of activity (average steps per day). Then record the number of steps you take during 10 minutes of brisk walking; three times that number would represent the Surgeon General's minimum of 30 minutes of brisk walking per day. With these numbers in mind, set a daily goal for physical activity, and continue to track and record your daily steps.

## Planning a Personal Exercise Program

Behavior Change Strategy

Although most people recognize the importance of incorporating exercise into their lives, many find it difficult to do. No single strategy will work for everyone, but the general steps outlined here should help you create an exercise program that fits your goals, preferences, and lifestyle. A carefully designed program plan can help you convert your vague wishes into a detailed plan of action.

### Step 1: Set Goals

Setting specific goals to accomplish by exercising is an important first step in a successful fitness program because it establishes the direction you want to take. Your goals might be specifically related to health, such as lowering your blood pressure and risk of heart disease, or they might relate to other aspects of your life, such as improving your tennis game or the fit of your clothes. If you can decide why you're starting to exercise, it can help you keep going.

Think carefully about your reasons for incorporating exercise into your life, and then fill in the goals portion of the Personal Fitness Contract in Wellness Worksheet S10 (see the Study Guide).

### Step 2: Select Activities

As discussed in the chapter, the success of your fitness program depends on the consistency of your involvement. Select activities that encourage your commitment: The right program will be its own incentive to continue; poor activity choices provide obstacles and can turn exercise into a chore.

When choosing activities for your fitness program, consider the following:

- Is this activity fun? Will it hold my interest over time?
- Will this activity help me reach the goals I have set?
- Will my current fitness and skill level enable me to participate fully in this activity?
- Can I easily fit this activity into my daily schedule? Are there any special requirements (facilities, partners, equipment, etc.) that I must plan for?
- Can I afford any special costs required for equipment or facilities?
- (If you have special exercise needs due to a particular health problem.) Does this activity conform to my special health needs? Will it enhance my ability to cope with my specific health problem?

Using the guidelines listed above, select a number of sports and activities. Fill in the Program Plan portion of the Fitness Contract.

### Step 3: Make a Commitment

Complete your Fitness Contract and Program Plan by signing your contract and having it witnessed and signed by someone who can help make you accountable for your progress. By completing a written contract, you will make a firm commitment and will be more likely to follow through until you meet your goals.

### Step 4: Begin and Maintain Your Program

Start out slowly to allow your body time to adjust. Be realistic and patient—meeting your goals will take time. The following guidelines may help you start and stick with your program:

- Set aside regular periods for exercise. Choose times that fit in best with your schedule, and stick to them. Allow an adequate amount of time for warm-up, cool-down, and a shower.
- Take advantage of any opportunity for exercise that presents itself (for example, walk to class, take the stairs instead of the elevator).
- Do what you can to avoid boredom. Do stretching exercises or jumping jacks to music, or watch the evening news while riding your stationary bicycle.
- Exercise with a group that shares your goals and general level of competence.
- Vary the program. Change your activities periodically. Alter your route or distance if biking or jogging. Change racquetball partners, or find a new volleyball court.

### Step 5: Record and Assess Your Progress

Keeping a record that notes the daily results of your program will help remind you of your ongoing commitment to your program and give you a sense of accomplishment. Create daily and weekly program logs that you can use to track your progress. Record the activity type, frequency, intensity, and time. Keep your log handy, and fill it in immediately after each exercise session. Post it in a visible place to remind you of your activity schedule and provide incentive for improvement.

SOURCE: Adapted from Kusinitz, I., and M. Fine. 1995. *Your Guide to Getting Fit,* 3rd ed. Mountain View, Calif.: Mayfield.

## For More Information

### Books


Anderson, B., and J. Anderson. 2003. *Stretching,* 20th anniv. ed. Bolinas, Calif.: Shelter Publications. *Updated edition of a classic, with more than 200 stretches for 60 sports and activities.*

Bahrke, M., and C. Yesalis. 2002. *Performance-Enhancing Substances in Sport Exercise.* Champaign, Ill.: Human Kinetics. *Provides up-to-date coverage of the issues surrounding supplements as well as the current state of research on major types of supplements and their effects on athletic performance.*

Fahey, T. 2005. *Weight Training Basics.* New York: McGraw-Hill. *Weight training and plyometric exercises for fitness, weight control, and improved sports performance.*

Fahey, T., P. Insel, and W. Roth. 2005. *Fit and Well: Core Concepts and Labs in Physical Fitness and Wellness,* 6th ed. New York: McGraw-Hill. *A comprehensive guide to developing a complete fitness program.*

## Organizations, Hotlines, and Web Sites

*American Academy of Orthopaedic Surgeons.* Provides fact sheets on many fitness and sports topics, including how to begin a program, how to choose equipment, and how to prevent and treat many types of injuries.
http://orthoinfo.aaos.org

*American College of Sports Medicine.* Provides brochures, publications, and videotapes on the positive effects of exercise.
317-637-9200
http://www.acsm.org

*American Council on Exercise.* Promotes exercise and fitness for all Americans; the Web site features fact sheets on many consumer topics, including choosing shoes, cross-training, steroids, and getting started on an exercise program.
800-529-8227
http://www.acefitness.org

*American Heart Association: Just Move.* Provides practical advice for people of all fitness levels plus an online fitness diary.
http://www.justmove.org

*Disabled Sports USA.* Provides sport and recreation services to people with physical or mobility disorders.
http://www.dsusa.org

*Exercise: A Guide from the National Institute on Aging and the National Aeronautics and Space Administration.* Provides practical advice on fitness for seniors; includes animated instructions for specific weight training and flexibility exercises.
http://weboflife.ksc.nasa.gov/exerciseandaging/toc.html

*Georgia State University: Exercise and Physical Fitness Page.* Provides information about the benefits of exercise and how to get started on a fitness program.
http://www.gsu.edu/~wwwfit

*MedlinePlus: Exercise and Physical Fitness.* Provides links to news and reliable information about fitness and exercise from government agencies and professional associations.
http://www.nlm.nih.gov/medlineplus/exercisephysicalfitness.html

*National Institute on Drug Abuse: Anabolic Steroid Abuse.* Provides information and links about anabolic steroids.
http://www.steroidabuse.org

*President's Council on Physical Fitness and Sports (PCPFS).* Provides information on PCPFS programs and publications.
http://www.fitness.gov
http://www.presidentschallenge.gov

*SmallStep.Gov.* Provides resources for increasing activity and improving diet through small changes in daily habits.
http://www.smallstep.gov

See also the listings for Chapters 9, 11, and 12.

## Selected Bibliography

American Cancer Society. 2005. *Cancer Prevention and Early Detection: Facts and Figures 2005.* Atlanta, Ga.: American Cancer Society.

American College of Sports Medicine. 2004. Position Stand: Physical activity and bone health. *Medicine and Science in Sports and Exercise* 36(11): 1985–1996.

American College of Sports Medicine. 2002. How much exercise is enough? Responding to the IOM report on dietary guidelines. *Sports Medicine Bulletin* 37(6): 5–6.

American Heart Association. 2005. *Heart Disease and Stroke Statistics—2005 Update.* Dallas: American Heart Association.

Brooks, G. A., et al. 2005. *Exercise Physiology: Human Bioenergetics and Its Applications,* 4th ed. New York: McGraw-Hill.

Brownson, R. C., T. K. Boehmer, and D. A. Luke. 2005. Declining rates of physical activity in the United States: What are the contributors? *Annual Review of Public Health* 26: 421–443.

Centers for Disease Control and Prevention. 2004. *Improving Nutrition and Increasing Physical Activity* (http://www.cdc.gov/nccdphp/bb_nutrition/index.htm; retrieved December 30, 2004).

Colbert, L. H., et al. 2004. Physical activity, exercise, and inflammatory markers in older adults: Findings from the health, aging and body composition study. *Journal of the American Geriatrics Society* 52: 1098–1104.

Cussler, E. C., et al. 2003. Weight lifted in strength training predicts bone change in postmenopausal women. *Medicine and Science in Sports and Exercise* 35(1): 10–17.

Dugan, S. 2005. Safe exercise for women. *ACSM Fit Society Page,* Winter.

Dunn, A. L., et al. 2005. Exercise treatment for depression: Efficacy and dose response. *American Journal of Preventive Medicine* 28(1): 1–8.

Fahey, T. D., P. M. Insel, and W. T. Roth. 2005. *Fit and Well: Core Concepts and Labs in Physical Fitness and Wellness,* 6th ed. New York: McGraw-Hill.

Fenicchia, L. M., et al. 2004. Influence of resistance exercise training on glucose control in women with type 2 diabetes. *Metabolism* 53(3): 284–289.

Food and Drug Administration. 2004. *Questions and Answers: Androstenedione* (http://cfsan.fda.gov/~androqa.html; retrieved April 8, 2004).

Gleeson, M., D. C. Nieman, and B. K. Pedersen. 2004. Exercise, nutrition, and immune function. *Journal of Sports Science* 22(1): 115–125.

John, E. M., P. L. Horn-Ross, and J. Koo. 2004. Lifetime physical activity and breast cancer risk in a multiethnic population. *Cancer Epidemiology, Biomarkers & Prevention* 12(11 Pt 1): 1143–1152.

Joint WHO/FAO Expert Consultation. 2003. *Diet, Nutrition, and the Prevention of Chronic Diseases.* Geneva: World Health Organization.

Le Masurier, G. C. 2004. Walk which way? *ACSM's Health and Fitness Journal,* January/February.

Pescatello, L. S., et al. 2004. American College of Sports Medicine Position Stand: Exercise and hypertension. *Medicine and Science in Sports and Exercise* 36(3): 533–553.

Sheel, A. W., et al. 2004. Sex differences in respiratory exercise physiology. *Sports Medicine* 34: 567–579.

Shekelle, P. G., et al. 2003. Efficacy and safety of ephedra and ephedrine for weight loss and athletic performance: A meta-analysis. *Journal of the American Medical Association* 289(12): 1537–1545.

Slattery, J. L. 2004. Physical activity and colorectal cancer. *Sports Medicine* 34(4): 239–252.

Stewart, K. J. 2004. Exercise training: Can it improve cardiovascular health in patients with type 2 diabetes? *British Journal of Sports Medicine* 38: 250–252.

Thacker, S. B., et al. 2004. The impact of stretching on sports injury risk: A systematic review of the literature. *Medicine and Science in Sports and Exercise* 36(3): 371–378.

U.S. Department of Health and Human Services. 2005. *Dietary Guidelines for Americans, 2005* (http://www.healthierus.gov/dietaryguidelines; retrieved February 12, 2005).

Weuve, J., et al. 2004. Physical activity, including walking, and cognitive function in older women. *Journal of the American Medical* Association 292(12): 1454–461.

Wong, S. L., et al. 2004. Cardiorespiratory fitness is associated with lower abdominal fat independent of body mass index. *Medicine and Science in Sports and Exercise* 36(2): 286–291.

World Health Organization. 2004. *Physical Activity* (http://www.who.int/dietphysicalactivity/publications/facts/pa/en; retrieved May 24, 2004).

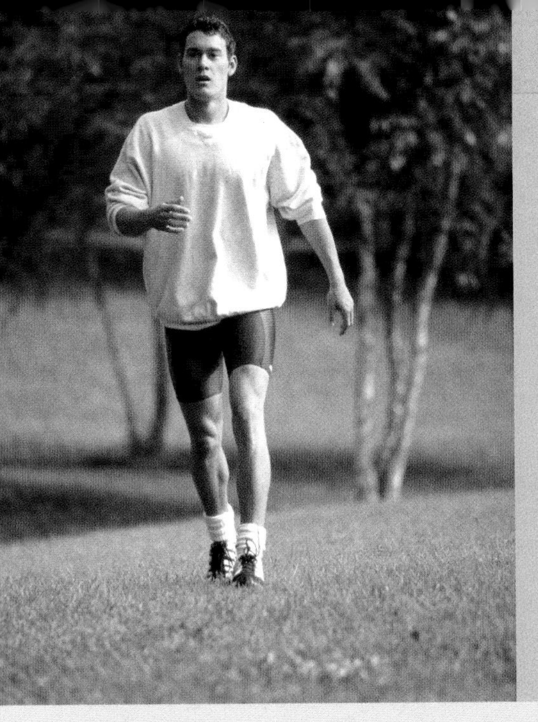

11

## Looking AHEAD

After reading this chapter, you should be able to

- Discuss different methods for assessing body weight and body composition
- Explain the health risks associated with overweight and obesity
- Explain factors that may contribute to a weight problem, including genetic, physiological, lifestyle, and psychosocial factors
- Describe lifestyle factors that contribute to weight gain and loss, including the role of diet, exercise, and emotional factors
- Identify and describe the symptoms of eating disorders and the health risks associated with them
- Design a personal plan for successfully managing body weight

# Weight Management

Achieving and maintaining a healthy body weight is a serious public health challenge in the United States and a source of distress for many Americans. Under standards developed by the National Institutes of Health, about 65% of American adults are overweight, including more than 30% who are obese (Figure 11-1). Lifestyle changes may be at the root of this increase (see the box "The Growing American Waistline" on p. 254). And while millions struggle to lose weight, others fall into dangerous eating patterns such as binge eating or self-starvation.

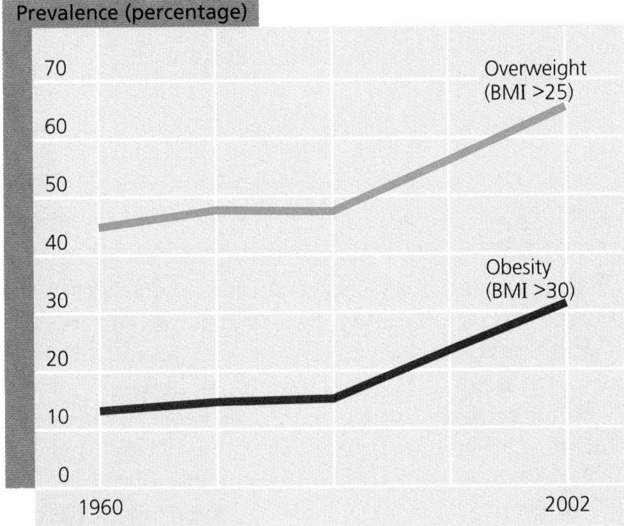


VITAL STATISTICS

**Figure 11-1 Prevalence of overweight and obesity among Americans.** SOURCE: National Center for Health Statistics. 2004. *Health, United States, 2004*. Hyattsville, Md.: National Center for Health Statistics.

Although not completely understood, managing body weight is not a mysterious process. The "secret" is balancing calories consumed with calories expended in daily activities—in other words, eating a moderate diet and exercising regularly. Successful weight management requires the long-term coordination of many aspects of a wellness lifestyle, including proper nutrition, adequate physical activity, and stress management.

This chapter explores the factors that contribute to the development of overweight and to eating disorders. It also takes a closer look at weight management through lifestyle behaviors and suggests specific strategies for reaching and maintaining a healthy weight. The information is designed to provide the tools necessary for integrating effective weight management into a wellness lifestyle.

## BASIC CONCEPTS OF WEIGHT MANAGEMENT

How many times have you or one of your friends said, "I'm too fat; I need to lose weight"? If you are like most people, you are concerned about what you weigh. But at

**Visit the *Core Concepts in Health* Online Learning Center (www.mhhe.com/inselbrief10e) for study aids and many additional resources.**

In the News

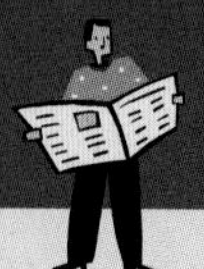

## The Growing American Waistline

By any measure, Americans are getting fatter. Since 1960, the average weight among adult men increased from 166 to 191 pounds; among women, from 140 to 164 pounds. The trend is also seen among young Americans, where the number of overweight and obese children has more than tripled since 1960.

Along with rising rates of obesity come increased rates of obesity-related health problems, including a more than 60% rise in rates of type 2 diabetes since 1990. Estimates vary, but inactivity and overweight may account for as many as 365,000 premature deaths annually in the United States, second only to tobacco-related deaths, and medical costs are more than $100 billion annually. Before long, rising rates of obesity may cut U.S. life expectancy.

### Contributing Factors

The basic facts of energy balance help explain the expanding American waistline: According to the CDC, average calorie intake among Americans has increased by about 250 calories per day since 1970, and levels of physical activity have declined. What are some of the factors underlying this change?

- *More meals eaten outside the home, especially fast-food meals:* The more people eat out, the more calories they consume, especially when they choose a fast-food restaurant. One-third of American children eat fast food on any given day, and children who eat fast food consume almost 200 more calories per day than those who don't.
- *Underestimation of portion sizes and food consumption:* When participants in one recent study were asked to report their food intake over the previous 24 hours, the majority underestimated their actual intake by about 600 calories!
- *Increased consumption of soft drinks and convenience snack foods:* Compared to 1970, Americans today consume significantly more carbohydrate, slightly more fat, and about the same amount of protein. These additional carbohydrate calories do not come from the fruits, vegetables, and whole grains recommended by health experts but rather from soft drinks, pizza, salty snacks, and desserts. Regular soft drinks are the leading source of calories in the American diet.
- *More time spend in sedentary activities:* Americans now spend far more time watching television and movies, sitting in cars, playing video games, and in other sedentary activities than they do in activities requiring more energy. For children, daily gym classes are no longer the norm.

### Possible Solutions

Some possible strategies for improving America's food choices were outlined in Chapter 9; these include making healthy foods more attractive from a price perspective, placing consumer-friendly nutrition and serving-size information in prominent locations, restricting food advertising aimed at children, and improving food options sold on school grounds.

Clear messages about physical activity and healthy food choices are needed from all sources, including public information campaigns, physicians, and school programs. Restaurants and food manufacturers should be encouraged to provide both more information and healthier choices and portion sizes. Support is also needed to get healthy food and activity options into communities that currently lack them. Residents of low-income and urban areas are less likely to have access to healthy foods and opportunities for safe physical activity.

As officials debate potential solutions, there are many actions you can take to manage your own weight and to promote healthy eating and activity habits among others. Refer to the suggestions in Chapters 9 and 10 as well as in this chapter.

SOURCES: Koplan, J. P., C. T. Liverman, and V. A. Kraak, eds. 2005. *Preventing Childhood Obesity: Health in the Balance.* Washington, D.C.: National Academy Press; Centers for Disease Control and Prevention. 2004. Mean body weight, height, and body mass index, United States 1960–2002. *Advance Data from Vital and Health Statistics* No. 347; Bowman, S. A., et al. 2004. Effects of fast-food consumption on energy intake and diet quality among children in a national household survey. *Pediatrics* 113(Pt 1): 112–118; Centers for Disease Control and Prevention. 2004. Trends in intake of energy and macronutrients—United States, 1971–2000. *Morbidity and Mortality Weekly Report* 53(4): 80–82.

what point does being overweight present a health risk? And how thin is too thin?

## Body Composition

The human body can be divided into fat-free mass and body fat. Fat-free mass is composed of all the body's nonfat tissues: bone, water, muscle, connective tissue, organ tissues, and teeth. Body fat includes both essential and nonessential body fat. (Remember that 1 pound of body fat is equal to 3500 calories.) **Essential fat** includes *lipids,* or fats, incorporated in the nerves, brain, heart, lungs, liver, and mammary glands. These fat deposits, crucial for normal body functioning, make up approximately 3–5% of total body weight in men and 8–12% in women. The larger percentage in women is due to fat deposits in the breasts, uterus, and other sites specific to females. It is normal for women to naturally have more body fat than men because of their ability to bear children.

**Nonessential (storage) fat** exists primarily within fat cells, or *adipose tissue,* often located just below the skin and around major organs. The amount of storage fat varies from person to person based on many factors, including gender, age, heredity, metabolism, diet, and activity level. When we talk about wanting to "lose weight," most of us are referring to storage fat.

What is most important for health is not total weight but rather the proportion of the body's total weight that is fat—the **percent body fat.** For example, two women may both be 5 feet, 5 inches tall and weigh 130 pounds. But one woman, an endurance runner, may have only 15% of her body weight as fat, whereas the second, sedentary woman could have 34% body fat. Although 130 pounds is not considered "overweight" for women of this height by most standards, the second woman may be overfat. Because most people use the word "overweight" to describe the condition of having too much body fat, we use it in this chapter, although "overfat" is actually a more accurate term.

## Energy Balance

The key to keeping a healthy ratio of fat to fat-free mass is maintaining an energy balance (Figure 11-2). You take in energy (calories) from the food you eat. Your body uses energy (calories) to maintain vital body functions (resting metabolism), to digest food, and to fuel physical activity. When energy in equals energy out, you maintain your current weight. To change your weight and body composition, you must tip the energy balance equation in a particular direction. If you take in more calories daily than your body burns, the excess calories will be stored as fat, and you will gain weight over time. If you eat fewer calories than you burn each day, you will lose some of that storage fat and probably lose weight.

The two parts of the energy balance equation over which you have the most control are the energy you take in as food and the energy you burn during physical activity. To create a negative energy balance and lose weight and body fat, you can increase the amount of energy you burn by increasing your level of physical activity and/or decrease the amount of energy you take in by consuming fewer calories.

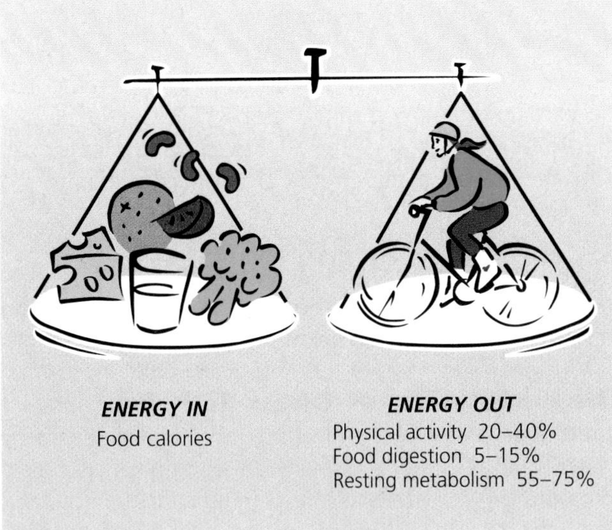


**Figure 11-2 The energy balance equation.** In order to maintain your current weight, you must burn up as many calories as you take in as food each day.

## Evaluating Body Weight and Body Composition

**Overweight** is usually defined as total body weight above the recommended range for good health (as determined by large-scale population surveys). **Obesity** is defined as a more serious degree of overweight. Many methods are available for measuring and evaluating body weight and percent body fat.

**Height-Weight Charts** In the past, many people relied on height-weight charts to evaluate body weight. Based on insurance company statistics, these charts list a range of "ideal" or "recommended" body weights associated with the lowest mortality for people of a particular sex, age, and height. Although easy to use, height-weight charts can be highly inaccurate for some people, and they provide only an indirect measure of body fatness.

**Body Mass Index** **Body mass index (BMI)** is a measure of body weight that is useful for classifying the health risks of body weight if you don't have access to more sophisticated methods. Though more accurate than height-weight tables, BMI is also based on the concept that weight should be proportional to height. Easy to calculate and rate, BMI is a fairly accurate measure of the health risks of body weight for average people. However, because BMI doesn't distinguish between fat weight and fat-free weight, it can be very inaccurate for some groups, including people of short stature, muscular athletes, and older adults with little muscle mass due to inactivity or an underlying disease. If you are in one of these groups, use one of the methods described below for estimating percent body fat to assess whether your current weight and body composition are healthy.

BMI is defined as body weight (in kilograms) divided by the square of height (in meters); this translates into multiplying your body weight in pounds by 704, and

### Terms

**essential fat** The fat in the body necessary for normal body functioning.

**nonessential (storage) fat** Extra fat or fat reserves stored in the body.

**percent body fat** The percentage of total body weight that is composed of fat.

**overweight** Body weight that falls above the range associated with minimum mortality.

**obesity** The condition of having an excess of nonessential body fat; having a body mass index of 30 or greater or having a percent body fat greater than about 24% for men and 38% for women.

**body mass index (BMI)** A measure of relative body weight that takes height into account and is highly correlated with more direct measures of body fat; calculated by dividing total body weight (in kilograms) by the square of height (in meters).

Vw

| | <18.5 Underweight | | 18.5–24.9 Normal | | | | | | 25–29.9 Overweight | | | | | 30–34.9 Obesity (Class I) | | | | | 35–39.9 Obesity (Class II) | | | | | ≥40 Extreme obesity |
|---|---|---|---|---|---|---|---|---|---|---|---|---|---|---|---|---|---|---|---|---|---|---|---|---|
| BMI | 17 | 18 | 19 | 20 | 21 | 22 | 23 | 24 | 25 | 26 | 27 | 28 | 29 | 30 | 31 | 32 | 33 | 34 | 35 | 36 | 37 | 38 | 39 | 40 |
| Height | | | | | | | | | | | | | Body Weight (pounds) | | | | | | | | | | | |
| 4' 10" | 81 | 86 | 91 | 96 | 101 | 105 | 110 | 115 | 120 | 124 | 129 | 134 | 139 | 144 | 148 | 153 | 158 | 163 | 168 | 172 | 177 | 182 | 187 | 192 |
| 4' 11" | 84 | 89 | 94 | 99 | 104 | 109 | 114 | 119 | 124 | 129 | 134 | 139 | 144 | 149 | 154 | 159 | 163 | 168 | 173 | 178 | 183 | 188 | 193 | 198 |
| 5' | 87 | 92 | 97 | 102 | 108 | 113 | 118 | 123 | 128 | 133 | 138 | 143 | 149 | 154 | 159 | 164 | 169 | 174 | 179 | 184 | 190 | 195 | 200 | 205 |
| 5' 1" | 90 | 95 | 101 | 106 | 111 | 117 | 122 | 127 | 132 | 138 | 143 | 148 | 154 | 159 | 164 | 169 | 175 | 180 | 185 | 191 | 196 | 201 | 207 | 212 |
| 5' 2" | 93 | 98 | 104 | 109 | 115 | 120 | 126 | 131 | 137 | 142 | 148 | 153 | 159 | 164 | 170 | 175 | 181 | 186 | 191 | 197 | 202 | 208 | 213 | 219 |
| 5' 3" | 96 | 102 | 107 | 113 | 119 | 124 | 130 | 136 | 141 | 147 | 153 | 158 | 164 | 169 | 175 | 181 | 186 | 192 | 198 | 203 | 209 | 215 | 220 | 226 |
| 5' 4" | 99 | 105 | 111 | 117 | 122 | 128 | 134 | 140 | 146 | 152 | 157 | 163 | 169 | 175 | 181 | 187 | 192 | 198 | 204 | 210 | 216 | 222 | 227 | 233 |
| 5' 5" | 102 | 108 | 114 | 120 | 126 | 132 | 138 | 144 | 150 | 156 | 162 | 168 | 174 | 180 | 186 | 192 | 198 | 204 | 210 | 216 | 222 | 229 | 235 | 241 |
| 5' 6" | 105 | 112 | 118 | 124 | 130 | 136 | 143 | 149 | 155 | 161 | 167 | 174 | 180 | 186 | 192 | 198 | 205 | 211 | 217 | 223 | 229 | 236 | 242 | 248 |
| 5' 7" | 109 | 115 | 121 | 128 | 134 | 141 | 147 | 153 | 160 | 166 | 173 | 179 | 185 | 192 | 198 | 204 | 211 | 217 | 224 | 230 | 236 | 243 | 249 | 256 |
| 5' 8" | 112 | 118 | 125 | 132 | 138 | 145 | 151 | 158 | 165 | 171 | 178 | 184 | 191 | 197 | 204 | 211 | 217 | 224 | 230 | 237 | 244 | 250 | 257 | 263 |
| 5' 9" | 115 | 122 | 129 | 136 | 142 | 149 | 156 | 163 | 169 | 176 | 183 | 190 | 197 | 203 | 210 | 217 | 224 | 230 | 237 | 244 | 251 | 258 | 264 | 271 |
| 5' 10" | 119 | 126 | 133 | 139 | 146 | 153 | 160 | 167 | 174 | 181 | 188 | 195 | 202 | 209 | 216 | 223 | 230 | 237 | 244 | 251 | 258 | 265 | 272 | 279 |
| 5' 11" | 122 | 129 | 136 | 143 | 151 | 158 | 165 | 172 | 179 | 187 | 194 | 201 | 208 | 215 | 222 | 230 | 237 | 244 | 251 | 258 | 265 | 273 | 280 | 287 |
| 6' | 125 | 133 | 140 | 148 | 155 | 162 | 170 | 177 | 184 | 192 | 199 | 207 | 214 | 221 | 229 | 236 | 243 | 251 | 258 | 266 | 273 | 280 | 288 | 295 |
| 6' 1" | 129 | 137 | 144 | 152 | 159 | 167 | 174 | 182 | 190 | 197 | 205 | 212 | 220 | 228 | 235 | 243 | 250 | 258 | 265 | 273 | 281 | 288 | 296 | 303 |
| 6' 2" | 132 | 140 | 148 | 156 | 164 | 171 | 179 | 187 | 195 | 203 | 210 | 218 | 226 | 234 | 242 | 249 | 257 | 265 | 273 | 281 | 288 | 296 | 304 | 312 |
| 6' 3" | 136 | 144 | 152 | 160 | 168 | 176 | 184 | 192 | 200 | 208 | 216 | 224 | 232 | 240 | 248 | 256 | 264 | 272 | 280 | 288 | 296 | 304 | 312 | 320 |
| 6' 4" | 140 | 148 | 156 | 164 | 173 | 181 | 189 | 197 | 206 | 214 | 222 | 230 | 238 | 247 | 255 | 263 | 271 | 280 | 288 | 296 | 304 | 312 | 321 | 329 |

**Figure 11-3 Body mass index (BMI).** To determine your BMI, find your height in the left column. Move across the appropriate row until you find the weight closest to your own. The number at the top of the column is the BMI at that height and weight. SOURCE: Ratings from National Heart, Lung, and Blood Institute. 1998. *Clinical Guidelines on the Identification, Evaluation, and Treatment of Overweight and Obesity in Adults: The Evidence Report.* Bethesda, Md.: National Institutes of Health.

then dividing the result by the square of your height in inches. Refer to Figure 11-3 for a chart of BMI values. Under standards issued by the National Institutes of Health (NIH), a BMI between 18.5 and 24.9 is considered healthy, a person with a BMI of 25 or above is classified as overweight; a person with a BMI of 30 or above is classified as obese. A person with a BMI below 18.5 is classified as underweight, although low BMI values may be healthy in some cases if they are not the result of smoking, an eating disorder, or an underlying disease. A BMI value of 17.5 or less is sometimes used as a diagnostic criterion for the eating disorder anorexia nervosa.

**Body Composition Analysis** The most accurate and direct way to evaluate body composition is to determine percent body fat; a variety of methods are available. Refer to Table 11-1 for body composition ratings based on percent body fat.

**HYDROSTATIC (UNDERWATER) WEIGHING** In this method, a person is submerged and weighed under water. Percent body fat can be calculated from body density. Muscle has a higher density and fat a lower density than water, so people with more fat tend to float and weigh less under water, while lean people tend to sink and weigh relatively more under water.

**SKINFOLD MEASUREMENTS** The skinfold thickness technique measures the thickness of fat under the skin. A technician grasps a fold of skin at a predetermined location and measures it using an instrument called a caliper. Measurements are taken at several sites and plugged into formulas that predict body fat percentages.

**ELECTRICAL IMPEDANCE ANALYSIS** In this method, electrodes are attached to the body and a harmless electrical current is transmitted from electrode to electrode. The electrical conduction through the body favors the path of the fat-free tissues over the fat tissues. A computer can calculate fat percentages from current measurements.

## Excess Body Fat and Wellness

The amount of fat in the body—and its location—can have profound effects on health.

**The Health Risks of Excess Body Fat** Obesity doubles mortality rates and can reduce life expectancy by 10–20 years. Obesity is associated with unhealthy cholesterol and triglyceride levels, impaired heart function, and death from cardiovascular disease. Other health risks associated with obesity include hypertension, many kinds of cancer, impaired immune function, gallbladder and kidney diseases, skin problems, impotence, sleep and

**Table 11-1 Percent Body Fat Classification**

| | Percent Body Fat (%) | | |
|---|---|---|---|
| | 20–39 Years | 40–59 Years | 60–79 Years |
| **Women** | | | |
| Essential[a] | 8–12 | 8–12 | 8–12 |
| Low/athletic[b] | 13–20 | 13–22 | 13–23 |
| Recommended | 21–32 | 23–33 | 24–35 |
| Overfat[c] | 33–38 | 34–39 | 36–41 |
| Obese[c] | ≥39 | ≥40 | ≥42 |
| **Men** | | | |
| Essential[a] | 3–5 | 3–5 | 3–5 |
| Low/athletic[b] | 6–7 | 6–10 | 6–12 |
| Recommended | 8–19 | 11–21 | 13–24 |
| Overfat[c] | 20–24 | 22–27 | 25–29 |
| Obese[c] | ≥25 | ≥28 | ≥30 |

The cutoffs for recommended, overfat, and obese ranges in this table are based on a study that linked body mass index classifications from the National Institutes of Health with predicted percent body fat (measured using dual energy X-ray absorptiometry).

[a]Essential body fat is necessary for the basic functioning of the body.
[b]Percent body fat in the low/athletic range may be appropriate for some people as long as it is not the result of illness or disordered eating habits.
[c]Health risks increase as percent body fat exceeds the recommended range.

SOURCES: Gallagher, D., et al. 2000. Healthy percentage body fat ranges: An approach for developing guidelines based on body mass index. *American Journal of Clinical Nutrition* 72: 694–701; American College of Sports Medicine. 2001. *ACSM's Resource Manual for Guidelines for Exercise Testing and Prescription,* 4th ed. Philadelphia: Lippincott, Williams and Wilkins.

breathing disorders, back pain, arthritis, and other bone and joint disorders. Obesity is also associated with complications of pregnancy, menstrual irregularities, urine leakage (stress incontinence), psychological disorders, and increased surgical risk.

Of particular note is the strong association between excess body fat and diabetes mellitus, a disease that causes a disruption of normal metabolism. The pancreas, a long, thin organ located behind the stomach, normally secretes the hormone insulin, which stimulates cells to take up glucose to produce energy (Figure 11-4). In a person with diabetes, this process is disrupted, causing a buildup of glucose in the bloodstream. Over the long term, diabetes is associated with kidney failure; nerve damage; circulation problems and amputations; retinal damage and blindness; and increased rates of heart attack, stroke, and hypertension (see the box "Diabetes" for more information).

The risks from obesity increase with its severity, and they are much more likely to occur in people who are more than twice their desirable body weight. The NIH recommends weight loss for people whose BMI places them in the obese category and for those who are overweight *and* have two or more major risk factors for disease such as tobacco use and high blood pressure. If your BMI is 25 or above, consult a physician for help in determining a healthy BMI for you.

Obesity can affect psychological as well as physical wellness. Being perceived as fat can be a source of ridicule, ostracism, and sometimes discrimination from others; it can contribute to psychological problems such as depression, anxiety, and low self-esteem (often caused by repeated failures at losing weight). For some, the stigma associated with obesity can give rise to a negative body image, body dissatisfaction, and eating disorders.

**Body Fat Distribution and Health** The distribution of body fat is also an important indicator of health. Men and postmenopausal women tend to store fat in the upper regions of their bodies, particularly in the abdominal area ("apples"). Premenopausal women usually store fat in hips, buttocks, and thighs ("pears"). Excess fat in the abdominal area, the apple shape, increases risk of high blood pressure, diabetes, early-onset heart disease, stroke, certain types of cancer, and mortality. It appears that abdominal fat is more easily mobilized and sent into the bloodstream, increasing disease-related blood fat levels.

The risks from body fat distribution are usually assessed by measuring waist circumference (the distance around the abdomen at the level of the hip bone, known as the iliac crest). A total waist measurement of more than 40 inches for men and 35 inches for women is associated with a significantly increased risk of disease. Large waist circumference can be a marker for increased risk of diabetes, high blood pressure, and CVD even in people with a BMI in the normal range.

**Body Image** The collective picture of the body as seen through the mind's eye, **body image** consists of perceptions, images, thoughts, attitudes, and emotions. A negative body image is characterized by dissatisfaction with the body in general or some part of the body in particular. Recent surveys indicate that the majority of Americans, many of whom are not actually overweight, are unhappy with their body weight or with some aspect of their appearance.

Losing weight or getting cosmetic surgery does not necessarily improve body image. On the other hand, improvements in body image may occur in the absence of changes in weight or appearance. Many experts now believe that body image issues must be dealt with as part of

**Term**

**body image** The mental representation a person holds about his or her body at any given moment in time, consisting of perceptions, images, thoughts, attitudes, and emotions about the body.

Vw

**Symptoms of diabetes:**

- Frequent urination
- Extreme thirst and hunger
- Unexplained weight loss
- Extreme fatigue
- Blurred vision
- Frequent infections
- Slow wound healing
- Tingling or numbness in hands and feet
- Dry, itchy skin

Note: In the early stages, diabetes often has no symptoms

Esophagus

Stomach

Pancreas

Small intestine

**Normal:**
Insulin binds to receptors on the surface of a cell and signals special transporters in the cell to transport glucose inside.

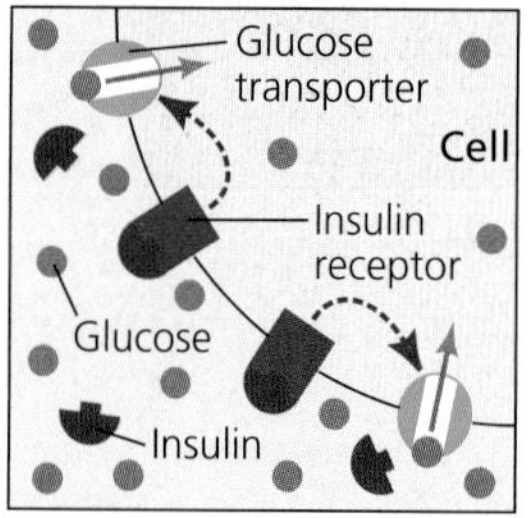


**Type 1 diabetes:**
The pancreas produces little or no insulin. Thus, no signal is sent instructing the cell to transport glucose, and glucose builds up in the bloodstream.

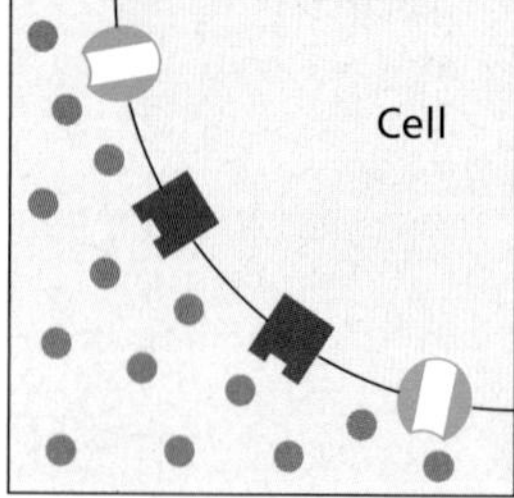


**Type 2 diabetes:**
The pancreas produces too little insulin and/or the body's cells are resistant to it. Some insulin binds to receptors on the cell's surface, but the signal to transport glucose is blocked. Glucose builds up in the bloodstream.

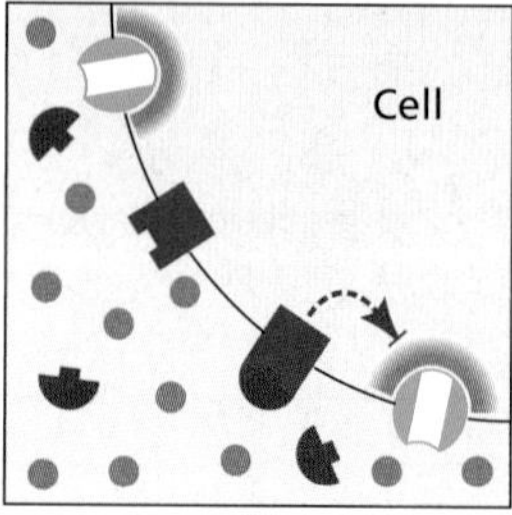


**Figure 11-4 Diabetes mellitus.** During digestion, carbohydrates are broken down in the small intestine into glucose, a simple sugar that enters the bloodstream. The presence of glucose signals the pancreas to release insulin, a hormone that helps cells take up glucose; once inside a cell, glucose can be converted to energy. In diabetes, this process is disrupted, resulting in a buildup of glucose in the bloodstream.

treating obesity and eating disorders. See pp. 269–273 for more information on body image and eating disorders.

**Problems Associated with Very Low Levels of Body Fat** Health experts have generally viewed very low levels of body fat—less than 8–12% for women and 3–5% for men—as a threat to wellness. Extreme leanness has been linked with reproductive, circulatory, and immune system disorders. Extremely lean people may experience muscle wasting and fatigue; they are also more likely to suffer from dangerous eating disorders.

In physically active women and girls, particularly those involved in sports where weight and appearance are important (ballet, gymnastics, skating, and distance running, for example), a condition called the **female athlete triad** may develop. The triad consists of three interrelated disorders: abnormal eating patterns (and excessive exercising), followed by **amenorrhea** (absence of menstruation), followed by decreased bone density (premature osteoporosis). Prolonged amenorrhea can cause bone density to erode to a point that a woman in her twenties will have the bone density of a woman in her sixties. Left untreated, the triad can lead to decreased physical performance, increased incidence of bone fractures, disturbances of heart rhythm and metabolism, and even death.

### Terms

Vw

**female athlete triad** A condition consisting of three interrelated disorders: abnormal eating patterns (and excessive exercising) followed by lack of menstrual periods (amenorrhea) and decreased bone density (premature osteoporosis).

**amenorrhea** The absence of menstruation.

## What Is the Right Weight for You?

For most of us, body weight and percentage of body fat fall somewhere below the levels associated with significant health risks. For us, these assessment tests do not really answer the question How much should I weigh? BMI, percent body fat, and waist measurement can best serve as general guides or estimates for body weight.

To answer the question of what you "should" weigh, let your lifestyle be your guide. Don't focus on a particular weight as your goal. Instead, focus on living a lifestyle that includes eating moderate amounts of healthful foods, getting plenty of exercise, thinking positively, and learning to cope with stress. Then let the pounds fall where they

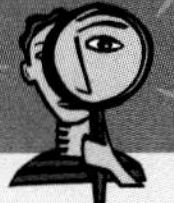

## Diabetes

### Types of Diabetes

Approximately 18 million (1 in 14) Americans have one of two major forms of diabetes. About 5–10% of people with diabetes have the more serious form, known as type 1 diabetes. In this type of diabetes, the pancreas produces little or no insulin, so daily doses of insulin are required. (Without insulin, a person with type 1 can lapse into a coma.) Type 1 diabetes occurs when the body's immune system, triggered by a viral infection or some other environmental factor, mistakenly destroys the insulin-producing cells in the pancreas. It usually strikes before age 30.

The remaining 90% of Americans with diabetes have type 2 diabetes. This condition can develop slowly, and about a third of affected individuals are unaware of their condition. In type 2 diabetes, the pancreas doesn't produce enough insulin, cells are resistant to insulin, or both. This condition is usually diagnosed in people over age 40, although there has been a tenfold increase in type 2 diabetes in children in the past two decades. About one-third of people with type 2 diabetes must take insulin; others may take medications that increase insulin production or stimulate cells to take up glucose.

A third type of diabetes occurs in about 2–5% of women during pregnancy. So-called *gestational diabetes* usually disappears after pregnancy, but more than half of women who experience it eventually develop type 2 diabetes.

In 2002, the U.S. Department of Health and Human Services and the American Diabetes Association adopted the term *pre-diabetes* to describe blood glucose levels that are higher than normal but not high enough for a diagnosis of full-blown diabetes. About 41 million Americans have pre-diabetes, and most people with the condition will develop type 2 diabetes within 10 years unless they adopt preventive lifestyle measures. Pre-diabetes poses a risk to health beyond just the development of diabetes: Blood glucose levels in the pre-diabetes range increase the risk of heart attack or stroke by 50%. The insulin resistance and elevated glucose levels associated with pre-diabetes (and diabetes) are one of the five defining risk factors of the condition known as metabolic syndrome, a collection of risk factors associated with heart disease; see Chapter 12 for more information on metabolic syndrome.

The major factors involved in the development of diabetes are age, obesity, physical inactivity, a family history of diabetes, and lifestyle. Excess body fat is a key risk factor because the cells of obese people are less responsive to insulin, and insulin resistance is almost always a precursor of type 2 diabetes. Ethnic background also plays a role. African Americans and people of Hispanic background are 55% more likely than non-Hispanic whites to develop type 2 diabetes; over 20% of Hispanics over age 65 have diabetes. Native Americans also have a higher-than-average incidence of diabetes.

### Prevention

It is estimated that 90% of cases of type 2 diabetes could be prevented if people adopted healthy lifestyle behaviors, including regular physical activity, a moderate diet, and modest weight loss. For people with pre-diabetes, lifestyle measures are more effective than medication for delaying or preventing the development of diabetes. Exercise (endurance and/or strength training) makes cells more sensitive to insulin and helps stabilize blood glucose levels; it also helps keep body fat at healthy levels.

A moderate diet to control body fat is perhaps the most important dietary recommendation for the prevention of diabetes. However, there is some evidence that the composition of the diet may also be important. Studies have linked diets low in fiber and high in sugar, refined carbohydrates, saturated fat, red meat, and high-fat dairy products to increased risk of diabetes; diets rich in whole grains, fruits, vegetables, legumes, fish, and poultry may be protective. The overall pattern of a person's diet is most important, but specific foods linked to higher risk of diabetes include regular (nondiet) soft drinks, white bread, white rice, french fries, processed meats (bacon, sausage, hot dogs), and sugary desserts. See Chapter 9 for information on different types of carbohydrates and strategies for increasing fiber and whole-grain intake.

### Treatment

There is no cure for diabetes, but it can be successfully managed. Treatment involves keeping blood sugar levels within safe limits through diet, exercise, and, if necessary, medication. Blood sugar levels can be monitored using a home test; close monitoring and control of glucose levels can significantly reduce the rate of serious complications among people with diabetes.

Nearly 90% of people with type 2 diabetes are overweight when diagnosed, including 55% who are obese, and an important step in treatment is to lose weight. Even a small amount of weight loss can be beneficial. People with diabetes should obtain carbohydrate from whole grains, fruits, vegetables, and low-fat dairy products; carbohydrate and monounsaturated fat together should provide 60–70% of total daily calories. Regular exercise and a healthy diet are often sufficient to control type 2 diabetes.

### Warning Signs and Testing

A wellness lifestyle that includes a healthy diet and regular exercise is the best strategy for preventing diabetes. If you do develop diabetes, the best way to avoid complications is to recognize the symptoms and get early diagnosis and treatment. Be alert for the warning signs listed in Figure 11-4. Pre-diabetes and type 2 diabetes are often asymptomatic in the early stages, and routine screening is recommended for people over age 45 and anyone younger who is at high risk, including anyone who is obese.

The Web site for the American Diabetes Association, listed in the For More Information section at the end of the chapter, includes an interactive diabetes risk assessment. Screening involves a blood test to check glucose levels after either a period of fasting or the administration of a set dose of glucose. A fasting glucose level of 126 mg/dl or higher indicates diabetes; a level of 100–125 mg/dl indicates pre-diabetes. If you are concerned about your risk for diabetes, talk with your physician about being tested.

may. For most people, the result will be close to the recommended weight ranges discussed earlier. For some, their weight will be somewhat higher than societal standards—but right for them. By letting a healthy lifestyle determine your weight, you can avoid developing unhealthy patterns of eating and a negative body image.

## FACTORS CONTRIBUTING TO EXCESS BODY FAT

Body weight and body composition are determined by multiple factors that may vary with each individual.

### Genetic Factors

Estimates of the genetic contribution to obesity vary widely, from about 25% to 40% of an individual's body fat. Genes influence body size and shape, body fat distribution, and metabolic rate. Genetic factors also affect the ease with which weight is gained as a result of overeating and where on the body extra weight is added. If both parents are overweight, their children are twice as likely to be overweight as are children who have only one overweight parent. In studies that compared adoptees and their biological parents, the weights of the adoptees were found to be more like those of the biological parents than the adoptive parents, again indicating a strong genetic link.

However, hereditary influences must be balanced against the contribution of environmental factors. Not all children of obese parents become obese, and normal-weight parents also have overweight children. The *tendency* to develop obesity may be inherited, but the expression of this tendency is affected by environmental influences.

The message you should take from this research is that genes are not destiny. It is true that some people have a harder time losing weight and maintaining weight loss than others. However, with increased exercise and attention to diet, even those with a genetic tendency toward obesity can maintain a healthy body weight.

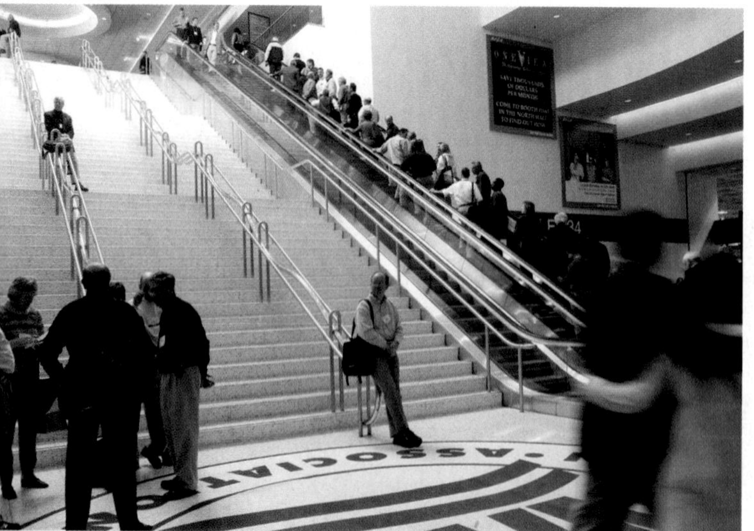

The typical American lifestyle does not lead naturally to healthy weight management. Labor-saving devices such as escalators help reinforce our sedentary habits.

### Metabolism

Metabolism is the sum of all the vital processes by which food energy and nutrients are made available to and used by the body. The largest component of metabolism, **resting metabolic rate (RMR),** is the energy required to maintain vital body functions, including respiration, heart rate, body temperature, and blood pressure, while the body is at rest. As shown in Figure 11-2, RMR accounts for about 55–75% of daily energy expenditure. The energy required to digest food accounts for an additional 5–15% of daily energy expenditure. The remaining 20–40% is expended during physical activity.

Both heredity and behavior affect metabolic rate. Men, who have a higher proportion of muscle mass than women, have a higher RMR (muscle tissue is more metabolically active than fat). Also, some individuals inherit a higher or lower RMR than others. A higher RMR means that a person burns more calories while at rest and can therefore take in more calories without gaining weight.

Weight loss or gain also affects metabolic rate. When a person loses weight, both RMR and the energy required to perform physical tasks decrease. The reverse occurs when weight is gained. Exercise has a positive effect on metabolism. When people exercise, they slightly increase their RMR—the number of calories their bodies burn at rest. They also increase their muscle mass, which is associated with a higher metabolic rate. The exercise itself also burns calories, raising total energy expenditure. The higher the energy expenditure, the more the person can eat without gaining weight.

### Lifestyle Factors

Although genetic and metabolism may increase risk for excess body fat, they are not sufficient to explain the increasingly high rate of obesity seen in the United States. The gene pool has not changed dramatically in the past 40 years, during which time the rate of obesity among Americans has more than doubled (see the box "Overweight and Obesity Among U.S. Ethnic Populations"). Clearly, other factors are at work—particularly lifestyle factors such as increased energy intake and decreased physical activity.

**Eating** Americans have access to an abundance of highly palatable and calorie-dense foods, and many have eating habits that contribute to weight gain. Most overweight adults will admit to eating more than they should of high-fat, high-sugar, high-calorie foods. Americans eat out more frequently now than in the past, and we rely more heavily on fast food and packaged convenience foods. Restaurant and convenience food portion sizes

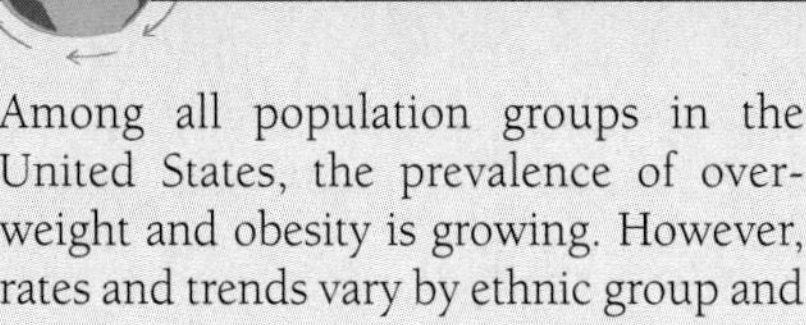

Dimensions of Diversity

## Overweight and Obesity Among U.S. Ethnic Populations

Among all population groups in the United States, the prevalence of overweight and obesity is growing. However, rates and trends vary by ethnic group and by other population characteristics:

- Certain groups, including African Americans, Latinos, and American Indians and Alaska Natives, have higher-than-average rates of obesity. Asian Americans have a low rate of obesity.
- There is considerable variation within populations grouped into general ethnic categories. For example, Asian Americans, Vietnamese Americans, and Chinese Americans have very low rates of obesity, and Asian Indians have much higher rates of obesity.
- Low socioeconomic status is associated with higher rates of overweight and obesity. Researchers theorize that people living in poor communities have fewer opportunities to purchase healthy foods and engage in regular physical activity. In addition, many foods low in price are high in calorie density (fast food, for example).
- Higher or increasing socioeconomic status is associated with lower rates of obesity among some groups and constant or increased rates of obesity among other groups. Groups that are transitioning from poverty, food scarcity, and jobs that require significant energy expenditure may not have good family or community models of reducing energy intake and increasing leisure-time physical activity.
- Acculturation boosts body weight. The longer a foreign-born person lives in the United States, the more likely she or he is to become obese.
- Cultural factors that influence dietary and exercise behaviors appear to play a role in the development of obesity. There are also cultural differences in acceptance of larger body size and in body image perception.
- Some studies have found that African Americans, on average, have lower resting metabolic rates than whites; in addition, weight loss may cause greater declines in RMR among African Americans.
- The health consequences of obesity affect ethnic populations in different ways. At a given level of BMI, Latinos are significantly more likely to have type 2 diabetes. Obesity in African Americans is associated with increased risk of developing hypertension at a younger age and in a more severe form.
- For Asian Americans or persons of Asian descent, waist circumference is a better indicator of relative disease risk than BMI, and disease risk goes up at a lower level of BMI than for individuals of other groups. For Asian populations, WHO guidelines have a lower BMI cutoff for defining overweight (BMI > 23).

SOURCES: Goel, M. S., et al. 2004. Obesity among U.S. immigrant subgroups by duration of residence. *Journal of the American Medical Association* 292(23): 2860–2867; Centers for Disease Control and Prevention. 2004. Prevalence of diabetes among Hispanics. *Morbidity and Mortality Weekly Report* 53(40): 941–944; Sanchez-Johnsen, L. A., et al. 2004. Ethnic differences in correlates of obesity between Latin-American and black women. *Obesity Research* 12(4): 652–660; Fitzgibbon, M. L., and M. R. Stolley. 2004. Environmental changes may be needed for prevention of overweight in minority children. *Pediatric Annals* 33(1): 45–49; American Obesity Association. 2004. *Obesity in Minority Populations* (http://www.obesity.org/subs/fastfacts/Obesity_Minority_Pop.shtml; September 29, 2004).

tend to be very large, and the foods themselves are more likely to be high in fat, sugar, and calories and low in nutrients. Studies have consistently found that people underestimate portion sizes by as much as 25%.

**Physical Activity** Activity levels among Americans are declining, beginning in childhood and continuing throughout the life cycle. Many schools have cut back on physical education classes and recess. Most adults drive to work, sit all day, and then relax in front of the TV at night. During leisure time, both children and adults surf the Internet, play video games, or watch TV rather than bicycle, participate in sports, or just do yardwork or chores around the house. On average, Americans exercise 15 minutes per day and watch 170 minutes of TV and movies. Modern conveniences such as remote controls, elevators, and power mowers have also reduced daily physical activity.

## Psychosocial Factors

Many people have learned to use food as a means of coping with stress and negative emotions. Eating can provide a powerful distraction from difficult feelings—loneliness, anger, boredom, anxiety, shame, sadness, inadequacy. It can be used to combat low moods, low energy levels, and low self-esteem. When food and eating become the primary means of regulating emotions, binge eating or other disturbed eating patterns can develop.

Obesity is strongly associated with socioeconomic status. The prevalence of obesity goes down as income level goes up. More women than men are obese at lower income levels, but men are somewhat more obese at higher levels. These differences may reflect the greater sensitivity and concern for a slim physical appearance among upper-income women, as well as greater access to nutrition information, to low-fat and low-calorie foods, and to opportunities for exercise. It may also reflect the greater acceptance of obesity among certain ethnic groups, as well as different cultural values related to food choices.

### Term

**resting metabolic rate (RMR)** The energy required to maintain vital body functions, including respiration, heart rate, body temperature, and blood pressure, while the body is at rest.

Vw

In some families and cultures, food is used as a symbol of love and caring. It is an integral part of social gatherings and celebrations. In such cases, it may be difficult to change established eating patterns because they are linked to cultural and family values.

## ADOPTING A HEALTHY LIFESTYLE FOR SUCCESSFUL WEIGHT MANAGEMENT

Permanent weight loss is not something you start and stop. You need to adopt healthy behaviors that you can maintain throughout your life.

### Diet and Eating Habits

In contrast to "dieting," which involves some form of food restriction, "diet" refers to your daily food choices. Everyone has a diet, but not everyone is dieting. You need to develop a diet that you enjoy and that enables you to maintain a healthy body composition. Use MyPyramid as the basis for planning a healthy diet (see Chapter 9). For weight management, you may need to pay special attention to total calories, portion sizes, energy density, fat and carbohydrate intake, and eating habits.

**Total Calories** As described in Chapter 9, MyPyramid suggests approximate daily energy intakes based on gender, age, and activity level (see Table 9-3). However, energy balance may be a more important consideration for weight management than total calories consumed (see Figure 11-2). To maintain your current weight, the total number of calories you eat must equal the number you burn. To lose weight, you must decrease your calorie intake and/or increase the number of calories you burn; to gain weight, the reverse is true. (One pound of body fat represents 3500 calories.)

The best approach for weight loss is combining an increase in physical activity with moderate calorie restriction. Don't go on a "crash diet." To maintain weight loss, you will probably have to maintain some degree of the calorie restriction you used to lose the weight. Therefore, you need to adopt a level of food intake that provides all the essential nutrients that you can live with over the long term. For most people, maintaining weight loss is more difficult than losing the weight in the first place.

**Portion Sizes** Overconsumption of total calories is closely tied to portion sizes. Most of us significantly underestimate the amount of food we eat. Limiting portion sizes is critical for maintaining good health. To counteract portion distortion, weigh and measure your food at home for a few days every now and then. In addition, check the serving sizes listed on packaged foods. When eating out, try to order the smallest-sized items on the menu. When a "small" isn't small enough, take half home or share it with a friend. It is especially important to limit serving sizes of foods that are high in calories and low in nutrients. Don't "supersize" your meals and snacks; although huge servings may seem like the best deal, it is more important to order just what you need.

**Energy (Calorie) Density** To cut back on calories and still feel full, then, you should favor foods with a low energy density—that is, those that are relatively heavy but have few calories. For example, for the same 100 calories, you could consume 21 baby carrots or 4 pretzel twists; you are more likely to feel full after eating the serving of carrots because it weighs 10 times that of the serving of pretzels (10 ounces versus 1 ounce). Fresh fruits and vegetables, with their high water and fiber content, are low in energy density, as are whole-grain foods. Meat, ice cream, potato chips, croissants, crackers, and low-fat cakes and cookies are examples of foods high in energy density. Strategies for lowering the energy density of your diet include the following:

- Eat fruit with breakfast and for dessert.
- Add extra vegetables to sandwiches, casseroles, stir-fry dishes, pizza, pasta dishes, and fajitas.
- Start meals with a bowl of broth-based soup; include a green salad or fruit salad.
- Snack on fresh fruits and vegetables rather than crackers, chips, or other energy-dense snack foods.
- Limit serving sizes of energy-dense foods such as butter, mayonnaise, cheese, chocolate, fatty meats, croissants, and snack foods that are fried or high in added sugars (including reduced-fat products).

**Fat Calories** Although some fat is needed in the diet to provide essential nutrients, you should avoid overeating fatty foods. Fat calories may be more easily converted to body fat than calories from protein or carbohydrate. Limiting fat in the diet can also help you limit your total calories. As described in Chapter 9, fat should supply no more than 35% of your average total daily calories, which translates into no more than 78 grams of fat in a 2000-calorie diet each day. Most of the fat in your diet should be in the form of unsaturated fats from plant and fish sources. Saturated and trans fats should be limited for weight control and disease prevention; foods high in unhealthy fats include full-fat dairy products, fatty meats, stick margarine, deep-fried foods, and other processed and fast foods.

Moving toward a diet strong in complex carbohydrates and fresh fruits and vegetables, and away from a reliance on meat and processed foods, is an effective approach to reducing fat consumption. Watch out for processed foods labeled "fat-free" or "reduced fat," as they may be high in calories (see the box "Evaluating Fat and Sugar Substitutes"). A low-fat diet that is high in calories will not lead to weight loss.

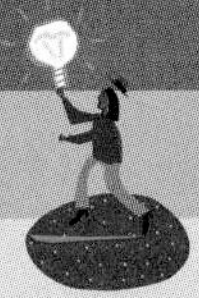

Critical Consumer

## Evaluating Fat and Sugar Substitutes

VW

For successful weight management, some people find it helpful to limit their intake of foods high in fat and simple sugars. Foods made with fat and sugar substitutes are often promoted for weight loss. However, whether fat and sugar substitutes help you achieve and maintain a healthy weight depends on your lifestyle—your overall eating and activity habits. When evaluating foods with fat and sugar substitutes, consider these issues:

- *Is the food lower in calories or just lower in fat?* Reduced-fat foods often contain extra sugar to improve the taste and texture lost when fat is removed, so such foods may be as high or even higher in total calories than their fattier counterparts. Limiting fat intake is an important goal for weight management, but so is controlling total calories.
- *Are you choosing foods with fat and/or sugar substitutes instead of foods you typically eat or in addition to foods you typically eat?* If you consume low-fat, no-sugar-added ice cream instead of regular ice cream, you may save calories. But if you add such ice cream to your daily diet simply because it is lower in fat and sugar, your overall calorie consumption—and your weight—may increase.
- *How many foods containing fat and sugar substitutes do you consume each day?* Although the FDA has given at least provisional approval to all the fat and sugar substitutes currently available, health concerns about some of these products linger. For example, the fat substitute Olestra, marketed under the trade name Olean, reduces the absorption of fat-soluble nutrients and certain antioxidants and causes gastrointestinal distress in some people. Sugar alcohols such as mannitol and sorbitol, used in sugar-free candies and some products marketed as low-carbohydrate foods, are digested in a way that can create gas, cramps, and diarrhea if they are consumed in large amounts—more than about 10 grams in one meal. One way to limit any potential adverse effects is to read labels and monitor how much of each product you consume.
- *Is an even healthier choice available?* Many of the foods containing fat and sugar substitutes are low-nutrient snack foods. Although substituting a lower-fat or lower-sugar version of the same food may be beneficial, fruits, vegetables, and whole grains are healthier snack choices.

**Carbohydrate** Americans currently consume most of their carbohydrate calories in the form of foods high in refined carbohydrates and added sugars—soft drinks and heavily sweetened fruit drinks, white rice, white potatoes, and breads, cereals, and snack foods made with refined grains. Such foods are typically high in calories and low in other essential nutrients; they also often cause dramatic swings in blood glucose and insulin levels and have been implicated in the development of type 2 diabetes and heart disease.

Foods high in whole grains and fiber are typically lower in calorie density, saturated fat, and added sugars and may promote feelings of satiety (fullness)—all characteristic features of a dietary pattern for successful weight management. They also help maintain normal blood glucose and insulin levels and reduce the risk of heart disease. For weight management and overall health, choose a diet with 45–65% of total daily calories as carbohydrate. Favor complex carbohydrates from whole grains, vegetables, and fruits; avoid high-fat toppings, added sugars (especially sugary soft drinks, fruit drinks, and desserts), and refined carbohydrates.

**Protein** The typical American consumes more than an adequate amount of protein. Foods high in protein are often also high in fat. Stick to the recommended protein intake of 10–35% of total daily calories. High-protein diets promoted for weight loss are discussed later in the chapter.

**Eating Habits** Equally important to weight management is eating small, frequent meals—three or more a day plus snacks—on a dependable, regular schedule. Skipping meals or banning certain foods leads to excessive hunger, feelings of deprivation, and increased vulnerability to binge eating or snacking on high-calorie, high-fat, or sugary foods. A regular pattern of eating, along with some personal "decision rules" governing food choices, is a way of thinking about and then internalizing the many details that go into a healthy, low-fat diet. Decision rules for breakfast might be these, for example: Choose a sugar-free, high-fiber cereal with fat-free milk on most days; once in a while (no more than once a week), have a hard-boiled egg; save pancakes and waffles for special occasions. Making the healthier choice more often than not is the essence of moderation.

## Physical Activity and Exercise

Physical activity and exercise burn calories and keep the metabolism geared to using food for energy instead of storing it as fat. Making significant cuts in food intake in order to lose weight is a difficult strategy to maintain; increasing your physical activity is a much better approach. The first step in becoming more active is to incorporate more physical activity into your daily life. Accumulate 30 minutes or more of moderate-intensity physical activity—walking, gardening, housework, and so on—on most, or preferably all, days of the week. In the long term, even a small increase in activity level can help maintain your current weight or help you lose a modest amount of weight. In fact, research suggests that fidgeting—stretching, squirming, standing up, and so on—may help prevent weight gain in some people.

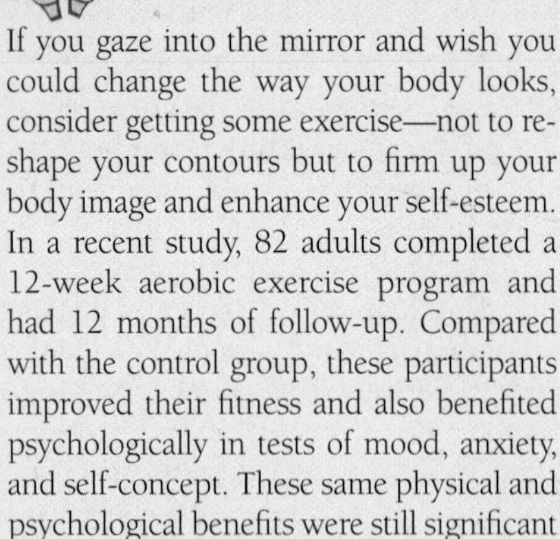


### Exercise, Body Image, and Self-Esteem

If you gaze into the mirror and wish you could change the way your body looks, consider getting some exercise—not to reshape your contours but to firm up your body image and enhance your self-esteem. In a recent study, 82 adults completed a 12-week aerobic exercise program and had 12 months of follow-up. Compared with the control group, these participants improved their fitness and also benefited psychologically in tests of mood, anxiety, and self-concept. These same physical and psychological benefits were still significant at the 1-year follow-up.

One reason for the findings may be that people who exercise regularly often gain a sense of mastery and competence that enhances their self-esteem and body image. In addition, exercise contributes to a more toned look, which many adults prefer. Research suggests that physically active people are more comfortable with their bodies and their image than sedentary people are. In one workplace study, 60 employees were asked to complete a 36-session stretching program whose main purpose was to prevent muscle strains at work. At the end of the program, besides the significant increase by all participants in measurements of flexibility, their perceptions of their bodies improved and so did their overall sense of self-worth.

Similar results were obtained in a Norwegian study, in which 219 middle-aged people at risk for heart disease were randomly assigned to one of four groups: diet, diet plus exercise, exercise, and no intervention. The greater the participation of individuals in the exercise component of the program, the higher were their scores in perceived competence/self-esteem and coping.

SOURCES: DiLorenzo, T. M., et al. 1999. Long-term effects of aerobic exercise on psychological outcomes. *Preventive Medicine* 28(1): 75–85; Sorensen, M., et al. 1999. The effect of exercise and diet on mental health and quality of life in middle-aged individuals with elevated risk factors for cardiovascular disease. *Journal of Sports Science* 17(5): 369–377; Moore, T. M. 1998. A workplace stretching program. *AAOHN Journal* 46(12): 563–568.

If you are overweight or obese and want to lose weight and keep it off, a greater amount of physical activity is necessary. People who lose weight and don't regain it typically burn at least 2800 calories per week in physical activity—the equivalent of about 1 hour of brisk walking per day. The 2005 Dietary Guidelines for Americans recommend at least 60 minutes of daily physical activity to avoid slow weight gain in adulthood, and at least 60–90 minutes of activity to lose weight or to prevent weight regain after losing weight.

Once you become more active every day, consider beginning a formal exercise program like that described in Chapter 10: cardiorespiratory endurance exercise, resistance training, and stretching exercises. The message about exercise is that regular exercise, maintained throughout life, makes weight management easier and improves quality of life (see the box "Exercise, Body Image, and Self-Esteem").

## Thinking and Emotions

The way you think about yourself and your world influences and is influenced by how you feel and how you act. Certain kinds of thinking produce negative emotions, which can undermine a healthy lifestyle. Research on people who have a weight problem indicates that low self-esteem and the negative emotions that accompany it are significant problems. This often results in part from mentally comparing the actual self to an internally held picture of the "ideal self." The greater the discrepancy, the larger the impact on self-esteem and the more likely the presence of negative emotions.

Often our internalized "ideal self" is the result of having adopted perfectionistic goals and beliefs about how we and others "should" be. Examples of such beliefs are "If I don't do things perfectly, I'm a failure" and "It's terrible if I'm not thin." These irrational beliefs may cause stress and emotional pain. The remedy is to challenge such beliefs and replace them with more realistic ones (see the discussion of self-talk in Chapter 3). A healthy lifestyle is supported by having realistic beliefs and goals and by engaging in positive self-talk and problem-solving efforts.

## Coping Strategies

Adequate and appropriate coping strategies for dealing with the stresses and challenges of life are another lifestyle factor in weight management. One strategy that some people adopt for coping is eating. Food may be used to alleviate loneliness or as a pickup for fatigue. Eating provides distraction from difficult problems and is a means of punishing the self or others for real or imagined transgressions.

People with a healthy lifestyle have more effective ways to get their needs met. Having learned to communicate assertively and to manage interpersonal conflict effectively, they don't shrink from problems or overreact. The person with a healthy lifestyle knows how to create and maintain relationships with others and has a solid network of friends and loved ones. Food is used appropriately—to fuel life's activities and gain personal satisfaction, not to manage stress.

Obtaining adequate amounts of sleep is important for stress management and may be a key component of successful weight management. A recent study found a link between sleep and body mass index: People with a healthy BMI slept more than people who were overweight and obese. The cause-and-effect relationship is not yet clear, but it is possible that insufficient sleep may affect hormones, metabolism, and appetite.

## APPROACHES TO OVERCOMING A WEIGHT PROBLEM

What should you do if you are overweight? Several options are available to you.

### Doing It Yourself

If you need to lose weight, focus on adopting the healthy lifestyle described throughout this book. The "right" weight for you will naturally evolve. Combine modest cuts in energy intake with exercise, and avoid very-low-calorie diets. By producing a negative energy balance of 250–1000 calories per day, you will produce the recommended weight loss of 0.5–2.0 pounds per week. Realize that most low-calorie diets cause a rapid loss of body water at first. When this phase passes, weight loss declines. But the smaller losses later in the diet are actually better than the initial big losses, because later loss is mostly fat loss, whereas initial loss is primarily fluid. Reasonable weight loss is 8–10% of body weight over 6 months. A registered dietitian or nutritionist can recommend an appropriate plan for you when you want to lose weight on your own. For more tips, refer to the box "Strategies for Successful Weight Management" and to the Behavior Change Strategy at the end of the chapter.

### Diet Books

Many people who try to lose weight by themselves fall prey to one or more of the dozens of diet books on the market. Although some contain useful advice and tips for motivation, most make empty promises. Some guidelines for evaluating and choosing a diet book follow:

- Reject books that advocate an unbalanced way of eating. These include books advocating a high-carbohydrate-only diet or those advocating low-carbohydrate, high-protein diets. Also reject books promoting a single food.
- Reject books that claim to be based on a "scientific breakthrough" or to have the "secret" to success.
- Reject books that use gimmicks, such as matching eating to blood type, hyping insulin resistance as the single cause of obesity, combining foods in special ways to achieve weight loss, rotating levels of calories, or purporting that a weight problem is due to food allergies, food sensitivities, yeast infections, or hormone imbalances.
- Reject books that promise quick weight loss or that limit the selection of foods.
- Accept books that advocate a balanced approach to diet plus exercise and sound nutrition advice.

Many "diets" can cause weight loss if maintained; the real difficulty is finding a safe and healthy pattern of food choices and physical activity that results in long-term maintenance of a healthy body weight and reduced risk of chronic disease (see the box "Is Any Diet Best for Weight Loss" on p. 267). Check the Online Learning Center for worksheets that can help you evaluate diet books and programs.

### Dietary Supplements and Diet Aids

Promoted in advertisements, magazines, direct mail campaigns, infomercials, and Web sites, diet supplements and aids typically promise a quick and easy path to weight loss. Most of these products are marketed as dietary supplements and so are subject to fewer regulations than OTC medications. A 2002 report from the Federal Trade Commission stated that more than half of advertisements for weight-loss products made representations that are very likely to be false. In addition, use of OTC products doesn't help in the adoption of lifestyle behaviors that can help people achieve and maintain a healthy weight over the long term.

The bottom line on nonprescription diet aids is caveat emptor—let the buyer beware. There is no quick and easy way to lose weight. The most effective approach is to develop healthy diet and exercise habits and make them a permanent part of your lifestyle. Some of the most commonly marketed OTC products for weight loss are described below.

**Formula Drinks and Food Bars** Canned diet drinks, powders used to make shakes, and diet food bars and snacks are designed to achieve weight loss by substituting for some or all of a person's daily food intake. However, most people find it difficult to use these products for long periods, and muscle loss and other serious health problems may result if they are used as the sole source of nutrition for an extended period. Use of such products sometimes results in rapid short-term weight loss, but the weight is typically regained because users don't learn to change the eating and lifestyle behaviors that caused the weight problem in the first place.

**Herbs and Herbal Products** As described in Chapter 9, herbs are marketed as dietary supplements, so there is little information about effectiveness, proper dosage, drug interactions, and side effects. In addition, labels may not accurately reflect the ingredients and dosages present, and safe manufacturing practices are not guaranteed. For example, the substitution of a toxic herb for another compound during the manufacture of a Chinese herbal weight-loss preparation caused more than 100 cases of kidney damage and cancer among users in Europe.

In 2004, the FDA banned the sale of ephedra (*ma huang*), stating that it presented a significant and unreasonable risk to human health. Ephedrine, the active ingredient in ephedra, is structurally similar to amphetamine and was widely used in weight-loss supplements. It may suppress appetite, but adverse effects have included elevated blood pressure, panic attacks, seizures, insomnia, and increased risk of heart attack or stroke, particularly in high doses or

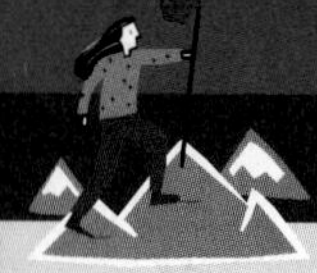

Take Charge

## Strategies for Successful Weight Management

### Food Choices

- Follow the recommendations in MyPyramid for eating a moderate, varied diet.
- Check food labels for serving sizes, calories, and nutrient levels. Favor foods with a low energy density and a high nutrient density.
- Watch for hidden calories. Reduced-fat foods often have as many calories as their full-fat versions. Condiments like butter, margarine, mayonnaise, and salad dressings provide about 100 calories per tablespoon; added sugars such as jams, jellies, and syrup are also packed with calories.
- Drink fewer calories. Many Americans consume high-calorie beverages such as soda, fruit drinks, sports drinks, alcohol, and specialty coffees and teas.
- For problem foods, try eating small amounts under controlled conditions. Go out for a scoop of ice cream, for example, rather than buying a half gallon for your freezer.

### Planning and Serving

- Keep a log of what you eat. Before you begin your program, your log will provide a realistic picture of your current diet. Once you start your program, a log will keep you focused on your food choices and portion sizes.
- Eat three meals a day, including breakfast. Replace impulse snacking with planned, healthy snacks. Keep low-calorie snacks on hand to combat the "munchies": baby carrots, popcorn, and fresh fruits and vegetables are good choices.
- When shopping, make a list and stick to it. Don't shop when you're hungry. Avoid aisles that contain problem foods.
- Use measuring cups and spoons and a food scale to become more familiar with appropriate portion sizes.
- Serve meals on small plates and in small bowls to help you eat smaller portions without feeling deprived.
- Eat only in specifically designated spots. Remove food from other areas of your house or apartment.
- When you eat, just eat—don't do anything else, such as read or watch TV.
- Eat more slowly. Take small bites and chew food thoroughly. Pay attention to every bite, and enjoy your food. Between bites, try putting down your fork or spoon and taking sips of water or another beverage.
- When you're done eating, remove your plate. Cue yourself that the meal is over—drink a glass of water, suck on a mint, chew gum, or brush your teeth.

### Special Occasions

- When you eat out, choose a restaurant where you can make healthy food choices. Ask the server not to put bread and butter on the table before the meal, and request that sauces and salad dressings be served on the side. If portion sizes are large, take half your food home for a meal later in the week.
- If you cook a large meal for friends, send leftovers home with your guests.
- If you're eating at a friend's, eat a little and leave the rest. Don't eat to be polite; if someone offers you food you don't want, thank the person and decline firmly: "No thank you, I've had enough" or "It's delicious, but I'm full."
- Take care during the winter holidays. Research indicates that people gain less than they think during the winter holidays (about a pound) but that the weight isn't lost during the rest of the year, leading to slow, steady weight gain.

### Physical Activity and Stress Management

- Increase your level of daily physical activity. Then begin a formal exercise program that includes cardiorespiratory endurance exercise, strength training, and stretching.
- Develop techniques for handling stress—go for a walk or use a relaxation technique. Practice positive self-talk.
- Develop strategies for coping with non-hunger cues to eat, such as boredom, sleepiness, or anxiety. Try calling a friend, taking a shower, or reading a magazine. Get adequate sleep.
- Tell family members and friends that you're making lifestyle changes, and ask them to be supportive.

For additional tips, visit the Department of Health and Human Services Small Steps Web site (www.smallstep.gov).

when combined with another stimulant, such as caffeine. The synthetic stimulant phenylpropanolamine was banned in 2000 for similar reasons. Other herbal stimulants include bitter orange extract, yerba mate (tea), guarana, and damiana.

So-called dieter's teas are made from botanical stimulant laxatives such as aloe, buckthorn, or senna. In excess amounts, these can cause diarrhea, vomiting, and potentially dangerous electrolyte imbalances.

**Other Supplements and Diet Aids** Fiber is another common ingredient in OTC diet aids, promoted for appetite control. However, dietary fiber acts as a bulking agent in the large intestine, not the stomach, so it doesn't have a pronounced effect on appetite. In addition, many diet aids contain only 3 or fewer grams of fiber, which does not contribute much toward the recommended daily intake of 25–38 grams. Other compounds marketed as diet aids include conjugated linoleic acid, carnitine, chromium, pyruvate, and a number of products labeled "fat absorbers," "fat blockers," and "starch blockers." Research has not found these products to be effective, and many have potentially adverse side effects.

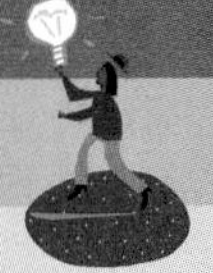



## Is Any Diet Best for Weight Loss?



Experts agree that reducing energy (calorie) intake promotes weight loss. However, many popular commercial and published weight-loss plans include special "hooks" and promote specific food choices and macronutrient (protein, fat, carbohydrate) combinations as best for weight loss. Research findings have been mixed, but two points are clear: Total calorie intake matters, and the best diet is probably the one that an individual can stick with.

### Low-Carbohydrate Diets

Recent popular diet books have advocated a diet very low in carbohydrate—with fewer than 10% of total calories from carbohydrate, compared with the 45–65% recommended by the Food and Nutrition Board. Some suggest daily carbohydrate intake below the 130 grams needed to provide essential carbohydrate in the diet. Small studies have found that low-carbohydrate diets can help with weight loss and be safe for relatively short periods of time—although unpleasant effects such as bad breath, constipation, and headache are fairly common.

Although low-carb diets are reasonably safe in the short term, there are concerns about their long-term effects because they tend to be very high in saturated fat and protein and low in fiber, whole grains, vegetables, fruits, and some vitamins, minerals, and phytochemicals. Over the long term, this dietary pattern has been linked to increased risk of heart disease, high blood pressure, and cancer. Diets very high in protein can also stress the kidneys.

### Low-Fat Diets

Many experts advocate diets that are relatively low in fat, high in carbohydrate, and moderate in protein. Critics of these diets blame them for rising rates of obesity and note that very-low-fat, very-high-carbohydrate diets can increase triglyceride levels and lower levels of good (HDL) cholesterol in some people. However, these negative effects can be counteracted with moderate-intensity exercise, and low-fat diets combined with physical activity can be safe and effective for many people.

Few experts take the position that low-fat, high-carbohydrate diets alone, separate from overall diet and activity patterns, are responsible for the increase in obesity among Americans. However, the debate has highlighted the importance of total calorie intake and the quality of carbohydrate choices. Most Americans consume large amounts of refined carbohydrates and added sugars from energy-dense, nutrient-poor foods; they do not consume the recommended whole grains, vegetables, and fruits. A low-fat diet is not a license to consume excess calories, even in the form of low-fat foods.

### How Do Popular Diets Measure Up?

In one recent study, obese people on a very-low-carbohydrate, high-fat diet lost more weight over a 6-month period than people following a moderate-fat diet. However, after a year, the difference in weight loss between the two groups was no longer significant, and the dropout rate from both groups was high.

A 2005 study followed participants in four popular diets that emphasize different strategies—Weight Watchers (restricted portion sizes and calories), Atkins (low-carbohydrate, high-fat), Zone (relatively high protein, moderate fat and carbohydrate), and Ornish (very low fat). Each of these diets modestly reduced body weight and heart disease risk factors. There was no significant difference in weight loss at 1 year among the diets, and the more closely people adhered to each diet, the more weight they lost. The dropout rates were very high—about 50% for Atkins and Ornish and about 35% for Weight Watchers and Zone. The message from this study? Finding a dietary approach that you can stick to is key to long-term success.

### Energy Balance Counts: The National Weight Control Registry

Future research may determine that certain macronutrient patterns may be somewhat more helpful for disease reduction in people with particular risk profiles. However, in terms of weight loss, such differences among diets are likely overshadowed by the importance of total calorie intake and physical activity. Important lessons about energy balance can be drawn from the National Weight Control Registry, an ongoing study of people who have lost significant amounts of weight and kept it off. The average participant in the registry has lost 71 pounds and kept the weight off for more than 5 years. Nearly all participants use a combination of diet and exercise to manage their weight. Most consumed diets moderate in calories and relatively low in fat and fried foods; they monitor their body weight and their food intake frequently. Participants engage in an average of 60 minutes of moderate physical activity daily. The National Weight Control Registry study illustrates that to lose weight and keep it off, you must decrease daily calorie intake and/or increase daily physical activity—and continue to do so over your lifetime.

### A Balanced Approach

For short-term weight loss, many types of diets can be safe and successful. However, long-term maintenance of healthy body weight and reduction of chronic disease risk requires permanent changes in lifestyle. Diets advocating strict limits on any nutrient or food group may be impractical and difficult to maintain over the long term. The latest USDA guidelines provide a good model for healthy food and activity choices. Basic guidelines for weight loss and risk reduction advocated by many experts include the following:

- Set reasonable goals; even small amounts of weight loss benefit health.
- Reduce your intake of saturated and trans fats, refined carbohydrates, and added sugars. Favor unsaturated fats, lean protein sources, whole grains, vegetables, and fruits. Select nutrient-dense choices within each food group.
- Incorporate 60 or more minutes of physical activity into your daily routine; begin a formal exercise program for even greater health and fitness benefits.
- Choose a healthy dietary pattern that works for you over the long term.

SOURCES: Dansinger, M. L., et al. 2005. Comparison of the Atkins, Ornish, Weight Watchers, and Zone diets for weight loss and heart disease risk reduction. *Journal of the American Medical Association* 293(1): 43–53; Hays, N. P., et al. 2004. Effects of an ad libitum low-fat, high-carbohydrate diet on body weight, body composition, and fat distribution in older men and women. *Archives of Internal Medicine* 164(2): 210–217; Hill, J., and R. Wing. 2003. The National Weight Control Registry. *The Permanente Journal* 7(3): 34–37; Bravata, D. M., et al. 2003. Efficacy and safety of low-carbohydrate diets. *Journal of the American Medical Association* 289: 1837–1850; Foster, G. D., et al. 2003. A randomized trial of low-carbohydrate diet for obesity. *New England Journal of Medicine* 348: 2082–2090; Samaha, F. F., et al. 2003. A low-carbohydrate as compared with a low-fat diet in severe obesity. *New England Journal of Medicine* 348: 2074–2081.

## Weight-Loss Programs

Weight-loss programs come in a variety of types, including noncommercial support organizations, commercial programs, Web sites, and clinical programs.

**Noncommercial Weight-Loss Programs** Noncommercial programs such as TOPS (Take Off Pounds Sensibly) and Overeaters Anonymous (OA) mainly provide group support. They do not advocate any particular diet but do recommend seeking professional advice for creating an individualized plan. These types of programs are generally free. Your physician or a registered dietitian can also provide information and support for weight loss.

**Commercial Weight-Loss Program** Commercial programs such as Weight Watchers, Jenny Craig, Diet Workshop, and Richard Simmons Slimmons typically provide group support, nutrition education, physical activity recommendations, and behavior modification advice for changing habits. Some also make available packaged foods to assist in following dietary advice. Many programs voluntarily belong to the Partnership for Healthy Weight Management established by the Federal Trade Commission in 1999. By doing so, they agree to provide clients with information on staff training and education, the risks associated with each program or product, the costs of the program, and the expected outcomes of the program, including rates of success. A responsible and safe weight-loss program should have the following features:

1. The recommended diet should be safe and balanced, include all the food groups, and meet the DRIs for all nutrients. Physical activity and exercise should be strongly encouraged.
2. The program should promote slow, steady weight loss averaging 0.5–2.0 pounds per week.
3. If a participant plans to lose more than 20 pounds, has any health problems, or is taking medication on a regular basis, physician evaluation and monitoring should be recommended. The staff of the program should include qualified counselors and health professionals.
4. The program should include plans for weight maintenance after the weight-loss phase is over.
5. The program should provide information on all fees and costs, including those of supplements and prepackaged foods, as well as data on risks and expected outcomes of participating in the program.

A plan for maintenance is especially important because only 10–15% of program participants maintain their weight loss—the rest gain back all or more than they have lost. One study of participants found that regular exercise was the best predictor of maintaining weight loss, whereas frequent television viewing was the best predictor of weight gain. Successful weight management requires long-term lifestyle changes.

**Online Weight-Loss Programs** A recent addition to the weight-loss program scene is the Internet-based program. Most such Web sites include a cross between self-help and group support through chat rooms, bulletin boards, and e-newsletters. Many sites offer online self-assessment for diet and physical activity habits as well as a meal plan; some provide access to a staff professional for individualized help. Many are free, but some charge a weekly or monthly fee. Research suggests that this type of program provides an alternative to in-person diet counseling and can lead to weight loss for some people. Weekly online contact in terms of behavior therapy proved most successful for weight loss. The criteria used to evaluate commercial programs can also be applied to Internet-based programs. In addition, check whether a program offers member-to-member support and access to staff professionals.

**Clinical Weight-Loss Programs** Medically supervised clinical programs are usually located in a hospital or other medical setting. Designed to help those who are severely obese, these programs typically involve a closely monitored very-low-calorie diet. The cost of a clinical program is usually high, but insurance will often cover part of the fee.

## Prescription Drugs

For a medicine to cause weight loss, it must reduce energy consumption, increase energy expenditure, and/or interfere with energy absorption. The medications most often prescribed for weight loss are appetite suppressants that reduce feelings of hunger or increase feelings of fullness. Most are approved by the FDA only for short-term use. Two drugs, however, are approved for longer-term use: sibutramine (Meridia) and orlistat (Xenical). Sibutramine is an appetite suppressant; its safety and efficacy record is good, but regular monitoring of blood pressure is required during therapy. Orlistat lowers calorie consumption by blocking fat absorption in the intestines; it prevents about 30% of the fat in food from being digested. Similar to the fat substitute olestra, orlistat reduces the absorption of fatsoluble vitamins and antioxidants. Side effects include diarrhea, cramping, and other gastrointestinal problems if users do not follow a low-fat diet.

Studies have generally found that appetite suppressants produce modest weight loss—about 5–22 pounds above the loss expected with nondrug obesity treatments. Individuals respond very differently, however, and some experience more weight loss than others. Unfortunately, weight loss tends to level off or reverse after 4–6 months on a medication, and many people regain the weight they've lost if they stop taking the drugs.

Side effects and risks are other concerns. In 1997, the FDA removed from the market two prescription weight-loss drugs, fenfluramine (Pondimin) and dexfenfluramine (Redux), after their use was linked to potentially life-threatening heart valve problems. It appears that people who took these drugs over a long period or at high dosages are at greatest risk for problems, but the FDA recommends that anyone who has taken either of these drugs be examined by a physician.

Prescription weight-loss drugs are not for people who want to lose a few pounds to wear a smaller size of jeans. The latest federal guidelines advise people to try lifestyle modification for at least 6 months before trying drug therapy. Prescription drugs are recommended—in conjunction with lifestyle changes—only in certain cases: for people who have been unable to lose weight with non-drug options and who have a BMI over 30 (or over 27 if two or more additional risk factors such as diabetes and high blood pressure are present).

### Surgery

About 3–5% of Americans are severely obese, meaning they have a BMI of 40 or higher or are 100 pounds or more over recommended weight. For such people, obesity is a serious medical condition that is often complicated by other health problems such as diabetes, sleep disorders, heart disease, and arthritis. Surgical intervention may be necessary as a treatment of last resort for those who have not been successful in permanently reducing weight through other methods. According to a National Institutes of Health (NIH) Consensus Conference, gastric bypass surgery is recommended for patients with a BMI greater than 40, or greater than 35 with obesity-related illnesses. Gastric bypass surgery modifies the gastrointestinal tract by changing either the size of the stomach or how the intestine drains, thereby reducing food intake.

Obesity-related health conditions, as well as risk of premature death, generally improve after surgical weight loss. However, surgery is not without risks and is not always successful.

## BODY IMAGE

As described earlier in the chapter, body image consists of perceptions, images, thoughts, attitudes, and emotions. Developing a positive body image is an important aspect of psychological wellness and an important component of successful weight management. See the box "Gender, Ethnicity, and Body Image" on page 270 for suggestions for developing a healthy body image.

### Severe Body Image Problems

Poor body image can cause significant psychological distress. A person can become preoccupied by a perceived defect in appearance, thereby damaging self-esteem and interfering with relationships. Adolescents and adults who have a negative body image are more likely to diet restrictively, eat compulsively, or develop some other form of disordered eating.

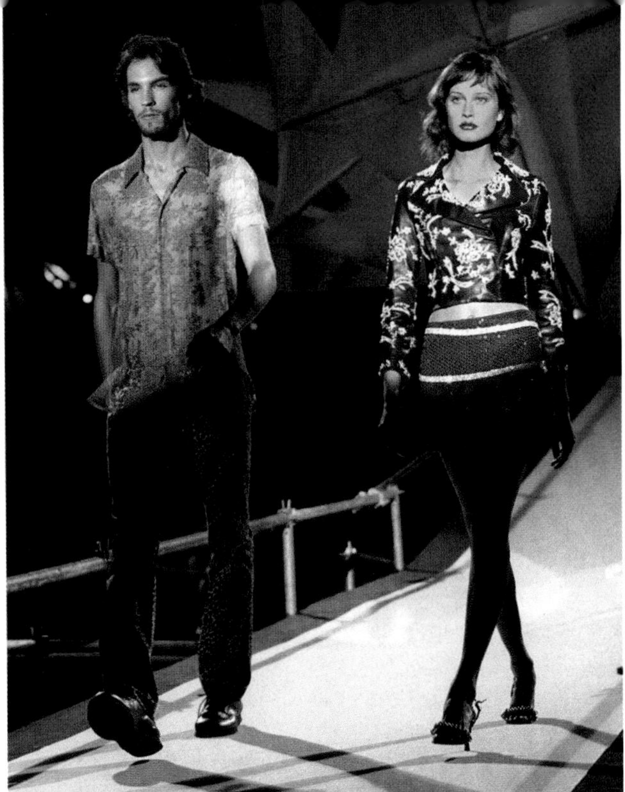

The image of the "ideal" body promoted by the fashion and fitness industries doesn't reflect the wide range of body shapes and sizes that are associated with good health. An overconcern with body image can contribute to low self-esteem and the development of eating disorders.

When dissatisfaction becomes extreme, the condition is called *body dysmorphic disorder* (BDD). BDD affects about 2% of Americans, males and females in equal numbers; BDD usually begins before age 18 but can begin in adulthood. Sufferers are overly concerned with physical appearance, often focusing on slight "flaws" of the face or head—things that are not obvious to others. Low self-esteem is common. Individuals with BDD may spend hours every day thinking about their defect and looking at themselves in mirrors; they may desire and seek repeated cosmetic surgeries. BDD is related to obsessive-compulsive disorder and can lead to depression, social phobia, and suicide if left untreated. An individual with BDD needs to get professional evaluation and treatment; medication and therapy can help people with BDD.

In some cases, body image may bear little resemblance to fact. A person suffering from the eating disorder anorexia nervosa typically has a severely distorted body image—she believes herself to be fat even when she has become emaciated. Distorted body image is also a hallmark of *muscle dysmorphia,* a disorder experienced by some bodybuilders and other active people in which they

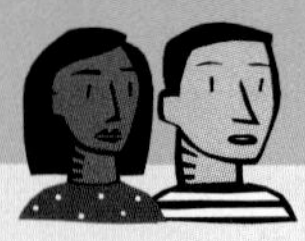

Gender Matters

## Gender, Ethnicity, and Body Image

### Body Image and Gender

Women are much more likely than men to be dissatisfied with their bodies, often wanting to be thinner than they are. In one study, only 30% of eighth-grade girls reported being content with their bodies, while 70% of their male classmates expressed satisfaction with their looks.

One reason that girls and women are dissatisfied with their bodies is that they are influenced by the media—particularly advertisements and women's fashion magazines. Most teen girls report that the media influence their idea of the perfect body and their decision to diet. In a study of adult women, viewing pictures of thin models in magazines had an immediate negative effect on their mood. Clearly, media images affect women's self-image and self-esteem. For American women of all ages, success is still too often equated with how we look rather than who we are.

It is important to note that the image of the "perfect" woman presented in the media is often unrealistic and even unhealthy. In a review of BMI data for Miss America pageant winners since 1922, researchers noted a significant decline in BMI over time, with an increasing number of recent winners having BMIs in the "underweight" category. The average fashion model is 4–7 inches taller and more than 25 pounds lighter than the average American woman.

Our culture may be promoting an unattainable masculine ideal as well. Researchers surveying male undergraduates found that media consumption was positively associated with a desire for thinness. Researchers studying male action figures such as GI Joe from the past 40 years noted that they have become increasingly muscular. A recent Batman action figure, if projected onto a man of average height, would result in someone with a 30-inch waist, 57-inch chest, and 27-inch biceps.

### Body Image and Ethnicity

Although some groups espouse thinness as an "ideal" body type, others do not. In many traditional African societies, for example, full-figured women's bodies are seen as symbols of health, prosperity, and fertility. African American teenage girls have a much more positive body image than do white girls; in one survey, two-thirds of them defined beauty as "the right attitude," whereas white girls were more preoccupied with weight and body shape.

A study of college students found that white and Latina students tend to have more body image problems than African American and Asian American students; black students had the most positive general body image among the groups of students in the study. Nevertheless, recent evidence indicates that African American women are as likely to engage in disordered eating behavior, especially binge eating and vomiting, as their Latina, American Indian, and white counterparts. These findings underscore the complex nature of eating disorders and body image.

### Avoiding Body Image Problems

To minimize your risk of developing a body image problem, keep the following strategies in mind:

- Focus on healthy habits and good physical health. Eat a moderate, balanced diet, and choose physical activities you enjoy. Avoid chronic or repetitive dieting.
- Focus on good psychological health and put concerns about physical appearance in perspective. Your worth as a human being is not dependent on how you look.
- Practice body acceptance. You can influence your body size and type to some degree through lifestyle, but the basic fact is that some people are genetically designed to be bigger or heavier than others. Focus on healthy lifestyle behaviors and accept your body as it is.
- Find things to appreciate in yourself besides an idealized body image. Men and women whose self-esteem is based primarily on standards of physical attractiveness can find it difficult to age gracefully. Those who can learn to value other aspects of themselves are more accepting of the physical changes that occur naturally with age.
- View food choices as morally neutral—eating dessert isn't "bad" and doesn't make you a bad person. Healthy eating habits are an important part of a wellness lifestyle, but the things you really care about and do are more important in defining who you are.
- Don't judge yourself or others based on appearance. Watch your attitudes toward people of differing body sizes and shapes, and don't joke about someone's body type. Take people seriously for what they say and do, not for their appearance. Body size is just one external characteristic; millions of happy and successful people also just happen to have a weight problem.
- See the beauty and fitness industries for what they are. Realize that one of their goals is to prompt dissatisfaction with yourself so that you will buy their products.

see themselves as small and out of shape despite being very muscular. Those who suffer from muscle dysmorphia may let obsessive bodybuilding interfere with their work and relationships. They may also use steroids and other potentially dangerous muscle-building drugs.

## Acceptance and Change

Most Americans, young and old, are unhappy with some aspect of their appearance and often their weight. The "can-do" attitude of Americans, together with the belief that there is a solution to this dissatisfaction, leads to even more problems with body image, as well as to dieting, disordered eating, and the desire for cosmetic surgery to "fix" perceived defects. In fact, there are limits to the changes that can be made to body weight and body shape, both of which are influenced by heredity. The changes that can and should be made are lifestyle changes—engaging in regular physical activity and maintaining healthy eating habits. With these changes, the body weight and shape that develop will be natural and appropriate for an individual's particular genetic makeup.

Knowing when the limits to healthy change have been reached—and learning to accept those limits—is crucial for overall wellness. Obesity is a serious health risk, but weight management needs to take place in a positive and realistic atmosphere. For an obese person, losing as few as 10 pounds can reduce blood pressure and improve mood. The hazards of excessive dieting and overconcern about body weight need to be countered by a change in attitude about what constitutes the perfect body and a reasonable body weight. A reasonable weight must take into account a person's weight history, social circumstances, metabolic profile, and psychological well-being.

## EATING DISORDERS

Problems with body weight and weight control are not limited to excessive body fat. A growing number of people, especially adolescent girls and young women, experience **eating disorders,** characterized by severe disturbances in eating patterns and eating-related behaviors. The major eating disorders are anorexia nervosa, bulimia nervosa, and binge-eating disorder. **Anorexia nervosa** is characterized by a refusal to maintain a minimally normal body weight. **Bulimia nervosa** is characterized by repeated episodes of binge eating followed by compensatory behaviors such as self-induced vomiting, the misuse of laxatives or diuretics, fasting, or excessive exercise. **Binge-eating disorder** is characterized by binge eating without regular use of compensatory behaviors.

At any given time, about 0.5–2.0% of Americans suffer from anorexia and 2.5% have bulimia. Research suggests that about 4% of college-aged women have bulimia. Binge-eating disorder may affect 2–5% of all adults and 8% of those who are obese. Many more people exhibit disordered eating behaviors that do not fully meet the criteria of the major eating disorders. Anorexia and bulemia affect far more women than men.

### Anorexia Nervosa

A person suffering from anorexia nervosa does not eat enough food to maintain a reasonable body weight. Anorexia affects 1–3 million Americans, 95% of them female. Although it can occur later, anorexia typically develops between the ages of 12 and 18.

**Characteristics of Anorexia Nervosa** People suffering from anorexia have an intense fear of gaining weight or becoming fat. Their body image is distorted, so that even when emaciated they think they are fat. People with anorexia may engage in compulsive behaviors or rituals that help keep them from eating, though some may also binge and purge. They often use vigorous and prolonged exercise to reduce body weight as well. Although they may express a great interest in food, even taking over the cooking responsibilities for the rest of the family, their own diet becomes more and more extreme. They often hide or hoard food without eating it.

Anorexic people are typically introverted, emotionally reserved, and socially insecure. They are often "model children" who rarely complain and are anxious to please others and win their approval. Although school performance is typically above average, they are often critical of themselves and not satisfied with their accomplishments. For people with anorexia nervosa, their entire sense of self-esteem may be tied up in their evaluation of their body shape and weight.

**Health Risks of Anorexia Nervosa** Because of extreme weight loss, females with anorexia often stop menstruating, become intolerant of cold, and develop low blood pressure and heart rate. They develop dry skin that is often covered by fine body hair like that of an infant. Their hands and feet may swell and take on a blue color.

Anorexia nervosa has been linked to a variety of medical complications, including disorders of the cardiovascular, gastrointestinal, endocrine, and skeletal systems. When body fat is virtually gone and muscles are severely wasted, the body turns to its own organs in a desperate search for protein. Death can occur from heart failure caused by electrolyte imbalances. About one in ten women with anorexia dies of starvation, cardiac arrest, or other medical complications—one of the highest death rates for any psychiatric disorder. Depression is also a serious risk, and about half the fatalities relating to anorexia are suicides.

### Bulimia Nervosa

A person suffering from bulimia nervosa engages in recurrent episodes of binge eating followed by **purging.** Bulimia is often difficult to recognize because sufferers

**Terms**

**eating disorder** A serious disturbance in eating patterns or eating-related behavior, characterized by a negative body image and concerns about body weight or body fat.

**anorexia nervosa** An eating disorder characterized by a refusal to maintain body weight at a minimally healthy level and an intense fear of gaining weight or becoming fat; self-starvation.

**bulimia nervosa** An eating disorder characterized by recurrent episodes of binge eating and purging—overeating and then using compensatory behaviors such as vomiting, laxatives, and excessive exercise to prevent weight gain.

**binge-eating disorder** An eating disorder characterized by binge eating and a lack of control over eating behavior in general.

**purging** The use of vomiting, laxatives, excessive exercise, restrictive dieting, enemas, diuretics, or diet pills to compensate for food that has been eaten and that the person fears will produce weight gain.

VW

conceal their eating habits and usually maintain a normal weight, although they may experience weight fluctuations of 10–15 pounds. Bulimia most often begins in adolescence or young adulthood.

**Characteristics of Bulimia Nervosa** During a binge, a bulimic person may rapidly consume anywhere from 1,000 to 60,000 calories. This is followed by an attempt to get rid of the food by purging, usually by vomiting or using laxatives or diuretics. During a binge, bulimics feel as though they have lost control and cannot stop or limit how much they eat. Some binge and purge only occasionally; others do so many times every day.

People with bulimia may appear to eat normally, but they are rarely comfortable around food. Binges usually occur in secret and can become nightmarish—ravaging the kitchen for food, going from one grocery store to another to buy food, or even stealing food. During the binge, all feelings are blocked out, and food acts as an anesthetic. Afterward, bulimics feel physically drained and emotionally spent. They usually feel deeply ashamed and disgusted with both themselves and their behavior and terrified that they will gain weight from the binge.

Major life changes such as leaving for college, getting married, having a baby, or losing a job can trigger a binge-purge cycle. At such times, stress is high and the person may have no good outlet for emotional conflict or tension. As with anorexia, bulimia sufferers are often insecure and depend on others for approval and self-esteem. They may hide difficult emotions such as anger and disappointment from themselves and others. Binge eating and purging become a way of dealing with feelings.

**Health Risks of Bulimia Nervosa** The binge-purge cycle of bulimia places a tremendous strain on the body. Contact with vomited stomach acids erodes tooth enamel. Repeated vomiting or the use of laxatives, in combination with deficient calorie intake, can damage the liver and kidneys and cause cardiac arrhythmia. Chronic hoarseness and esophageal tearing with bleeding may also result from vomiting. More rarely, binge eating can lead to rupture of the stomach. Although many bulimic women maintain normal weight, even small amounts of weight loss can cause menstrual problems. And although less often associated with suicide or premature death than anorexia, bulimia is associated with increased depression, excessive preoccupation with food and body image, and sometimes disturbances in cognitive functioning.

## Binge-Eating Disorder

Binge-eating disorder is characterized by uncontrollable eating, usually followed by feelings of guilt and shame with weight gain. Common eating patterns are eating more rapidly than normal, eating until uncomfortably full, eating when not hungry, and preferring to eat alone. Binge eaters may eat large amounts of food throughout the day, with no planned mealtimes. Many people with binge-eating disorder mistakenly see rigid dieting as the only solution to their problem. However, rigid dieting usually causes feelings of deprivation and a return to overeating.

Compulsive overeaters rarely eat because of hunger. Instead, food is used as a means of coping with stress, conflict, and other difficult emotions or to provide solace and entertainment. People who do not have the resources to deal effectively with stress may be more vulnerable to binge-eating disorder. Inappropriate overeating often begins during childhood. In some families, eating may be used as an activity to fill otherwise empty time. Parents may reward children with food for good behavior or withhold food as a means of punishment, thereby creating distorted feelings about the use of food.

Binge eaters are almost always obese, so they face all the health risks associated with obesity. In addition, binge eaters may have higher rates of depression and anxiety.

## Borderline Disordered Eating

Eating habits and body image run a continuum from healthy to seriously disordered. Where each of us falls along that continuum can change depending on life stresses, illnesses, and many other factors. People with borderline disordered eating have some symptoms of eating disorders but do not meet the full diagnostic criteria for anorexia, bulimia, or binge-eating disorder. Behaviors such as excessive dieting, occasional bingeing or purging, or the inability to control eating turn food into the enemy and create havoc in the lives of millions of Americans.

How do you know if you have disordered eating habits? When thoughts about food and weight dominate your life, you have a problem. If you're convinced that your worth as a person hinges on how you look and how much you weigh, it's time to get help. Other danger signs include frequent feelings of guilt after a meal or snack, any use of vomiting or laxatives after meals, or overexercising or severely restricting your food intake to compensate for what you've eaten.

If you suspect you have an eating problem, don't go it alone or delay getting help, as disordered eating habits can develop into a full-blown eating disorder. Check with your student health or counseling center—nearly all colleges have counselors and medical personnel who can help you or refer you to a specialist if needed. If you are concerned about the eating behaviors of a friend or family member, refer to the suggestions in the box "If Someone You Know Has an Eating Disorder . . ."

## Treating Eating Disorders

The treatment of eating disorders must address both problematic eating behaviors and the misuse of food to

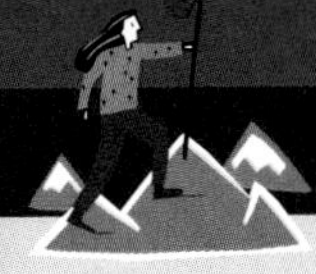

Take Charge

## If Someone You Know Has an Eating Disorder . . .

- Educate yourself about eating disorders and their risks and about treatment resources in your community. (See the For More Information section for suggestions.)
- Write down specific ways the person's eating problem is affecting you or others in the household. Call a house meeting to talk about how others are affected by the problem and how to take action.
- Consider consulting a professional about the best way to approach the situation. Research how and where your friend can get help. Attend a local support group.
- Arrange to speak privately with the person, along with other friends or family members. Let one person lead the group and do most of the talking. Discuss specific incidents and the consequences of disordered eating.
- If you are going to speak with your friend, write down ahead of time what your concerns are and what you would like to say. Expect that the person you are concerned about will deny there is a problem, minimize it, or become angry with you. Remain calm and nonjudgmental, and continue to express your concern.
- Avoid giving simplistic advice about eating habits. Gently encourage your friend to eat properly.
- Take time to listen to your friend, and express your support and understanding. Encourage honest communication. Emphasize your friend's good characteristics and compliment all her or his successes.
- Help maintain the person's sense of dignity by encouraging personal responsibility and decision making. Be patient and realistic; recovery is a long process. Continue to love and support your friend.
- If the situation is an emergency—if the person has fainted or attempted suicide, for example—take immediate action. Call 911 for help.
- If you feel very upset about the situation, seek professional help. Remember, you are not to blame for another person's eating disorder.

manage stress and emotions. Anorexia nervosa treatment first involves averting a medical crisis by restoring adequate body weight; then the psychological aspects of the disorder can be addressed. The treatment of bulimia nervosa or binge-eating disorder involves first stabilizing the eating patterns and then identifying and changing the patterns of thinking that lead to disordered eating and improving coping skills. Concurrent problems, such as depression or anxiety, must also be addressed. In 1996, the antidepressant Prozac became the first medication approved by the FDA for the treatment of bulimia.

Treatment of eating disorders usually involves a combination of psychotherapy and medical management. The therapy may be carried out individually or in a group; sessions involving the entire family may be recommended. A support or self-help group can be a useful adjunct to such treatment. Depending on the severity of the disorder, treatment may last from a few months to several years.

## Today's Challenge

Eating disorders can be seen as the logical extension of the concern with weight that pervades American society. Although most people don't succumb to irrational or distorted ideas about their bodies, many do become obsessed with dieting. The challenge facing Americans today is achieving a healthy body weight without excessive dieting—by adopting and maintaining sensible eating habits, an active lifestyle, realistic and positive attitudes and emotions, and creative ways of handling stress.

Tips for Today

Maintaining a healthy weight means balancing calories in with calories out. Many forces and factors in contemporary society work against a healthy balance, so it's imperative that individuals take active control of managing their weight. Many approaches work, but the simplest formula is moderate food intake coupled with regular exercise.

*Right now you can*

- Drink a glass of water instead of a soda.
- Throw away any high-calorie, low-nutrient snack foods in your kitchen and start a list of fruits and vegetables you can buy as snacks instead.
- Put a sign on your refrigerator reminding you of your weight-management goals.
- Go outside and walk or jog for 15 minutes or take a 15-minute bike ride.
- Review the information on portion sizes in Chapter 9 and consider whether the portions you usually take at meals are larger than they need to be.

## SUMMARY

- Body composition is the relative amounts of fat-free mass and fat in the body. *Overweight* and *obesity* refer to body weight or the percentage of body fat that exceeds what is associated with good health.
- The key to weight management is maintaining a balance of calories in (food) and calories out (resting metabolism, food digestion, and physical activity).
- Standards for assessing body weight and body composition include body mass index (BMI) and percent body fat.
- Too much or too little body fat is linked to health problems; the distribution of body fat can also be a significant risk factor.
- An inaccurate or negative body image is common and can lead to psychological distress.
- Factors involved in the regulation of body weight and body fat include heredity and metabolic rate.
- Nutritional guidelines for weight management include consuming a moderate number of calories; limiting portion sizes, energy density, and the intake of fat, simple sugars, refined carbohydrates, and protein to recommended levels; and developing an eating schedule and decision rules for food choices.
- Activity guidelines for weight management emphasize daily physical activity and regular sessions of cardiorespiratory endurance exercise and strength training.
- Weight management requires developing positive, realistic self-talk and self-esteem and a repertoire of appropriate techniques for handling stress and other emotional and physical challenges.
- People can be successful at long-term weight loss on their own, by combining diet and exercise.
- Diet books, OTC diet aids and supplements, and formal weight-loss programs should be assessed for safety and efficacy.
- Professional help is needed in cases of severe obesity; medical treatments include prescription drugs, surgery, and psychological therapy.
- Dissatisfaction with weight and shape are common to all eating disorders. Anorexia nervosa is characterized by self-starvation, distorted body image, and an intense fear of gaining weight. Bulimia nervosa is characterized by recurrent episodes of uncontrolled binge eating and frequent purging. Binge-eating disorder involves binge eating without regular use of compensatory purging.

## Take Action

1. **Interview a successful dieter:** Identify some people who have successfully lost weight and kept it off, and interview them. What were their strategies and techniques? In what ways did they change their exercise and eating habits? Do you think their approach would work for others?

2. **Assess your body composition:** Find out what percentage of your body weight is fat by taking one of the tests described in this chapter at your campus health clinic, sports medicine clinic, or health club. If you have too high or too low a proportion of body fat, consider taking steps to change it.

## For More Information

### Books

Beck, C. 2003. *Anorexia and Bulimia for Dummies.* Hoboken, N.J.: John Wiley & Sons. *An easy-to-understand guide to eating disorders.*

Ferguson, J. M., and C. Ferguson. 2003. *Habits Not Diets,* 4th ed. Boulder, Colo.: Bull. *A behavior-change approach to changing diet and activity habits that includes many helpful practical tips, assessment worksheets, and tracking forms.*

Hensrud, D. D. 2005. *Mayo Clinic Healthy Weight for Everyone.* Rochester, Minn.: Mayo Clinic. *Provides guidelines for successful weight management.*

Milchovich, S. K., and B. Dunn-Long. 2003. *Diabetes Mellitus: A Practical Handbook,* 8th. ed. Boulder, Colo.: Bull. *A user-friendly guide to diabetes.*

Nash, J. D. 2003. *Maximize Your Body Potential: Lifetime Skills for Successful Weight Management.* Boulder, Colo.: Bull. *A do-it-yourself guide that provides self-assessment tools and guidelines for setting realistic goals and developing an individualized weight management plan.*

Pope, H. G., K. A. Phillips, and R. Olivardia. 2000. *Adonis Complex: The Secret Crisis of Male Body Obsession.* New York: Free Press. *Provides a historical review of the changing fashions in male body type and information about body image problems.*

### Organizations, Hotlines, and Web Sites

*American Diabetes Association.* Provides information, a free newsletter, and referrals to local support groups; the Web site includes an online diabetes risk assessment.
800-342-2383
http://www.diabetes.org

*Calorie Control Council.* Site includes a variety of interactive calculators, including an Exercise Calculator that estimates the calories burned from various forms of physical activity.
http://www.caloriecontrol.org

*Cyberdiet.* Provides a variety of assessment and planning tools as well as practical tips for adopting a healthy lifestyle.
http://www.cyberdiet.com

*FDA Center for Food Safety and Applied Nutrition: Dietary Supplements.* Provides background facts and information on the current regulatory status of dietary supplements, including compounds marketed for weight loss.
http://www.cfsan.fda.gov/~dms/supplmnt.html

## A Weight-Management Program

The behavior management plan described in Chapter 1 provides an excellent framework for a weight-management program. Following are some suggestions about specific ways you can adapt that general plan to controlling your weight.

### Motivation and Commitment

Make sure you are motivated and committed before you begin. Failure at weight loss is a frustrating experience that can make it more difficult to lose weight in the future. Think about the reasons you want to lose weight. Self-focused reasons, such as to feel good about yourself or to have a greater sense of well-being, are often associated with success. Trying to lose weight for others or out of concern for how others view you is a poor foundation for a weight-loss program. Make a list of your reasons for wanting to lose weight, and post it in a prominent place.

### Setting Goals

Choose a reasonable weight you think you would like to reach over the long term, and be willing to renegotiate it as you get further along. Break down your long-term weight and behavioral goals into a series of short-term goals. Develop a new way of behaving by designing small, manageable steps that will get you to where you want to go.

### Creating a Negative Energy Balance

When your weight is constant, you are burning approximately the same number of calories as you are taking in. To tip the energy balance toward weight loss, you must either consume fewer calories or burn more calories through physical activity, or both. One pound of body fat represents 3500 calories. To lose weight at the recommended rate of 0.5–2.0 pounds per week, you must create a negative energy balance of 1750–7000 calories per week or 250–1000 calories per day. To generate your negative energy balance, it's usually best to begin by increasing your activity level rather than decreasing your calorie consumption.

### Physical Activity

Consider how you can increase your energy output simply by increasing routine physical activity, such as walking or taking the stairs. (Figure 10-2 shows activities that use about 150 calories.) If you are not already involved in a regular exercise routine aimed at increasing endurance and building or maintaining muscle mass, seek help from someone who is competent to help you plan and start an appropriate exercise routine. If you are already doing regular physical exercise, evaluate your program according to the guidelines in Chapter 10.

Don't try to use exercise to "spot reduce." Leg lifts, for example, contribute to fat loss only to the extent that they burn calories; they don't burn fat just from your legs. You can make parts of your body appear more fit by exercising them, but the only way you can reduce fat in any specific part of your body is to create an overall negative energy balance.

### Diet and Eating Habits

If you can't generate a large enough negative energy balance solely by increasing physical activity, you may want to supplement exercise with modest cuts in your calorie intake. Don't think of this as "going on a diet"; your goal is to make small changes in your diet that you can maintain for a lifetime. Focus on cutting your intake of saturated and trans fats and added sugars and on eating a variety of nutritious foods in moderation. Don't try skipping meals, fasting, or going on a very-low-calorie diet or a diet that is unbalanced.

Making changes in eating habits is another important strategy for weight management. If your program centers on a conscious restriction of certain food items, you're likely to spend all your time thinking about the forbidden foods. Focus on *how* to eat rather than *what* to eat. Refer to the box "Strategies for Successful Weight Management" for suggestions.

### Self-Monitoring

Keep a record of your weight and behavior change progress. Try keeping a record of everything you eat. Write down what you plan to eat, in what quantity, *before* you eat. You'll find that just having to record something that is "not OK" to eat is likely to stop you from eating it. If you also note what seems to be triggering your urges to eat (for example, you feel bored, or someone offered you something), you'll become more aware of your weak spots and be better able to take corrective action. Also, keep track of your daily activities and your formal exercise program so you can monitor increases in physical activity.

### Putting Your Plan into Action

- Examine the environmental cues that trigger poor eating and exercise habits, and devise strategies for dealing with them. For example, you may need to remove "problem" foods from your house temporarily or put a sign on the refrigerator reminding you to go for a walk instead of having a snack. Anticipate problem situations, and plan ways to handle them more effectively.
- Create new environmental cues that will support your new healthy behaviors. Put your walking shoes by the front door. Move fruits and vegetables to the front of the refrigerator.
- Get others to help. Talk to friends and family members about what they can do to support your efforts. Find a buddy to join you in your exercise program.
- Give yourself lots of praise and rewards. Think about your accomplishments and achievements and congratulate yourself. Plan special nonfood treats for yourself, such as a walk or a movie. Reward yourself often and for anything that counts toward success.
- If you do slip, tell yourself to get back on track immediately, and don't waste time on self-criticism. Think positively instead of getting into a cycle of guilt and self-blame. Don't demand too much of yourself.
- Don't get discouraged. Be aware that although weight loss is bound to slow down after the first loss of body fluid, the weight loss at this slower rate is more permanent than earlier, more dramatic losses.
- Remember that weight management is a lifelong project. You need to adopt reasonable goals and strategies that you can maintain over the long term.

*Federal Trade Commission (FTC): Project Waistline.* Provides advice for evaluating advertising about weight-loss products.
http://www.ftc.gov/bcp/conline/edcams/waistline

*National Heart, Lung, and Blood Institute (NHLBI): Aim for a Healthy Weight.* Provides information and tips on diet and physical activity, as well as a BMI calculator.
http://www.nhlbi.nih.gov/health/public/heart/obesity/lose_wt

*National Institute of Diabetes and Digestive and Kidney Diseases (NIDDK).* Provides information and referrals for problems related to obesity, weight control, and nutritional disorders.
877-946-4627
http://win.niddk.nih.gov

*Partnership for Healthy Weight Management.* Provides information on evaluating weight-loss programs and advertising claims.
http://www.consumer.gov/weightloss

*USDA Food and Nutrition Information Center: Reports and Studies on Obesity.* Provides links to recent reports and studies on the issue of obesity among Americans.
http://www.nal.usda.gov/fnic/reports/obesity.html

Resources for people concerned about eating disorders:

*Eating Disorder Referral and Information Center*
http://www.edreferral.com

*Eating Disorders Shared Awareness*
http://www.something-fishy.org

*MedlinePlus: Eating Disorders*
http://www.nlm.nih.gov/medlineplus/eatingdisorders.html

*National Eating Disorders Association*
http://www.nationaleatingdisorders.org

*National Association of Anorexia Nervosa and Associated Disorders*
847-831-3438 (referral line)
http://www.anad.org

See also the listings in Chapters 9 and 10.

## Selected Bibliography


American Diabetes Association. 2004. *How to Tell if You Have Pre-Diabetes* (http://www.diabetes.org/pre-diabetes/pre-diabetes-symptoms.jsp; retrieved March 27, 2005).

Bowman, S. A., et al. 2004. Effects of fast-food consumption on energy intake and diet quality among children in a national household survey. *Pediatrics* 113(1 Pt 1): 112–118.

Buchwald, H., et al. 2004. Bariatric surgery: A systematic review and meta-analysis. *Journal of the American Medical Association* 292(14): 1724–1737.

Centers for Disease Control and Prevention. 2004. Prevalence of diabetes among Hispanics—selected areas, 1998–2002. *Morbidity and Mortality Weekly Report* 53(40): 941–944.

Centers for Disease Control and Prevention. 2004. *Overweight and Obesity: Economic Consequences* (http://www.cdc.gov/nccdphp/dnpa/obesity/economic_consequences.htm; retrieved January 3, 2005).

Dong, L., G. Block, and S. Mandel. 2004. Activities contributing to total energy expenditure in the United States: Results from the NHAPS Study. *International Journal of Behavioral Nutrition and Physical Activity* 1(4).

Farshchi, H. R., M. A. Taylor, and I. A. Macdonald. 2005. Deleterious effects of omitting breakfast on insulin sensitivity and fasting lipid profiles in healthy lean women. *American Journal of Clinical Nutrition* 81(2): 388–396.

Fenicchia, L. M., et al. 2004. Influence of resistance exercise training on glucose control in women with type 2 diabetes. *Metabolism* 53(3): 284–289.

Fontaine, K. R., et al. 2003. Years of life lost due to obesity. *Journal of the American Medical Association* 289(2): 187–193.

Fung, T. T., et al. 2004. Dietary patterns, meat intake, and the risk of type 2 diabetes in women. *Archives of Internal Medicine* 164(20): 2235–2240.

Graves, B. S., and R. L. Welsh. 2004. Recognizing the signs of body dysmorphic disorder and muscle dysmorphia. *ACSM's Health and Fitness Journal,* January/February.

Hu, F. B., et al. 2003. Television watching and other sedentary behaviors in relation to risk of obesity and type 2 diabetes mellitus in women. *Journal of the American Medical Association* 289(14): 1785–1791.

Hu, F. B., et al. 2004. Adiposity as compared with physical activity in predicting mortality among women. *New England Journal of Medicine* 351(26): 2694–2703.

Ma, Y., et al. 2005. Association between dietary carbohydrates and body weight. *American Journal of Epidemiology* 161(4): 359–367.

Mokdad, A. H., et al. 2005. Correction: Actual causes of death in the United States, 2000. *Journal of the American Medical Association* 293(3): 293–294.

Mokdad, A. H., et al. 2003. Prevalence of obesity, diabetes, and obesity-related health risk factors, 2001. *Journal of the American Medical Association* 289: 76–79.

Nicklas, B. J., et al. 2004. Association of visceral adipose tissue with incident myocardial infarction in older men and women: The Health, Aging and Body Composition Study. *American Journal of Epidemiology* 160(8): 741–749.

Nielsen, S. J., and B. M. Popkin. 2003. Patterns and trends in food portion sizes, 1977–1996. *Journal of the American Medical Association* 289(4): 450–453.

Olshansky, S. J., et al. 2005. A potential decline in life expectancy in the United States in the 21st century. *New England Journal of Medicine* 352(11): 1138–1145.

Schulze, M. B., et al. 2004. Sugar-sweetened beverages, weight gain, and incidence of type 2 diabetes in young and middle-aged women. *Journal of the American Medical Association* 292(8): 927–934.

Sweeteners can sour your health. 2005. *Consumer Reports on Health,* January.

Tsai, A. G., and T. A. Wadden. 2005. Systematic review: An evaluation of major commercial weight loss programs in the United States. *Annals of Internal Medicine* 142(1): 56–66.

U.S. Department of Health and Human Services. 2005. *Dietary Guidelines for Americans* (http://www.healthierus.gov/dietaryguidelines; retrieved January 15, 2005).

Vorona, R. D., et al. 2005. Overweight and obese patients in a primary care population report less sleep than patients with a normal body mass index. *Archives of Internal Medicine* 165: 25–30.

Weinstein, A. R., et al. 2004. Relationship of physical activity vs. body mass index with type 2 diabetes in women. *Journal of the American Medical Association* 292(10): 1188–1194.

Wong, S. L., et al. 2004. Cardiorespiratory fitness is associated with lower abdominal fat independent of body mass index. *Medicine and Science in Sports and Exercise* 36(2): 286–291.

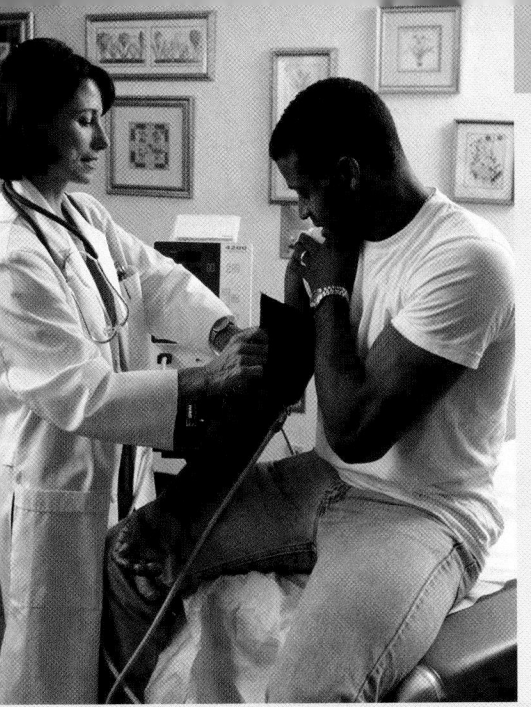

## Looking AHEAD

After reading this chapter, you should be able to

- List the major components of the cardiovascular system and describe how blood is pumped and circulated throughout the body
- Describe the controllable and uncontrollable risk factors associated with cardiovascular disease
- Discuss the major forms of cardiovascular disease and how they develop
- Explain what cancer is and how it spreads
- List and describe common cancers—their risk factors, signs and symptoms, treatments, and approaches to prevention
- List specific actions you can take to lower your risk of CVD and cancer

12

# Cardiovascular Disease and Cancer

**Cardiovascular disease (CVD)** is the leading cause of death in the United States, accounting for nearly half of all deaths. Cancer is the second leading cause, accounting for nearly a quarter of all deaths; it is the leading cause of death among people under age 85. Although age, genetics, and the physical environment play roles in the development of CVD and cancer, these diseases are primarily lifestyle diseases, linked to many controllable lifestyle factors. This chapter describes the forms and causes of these two killers and provides information about how you can reduce your risk of developing and dying from CVD or cancer.

## THE CARDIOVASCULAR SYSTEM

The cardiovascular system consists of the heart and blood vessels (veins, arteries, and capillaries); together, they pump and circulate blood throughout the body. A person weighing 150 pounds has about 5 quarts of blood, which circulates about once every minute.

The heart is a four-chambered, fist-size muscle located just beneath the ribs under the left breast (Figure 12-1). Its role is to pump deoxygenated (oxygen-poor) blood to the lungs and oxygenated (oxygen-rich) blood to the rest of the body. Blood actually travels through two separate circulatory systems: The right side of the heart pumps blood to and from the lungs in what is called the *pulmonary circulation*, and the left side pumps blood through the rest of the body in the *systemic circulation*.

Used, oxygen-poor blood enters the right upper chamber, or **atrium**, of the heart through the **vena cava**, the largest vein in the body (Figure 12-2). Valves prevent the blood from flowing the wrong way. As the right atrium fills, it contracts and pumps blood into the right lower chamber, or **ventricle**, which, when it contracts, pumps blood through the pulmonary artery into the lungs. There, blood picks up oxygen and discards carbon dioxide.

### Terms

**cardiovascular disease (CVD)** The collective term for various forms of diseases of the heart and blood vessels.

**atria** The two upper chambers of the heart in which blood collects before passing to the ventricles.

**vena cava** The large vein through which blood is returned to the right atrium of the heart.

**ventricles** The two lower chambers of the heart that pump blood through arteries to the lungs and other parts of the body.

Vw

**Vw Visit the *Core Concepts in Health* Online Learning Center (www.mhhe.com/inselbrief10e) for study aids and many additional resources.**

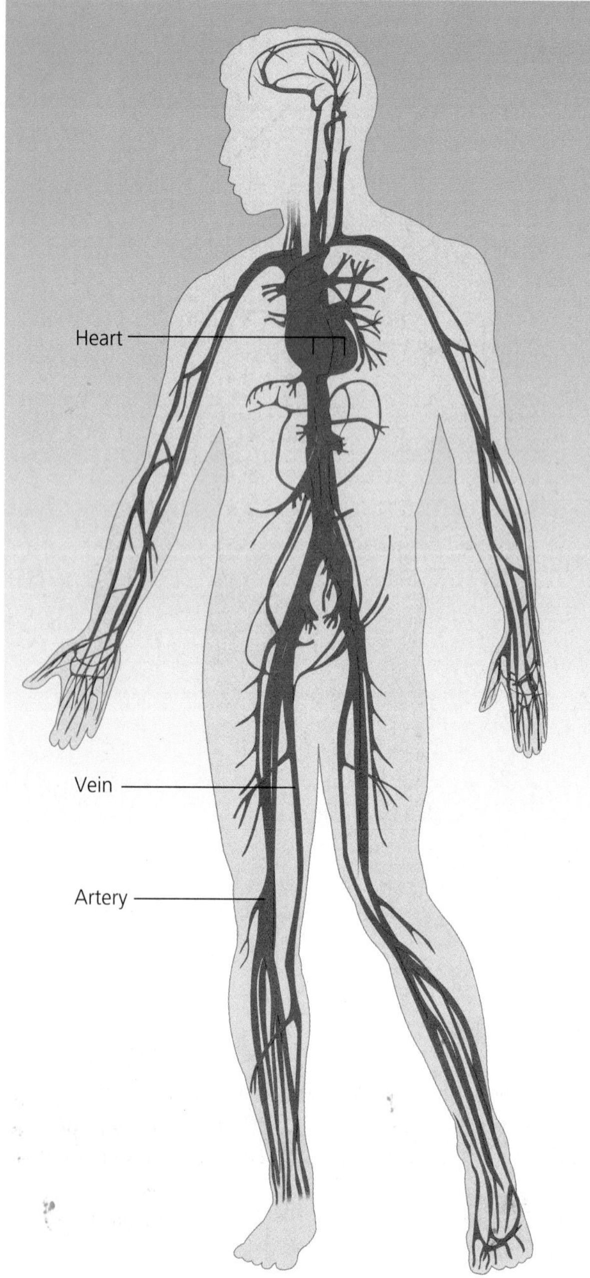


**Figure 12-1 The cardiovascular system.**

Cleaned, oxygenated blood then flows through the pulmonary veins into the left atrium. As this chamber fills, it contracts and pumps blood into the powerful left ventricle, which pumps it through the **aorta**, the body's largest artery, to be fed into the rest of the body's blood vessels. The period of the heart's contraction is called *systole*; the period of relaxation is called *diastole*.

The heartbeat—the split-second sequence of contractions of the heart's four chambers—is controlled by electrical impulses. These signals originate in a bundle of specialized cells in the right atrium called the *sinus node*. Unless the pace is speeded up or slowed down by the brain in response to stimuli such as danger or exhaustion, the heart produces electrical impulses at a steady rate.

Blood vessels are classified by size and function. **Veins** carry blood to the heart; **arteries** carry blood away from the heart. Veins have thin walls; arteries have thick elastic walls that enable them to expand or contract with the volume of the blood being pumped through them. After leaving the heart, the aorta branches into smaller and smaller vessels. Two vital arteries, called the left and right coronary arteries, branch off the aorta to carry blood back to the heart muscle itself.

The smallest arteries branch still further into **capillaries**, tiny vessels only one cell thick. The capillaries deliver oxygen and nutrient-rich blood to the tissues and receive oxygen-poor, waste-carrying blood. From the capillaries, this blood empties into small veins and then into larger veins that return it to the heart. From there the cycle is repeated.

## RISK FACTORS FOR CARDIOVASCULAR DISEASE

Researchers have identified a variety of factors associated with an increased risk of developing cardiovascular disease. They are grouped into two categories: major risk factors and contributing risk factors. Some risk factors, such as diet, exercise habits, and use of tobacco, are linked to controllable aspects of lifestyle and can therefore be changed. Others, such as age, sex, and heredity, are beyond an individual's control.

### Major Risk Factors That Can Be Changed

The American Heart Association (AHA) has identified six major risk factors for CVD that can be changed: tobacco use, high blood pressure, unhealthy blood cholesterol levels, physical inactivity, obesity, and diabetes.

**Tobacco Use** About one in five deaths from CVD is attributable to smoking. People who smoke a pack of cigarettes a day have twice the risk of heart attack that nonsmokers have; smoking two or more packs a day triples the risk. And when smokers do have heart attacks, they are 2 to 4 times more likely than nonsmokers to die from them. Women who smoke heavily and use oral contraceptives are up to 32 times more likely to have a heart attack and up to 20 times more likely to have a stroke than women who don't smoke and take the pill.

Smoking harms the cardiovascular system and raises the risk for CVD in several ways. Nicotine, a central nervous system stimulant, increases blood pressure and heart rate; the carbon monoxide in cigarette smoke displaces oxygen in the blood, reducing the amount of oxygen available to the heart and other parts of the body. Smoking

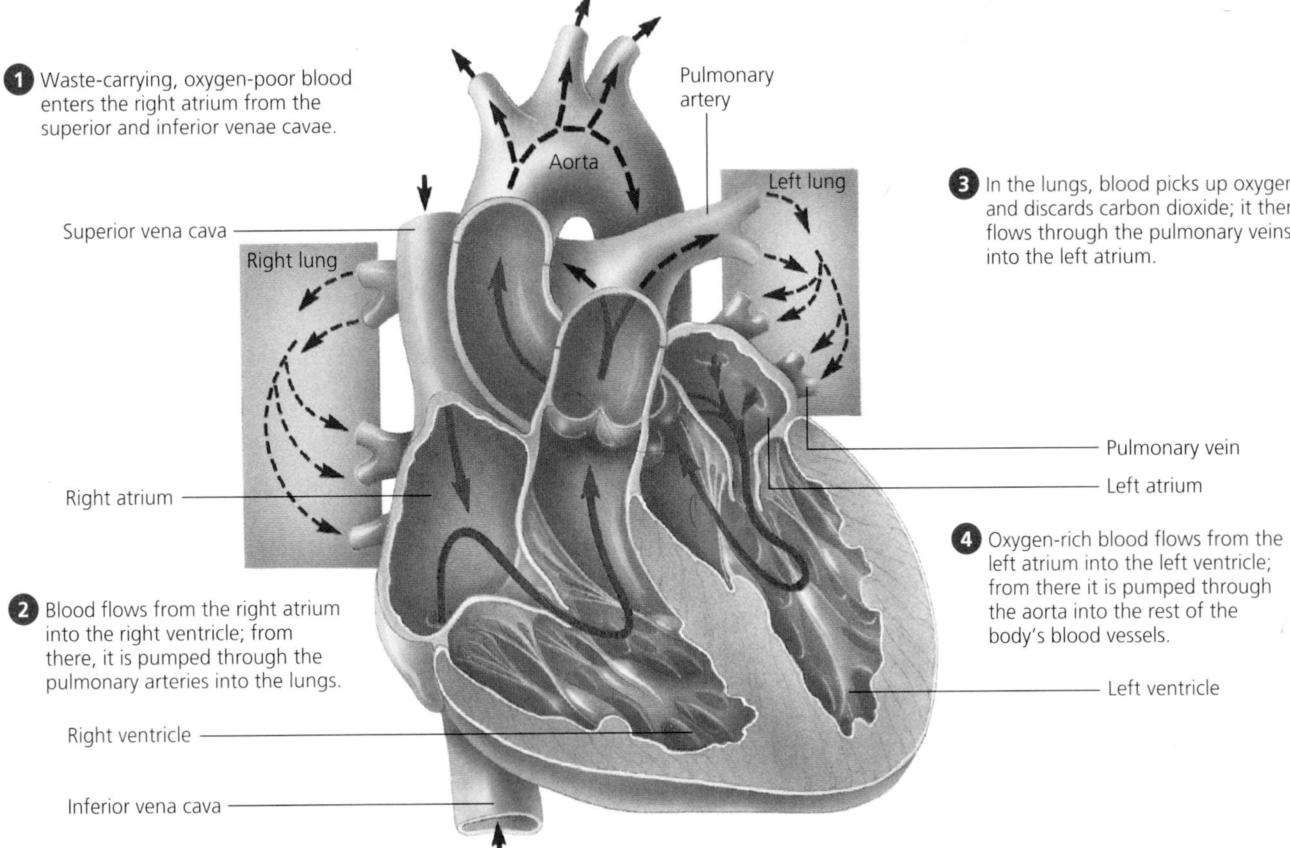


**Figure 12-2 Circulation in the heart.**

damages the linings of arteries, and it contributes to unhealthy blood fat levels by reducing levels of high-density lipoproteins (HDL), "good" cholesterol, and raising levels of triglycerides and low-density lipoproteins (LDL), "bad" cholesterol. It causes the **platelets** in blood to become sticky and cluster, promoting clotting. Smoking also permanently accelerates the rate at which fatty deposits are laid down in arteries.

You don't have to smoke to be affected. The risk of death from coronary heart disease increases up to 30% among those exposed to environmental tobacco smoke (ETS) at home or at work. Researchers estimate that as many as 62,000 nonsmokers die from CVD each year as a result of exposure to ETS.

**High Blood Pressure** High blood pressure, or **hypertension,** is a risk factor for many forms of cardiovascular disease, including heart attacks and strokes, and is itself considered a form of CVD. Hypertension can also cause kidney failure and damage to nearly every organ in the body. Blood pressure, the force exerted by the blood on the vessel walls, is created by the pumping action of the heart. When the heart contracts (systole), blood pressure increases. When the heart relaxes (diastole), pressure decreases. High blood pressure occurs when too much force is exerted against the walls of the arteries. Short periods of high blood pressure are normal, such as during exercise, but blood pressure that is continually at an abnormally high level constitutes hypertension.

Blood pressure is measured with a stethoscope and an instrument called a sphygmomanometer. It is expressed as two numbers—for example, 120 over 80—and measured in millimeters of mercury. The first and larger number is the systolic blood pressure; the second is the diastolic blood pressure. A normal blood pressure reading for a healthy young adult is 115 systolic over 75 diastolic; CVD

## Terms

VW

**aorta** The large artery that receives blood from the left ventricle and distributes it to the body.

**veins** Vessels that carry blood to the heart.

**arteries** Vessels that carry blood away from the heart.

**capillaries** Very small blood vessels that serve to exchange oxygen and nutrients between the blood and the tissues.

**platelets** Microscopic disk-shaped cell fragments in the blood that disintegrate on contact with foreign objects and release chemicals that are necessary for the formation of blood clots.

**hypertension** Sustained abnormally high blood pressure.

## Table 12-1 Blood Pressure Classification for Healthy Adults

| Category[a] | Systolic (mm Hg) | | Diastolic (mm Hg) |
|---|---|---|---|
| Normal[b] | below 120 | and | below 80 |
| Prehypertension | 120–139 | or | 80–89 |
| Hypertension[c] | | | |
| Stage 1 | 140–159 | or | 90–99 |
| Stage 2 | 160 and above | or | 100 and above |

[a]When systolic and diastolic pressure fall into different categories, the higher category should be used to classify blood pressure status.

[b]The risk of death from heart attack and stroke begins to rise when blood pressure is above 115/75.

[c]Based on the average of two or more readings taken at different physician visits. In persons older than 50 years, systolic blood pressure greater than 140 is a much more significant CVD risk factor than diastolic blood pressure.

SOURCE: *The Seventh Report of the Joint National Committee on Prevention, Detection, Evaluation, and Treatment of High Blood Pressure.* 2003. Bethesda, Md.: National Heart, Lung, and Blood Institute National Institutes of Health (NIH Publication No. 03-5233).

risk increases when blood pressure rises above this level. High blood pressure in adults is defined as equal to or greater than 140 over 90 (Table 12-1).

High blood pressure results from either an increased output of blood by the heart or, most often, increased resistance to blood flow in the arteries. The latter condition can be caused by **atherosclerosis,** discussed later in the chapter, or by constriction of smooth muscle surrounding the arteries. When a person has high blood pressure, the heart must work harder than normal to force blood through the narrowed arteries, thereby straining both the heart and arteries. High blood pressure is often called a "silent killer," because it usually has no symptoms. A person may have high blood pressure for years without realizing it. But during that time, it damages vital organs and increases the risk of heart attack, congestive heart failure, stroke, kidney failure, and blindness.

### Terms

VW

**atherosclerosis** A form of CVD in which the inner layers of artery walls are made thick and irregular by plaque deposits; arteries become narrow, and blood supply is reduced.

**low-density lipoproteins (LDL)** Blood fat that transports cholesterol from the liver to organs and tissues; excess is deposited on artery walls, where it can eventually block the flow of blood to the heart and brain; "bad" cholesterol.

**high-density lipoproteins (HDL)** Blood fat that helps transport cholesterol out of the arteries and thus protects against heart diseases; "good" cholesterol.

Hypertension is common, and its incidence rises dramatically with increasing age. The risk of developing hypertension is highest in African Americans, in whom, compared with other groups, the disorder is often more severe, more resistant to treatment, and more likely to be fatal at an early age. Overall, about 30% of adults have hypertension, 30% have prehypertension, and 40% have normal blood pressure.

In most cases, hypertension cannot be cured, but it can be controlled. Because hypertension has no early warning signs, it's crucial to have your blood pressure tested at least once every 2 years (more often if you have other CVD risk factors). Lifestyle changes are recommended for everyone with prehypertension and hypertension (see Table 12-1). These lifestyle changes include weight reduction, regular physical activity, a healthy diet, and moderation of alcohol consumption. The DASH diet is recommended; it emphasizes fruits, vegetables, and whole grains, foods that are rich in potassium and fiber (see p. 293). Sodium restriction is also helpful. Many people are "salt-sensitive," meaning that their blood pressure will decrease significantly when salt intake is restricted. The 2005 Dietary Guidelines for Americans recommend that Americans consume less than 2300 mg of sodium (about 1 teaspoon of salt) per day. People with hypertension, African Americans, and middle-aged and older adults should aim to consume no more than 1500 mg of sodium per day. Adequate potassium intake is also important. For people whose blood pressure isn't adequately controlled with lifestyle changes, medication is prescribed.

### High Levels of Cholesterol

Cholesterol is a fatty, waxlike substance that circulates through the bloodstream and is an important component of cell membranes, sex hormones, vitamin D, the fluid that coats the lungs, and the protective sheaths around nerves. Adequate cholesterol is essential for the proper functioning of the body. However, excess cholesterol can clog arteries and increase the risk of cardiovascular disease. Our bodies obtain cholesterol in two ways: from the liver, which manufactures it, and from the foods we eat. Cholesterol levels vary depending on diet, age, sex, heredity, and other factors.

**GOOD VERSUS BAD CHOLESTEROL** Cholesterol is carried in the blood in protein-lipid packages called lipoproteins. Lipoproteins can be thought of as shuttles that transport cholesterol to and from the liver through the circulatory system. **Low-density lipoproteins (LDLs)** shuttle cholesterol from the liver to the organs and tissues that require it. LDL is known as "bad" cholesterol because if there is more than the body can use, the excess is deposited in the blood vessels. If coronary arteries are blocked, the result may be a heart attack; if an artery carrying blood to the brain is blocked, a stroke may occur. **High-density lipoproteins (HDLs),** or "good" cholesterol, shuttle unused cholesterol back to the liver for recycling. By removing cholesterol from blood vessels, HDL helps protect against atherosclerosis.

**RECOMMENDED BLOOD CHOLESTEROL LEVELS** The risk for CVD increases with increasing blood cholesterol levels, especially LDL. The National Cholesterol Education Program (NCEP) recommends lipoprotein testing at least once every 5 years for all adults, beginning at age 20. The recommended test is a fasting lipoprotein profile that measures total cholesterol, LDL cholesterol, HDL cholesterol, and triglycerides (another blood fat). General cholesterol and triglyceride guidelines are given in Table 12-2. In general, high LDL levels and low HDL levels are associated with a high risk for CVD; low levels of LDL and high levels of HDL are associated with lower risk. HDL is important because a high HDL level seems to offer protection from CVD even in cases where total cholesterol is high. This seems to be especially true for women.

**Table 12-2 Cholesterol Guidelines**

| | |
|---|---|
| **LDL cholesterol (mg/dl)*** | |
| Less than 100 | Optimal |
| 100–129 | Near optimal/above optimal |
| 130–159 | Borderline high |
| 160–189 | High |
| 190 or more | Very high |
| **Total cholesterol (mg/dl)** | |
| Less than 200 | Desirable |
| 200–239 | Borderline high |
| 240 or more | High |
| **HDL cholesterol (mg/dl)** | |
| Less than 40 | Low (undesirable) |
| 60 or more | High (desirable) |
| **Triglycerides (mg/dl)** | |
| Less than 150 | Normal |
| 150–199 | Borderline high |
| 200–499 | High |
| 500 or more | Very high |

*These are general goals for LDL; specific LDL goals depend on a person's other risk factors (see p. 294 for more information); for people at very high risk, an LDL goal of less than 70 mg/dl may be appropriate.

SOURCES: Grundy, S. M., et al. 2004. Implications of recent clinical trials for the National Cholesterol Education Program Adult Treatment Panel III Guidelines. *Circulation* 110: 227–239; Expert Panel on Detection, Evaluation, and Treatment of High Blood Cholesterol in Adults. 2001. Executive Summary of the Third Report of the National Cholesterol Education Program (NCEP) Expert Panel on Detection, Evaluation, and Treatment of High Blood Cholesterol in Adults (Adult Treatment Panel III). *Journal of the American Medical Association* 285(19).

As shown in Table 12-2, LDL levels below 100 mg/dl (milligrams per deciliter) and total cholesterol levels below 200 mg/dl are desirable. An estimated 107 million American adults—over half the population—have total cholesterol levels of 200 mg/dl or higher. The CVD risk associated with elevated cholesterol levels also depends on other factors. For example, a high LDL level would be of more concern for an individual who also smokes and has high blood pressure than for an individual without these additional risk factors, and it is especially a concern for diabetics.

**IMPROVING CHOLESTEROL LEVELS** Your primary goal should be to reduce LDL to healthy levels. Important dietary changes for reducing LDL levels include substituting unsaturated for saturated and trans fats and increasing fiber intake. Decreasing your intake of saturated and trans fats is particularly important because they promote the production and excretion of cholesterol by the liver. Exercising regularly and eating more fruits, vegetables, and whole grains also help. You can raise your HDL levels by exercising regularly, losing weight if you are overweight, quitting smoking, and altering the amount and type of fat you consume.

### Physical Inactivity

Regular physical activity has direct and indirect benefits on the heart. Directly, it lowers heart rate and blood pressure, while improving the strength with which the heart pumps blood to the body and the ability of the tissues to extract oxygen from that blood. Indirectly, physical activity positively affects almost every risk factor for CVD. It helps decrease blood pressure, increase HDL levels, maintain desirable weight, and prevent or control diabetes. Exercise also improves the functioning of the endothelial cells that line coronary arteries and decreases platelet aggregation, which can lead to clot formation in the coronary arteries.

In general, the more physical activity you engage in, the more cardiovascular benefit you derive. A minimum of 30–60 minutes per day of moderate physical activity is recommended. More intense or longer-duration exercise has even greater health benefits.

### Obesity

The risk of death from CVD is two to three times higher in obese people (BMI $\geq$ 30 ) than it is in lean people (BMI 18.5–24.9), and for every 5-unit increment of BMI, a person's risk of death from coronary heart disease increases by 30%. The increased risk of CVD associated with overweight is present even if a person has no other risk factors, but unfortunately, overweight people usually do have other CVD risk factors. Excess body fat is strongly associated with hypertension, high cholesterol levels, insulin resistance, diabetes, and other problems with blood flow and the function of arteries.

As discussed in Chapter 11, the distribution of body fat is significant: Fat that collects in the torso is more dangerous than fat that collects around the hips. Obesity in general, and abdominal obesity in particular, is significantly associated with narrowing of the coronary arteries, even in young adults in their twenties. Having abdominal obesity can increase your risk even if your weight is normal. A sensible diet and regular exercise are the best ways to achieve and maintain a healthy body weight. For someone who is overweight, even modest weight reduction—5–10% of body weight—can reduce CVD risk by lowering blood pressure, improving cholesterol levels, and reducing diabetes risk.

**Diabetes** As described in Chapter 11, diabetes is a disorder characterized by elevated blood glucose levels due to insufficient supply or action of insulin. Having diabetes doubles the risk of CVD for men and triples the risk for women. Diabetics have higher rates of other CVD risk factors, including hypertension, obesity, and unhealthy blood lipid levels (typically, high triglyceride levels and low HDL levels). The elevated blood glucose and insulin levels that occur in diabetes can damage the cells that line the arteries, making them more vulnerable to atherosclerosis; diabetics also often have platelet and blood coagulation abnormalities that increase the risk of heart attacks and strokes. People with pre-diabetes also face a significantly increased risk of CVD.

For people with diabetes, a healthy diet, exercise, and careful control of glucose levels is recommended to decrease chances of developing CVD and other problems, but even people whose diabetes is under control face a high risk of CVD. For that reason, careful control of other CVD risk factors is critical for people with diabetes.

## Contributing Risk Factors That Can Be Changed

Various other factors that can be changed have been identified as contributing to CVD risk, including triglyceride levels and psychological and social factors.

**High Triglyceride Levels** Like cholesterol, triglycerides are blood fats that are obtained from food and manufactured by the body. High triglyceride levels are a reliable predictor of heart disease, especially if associated with other risk factors, such as low HDL levels, obesity, and diabetes. Factors contributing to elevated triglyceride levels include excess body fat, physical inactivity, cigarette smoking, type 2 diabetes, excess alcohol intake, very high carbohydrate diets, and certain diseases and medications.

A full lipid profile should include testing and evaluation of triglyceride levels (see Table 12-2). For people with borderline high triglyceride levels, increased physical activity, reduced intake of added sugars and starches, and weight reduction can help bring levels down into the healthy range; for people with high triglyceride levels, drug therapy may be recommended. Being moderate in the use of alcohol and quitting smoking are also important.

**Psychological and Social Factors** Many of the psychological and social factors that influence other areas of wellness are also important risk factors for CVD. The idea that the mind and the body are connected certainly seems to be true when it comes to the heart. When you become excited or stressed or angry, you can probably feel your heart pounding harder and faster. The cardiovascular system is affected by both sudden, acute episodes of mental stress and the more chronic, underlying emotions of anger, anxiety, and depression.

- *Stress:* Excess stress can strain the heart and blood vessels over time and contribute to CVD. A full-blown stress response causes blood pressure and levels of blood glucose and cholesterol to rise; blood platelets become more likely to cluster, possibly enhancing the formation of artery-clogging clots. Stress can also trigger abnormal heart rhythms (arrhythmias), with potentially fatal consequences.
- *Chronic hostility and anger:* Certain traits in the hard-driving "Type A" personality—hostility, cynicism, and anger—are associated with increased risk of heart disease. Men prone to anger have two to three times the heart attack risk of calmer men and are much more likely to develop CVD at young ages. See the box "Anger, Hostility, and Heart Disease" for more information.
- *Suppressing psychological distress:* Suppressing anger and other negative emotions may also be hazardous. People who hide psychological distress appear to have higher rates of heart disease than people who experience similar distress but share it with others. People with so-called Type D personalities tend to be pessimistic, negative, and unhappy and to suppress these feelings.
- *Depression and anxiety:* Depression increases the risk of CVD in healthy individuals and the risk of adverse cardiac events in those who already have heart disease. Depression can cause physiological changes, such as increases in stress hormones, and may also affect lifestyle in ways that are not heart-healthy. Chronic anxiety and anxiety disorders are associated with up to a three-fold increased risk of heart attack.
- *Social isolation:* People with little social support are at higher risk for dying from CVD than people with close ties to others. A strong social support network is a major antidote to stress. Friends and family members can also promote and support a healthy lifestyle.
- *Low socioeconomic status:* Poverty and low educational attainment also increase risk for CVD. These associations are probably due to a variety of factors, including lifestyle and access to health care.

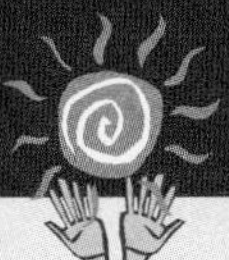

## Anger, Hostility, and Heart Disease

Current research suggests that people with a quick temper, a persistently hostile outlook, and a cynical, mistrusting attitude toward life are more likely to develop heart disease than those with a calmer, more trusting attitude. People who are angry frequently, intensely, and for long periods experience the stress response—and its accompanying boosts in heart rate, blood pressure, and stress hormone levels—much more often than more relaxed individuals. Over the long term, these effects may damage arteries and promote CVD.

### Are You Too Hostile?

To help answer that question, Duke University researcher Redford Williams, M.D., has devised a short self-test. It's not a scientific evaluation, but it does offer a rough measure of hostility. Are the following statements true or false for you?

1. I often get annoyed at checkout cashiers or the people in front of me when I'm waiting in line.
2. I usually keep an eye on the people I work or live with to make sure they do what they should.
3. I often wonder how homeless people can have so little respect for themselves.
4. I believe that most people will take advantage of you if you let them.
5. The habits of friends or family members often annoy me.
6. When I'm stuck in traffic, I often start breathing faster and my heart pounds.
7. When I'm annoyed with people, I really want to let them know it.
8. If someone does me wrong, I want to get even.
9. I'd like to have the last word in any argument.
10. At least once a week, I have the urge to yell at or even hit someone.

According to Williams, five or more "true" statements suggest that you're excessively hostile and should consider taking steps to mellow out.

### Managing Your Anger

Begin by monitoring your angry responses and looking for triggers—people or situations that typically make you angry. Familiarize yourself with the patterns of thinking that lead to angry or hostile feelings, and then try to head them off before they develop into full-blown anger. If you feel your anger starting to build, try reasoning with yourself by asking the following questions:

1. *Is this really important enough to get angry about?* For example, is having to wait an extra 5 minutes for a late bus so important that you should stew about it for the entire 15-minute ride?
2. *Am I really justified in getting angry?* Is the person in front of you really driving slowly, or are you trying to speed?
3. *Is getting angry going to make a real and positive difference in this situation?* Will yelling and slamming the door really help your friend find the concert tickets he misplaced?

If you answer yes to all three questions, then calm but assertive communication may be an appropriate response. If your anger isn't reasonable, try distracting yourself or removing yourself from the situation. Exercise, humor, social support, and other stress-management techniques can also help (see Chapter 3 for additional anger-management tips). Your heart—and the people around you—will benefit from your calmer, more positive outlook.

SOURCES: Take it to heart: "Chill out." 2000. *Mind/Body Health Newsletter* 9(2): 1–2; Anger and heart-disease risk. 2000. *Harvard Heart Letter,* July. QUIZ SOURCE: Williams, Virginia, and Redford Williams. *Life Skills.* New York: Times Books. Reprinted by permission of the authors.

**Alcohol and Drugs** Although moderate drinking may have health benefits for some people, drinking too much alcohol raises blood pressure and can increase the risk of stroke and heart failure. Stimulant drugs, particularly cocaine, can also cause serious cardiac problems, including heart attack, stroke, and sudden cardiac death. The risk increases if cocaine use is combined with use of tobacco or another drug. Injection drug use can cause infection of the heart and stroke.

## Major Risk Factors That Can't Be Changed

A number of major risk factors for CVD cannot be changed: heredity, aging, being male, and ethnicity.

**Heredity** CVD is considered a genetically complex disease because there is no one gene that causes it. Instead, multiple genes contribute to the development of CVD and its associated risk factors, such as high cholesterol, hypertension, diabetes, and obesity. Having a favorable set of genes decreases your risk of developing CVD; having an unfavorable set of genes increases your risk. Risk, however, is modifiable by lifestyle factors such as whether you smoke, exercise, or eat a healthy diet.

**Aging** The risk of heart attack increases dramatically after age 65. About 70% of all heart attack victims are age 65 or older, and more than four out of five who suffer fatal heart attacks are over 65. For people over 55, the incidence of stroke more than doubles in each successive decade. However, many people in their thirties and forties, especially men, have heart attacks.

**Being Male** Although CVD is the leading killer of both men and women in the United States, men face a

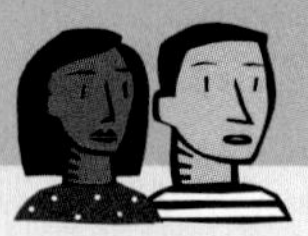

Gender Matters

## Women and CVD

On average, women live 10–15 more years free of coronary heart disease than men do. But heart disease is the leading cause of death among women, and it has killed more women than men every year since 1984.

Polls indicate that women vastly underestimate their risk of dying of a heart attack and, in turn, overestimate their risk of dying of breast cancer. In reality, nearly 1 in 2 women dies of CVD, whereas 1 in 30 dies of breast cancer. Minority women face the highest risk of developing CVD, but their awareness of heart disease as a killer of women is lower than among white women. To help raise awareness of CVD in women, the American Heart Association launched the "Go Red for Women" campaign in 2004; visit their Web site for more information (www.americanheart.org).

Risk factors for CVD are similar for men and women, but there are some gender differences. HDL appears to be an even more powerful predictor of CVD risk in women than it is in men. Also, women with diabetes have a greater risk of CVD, so much so that diabetes appears to eliminate the 10- to 15-year advantage women traditionally have had over men for CVD.

### Estrogen: A Heart Protector?

The hormone estrogen, produced naturally by a woman's ovaries until menopause, improves blood lipid concentrations and other CVD risk factors. For the past several decades, many U.S. physicians encouraged menopausal women to take hormone replacement therapy (HRT) to relieve menopause symptoms and presumably reduce the risk of CVD. However, recent studies have found that HRT may actually *increase* a woman's risk for heart disease and certain other health problems, and the U.S. Preventive Services Task Force currently recommends against the use of HRT for the prevention of chronic diseases such as CVD.

For younger women, the most common form of hormonal medication is oral contraceptives (OCs). Typical OCs contain estrogen and progestin in relatively low doses and are generally considered safe for most nonsmoking women. But women who smoke and use OCs are up to 32 times more likely to have a heart attack than nonsmoking OC users.

### Postmenopausal Women: At Risk

When women do have heart attacks, they are more likely than men to die within a year. One reason is that because women develop heart disease at older ages, they are more likely to have other health problems that complicate treatment. Women also have smaller hearts and arteries than men, possibly making diagnosis and treatment more difficult. There may also be unknown biological or psychosocial risk factors contributing to increased mortality among women.

Another reason is that medical personnel appear to evaluate and treat women less aggressively than men. Women with positive stress tests and those with a recent MI are less likely to be referred to catheterization than are men with similar findings, and coronary angiography is performed more often in men than in women.

Studies of heart attack patients have found that women usually have to wait longer than men to receive clot-dissolving drugs in an emergency room. Women are more likely than men to have a heart attack *without* chest pain. In one study, many women reported severe fatigue and disturbed sleep in the month leading up to the attack, and fatigue, weakness, and shortness of breath during the attack. Women are also more likely than men to report nausea and pain in the abdomen, back, neck, and/or jaw.

Careful diagnosis of cardiac symptoms is also key in cases of stress cardiomyopathy ("broken heart syndrome"), which occurs much more commonly in women. In this condition, exposure to hormones and neurotransmitters associated with a severe stress response stun the heart and produce heart-attack-like symptoms without any corresponding damage to the heart muscle. Typically, the condition can be reversed quickly, and correct diagnosis is important to avoid unnecessary invasive procedures.

Researchers are now focusing more attention on the health problems of women, and more accurate diagnostic techniques may soon be in use. And of course, positive lifestyle choices such as physical activity, quitting smoking, and management of risk factors like blood pressure and cholesterol levels are recommended for women of all ages.

greater risk of heart attack than women, especially earlier in life. Until age 55, men also have a greater risk of hypertension than women. By age 75, the gender gap nearly disappears (see the box "Women and CVD").

**Ethnicity** Death rates from heart disease vary among ethnic groups in the United States, with African Americans having much higher rates of hypertension, heart disease, and stroke than other groups (see the box "Ethnicity and CVD"). Puerto Rican Americans, Cuban Americans, and Mexican Americans are also more likely to suffer from high blood pressure and angina (a warning sign of heart disease) than non-Hispanic white Americans. These differences may be due in part to differences in education, income, and other socioeconomic factors. Asian Americans historically have had far lower rates of CVD than white Americans. However, cholesterol levels among Asian Americans appear to be rising, presumably because of the adoption of a high-fat American diet.

## Possible Risk Factors Currently Being Studied

In recent years, a number of other possible risk factors for CVD have been identified. Some of the most studied are described in this section.

**Inflammation and C-Reactive Protein** Inflammation plays a key role in the development of CVD. When an artery is injured by smoking, cholesterol, infectious

Dimensions of Diversity

## Ethnicity and CVD

African Americans are at substantially higher risk for death from CVD than other groups. The rate of hypertension among African Americans is among the highest of any group in the world. Blacks tend to develop hypertension at an earlier age than whites, and their average blood pressures are much higher. African Americans have a higher risk of stroke, have strokes at younger ages, and, if they survive, have more significant stroke-related disabilities. Some experts recommend that blacks be treated with antihypertensive drugs at an earlier stage—when blood pressure reaches 130/80 rather than the typical 140/90 cutoff for hypertension.

A number of genetic and biological factors may contribute to CVD in African Americans. They may be more sensitive to dietary sodium, leading to greater blood pressure elevation in response to a given amount of sodium. African Americans may also experience less dilation of blood vessels in response to stress, an attribute that also raises blood pressure.

Heredity also plays a large role in the tendency to develop diabetes, another important CVD risk factor that is more common in blacks than whites. However, Latinos are even more likely to develop diabetes and insulin resistance, and at a younger age, than blacks. There is variation within the Latino population, however, with a higher prevalence of diabetes occurring among Mexican Americans and Puerto Ricans and a relatively lower prevalence among the Cuban Americans.

Another factor that likely contributes to the high incidence of CVD among ethnic minority groups is low income. Economic deprivation usually means reduced access to adequate health care and health insurance. Also associated with low income is low educational attainment, which often mean less information about preventive health measures, such as diet and stress management. And people with low incomes tend to smoke more, use more salt, and exercise less than those with higher incomes.

Discrimination may also play a role in CVD. Physicians and hospitals may treat the medical problems of ethnic minorities differently than those of whites. Discrimination, along with low income and other forms of deprivation, may also increase stress, which is linked with hypertension and CVD. In terms of access to care, factors such as insurance coverage and availability of high-tech cardiac equipment in hospitals used most often by minorities may also play a role.

CVD risk in ethnic groups is further affected by immigration and one's place of birth. Upon immigration to the United States, an Asian's risk for CVD tends to increase and reflect that of a typical American more than a typical Asian, perhaps in part because Asian immigrants often abandon their traditional (and healthier) diets.

However, birthplace (and its associated lifestyle factors) also seems to be a strong determinant of risk. One study found that among New Yorkers born in the Northeast, blacks and whites have nearly identical risk of CVD. But black New Yorkers who were born in the South have a sharply higher risk, and black New Yorkers born in the Caribbean have a significantly lower risk. Researchers speculate that instead of abandoning their traditional diets and lifestyles, blacks from the South instead bring these traditions with them. Some risk factors for CVD, including smoking and a high-fat diet, are more common in the South. When combined with urban stress, these factors create a lifestyle that is far from heart-healthy.

All Americans are advised to have their blood pressure checked regularly, exercise, eat a healthy diet, manage stress, and avoid smoking. These general preventive strategies may be particularly helpful for ethnic minorities. Tailoring your lifestyle to your particular ethnic risk may also be helpful in some cases. For example, studies have found that diets high in potassium and calcium may be particularly helpful in improving blood pressure in African Americans; fruits, vegetables, grains, and nuts are rich in potassium, and dairy products are high in calcium. Latinos, who are at greater risk for insulin resistance, may benefit from lifestyle strategies targeting metabolic syndrome. Discuss your particular risk profile with your physician to help identify lifestyle changes most appropriate for you.

agents, or other factors, the body's response produces inflammation. A substance called C-reactive protein (CRP) is released into the bloodstream during the inflammatory response, and studies suggest that high levels of CRP indicate a substantially elevated risk of heart attack and stroke.

In 2003, the CDC and the American Heart Association jointly recommended testing of CRP levels for people at intermediate risk for CVD because people in this risk category who are found to also have high CRP levels may benefit from additional CVD testing or treatment. (This guideline assumes that people at high risk for CVD are already receiving treatment.) Lifestyle changes and certain drugs can reduce CRP levels. Statin drugs, widely prescribed to lower cholesterol, also decrease inflammation and reduce CRP levels; this may be one reason why statin drugs seem to lower CVD risk even in people with normal blood lipid levels.

### Insulin Resistance and Metabolic Syndrome

As described in Chapter 9, when you consume carbohydrate, your blood glucose level increases. This stimulates the pancreas to secrete insulin, which allows body cells to pick up glucose to use for energy. As people gain weight and engage in less physical activity, their muscles, fat, and liver become less sensitive to the effect of insulin—a condition known as insulin resistance (or pre-diabetes). As the body becomes increasingly insulin resistant, the pancreas must secrete more and more insulin to keep glucose levels within a normal range (hyperinsulinemia). Eventually,

**Table 12-3 Defining Characteristics of Metabolic Syndrome***

| | |
|---|---|
| Abdominal obesity (waist circumference) | |
| Men | >40 in (>102 cm) |
| Women | >35 in (>88 cm) |
| Triglycerides | ≥150 mg/dl |
| HDL cholesterol | |
| Men | <40 mg/dl |
| Women | <50 mg/dl |
| Blood pressure | ≥130/≥85 mm Hg |
| Fasting glucose | ≥110 mg/dl |

*A person is diagnosed with metabolic syndrome if she or he has three or more of the risk factors listed here.

SOURCE: National Cholesterol Education Program. 2001. *ATP III Guidelines At-A-Glance Quick Desk Reference.* Bethesda, Md.: National Heart, Lung, and Blood Institute. NIH Publication No. 01-3305.

however, even high levels of insulin may become insufficient, and blood glucose levels will also start to rise (hyperglycemia), resulting in type 2 diabetes.

Those who have insulin resistance tend to have several other related risk factors; as a group, this cluster of abnormalities is called metabolic syndrome, insulin resistance syndrome, or syndrome X (Table 12-3). Having metabolic syndrome significantly increases the risk of CVD—up to three times in men and six times in women. It is estimated that nearly 25% of the U.S. population has metabolic syndrome. Rates are highest among Mexican Americans, especially women. Among whites, the prevalence is similar in men and women, but among African Americans, the prevalence among women is 57% higher than in men.

To reduce your risk for metabolic syndrome, choose a healthy diet and get plenty of exercise. Regular physical activity increases your body's sensitivity to insulin in addition to improving cholesterol levels and decreasing blood pressure. Reducing calorie intake to prevent weight gain or losing weight if needed will also reduce insulin resistance. The amount and type of carbohydrate intake is also important: Diets very high in carbohydrates, especially high-glycemic-index foods, can raise levels of glucose and triglycerides and lower HDL, thus contributing to the development or worsening of metabolic syndrome and CVD, particularly in people who are already sedentary and overweight. For people prone to insulin resistance, eating more unsaturated fats, protein, vegetables, and fiber while limiting added sugars and starches may be beneficial.

**Homocysteine** Elevated levels of homocysteine, an amino acid circulating in the blood, are associated with an increased risk of CVD. Homocysteine appears to damage the lining of blood vessels, resulting in inflammation and the development of fatty deposits in artery walls. These changes can lead to the formation of clots and blockages in arteries, which in turn can cause heart attacks and strokes. Men generally have higher homocysteine levels than women, as do individuals with diets low in folic acid, vitamin B-12, and vitamin B-6. Most people can lower homocysteine levels easily by adopting a healthy diet rich in fruits, vegetables, and grains and by taking supplements if needed.

## MAJOR FORMS OF CARDIOVASCULAR DISEASE

Collectively, the various forms of CVD kill more Americans than the next four leading causes of death combined. The financial burden of CVD, including the costs of medical treatments and lost productivity, is nearly $400 billion annually. The main forms of CVD are interrelated and have elements in common; we treat them separately here for the sake of clarity. Hypertension, which is both a major risk factor and a form of CVD, was described earlier in the chapter.

### Atherosclerosis

Atherosclerosis is a form of arteriosclerosis, or thickening and hardening of the arteries. In atherosclerosis, arteries become narrowed by deposits of fat, cholesterol, and other substances. The process begins when the cells that line the arteries (endothelial cells) become damaged, most likely through a combination of factors such as smoking, high blood pressure, high insulin or glucose levels, deposits of oxidized LDL particles, and high homocysteine levels. The body's response to this damage results in inflammation and changes in the artery lining that create a sort of magnet for LDL, platelets, and other cells; these cells build up and cause a bulge in the wall of the artery. As these deposits, called **plaques,** accumulate on artery walls, the arteries lose their elasticity and their ability to expand and contract, restricting blood flow. Once narrowed by a plaque, an artery is vulnerable to blockage by blood clots (Figure 12-3).

If the heart, brain, and/or other organs are deprived of blood, and thus the vital oxygen it carries, the effects of

### Terms

VW

**plaque** A deposit of fatty (and other) substances on the inner wall of the arteries.

**coronary heart disease (CHD)** Heart disease caused by atherosclerosis in the arteries that supply oxygen to the heart muscle; also called *coronary artery disease.*

**heart attack** Damage to, or death of, heart muscle, sometimes resulting in a failure of the heart to deliver enough blood to the body; also known as *myocardial infarction (MI).*

**coronary thrombosis** A clot in a coronary artery, often causing sudden death.

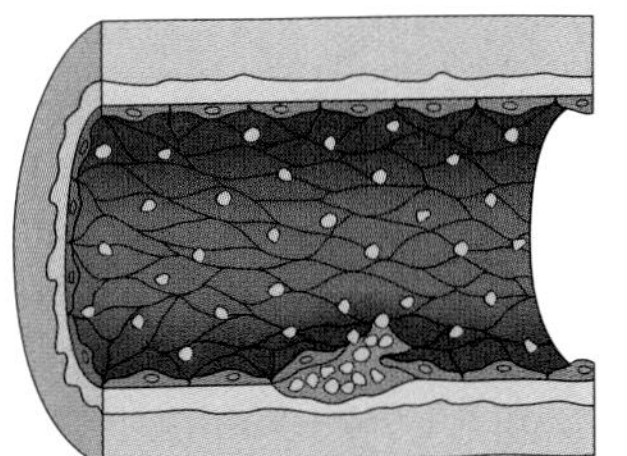

Plaque buildup begins when endothelial cells lining the arteries are damaged by smoking, high blood pressure, oxidized LDL, and other causes; excess cholesterol particles collect beneath these cells.

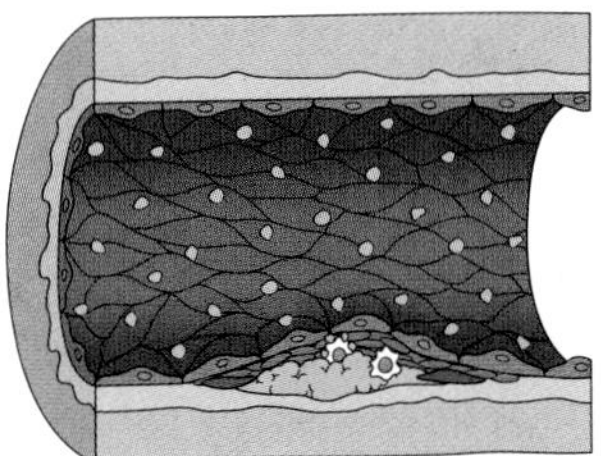

In response to the damage, platelets and other types of cells collect at the site; a fibrous cap forms, isolating the plaque within the artery wall. An early-stage plaque is called a fatty streak.

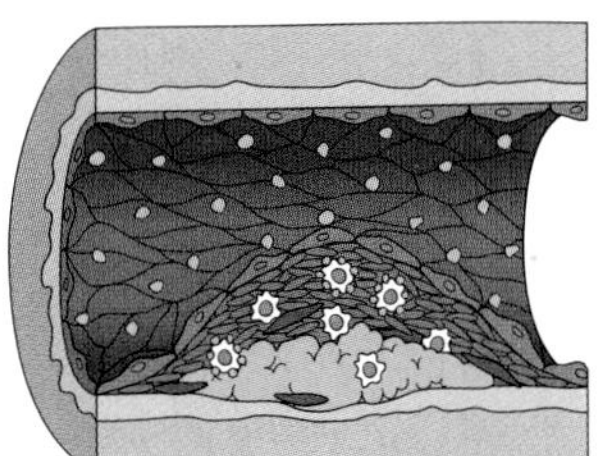

Chemicals released by cells in and around the plaque cause further inflammation and buildup; an advanced plaque contains LDL, white blood cells, connective tissue, smooth muscle cells, platelets, and other compounds.

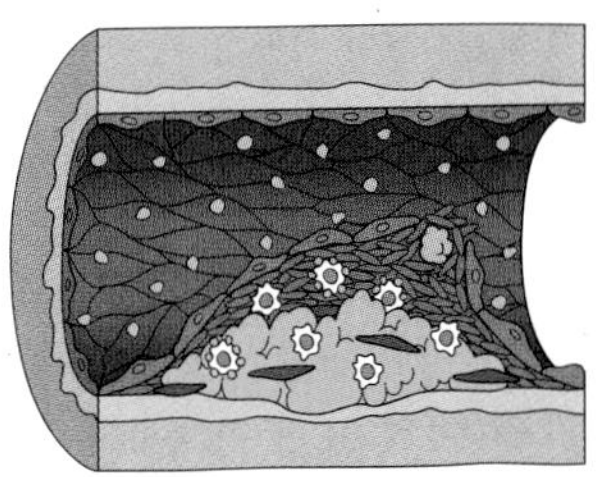

The narrowed artery is vulnerable to blockage by clots. The risk of blockage and heart attack rises if the fibrous cap cracks (probably due to destructive enzymes released by white blood cells within the plaque).

**Figure 12-3 Stages of plaque development.**

atherosclerosis can be deadly. Coronary arteries, which supply the heart with blood, are particularly susceptible to plaque buildup, a condition called **coronary heart disease (CHD),** or *coronary artery disease (CAD).* The blockage of a coronary artery causes a heart attack. If a cerebral artery (leading to the brain) is blocked, the result is a stroke. If an artery in a limb becomes narrowed or blocked, it causes *peripheral arterial disease,* a condition that causes pain and sometimes loss of the affected limb.

The main risk factors for atherosclerosis are cigarette smoking, physical inactivity, high levels of blood cholesterol, high blood pressure, and diabetes. Atherosclerosis often begins in childhood.

## Heart Disease and Heart Attack

Every year, about 1.2 million Americans have a heart attack (Figure 12-4). Although a **heart attack,** or myocardial infarction (MI), may come without warning, it is usually the end result of a long-term disease process. When one of the coronary arteries, the arteries that branch off the aorta and supply blood directly to the heart muscle, becomes blocked, a heart attack results. A heart attack caused by a clot is called a **coronary thrombosis.** During a heart attack, part of the heart muscle (myocardium) may die from lack of oxygen. If an MI is not fatal, the heart muscle may sometimes partially repair itself.

Symptoms of MI may include chest pain or pressure; arm, neck, or jaw pain; difficulty breathing; excessive sweating; nausea and vomiting; and loss of consciousness. Although chest pain occurs in the majority of MI victims, a recent study of over 750,000 MI patients revealed that about one-third of people having a heart attack do not experience chest pain. Women, ethnic minorities, older adults, and people with diabetes were the most likely groups to experience heart attack without chest pain or to have several other accompanying symptoms.

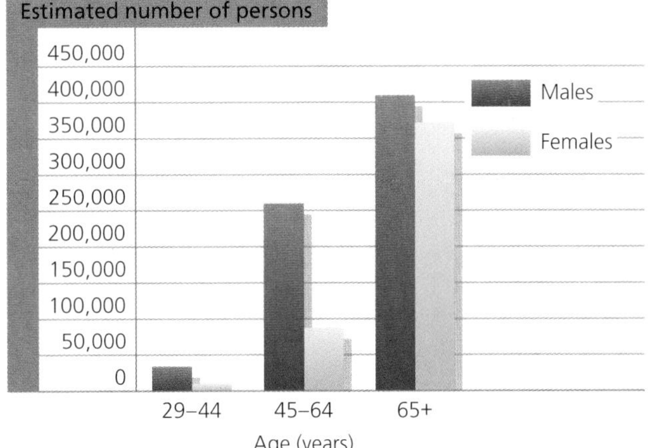


(a) Annual incidence of heart attack

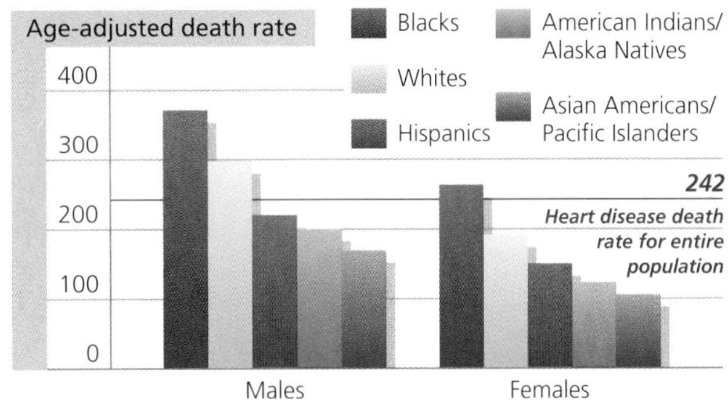


(b) Heart disease death rates

VITAL STATISTICS

**Figure 12-4 A statistical look at cardiovascular disease in the United States.** (a) Estimated numbers of Americans who have a heart attack each year. Among heart attack victims under age 65, men significantly outnumber women; after age 65, women start to catch up. (b) Heart disease death rates by gender and ethnicity.

SOURCES: American Heart Association. 2005. *2005 Heart and Stroke Facts Statistical Update.* Dallas, Tex.: American Heart Association; National Center for Health Statistics. 2004. *Health, United States, 2004.* Hyattsville, Md.: U.S. Public Health Service.

**Angina** Arteries narrowed by disease may still be open enough to deliver blood to the heart. At times, however—primarily during emotional excitement, stress, or physical exertion—the heart requires more oxygen than narrowed arteries can accommodate. When the need for oxygen exceeds the supply, chest pain, called **angina pectoris,** may occur. Angina pain is felt as an extreme tightness in the chest and heavy pressure behind the breastbone or in the shoulder, neck, arm, hand, or back. Angina may be controlled in a number of ways (with drugs and surgical or nonsurgical procedures), but its course is unpredictable. Over a period ranging from hours to years, the narrowing may go on to full blockage and a heart attack.

**Arrhythmias and Sudden Cardiac Death** The pumping of the heart is controlled by electrical impulses from the sinus node that maintain a regular heartbeat of 60–100 beats per minute. If this electrical conduction system is disrupted, the heart may beat too quickly, too slowly, or in an irregular fashion, a condition known as **arrhythmia.** Arrhythmia can cause symptoms ranging from imperceptible to severe and even fatal.

**Sudden cardiac death,** also called cardiac arrest, is most often caused by an arrhythmia called ventricular fibrillation, a kind of quivering of the ventricle that makes it ineffective in pumping blood. If ventricular fibrillation continues for more than a few minutes, it is fatal. Cardiac defribrillation, in which an electrical shock is delivered to the heart, can be effective in jolting the heart into a more efficient rhythm. Some arrhythmias cause no problems and resolve without treatment; more serious arrhythmias are usually treated with medication or a surgically implanted pacemaker or defibrillator that delivers electrical stimulation to the heart to create a more normal rhythm.

## Terms

VW

**angina pectoris** Pain in the chest, and often in the left arm and shoulder, caused by the heart muscle not receiving enough blood.

**arrhythmia** A change in the normal pattern of the heartbeat.

**sudden cardiac death** A nontraumatic, unexpected death from sudden cardiac arrest, most often due to arrhythmia; in most instances, victims have underlying heart disease.

**cardiopulmonary resuscitation (CPR)** A technique involving mouth-to-mouth breathing and chest compression to keep oxygen flowing to the brain.

**electrocardiogram (ECG or EKG)** A test to detect abnormalities by measuring the electrical activity in the heart.

**stroke** An impeded blood supply to some part of the brain resulting in the destruction of brain cells; also called *cerebrovascular accident.*

**ischemic stroke** Impeded blood supply to the brain caused by the obstruction of a blood vessel by a clot.

**hemorrhagic stroke** Impeded blood supply to the brain caused by the rupture of a blood vessel.

**Helping a Heart Attack Victim** Most people who die from a heart attack do so within 2 hours from the time they experience the first symptoms. If you or someone you are with has any of the warning signs of heart attack listed in the box "What to Do in Case of a Heart Attack, Cardiac Arrest, or Stroke," take immediate action. Get help even if the person denies there is something wrong. One additional step recommended by many experts is for the affected individual to chew and swallow one adult aspirin tablet (325 mg); aspirin has an immediate anticlotting effect.

If the person loses consciousness, emergency **cardiopulmonary resuscitation (CPR)** should be initiated by a qualified person. If the victim receives emergency care quickly enough, a clot-dissolving agent can be injected to break up a clot in the coronary artery. These clot-busting drugs are being used successfully to treat not only heart attacks but also some types of stroke.

**Detecting and Treating Heart Disease** Currently, the most common initial screening tool for heart disease is the stress, or exercise, test, in which a patient runs or walks on a treadmill or pedals a stationary cycle while being monitored for abnormalities with an **electrocardiogram (ECG** or **EKG).** Certain characteristic changes in the heart's electrical activity while under stress can reveal particular heart problems, such as restricted blood flow. Exercise testing can also be performed in conjunction with techniques such as nuclear medicine that provide further information about the heart and arteries. Other non-invasive tests for evaluating CVD include electron-beam computed tomography (EBCT), which detects calcium in the arteries, a marker for atherosclerosis; echocardiographic equipment, which utilizes sound waves to examine the heart; and magnetic resonance imaging, which uses powerful magnets to generate pictures of the heart and blood vessels. If symptoms or non-invasive tests suggest coronary artery disease, the next step is usually a coronary angiogram. In this test, a catheter (small plastic tube) is threaded into the opening of the coronary artery and a special dye is njected. The dye can be seen moving through the arteries under moving X ray, and any narrowings or blockages can be identified.

Treatments ranging from changes in diet to major surgery are available if a problem is detected. Along with a low-fat diet, regular exercise, and smoking cessation, one frequent nonsurgical recommendation for people at high risk for CVD is to take an aspirin tablet every day. (Low-dose aspirin therapy appears to help prevent first heart attacks in men, second heart attacks in men and women, and strokes in women over age 65.) Prescription drugs can help control heart rate, dilate arteries, lower blood pressure, and reduce the strain on the heart.

A common procedure for treating heart disease is *balloon angioplasty*. This technique involves threading a

Take Charge

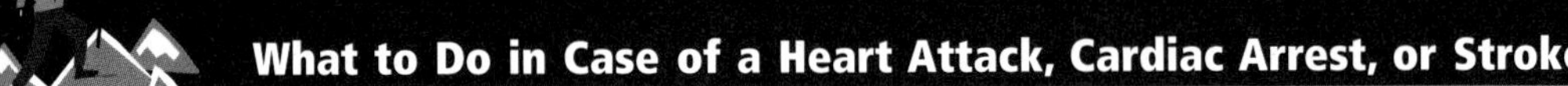

## What to Do in Case of a Heart Attack, Cardiac Arrest, or Stroke

### Heart Attack Warning Signs

Some heart attacks are sudden and intense—the "movie heart attack," where no one doubts what's happening. But most heart attacks start slowly, with mild pain or discomfort. Often people affected aren't sure what's wrong and wait too long before getting help. Here are signs that can mean a heart attack is happening:

- **Chest discomfort.** Most heart attacks involve discomfort in the center of the chest that lasts more than a few minutes, or that goes away and comes back. It can feel like uncomfortable pressure, squeezing, fullness, or pain.
- **Discomfort in other areas of the upper body.** Symptoms can include pain or discomfort in one or both arms, the back, neck, jaw or stomach.
- **Shortness of breath.** May occur with or without chest discomfort.
- **Other signs:** These may include breaking out in a cold sweat, nausea, or lightheadedness.

If you or someone you're with has chest discomfort, especially with one or more of the other signs, don't wait longer than a few minutes (no more than 5) before calling for help. Call 9-1-1 . . . Get to a hospital right away.

Calling 9-1-1 is almost always the fastest way to get lifesaving treatment. Emergency medical services staff can begin treatment when they arrive—up to an hour sooner than if someone gets to the hospital by car. The staff are also trained to revive someone whose heart has stopped. Patients with chest pain who arrive by ambulance usually receive faster treatment at the hospital, too.

If you can't access the emergency medical services (EMS), have someone drive you to the hospital right away. If you're the one having symptoms, don't drive yourself, unless you have absolutely no other option.

### Stroke Warning Signs

The American Stroke Association says these are the warning signs of stroke:

- Sudden numbness or weakness of the face, arm, or leg, especially on one side of the body
- Sudden confusion, trouble speaking or understanding
- Sudden trouble seeing in one or both eyes
- Sudden trouble walking, dizziness, or loss of balance or coordination
- Sudden, severe headache with no known cause

If you or someone with you has one or more of these signs, don't delay! Immediately call 9-1-1 or the emergency medical services (EMS) number so an ambulance (ideally with advanced life support) can be sent for you. Also, check the time so you'll know when the first symptoms appeared. It's very important to take immediate action. If given within three hours of the start of symptoms, a clot-busting drug can reduce long-term disability for the most common type of stroke.

### Cardiac arrest strikes immediately and without warning.

Here are the signs:

- Sudden loss of responsiveness. No response to gentle shaking.
- No normal breathing. The victim does not take a normal breath when you check for several seconds.
- No signs of circulation. No movement or coughing.

If cardiac arrest occurs, call 9-1-1 and begin CPR immediately. If an automated external defibrillator (AED) is available and someone trained to use it is nearby, involve her or him.

SOURCE: American Heart Association. 2005. Heart Attack, Stroke, and Cardiac Arrest Warning Signs. Reproduced with permission. www.americanheart.org. 

catheter with a deflated balloon on it through the artery until it reaches the area of blockage. The balloon is then inflated, flattening the fatty plaque and widening the arterial opening. This is generally followed by placement of a stent, a small metal tube that helps keep the artery open. Repeat clogging of the artery, known as restenosis, can occur, but the introduction of stents coated in medication, which is slowly released over a few months, significantly decreases the chance of restenosis. Every year, coronary bypass surgery is performed on over 300,000 people, about half of whom are under age 65. Cardiothoracic surgeons remove a healthy blood vessel, usually a vein from one of the patient's legs, and graft it from the aorta to one or more coronary arteries to bypass a blockage.

## Stroke

For brain cells to function as they should, they must have a continuous and ample supply of oxygen-rich blood. If brain cells are deprived of blood for more than a few minutes, they die. A **stroke**, also called a *cerebrovascular accident (CVA)*, occurs when the blood supply to the brain is cut off. Many experts now refer to strokes as "brain attacks" to emphasize their similarity to heart attacks and the importance of early treatment.

**Types of Strokes** There are two major types of strokes: **ischemic strokes**, which are caused by blockages in blood vessels, and **hemorrhagic strokes**, which are caused by rupture of blood vessels, leading to bleeding into

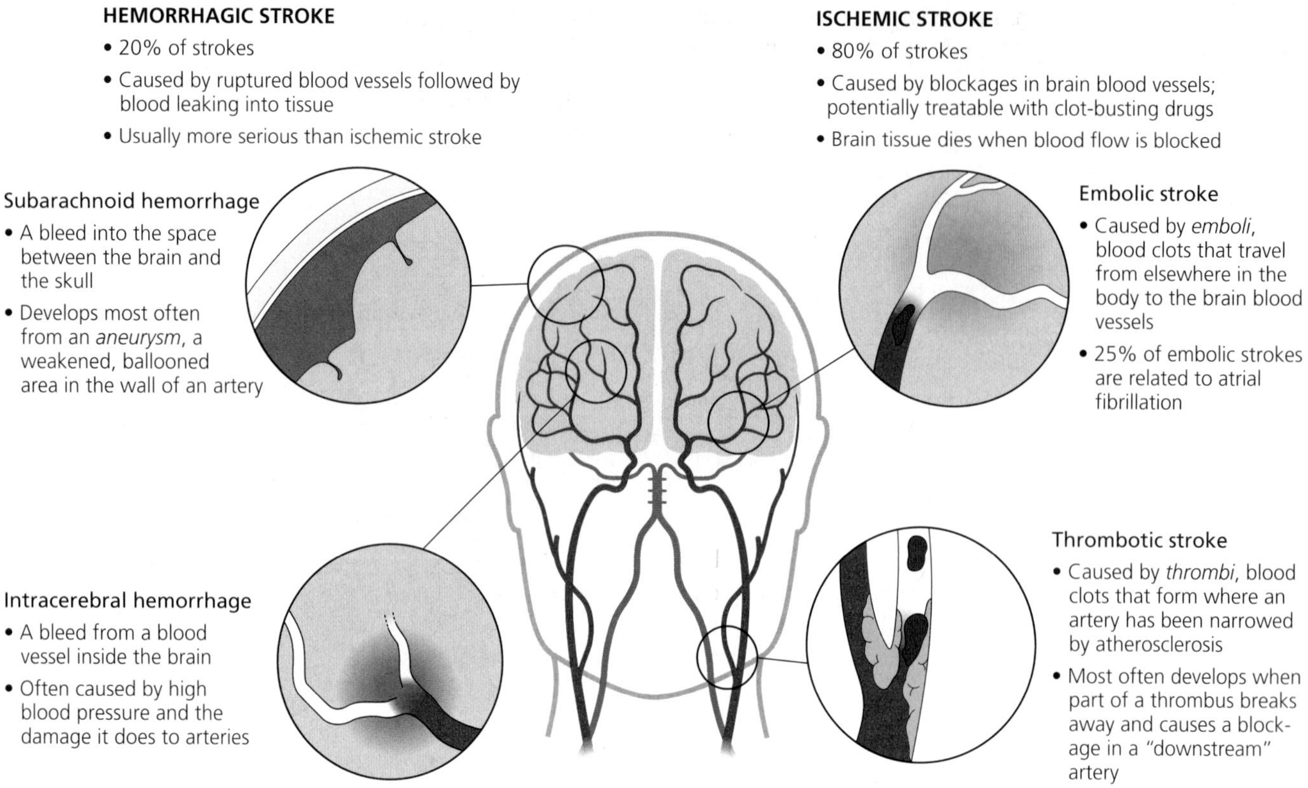

**HEMORRHAGIC STROKE**
- 20% of strokes
- Caused by ruptured blood vessels followed by blood leaking into tissue
- Usually more serious than ischemic stroke

Subarachnoid hemorrhage
- A bleed into the space between the brain and the skull
- Develops most often from an *aneurysm*, a weakened, ballooned area in the wall of an artery

Intracerebral hemorrhage
- A bleed from a blood vessel inside the brain
- Often caused by high blood pressure and the damage it does to arteries

**ISCHEMIC STROKE**
- 80% of strokes
- Caused by blockages in brain blood vessels; potentially treatable with clot-busting drugs
- Brain tissue dies when blood flow is blocked

Embolic stroke
- Caused by *emboli*, blood clots that travel from elsewhere in the body to the brain blood vessels
- 25% of embolic strokes are related to atrial fibrillation

Thrombotic stroke
- Caused by *thrombi*, blood clots that form where an artery has been narrowed by atherosclerosis
- Most often develops when part of a thrombus breaks away and causes a blockage in a "downstream" artery

**Figure 12-5 Types of stroke.** SOURCE: Types of stroke. 2000. *Harvard Health Letter*, April. Copyright © 2000 by Harriet R. Greenfield. Used by permission.

the brain (Figure 12-5). One type of ischemic stroke, the *thrombotic stroke*, is caused by a **thrombus**, a blood clot that forms in a cerebral artery that has been narrowed or damaged by atherosclerosis. The second type of ischemic stroke, called an *embolic stroke*, is caused by an **embolus**, a wandering blood clot that is carried in the bloodstream and may become wedged in one of the cerebral arteries. Many embolic strokes are linked to a type of abnormal heart rhythm called atrial fibrillation.

The other type of stroke, less common but more severe, is the hemorrhagic stroke. It occurs when a blood vessel in the brain bursts, spilling blood into the surrounding tissue. Cells normally nourished by the artery are deprived of blood and cannot function. In addition, accumulated blood from the burst vessel may put pressure on surrounding brain tissue, causing damage and even death. Hemorrhages can be caused by head injuries or the bursting of a malformed blood vessel or an **aneurysm**, a blood-filled pocket that bulges out from a weak spot in an artery wall. Aneurysms in the brain may remain stable and never break. But when they do, the result is a stroke. Aneurysms may be caused or worsened by high blood pressure.

**The Effects of a Stroke** The interruption of the blood supply to any area of the brain prevents the nerve cells there from functioning—in some cases causing death. Of the 700,000 Americans who have strokes each year, nearly one-third die within a year. Those who survive usually have some lasting disability. A stroke may cause paralysis, walking disability, speech impairment, memory loss, and changes in behavior. The severity of the stroke and its long-term effects depend on which brain cells have been injured, how widespread the damage is, how effectively the body can restore the blood supply, and how rapidly other areas of the brain can take over.

**Detecting and Treating Stroke** Effective treatment requires the prompt recognition of symptoms and correct diagnosis of the type of stroke that has occurred. Some stroke victims have a **transient ischemic attack (TIA)**, or ministroke, days, weeks, or months before they have a full-blown stroke. A TIA produces temporary strokelike symptoms, such as weakness or numbness in an arm or a leg, speech difficulty, or dizziness; but these symptoms are brief, often lasting just a few minutes, and do not cause permanent damage. However, TIAs should be taken as warning signs of a stroke, and anyone with a suspected TIA should get immediate medical help.

Strokes should be treated with the same urgency as heart attacks. A person with stroke symptoms should be rushed to the hospital. A **computed tomography (CT)** scan, which uses a computer to construct an image of the brain from X rays, can assess brain damage and determine the type of stroke. Newer techniques using MRI and ultrasound are becoming increasingly available and should improve the speed and accuracy of stroke diagnosis.

If tests reveal that a stroke is caused by a blood clot—and if help is sought within a few hours of the onset of symptoms—the person can be treated with the same kind of clot-dissolving drugs that are used to treat coronary artery blockages. If the clot is dissolved quickly enough, brain damage is minimized and symptoms may disappear. (The longer the brain goes without oxygen, the greater the risk of permanent damage.) People who have had TIAs or who are at high risk for stroke due to narrowing of the carotid arteries may undergo a surgical procedure called *carotid endarterectomy,* in which plaque is removed. There is also a nonsurgical procedure, similar to coronary angioplasty and stenting, that can be done in the carotid arteries.

If tests reveal that a stroke was caused by a cerebral hemorrhage, drugs may be prescribed to lower the blood pressure, which will usually be high. Careful diagnosis is crucial, because administering clot-dissolving drugs to a person suffering a hemorrhagic stroke would cause more bleeding and potentially more brain damage.

If detection and treatment of stroke come too late, rehabilitation is the only treatment. Although damaged or destroyed brain tissue does not normally regenerate, nerve cells in the brain can make new pathways, and some functions can be taken over by other parts of the brain. Some people recover completely in a matter of days or weeks, but most stroke victims who survive must adapt to a lifelong disability.

## Congestive Heart Failure

A number of conditions—high blood pressure, heart attack, atherosclerosis, alcoholism, viral infections, rheumatic fever, birth defects—can damage the heart's pumping mechanism. When the heart cannot maintain its regular pumping rate and force, fluids begin to back up. When extra fluid seeps through capillary walls, edema (swelling) results, usually in the legs and ankles, but sometimes in other parts of the body as well. Fluid can collect in the lungs and interfere with breathing, particularly when a person is lying down. This condition is called *pulmonary edema,* and the entire process is known as **congestive heart failure.** Treatment includes reducing the workload on the heart, modifying salt intake, and using drugs that help the body eliminate excess fluid. Heart transplant is a solution for some patients with severe heart failure, but the need greatly exceeds the number of hearts available.

The risk of heart failure increases with age, and being overweight is a significant independent risk factor. Experts fear that the incidence of heart failure will increase dramatically over the next few decades as our population ages and becomes increasingly obese.

## Other Forms of Heart Disease

Other, less common forms of heart disease include congenital heart disease, rheumatic heart disease, and heart valve disorders.

**Congenital Heart Disease** About 40,000 children born each year in the United States have a defect or malformation of the heart or major blood vessels. These conditions are collectively referred to as **congenital heart disease,** and they cause about 4300 deaths a year. The most common congenital defects are holes in the wall that divides the chambers of the heart and *coarctation of the aorta,* a narrowing, or constriction, of the aorta. Most congenital defects can be accurately diagnosed and treated with medication or surgery.

**Hypertrophic cardiomyopathy (HCM)** occurs in 1 out of every 500 people and is the most common cause of sudden death among athletes younger than age 35. It is an inherited condition that causes the heart muscle to become hypertrophic (enlarged), primarily in the septum, which is the area between the two ventricles. Young children with this disorder usually have no obvious symptoms; the hypertrophy generally develops gradually between ages 5 and 15. People with hypertrophic cardiomyopathy are at high risk for sudden death, mainly due to serious arrhythmias. A new test for hypertrophic cardiomyopathy using echocardiography may help health care providers diagnose the problem earlier, before serious problems arise. Individuals with hypertrophic cardiomyopathy should usually not participate in competitive sports because of the high risk of sudden death.

### Terms

**thrombus** A blood clot in a blood vessel that usually occurs at the point of its formation.

**embolus** A blood clot that breaks off from its place of origin in a blood vessel and travels through the bloodstream.

**aneurysm** A sac formed by a distention or dilation of the artery wall.

**transient ischemic attack (TIA)** A small stroke; usually a temporary interruption of blood supply to the brain, causing numbness or difficulty with speech.

**computed tomography (CT)** The use of computerized X ray images to create a cross-sectional depiction (scan) of tissue density.

**congestive heart failure** A condition resulting from the heart's inability to pump out all the blood that returns to it; blood backs up in the veins leading to the heart, causing an accumulation of fluid in various parts of the body.

**congenital heart disease** A defect or malformation of the heart or its major blood vessels present at birth.

**hypertrophic cardiomyopathy (HCM)** An inherited condition in which there is an enlargement of the heart muscle, especially between the two ventricles.

**Rheumatic Heart Disease** Worldwide, a leading cause of heart trouble is **rheumatic fever,** a consequence of certain types of untreated streptococcal throat infections (group A beta-hemolytic). Rheumatic fever can permanently damage the heart muscle and heart valves, a condition called rheumatic heart disease (RHD). Symptoms of strep throat include the sudden onset of a sore throat, painful swallowing, fever, swollen glands, headache, nausea, and vomiting. Rheumatic fever can be prevented by treating strep throat, when it occurs, with antibiotics.

**Heart Valve Disorders** Congenital defects and certain types of infections can cause abnormalities in the valves between the chambers of the heart. The most common heart valve disorder is **mitral valve prolapse (MVP),** which occurs in about 4% of the population. MVP is characterized by a "billowing" of the mitral valve, which separates the left ventricle and left atrium, during ventricular contraction; in some cases, blood leaks from the ventricle into the atrium. Most people with MVP have no symptoms, and treatment is usually unnecessary. Experts disagree over whether patients with MVP should take antibiotics prior to dental procedures to prevent infection of the defective valve; most often, only those patients with significant leakage of the valve are advised to take antibiotics.

## PROTECTING YOURSELF AGAINST CARDIOVASCULAR DISEASE

There are several important steps you can take now to lower your risk of developing CVD in the future.

### Eat Heart-Healthy

For most Americans, changing to a heart-healthy diet involves many of the changes suggested in the 2005 Dietary Guidelines for Americans: substituting unsaturated fats for saturated and trans fats and increasing intake of whole grains and fiber.

**Decreased Fat and Cholesterol Intake** The National Cholesterol Education Program (NCEP) recommends that all Americans over the age of 2 adopt a diet in which total fat consumption is no more than 30% of total daily calories, with no more than one-third of those fat calories (10% of total daily calories) coming from saturated fat. For people with heart disease or high LDL levels, the NCEP recommends a total fat intake of 25–35% of total daily calories and a saturated fat intake of less than 7% of total calories.

**Terms**

**rheumatic fever** A disease, mainly of children, characterized by fever, inflammation, and pain in the joints; often damages the heart muscle, a condition called rheumatic heart disease.

**mitral valve prolapse (MVP)** A condition in which the mitral valve "billows" out during ventricular contraction, possibly allowing leakage of blood from the left ventricle into the left atrium; often asymptomatic and usually requiring treatment only in cases of significant leakage.

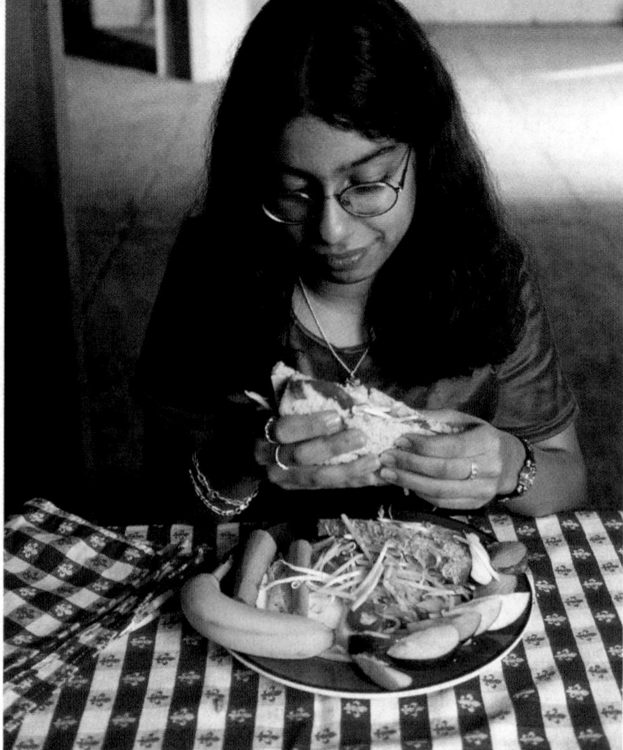

A diet high in fiber and low in saturated and trans fats can help lower levels of total cholesterol and LDL. This young woman is eating a vegetable sandwich on whole-grain bread with fresh fruit for lunch.

Saturated fats are found in animal products; palm and coconut oil; and hydrogenated vegetables oils, which are also high in trans fats. Choose unsaturated fats, especially monounsaturated fats and omega-3 polyunsaturated fats, over saturated and trans fats. Animal products contain cholesterol as well as saturated fat; vegetable products do not contain cholesterol. The NCEP recommends that most Americans limit dietary cholesterol intake to no more than 300 mg per day; for people with heart disease or high LDL levels, the suggested daily limit is 200 mg. The cholesterol content of packaged foods is provided on food labels, along with their total, saturated, and (beginning in 2006) trans fat content.

**Increased Fiber Intake** Fiber traps the bile acids the liver needs to manufacture cholesterol and carries them to the large intestine, where they are excreted. It slows the production of proteins that promote blood clotting. Fiber may also interfere with the absorption of dietary fat and may help you cut total food intake because foods rich in fiber tend to be filling. To obtain the recommended 25–38 grams of dietary fiber per day, choose a diet rich in whole grains, fruits, and vegetables. Good sources of fiber include oatmeal, some breakfast cereals, barley, legumes, and most fruits and vegetables.

**Decreased Sodium Intake and Increased Potassium Intake** The recommended limit for sodium intake is 2300 mg per day; for population groups at special risk, including those with hypertension, middle-aged and older adults, and African Americans, the recommended limit is 1500 mg per day. To limit sodium intake, read food labels carefully, and avoid foods particularly high in sodium; foods that are fresh, less processed, and less sodium-dense are good choices. Adequate potassium intake is also important in control of blood pressure. Good food sources include leafy green vegetables like spinach and beet greens, root vegetables like white and sweet potatoes, vine fruits like cantaloupe and honeydew melon, winter squash, bananas, many dried fruits, and tomato sauce.

**Moderate Alcohol Consumption (For Some)** The Dietary Guidelines for Americans state that moderate alcohol consumption may lower the risk of CHD among middle-aged and older adults. (Moderate means no more than one drink per day for women and two drinks per day for men.) For most people under age 45, however, the risks of alcohol use probably outweigh any health benefit. If you do drink, do so moderately, with food, and at times when drinking will not put you or others at risk.

**Other Dietary Factors** Researchers have identified other dietary factors that may affect CVD risk:

- *Omega-3 fatty acids.* Found in fish, shellfish, and some plant foods (nuts and canola, soybean, and flaxseed oils), omega-3 fatty acids may reduce clotting, abnormal heart rhythms, and inflammation and have other heart-healthy effects. The American Heart Association recommends eating fish two or more times a week.
- *Plant stanols and sterols.* Plant stanols and sterols, found in some new types of trans fat–free margarines and other products, reduce the absorption of cholesterol in the body and help lower LDL levels.
- *Folic acid, vitamin B-6, and vitamin B-12.* These vitamins affect CVD risk by lowering homocysteine levels.
- *Calcium.* Diets rich in calcium may help prevent hypertension and possibly stroke by reducing insulin resistance and platelet aggegration.
- *Soy protein.* Replacing some animal proteins with soy protein may lower LDL cholesterol. Soy-based foods include tofu and tempeh.
- *Healthy carbohydrates.* Most of the carbohydrates in the current American diet come from added sugars, refined grains, and starchy foods, including soft drinks, sweets, white potatoes (including those served as french fries), white bread, and refined ready-to-eat cereals; these foods are often relatively low in nutrients and have a high glycemic index. Healthier carbohydrates choices, including whole grains, fruits, and nonstarchy vegetables, typically provide more nutrients and have a lower glycemic index. Choosing healthy carbohydrates may be of particular importance for people with insulin resistance.
- *Total calories.* Reducing energy intake may improve cholesterol and triglyceride levels as much as reducing fat intake does. Reduced calorie intake also helps control body weight.

**DASH** A dietary plan that reflects many of the suggestions described here was released as part of a study called Dietary Approaches to Stop Hypertension, or DASH. The DASH diet plan is as follows:

- 7–8 servings per day of grains and grain products
- 4–5 servings per day of vegetables
- 4–5 servings per day of fruits
- 2–3 servings per day of low-fat or fat-free dairy products
- 2 or fewer servings per day of meats, poultry, and fish
- 4–5 servings per *week* of nuts, seeds, and legumes
- 2–3 servings per day of added fats, oils, and salad dressings
- 5 servings per *week* of snacks and sweets

## Exercise Regularly

You can significantly reduce your risk of CVD with a moderate amount of physical activity. Begin by accumulating at least 30 minutes of moderate-intensity physical activity each day. Activities like brisk walking, gardening, and stair climbing are appropriate. Increasing the duration or intensity of exercise can provide even greater health benefits. The American Heart Association recently recommended strength training in addition to aerobic exercise for building and maintaining cardiovascular health.

## Avoid Tobacco

Remember: The number-one risk factor for CVD that you can control is smoking. If you smoke, quit. If you don't, don't start. If you live or work with people who smoke, encourage them to quit—for their sake and yours. If you find yourself breathing in smoke, take steps to prevent or stop this exposure. Quitting smoking significantly reduces CVD risk, but smoking and exposure to ETS may permanently increase the rate of plaque formation in arteries. Quitting smoking is highly beneficial, but abstaining from cigarette smoking and avoiding ETS throughout your entire life is even better.

## Know and Manage Your Blood Pressure

If you have no CVD risk factors, have your blood pressure measured by a trained professional at least once every 2 years; yearly tests are recommended if you have other risk factors. If your blood pressure is high, follow your physician's advice on how to lower it.

## Know and Manage Your Cholesterol Levels

All people age 20 and over should have their cholesterol checked at least once every 5 years. Your LDL goal depends in part on how many of the following major risk factors you have: cigarette smoking, high blood pressure, low HDL cholesterol (less than 40 mg/dl), a family history of heart disease, and age (45 years and older for men, 55 years and older for women). An HDL level of 60 mg/dl or higher is protective and counts as a "negative" risk factor, meaning it removes one risk factor from your total count of risk factors.

Depending on your LDL level and other risk factors, your physician may recommend changes in lifestyle alone or lifestyle changes in combination with drug therapy. The lifestyle modifications recommended by the 2001 NCEP guidelines, known collectively as "Therapeutic Lifestyle Changes," or TLC, include the TLC diet, weight management, and increased physical activity. The TLC diet includes total fat intake of 25–35% of total daily calories, saturated fat intake less than 7% of total calories, and, for some people, 10–25 grams per day of viscous (soluble) fiber and 2 grams per day of plant stanols and sterols.

- If you have one or no risk factors, the NCEP sets an LDL goal of less than 160 mg/dl. If your LDL is below that level, maintain a healthy lifestyle by eating a heart-healthy diet, getting regular exercise, maintaining a healthy body weight, and not smoking. If your LDL is 160 mg/dl or higher, you should begin TLC; you may also need medication to bring your LDL into the healthy range.
- If you have two or more risk factors for heart disease, the NCEP sets an LDL goal of less than 130 mg/dl. If your LDL level is 130 or above, begin TLC; if your LDL level remains above the goal and your risk for CVD is fairly high, your physician may recommend medication.
- If you have heart disease or a condition such as diabetes that the NCEP considers the risk equivalent of heart disease, your goal for LDL is less than 100 mg/dl. For very high-risk patients, the goal was recently changed to less than 70 mg/dl. TLC is recommended for all people in this risk category. In addition, a variety of medications are available to lower LDL and improve other blood fat levels.

## Develop Effective Ways to Handle Stress and Anger

To reduce the psychological and social risk factors for CVD, develop effective strategies for handling the stress in your life. Shore up your social support network, and try some of the techniques described in Chapter 2 for managing stress.

## Manage Other Risk Factors and Medical Conditions

Know your CVD risk factors and follow your physician's advice for testing, lifestyle modification, and any drug treatments. If you are at high risk for CVD, consult a physician about taking small doses of aspirin. Low doses of aspirin (50–325 mg) are recommended for men and women to treat TIA, stroke, angina, heart attack, and certain other cardiovascular problems. Because of possible side effects, including gastrointestinal bleeding and increased risk of certain types of strokes, the FDA cautions people to consult with their physician before taking aspirin regularly.

# WHAT IS CANCER?

**Cancer** is the abnormal, uncontrolled growth of cells, which, if left untreated, can ultimately cause death.

## Benign Versus Malignant Tumors

Most cancers take the form of tumors, although not all tumors are cancerous. A tumor is simply a mass of tissue that serves no physiological purpose. It can be benign, like a wart, or malignant, like most lung cancers. The term **malignant tumor** (or *neoplasm*) is synonymous with cancer. **Benign tumors** are made up of cells similar to the surrounding normal cells and are enclosed in a membrane that prevents them from penetrating neighboring tissues. They are dangerous only if their physical presence interferes with body functions. A benign brain tumor, for example, can cause death if it blocks the blood supply to the brain.

### Terms

VW

**cancer** Abnormal, uncontrolled cellular growth.

**malignant tumor** A tumor that is cancerous and capable of spreading.

**benign tumor** A tumor that is not cancerous.

**lymphatic system** A system of vessels that returns proteins, lipids, and other substances from fluid in the tissues to the circulatory system.

**biopsy** The removal and examination of a small piece of body tissue; a needle biopsy uses a needle to remove a small sample; some biopsies require surgery.

**metastasis** The spread of cancer cells from one part of the body to another.

A malignant tumor, or cancer, is capable of invading surrounding structures, including blood vessels, the **lymphatic system,** and nerves. It can also spread to distant sites via the blood and lymphatic circulation, thereby producing invasive tumors in almost any part of the body. A few cancers, like leukemia, or cancer of the blood, do not produce a mass and therefore are not properly called tumors. But because leukemia cells do have the fundamental property of rapid, uncontrolled growth, they are still malignant and therefore cancers.

Every case of cancer begins as a change in a cell that allows it to grow and divide when it should not. Normally (in adults), cells divide and grow at a rate just sufficient to replace dying cells. In contrast, a malignant cell divides without regard for normal control mechanisms and gradually produces a mass of abnormal cells, or a tumor. It takes about a billion cells to make a mass the size of a pea, so a single tumor cell must go through many divisions, often taking years, before the tumor grows to a noticeable size.

Eventually a tumor produces a sign or symptom. In the breast, for example, a tumor may be felt as a lump and diagnosed as cancer by an X ray or **biopsy.** In less accessible locations, like the lung, ovary, or intestine, a tumor may be noticed only after considerable growth has taken place and may then be detected only by an indirect symptom—for instance, a persistent cough or unexplained bleeding or pain. In the case of leukemia, there is no lump, but the changes in the blood will eventually be noticed as increasing fatigue, infection, or abnormal bleeding.

## How Cancer Spreads: Metastasis

**Metastasis,** the spreading of cancer cells, occurs because cancer cells do not stick to each other as strongly as normal cells do and therefore may not remain at the site of the *primary tumor,* the original location. They break away and can pass through the lining of lymph or blood vessels to invade nearby tissue. They can also drift to distant parts of the body, where they establish new colonies of cancer cells. This traveling and seeding process is called metastasizing, and the new tumors are called *secondary tumors,* or *metastases.* This ability of cancer cells to metastasize makes early cancer detection critical. To control the cancer and prevent death, every cancerous cell must be removed. Once cancer cells enter either the lymphatic system or the bloodstream, it is extremely difficult to stop their spread to other organs of the body.

## Types of Cancer

The behavior of tumors arising in different body organs is characteristic of the tissue of origin. (Figure 12-6 shows

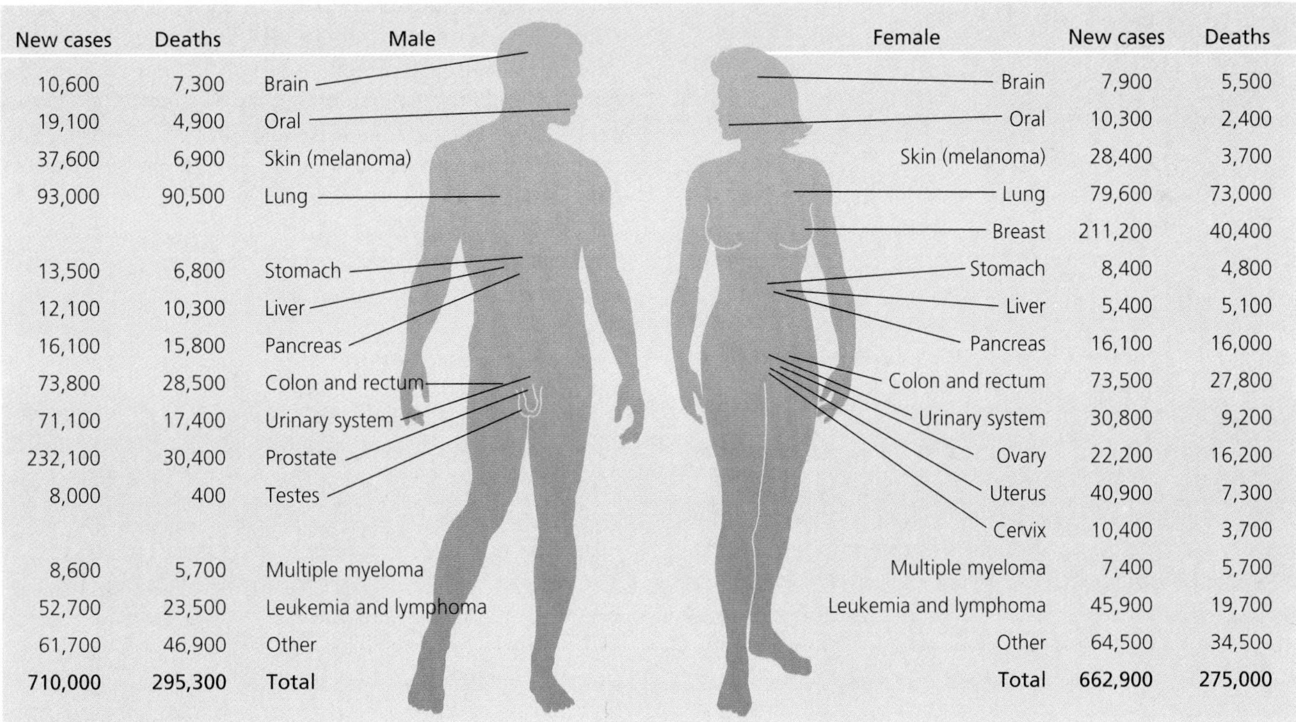


VITAL STATISTICS

**Figure 12-6 Cancer cases and deaths by site and sex.** The New cases column indicates the number of cancers that occurred in each site; the Deaths column indicates the number of cancer deaths that were attributed to each type. SOURCE: American Cancer Society. 2005. *Cancer Facts and Figures, 2005.* Atlanta: American Cancer Society.

the major cancer sites and the incidence of each type.) Malignant tumors are classified according to the types of cells that give rise to them:

- *Carcinomas* arise from epithelia, tissues that cover external body surfaces, line internal tubes and cavities, and form the secreting portion of glands. They are the most common type of cancers; major sites include the skin, breast, uterus, prostate, lungs, and gastrointestinal tract.
- *Sarcomas* arise from connective and fibrous tissues such as muscle, bone, cartilage, and the membranes covering muscles and fat.
- *Lymphomas* are cancers of the lymph nodes, part of the body's infection-fighting system.
- *Leukemias* are cancers of the blood-forming cells, which reside chiefly in the **bone marrow.**

There is a great deal of variation in how easily different cancers can be detected and how well they respond to treatment. For example, certain types of skin cancer are easily detected, grow slowly, and are very easy to remove; virtually all of the 1 million cases that occur each year in the United States are cured. Cancer of the pancreas, on the other hand, is very difficult to detect or treat, and very few patients survive the disease.

### The Incidence of Cancer

Each year, about 1.4 million people in the United States are diagnosed with cancer. Most will be cured, but about 36% will die as a result of their cancer within 5 years of diagnosis. These grim statistics exclude more than 1 million cases of the curable types of skin cancer. At current U.S. rates, nearly 1 in 2 men and more than 1 in 3 women will develop cancer at some point in their lives.

Are cancer deaths increasing in the United States? Until 1991, the answer was yes, largely due to a wave of lethal lung cancers among men caused by smoking. In 1991, the death rate stopped increasing and began to fall slowly. This is a very promising trend, as it suggests that efforts at prevention, early detection, and improved therapy are all bearing fruit. However, death rates from cancer are not declining as fast as those from heart disease, in large part because of the differing effects that quitting smoking has on disease risk: Heart-related damage of smoking reverses more quickly and more significantly than the cancer-related damage from smoking; smoking-related gene mutations cannot be reversed, although other mechanisms can sometimes control cellular changes. If heart disease death rates continue to decline faster than cancer death rates, cancer may overtake heart disease as the leading cause of death among Americans.

The American Cancer Society (ACS) estimates that 90% of skin cancer could be prevented by protecting the skin from the rays of the sun and 87% of lung cancer could be prevented by avoiding exposure to tobacco smoke. Thousands of cases of colon, breast, and uterine cancer could be prevented by improving the diet and controlling body weight. Regular screenings and self-examinations have the potential to save an additional 100,000 lives per year. There are many concrete strategies you can adopt to reduce your risk.

## COMMON CANCERS

A discussion of all types of cancer is beyond the scope of this book. In this section we look at some of the most common cancers and their causes, prevention, and treatment.

### Lung Cancer

Lung cancer is the most common cause of cancer death in the United States, responsible for about 163,000 deaths each year. For over 40 years, breast cancer was the major cause of cancer death in women, but since 1987 lung cancer has surpassed breast cancer as a killer of women.

**Risk Factors** The chief risk factor for lung cancer is tobacco smoke, which accounts for 87% of cancers. When smoking is combined with exposure to other **carcinogens,** such as asbestos particles or certain pollutants, the risk of cancer can be multiplied by a factor of 10 or more. Long-term exposure to ETS also increases the risk of lung cancer. Secondhand smoke, the smoke from the burning end of the cigarette, has significantly higher concentrations of the toxic and carcinogenic compounds found in mainstream smoke. It is estimated that ETS causes about 3000 lung cancer deaths each year.

**Detection and Treatment** Lung cancer is difficult to detect at an early stage and hard to cure even when detected early. Symptoms of lung cancer do not usually appear until the disease has advanced to the invasive stage. Signals such as a persistent cough, chest pain, or recurring bronchitis may be the first indication of a tumor's presence. A diagnosis can usually be made by CT scanning or chest X ray or by studying the cells in sputum. Tumors can sometimes be visualized by fiber-optic bronchoscopy, a test in which a flexible lighted tube is inserted into the windpipe and the surfaces of the lung passages are directly inspected.

If caught early, localized cancers can be treated with surgery. But because only about 16% of lung cancers are detected before they spread, radiation and **chemotherapy** are often used in addition to surgery. For cases detected early, 49% of patients are alive 5 years after diagnosis; but overall, the survival rate is only 15%. One form of lung cancer, known as small-cell lung cancer and accounting for about 20% of cases, can be treated fairly successfully with chemotherapy—alone or in combination with radiation.

A large percentage of cases respond with **remission**, which in some cases lasts for years.

## Colon and Rectal Cancer

Colon and rectal cancer (also called colorectal cancer) is the second leading cause of cancer death.

**Risk Factors** Age is a key risk factor for colon and rectal cancer, with more than 90% of cases diagnosed in people age 50 and older. Heredity also plays a role: Many cancers arise from preexisting polyps, small growths on the wall of the colon that may gradually develop into malignancies. The tendency to form colon polyps appears to be determined by specific genes, and 15–30% of colon cancers may be due to inherited gene mutations. Chronic inflammation of the colon as a result of disorders such as ulcerative colitis also increases the risk of colon cancer.

Lifestyle is also a risk factor for colon and rectal cancer. Regular physical activity appears to reduce a person's risk, whereas obesity increases risk. A diet rich in red and processed meat increases risk, although it is unclear whether fat or some other component of meat is the culprit. A diet rich in fruits, vegetables, and whole grains is associated with lower risk. Studies have also suggested a protective role for folic acid, magnesium, vitamin D, and calcium; in contrast, high intake of refined carbohydrates, simple sugars, and smoked meats and fish may increase risk.

Other lifestyle factors that may increase the risk of colon and rectal cancer include excessive alcohol consumption and smoking. Use of oral contraceptives or hormone replacement therapy may reduce risk in women. Regular use of nonsteroidal anti-inflammatory drugs such as aspirin and ibuprofen decreases the risk of developing colon cancer and other cancers of the digestive tract.

**Detection and Treatment** If identified early, precancerous polyps and early-stage cancers can be removed before they become malignant or spread. Because polyps may bleed as they progress, the standard warning signs of colon cancer are bleeding from the rectum and a change in bowel habits. Regular screening tests are recommended beginning at age 50 (earlier for people with a family history of the disease). A yearly stool blood test can detect small amounts of blood in the stool long before obvious bleeding would be noticed. More involved screening tests are recommended at 5- or 10-year intervals. In sigmoidoscopy or colonoscopy, a flexible fiber-optic device is inserted through the rectum; part or all of the colon can be examined, and polyps can be biopsied or even removed without major surgery.

Surgery is the primary treatment for colon and rectal cancer. Radiation and chemotherapy may be used before surgery to shrink a tumor or after surgery to destroy any remaining cancerous cells. The survival rate is 90% for colon and rectal cancers detected early and 63% overall.

## Breast Cancer

Breast cancer is the most common cancer in women and causes almost as many deaths in women as lung cancer. In men, breast cancer occurs only rarely. In the United States, about 1 woman in 7 will develop breast cancer during her lifetime, and about 1 woman in 30 will die from the disease. About 210,000 American women are diagnosed with breast cancer each year. Although mortality rates declined during the early 1990s, about 40,000 women die from breast cancer each year.

Less then 1% of breast cancer cases occur in women under age 30, but a woman's risk doubles every 5 years between the ages of 30 and 45 and then increases more slowly, by 10–15% every 5 years after age 45. More than 75% of breast cancers are diagnosed in women over 50. White women have a higher incidence of breast cancer, but African American women are more likely to have aggressive tumors and they have a higher death rate from the disease.

**Risk Factors** There is a strong genetic factor in breast cancer. A woman who has two close relatives with breast cancer is four to six times more likely to develop the disease than a woman who has no close relatives with it. However, even though genetic factors are important, only about 15% of cancers occur in women with a family history of breast cancer.

Other risk factors include early onset of menstruation, late onset of menopause, having no children or having a first child after age 30, current use of hormone replacement therapy, obesity, and alcohol use. The unifying factor for many of these risk factors may be the female sex hormone estrogen, which circulates in a woman's body in high concentrations between puberty and menopause. Fat cells also produce estrogen, and estrogen levels are higher in obese women. Alcohol can interfere with estrogen metabolism in the liver and increase estrogen levels in the blood. Estrogen promotes the growth of cells in responsive sites, including the breast and the uterus, so any factor that increases estrogen exposure may raise breast cancer risk. In addition, pregnancy and breastfeeding trigger changes in breast cells that make them less susceptible to cancerous changes.

Diet and exercise habits may play a role: Monounsaturated fats have been linked with reduced risk, and certain

### Terms

VW

**bone marrow** Soft vascular tissue in the interior cavities of bones that produces blood cells.

**carcinogen** Any substance that causes cancer.

**chemotherapy** The treatment of cancer with chemicals that selectively destroy cancerous cells.

**remission** A period during the course of cancer in which there are no symptoms or other evidence of disease.

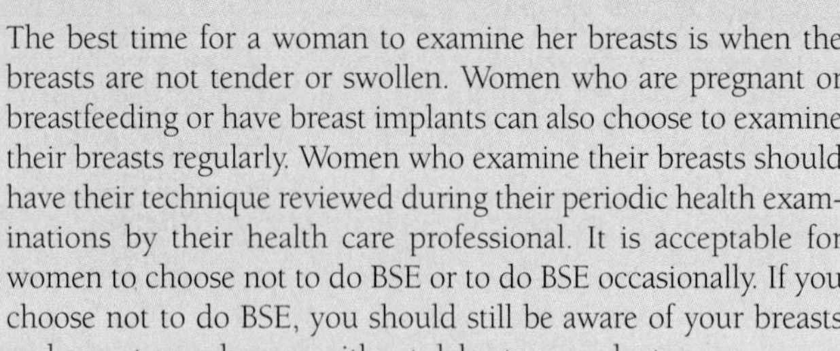

## Breast Self-Examination

Take Charge

The best time for a woman to examine her breasts is when the breasts are not tender or swollen. Women who are pregnant or breastfeeding or have breast implants can also choose to examine their breasts regularly. Women who examine their breasts should have their technique reviewed during their periodic health examinations by their health care professional. It is acceptable for women to choose not to do BSE or to do BSE occasionally. If you choose not to do BSE, you should still be aware of your breasts and report any changes without delay to your doctor.

### How to Examine Your Breasts

- Lie down and place your right arm behind your head. The exam is done while lying down, not standing up, because the breast tissue then spreads evenly over the chest wall and is as thin as possible, making it much easier to feel all the breast tissue.
- Use the finger pads of the three middle fingers on your left hand to feel for lumps in the right breast. Use overlapping dime-size circular motions of the finger pads to feel the breast tissue.

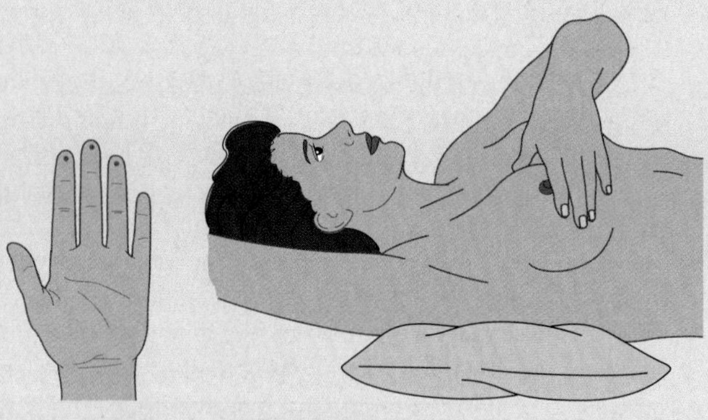

- Use three different levels of pressure to feel all the breast tissue. Light pressure is needed to feel the tissue closest to the skin; medium pressure to feel a little deeper; and firm pressure to feel the tissue closest to the chest and ribs. A firm ridge in the lower curve of each breast is normal. If you're not sure how hard to press, talk with your doctor or nurse. Use each pressure level to feel the breast tissue before moving on to the next spot.
- Move around the breast in an up-and-down pattern starting at an imaginary line drawn straight down your side from the underarm and moving across the breast to the middle of the chest bone (the sternum, or breastbone). Be sure to check the entire breast area, going down until you feel only ribs and going up to the neck or collar bone (clavicle).
- Repeat the exam on your left breast, using the finger pads of the right hand. Some evidence suggests that the up-and-down pattern (sometimes called the vertical pattern) is the most effective pattern for covering the entire breast, without missing any breast tissue.

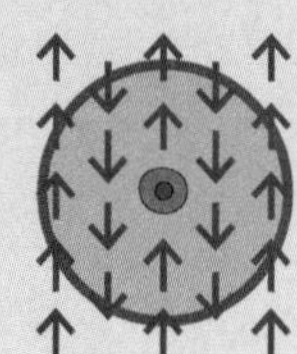

- While standing in front of a mirror with your hands pressing firmly down on your hips, look at your breasts for any changes of size, shape, contour, or dimpling. (Pressing down on the hips contracts the chest wall muscles and enhances any breast changes.)
- Examine each underarm while sitting up or standing and with your arm only slightly raised so you can easily feel in this area. Raising your arm straight up tightens the tissue in this area and makes it difficult to examine.

SOURCE: American Cancer Society's web site www.cancer.org, 2005. 

types of polyunsaturated fat may increase risk. A diet rich in vegetables may also have a protective effect. Vigorous exercise may reduce estrogen levels in the blood, and physical activity of all intensities helps control body weight. Both obesity and significant weight gain during adulthood are linked to increased risk of breast cancer.

**Early Detection** A cure is most likely if breast cancer is detected early, so regular screening is a good investment, even for younger women. The ACS advises a three-part personal program for the early detection of breast cancer:

- *Mammography:* The ACS recommends a **mammogram** (low-dose breast X ray) every year for women over 40. Mammography is especially valuable as an early detection tool because it can identify breast abnormalities that may be cancer at an early stage, before physical symptoms develop. (Some physicians consider individual risk factors in determining a recommended frequency of mammograms.)
- *Clinical breast exam:* Women between the ages of 20 and 39 should have a clinical breast exam every 3 years, and women age 40 and older should have a breast exam by a health professional every year before their scheduled mammogram.
- *Breast self-exams:* Breast self-exam (BSE) allows a woman to become familiar with her own breasts, so she can alert her health care provider to any changes. Starting at age 20, women should consider BSE an option for early detection (see the box "Breast Self-Examination").

**Treatment** If a lump is detected, it may be scanned by **ultrasonography** and biopsied to see if it is cancerous. The biopsy may be done either by needle in the physician's office or surgically. In 90% of cases, the lump is found to be a cyst or other harmless growth, and no further treatment is needed. If the lump does contain cancer cells, a variety of surgeries may be called for, ranging from a lumpectomy (removal of the lump and surrounding tissue) to a mastectomy (removal of the breast). For small tumors, lumpectomy is as effective as mastectomy.

If the tumor is discovered early, before it has spread to the adjacent lymph nodes, the patient has about a 98% chance of surviving more than 5 years. The survival rate for all stages is 88% at 5 years and 77% at 10 years.

**New Strategies for Treatment and Prevention** A number of new drugs have been developed for the treatment or prevention of breast cancer. A family of drugs called selective estrogen-receptor modulators, or SERMs, act like estrogen in some tissues of the body but block estrogen's effects in others. One SERM, tamoxifen, has long been used in breast cancer treatment because it blocks the action of estrogen in breast tissue. In 1998, the FDA approved the use of tamoxifen to reduce the risk of breast cancer in healthy women who are at high risk for the disease. Another SERM currently being tested as a potential preventive agent is raloxifene, a drug used to treat osteoporosis that has fewer side effects than tamoxifen.

Women may take tamoxifen or other drugs or undergo chemotherapy to help reduce the risk of recurrence. For advanced cancer, treatment with trastuzumab (Herceptin), a monoclonal antibody, is an option for some women. Monoclonal antibodies are a special type of antibody that is produced in the laboratory and designed to bind to a specific cancer-related target. About 30% of metastatic breast cancer tumors produce excess amounts of a growth-promoting protein called HER2. Herceptin binds to the excess HER2, thus blocking its action and slowing tumor growth.

## Prostate Cancer

The prostate gland is situated at the base of the bladder in men. It produces seminal fluid; if enlarged, it can block the flow of urine. Prostate cancer is the most common cancer in men and, after lung cancer, the cause of the most deaths. More than 230,000 new cases are diagnosed each year, and about 30,000 American men die from the disease each year.

**Risk Factors** Age is the strongest predictor of the risk, with about 75% of cases of prostate cancer diagnosed in men over age 65. Inherited genetic predisposition may be responsible for 5–10% of cases, and men with a family history of the disease should be particularly vigilant about screening. African American men have the highest rate of prostate cancer of any group in the world; both genetic and lifestyle factors may be involved. Diets high in calories, dairy products, and animal fats and low in plant foods have also been implicated as possible culprits, as have obesity, inactivity, and a history of sexually transmitted diseases. Compounds in soy foods, tomatoes, and cruciferous vegetables are being investigated for their possible protective effects.

**Detection** Early prostate cancer usually has no symptoms. Warning signs can include changes in urinary frequency, weak or interrupted urine flow, painful urination, and blood in the urine. Screening tests for early detection are recommended annually for men age 50 and over—earlier for African Americans and those with a strong family history of the disease. Techniques for early detection include a digital rectal examination and the **prostate-specific antigen (PSA) blood test.**

During a digital rectal exam, a physician feels the prostate gland through the rectum to determine if the gland is enlarged or if lumps are present. For the PSA blood test, an elevated level or a rapid increase in PSA can signal trouble. The PSA test can help catch early prostate cancer, but it also registers benign conditions (more than half of men over 50 have benign prostate disease) and very slow-growing cancers that are unlikely to kill affected individuals. In addition, prostate cancer is not rare in men with normal PSA levels.

Ultrasound is used increasingly as a follow-up, to detect lumps too small to be felt and to determine their size, shape, and properties. A needle biopsy of suspicious lumps can be performed to determine if biopsied cells are malignant.

**Treatment** Treatments vary based on the stage of the cancer and the age of the patient. A small, slow-growing tumor in an older man may be treated with "watchful waiting" because he is more likely to die from another cause before his cancer becomes life threatening. More aggressive treatment would be indicated for younger men or those with more advanced cancers. Treatment usually involves radical prostatectomy, in which the prostate is removed surgically. Although radical surgery has an excellent cure rate, it is major surgery and often results in incontinence and impotence. A less-invasive alternative involves surgical implantation of radioactive seeds. Alternative or additional treatments include external radiation, hormones that shrink tumors, cryotherapy, and anti-cancer

### Terms

**mammograms** Low-dose X rays of the breasts used to check for early signs of breast cancer.

**ultrasonography** An imaging method in which sound waves are bounced off body structures to create an image on a TV monitor; also called *ultrasound.*

**prostate-specific antigen (PSA) blood test** A diagnostic test for prostate cancer that measures blood levels of prostate-specific antigen (PSA).

drugs. Survival rates for all stages of this cancer have improved steadily since 1940; the 5-year survival rate is currently about 99%.

## Cancers of the Female Reproductive Tract

Because the uterus, cervix, and ovaries are subject to similar hormonal influences, the cancers of these organs can be discussed as a group.

**Cervical Cancer** Cervical cancer is at least in part a sexually transmitted disease. Probably more than 80% of cervical cancer stems from infection by the human papillomavirus (HPV), a large group of related viruses that cause both common warts and genital warts. When certain types of HPV are introduced into the cervix, usually by an infected sex partner, the virus infects cervical cells, causing the cells to divide and grow. If unchecked, this growth can develop into cervical cancer. Cervical cancer is associated with multiple sex partners. The regular use of condoms can reduce the risk of transmitting HPV. Studies also suggest that women whose sexual partners are circumcised may be at reduced risk because circumcised men are less likely to be infected with HPV and to pass it to their partners.

Because only a very small percentage of HPV-infected women ever get cervical cancer, other factors must be involved. Two of the most important seem to be smoking and infection with genital herpes. Exposure to environmental tobacco smoke also appears to increase risk, as does past exposure to the bacterium that causes the STD chlamydia.

Screening for the changes in cervical cells that precede cancer is done chiefly by means of the **Pap test.** During a pelvic exam, loose cells are scraped from the cervix, spread on a slide, stained for easier viewing, and examined under a microscope to see whether they are normal in size and shape. If cells are abnormal, a condition commonly referred to as *cervical dysplasia,* the Pap test is repeated at intervals. Sometimes cervical cells spontaneously return to normal, but in about one-third of cases, the cellular changes progress toward malignancy. If this happens, the abnormal cells must be removed, either surgically or by destroying them with a cryoscopic (ultracold) probe or localized laser treatment. Without timely surgery, the malignant patch of cells goes on to invade the wall of the cervix and spreads to adjacent lymph nodes and to the uterus. At this stage, chemotherapy may be used with radiation to kill the fast-growing cancer cells, but chances for a complete cure are lower.

Because the Pap test is highly effective, all sexually active women and women between the ages of 18 and 65 should be tested. The recommended schedule for testing depends on risk factors, the type of Pap test performed, and whether the Pap test is combined with HPV testing. Unlike most cancers, cancer of the cervix occurs frequently in women in their thirties or even twenties. Although screening can clearly save lives, *Healthy People 2010* reports lower-than-average rates of Pap testing for certain groups, including Latinas, women of low socioeconomic status, and women with less than a high school education. Mortality rates for cervical cancer are twice as high for black women as for white women. Worldwide, cervical cancer kills about 230,000 women each year.

Encouraging results have been seen in studies of a vaccine designed to protect women from infection with HPV. A vaccine may be available in the United States by 2006; if effective, it could dramatically reduce rates of cervical cancer by preventing HPV infection.

**Uterine, or Endometrial, Cancer** Cancer of the lining of the uterus, or endometrium, most often occurs after the age of 55. The risk factors are similar to those for breast cancer: prolonged exposure to estrogen, early onset of menstruation, late menopause, never having been pregnant, and obesity; type 2 diabetes is also associated with increased risk. The use of oral contraceptives, which combine estrogen and progestin, appears to provide protection.

Endometrial cancer is usually detectable by pelvic examination. It is treated surgically, commonly by hysterectomy, or removal of the uterus; radiation treatment, hormones, and chemotherapy may be used in addition to surgery. When the tumor is detected at an early stage, about 96% of patients are alive and disease-free 5 years later. When the disease has spread beyond the uterus, the 5-year survival rate is less than 67%.

**Ovarian Cancer** Although ovarian cancer is rare compared with cervical or uterine cancer, it causes more deaths than the other two combined. It cannot be detected by Pap tests or any other simple screening method and is often diagnosed only late in its development, when surgery and other therapies are unlikely to be successful. The risk factors are similar to those for breast and endometrial cancer: increasing age, never having been pregnant, a family history of breast or ovarian cancer, obesity, and specific genetic mutations. A high number of ovulations appears to increase the chance that a cancer-causing genetic mutation will occur, so anything that lowers the number of lifetime ovulation cycles—pregnancy, breastfeeding, or use of oral contraceptives—reduces a woman's risk of ovarian cancer. A diet rich in fruits and vegetables may be associated with reduced risk.

There are often no warning signs of developing ovarian cancer. Early clues may include increased abdominal size and bloating, urinary urgency, and pelvic pain. Women with symptoms or who are at high risk because of family history or because they harbor a mutant gene should have thorough pelvic exams at regular intervals. Blood tests for a tumor marker called CA-125 and for a group of protein markers are being investigated as possible screening tests.

Ovarian cancer may be treated by surgical removal of the uterus, ovaries, and oviducts. Radiation and chemotherapy may be used in addition to surgery.

**Other Female Reproductive Tract Cancers** From 1938 to 1971, millions of women were given a synthetic hormone called DES (diethylstilbestrol), which was thought to help prevent miscarriage. It was later discovered that daughters born to these women (DES daughters) have an increased risk, about 1 in 1000, of a vaginal or cervical cancer called clear cell cancer. There is also some risk to DES sons, who may have an increased risk of abnormalities of the reproductive tract, including undescended testicles, a risk factor for testicular cancer. A DES daughter should find a physician who is familiar with the problems of DES exposure; more frequent and more thorough pelvic exams are recommended. A recent animal study suggested the possibility of an increased third-generation cancer risk from DES, but further research is needed to determine if the finding applies to DES granddaughters.

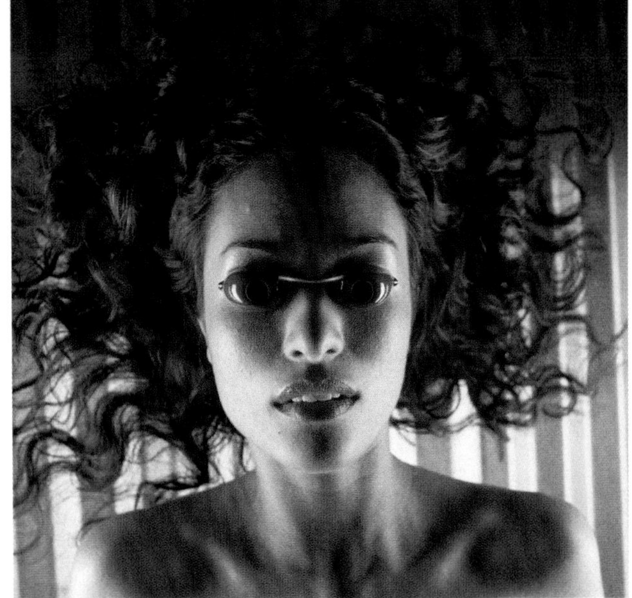

The UVA radiation emitted by most tanning-salon beds doesn't usually cause an immediate sunburn, but it does cause premature wrinkling and aging of the skin and skin cancer.

## Skin Cancer

Skin cancer is the most common cancer of all when cases of the highly curable forms are included in the count. Of the more than 1 million cases of skin cancer diagnosed each year, 54,000 are of the most serious type, **melanoma.** Treatments are usually simple and successful when the cancers are caught early.

**Risk Factors** Almost all cases of skin cancer can be traced to excessive exposure to **ultraviolet (UV) radiation** from the sun, including longer-wavelength ultraviolet A (UVA) and shorter-wavelength ultraviolet B (UVB) radiation. UVB radiation causes sunburns and can damage the eyes and the immune system. UVA is less likely to cause an immediate sunburn, but by damaging connective tissue it leads to premature aging of the skin. (Tanning lamps and tanning-salon beds emit mostly UVA radiation.) Both UVA and UVB radiation have been linked to the development of skin cancer, and the National Toxicology Program has declared both solar and artificial sources of UV radiation to be known human carcinogens.

Both severe, acute sun reactions (sunburns) and chronic low-level sun reactions (suntans) can lead to skin cancer. People with fair skin have less natural protection against skin damage from the sun and a higher risk of developing skin cancer; people with naturally dark skin have a considerable degree of protection: Caucasians are about 20 times more likely than African Americans to develop melanoma, but African Americans and Latinos are still at risk. Severe sunburns in childhood have been linked to a greatly increased risk of skin cancer in later life, so children in particular should be protected. Because of damage to the ozone layer of the atmosphere, there is a chance that we may all be exposed to increasing amounts of UV radiation in the future. Other risk factors for skin cancer include having many moles, particularly large ones; spending time at high altitudes; and a family history of the disease.

**Types of Skin Cancer** There are three main types of skin cancer, named for the types of skin cells from which they develop. **Basal cell** and **squamous cell carcinomas** together account for about 95% of the skin cancers diagnosed each year. They are usually found in chronically sun-exposed areas, such as the face, neck, hands, and arms. They usually appear as pale, waxlike, pearly nodules or red, scaly, sharply outlined patches. These cancers are often painless, although they may bleed, crust, and form an open sore on the skin.

Melanoma is by far the most dangerous skin cancer because it spreads so rapidly. It is the most common cancer among women age 25–29 years. It can occur anywhere on the body, but the most common sites are the back, chest, abdomen, and lower legs. A melanoma usually appears at

### Terms

VW

**Pap test** A scraping of cells from the cervix for examination under a microscope to detect cancer.

**melanoma** A malignant tumor of the skin that arises from pigmented cells, usually a mole.

**ultraviolet (UV) radiation** Light rays of a specific wavelength emitted by the sun; most UV rays are blocked by the ozone layer in the upper atmosphere.

**basal cell carcinoma** Cancer of the deepest layers of the skin.

**squamous cell carcinoma** Cancer of the surface layers of the skin.

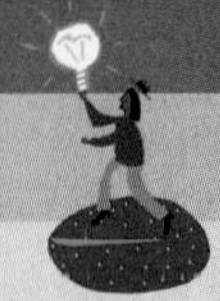

Critical Consumer

## Choosing and Using Sunscreens and Sun-Protective Clothing

VW

With consistent use of the proper clothing, sunscreens, and common sense, you can lead an active outdoor life *and* protect your skin against most sun-induced damage. Clothing should be your first and best line of defense. Sun-protective clothing can effectively block nearly all UVA and UVB rays. Sunscreens do provide protection, but many allow considerable UVA radiation to pass through to your skin. And even the best sunscreens are effective only when applied properly and reapplied frequently—something most people fail to do.

### Clothing

- Wear long-sleeved shirts and long pants. Dark-colored, tightly woven fabrics provide reasonable protection from the sun. Another good choice is clothing made from special sun-protective fabrics; these garments have an Ultraviolet Protection Factor (UPF) rating, similar to the SPF for sunscreens. For example, a fabric with a UPF rating of 20 allows only one-twentieth of the sun's UV radiation to pass through. There are three categories of UPF protection: A UPF of 15–24 provides "good" UV protection, a UPF of 25–39 provides "very good" protection, and a UPF of 40–50 provides "excellent" protection. By comparison, typical shirts provide a UPF of only 5–9, a value that drops when clothing is wet.
- Consider washing some extra sun protection into your current wardrobe. A new laundry additive adds UV protection to ordinary fabrics and is recommended by the Skin Cancer Foundation.
- Put on a hat. Your face, ears, neck, and scalp are especially vulnerable to the sun's harmful effects, making hats an essential weapon in the battle against sun damage. Baseball caps are popular, but they don't protect the ears, the back of the neck and the lower face. A better choice is a broad-brimmed hat or a legionnaire-style cap that covers the ears and neck. You still need to wear sunscreen on your face even if you are wearing a hat, because sand, water, rocks, concrete, and snow all reflect the sun's rays back up onto your face.

### Sunscreen

- Use a sunscreen and lip balm with a sun protection factor (SPF) of 15 or higher. (An SPF rating refers to the amount of time you can stay out in the sun before you burn, compared with not using sunscreen; for example, a product with an SPF of 15 would allow you to remain in the sun without burning 15 times longer, on average, than if you didn't apply sunscreen.) If you're fair-skinned, have a family history of skin cancer, are at high altitude, or will be outdoors for many hours, use a sunscreen with a high SPF (30+).
- Choose a "broad-spectrum" sunscreen that protects against both UVA and UVB radiation. The SPF rating of a sunscreen currently applies only to UVB, but a number of ingredients, especially titanium dioxide and zinc oxide, are effective at blocking most UVA radiation. Use a water-resistant sunscreen if you swim or sweat quite a bit. If you have sensitive skin, you may need to try several brands before finding one that doesn't irritate your skin. If you have acne, look for a sunscreen that is labeled "noncomedogenic," which means that it will not cause pimples.
- Apply sunscreen 30 minutes before exposure to allow it time to penetrate the skin; shake it before applying. Reapply sunscreen frequently and generously to all sun-exposed areas (many people overlook their temples, ears, and sides and backs of their necks). Most people use less than half as much as they would need to attain the full SPF rating. One ounce of sunscreen—one-fourth of a 4-ounce container—is about enough to provide one application for an average-size adult in a swimsuit. Reapply sunscreen 15–30 minutes after sun exposure begins and then every few hours after that and/or following activities such as swimming or toweling that could remove sunscreen.
- If you're taking medications, ask your physician or pharmacist about possible reactions to sunlight or interactions with sunscreens. Medications for acne, allergies, and diabetes are just a few of the products that can trigger reactions. If you're using sunscreen and an insect repellent containing DEET, use extra sunscreen (DEET may decrease sunscreen effectiveness).
- Don't let sunscreens give you a false sense of security. Most of the sunscreens currently on the market allow considerable UVA radiation to penetrate the skin, with the potential for causing skin cancers (especially melanoma) as well as wrinkles and other forms of skin damage. Experts worry that our use of sunscreens may sometimes backfire by allowing us to spend many more hours in the sun than we would if we had to worry about getting a sunburn.

### Time of Day and Location

- Avoid sun exposure between 10 A.M. and 4 P.M., when the sun's rays are most intense. Clouds allow as much as 80% of UV rays to reach your skin. Stay in the shade when you can.
- Consult the day's UV Index, which predicts UV levels on a 0–10+ scale, to get a sense of the amount of sun protection you'll need; take special care on days with a rating of 5 or above. UV Index ratings are available in local newspapers, from the weather bureau, or from certain Web sites. Also take special care in locations near the equator or at high altitudes, where the sun is more intense; use a stronger sunscreen and apply it more frequently.
- UV rays can penetrate at least 3 feet in water, so swimmers should wear water-resistant sunscreens. Snow reflects the sun's rays, so don't forget to apply sunscreen before skiing and other snow activities. Sand and water also reflect the sun's rays, so you still need to apply a sunscreen if you are under a beach umbrella. Concrete and white-painted surfaces are also highly reflective.

### Tanning Salons

- Stay away from tanning salons! Despite advertising claims to the contrary, the lights used in tanning parlors are damaging to your skin. Tanning beds and lamps emit mostly UVA radiation, increasing your risk of premature skin aging (such as wrinkles) and skin cancer. If you *must* have a tan, consider using sunless self-tanning lotions. These can provide that bronzed look without the risks of UV radiation.

the site of a preexisting mole. The mole may begin to enlarge, become mottled or varied in color (colors can include blue, pink, and white), or develop an irregular surface or irregular borders. Tissue invaded by melanoma may also itch, burn, or bleed easily.

**Prevention** One of the major steps you can take to protect yourself against all forms of skin cancer is to avoid lifelong overexposure to sunlight. Blistering, peeling sunburns from unprotected sun exposure are particularly dangerous, but suntans—whether from sunlight or tanning lamps—also increase your risk of developing skin cancer later in life. People of every age, including babies and children, need to be protected from the sun with sunscreens and protective clothing. For a closer look at sunlight and skin cancer, see the box "Choosing and Using Sunscreens and Sun-Protective Clothing."

**Detection and Treatment** Make it a habit to examine your skin regularly. Most of the spots, freckles, moles, and blemishes on your body are normal; you were born with some of them, and others appear and disappear throughout your life. But if you notice an unusual growth, discoloration, sore that does not heal, or mole that undergoes a sudden or progressive change, see your physician or a dermatologist immediately.

The characteristics that may signal that a skin lesion is a melanoma—asymmetry, border irregularity, color change, and a diameter greater than ¼ inch—are illustrated in Figure 12-7. A mole that changes in size, shape, or color is also of concern. In addition, if someone in your family has had numerous skin cancers or melanomas, you may want to consult a dermatologist for a complete skin examination and discussion of your particular risk. If you do have an unusual skin lesion, your physician will examine it and possibly perform a biopsy. If the lesion is cancerous, it is usually removed surgically, a procedure that can almost always be performed in the physician's office using a local anesthetic.

A—Asymmetry: Is one half unlike the other?

B—Border irregularity: Does it have an uneven, scalloped edge rather than a clearly defined border?

C—Color variation: Is the color uniform, or does it vary from one area to another, from tan to brown to black, or from white to red to blue?

¼ in.

D—Diameter larger than ¼ inch: At its widest point, is the growth as large as, or larger than, a pencil eraser?

**Figure 12-7 The ABCD test for melanoma.** To see a variety of photos of melanoma and benign moles, visit the National Cancer Institute's Visuals Online site (http://visualsonline.cancer.gov).

## Oral Cancer

Oral cancer—cancers of the lip, tongue, mouth, and throat—can be traced principally to cigarette, cigar, or pipe smoking, the use of spit tobacco, and the excessive consumption of alcohol. The incidence of oral cancer is twice as great in men as in women and most frequent in men over 40. Oral cancers are fairly easy to detect, but they are often hard to cure. Furthermore, among those who survive, a significant number will develop another primary cancer of the head and neck. The primary methods of treatment are surgery and radiation.

## Testicular Cancer

Testicular cancer is relatively rare, accounting for only 1% of cancer in men (about 7600 cases per year), but it is the most common cancer in men age 20–35. It is much more common among white Americans than Latinos, Asian Americans, or African Americans and among men whose fathers had testicular cancer. Men with undescended testicles are at increased risk for testicular cancer, and for this reason the condition should be corrected in early childhood. Men whose mothers took DES during pregnancy have an increased risk of undescended testicles and other genital anomalies. For this reason, they may have a higher risk of testicular cancer. Self-examination may help in the early detection of testicular cancer (see the box "Testicle Self-Examination" on p. 304). Tumors are treated by surgical removal of the testicle and, if the tumor has spread, by chemotherapy.

# THE CAUSES OF CANCER

Although scientists do not know everything about what causes cancer, they have identified genetic, environmental, and lifestyle factors. There are usually several steps in the transformation of a normal cell into a cancer cell, and in many cases different factors may work together in the development of cancer.

## The Role of DNA

Heredity and genetics are becoming increasingly important factors in assessing a person's risk of cancer. The inheritance of certain genes may predispose some people

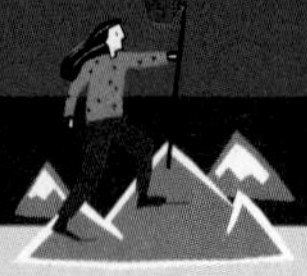

Take Charge

## Testicle Self-Examination

The best time to perform a testicular self-exam is after a warm shower or bath, when the scrotum is relaxed. First, stand in front of a mirror and look for any swelling of the scrotum. Then examine each testicle with both hands. Place the index and middle fingers under the testicle and the thumbs on top; roll the testicle gently between the fingers and thumbs. Don't worry if one testicle seems slightly larger than the other—that's common. Also, expect to feel the epididymis, the soft, sperm-carrying tube at the rear of the testicle.

Perform the self-exam each month. If you find a lump, swelling, or nodule, consult a physician right away. The abnormality may not be cancer, but only a physician can make a diagnosis. Other possible signs of testicular cancer include a change in the way a testicle feels, a sudden collection of fluid in the scrotum, a dull ache in the lower abdomen or groin, a feeling of heaviness in the scrotum, or pain in a testicle or the scrotum.

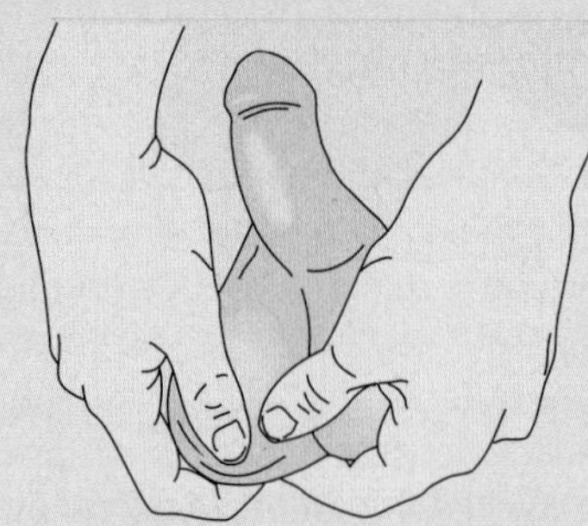

SOURCES: Testicular Cancer Resource Center. 2001. *How to Do a Testicular Self Examination* (http://www.acor.org/TCRC/tcexam.html; retrieved February 14, 2001); National Cancer Institute. 2000. *Questions and Answers About Testicular Cancer* (http://cis.nci.nih.gov/fact/6_34.htm; retrieved February 14, 2001).

to develop cancers at a younger age, and various DNA techniques are used to identify specific genetic mutations associated with such cancers.

**DNA Basics** The nucleus of each cell in your body contains 23 pairs of **chromosomes,** which are made up of tightly packed coils of **DNA** (deoxyribonucleic acid). Each chromosome contains hundreds, and in some cases thousands, of **genes;** you have about 25,000 genes in all. Each of your genes controls the production of a particular protein. By making different proteins at different times, genes can act as switches to alter the ways a cell works. Genes that control the rate of cell division often play a critical role in the development of cancer.

**DNA Mutations and Cancer** A mutation is any change in the makeup of a gene. Some mutations are inherited; others occur during cell division, and still others are caused by environmental agents known as *mutagens.* Examples of mutagens are radiation, certain viruses, and chemical substances in the air we breathe. (When a mutagen also causes cancer, it is called a carcinogen.)

A mutated gene no longer contains the proper code for producing its protein. It usually requires several mutational changes over a period of years before a normal cell takes on the properties of a cancer cell. Genes in which mutations are associated with the conversion of a normal cell into a cancer cell are known as **oncogenes.** In their undamaged form, many oncogenes play a role in controlling or restricting cell growth; these are called tumor suppressor genes. Mutational damage to these genes releases the brake on growth and leads to rapid and uncontrolled cell division—a precondition for the development of cancer.

An example of an inherited mutated oncogene is an alteration in a suppressor gene vital for controlling the growth of colon cells. Children who inherit the altered gene are thought to face a 70–80% chance of developing the disease. Another example is BRCA1 (breast cancer gene 1): Women who inherit a damaged copy of this suppressor gene face a significantly increased risk of breast and ovarian cancer.

It is important to remember, however, that most cancers are not linked to heredity; mutational damage usually occurs after birth. For example, only about 5–10% of breast cancer cases can be traced to inherited copies of a damaged BRCA1 gene. In addition, lifestyle is important even for those who have inherited a damaged suppressor gene: Eating plenty of fruits and vegetables, exercising regularly, and maintaining a healthy body weight may protect against breast cancer. Testing and identification of hereditary cancer risks can be helpful for some people, especially if it leads to increased attention to controllable risk factors and better medical screening.

### Terms

VW

**chromosomes** The threadlike bodies in a cell nucleus that contain molecules of DNA; most human cells contain 23 pairs of chromosomes.

**DNA** Deoxyribonucleic acid, a chemical substance that carries genetic information.

**gene** A section of a chromosome that contains the nucleotide base sequence for making a particular protein; the basic unit of heredity.

**oncogene** A gene involved in the transformation of a normal cell into a cancer cell.

**Cancer Promoters** Substances known as cancer promoters make up another important piece of the cancer puzzle. Cancer promoters don't directly produce DNA mutations, but they accelerate the growth of cells, leaving less time for a cell to repair DNA damage caused by other factors. Estrogen, which stimulates cellular growth in the female reproductive organs, is an example of a cancer promoter. Cigarette smoke is a complete carcinogen because it acts as both an initiator and a promoter.

## Dietary Factors

Diet is one of the most important factors in cancer prevention (Figure 12-8). It is also one of the most complex and controversial. Diets high in meat, fast food, refined carbohydrates, and simple sugars and low in fruits and vegetables are associated with a higher risk of cancer than are plant-based diets rich in whole grains, fruits, and vegetables. The picture becomes less clear, however, when researchers attempt to identify the particular constituents of foods that affect cancer risk.

**Dietary Fat and Meat** In general, diets high in fat and meat have been associated with higher rates of certain cancers, including those of the colon, esophagus, stomach, and prostate. Dietary fat may promote colon cancer by stimulating the production of bile acids, which are necessary to break down and digest material in the colon. Once produced, these bile acids remove layers of cells from the intestinal epithelium, which in turn are replaced by new cells. Newly formed and rapidly growing cells are particularly susceptible to carcinogens. Diets high in animal fats and low in plant fats may also increase the risk of aggressive forms of prostate cancer, possibly by affecting hormone levels.

Diets favoring omega-6 polyunsaturated fats over the omega-3 forms commonly found in fish may be associated with a higher risk of certain cancers, while monounsaturated fats may have a protective effect. Omega-3 fatty acids appear to slow the growth of colon cancer cells and may have protective factors against breast, prostate, and pancreatic cancers. The association between meat and cancer may be linked to the particular mix of fatty acids found in meat and how those fats are digested; in addition, high consumption of the iron in meat may promote the formation of free radicals. Curing, smoking, and grilling and other cooking methods utilizing a direct flame or high temperatures may also produce carcinogenic compounds. (Grilling vegetables does not produce these compounds.)

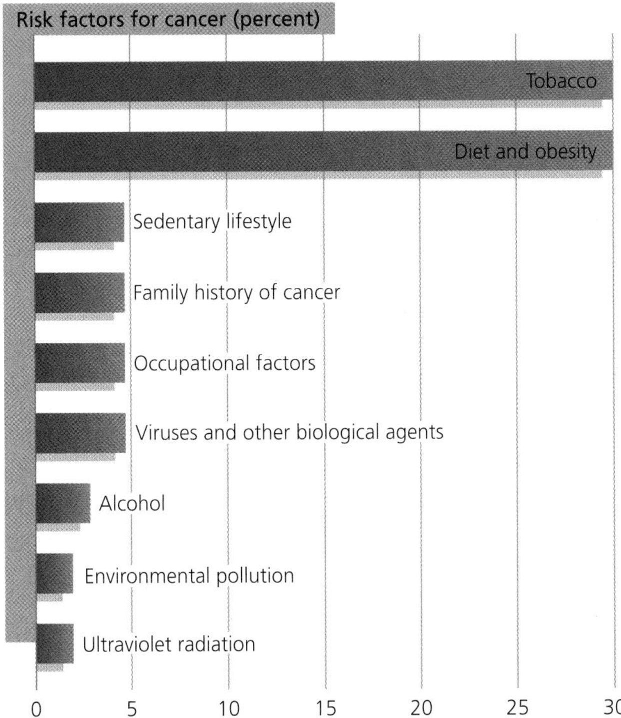


VITAL STATISTICS

**Figure 12-8 Percentage of all cancer deaths linked to risk factors.** SOURCE: Harvard Center for Cancer Prevention. 1996. Harvard Report on Cancer Prevention. Vol. 1: Causes of Human Cancer. *Cancer Causes and Control* 7(Suppl).

**Alcohol** Alcohol is associated with an increased incidence of several cancers. An average alcohol intake of three drinks per day is associated with a doubling in the risk of breast cancer; alcohol also increases the risk of colon cancer. Alcohol and tobacco interact as risk factors for oral cancer.

**Fried Foods** In 2002, scientists in Sweden reported finding high levels of the chemical acrylamide in starch-based foods that had been fried or baked at high temperatures, including french fries and certain types of snack chips and crackers. At high doses, acrylamide is toxic to humans and can induce mutations and cancer in lab animals; it is classified as a probable human carcinogen.

Studies are ongoing, but in 2005, WHO urged food companies to work to lower the acrylamide content of foods to reduce any risk to public health. Acrylamide levels vary widely in foods, and there are currently no warnings against eating specific foods. The wisest course may be to consume a variety of foods and avoid overindulging in any single class of foods, particularly foods like french fries and potato chips, which may contain other unhealthy substances such as saturated and trans fats. You can also limit your exposure to acrylamide by not smoking—you would get much more of the chemical from smoking than from food.

**Fiber** Determining the effects of fiber intake on cancer risk is complicated by the fact that fiber is found in foods that also contain many other potential anti-cancer agents—fruits, vegetables, and whole grains. Various potential cancer-fighting actions have been proposed for fiber, but none of these actions has been firmly established. Further study is needed to clarify the relationship between fiber intake and cancer risk, and experts still recommend a high-fiber diet for its overall positive effect on health.

**Fruits and Vegetables** Exactly which constituents of fruits and vegetables are responsible for reducing cancer risk is not clear, but researchers have identified many mechanisms by which food components may act against cancer.

Some essential nutrients act against cancer. For example, vitamin C, vitamin E, selenium, and the **carotenoids** (vitamin A precursors) may help block the initiation of cancer by acting as **antioxidants.** As described in Chapter 9, antioxidants prevent **free radicals** from damaging DNA. Vitamin C may also block the conversion of nitrites (food preservatives) into cancer-causing agents. Folic acid may inhibit the transformation of normal cells into malignant cells and strengthen immune function. Calcium inhibits the growth of cells in the colon and may slow the spread of potentially cancerous cells. Many other anti-cancer agents in the diet fall under the broader heading of **phytochemicals,** substances in plants that help protect against chronic diseases. One of the first to be identified was sulforaphane, a potent anticarcinogen found in broccoli.

To increase your intake of phytochemicals, eat a wide variety of fruits, vegetables, legumes, and grains. Don't try to rely on supplements. Many of these compounds are not yet available in supplement form, and optimal intakes have not been determined. Like many vitamins and minerals, isolated phytochemicals may be harmful if taken in high doses. Beta-carotene pills, for example, may increase smokers' risk of lung cancer. In addition, it is likely that the anti-cancer effects of many foods are the result of many chemical substances working in combination. Some practical suggestions for maximizing your intake of anti-cancer agents are included in the Behavior Change Strategy at the end of the chapter.

## Terms

VW

**carotenoid** Any of a group of yellow-to-red plant pigments that can be converted to vitamin A by the liver; many act as antioxidants or have other anti-cancer effects. The carotenoids include beta-carotene, lutein, lycopene, and zeaxanthin.

**antioxidant** A substance that can lessen the breakdown of food or body constituents; actions include binding oxygen and donating electrons to free radicals.

**free radicals** Electron-seeking compounds that can react with fats, proteins, and DNA, damaging cell membranes and mutating genes in their search for electrons; produced through chemical reactions in the body and by exposure to environmental factors such as sunlight and tobacco smoke.

**phytochemical** A naturally occurring substance found in plant foods that may help prevent chronic diseases such as cancer and heart disease; *phyto* means "plant."

## Inactivity and Obesity

There is good evidence that exercise reduces the risk of colon cancer; and when young girls get adequate exercise, they tend to gain weight more slowly, menstruation begins later, and their risk of breast and ovarian cancers is reduced. In addition, exercise is important because it helps prevent obesity, an independent risk factor for cancer. A high percentage of body fat appears to increase the risk of cancers of the prostate, breast, female reproductive tract, and kidney and possibly the colon and gallbladder.

## Microbes

It is estimated that about 15% of the world's cancers are caused by microbes, including viruses, bacteria, and parasites, although the percentage is much lower in developed countries like the United States. As discussed earlier, certain types of human papillomavirus cause many cases of cervical cancer. The *Helicobacter pylori* bacterium, which causes ulcers, has been definitely linked to stomach cancer. The Epstein-Barr virus, best known for causing mononucleosis, is also suspected of contributing to Hodgkin's disease, cancer of the pharynx, and some stomach cancers. Human herpesvirus 8 has been linked to Kaposi's sarcoma and certain types of lymphoma. Hepatitis viruses B and C together cause as many as 80% of the world's liver cancers.

## Carcinogens in the Environment

Some carcinogens occur naturally in the environment, like the sun's UV rays. Others are synthetic substances that show up occasionally in the general environment but more often in the work environments of specific industries.

**Ingested Chemicals** The food industry uses preservatives and other additives to prevent food from becoming spoiled or stale. Some of these compounds are antioxidants and may actually decrease any cancer-causing properties the food might have. Other compounds, like the nitrates and nitrites found in processed meat, are potentially more dangerous. Although nitrates and nitrites are not themselves carcinogenic, they can combine with dietary substances in the stomach and be converted to nitrosamines, highly potent carcinogens. Foods cured with nitrites, as well as those cured by salt or smoke, have been linked to esophageal and stomach cancer, and they should be eaten only in modest amounts.

**Environmental and Industrial Pollution** Pollutants in urban air appear to have a measurable but limited role in causing lung cancer. The best available data indicate that less than 2% of cancer deaths are caused by general environmental pollution, such as substances in our air and water (see the box "Putting Cancer Risks in Perspective"). Exposure to carcinogenic materials in the workplace is a more serious problem and may account for up to 5% of

In the News

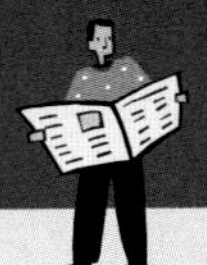

## Putting Cancer Risks in Perspective

WW

In surveys, about one in four Americans agree with the statement that there is nothing a person can do to keep from getting cancer. Many more focus most of their worry and attention on risk factors that account for relatively few cases of cancer—inherited gene mutations and chemicals in food, for example.

As in the case of heart disease—the other major killer of Americans—it is true that some cancer risk factors, such as age, are out of your control. However, you can significantly reduce your risk of cancer by making certain lifestyle changes.

### Cancer—A Complex Disease

One of the reasons people may feel powerless to protect themselves from cancer is that cancer is such a complex group of diseases, caused by the long-term interplay of genetic, environmental, and lifestyle factors. Some people engage in many unhealthy habits and never develop cancer; yet others seem to have near-ideal lifestyles but do develop cancer, possibly because they are more sensitive than others to cancer-causing agents.

In a relatively small proportion of cases, an inherited gene mutation may increase cancer risk; a family health history can help identify these situations and, in some cases, lead to increased screening and/or preventive therapies such as tamoxifen. In most cases, however, cancer develops from a series of gene mutations that occur after birth. Until researchers can pinpoint and test for elevated risk in the general population, the best cancer prevention strategy for most people is to follow the general advice for lifestyle changes and screening from major health organizations.

### Cancer in the News

With new risk factors reported by the media nearly every week, it is difficult to know what to take seriously and act on and what to ignore. It also seems like the findings are constantly changing—one week, a specific dietary component is touted as a cancer protector, and a month later, a different study finds that it has no benefit. Some of the apparent flip-flops reflect the nature of science, because it often takes many studies to pinpoint the effects of a particular risk factor.

Often, too, the media may oversimplify the results of a study or exaggerate what it means for the average person. It is important to use your critical thinking skills when evaluating cancer news. In particular, consider whether a news story is a finding from a single research study or new health advice from a reputable source. Health behavior guidelines offered by government agencies or national research foundations are typically based on many long-term research studies and can be seen as the best available advice.

### Putting Risks into Perspective—and Taking Action

It is estimated that more than half of all cancer deaths could be prevented through individual action. On the positive side, surveys show that most Americans identify tobacco use and sun exposure as causes of cancer, and that declines in smoking rates are now being mirrored in declines in lung cancer deaths. Pap tests to detect early cervical cancer are widely performed and have significantly reduced deaths from cervical cancer.

However, the same surveys indicate that more than half of Americans overlook other lifestyle factors that have been linked to more than a third of all cancer deaths—dietary choices, inactivity, obesity, and excessive consumption of alcohol. Instead, they focus attention on environmental carcinogens like food additives and pollutants that scientists believe are responsible for less than 5% of all cancers. In addition, many Americans do not keep up with recommended screening tests like colonoscopy and mammography that can detect cancer in its early, most treatable stage.

Don't let cancer's complexity make you feel powerless and unmotivated to act. Perhaps the best advice is to focus your energy on the most significant risk factors and the known ways of reducing cancer risk: Don't use tobacco; be physically active; eat a diet rich in fruits, vegetables, and whole grains; and obtain recommended screening tests. These strategies may not seem as simple and "sexy" as the latest supplement or fad diet you see in a magazine, but they are based on the best available information and have the added benefit of improving quality of life and reducing the risk of many other chronic diseases.

SOURCES: American Cancer Society. 2005. *Cancer Facts and Figures 2005.* Atlanta: American Cancer Society; National Cancer Institute. 2002. *Possible Causes and Prevention of Cancer* (http://www.cancer.gov/cancertopics/wyntk/overview/page3; retrieved January 27, 2005); American Institute for Cancer Research. 2001. *New Survey of Americans Uncovers Widespread Fear of Cancer, But Little Knowledge About Reducing Risk* (http://www.aicr.org/press/pubsearchdetail.lasso?index=1318; retrieved January 27, 2005).

cancer deaths. For example, diesel exhaust may contribute to lung cancer in truck operators and railroad workers. With increasing industry and government regulation, industrial sources of cancer risk should continue to diminish.

**Radiation** All sources of radiation are potentially carcinogenic, including medical X rays, radioactive substances (radioisotopes), and UV rays from the sun. Successful efforts have been made to reduce the amount of radiation needed for mammograms, dental X rays, and other necessary medical X rays. Full-body CT scans are sometimes advertised for routine screening in otherwise well individuals in order to look for tumors. Such screening is not recommended; it is typically expensive and may have false-positive findings that lead to unnecessary and invasive additional tests. Also, the radiation in these full-body X rays may itself raise the risk of cancer; the radiation dose of one full-body CT scan is nearly 100 times that of a typical mammogram.

Another source of environmental radiation is radon gas. Radon is a radioactive decomposition product of radium, which is found in small quantities in some rocks and soils. In most of our homes and classrooms, radon is rapidly dissipated into the atmosphere, and very low levels of radon do not appear to increase cancer risk. But in certain kinds of enclosed spaces, such as mines, some basements, and airtight houses built of brick or stone, it can rise to dangerous levels (see Chapter 17).

Sunlight is a very important source of radiation, but because its rays penetrate only a millimeter or so into the skin, it could be considered a "surface" carcinogen. Most cases of skin cancer are the relatively benign and highly curable basal cell carcinomas, but a substantial minority are the potentially deadly malignant melanomas.

Cell phones generate low levels of non-ionizing radiation, a different type of radiation from that used for medical X rays. Studies of the effects of exposure to non-ionizing radiation from cell phones have had mixed results, and researchers have found no conclusive link between cell phone use and brain cancer. Research is ongoing, however, and until the effects of such radiation exposure have been determined, some health professionals suggest discouraging children from using mobile phones excessively because their brains are more susceptible to radiation than are those of adults.

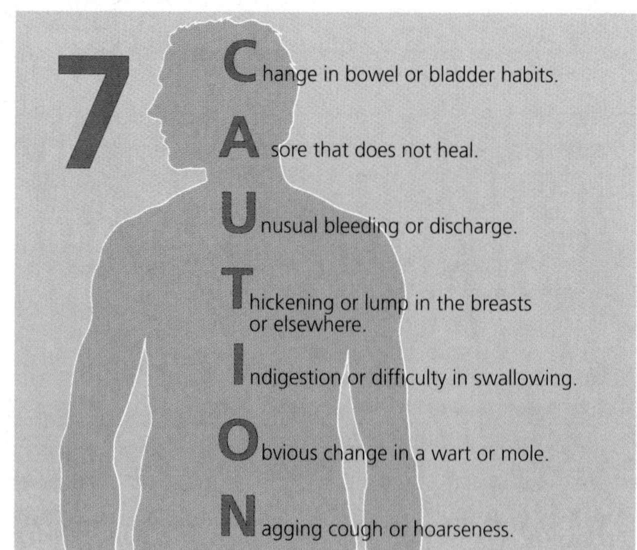


**Figure 12-9 The seven major warning signs of cancer.**

## DETECTING, DIAGNOSING, AND TREATING CANCER

Early cancer detection often depends on our willingness to be aware of changes in our own body and to make sure we keep up with recommended diagnostic tests. Although treatment success varies with individual cancers, cure rates have increased—sometimes dramatically—in this century.

### Detecting Cancer

Early signs of cancer are usually not apparent to anyone but the person who has them. The American Cancer Society recommends that you watch for the seven major warning signs shown in Figure 12-9. Remember them by the acronym CAUTION.

Although none of the warning signs is a sure indication of cancer, the appearance of any one should send you to see your physician. By being aware yourself of the risk factors in your own life, including the cancer history of your immediate family and your own past history, you can often bring a problem to the attention of a physician long before it would have been detected at a routine physical.

In addition to self-monitoring, the ACS recommends routine cancer checkups, as well as specific screening tests for certain cancers (Table 12-4).

### Diagnosing and Treating Cancer

Imaging studies or exploratory surgery may be performed to identify a cancer's *stage*—a designation based on a tumor's size, location, and spread that helps determine appropriate treatment. A biopsy may be performed to confirm the type of tumor. New diagnostic imaging techniques have replaced exploratory surgery for some patients. In magnetic resonance imaging (MRI), a huge electromagnet is used to detect hidden tumors by mapping, on a computer screen, the vibrations of different atoms in the body. Computed tomography (CT) scanning uses X rays to examine the brain and other parts of the body. The process allows the construction of cross sections, which show a tumor's shape and location more accurately than is possible with conventional X rays. Ultrasonography has also been used increasingly in the past few years to view tumors.

The primary treatment methods for cancer are surgery, chemotherapy, and radiation therapy. In chemotherapy, cancer cells that can't be surgically removed are killed by interfering chemically with their growth; in radiation therapy, they are killed directly with concentrated ionizing radiation. Newer and still experimental methods are also showing promise. In gene therapy, scientists can compare normal DNA sequences with the sequences found in tumor cells; using this approach, they hope to develop a variety of powerful, targeted therapies for use in treatment of specific cancers. Bone marrow and stem cell transplants are used in cancers of the blood-forming or lymph cells. Biological therapies are used to enhance the immune system's reaction to a tumor. New drugs are being developed to block cancer cells' ability to invade normal tissue and metastasize, to prevent their growth, and to keep them from dividing.

Because of successful treatment of cancer, survival has become the norm. However, cancer survivors must live with the fear of recurrence. They may also suffer

## Table 12-4 Screening Guidelines for the Early Detection of Cancer in Asymptomatic People

| Site | Recommendation |
|---|---|
| *Breast* | • Yearly mammograms are recommended starting at age 40. The age at which screening should be stopped should be individualized by considering the potential risks and benefits of screening in the context of overall health status and longevity.<br>• Clinical breast exam should be part of a periodic health exam, about every 3 years for women age 20–39, and every year for women age 40 and older.<br>• Women should know how their breasts normally feel and report any breast change promptly to their health care providers. Breast self-exam is an option for women starting at age 20.<br>• Women at increased risk (e.g., family history, genetic tendency, past breast cancer) should talk with their doctors about the benefits and limitations of starting mammography screening earlier, having additional tests (i.e., breast ultrasound and MRI), or having more frequent exams. |
| *Colon and rectum* | Beginning at age 50, men and women should begin screening with one of the examination schedules below.<br>• A fecal occult blood test (FOBT) or fecal immunochemical test (FIT) every year<br>• A flexible sigmoidoscopy (FSIG) every 5 years<br>• Annual FOBT or FIT and flexible sigmoidoscopy every 5 years*<br>• A double-contrast barium enema every 5 years<br>• A colonoscopy every 10 years<br>**Combined testing is preferred over either annual FOBT or FIT, or FSIG every 5 years, alone. People who are at moderate or high risk for colorectal cancer should talk with a doctor about a different testing schedule.* |
| *Prostate* | The PSA test and the digital rectal examination should be offered annually, beginning at age 50, to men who have a life expectancy of at least 10 years. Men at high risk (African American men and men with a strong family history of one or more first-degree relatives diagnosed with prostate cancer at an early age) should begin testing at age 45. For men at both average risk and high risk, information should be provided about what is known and what is uncertain about the benefits and limitations of early detection and treatment of prostate cancer so that they can make an informed decision about testing. |
| *Uterus* | ***Cervix:*** Screening should begin approximately 3 years after a woman begins having vaginal intercourse, but no later than age 21. Screening should be done every year with regular Pap tests or every 2 years using liquid-based tests. At or after age 30, women who have had three normal test results in a row may get screened every 2 to 3 years. Alternatively, cervical cancer screening with HPV DNA testing and conventional or liquid-based cytology could be performed every 3 years. However, doctors may suggest a woman get screened more often if she has certain risk factors, such as HIV infection or a weak immune system. Women 70 years and older who have had three or more consecutive normal Pap tests in the last 10 years may choose to stop cervical cancer screening. Screening after total hysterectomy (with removal of the cervix) is not necessary unless the surgery was done as a treatment for cervical cancer.<br>***Endometrium:*** The American Cancer Society recommends that at the time of menopause all women should be informed about the risks and symptoms of endometrial cancer, and strongly encouraged to report any unexpected bleeding or spotting to their physicians. Annual screening for endometrial cancer with endometrial biopsy beginning at age 35 should be offered to women with or at risk for hereditary nonpolyposis colon cancer (HNPCC). |
| *Cancer-related checkup* | For individuals undergoing periodic health examinations, a cancer-related checkup should include health counseling and, depending on a person's age and gender, might include examinations for cancers of the thyroid, oral cavity, skin, lymph nodes, testes, and ovaries, as well as for some nonmalignant diseases. |

SOURCE: American Cancer Society's *Cancer Facts and Figures 2005*. Copyright © 2005 American Cancer Society, Inc. www.cancer.org. Reprinted with permission.

from discrimination from insurers, although some states have passed legislation to prevent this.

For cancer patients, psychological support is an important part of treatment and recovery. Family and friends, concerned health care providers, and organized support groups can all play roles in the lives of cancer patients. Support groups can have an especially positive impact on the emotional wellness of both patients and families.

## PREVENTING CANCER

Your lifestyle choices can radically lower your cancer risks, so you *can* take a very practical approach to cancer prevention.

- *Avoid tobacco.* Smoking is responsible for about 30% of all cancer deaths. People who smoke two or more packs of cigarettes a day have lung cancer mortality rates 15–25 times greater than those of nonsmokers. The carcinogenic chemicals in smoke are transported throughout the body in the bloodstream, making smoking a carcinogen for many forms of cancer other than lung cancer. ETS is dangerous to nonsmokers. The use of spit tobacco increases the risk of cancers of the mouth, larynx, throat, and esophagus.

- *Control diet and weight.* About one-third of all cancers are in some way linked to what we eat. Choose a low-fat, plant-based diet containing a wide variety of fruits, vegetables, and whole grains rich in phytochemicals. Drink alcohol only in moderation, if at all. Maintain a healthy weight.
- *Exercise regularly.* Regular exercise is linked to lower rates of colon and other cancers. It also helps control weight.
- *Protect skin from the sun.* Almost all cases of skin cancer are considered to be sun-related. Wear protective clothing when you're out in the sun, and use a sunscreen with an SPF rating of 15 or higher. Don't go to tanning salons.
- *Avoid environmental and occupational carcinogens.* Try to avoid occupational exposure to carcinogens, and don't smoke; the cancer risks of many of these agents increase greatly when combined with smoking.
- *Have recommended screening tests.* Stay alert for the signs and symptoms that could indicate cancer, and follow the American Cancer Society screening guidelines listed in Table 12-4. Both lifestyle changes and a program of early detection are important to your long-term health.

**Tips for Today**

Cardiovascular disease and cancer are both "lifestyle diseases"—that is, although there are contributing factors that are beyond our control, including genetic factors, age, and ethnicity, there are also many lifestyle factors that have an impact on our risk. Choices we make every day—especially about tobacco, diet, and physical activity—can help us stay free of these diseases over the long term.

*Right now you can*

- Plan to have fish for dinner two times this week.
- Go to the gym or fitness facility on your campus and get started on an aerobic exercise program.
- Do a breast self-exam, if you are a woman, or a testicular self-exam, if you are a man.
- Plan to have two vegetables with dinner tonight, one of them broccoli, cauliflower, brussels sprouts, or kale.
- Put your sunscreen by the front door so you'll remember to apply it the next time you go out in the sun, or put a brimmed hat by the door or in the car.

## SUMMARY

- The cardiovascular system pumps and circulates blood throughout the body. The heart pumps blood to the lungs via the pulmonary artery and to the body via the aorta.
- The six major risk factors that can be changed are smoking, high blood pressure, unhealthy cholesterol levels, inactivity, obesity, and diabetes.
- Hypertension occurs when blood pressure exceeds normal limits most of the time. It weakens the heart, scars and hardens arteries.
- Contributing risk factors that can be changed include high triglyceride levels and psychological and social factors.
- Risk factors for CVD that can't be changed include being over 65, being male, being African American, and having a family history of CVD.
- Atherosclerosis is a progressive hardening and narrowing of arteries that can lead to restricted blood flow and even complete blockage.
- Heart attacks are usually the result of a long-term disease process.
- A stroke occurs when the blood supply to the brain is cut off by a blood clot or hemorrhage.
- Congestive heart failure occurs when the heart's pumping action becomes less efficient and fluid collects in the lungs or in other parts of the body.
- CVD risk can be reduced by improving diet, engaging in regular exercise, not smoking cigarettes and avoiding environmental tobacco smoke, knowing and managing your blood pressure and cholesterol levels, developing effective ways of handling stress and anger, and managing other risk factors and medical conditions.
- A malignant tumor can invade surrounding structures and spread to distant sites via the blood and lymphatic system, producing additional tumors.
- Lung cancer kills more people than any other type of cancer. Tobacco smoke is the primary cause.
- Colon and rectal cancer is linked to age, heredity, obesity, and a diet rich in red meat and low in fruits and vegetables. Most colon cancers arise from preexisting polyps.
- Breast cancer affects about one in seven women in the United States. Although there is a genetic component to breast cancer, diet and hormones are also risk factors.
- Prostate cancer is chiefly a disease of aging; diet and lifestyle probably are factors in its occurrence.
- Cancers of the female reproductive tract include cervical, uterine, and ovarian cancer. The Pap test is an effective screening test for cervical cancer.
- Skin cancers occur as basal cell carcinoma, squamous cell carcinoma, and melanoma.
- Oral cancer is caused primarily by smoking, excess alcohol consumption, and use of spit tobacco.

## Modifying Your Diet for Heart Health and Cancer Prevention

Behavior Change Strategy

Gradually modifying your diet to include less saturated and trans fat and more fruits and vegetables can help you avoid both CVD and cancer in the future. Begin by assessing your current diet: Keep a record in your health journal of everything you eat for a week. At the end of the week, you can evaluate your diet and start taking steps to modify it.

### Reducing Saturated and Trans Fat in Your Diet

The American Heart Association recommends that no more than 10% of the calories in your diet come from saturated and trans fat. Foods high in these fats include meat, poultry skin, full-fat dairy products, coconut and palm oils, and products made with hydrogenated vegetable oils, such as deep-fried fast food and packaged baked goods. To find out if your diet is within the 10% recommendation, at the end of the week, record the grams of saturated and trans fat next to the foods you've listed in your health journal. This information is available on many food labels, in books, and on the Internet. For fast foods, use the Appendix. Trans fat content can be more difficult to determine. Here are the average values per serving for a few trans fat–rich foods: french fries (large), 5 g; pound cake, 5 g; doughnut, 4 g; fried breaded chicken, 3 g; Danish pastry, 3 g; vegetable shortening, 3 g; sandwich cookies, 2 g; crackers, 2 g; margarine (stick), 2 g; margarine (tub), 1 g.

Once you have the grams of fat listed, add up what you consumed each day. For a 1600-calorie diet, the 10% limit corresponds to 18 grams of saturated and trans fat; for a 2200-calorie diet, it corresponds to 24 grams; and for a 2800-calorie diet, it corresponds to 31 grams. (If you have high cholesterol, you may want to follow the 7% limit set by the NCEP, which corresponds to 12 grams of saturated and trans fat in a 1600-calorie diet, 17 grams in a 2200-calorie diet, and 22 grams in a 2800-calorie diet.) If you're not able to get all the data you need, estimate by looking at the number of servings of food high in saturated or trans fat you consume in a day.

If your diet is higher in these fats than it should be, look at your food record to see if you are choosing high-fat foods more often than you should. To reduce your intake of saturated and trans fats, try making healthy substitutions:

- Vegetable oils or trans fat–free tub margarine rather than butter, stick margarine, or vegetable shortening
- Fruits, vegetables, rice cakes, unbuttered popcorn, or pretzels instead of chips, crackers, or cheese puffs
- Low-fat or fat-free milk, cheese, yogurt, or mayonnaise instead of the full-fat versions
- Fruit or a low-fat sweet (angel food cake, frozen yogurt, sorbet) instead of cakes, cookies, pastries, or regular ice cream
- Whole-grain breads and rolls, English muffins, or bagels instead of croissants, muffins, or coffee cake
- Lean meat, skinless poultry, or a veggie burger instead of ground beef, fried chicken, or lunch meats
- Baked potato or rice instead of french fries or onion rings
- Vegetarian chili or pasta with vegetables instead of pizza or macaroni and cheese

When you do eat high-fat foods, eat smaller portions, and balance your higher-fat choices with low-fat choices over the course of the day.

### Increasing Fruits and Vegetables in Your Diet

Many fruits and vegetables contain phytochemicals, compounds that help slow, stop, or even reverse the process of cancer. For this reason, the National Cancer Institute (NCI) has developed the "Eat 5 to 9 a Day for Better Health" program to help Americans increase their consumption of fruits and vegetables to health-promoting levels. Take a look at the foods you've listed in your health journal for a week. Have you included five or more fruits and vegetables each day? If not, here are some tips from the NCI:

- Drink 100% juice every morning.
- Add raisins, berries, or sliced fruit to cereal; top bagels with tomato slices.
- Make a fruit smoothie from fresh or frozen fruit and orange juice or low-fat yogurt.
- Have vegetable soup or a salad with your lunch.
- Replace french fries or potato chips with cut-up vegetables.
- Try adding vegetables such as roasted peppers, cucumber slices, shredded carrots, avocado, or salsa to sandwiches.
- Drink tomato or vegetable juice instead of soda (monitor the sodium content of vegetable juices).
- Microwave vegetables and sprinkle them with a little bit of Parmesan cheese.
- At the salad bar, pile your plate with healthy fruits and vegetables and use low-fat or fat-free dressing.
- At dinner, choose a vegetarian main dish, such as stir-fry, or include two servings of vegetables.
- Substitute vegetables for meat in pasta, chili, and casseroles.
- Keep raw fruits and vegetables (apples, plums, carrots) on hand for snacks.
- Try buying a new fruit or vegetable at the store every week.

Stock up on canned, frozen, and dried fruits and vegetables when they go on sale. Buy fresh fruits and vegetables in season; they'll taste best and be less expensive.

Some fruits and vegetables are particularly rich in phytochemicals; choose them as often as you can. They include cruciferous vegetables (e.g., broccoli, cauliflower, cabbage, bok choy, brussels sprouts); citrus fruits (e.g., oranges, lemons, grapefruit); berries (e.g., strawberries, raspberries); dark-green leafy vegetables (e.g., spinach, chard, romaine lettuce); and deep-yellow, orange, and red fruits and vegetables (e.g., carrots, red and yellow bell peppers, winter squash, cantaloupe, apricots).

With a little attention and effort, you can modify your diet now, with steps like these, to help safeguard yourself from CVD and cancer in the future.

SOURCES: American Heart Association. 2000. *An Eating Plan for Healthy Americans: The New 2000 Food Guidelines.* Dallas, Tex.: American Heart Association; Food and Drug Administration. 1999. *Questions and Answers on Trans Fat Proposed Rule* (http://vm.cfsan.fda.gov/~dms/qa-trans.html); Center for Science in the Public Interest. 1997. The sat fat switch. *Nutrition Action Healthletter,* January/February; National Cancer Institute. 2000. *Eat 5 to 9 A Day for Better Health* (http://www.5aday.gov; retrieved March 25, 2005); Welland, D. 1999. Fruits and vegetables: Easy ways to five-a-day. *Environmental Nutrition,* June.

- Testicular cancer can be detected early through self-examination.
- Mutational damage to a cell's DNA can lead to rapid and uncontrolled growth of cells.
- Cancer-promoting dietary factors include meat, certain types of fats, and alcohol. Diets high in fruits and vegetables are linked to a lower risk of cancer.
- Other possible causes of cancer include inactivity and obesity, certain types of infections and chemicals, and radiation.
- Self-monitoring and regular screening tests are essential to early cancer detection.
- Treatment methods usually consist of some combination of surgery, chemotherapy, and radiation.
- Strategies for preventing cancer include avoiding tobacco; eating a varied, moderate diet and controlling weight; exercising regularly; protecting skin from the sun; avoiding exposure to environmental and occupational carcinogens; and getting recommended cancer screening tests.

## Take Action

1. **Learn CPR:** The CPR courses given by the American Red Cross and other groups provide invaluable training that may help you save a life some day. Anyone can take these courses and become qualified to perform CPR and possibly use AED equipment. Investigate CPR courses in your community, and sign up to take one.

2. **Investigate your family's CVD and cancer history:** Do some research into your family medical history. Is there CVD or cancer in your family, as indicated by premature deaths from heart attack, stroke, heart failure, or any type of cancer? Is there a family history of diabetes? Keep your family health history in mind as you consider whether you need to make lifestyle changes to avoid CVD and cancer.

3. **Do a self-exam:** Devise a plan for incorporating regular self-examinations for cancer (breast self-examination or testicle self-examination) into your life. What strategies will help you remember to do your monthly exam? How can you keep yourself motivated?

## For More Information

### Books


American Cancer Society. 2003. *Cancer: What Causes It. What Doesn't.* Atlanta, Ga.: American Cancer Society. *Provides basic background information about cancer and its causes.*

American Institute for Cancer Research. 2005. *The New American Plate Cookbook.* Berkeley, Calif.: U.C. Berkeley Press. *Provides guidelines and recipes for healthy eating to prevent cancer and other chronic diseases.*

Freeman, M. W., and C. E. Junge. 2005. *Harvard Medical School Guide to Lowering Your Cholesterol.* New York: McGraw-Hill. *Information about cholesterol, including lifestyle changes and medication for improving cholesterol levels.*

Nelson, M. E., and A. Lichtenstein. 2005. *Strong Women, Strong Hearts.* New York: Putnum Adult. *Lifestyle advice for women to prevent heart disease.*

Romaine, D. S., and O. S. Randall. 2005. *The Encyclopedia of Heart and Heart Disease.* New York: Facts on File. *Includes entries on the functioning of the cardiovascular system, types and causes of heart disease, and prevention and treatment.*

Runkington, C., and J. J. Straus. 2005. *The Encyclopedia of Cancer.* New York: Facts on File. *Includes entries on a variety of topics relating to cancer causes, prevention, diagnosis, and treatment.*


### VW Organizations, Hotlines, and Web Sites

*American Academy of Dermatology.* Provides information on skin cancer prevention.
888-462-DERM
http://www.aad.org

*American Cancer Society.* Provides a wide range of free materials on the prevention and treatment of cancer.
800-ACS-2345
http://www.cancer.org

*American Heart Association.* Provides information on hundreds of topics relating to the prevention and control of cardiovascular disease; sponsors a general Web site as well as several sites focusing on specific topics.
800-AHA-USA1 (general information)
http://www.americanheart.org (general information)
http://www.deliciousdecisions.org (dietary advice)
http://www.justmove.org (fitness advice)

*American Institute for Cancer Research.* Provides information on lifestyle and cancer prevention, especially nutrition.
800-843-8114
http://www.aicr.org

*Cancer Guide: Steve Dunn's Cancer Information Page.* Links to many good cancer resources on the Internet and advice about how to make best use of information.
http://www.cancerguide.org

*Clinical Trials.* Information about clinical trials for new cancer treatments can be accessed at the following sites:
http://www.cancer.gov/clinicaltrials
http://www.centerwatch.com

*Franklin Institute Science Museum/The Heart:An On-Line Exploration.* An online museum exhibit containing information on the structure and function of the heart, how to monitor your heart's health, and how to maintain a healthy heart.
http://www.fi.edu/biosci/heart.html

*Harvard Center for Cancer Prevention: Your Disease Risk.* Includes interactive risk assessments as well as tips for preventing common cancers.
http://www.yourcancerrisk.harvard.edu

*MedlinePlus: Heart and Circulation Topics.* Provides links to reliable sources of information on many topics relating to cardiovascular health.
http://www.nlm.nih.gov/medlineplus/heartandcirculation.html

*National Cancer Institute.* Provides information on treatment options, screening, and clinical trials and on the national "5 to 9 A Day for Better Health Program" that promotes greater consumption of fruits and vegetables.

800-4-CANCER
http://www.cancer.gov
http://5aday.nci.nih.gov

*National Heart, Lung, and Blood Institute.* Provides information on and interactive applications for a variety of topics relating to cardiovascular health and disease, including cholesterol, smoking, obesity, hypertension, and the DASH diet.

800-575-WELL
http://www.nhlbi.nih.gov
http://rover.nhlbi.nih.gov/chd

*National Stroke Association.* Provides information and referrals for stroke victims and their families; the Web site has a stroke risk assessment.

800-STROKES
http://www.stroke.org

*Oncolink/The University of Pennsylvania Cancer Center Resources.* Contains information on different types of cancer and answers to frequently asked questions.

http://www.oncolink.org

See also the listings for Chapters 2, 3, and 9–11.

## Selected Bibliography


American Cancer Society. 2005. *Cancer Facts and Figures, 2005.* Atlanta: American Cancer Society.

American Heart Association. 2005. *Heart and Stroke Statistical Update, 2005.* Dallas, Tex.: American Heart Association.

Brenner, D. J., et al. 2004. Estimated radiation risks potentially associated with full-body CT screening. *Radiology* 232(3): 735–738.

Calle, E. E., et al. 2003. Overweight, obesity, and mortality from cancer in a prospectively studied cohort of U.S. adults. *New England Journal of Medicine* 348: 1625–1638.

Chia, K. S., et al. 2005. Profound changes in breast cancer incidence may reflect changes into a Westernized lifestyle: A comparative population-based study in Singapore and Sweden. *International Journal of Cancer* 113(2): 302–306.

Daviglus, M. L., et al. 2004. Favorable cardiovascular risk profile in young women and long-term risk of cardiovascular and all-cause mortality. *Journal of the American Medical Association* 292(13): 1588–1592.

Douglas, J. G., et al. 2003. Management of high blood pressure in African Americans: Consensus statement of the Hypertension in African Americans Working Group of the International Society on Hypertension in Blacks. *Archives of Internal Medicine* 163(5): 525–541.

Eaker, E., et al. 2004. Anger and hostility predict the development of atrial fibrillation in men in the Framingham Offspring Study. *Circulation* 109: 1267–1271.

Elmore, J. G., et al. 2005. Screening for breast cancer. *Journal of the American Medical Association* 293(10): 1245–1256.

Flood, A., et al. 2005. Calcium from diet and supplements is associated with reduced risk of colorectal cancer in a prospective cohort of women. *Cancer Epidemiology, Biomarkers and Prevention* 14(1): 126–132.

Food and Agriculture Organization and World Health Organization. 2005. *Joint FAO/WHO Expert Committee on Food Additives: Summary and Conclusions* (http://www.who.int/ipcs/food/jecfa/summaries/en; retrieved March 29, 2005).

Goff, B. A., et al. 2004. Frequency of symptoms of ovarian cancer in women presenting to primary care clinics. *Journal of the American Medical Association* 291(22): 2705–2712.

Jemal, A., et al. 2005. Cancer Statistics, 2005. *CA: A Cancer Journal for Clinicians* 55(1): 10–30.

Jensen, M. K., et al. 2004. Intakes of whole grains, bran, and germ and the risk of coronary heart disease in men. *American Journal of Clinical Nutrition* 80(6): 1492–1499.

Kelemen, L. E., et al. 2005. Associations of dietary protein with disease and mortality in a prospective study of postmenopausal women. *American Journal of Epidemiology* 161(3): 239–249.

Kroenke, C. H., et al. 2005. Weight, weight gain, and survival after breast cancer diagnosis. *Journal of Clinical Oncology* 23(7): 1370–1378.

Martinez, M. E. 2005. Primary prevention of colorectal cancer: Lifestyle, nutrition, exercise. *Recent Results in Cancer Research* 166: 177–211.

Meadows, M. 2005. Brain attack: A look at stroke prevention and treatment. *FDA Consumer,* March/April.

Mor, G., et al. 2005. Serum protein markers for early detection of ovarian cancer. *Proceedings of the National Academy of Sciences USA,* epub May 12.

Mozaffarian, D., et al. 2005. Interplay between different polyunsaturated fatty acids and risk of coronary heart disease in men. *Circulation,* 111(2): 157–164.

National Toxicology Program. 2005. *Report on Carcinogens,* Eleventh Edition. Research Triangle Park, N. C.: National Toxicology Program.

Nissen, S. E., et al. 2005. Statin therapy, LDL cholesterol, C-reactive protein, and coronary artery disease. *New England Journal of Medicine* 352(1): 29–38.

Ridker, P. M., et al. 2005. C-reactive protein levels and outcomes after statin therapy. *New England Journal of Medicine* 352(1): 20–28.

Ridker, P. M., et al. 2005. A randomized trial of low-dose aspirin in the primary prevention of cardiovascular disease in women. *New England Journal of Medicine,* epub, March 7.

Roden, R. B., et al. 2004. Vaccination to prevent and treat cervical cancer. *Human Pathology* 35(8): 971–982.

Rothwell, P. M., and C. P. Warlow. 2005. Timing of TIAs preceding stroke: time window for prevention is very short. *Neurology* 64(5): 817–820.

Rozanski, A. S., et al. 2005. The epidemiology, pathophysiology, and management of psychosocial risk factors in cardiac practice: The emerging field of behavioral cardiology. *Journal of the American College of Cardiology* 45(5): 637–651.

Shai, I., et al. 2004. Homocysteine as a risk factor for coronary heart diseases and its association with inflammatory biomarkers, lipids and dietary factors. *Atherosclerosis* 177(2): 375–381.

Thompson, I. M., et al. 2004. Prevalence of prostate cancer among men with prostate-specific antigen level < or =4.0 ng per milliliter. *New England Journal of Medicine* 350(22): 2239–2246.

Weinstein, S. J., et al. 2005. Serum alpha-tocopherol and gamma-tocopherol in relation to prostate cancer risk in a prospective study. *Journal of the National Cancer Institute* 97(5): 396–399.

Willingham, S. A., and E. S. Kilpatrick. 2005. Evidence of gender bias when applying the new diagnostic criteria for myocardial infarction. *Heart* 91(2): 237–238.

Wittstein, I. S., et al. 2005. Neurohumoral features of myocardial stunning due to sudden emotional stress. *New England Journal of Medicine* 352(6): 539–548.

World Health Organization. 2005. *Cancer: Diet and Physical Activity's Impact* (http://www.who.int/dietphysicalactivity/publications/facts/cancer/en/; retrieved January 20, 2005).

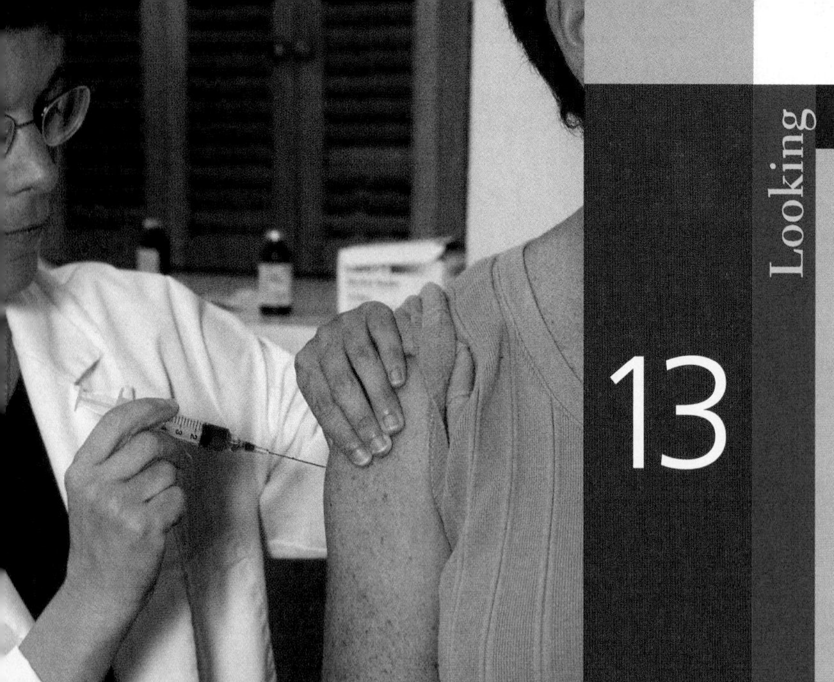

13

# Looking AHEAD

After reading this chapter, you should be able to

- Describe the step-by-step process by which infectious diseases are transmitted
- Explain how the immune system responds to an invading microorganism
- List the major types of pathogens and describe the common diseases they cause
- Explain how HIV infection and other STDs affect the body and how they are transmitted, diagnosed, and treated
- Discuss steps you can take to prevent infections, including STDs, and strengthen your immune system

# Immunity and Infection

The immune system works continuously to keep the body from being overwhelmed by external invaders that cause **infections** and from internal changes such as cancer. Most people don't pay much attention to these internal skirmishes unless they become sick and find themselves deprived of their usual feelings of well-being. But many people today are more knowledgeable about the complexities of immunity because they have heard about, or had experience with, HIV infection, which directly attacks the immune system. This chapter provides information that will help you understand immunity, infection, and how to keep yourself well in a world of disease-causing microorganisms.

## THE CHAIN OF INFECTION

Infectious diseases are transmitted from one person to another through a series of steps—a chain of infection. The infectious disease cycle begins with a **pathogen,** a microorganism that causes disease. HIV, the virus that causes AIDS, and the tuberculosis bacterium are examples of pathogens. The pathogen has a natural environment in which it typically resides. This so-called *reservoir* can be a person, an animal, or an environmental component like soil or water. To transmit infection, the pathogen must leave the reservoir through some *portal of exit.* In the case of a human reservoir, portals of exit include saliva (for mumps, for example), the mucous membranes (for many sexually transmitted diseases), blood (for HIV and hepatitis), feces (for intestinal infections), and nose and throat discharges (for colds and influenza).

*Transmission* can occur directly—from one person to another—or indirectly—through an insect or animal, through contaminated soil, food, or water, or from inanimate objects, such as eating utensils. To infect a new host, a pathogen must have a *portal of entry* into the body. Pathogens can enter via penetration of the skin or direct contact, inhalation through the mouth or nose, or ingestion of contaminated food or water. Pathogens that enter the skin or mucous membranes can cause a local infection of the tissue, or they may penetrate into the bloodstream or **lymphatic system,** thereby causing a more extensive **systemic infection.** Agents that cause STDs usually enter the body through the mucous membranes lining the urethra (in males) or the cervix (in females). Organisms that are transmitted via respiratory secretions may cause upper respiratory infections or pneumonia, or they may enter the bloodstream and cause systemic infection. Foodborne and waterborne organisms enter the mouth and may attack the cells of the small intestine or the colon, causing diarrhea, or they may enter the bloodstream via the digestive system and travel to other parts of the body.

Once in the new host, a variety of factors determine whether the pathogen will be able to establish itself and cause infection. People with a strong immune system or

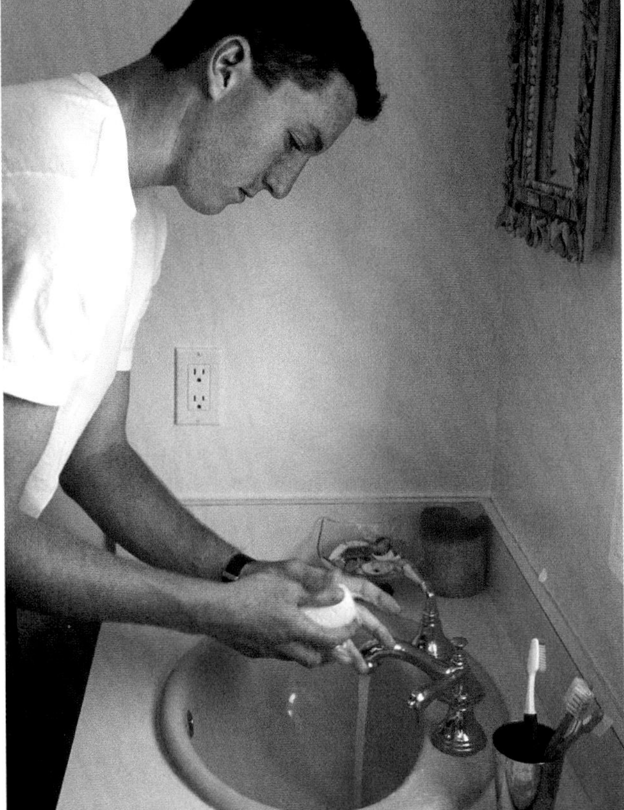

Hand washing is one of the best ways to prevent the spread of infectious diseases. Always wash your hands before, during, and after preparing food; before eating; and after using the bathroom. Wet your hands, apply soap, and rub vigorously for 10–20 seconds.

resistance to a particular pathogen will be less likely to become ill than people with poor immunity. If conditions are right, the pathogen will multiply and produce disease in the new host. In such a case, the new host may become a reservoir from which a new chain of infection can be started.

Interruption of the chain of infection at any point can prevent disease. Strategies for breaking the chain include a mix of public health measures and individual action. For example, a pathogen's reservoir can be isolated or destroyed, as when a sick individual is placed under quarantine or when insects or animals carrying pathogens are killed. Public sanitation practices, such as sewage treatment and the chlorination of drinking water, can also kill pathogens. Transmission can be disrupted through strategies like hand washing and the use of facemasks. Immunization and the treatment of infected hosts can stop the pathogen from multiplying, producing a serious disease, and being passed on to a new host.

## THE BODY'S DEFENSE SYSTEM

Our bodies have very effective ways of protecting themselves against invasion by pathogens. The body's first line of defense is a formidable array of physical and chemical barriers. When these barriers are breached, the body's immune system comes into play.

### Physical and Chemical Barriers

The skin, the body's largest organ, prevents many microorganisms from entering the body. Although many bacterial and fungal organisms live on the surface of the skin, very few can penetrate it except through a cut or break. Wherever there is an opening in the body, or an area without skin, other barriers exist. The mouth, the main entry to the gastrointestinal system, is lined with mucous membranes, which contain cells designed to prevent the passage of unwanted organisms and particles. Body openings and the fluids that cover them (for example, tears, saliva, and vaginal secretions) are rich in antibodies (discussed in detail later in the chapter) and in enzymes that break down and destroy many microorganisms.

The respiratory tract is lined not only with mucous membranes but also with cells having hairlike protrusions called cilia. The cilia sweep foreign matter up and out of the respiratory tract. Particles that are not caught by this mechanism may be expelled from the system by a cough. If the ciliated cells are damaged or destroyed, as they are by smoking, a cough is the body's only way of ridding the airways of foreign particles.

### The Immune System

Once the body has been invaded by a foreign organism, an elaborate system of responses is activated. We discuss here two of the body's responses: the inflammatory response and the immune response. But before we cover these specific defenses, we briefly describe the defenders themselves and the mechanisms by which they work.

**Immunological Defenders** The immune response is carried out by different types of white blood cells, all of which are continuously being produced in the bone marrow. **Neutrophils**, one type of white blood cell, travel in the bloodstream to areas of invasion, attacking and ingesting pathogens. **Macrophages**, or "big eaters," take up stations in tissues and act as scavengers, devouring

**Terms**

VW

**infection** Invasion of the body by a microorganism.

**pathogen** An organism that causes disease.

**lymphatic system** A system of vessels and organs that picks up excess fluid, proteins, lipids, and other substances from the tissues; filters out pathogens and other waste products; and returns the cleansed fluid to the general circulation.

**systemic infection** An infection spread by the blood or lymphatic system to large portions of the body.

**neutrophil** A type of white blood cell that engulfs foreign organisms and infected, damaged, or aged cells; particularly prevalent during the inflammatory response.

**macrophage** A large phagocytic (cell-eating) cell that devours foreign particles.

pathogens and worn-out cells. **Natural killer cells** directly destroy virus-infected cells and cells that have turned cancerous. **Dendritic cells,** which reside in tissues, eat pathogens and activate lymphocytes. **Lymphocytes,** of which there are several types, are white blood cells that travel in both the bloodstream and the lymphatic system. At various places in the lymphatic system there are lymph nodes (or glands), where macrophages and dendritic cells congregate and filter bacteria and other substances from the lymph. When these nodes are actively involved in fighting an invasion of microorganisms, they fill with cells; physicians use the location of swollen lymph nodes as a clue to the location and cause of an infection.

The two main types of lymphocytes are known as **T cells** and **B cells.** T cells are further differentiated into **helper T cells, killer T cells,** and **suppressor T cells.** B cells are lymphocytes that produce **antibodies.** The first time T cells and B cells encounter a specific invader, some of them are reserved as **memory T and B cells,** enabling the body to mount a rapid response should the same invader appear again in the future.

## Terms

VW

**natural killer cell** A type of white blood cell that directly destroys virus-infected cells and cancer cells.

**dendritic cell** A white blood cell specialized to activate T and B cells.

**lymphocyte** A white blood cell continuously made in lymphoid tissue as well as in bone marrow.

**T cell** A lymphocyte that arises in bone marrow and matures in the thymus (thus its name).

**B cell** A lymphocyte that matures in the bone marrow and produces antibodies.

**helper T cell** A lymphocyte that helps activate other T cells and may help B cells produce antibodies.

**killer T cell** A lymphocyte that kills body cells that have been invaded by foreign organisms; also can kill cells that have turned cancerous.

**suppressor T cell** A lymphocyte that inhibits the growth of other lymphocytes.

**antibody** A specialized protein, produced by white blood cells, that can recognize and neutralize specific microbes.

**memory T and B cells** Lymphocytes generated during an initial infection that circulate in the body for years, "remembering" the specific antigens that caused the infection and quickly destroying them if they appear again.

**autoimmune disease** A disease in which the immune system attacks the person's own body.

**antigen** A marker on the surface of a foreign substance that immune system cells recognize as nonself and that triggers the immune response.

**histamine** A chemical responsible for the dilation and increased permeability of blood vessels in allergic reactions.

**immunity** Mechanisms that defend the body against infection; specific defenses against specific pathogens.

The immune system is built on a remarkable feature of these defenders: the ability to distinguish foreign cells from the body's own cells. Because lymphocytes are capable of great destruction, it is essential that they not attack the body itself. When they do, they cause **autoimmune diseases,** such as lupus and rheumatoid arthritis.

How do lymphocytes know when they have encountered foreign substances? All the cells of an individual's body display markers on their surfaces—tiny molecular shapes—that identify them as "self" to lymphocytes that encounter them. Invading microorganisms also display markers on their surface; lymphocytes identify these as foreign, or "nonself." Nonself markers that trigger the immune response are known as **antigens.** Antibodies have complementary surface markers that work with antigens like a lock and key. When an antigen appears in the body, it eventually encounters an antibody with a complementary pattern; the antibody locks onto the antigen, triggering a series of events designed to destroy the invading pathogen.

**The Inflammatory Response** When the body has been injured or infected, one of the body's responses is the inflammatory response. Special cells in the area of invasion or injury release **histamine** and other substances that cause blood vessels to dilate and fluid to flow out of capillaries into the injured tissue. This produces increased heat, swelling, and redness in the affected area. White blood cells, including neutrophils, dendritic cells, and macrophages, are drawn to the area and attack the invaders—in many cases, destroying them.

**The Immune Response** Another body reaction to infection is the immune response (Figure 13-1). For convenience, we can think of the immune response as having four phases: (1) recognition of the invading pathogen, (2) amplification of defenses, (3) attack, and (4) slowdown.

- *Phase 1.* Dendritic cells are drawn to the site of the injury and consume the foreign cells; they then provide information about the pathogen by displaying its antigen on their surfaces. Helper T cells "read" this information and rush to respond.
- *Phase 2.* Helper T cells multiply rapidly and trigger the production of killer T cells and B cells in the spleen and lymph nodes. Cytokines, chemical messengers secreted by lymphocytes, help regulate and coordinate the immune response; *interleukins* and *interferons* are two examples of cytokines. They stimulate increased production of T cells, B cells, and antibodies; promote the activities of natural killer cells; produce fever; and have special antipathogenic properties themselves.
- *Phase 3.* Killer T cells strike at foreign cells and body cells that have been invaded and infected, identifying

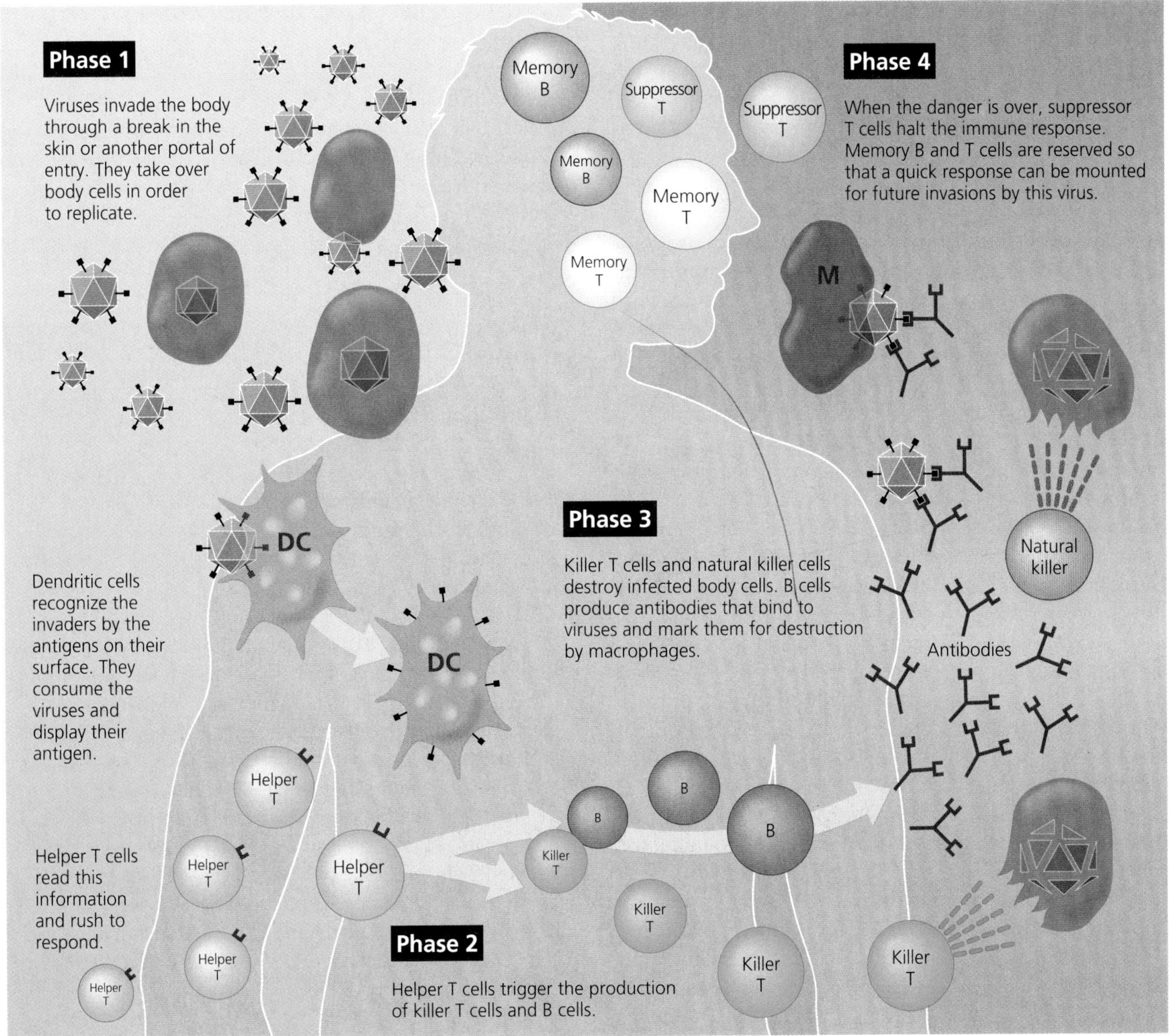


**Figure 13-1 The immune response.** Once invaded by a pathogen, the body mounts a complex series of reactions to eliminate the invader. Pictured here are the principal elements of the immune response to a virus.

them by the antigens displayed on the cell surfaces. Puncturing the cell membrane, they sacrifice body cells in order to destroy the foreign organism within.

B cells work in a different way. Stimulated to multiply by helper T cells, they produce large quantities of antibody molecules, which are released in the bloodstream and tissues. Antibodies are Y-shaped protein molecules that bind to antigen-bearing targets and mark them for destruction by macrophages. Antibodies work against bacteria and against viruses and other substances when they are in the body but outside cells.

- *Phase 4.* The last phase of the immune response is a slowdown of activity. When the danger is over, suppressor T cells halt the immune response and restore stability, or homeostasis. The dead cells, killed pathogens, and other debris that result from the immune response are filtered out of circulation and excreted from the body.

**Immunity** After an infection, survival often confers **immunity;** that is, an infected person will never get the same illness again. This is because some of the lymphocytes created during the amplification phase of the immune response are reserved as memory T and B cells. If the same antigen enters the body again, the memory T and B cells recognize and destroy it before it can cause illness. The ability of memory lymphocytes to remember previous infections is known as *acquired immunity.*

**Symptoms and Contagion** The immune system is operating at the cellular level at all times, maintaining its vigilance when you're well and fighting invaders when you're sick. During **incubation,** when pathogens are actively multiplying before the immune system has gathered momentum, you may not have any symptoms of the illness, but you may be contagious. During the second and third phases of the immune response, you may still be unaware of the infection, or you may "feel a cold coming on." Symptoms first appear during the **prodromal period,** which follows incubation. If the infected host has acquired immunity, the infection may be eradicated during the incubation period or the prodromal period. In this case, although you may have felt you were coming down with a cold, for example, it does not develop into a full-blown illness.

Many symptoms of an illness are actually due to the immune response of the body rather than to the actions or products of the invading organism. For example, fever is caused by the release and activation of certain cytokines during the immune response. These cytokines travel in the bloodstream to the brain and cause the body's thermostat to be "reset" to a higher level. The resulting elevated temperature helps the body in its fight against pathogens by enhancing immune responses. (During an illness, it is necessary to lower a fever only if it is uncomfortably high [over 101.5°F] or if it occurs in an infant who is at risk for seizures from fever.)

Similarly, you get a runny nose when your lymphocytes destroy infected mucosal cells, leading to increased mucus production. You get a sore throat when your lymphocytes destroy infected throat cells, and the malaise and fatigue of the flu may be caused by interferons.

You are contagious when there are infectious microbes in your body and they can gain access to another person. This may be before a vigorous immune response has occurred, so at times you may be contagious before experiencing any symptoms. This means that you can transmit an illness without knowing you're infected or catch an illness from someone who doesn't appear to be sick. On the other hand, your symptoms may continue after the pathogens have been mostly destroyed, when you are no longer infectious.

## Immunization

The ability of the immune system to remember previously encountered organisms and retain its strength against them is the basis for immunization. When a person is immunized, the immune system is "primed" with an antigen similar to the pathogenic organism but not as dangerous. The body responds by producing antibodies, which prevent serious infection when and if the person is exposed to the disease organism itself. These preparations used to manipulate the immune system are known as **vaccines.** Most vaccines are made from microbes that have been weakened or killed in the laboratory but still retain their ability to stimulate the production of antibodies.

Vaccines confer what is known as *active immunity*—that is, the vaccinated person produces his or her own antibodies to the microorganism. Another type of injection confers *passive immunity.* In this case, a person exposed to a disease is injected with the antibodies themselves, produced by other human beings or animals who have recovered from the disease. Injections of gamma globulin—a product made from the blood plasma of many individuals containing all the antibodies they have ever made—are sometimes given to people exposed to a disease against which they have not been immunized. Such injections create a rapid but temporary immunity and are useful against certain viruses, such as hepatitis A.

For information on current vaccination recommendations for children, adults, and travelers, visit the web site for the CDC National Immunization Program (www.cdc.gov/nip).

## Allergy: The Body's Defense System Gone Haywire

Are you among the estimated 50 million Americans affected by **allergies?** Allergies result from a hypersensitive and overactive immune system. The immune system typically defends the body against only genuinely harmful pathogens such as viruses and bacteria. However, in someone with an allergy, the immune system also mounts a response to a harmless substance such as pollen or animal dander. The unpleasant and potentially serious symptoms of an allergy—stuffy nose, sneezing, wheezing, skin rashes, and so on—result primarily from the immune response rather than from the **allergens,** the substances that provoke the response. Different people have

### Terms

**incubation** The period when bacteria or viruses are actively multiplying inside the body's cells; usually a period without symptoms of illness.

**prodromal period** The stage of an infection following incubation, during which initial symptoms begin to appear but the host does not feel ill; a highly contagious period.

**vaccine** A preparation of killed or weakened microorganisms, inactivated toxins, or components of microorganisms that is administered to stimulate an immune response; a vaccine protects against future infection by the pathogen.

**allergy** A disorder caused by the body's exaggerated response to foreign chemicals and proteins; also called *hypersensitivity*.

**allergen** A substance that triggers an allergic reaction.

**anaphylaxis** A severe systemic hypersensitive reaction to an allergen characterized by difficulty breathing, low blood pressure, heart arrhythmia, seizure, and sometimes death.

allergic reactions to different substances. Common allergens include pollen, animal dander, dust mites, cockroaches, molds, mildew, foods, and insect stings. People may also be allergic to certain medications, plants such as poison oak, latex, metals such as nickel, and compounds found in cosmetics.

**The Allergic Response** Most allergic reactions are due to the production of a special type of antibody known as immunoglobulin E (IgE). Initial exposure to a particular allergen may cause little response, but it sensitizes the immune system. When the body is subsequently exposed to the allergen, the allergen binds to IgE, causing the release of large amounts of histamine and other compounds into surrounding tissues. Histamine has many effects, including increasing the inflammatory response and stimulating mucus production. In the nose, histamine may cause congestion and sneezing; in the eyes, itchiness and tearing; in the skin, redness, swelling, and itching; in the intestines, bloating and cramping; and in the lungs, coughing, wheezing, and shortness of breath. In some people, an allergen can trigger an asthma attack.

The most serious, but rare, kind of allergic reaction is **anaphylaxis,** which results from a release of histamine throughout the body. Anaphylactic reactions can be life-threatening because symptoms may include swelling of the throat, extremely low blood pressure, fainting, heart arrhythmia, and seizures. Anaphylaxis is a medical emergency and requires immediate injection of epinephrine.

**Dealing with Allergies** If you suspect you might have an allergy, visit your physician or an allergy specialist. You may be asked to keep a diary to help identify allergens to which you are susceptible, or you may undergo allergy skin tests or blood tests. There are three general strategies for dealing with allergies:

- *Avoidance:* You may be able to avoid or minimize exposure to allergens by making changes in your environment or behavior. For example, removing carpets from the bedroom and using special bedding can reduce dust mite contact.
- *Medication:* Many over-the-counter (OTC) antihistamines are effective at controlling symptoms. Prescription corticosteroids markedly reduce allergy symptoms, but they have significant side effects.
- *Immunotherapy:* Referred to as "allergy shots," immunotherapy desensitizes a person to a particular allergen through the administration of gradually increasing doses of the allergen over a period of months or years.

**Asthma** More than 30 million Americans have asthma, which causes more than 4000 U.S. deaths each year. Particularly affected are African Americans, American Indians and Alaska Natives, people living in inner cities, children, and people older than age 65. Asthma is caused by both inflammation of the airways and spasm of the muscles surrounding the airways. The spasm causes constriction, and the inflammation causes the airway linings to swell and secrete extra mucus, which further obstructs the passages. The result is wheezing, tightness in the chest, and shortness of breath. An attack begins when something sets off inflammation of the bronchial tubes; usually it's an allergic reaction to an inhaled allergen such as pollen, but anything that irritates the airways can trigger spasms, including exercise, cold air, tobacco smoke, and stress. Some of the same strategies that help control allergies—including avoidance of allergens and regular use of medication—are recommended for asthma.

## THE TROUBLEMAKERS: PATHOGENS AND DISEASE

Now that we've discussed the intricate system that protects us from disease, let's consider some pathogens, the disease-producing organisms that live within us and around us. When they succeed in gaining entry to body tissue, they can cause illness and sometimes death to the unfortunate host. Worldwide, infectious diseases are responsible for more than 10 million deaths each year (Table 13-1). Pathogens include bacteria, viruses, fungi, protozoa, parasitic worms, and prions (Figure 13-2).

VITAL STATISTICS

**Table 13-1 Top Infectious Diseases Worldwide**

| Disease | Approximate Number of Deaths per Year |
|---|---|
| Pneumonia | 3,884,000 |
| HIV/AIDS | 2,777,000 |
| Diarrheal diseases | 1,798,000 |
| Tuberculosis | 1,566,000 |
| Malaria | 1,272,000 |
| Measles | 611,000 |
| Pertussis (whooping cough) | 294,000 |
| Tetanus | 214,000 |
| Meningitis | 173,000 |
| Syphilis | 157,000 |

Many of the 618,000 deaths from liver cancer each year can be traced to viral hepatitis. Overall, infectious diseases kill more than 11 million people each year, representing nearly 19% of all deaths.

SOURCE: World Health Organization. 2004. *The World Health Report 2004*. Geneva: World Health Organization.

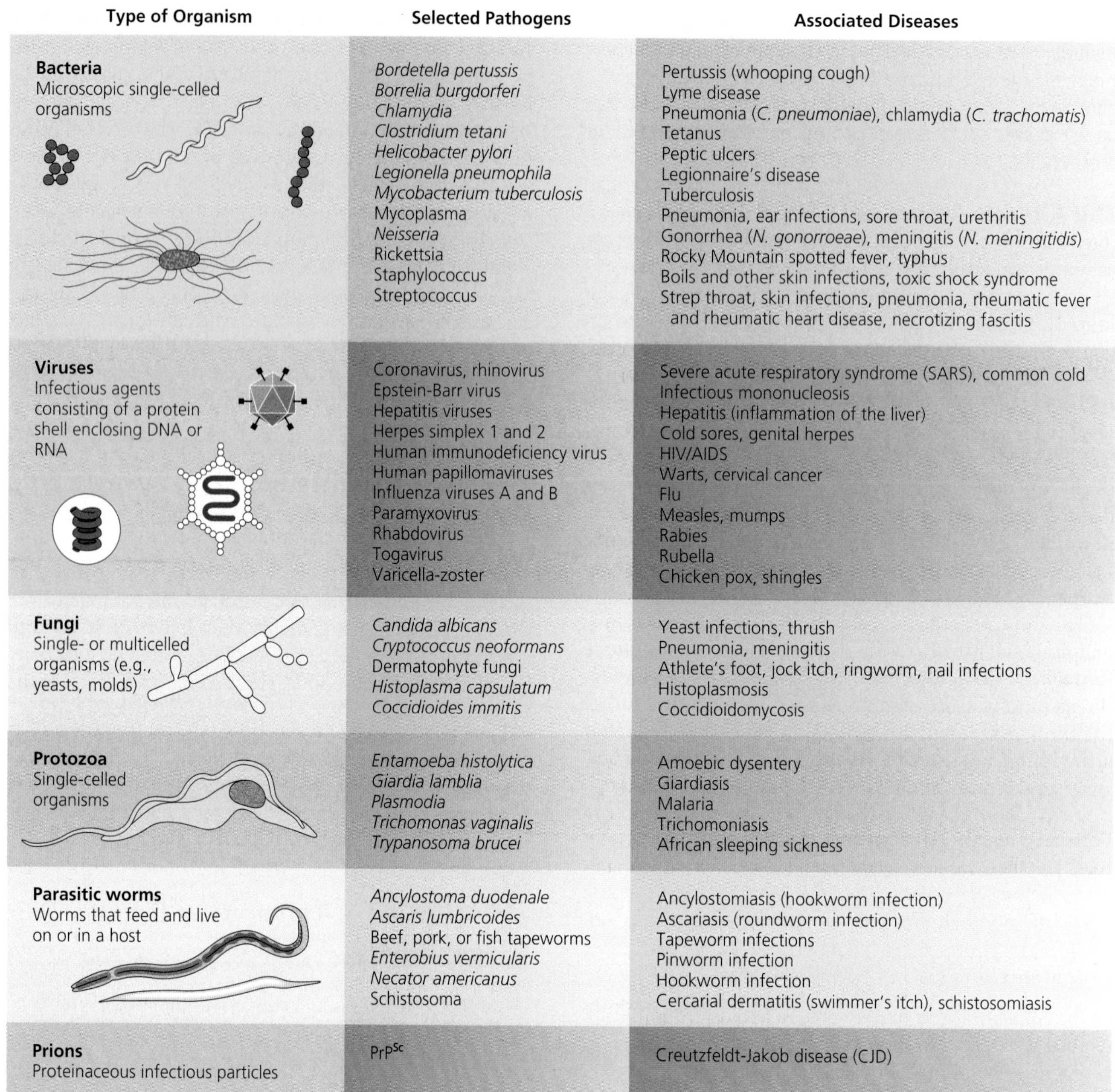

| Type of Organism | Selected Pathogens | Associated Diseases |
|---|---|---|
| **Bacteria**<br>Microscopic single-celled organisms | *Bordetella pertussis*<br>*Borrelia burgdorferi*<br>*Chlamydia*<br>*Clostridium tetani*<br>*Helicobacter pylori*<br>*Legionella pneumophila*<br>*Mycobacterium tuberculosis*<br>Mycoplasma<br>*Neisseria*<br>Rickettsia<br>Staphylococcus<br>Streptococcus | Pertussis (whooping cough)<br>Lyme disease<br>Pneumonia (*C. pneumoniae*), chlamydia (*C. trachomatis*)<br>Tetanus<br>Peptic ulcers<br>Legionnaire's disease<br>Tuberculosis<br>Pneumonia, ear infections, sore throat, urethritis<br>Gonorrhea (*N. gonorroeae*), meningitis (*N. meningitidis*)<br>Rocky Mountain spotted fever, typhus<br>Boils and other skin infections, toxic shock syndrome<br>Strep throat, skin infections, pneumonia, rheumatic fever and rheumatic heart disease, necrotizing fascitis |
| **Viruses**<br>Infectious agents consisting of a protein shell enclosing DNA or RNA | Coronavirus, rhinovirus<br>Epstein-Barr virus<br>Hepatitis viruses<br>Herpes simplex 1 and 2<br>Human immunodeficiency virus<br>Human papillomaviruses<br>Influenza viruses A and B<br>Paramyxovirus<br>Rhabdovirus<br>Togavirus<br>Varicella-zoster | Severe acute respiratory syndrome (SARS), common cold<br>Infectious mononucleosis<br>Hepatitis (inflammation of the liver)<br>Cold sores, genital herpes<br>HIV/AIDS<br>Warts, cervical cancer<br>Flu<br>Measles, mumps<br>Rabies<br>Rubella<br>Chicken pox, shingles |
| **Fungi**<br>Single- or multicelled organisms (e.g., yeasts, molds) | *Candida albicans*<br>*Cryptococcus neoformans*<br>Dermatophyte fungi<br>*Histoplasma capsulatum*<br>*Coccidioides immitis* | Yeast infections, thrush<br>Pneumonia, meningitis<br>Athlete's foot, jock itch, ringworm, nail infections<br>Histoplasmosis<br>Coccidioidomycosis |
| **Protozoa**<br>Single-celled organisms | *Entamoeba histolytica*<br>*Giardia lamblia*<br>*Plasmodia*<br>*Trichomonas vaginalis*<br>*Trypanosoma brucei* | Amoebic dysentery<br>Giardiasis<br>Malaria<br>Trichomoniasis<br>African sleeping sickness |
| **Parasitic worms**<br>Worms that feed and live on or in a host | *Ancylostoma duodenale*<br>*Ascaris lumbricoides*<br>Beef, pork, or fish tapeworms<br>*Enterobius vermicularis*<br>*Necator americanus*<br>Schistosoma | Ancylostomiasis (hookworm infection)<br>Ascariasis (roundworm infection)<br>Tapeworm infections<br>Pinworm infection<br>Hookworm infection<br>Cercarial dermatitis (swimmer's itch), schistosomiasis |
| **Prions**<br>Proteinaceous infectious particles | $PrP^{Sc}$ | Creutzfeldt-Jakob disease (CJD) |

**Figure 13-2 Pathogens and associated infectious diseases.**

## Bacteria

The most abundant living things on earth are **bacteria,** single-celled organisms that usually reproduce by splitting in two to create a pair of identical cells. We harbor both helpful and harmful bacteria on our skin and in our gastrointestinal and reproductive tracts. The human colon contains "friendly" bacteria that produce certain vitamins and help digest nutrients. (A large portion of feces consists of bacteria.) Friendly bacteria also keep harmful bacteria in check by competing for food and resources and secreting substances toxic to pathogenic bacteria. Not all bacteria found in the body are beneficial, however. Some bacterial infections of concern are described on the following pages.

**Pneumonia** Inflammation of the lungs, called **pneumonia,** may be caused by infection with bacteria, viruses, or fungi or by contact with chemical toxins or irritants. Pneumonia often follows another illness, such as a cold or the flu, but the symptoms are typically more severe—fever, chills, shortness of breath, increased mucus production, and cough. Pneumonia ranks seventh among the leading causes of death for Americans.

Pneumococcus bacteria are the most common cause of bacterial pneumonia; a vaccine is available and recommended for all adults age 65 and older and others at risk. Other bacteria that may cause pneumonia include *Streptococcus pneumoniae, Chlamydia pneumoniae,* and *mycoplasmas.* Outbreaks of infection with mycoplasmas are relatively common among young adults, especially in crowded settings such as dormitories.

**Meningitis** Infection of the *meninges,* the membranes covering the brain and spinal cord, is called **meningitis.** Viral meningitis is usually mild and goes away on its own; bacterial meningitis, however, can be life-threatening and requires immediate treatment with antibiotics. Symptoms of meningitis include fever, a severe headache, stiff neck, sensitivity to light, and confusion. The disease is fatal in 10% of cases, and about 10–20% of people who recover have permanent hearing loss or other serious effects. A vaccine is available, but it is not effective against all strains of meningitis-causing bacteria. The CDC recommends routine vaccination of children 11–12 years old, previously unvaccinated adolescents at high school entry, and first-year college students who live in dormitories.

**Strep Throat and Other Streptococcal Infections** The **streptococcus** bacterium can cause streptococcal pharyngitis, or strep throat, characterized by a red, sore throat with white patches on the tonsils, swollen lymph nodes, fever, and headache. It is typically spread through close contact with an infected person via respiratory droplets (sneezing or coughing). If left untreated, strep throat can develop into the more serious rheumatic fever. A particularly virulent type of streptococcus can invade the bloodstream, spread, and produce dangerous systemic illness. It can also cause a serious but rare infection of the deeper layers of the skin, a condition called necrotizing fascitis or "flesh-eating strep."

**Toxic Shock Syndrome and Other Staphylococcal Infections** The spherical-shaped **staphylococcus** bacterium can cause infections ranging from minor skin infections such as boils to very serious conditions such as blood infections and pneumonia. A particular species of the bacteria, *Staphylococcus aureus,* is responsible for many cases of **toxic shock syndrome (TSS).** The bacteria produce a deadly toxin that causes shock (potentially life-threatening low blood pressure), high fever, a peeling skin rash, and inflammation of several organ systems.

**Tuberculosis** Caused by the bacterium *Mycobacterium tuberculosis,* **tuberculosis (TB)** is a chronic bacterial infection that usually affects the lungs. TB is spread via the respiratory route through prolonged contact with someone who has the disease in its active form. Symptoms include coughing, fatigue, night sweats, weight loss, and fever. Ten to 15 million Americans have been infected with, and therefore continue to carry, *M. tuberculosis.* However, only about 10% of people with so-called latent TB infections actually develop an active case of the disease during their lifetime. In the United States, active TB is most common among people infected with HIV, recent immigrants from countries where TB is **endemic,** and those who live in the inner cities. Many strains of tuberculosis respond to antibiotics, but only over a long course of treatment lasting 6–12 months. Failure to complete treatment can lead to relapse and the development of strains of antibiotic-resistant bacteria.

**Lyme Disease** Lyme disease is spread by the bite of a tick of the genus *Ixodes* that is infected with the spiral-shaped bacterium *Borrelia burgdorferi.* Symptoms of Lyme disease vary but typically occur in stages, beginning with a bull's-eye-shaped rash in the area of the bite; later symptoms can include impaired coordination and chronic or recurrent arthritis. Lyme disease is preventable by avoiding contact with ticks or by removing a tick before it has had the chance to transmit the infection (see the box "Protecting Yourself Against Tickborne and Mosquitoborne Infections"). Lyme disease is treatable at all stages, although arthritis symptoms may not completely resolve.

**Ulcers** About 25 million Americans suffer from ulcers, sores or holes in the lining of the stomach or the first part of the small intestine. It used to be thought that spicy food and stress were major causes of ulcers, but it is now known that as many as 90% of ulcers are caused by infection with *Helicobacter pylori.* Ulcer symptoms include gnawing or burning pain in the abdomen, nausea, and loss of appetite. If tests show the presence of *H. pylori,* treatment with antibiotics often cures the infection and the ulcers.

## Terms

**bacterium** (plural, **bacteria**) A microscopic single-celled organism; about 100 bacterial species can cause disease in humans.

**pneumonia** Inflammation of the lungs, typically caused by infection or exposure to chemical toxins or irritants.

**meningitis** Infection of the membranes covering the brain and spinal cord (meninges).

**streptococcus** Any of a genus *(Streptococcus)* of spherical bacteria; streptococcal species can cause skin infections, strep throat, rheumatic fever, pneumonia, scarlet fever, and other diseases.

**staphylococcus** Any of a genus *(Staphylococcus)* of spherical, clustered bacteria commonly found on the skin or in the nasal passages; staphylococcal species may enter the body and cause conditions such as boils, pneumonia, and toxic shock syndrome.

**toxic shock syndrome (TSS)** Sudden onset of fever, aches, vomiting, and peeling rash, followed in some cases by shock and inflammation of multiple organs; often caused by a toxin produced by *Staphylococcus aureus.*

**tuberculosis (TB)** A chronic bacterial infection that usually affects the lungs.

**endemic** Persistent and relatively widespread in a given population.

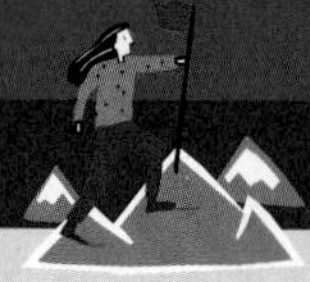

Take Charge

## Protecting Yourself Against Tickborne and Mosquitoborne Infections

### Avoid Tick Habitat

When possible, avoid areas that are likely to be infested with ticks, particularly in spring and summer, when the immature ticks, called nymphs, are most likely to feed. Ticks favor moist, shaded habitats, especially as provided by leaf litter and low-lying vegetation in wooded, brushy, or overgrown grassy habitats. Don't sit on logs or lean against trees. State and local health departments, park personnel, and agricultural extension services can provide information on the distribution of ticks in your area.

### Avoid Mosquitoes

Dawn, dusk, and early evening are times of major mosquito activity, so limit your outdoor activities during these periods or take special care to wear appropriate clothing and use insect repellent (see below). Installing or repairing window and door screens can help keep insects outside. Place mosquito netting over infant carriers when you are outdoors with infants.

Eliminate any standing water near your home to prevent mosquitoes from breeding. Drain or upend containers (flower pots, pet dishes, and so on), change birdbath water weekly, and drill holes in the bottom of containers and tire swings that are left outside. Report dead birds to state and local health departments; birds are particularly susceptible to West Nile virus, and dead ones may indicate local infection.

### Wear Protective Clothing and Apply Insect Repellent

Wear light-colored clothing so that insects can be spotted more easily. Wear long-sleeved shirts and tuck pants into socks or the tops of boots to help keep ticks from reaching your skin. Ticks are usually located close to the ground, so wearing high boots may provide additional protection. In 2005, the CDC expanded its list of recommended mosquito repellents to include DEET (n,n-diethyl-m-toluamide), picaridin (KBR 3023), and oil of lemon eucalyptus (PMD); the repellent permethrin can be applied to clothing but not skin. All repellents should be used carefully and as described on the product label.

### Remove Attached Ticks

Transmission of an infectious agent is unlikely to occur until a tick has fed on you for several hours (36 hours in the case of Lyme disease), so daily checks for ticks and their prompt removal will help prevent infection. Search your entire body for ticks, using a handheld or full-length mirror; also check children and pets. Ticks are small; in the nymph phase, they may resemble poppy seeds (see figure).

Deer tick (actual size)

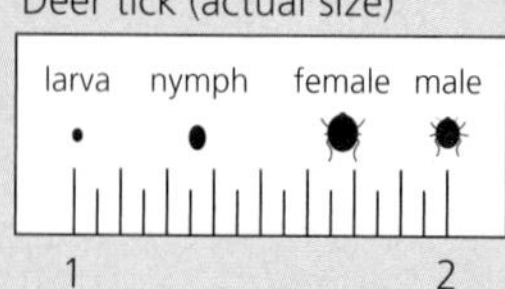


To remove a tick, use blunt-tipped tweezers and shield your fingers with rubber gloves or a paper towel. Grasp the tick as close to the skin surface as possible and pull upward (away from the skin) with steady, even pressure. Do not twist or jerk the tick, as this may cause the mouthparts to break off and remain in the skin. If this happens, remove the mouthparts with tweezers. Do not squeeze, crush, or puncture the body of the tick because its fluids may contain infectious organisms. After removing the tick, disinfect the bite site and wash your hands with soap and water. Save ticks for identification in case you become ill. Place the tick in a plastic bag in your freezer, and note the date of the bite.

SOURCES: Centers for Disease Control and Prevention. 2005. *Updated Information Regarding Mosquito Repellents* (http://www.cdc.gov/ncidod/dvbid/westnile/RepellentUpdates.htm; retrieved May 13, 2005). West Nile: Behind the buzz. 2004. *UC Berkeley Wellness Letter*, July; Centers for Disease Control and Prevention. 2003. *West Nile Virus Prevention* (http://www.cdc.gov/ncidod/dvbid/westnile/qa/prevention.htm; retrieved January 31, 2005); Centers for Disease Control and Prevention. 2002. *Lyme Disease: Prevention and Control* (http://www.cdc.gov/ncidod/dvbid/lyme; retrieved December 10, 2002).

**Antibiotic Treatments** Antibiotics are both naturally occurring and synthetic substances having the ability to kill bacteria. Most antibiotics work in a similar fashion: They interrupt the production of new bacteria by damaging some part of their reproductive cycle or by causing faulty parts of new bacteria to be made. Antibiotics are among the most widely prescribed and effective prescription drugs.

When antibiotics are misused or overused, the pathogens they are designed to treat can become resistant to their effects. A bacterium can become resistant from a chance genetic mutation or through the transfer of genetic material from one bacterium to another. When exposed to antibiotics, resistant bacteria can grow and flourish, while the antibiotic-sensitive bacteria die off. Antibiotic-resistant strains of many common bacteria have developed, including strains of gonorrhea (an STD) and salmonellosis (a foodborne illness). One strain of tuberculosis is resistant to seven different antibiotics. Antibiotic resistance is a major factor contributing to the recent rise in problematic infectious diseases.

You can help prevent the development of antibiotic-resistant strains of bacteria by using antibiotics properly:

- Don't expect to take an antibiotic every time you get sick. They are mainly helpful for bacterial infections; against viruses, they are ineffective.
- Use antibiotics as directed, and finish the full course of medication even if you begin to feel better. This helps ensure that all targeted bacteria are killed off.
- Never take an antibiotic without a prescription. If you take an antibiotic for a viral infection, take the wrong one, or take an insufficient dose, your illness will not improve, and you'll give bacteria the opportunity to develop resistance.

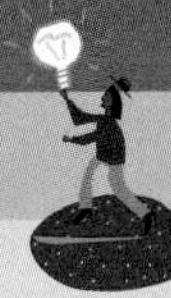

Critical Consumer

## Preventing and Treating the Common Cold

VW

### Prevention

Colds are usually spread by hand-to-hand contact with another person or with objects such as doorknobs and telephones, which an infected person may have handled. The best way to avoid transmission is to wash your hands frequently with warm water and soap. Keeping your immune system strong is another good prevention strategy (see the guidelines provided later in the chapter).

### Home Treatments

- Get some extra rest. It isn't usually necessary to stay home in bed, but you will need to slow down a little from your usual routine to give your body a chance to fight the infection.
- Drink plenty of liquids to prevent dehydration. Hot liquids such as herbal tea and clear chicken soup will soothe a sore throat and loosen secretions; gargling with a glass of slightly salty water may also help. Avoid alcoholic beverages when you have a cold.
- Hot showers or the use of a humidifier can help eliminate nasal stuffiness and soothe inflamed membranes.

### Over-the-Counter Treatments

Avoid multisymptom cold remedies. Because these products include drugs to treat symptoms you may not even have, you risk suffering from side effects from medications you don't need. It's better to treat each symptom separately:

- *Analgesics*—aspirin, acetaminophen (Tylenol), ibuprofen (Advil or Motrin), and naproxen sodium (Aleve)—all help lower fever and relieve muscle aches. Use of aspirin is associated with an increased risk of a serious condition called Reye's syndrome in children and teenagers; for this reason, aspirin should be given only to adults.
- *Decongestants* shrink nasal blood vessels, relieving swelling and congestion. However, they may dry out mucous membranes in the throat and make a sore throat worse. Nasal sprays shouldn't be used for more than 2–3 days to avoid "rebound" congestion.
- *Cough medicines* may be helpful when your cough is nonproductive (not bringing up mucus) or if it disrupts your sleep or work. Expectorants make coughs more productive by increasing the volume of mucus and decreasing its thickness, thereby helping remove irritants from the respiratory airways. Suppressants (antitussives) reduce the frequency of coughing.
- *Antihistamines* decrease nasal secretions caused by the effects of histamine, so they are much more useful in treating allergies than colds. *Caution:* Many antihistamines can make you drowsy.

Antibiotics will not help a cold unless a bacterial infection such as strep throat is also present, and overuse of antibiotics leads to the development of drug resistance. The jury is still out on whether other remedies, including zinc gluconate lozenges, echinacea, and vitamin C, will relieve symptoms or shorten the duration of a cold. Researchers are also studying antiviral drugs that target the most common types of cold viruses.

Sometimes a cold leads to a more serious complication, such as bronchitis, pneumonia, or strep throat. If a fever of 102°F or higher persists, or if cold symptoms don't get better after 2 weeks, see your physician.

## Viruses

**Viruses** are on the borderline between living and nonliving matter. They lack all the enzymes essential to energy production and protein synthesis in normal animal cells, and they cannot grow or reproduce by themselves; they use what they need for growth and reproduction from the cells they invade. Once a virus is inside the host cell, it sheds its protein covering, and its genetic material takes control of the cell and manufactures more viruses like itself. The normal functioning of the host cell is thereby disrupted. Illnesses caused by viruses are the most common forms of **contagious disease.**

**The Common Cold** Although generally brief, lasting only 4–7 days, colds are nonetheless irritating and often interfere with one's normal activities. A cold may be caused by any of more than 200 different viruses that attack the lining of the nasal passages. Cold viruses are almost always transmitted by hand-to-hand contact. To lessen your risk of contracting a cold, wash your hands frequently; if you touch someone else, avoid touching your face until after you've washed your hands. If you do catch a cold, over-the-counter cold remedies may help treat your symptoms but do not directly attack the viral cause (see the box "Preventing and Treating the Common Cold").

**Influenza** Commonly called "the flu," **influenza** is an infection of the respiratory tract caused by the influenza

### Terms

VW

**virus** A very small infectious agent composed of nucleic acid (DNA or RNA) surrounded by a protein coat; lacks an independent metabolism and reproduces only within a host cell.

**contagious disease** A disease that can be transmitted from one person to another; most are viral diseases, such as the common cold and flu.

**influenza** Infection of the respiratory tract by the influenza virus, which is highly infectious and adaptable; the form changes so easily that every year new strains arise, making treatment difficult; commonly known as the flu.

In the News

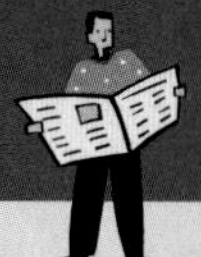

## The Next Influenza Pandemic—When, Not If?

There are three main types of influenza viruses, designated A, B, and C. Influenza C usually causes only mild illness and has not been associated with widespread outbreaks. Types A and B, however, are responsible for **epidemics** of respiratory illness that occur almost every winter.

Through replication errors and gene sharing, influenza viruses undergo constant change, enabling them to evade the immune system and thereby make people susceptible to influenza throughout life. A person infected with influenza does develop antibodies, but as the antigens change, the antibodies no longer recognize the virus, and reinfection can occur. Small changes in antigens are why the flu vaccine is reformulated each year. Fortunately, if the changes are small, the immune system may at least partially recognize the virus, giving many people some immune protection against the new strain.

Occasionally, an influenza A virus undergoes a sudden, dramatic change. If the new virus spreads easily from person to person, a worldwide epidemic, called a **pandemic**, can occur because few people have any antibody protection against the virus. Influenza pandemics usually occur about every 30 years or so. During the twentieth century, three major influenza pandemics occurred in humans:

- 1918–1919 ("Spanish flu"): About 20–40% of the world's population became ill, and as many as 40 million people died, including more than 500,000 Americans.
- 1957–1958 ("Asian flu")
- 1968–1969 ("Hong Kong flu")

Many experts believe that an influenza pandemic is overdue, inevitable, and possibly imminent. Conditions that allow the mingling of flu viruses—including wild and domestic birds, humans, and other flu carriers living in crowded conditions and close proximity—exist in many parts of the world. This mingling of viruses increases the likelihood of significant changes to flu antigens.

Scientists have been monitoring the progress of a strain of avian influenza A(H5N1) in Asia that has caused a small but deadly number of cases in humans. The H5N1 strain doesn't pass easily to or between humans. However, when it infects humans, it is deadly—as of April 2005, there had been 79 confirmed cases and 50 deaths.

Scientists are studying the virus to determine how many mutations it would take to allow H5N1 to pass easily between humans. Attempts are also being made to develop a vaccine ahead of a pandemic; however, the long lag time in flu vaccine production presents a major challenge. Close monitoring and quick action may be the world's best protection.

SOURCES: Orent, W. 2005. Worrying about killer flu. *Discover,* February; Taubenberger, J. K., A. H. Reid, and T. G. Fanning. 2005. Capturing a killer flu virus. *Scientific American,* January; U.S. Department of Health and Human Services. 2004. *National Vaccine Program Office: Influenza* (http://www.hhs.gov/nvpo/pandemics/fluprint.htm; retrieved February 3, 2005).

virus. Compared to the common cold, influenza is a more serious illness, usually including a fever and extreme fatigue. Most people who get the flu recover within 1–2 weeks, but some develop potentially life-threatening complications, such as pneumonia. Influenza is highly contagious and is spread via respiratory droplets.

The most effective way of preventing the flu is through annual vaccination. The influenza vaccine consists of killed virus and provides protection against the strains of the virus currently circulating; it is updated each year in response to changes in the virus (see the box "The Next Influenza Pandemic—When, Not If?"). Vaccination can be appropriate for anyone age 6 months or older who wants to reduce his or her risk of the flu. A number of medications are also available to treat influenza and to reduce the risk of serious illness from influenza.

**Chicken Pox, Cold Sores, and Other Herpesvirus Infections** The **herpesviruses** are a large group of viruses. Once infected, the host is never free of the virus. The virus lies latent within certain cells and becomes active periodically, producing symptoms. The family of herpesviruses includes varicella-zoster virus, which causes chicken pox and shingles; herpes simplex virus (HSV) types 1 and 2, which cause cold sores and the STD herpes; and Epstein-Barr virus (EBV), which causes infectious mononucleosis. Two herpesviruses that can cause severe infections in people with a suppressed immune system are cytomegalovirus (CMV), which infects the lungs, brain, colon, and eyes, and human herpesvirus 8 (HHV-8), which has been linked to Kaposi's sarcoma.

**Viral Hepatitis** Viral **hepatitis** is a term used to describe several different infections that cause inflammation of the liver. Hepatitis is usually caused by one of the three most common hepatitis viruses. Hepatitis A virus (HAV) causes the mildest form of the disease and is usually transmitted by food or water contaminated by sewage or an infected person. Hepatitis B virus (HBV) is usually transmitted sexually (see p. 340). Hepatitis C virus (HCV) can also be transmitted sexually, but it is much more commonly passed through direct contact with infected blood via injection drug use or, prior to the development of screening tests, blood transfusions. HBV and, to a lesser extent, HCV can also be passed from a pregnant woman to her child. There are effective vaccines for hepatitis A and B.

Symptoms of acute hepatitis infection can include fatigue, jaundice, abdominal pain, loss of appetite, nausea,

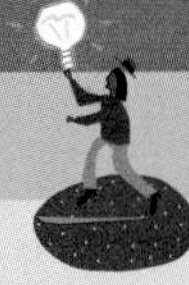

## Tattoos and Body Piercing

Careful selection of a body artist and attention to aftercare instructions can help improve safety and satisfaction following tattooing or piercing.

### Potential Health Issues

- ***Infection:*** There is a risk of transmission of bloodborne infectious agents, including hepatitis B and C and HIV, if instruments are not sterilized properly; however, no cases of HIV infection have been traced to tattooing or piercing. The risk of infection is much higher if body art is applied by untrained individuals or if people fail to follow aftercare instructions. Any unexpected degree of pain or swelling should be promptly evaluated by a physician. Due to the potential risks, people currently cannot donate blood for 12 months following application of body art, including tattoos and some body piercings. People with heart valve problems should check with a physician prior to body piercing to determine if they should take antibiotics in advance of the procedure in order to prevent infection of the heart.
- ***Allergic reactions:*** Some people may be allergic to pigments used in tattooing or to metals used in body-piercing jewelry. All jewelry should be of noncorrosive materials such as stainless steel or titanium; avoid jewelry that contains nickel.
- ***Nodules and scars:*** Some people may develop granulomas (nodules) or keloids (a type of scar) following tattooing or body piercing.
- ***Problems relating to placement:*** Tattoos may become swollen or burned if people undergo magnetic resonance imaging (MRI), and tattoos may also interfere with the quality of MRI images. Oral ornaments may obscure dental problems in dental X rays; they may also damage teeth and fillings and interfere with speech and chewing. Women who breastfeed should remove nipple ornaments before doing so. Navel piercings may become infected more easily because tight-fitting clothes allow moisture to collect in the area.
- ***Dissatisfaction:*** The most common problem with body art is dissatisfaction. Tattoos are meant to be permanent and so are expensive and very difficult (or impossible) to remove completely. Body piercings may close and heal once the jewelry is removed, but they may leave a permanent scar.

### Choosing a Body Artist and Studio

Ask about experience and infection-control procedures. *Remember:* You could be wearing someone else's mistake for the rest of your life. A body art studio should be clean and have an autoclave for sterilizing instruments. Needles should be sterilized and disposable; piercing guns should not be used, as they cannot be adequately sterilized. The body artist should wear disposable latex gloves throughout the procedure. Leftover tattoo ink should be thrown away and not reused. Ask to see references and aftercare instructions beforehand.

Some states and local health departments regulate body art facilities. In addition, you can ask if the studio and/or artist are members of the Alliance for Professional Tattooists (http://www.safe-tattoos.com) or the Association of Professional Piercers (http://www.safepiercing.org); these organizations have developed infection-control and other guidelines for their members to follow.

and diarrhea. Most people recover from hepatitis A within a month or so. However, 5–10% of people infected with HBV and 85–90% of people infected with HCV become chronic carriers of the virus, capable of infecting others for the rest of their lives. Some chronic carriers remain asymptomatic, while others slowly develop chronic liver disease, cirrhosis, or liver cancer. An estimated 4 million Americans and 500 million people worldwide may be chronic carriers of hepatitis.

The extent of HCV infection has only recently been recognized, and most infected people are unaware of their condition. To ensure proper treatment and prevention, testing for HCV may be recommended for people at risk, including people who have ever injected drugs (even once), who received a blood transfusion or a donated organ prior to July 1992, who have engaged in high-risk sexual behavior, or who have had body piercing, tattoos, or acupuncture involving unsterile equipment. (See the box "Tattoos and Body Piercing" for information on improving safety and satisfaction related to body art.)

**Warts** Infection by the human papillomavirus (HPV), which causes cell proliferation, can cause warts (noncancerous skin tumors). The more than 100 different types of HPV cause a variety of warts, including common warts on the hands, plantar warts on the soles of the feet, and genital warts around the genitalia. Depending on

### Terms

**epidemic** The occurrence in a particular community or region of more than the expected number of cases of a particular disease.

**pandemic** A disease epidemic that is unusually severe or widespread; often used to refer to worldwide epidemics affecting a large proportion of the population.

**herpesvirus** A family of viruses responsible for cold sores, mononucleosis, chicken pox, and the STD known as herpes; frequently causes latent infections.

**hepatitis** Inflammation of the liver, which can be caused by infection, drugs, or toxins.

their location, warts may be removed using over-the-counter preparations or professional methods such as laser surgery or cryosurgery. Because HPV infection is chronic, warts can reappear despite treatment.

**Treating Viral Illnesses** Although many viruses cannot be treated medically, researchers have recently begun to develop antiviral drugs. These typically work by interfering with some part of the viral life cycle; for example, they may prevent a virus from entering body cells or from successfully reproducing within cells. Antivirals are currently available to fight infections caused by HIV, influenza, herpes simplex, varicella-zoster, HBV, and HCV. Most other viral diseases must simply run their course.

## Fungi

A **fungus** is an organism that absorbs food from organic matter. Mushrooms and the molds that form on bread and cheese are all examples of fungi. Only about 50 fungi out of many thousands of species cause disease in humans, and these diseases are usually restricted to the skin, mucous membranes, and lungs.

*Candida albicans* is a common fungus found naturally in the vagina of most women. In normal amounts, it causes no problems, but when excessive growth occurs, the result is itching and discomfort, commonly known as a yeast infection. Other common fungal conditions, including athlete's foot, jock itch, and ringworm, a disease of the scalp, affect the skin. Fungi can also cause systemic diseases that are severe, life-threatening, and extremely difficult to treat. Fungal infections can be especially deadly in people with an impaired immune system.

## Protozoa

Another group of pathogens is single-celled organisms known as **protozoa.** Many protozoal diseases are recurrent: The pathogen remains in the body, alternating between activity and inactivity. Hundreds of millions of people in developing countries suffer from protozoal infections. For example, each year, there are more than 500 million new cases of malaria and more than 1 million deaths, mostly among infants and children. Other protozoal diseases include giardiasis, an intestinal infection characterized by nausea and diarrhea; trichomoniasis ("trich"), a treatable vaginal infection; trypanosomiasis, known as African sleeping sickness; and amoebic dysentery.

## Parasitic Worms

The **parasitic worms** are the largest organisms that can enter the body to cause infection. The tapeworm, for example, can grow to a length of many feet. Worms cause a great variety of relatively mild infections. Pinworm, the most common worm infection in the United States, primarily affects young children. Generally speaking, worm infections originate from contaminated food or drink and can be controlled by careful attention to hygiene.

## Prions

In recent years, several fatal degenerative disorders of the central nervous system have been linked to "proteinaceous infectious particles," or **prions.** Unlike all other infectious agents, prions appear to lack DNA or RNA and to consist only of protein; their presence in the body does not trigger an immune response. Prions have an abnormal shape and form deposits in the brain. Prions are associated with a class of diseases known as *transmissible spongiform encephalopathies (TSEs),* which are characterized by sponge-like holes in the brain; symptoms of TSEs include loss of coordination, weakness, dementia, and death. Known prion diseases include Creutzfeldt-Jakob disease (CJD) in humans; bovine spongiform encephalopathy (BSE), or "mad cow disease," in cattle; and scrapie in sheep. Some prion diseases are inherited or the result of spontaneous genetic mutations, whereas others are the result of eating infected tissue or being exposed during medical procedures such as organ transplants.

## Emerging Infectious Diseases

The reduction in deaths from infectious diseases in the United States is one of the major public health achievements of the past century. Improvements in sanitation, hygiene, and water quality and the development of antibiotics all contributed to reduced death rates from tuberculosis, pneumonia, diarrhea, and other infections. However, after decades of decline, the U.S. death rate from infectious disease began to climb in 1981, largely due to the AIDS epidemic. Globally, infectious diseases remain a major killer, and new areas of concern have emerged in the past 20 years. Emerging infectious diseases are diseases of infectious origin whose incidence in humans has increased or threatens to increase in the near future. They include both known diseases that have experienced a resurgence, and diseases that were previously unknown or confined to specific areas.

**Selected Infections of Concern** Although the chances of the average American contracting an exotic infection are very low, emerging infections are a concern to public health officials and represent a challenge to all nations in the future. Some emerging infections, including avian influenza and mad cow disease, were discussed earlier; other infections of concern include the following.

**WEST NILE VIRUS** A mini-outbreak of encephalitis in New York in 1999 led to identification of this virus, which had previously been restricted to Africa, the Middle East, and parts of Europe. Since that time, the virus has spread across the United States and caused more than 17,000 illnesses and 650 deaths. West Nile virus is carried by birds and then passed to humans when mosquitoes bite first an infected bird and then a person. A few cases have also been traced to blood transfusions from infected donors. Most people have few or no symptoms, but the virus can cause permanent brain damage or death in some cases.

**SEVERE ACUTE RESPIRATORY SYNDROME (SARS)** In late 2002, SARS appeared in southern China and quickly spread to more than 15 countries; it is a form of pneumonia that is fatal in about 5–15% of cases. SARS is caused by a new type of coronavirus found in wildlife that may have crossed the species barrier when certain wildlife species were consumed as delicacies. It has reemerged several times since 2002, and by 2005 had been responsible for more than 8000 illnesses and 800 deaths.

**ESCHERICHIA COLI O157:H7** This potentially deadly strain of *E. coli,* transmitted in contaminated food, can cause bloody diarrhea and kidney damage. The first major outbreak occurred in 1993, when over 600 people became ill and 4 children died after eating contaminated and undercooked fast-food hamburgers. Additional outbreaks have been linked to lettuce, alfalfa sprouts, unpasteurized juice, contaminated public swimming pools, and petting zoos. An estimated 70,000 cases and 6 deaths occur in the United States each year.

**HANTAVIRUS** Since first being recognized in 1993, over 300 cases of hantavirus pulmonary syndrome (HPS) have been reported in the United States. HPS is caused by the rodentborne Sin Nombre virus (SNV) and is spread primarily through airborne viral particles from rodent urine, droppings, or saliva. It is characterized by a dangerous fluid buildup in the lungs and is fatal in about 45% of cases.

**EBOLA** So far, outbreaks of the often fatal Ebola hemorrhagic fever (EHF) in humans have occurred only in Africa. The Ebola virus is transmitted by direct contact with infected blood or other body secretions, and many cases of EHF have been linked to unsanitary conditions in medical facilities. Because symptoms appear quickly and 70% of victims die, usually within a few days, the virus tends not to spread widely (unlike HIV or hepatitis, which can infect a person for years before any symptoms appear). Also of concern is the potential use of the Ebola virus by bioterrorists.

## Factors Contributing to Emerging Infections

What's behind this rising tide of infectious diseases? Contributing factors are complex and interrelated:

- *Drug resistance.* New or increasing drug resistance has been found in organisms that cause malaria, tuberculosis, gonorrhea, influenza, AIDS, and pneumococcal and staphylococcal infections. Some bacterial strains now appear to be resistant to all available antibiotics.
- *Poverty.* More than 1 billion people live in extreme poverty, and half the world's population have no regular access to essential drugs. Population growth, urbanization, overcrowding, and migration (including the movement of refugees) also spread infectious diseases.
- *Breakdown of public health measures.* A poor public health infrastructure is often associated with poverty and social upheaval, but problems such as contaminated water supplies and inadequate vaccination can occur even in industrial countries. Natural disasters such as the 2004 tsunami also disrupt the public health infrastructure, leaving survivors with contaminated water and food supplies and no shelter from disease-carrying insects.
- *Environmental changes.* Changes in land use—deforestation, the damming of rivers, the spread of ranching and farming—alter the distribution of disease vectors and bring people into contact with new pathogens. A shift in rainfall patterns caused by global warming may allow mosquitoborne diseases such as malaria to spread from the tropics into the temperate zones.
- *Travel and commerce.* More than 500 million travelers cross national borders each year, and international tourism and trade open the world to infectious agents. SARS was quickly spread throughout the world by infected air travelers. The reintroduction of cholera into the Western Hemisphere is another example—it is thought to have occurred through the discharge of bilge water from a Chinese freighter into the waters off Peru.
- *Mass food production and distribution.* Food now travels long distances to our table, and microbes are transmitted along with it. Mass production of food increases the likelihood that a chance contamination can lead to mass illness.
- *Human behaviors.* The widespread use of injectable drugs rapidly transmits HIV infection and hepatitis. Changes in sexual behavior over the past 30 years have led to a proliferation of new and old STDs. The use of day-care facilities for children has led to increases in the incidence of infections that cause diarrhea.

### Terms

VW

**fungus** A single-celled or multicelled organism that absorbs food from living or dead organic matter; examples include molds, mushrooms, and yeasts. Fungal diseases include yeast infections, athlete's foot, and ringworm.

**protozoan** (plural, **protozoa**) A microscopic single-celled organism that often produces recurrent, cyclical attacks of disease.

**parasitic worm** A pathogen that causes intestinal and other infections; includes tapeworms, hookworms, pinworms, and flukes.

**prion** Proteinaceous infectious particles thought to be responsible for a class of neurodegenerative diseases known as transmissible spongiform encephalopathies; Creutzfeldt-Jakob disease in humans and bovine spongiform encephalopathy ("mad cow disease") are examples of prion diseases.

- *Bioterrorism.* The deliberate release of deadly infectious agents is an ongoing concern. In 2001, infectious anthrax spores placed in mailing envelopes sickened 11 and killed 5 people in the United States. Potential bioterrorism agents that the CDC categorizes as a highest concern are those that can be easily disseminated or transmitted from person to person and that have a high mortality rate and the potential for a major public health impact; these include anthrax, smallpox, plague, botulism, and viral hemorrhagic fevers such as Ebola.

International efforts at monitoring, preventing, and controlling the spread of emerging infections are under way. Microbes do not respect national borders, so only a global response can make the world a safer and healthier place for everyone.

### Other Immune Disorders: Cancer and Autoimmune Diseases

Sometimes, as in the case of cancer, the body comes under attack by its own cells. The immune system can often detect cells that have recently become cancerous and then destroy them just as it would a foreign microorganism. But if the immune system breaks down, the cancer cells may multiply out of control before the immune system recognizes the danger.

Another immune disorder occurs when the body confuses its own cells with foreign organisms. This is what happens in so-called autoimmune diseases such as rheumatoid arthritis and systemic lupus erythematosus. In this type of malady, the immune system seems to be a bit too sensitive and begins to misapprehend itself as "nonself." For reasons not well understood, these conditions are much more common in women than in men.

## GIVING YOURSELF A FIGHTING CHANCE: HOW TO SUPPORT YOUR IMMUNE SYSTEM

Pathogens pose a formidable threat to wellness, but you can take many steps to prevent them from getting control of your body and compromising your health. Public health measures protect people from many diseases that are transmitted via water, food, or insects. A clean water supply and adequate sewage treatment help control typhoid fever and cholera, for example, and mosquito eradication programs control malaria and encephalitis. Proper food inspection and preparation prevent illness caused by foodborne pathogens.

But what can you do as an individual to strengthen your immune system to help prevent infection? The most important thing you can do is to take good care of your body:

- Eat a balanced diet, and maintain a healthy weight.
- Get enough sleep, 6–8 hours every night.
- Exercise (but not while you're sick).
- Don't smoke, and drink alcohol only in moderation.
- Wash your hands frequently and thoroughly.
- Handle and prepare foods safely.
- Avoid contact with mosquitoes, ticks, rodents, and other potential disease carriers.
- Practice safer sex and don't inject drugs.
- Get all appropriate immunizations, and use antibiotics appropriately.

Stress influences the immune response and is affected by lifestyle and attitudes. Research has shown that the actual number of helper T cells rises and falls inversely with stress; that is, the higher the stress, the lower the T-cell count (see the box "Immunity and Stress"). Developing effective ways of coping with stress can improve many of the dimensions of wellness.

## SEXUALLY TRANSMITTED DISEASES

The United States has the highest rate of **sexually transmitted diseases (STDs)** of any developed nation; at current U.S. rates, half of all young people will acquire an STD by age 25. Worldwide, more than 340 million people are affected by STDs each year. Seven different STDs pose major health threats: HIV/AIDS, hepatitis, syphilis, chlamydia, gonorrhea, herpes, and HPV infection (genital warts). These diseases are considered major because they are serious in themselves, cause serious complications if left untreated, and/or pose risks to a fetus or newborn. In addition, pelvic inflammatory disease (PID) is a common complication of gonorrhea and chlamydia and merits discussion as a separate disease.

The bacterial STDs, including chlamydia, gonorrhea, and syphilis, are curable with antibiotics. Unfortunately, previous infection does not confer immunity, so a person can be reinfected despite treatment. The viral STDs—herpes, genital HPV infection (warts), hepatitis, and HIV infection—are not curable with current therapies. Although antiviral drugs and other medications can help target the effects of these STDs, the virus remains in the body and may cause chronic or recurrent infection. A further risk of all STDs is that the associated sores and inflammation caused by STDs allow HIV to pass more easily from one person to another.

### HIV Infection and AIDS

**Acquired immunodeficiency syndrome (AIDS)** is a leading cause of death in many parts of the world. Most of

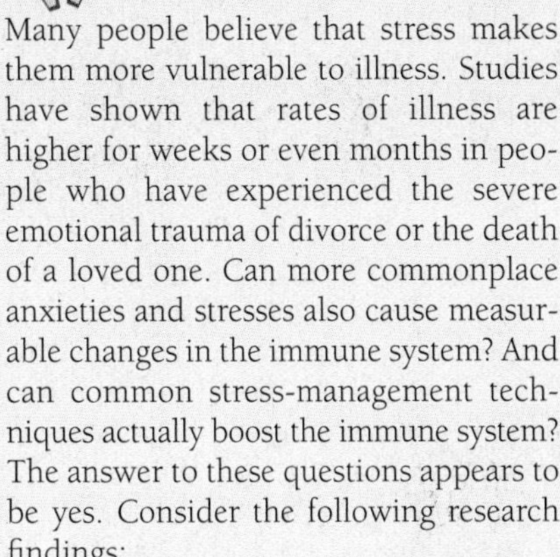

Mind/Body/Spirit

## Immunity and Stress

Many people believe that stress makes them more vulnerable to illness. Studies have shown that rates of illness are higher for weeks or even months in people who have experienced the severe emotional trauma of divorce or the death of a loved one. Can more commonplace anxieties and stresses also cause measurable changes in the immune system? And can common stress-management techniques actually boost the immune system? The answer to these questions appears to be yes. Consider the following research findings:

- Medical students taking final exams showed a much weaker immune response to a hepatitis vaccination than unstressed students. In other studies, stress was associated with lower T-cell responses and antibody levels following influenza vaccinations.
- Individuals who had higher levels of stress and who had a negative or pessimistic outlook developed more colds over the course of a yearlong study than individuals with lower levels of stress and a more positive outlook.
- In a study of caregivers, relaxation sessions were associated with increased secretion of cytokines in minor wounds, thus speeding healing. Relaxation and imagery have also been shown to increase T-cell levels in some people.
- A study comparing parents of children with cancer (who presumably had high stress levels) with parents of healthy children found that stress appears to interfere with the body's ability to shut down the inflammatory response after it gets started. Continuing high levels of cytokines and inflammation could harm health. The same study found that social support improves the immune response.

In seeking to explain these effects, researchers are looking at the connections between stress, hormones, and immunity. Some hormones, such as cortisol, appear to impair the ability of immune cells to multiply and function. Others, such as prolactin, seem to give immune cells a boost. By matching stress levels and hormonal changes to the ups and downs of immune function, researchers hope to learn more about the shifting chemistry of mind and immunity.

SOURCES: Miller, G. E., S. Cohen, and A. K. Ritchey. 2002. Chronic psychological stress and the regulation of pro-inflammatory cytokines: A glucocorticoid-resistance model. *Health Psychology* 21(6): 531–541; Takkouche, B., et al. 2001. A cohort study of stress and the common cold. *Epidemiology* 12: 345–349; Bauer, M. E., et al. 2000. Chronic stress in caregivers of dementia patients is associated with reduced lymphocyte sensitivity to glucocorticoids. *Journal of Neuroimmunology* 103(1): 84–92; Cohen, S., W. J. Doyle, and D. P. Skoner. 1999. Psychological stress, cytokine production, and severity of upper respiratory illness. *Psychosomatic Medicine* 61(2): 175–180.

the nearly 40 million people around the world who are infected with **human immunodeficiency virus (HIV),** the virus that causes AIDS, will likely die within the next 10 years. Although the death rate from AIDS in the United States began to decline in 1996, more than 500,000 of the approximately 1.5 million Americans who have been infected with HIV have died from the disease, and it remains a major killer.

Worldwide, it is estimated that more than 60 million people have been infected since the epidemic began—nearly 1% of the world's population—and that more than 20 million have died (see the box "HIV Infection Around the World" on p. 330). About 10 people are infected every minute—5 million per year—and half of these new infections are in people age 15–24. By 2004, nearly 1 million Americans were believed to be living with HIV—about 1 in 160 males and 1 in 800 females over age 12. Although the death rate from AIDS among Americans has declined, new infections are holding steady at about 40,000 per year, meaning the number of Americans living with HIV infection is growing. About one-quarter of HIV-infected Americans are unaware they are infected.

**What Is HIV Infection?** **HIV infection** is a chronic disease that progressively damages the body's immune system, making an otherwise healthy person less able to resist a variety of infections and disorders. Normally, when a virus or other pathogen enters the body, it is targeted and destroyed by the immune system. But the human immunodeficiency virus (HIV) attacks the immune system itself, invading and taking over **CD4 T cells,** monocytes, and macrophages, which are essential elements of the immune system. HIV enters a human cell and converts its own genetic material, RNA, into DNA. It then inserts this DNA into the chromosomes of the host cell. The viral DNA takes over the CD4 cell, causing it to produce new copies of HIV; it also makes the CD4 cell incapable of performing its immune functions.

Immediately following infection with HIV, billions of infectious particles are produced every day. For a time,

### Terms

**sexually transmitted disease (STD)** A disease that can be transmitted by sexual contact; some STDs can also be transmitted by other means.

**acquired immunodeficiency syndrome (AIDS)** A generally fatal, incurable, sexually transmitted viral disease.

**human immunodeficiency virus (HIV)** The virus that causes HIV infection and AIDS.

**HIV infection** A chronic, progressive viral infection that damages the immune system.

**CD4 T cell** A type of white blood cell that helps coordinate the activity of the immune system; the primary target for HIV infection. A decrease in the number of these cells correlates with the risk and severity of HIV-related illness.

## HIV Infection Around the World

Although first detected among heterosexuals in Africa, AIDS captured world attention in the early 1980s as a disease occurring primarily among homosexual men in the United States and Europe. Since then, AIDS has spread around the world. More than 60 million people worldwide have been infected with HIV since the epidemic began, and more than 20 million have died. The United Nations has declared the spread of HIV infection a threat to world peace.

The vast majority of cases—95%—have occurred in developing countries, where heterosexual contact is the primary means of transmission, responsible for 85% of all adult infections. In the developed world, HIV is increasingly becoming a disease that disproportionately affects the poor and ethnic minorities. Worldwide, women are the fastest-growing group of newly infected people, and more than half the new cases of HIV infection in 2004 occurred in women and children. In addition, an estimated 2.2 million children are living with HIV infection and about 15 million children are AIDS orphans.

Sub-Saharan Africa remains the hardest hit of all areas of the world; in some countries, 20–40% of adults carry the virus, and overall life expectancy has begun to decline dramatically. However, because the epidemic started about 10 years later in Asia than in Africa, experts expect an explosion of new cases in Asia. And because Asia accounts for more than 50% of the world's population, the pool of people at risk is much larger than in Africa. HIV is also spreading rapidly in Eastern Europe, where injection drug use and commercial sex are increasing. The former Soviet countries have seen a 50-fold increase in HIV infection in 8 years.

Efforts to combat AIDS are complicated by political, economic, and cultural barriers. Education and prevention programs are often hampered by resistance from social and religious institutions and by the taboo on openly discussing sexual issues. Condoms are unfamiliar in many countries, and women in many societies do not have sufficient control over their lives to demand that men use condoms during sex. Prevention approaches that have had success include STD treatment and education, public education campaigns about safer sex, and syringe exchange programs for injection drug users.

In countries where there is a substantial imbalance in the social power of men and women, focusing prevention efforts on men is an essential step. In some cultures, older men choose young women and children as sexual partners, believing that they are less likely to be infected or that an HIV carrier who rapes a virgin will be cured, an unfortunately prevalent myth. Sexual violence and traditional practices such as very early marriage and widows being "inherited" by their husband's male relatives increase women's exposure to HIV.

International efforts are under way to make condoms more available by lowering their price and to develop effective antiviral creams that women can use without the knowledge of their partners. Education and other public health measures have been successful in slowing rates of new infection in some countries. In developed nations such as the United States, new drugs are easing AIDS symptoms and lowering viral levels dramatically for some patients. In the past few years, a small but growing number of people in poor countries have gained access to antiviral drugs because of the introduction of inexpensive generic drugs and increasing international funding for HIV treatment. Still, the vast majority of people with HIV remain untreated. Ultimately what we need is an effective vaccine. But until vaccines or a low-cost cure is developed, efforts must continue to focus on widespread educational campaigns and prevention through behavior change.

SOURCE: Joint United Nations Programme on HIV/AIDS (UNAIDS). 2004. *AIDS Epidemic Update: December 2004*. Geneva: UNAIDS/WHO.

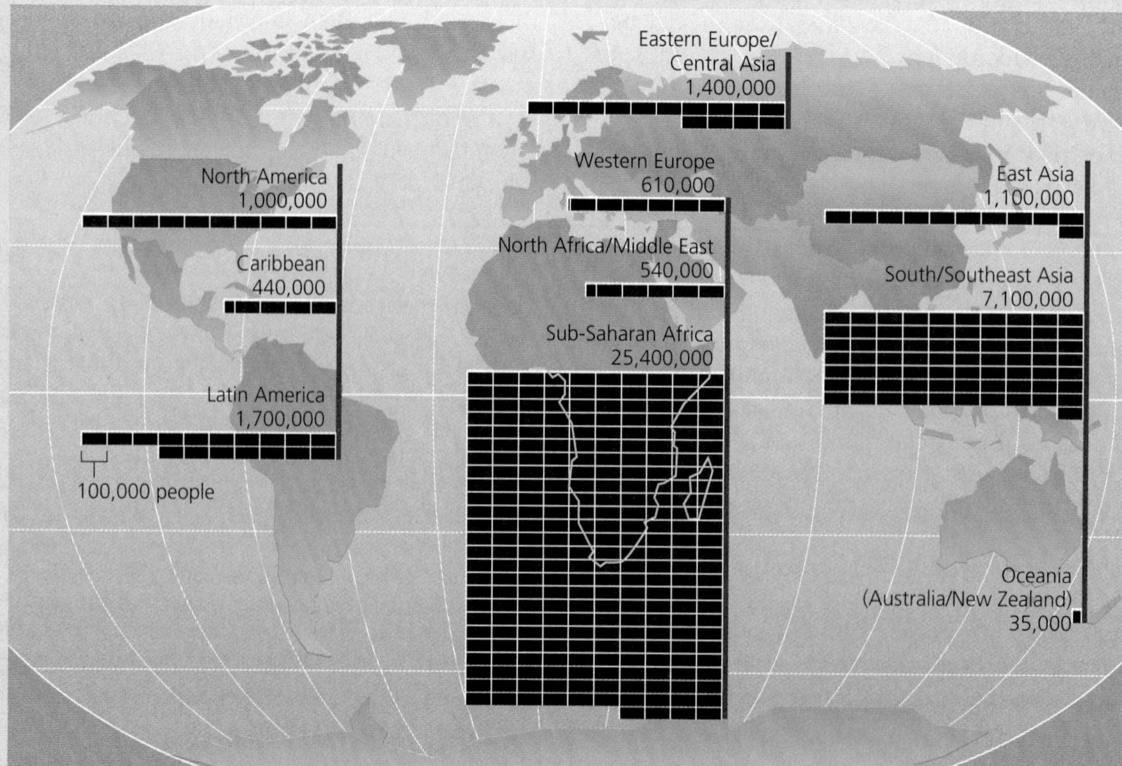


Approximate number of people living with HIV/AIDS at the beginning of 2005.

the immune system keeps pace, also producing billions of new cells. Unlike the virus, however, the immune system cannot make new cells indefinitely; as long as the virus keeps replicating, it wins in the end. The destruction of the immune system is signaled by the loss of CD4 T cells. As the number of CD4 cells declines, an infected person may begin to experience mild to moderately severe symptoms. A person is diagnosed with full-blown AIDS when he or she develops one of the conditions defined as a marker for AIDS or when the number of CD4 cells in the blood drops below a certain level (200/μl). People with AIDS are vulnerable to a number of serious—often fatal—secondary, or opportunistic, infections.

The first weeks after being infected with HIV are called the *primary infection* phase. About half of infected people develop flu-like symptoms during this time. During primary HIV infection, people have large amounts of HIV in the bloodstream, making them much more infectious than they will be several months later when they enter the chronic infection stage. The vast majority of people with primary infection have no idea they are infected, and even if they suspect infection and get tested, the most commonly used tests for HIV will be negative in this stage. Special tests (see below) are needed to detect primary infection.

The next phase of HIV infection is the chronic asymptomatic (symptom-free) stage. This period can last from 2 to 20 years, with an average of 11 years in untreated adults. During this time the virus is progressively infecting and destroying the cells of the immune system. People infected with HIV can transmit the disease to others, even if they are symptom-free.

**Transmitting the Virus** HIV lives only within cells and body fluids, not outside the body. It is transmitted by blood and blood products, semen, vaginal and cervical secretions, and breast milk. It cannot live in air, in water, or on objects or surfaces such as toilet seats, eating utensils, or telephones. The three main routes of HIV transmission are (1) from specific kinds of sexual contact, (2) from direct exposure to infected blood, and (3) from an HIV-infected woman to her fetus during pregnancy or childbirth or to her infant during breastfeeding.

HIV is more likely to be transmitted by unprotected anal or vaginal intercourse than by other sexual activities. Being the receptive partner during unprotected anal intercourse is the riskiest of all sexual activities. Oral-genital contact carries some risk of transmission, although less than anal or vaginal intercourse. Oral sex is responsible for a small but significant number of cases of HIV transmission. HIV can be transmitted through tiny tears in the fragile lining of the vagina, cervix, penis, anus, and mouth and through direct infection of cells in some of these areas.

The presence of lesions, blisters, or inflammation from other STDs in the genital, anal, or oral areas makes it two to nine times easier for the virus to be passed. In addition, any trauma or irritation of tissues, such as might occur from rough or unwanted intercourse or the use of enemas prior to anal intercourse, increases the risk. Spermicides containing nonoxynol-9 may also cause irritation and increase the risk of HIV transmission. The risk of HIV transmission during oral sex increases if a person has poor oral hygiene, has oral sores, or has brushed or flossed just before or after oral sex. During vaginal intercourse, male-to-female transmission is more likely to occur than female-to-male transmission. HIV has been found in preejaculatory fluid, so transmission can occur before ejaculation.

Direct contact with the blood of an infected person is the second major route of HIV transmission. Needles used to inject drugs (including heroin, cocaine, and anabolic steroids) are routinely contaminated by the blood of the user. If needles are shared, small amounts of one person's blood are directly injected into another person's bloodstream. HIV may be transmitted through subcutaneous and intramuscular injection as well, from needles or blades used in acupuncture, tattooing, ritual scarring, and piercing of the earlobes, nose, lip, nipple, navel, or other body part.

HIV has been transmitted in blood and blood products used in the medical treatment of injuries, serious illnesses, and **hemophilia,** resulting in about 14,000 cases of AIDS in the United States. Nearly all of these cases occurred in the early days of the AIDS epidemic, before effective screening tests were available. All blood in licensed U.S. blood banks and plasma centers is now thoroughly screened for HIV. The American Blood Bank Association estimates that fewer than 1 in 2 million units of blood products is capable of transmitting HIV.

The final major route of HIV transmission is mother-to-child, also called *vertical,* or *perinatal, transmission,* which can occur during pregnancy, childbirth, or breastfeeding. About 25–30% of infants born to untreated HIV-infected mothers are also infected with the virus; treatment can dramatically lower this infection rate. Worldwide, about two-thirds of vertical transmission occurs during pregnancy and childbirth and one-third through breastfeeding. About 600,000 infants are infected each year.

A person is *not* at risk of getting HIV infection by being in the same classroom, dining room, or even household with someone who is infected. Before this was generally known, many people with HIV infection, including children, were the targets of ostracism, hysteria, and outright violence. Today, it is an acknowledged responsibility of everyone to treat people with HIV infection with respect and compassion, regardless of their age or how they became infected.

**Term**

**hemophilia** A hereditary blood disease in which blood fails to clot and abnormal bleeding occurs, requiring transfusions of blood products with a specific factor to aid coagulation.

Vw

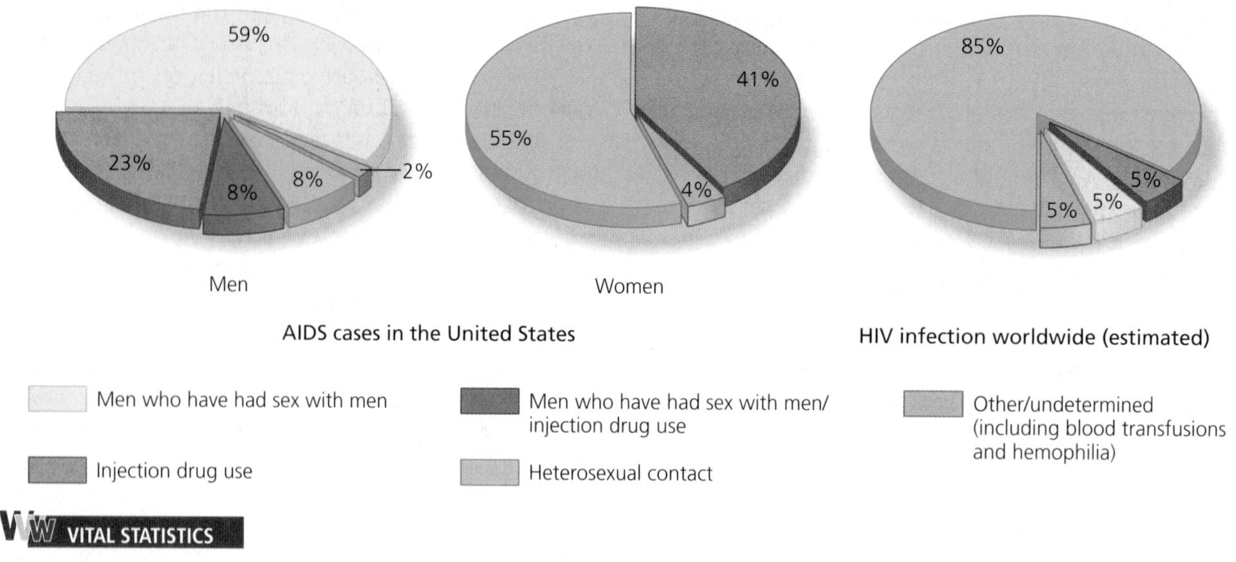


**Figure 13-3 Routes of HIV transmission among adults.** SOURCES: Centers for Disease Control and Prevention. 2004. *HIV/AIDS Surveillance Report* 15; Joint United Nations Programme on HIV/AIDS (UNAIDS). 2004. *AIDS Epidemic Update, December 2004*. Geneva: UNAIDS; World Health Organization. 2001. Global AIDS surveillance. *Weekly Epidemiological Record* 76(50): 389–400.

**Populations of Special Concern for HIV Infection** Among Americans with AIDS, the most common means of exposure to HIV has been sexual activity between men; injection drug use (IDU) and heterosexual contact are the next most common (Figure 13-3). Although the transmission of HIV occurs through specific individual behaviors, disproportionately high rates of infection in certain groups are tied to social, cultural, and economic factors. HIV in the United States is increasingly becoming a disease that affects ethnic minorities, women, and the poor. Women, especially African American women and Latinas, make up an increasingly large proportion of all U.S. AIDS cases. Overall, African American men and women are vastly overrepresented among people newly diagnosed with AIDS. African Americans represent 12.6% of the U.S. population but account for 40% of all AIDS cases diagnosed since the start of the epidemic and nearly 50% of new cases diagnosed in 2003.

Another group of people at increased risk for HIV infection are young men who have sex with men. There are probably several factors underlying this trend. Young gay men are less likely than older men to have had the experience of watching friends die from AIDS and thus are more removed from the reality of the disease. They may be less afraid of acquiring HIV because of less direct experience with friends with AIDS and because of advances in treatment and a false belief that a cure is just around the corner. Drug use and the practice of meeting sex partners over the Internet are also associated with increased rates of HIV infection among men who have sex with men.

There also appears to be a growing number of cases among men who acquire HIV through sex with other men but who do not identify themselves as gay. Particularly among minorities, many men who have sex with men also have sex with women, and they identify themselves as heterosexual, not gay or bisexual. Men who have sex with men and who do not disclose their sexual orientation are just as likely to be infected with HIV as are gay and bisexual men who are "out," but they are much less likely to know their HIV status and so may be more likely to transmit HIV to a male or female partner.

These patterns of HIV infection reflect complex social, economic, and behavioral factors. Reducing the rates of HIV transmission and AIDS death in minorities, women, and other groups at risk will require dealing with the difficult problems of drug abuse, poverty, and discrimination. HIV prevention programs must be tailored to meet the special needs of minority communities.

**Symptoms of HIV Infection** Within a few days or weeks of infection with HIV, about half of people will develop the flulike symptoms of primary HIV infection. Diagnosis of HIV at this very early stage of infection, although uncommon, is extremely beneficial. People who have engaged in behavior that places them at risk for HIV infection and who then experience symptoms of primary HIV infection should immediately inform their physician of their risk status. Standard tests for HIV will usually be negative in the very early stages of infection, so specialized tests such as the **HIV RNA assay**, which directly measures the amount of virus in the body, must be used.

Other than the initial flulike symptoms associated with primary HIV infection, most people in the first months or years of HIV infection have few if any symptoms. As the immune system weakens, however, a variety of symptoms can develop—ranging from persistent swollen lymph nodes and night sweats to memory loss and seizures.

Because the immune system is weakened, people with HIV infection are highly susceptible to infections, both common and uncommon. The infection most often seen in the United States among people with HIV is *Pneumocystis carinii* pneumonia, a protozoal infection. Kaposi's sarcoma, a previously rare form of cancer, is common in HIV-infected men. Women with HIV infection often have frequent and difficult-to-treat vaginal yeast infections. Cases of tuberculosis (TB) are also increasingly being reported in people with HIV.

**Diagnosing HIV Infection and AIDS** Early diagnosis of HIV infection is important to minimize the impact of the disease and reduce the risk of infecting others. The most common tests are **HIV antibody tests.** Standard testing involves an initial test called an **ELISA;** if it is positive, a second test called a **Western blot** is done to confirm the results (see the box "Getting an HIV Test" on p. 334). Not everyone with HIV infection will test positive on antibody tests, however. Antibodies may not appear in the blood for weeks or months after infection, so people who are newly infected are likely to have a negative antibody test. The infection can be detected with the more expensive HIV RNA assay.

If a person is diagnosed as **HIV-positive,** the next step is to determine the current severity of the disease. The status of the immune system can be gauged by taking CD4 T-cell measurements every few months. The infection itself can be monitored by tracking the amount of virus in the body (the "viral load") through HIV RNA assay. A new diagnostic test that may help guide treatment decisions is called HIV Replication Capacity; this test shows how fast HIV from a patient's blood sample can reproduce itself.

The CDC's criteria for a diagnosis of AIDS reflect the stage of HIV infection at which a person's immune system becomes dangerously compromised. Since January 1993, a diagnosis of AIDS has been made if a person is HIV-positive and either has developed an infection defined as an AIDS indicator or has a severely damaged immune system (as measured by CD4 T-cell counts).

**Treatment** There is no known cure for HIV infection, but medications can significantly alter the course of the disease and extend life. The drop in the number of U.S. AIDS deaths that has occurred since 1996 is in large part due to the increasing use of combinations of new drugs.

**ANTIVIRAL DRUGS** Current antiviral drugs to combat HIV fall into three major categories: reverse transcriptase inhibitors, protease inhibitors, and fusion inhibitors. These medications inhibit the ability of the virus to replicate itself. Treatment with a combination of drugs, referred to as highly active antiretroviral therapy, or HAART, can reduce HIV in the blood to undetectable levels in some people. However, latent virus is still present in the body, and HIV-infected men on HAART carry potentially transmissible HIV in their semen. Researchers are looking for different ways to attack HIV. People who carry a particular genetic mutation have been found to be resistant to infection, and scientists hope to develop a drug that will mimic the effects of this mutation, which blocks HIV from entering cells.

**POSTEXPOSURE PROPHYLAXIS (PEP)** Antiviral medications are being used in some cases in an attempt to prevent infection in people who have been exposed to HIV. The CDC has long recommended that health care workers who have significant exposure to HIV-infected blood or body fluids via a needle stick or other mishap consider starting antiviral medication as soon as possible (preferably within a few hours of exposure) to decrease the risk of infection. PEP is also often recommended for victims of sexual assault. In 2005, the CDC for the first time recommended PEP for people who are at risk for HIV infection from recent nonoccupational exposure to blood, genital secretions, or other potentially infectious body fluids of a person known to have HIV. Nonoccupational exposure refers to situations such as unprotected sex or contact with a contaminated needle. PEP consists of 28 days of HAART, which should begin as soon as possible after exposure, but always within 72 hours.

**TREATMENTS FOR OPPORTUNISTIC INFECTIONS** In addition to antiviral drugs, most patients with low CD4 T-cell counts also take a variety of antibiotics to help prevent opportunistic infections such as *Pneumocystis carinii* pneumonia and tuberculosis. A person with advanced HIV infection may need to take 20 or more pills every day.

**HIV AND PREGNANCY** Early-stage HIV infection does not appear to significantly affect a woman's chance of becoming pregnant. Without treatment, 25–30% of infants born to HIV-infected women are themselves infected with the virus. The risk of transmitting HIV from an infected mother to her baby can be reduced to less than 2% by treating the mother during her pregnancy and labor, giving the baby antiretroviral drugs during the first weeks

## Terms

**HIV RNA assay** A test used to determine the amount of HIV in the blood (the "viral load").

**HIV antibody test** A blood test to determine whether a person has been infected by HIV; becomes positive within weeks or months of exposure.

**ELISA (enzyme-linked immunosorbent assay)** A blood test that detects the presence of antibodies to HIV.

**Western blot** A blood test that detects the presence of HIV antibodies; a more accurate and more expensive test used to confirm positive results from an ELISA test.

**HIV-positive** A diagnosis resulting from the presence of HIV in the bloodstream; also referred to as *seropositive.*

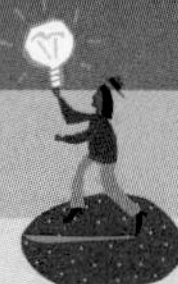

Critical Consumer

## Getting an HIV Test

Some experts recommend HIV testing for all Americans. An individual should strongly consider being tested if any of the following apply to him or her or to any past or current sexual partner: you have had unprotected sex (vaginal, anal, or oral) with more than one partner or with a partner who was not in a mutually monogamous relationship with you; you have used or shared needles, syringes, or other paraphernalia for injecting drugs (including steroids); you received a transfusion of blood or blood products between 1978 and 1985; or you have been diagnosed with an STD.

### Testing Options

If you decide to get an HIV test, either you can visit a physician or health clinic or you can take a home test. A big advantage to having the test performed by a physician or clinician is that you will get one-on-one counseling about the test, your results, and ways to avoid future infection or spreading the disease. The home test is a good alternative for people at low risk who just want to be sure.

### Physician or Clinic Testing

Your physician, student health clinic, Planned Parenthood, public health department, or local AIDS association can arrange your HIV test. It usually costs \$50–\$100, but public clinics often charge little or nothing. The standard test involves drawing a sample of blood that is sent to a laboratory for analysis for the presence of antibodies; if the first stage of testing is positive, a confirmatory test is done. This standard test takes 1–2 weeks, and you'll be asked to phone or come in personally to obtain your results, which should also include appropriate counseling.

Alternative tests are available at some clinics. The Orasure test uses oral fluid, which is collected by placing a treated cotton pad in the mouth; urine tests are also available. Oral fluid and urine tests may be helpful for people who avoid blood tests due to fear of needles; they also protect health care workers from needlestick exposure to potentially infected blood. If you suspect you have been recently exposed to HIV and might have primary infection, see your physician and ask about an HIV RNA test.

New rapid tests are now also available at some locations. These tests involve the use of blood or oral fluid and can provide results in as little as 20 minutes. If a rapid test is positive for HIV infection, a confirmatory test will be performed.

Before you get an HIV test, be sure you understand what will be done with the results. Results from confidential tests may still become part of your medical record and/or be reported (with your name or some other identifier) to state and federal public health agencies. If you decide you want to be tested anonymously—in which case the results will not be reported to anyone but yourself—check with your physician or counselor about how to obtain an anonymous test or use a home test.

### Home Testing

Home test kits for HIV are now available; they cost about \$40–60. (Take care to avoid testing kits that are not FDA-approved; many such unapproved kits are being sold over the Internet.) To use a home test, you prick a finger with a supplied lancet, blot a few drops of blood onto blotting paper, and mail it to the company's laboratory. In about a week, you call a toll-free number to find out your results. Anyone testing positive is routed to a trained counselor, who can provide emotional and medical support. The results of home test kits are anonymous.

### Understanding the Results

A negative test result means that no antibodies were found in your sample. However, it usually takes at least a month (and possibly as long as 6 months in some people) after exposure to HIV for antibodies to appear, a process called **seroconversion.** Therefore, an infected person may get a false-negative result. If you think you've been exposed to HIV, get a test immediately; if it's negative but your risk of infection is high, ask about obtaining an HIV RNA assay, which allows very early diagnosis, and about the appropriateness of retesting in a few months. If you test negative, you'll also receive information about how to avoid infection.

A positive result means that you are infected. It is important to seek medical care and counseling immediately. You need to know more about your medical options; the possible psychological, social, and financial repercussions; and how to avoid spreading the disease. Rapid progress is being made in treating HIV, and treatments are potentially much more successful when begun early.

For more information about HIV testing and a national directory of testing sites, visit the CDC National HIV Testing Resources site (www.hivtest.org).

of life, avoiding breastfeeding, and delivering the baby by cesarean section if the mother has high blood levels of HIV. Because treatment can make such a dramatic difference in the health of the baby, HIV testing is strongly recommended for all pregnant women.

**Term**

**seroconversion** The appearance of antibodies to HIV in the blood of an infected person; usually occurs 1–6 months after infection.

**TREATMENT CHALLENGES** The average cost of treatment for HIV is \$14,000–35,000 per year. These costs are tremendous even for relatively wealthy countries. But 95% of people with HIV infection live in developing countries, where these treatments are unlikely to be available to anyone except the wealthiest few. Long-term use of HAART can also cause a number of serious effects. For this reason, the National Institutes of Health issued new HIV treatment guidelines in 2001 that recommend that asymptomatic patients hold off on treatment until they are at a more advanced stage of the disease.

Even for those who have access to the drugs and can tolerate the side effects, treatment is difficult. Some people cannot tolerate the toxic side effects of these powerful drugs, and the drugs are much more effective for some people than for others. Currently available antiviral drugs do not appear able to completely eliminate the virus from the body. It is also unclear to what degree a damaged immune system can rebound from the effects of long-term HIV infection.

If an effective, safe, affordable vaccine against HIV could be developed, it might be possible to stop the worldwide HIV epidemic in its tracks. Many different approaches to the development of an AIDS vaccine are currently under investigation, and human trials have begun on several vaccines. Unfortunately, no vaccine is likely to be ready for widespread use within the next 5 years. Researchers are making more rapid progress in producing a microbicide that could be used to prevent HIV and other STDs. A microbicide in the form of a cream, gel, sponge, or suppository that could be inserted into the vagina or rectum could function as a kind of chemical condom.

### How Can You Protect Yourself?

Although AIDS is currently incurable, it is preventable. You can protect yourself by avoiding behaviors that may bring you into contact with HIV.

**MAKE CAREFUL CHOICES ABOUT SEXUAL ACTIVITY** In a sexual relationship, the current and past behaviors of you and your partner determine the amount of risk involved. If you are uninfected and in a mutually monogamous relationship with another uninfected person, you are not at risk for HIV. Of course, it is often hard to know for sure whether your partner is completely faithful and is truly uninfected. Having a series of monogamous relationships is not a safe prevention strategy.

For anyone not involved in a long-term, mutually monogamous relationship, abstinence from any sexual activity that involves the exchange of body fluids is the only sure way to prevent HIV infection (Figure 13-4). Safer sex includes many activities that carry virtually no risk of HIV infection, such as hugging, massaging, closed-lip kissing, rubbing clothed bodies together, kissing your partner's skin, and mutual masturbation.

Anal and vaginal intercourse are the sexual activities associated with the highest risk of HIV infection. If you have intercourse, always use a condom. Use of a lubricated condom reduces the risk of transmitting HIV during all forms of intercourse. Condoms are not perfect, and they do not provide risk-free sex; however, used properly, a condom provides a high level of protection against HIV. Condoms should also be worn during oral sex. Experts also suggest the use of latex squares and dental dams, rubber devices that can be used as barriers during oral-genital or oral-anal sexual contact.

High Risk
**Unprotected anal sex** is the riskiest sexual behavior, especially for the receptive partner.
**Unprotected vaginal intercourse** is the next riskiest, especially for women, who are much more likely to be infected by an infected male partner than vice versa.
**Oral sex** is probably considerably less risky than anal and vaginal intercourse but can still result in HIV transmission.
**Sharing of sex toys** can be risky because they can carry blood, semen, or vaginal fluid.
**Use of a condom** reduces risk considerably but not completely for any type of intercourse. Anal sex with a condom is riskier than vaginal sex with a condom; oral sex with a condom is less risky, especially if the man does not ejaculate.
**Hand-genital contact and deep kissing** are less risky but could still theoretically transmit HIV; the presence of cuts or sores increases risk.
**Sex with only one uninfected and totally faithful partner** is without risk, but effective only if both partners are uninfected and completely monogamous.
**Activities that don't involve the exchange of body fluids** carry no risk: hugging, massage, closed-mouth kissing, masturbation, phone sex, and fantasy.
**Abstinence** is completely without risk. For many people, it can be an effective and reasonable method of avoiding HIV infection and other STDs during certain periods of life.
No Risk

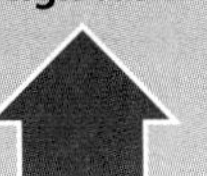

**Figure 13-4 What's risky and what's not: The approximate relative risk of HIV transmission of various sexual activities.** Safer sex strategies that reduce the risk of HIV infection will also help protect you against other STDs. The main point to remember is that any activity that involves contact with blood, semen, or vaginal fluid can transmit HIV.

Limiting the number of partners you have—particularly those who have engaged in risky sexual behaviors in the past—can also lower your risk of exposure to HIV. Take the time to talk with a potential new partner about HIV and safer sex. Talking about sex may seem embarrassing and uncomfortable, but good communication is critical for your health.

Removing alcohol and other drugs from sexual activity is another crucial component of safer sex. The use of alcohol and mood-altering drugs may lower inhibitions and affect judgment, making you more likely to engage in unsafe sex. The use of drugs is also associated with sexual activity with multiple partners. Some experts attribute much of the recent increase in rates of syphilis and HIV infection among U.S. gay and bisexual men to the nonmedical use of anti-impotence drugs such as Viagra in combination with crystal methamphetamine.

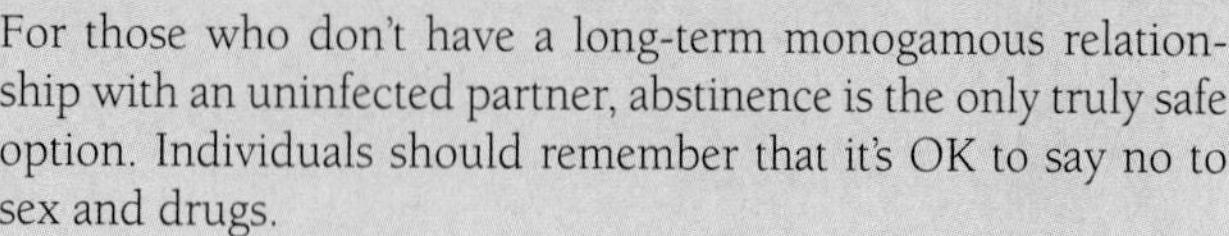

## Take Charge: Preventing HIV Infection and Other STDs

For those who don't have a long-term monogamous relationship with an uninfected partner, abstinence is the only truly safe option. Individuals should remember that it's OK to say no to sex and drugs.

Safer sexual activities that allow close person-to-person contact with almost no risk of contracting STDs or HIV include fantasy, hugging, massage, rubbing clothed bodies together, self-stimulation by both partners, and kissing with lips closed.

If you choose to be sexually active, talk with potential partners about HIV, safer sex, and the use of condoms before you begin a sexual relationship. The following behaviors will help lower your risk of exposure to HIV during sexual activities:

- Don't drink alcohol or use drugs in sexual situations. Mood-altering drugs can affect your judgment and make you more likely to engage in risky behaviors.
- Limit the number of partners. Avoid sexual contact with people who have HIV or an STD or who have engaged in risky behaviors in the past, including unprotected sex and injection drug use.
- Use condoms during every act of intercourse and oral sex. Many STDs are not easy to diagnose in their asymptomatic stage, which can last for years, and asymptomatic individuals can still infect others. Even if your partner claims to have been tested for HIV and STDs, you have no guarantee that you will not contract an STD during any sexual encounter. If you choose to have intercourse, your best protection is to *always* use a condom. Condoms do not provide perfect protection, but they greatly reduce your risk of contracting an infection.
- Use condoms properly to obtain maximum protection (refer to the instructions for condom use in Chapter 6). Use a water-based lubricant; don't use oil-based lubricants such as petroleum jelly or baby oil or any vaginal product containing mineral or vegetable oil. Avoid using lubricants or condoms containing nonoxynol-9, particularly for anal intercourse. Unroll condoms gently to avoid tearing them, and smooth out any air bubbles.
- Avoid sexual contact that could cause cuts or tears in the skin or tissue. Using extra lubricant (water-based) can help prevent damage to delicate tissues.
- Get periodic screening tests for STDs and HIV. Young women need yearly pelvic exams and Pap tests. Get prompt treatment for any STDs you contract.
- Get vaccinated for hepatitis B.

If you inject drugs of any kind, don't share needles, syringes, or anything that might have blood on it. If your community has a syringe exchange program, use it. Seek treatment; stop using injectable drugs.

If you are at risk for HIV infection, don't donate blood, sperm, or body organs. Don't have unprotected sex or share needles or syringes. Get tested for HIV soon, and get treated. HIV-infected people who get early treatment generally feel better and live longer than those who delay.

Surveys of college students indicate that the majority of students are not engaging in safer sex. Although most students know that condom use can protect against HIV infection, this knowledge is often not translated into action. Many students also report a willingness to lie about past sexual activity in order to obtain sex. In addition, many students believe their risk of contracting HIV depends on "who they are" rather than on their sexual behavior. These attitudes and behaviors place college students at continued high risk for contracting HIV. (see the box "Preventing HIV Infection and Other STDs").

**DON'T SHARE DRUG NEEDLES** People who inject drugs should avoid sharing needles, syringes, or anything that might have blood on it. Needles can be decontaminated with a solution of bleach and water, but it is not a foolproof procedure, and HIV can survive in a syringe for a month or longer. (Boiling needles and syringes does not necessarily destroy HIV either.) If you are an injection drug user, your best protection against HIV is to obtain treatment and refrain from using drugs.

## Chlamydia

*Chlamydia trachomatis* causes **chlamydia,** the most prevalent bacterial STD in the United States. About 3 million new cases occur each year. An estimated 5–15% of all sexually active young American women are infected with chlamydia; rates among men are similar. The highest rates of infection occur in single people between ages 18 and 24. *C. trachomatis* can be transmitted by oral sex as well as by other forms of sexual intercourse.

Both men and women are susceptible to chlamydia, but, as with most STDs, women bear the greater burden because of possible complications and consequences of the disease. If left untreated, chlamydia can lead to pelvic inflammatory disease (PID), a serious infection involving the oviducts (fallopian tubes) and uterus that can lead to infertility. Chlamydia also greatly increases a woman's risk for ectopic (tubal) pregnancy. The U.S. Preventive Services Task Force currently recommends routine screening for all sexually active women age 25 or younger and for older women who are at increased risk (such as those who have multiple sex partners).

Chlamydia can also lead to infertility in men, although not as often as in women. In men under age 35, chlamydia is the most common cause of epididymitis, inflammation of the sperm-carrying ducts. And up to half of all cases of urethritis, inflammation of the urethra, in men are caused by chlamydia. Despite these statistics, many infected men have no symptoms.

Infants of infected mothers can acquire the infection through contact with the pathogen in the birth canal during delivery. Every year, over 150,000 newborns suffer from eye infections and pneumonia as a result of untreated maternal chlamydial infections.

**Symptoms** Most people experience few or no symptoms of chlamydia, increasing the likelihood that they will inadvertently spread the infection to their partners. In men, chlamydia symptoms can include painful urination, a slight watery discharge from the penis, and sometimes pain around the testicles. Women may notice increased vaginal discharge, burning with urination, pain or bleeding with intercourse, and lower abdominal pain.

**Diagnosis and Treatment** Chlamydia is typically diagnosed through laboratory tests on a urine sample or a small amount of fluid from the urethra or cervix. Once chlamydia has been diagnosed, the infected person and his or her partner(s) are given antibiotics—usually doxycycline, erythromycin, or a newer drug, azithromycin, which can cure infection in one dose.

## Gonorrhea

In the United States, an estimated 700,000 new cases of **gonorrhea** are diagnosed every year. The highest incidence is among 15–24-year-olds. Like chlamydia, untreated gonorrhea can cause PID in women and urethritis and epididymitis in men. It can also cause arthritis, rashes, and eye infections, and it occasionally involves internal organs. A woman who is infected during pregnancy is at risk for preterm delivery and for having a baby with life-threatening gonorrheal infection of the blood or joints. An infant passing through the birth canal of an infected mother may contract an infection in the eyes that can cause blindness if not treated. Gonorrhea is caused by the bacterium *Neisseria gonorrhoeae*, which flourishes in mucous membranes.

**Symptoms** In males, the incubation period for gonorrhea is brief, generally 2–7 days. The first symptoms are due to urethritis, which causes urinary discomfort and a thick, yellowish white or yellowish green discharge from the penis. The lips of the urethral opening may become inflamed and swollen. In some cases, the lymph glands in the groin become enlarged and swollen. Up to half of males have very minor symptoms or none at all.

Most females with gonorrhea are asymptomatic. Those who do have symptoms often experience pain with urination, increased vaginal discharge, and severe menstrual cramps. Up to 40% of women with untreated gonorrhea develop PID. Women may also develop painful abscesses in the Bartholin's glands, a pair of glands located on either side of the opening of the vagina.

Gonorrhea can also infect the throat or rectum of people who engage in oral or anal sex. Gonorrhea symptoms in the throat may be a sore throat or pus on the tonsils, and those in the rectum may be pus or blood in the feces or rectal pain and itching.

**Diagnosis and Treatment** Several tests—gram stain, detection of bacterial genes or DNA, or culture—may be performed; depending on the test, samples of urine or cervical, urethral, throat, or rectal fluids may be collected. A variety of new and relatively expensive antibiotics are usually effective in curing gonorrhea. Older, less expensive antibiotics such as penicillin and tetracycline are not currently recommended for treating gonorrhea because of widespread drug resistance.

## Pelvic Inflammatory Disease

A major complication in 10–40% of women who have been infected with either gonorrhea or chlamydia and have not received adequate treatment is **pelvic inflammatory disease (PID).** PID occurs when the initial infection with gonorrhea and/or chlamydia travels upward, often along with other bacteria, beyond the cervix into the uterus, oviducts, ovaries, and pelvic cavity. PID is often serious enough to require hospitalization and sometimes surgery. Even if the disease is treated successfully, about 25% of affected women will have long-term problems such as a continuing susceptibility to infection, ectopic pregnancy, infertility, and chronic pelvic pain. PID is the leading cause of infertility in young women; infertility occurs in 8% of women after one episode of PID, 20% after two episodes, and 40% after three episodes.

Young women under age 25 are much more likely to develop PID than are older women. As with all STDs, the more sex partners a woman has had, the greater her risk of PID. Smokers have twice the risk of PID as nonsmokers. Using IUDs for contraception also increases the risk of PID. Research into whether the use of other contraceptives protects against PID has yielded mixed results; OC use may reduce the severity of PID symptoms.

### Terms

**chlamydia** An STD transmitted by the pathogenic bacterium *Chlamydia trachomatis*.

**gonorrhea** A sexually transmitted bacterial infection that usually affects mucous membranes.

**pelvic inflammatory disease (PID)** An infection that progresses from the vagina and cervix to the uterus, oviducts, and pelvic cavity.

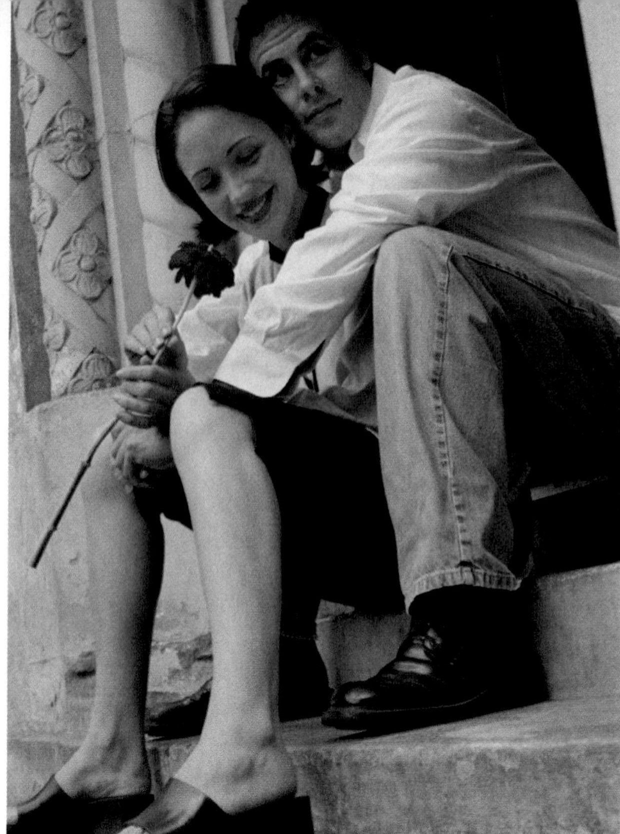

By taking a responsible attitude toward STDs, people show respect and concern for themselves and their partners. This couple's plans for the future could be seriously disrupted if one of them contracted an STD like gonorrhea or chlamydia. Either of these diseases, if untreated, could result in PID, the leading cause of infertility in young women.

**Symptoms** Some women may be asymptomatic; others may feel very ill with abdominal pain, fever, chills, nausea, and vomiting. Early symptoms are essentially the same as those described earlier for chlamydia and gonorrhea. Symptoms often begin or worsen during or soon after a woman's menstrual period. Many women have abnormal vaginal bleeding—either bleeding between periods or heavy and painful menstrual bleeding.

**Diagnosis and Treatment** Diagnosis of PID is made on the basis of symptoms, physical examination, ultrasound, and laboratory tests. Laparoscopy may be used to confirm the diagnosis and obtain material for cultures.

### Terms

VW

**human papillomavirus (HPV)** The pathogen that causes human warts, including genital warts.

**genital warts** A sexually transmitted viral infection characterized by growths on the genitals; also called *genital HPV infection* or *condyloma*.

**genital herpes** A sexually transmitted infection caused by the herpes simplex virus.

Antibiotics are usually started immediately; in severe cases, the woman may be hospitalized and antibiotics given intravenously. Prompt treatment can help minimize organ damage. It is especially important that an infected woman's partners be treated. As many as 60% of the male contacts of women with PID are infected but asymptomatic.

## Human Papillomavirus Infection (Genital Warts)

**Human papillomavirus (HPV)** infection is one of the most common STDs in the United States. All human warts, including **genital warts,** as well as almost all cases of cervical cancer are caused by HPV infection. The CDC estimates that more than 20 million people in the United States have this persistent genital viral infection, and another 6.2 million people are infected each year. Nearly 20% of Americans age 15–59 years have genital HPV infection and are potentially contagious. The vast majority of these people have no visible warts and have no idea that they are infected. Rates are even higher among college students. Many young women contract HPV infection within 3 months of becoming sexually active (see the box "Women Are Hard Hit by STDs").

A precancerous condition known as cervical dysplasia often occurs among women with genital HPV infection. If untreated, women with this condition sometimes develop cervical cancer. Recent evidence suggests that HPV infection also increases the risk of HIV transmission. More than 30 strains of HPV are likely to cause genital infections, and 5 of these are often implicated in cervical cancer; other strains are linked to anal, penile, and other genital cancers. The good news is that a vaccine to prevent HPV infection and cervical cancer may soon be available.

Genital HPV infection is quite contagious. Condoms and other barrier methods can help prevent the transmission of HPV, but HPV infection frequently occurs in areas where condoms are not fully protective. These areas are the labia in women, the base of the penis and the scrotum in men, and around the anus in both men and women.

**Symptoms** HPV-infected tissue often appears normal; it may also look like anything from a small bump on the skin to a large, warty growth. Depending on location and size, genital warts are sometimes painful. Untreated warts can grow together to form a cauliflower-like mass. In males, they appear on the penis and often involve the urethra, appearing first at the opening and then spreading inside. The growths may cause irritation and bleeding, leading to painful urination and a urethral discharge. Warts may also appear around the anus or within the rectum. In women, warts may appear on the labia or vulva and may spread to the perineum, the area between the vagina and the rectum. If warts occur only on the cervix, the woman will generally have no symptoms or awareness that she has HPV.

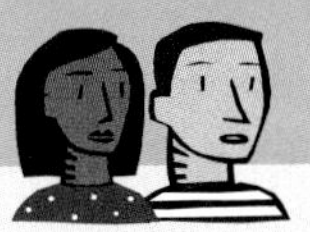

## Women Are Hit Hard by STDs

STDs cause suffering for all who are infected, but in many ways, women and girls are the hardest hit, for both biological and social reasons. Among Americans, 62% of all cases of adverse health problems from STDs occur in women. Worldwide, as many women as men now die from AIDS each year.

Male-to-female transmission of many infections is more likely to occur than female-to-male transmission. This is particularly true of HIV: Studies show that it is three to eight times easier for an HIV-positive man to transmit the virus to a woman than it is for an HIV-positive woman to infect a man.

Young women are even more vulnerable to STDs than older women because the less-mature cervix is more susceptible to injury and infection. As a woman ages, the cells at the opening of the cervix become more resistant to infection. If an 18-year-old woman and a 30-year-old woman are exposed to the same pathogen, the younger woman is far more likely to develop a serious STD. Young women are also more vulnerable for social and emotional reasons: Lack of control in relationships, fear of discussing condom use, and having an older sex partner are all linked to increased STD risk.

Once infected, women tend to suffer more consequences of STDs than men. For example, gonorrhea and chlamydia can cause PID and permanent damage to the oviducts in women, but these infections tend to have less serious effects in men. HPV infection causes nearly all cases of cervical cancer. Women also have the added concern of the potential effects of STDs during pregnancy.

Between 1985 and 2003, the proportion of new U.S. AIDS cases in women increased from 7% to 28%. Women may become sicker at lower viral loads compared with men. Women and men with HIV do about equally well if they have similar access to treatment, but in many cases women are diagnosed later in the course of HIV infection, receive less treatment, and die sooner.

Worldwide, social and economic factors play a large role in the transmission and consequences of STDs for women. Violence against women is spreading AIDS, as are such practices as very early marriage for women, often to much older men who have had many sexual partners. For many women, being vulnerable to HIV can simply mean being married. Cultural gender norms that promote premarital and extramarital relationships for men, combined with women's lack of power to negotiate safe sex, make HIV a risk even for women who are married and monogamous. In addition, lack of education and limited economic opportunities can force women into commercial sex work, placing them at high risk for all STDs.

SOURCES: Ebrahim, S. H., M. T. McKenna, and J. S. Marks. 2005. Sexual behaviour: Related adverse health burden in the United States. *Sexually Transmitted Infection* 81(1): 38–40; Dunkle, K. M., et al. 2004. Gender-based violence, relationship power, and risk of HIV infection in women attending antenatal clinics in South Africa. *Lancet* 363(9419): 1415–1421; Joint United Nations Programme on HIV/AIDS. 2004. *AIDS Epidemic Update, December 2004.* Geneva: UNAIDS; World Health Organization. 2003. *Gender and HIV/AIDS.* Geneva: World Health Organization.

The incubation period ranges from 1 month to 2 years from the time of contact. People can be infected with the virus and be capable of transmitting it to their sex partners without having any symptoms at all. The vast majority of people with HPV infection have no visible warts or symptoms of any kind.

**Diagnosis and Treatment** Genital warts are usually diagnosed based on the appearance of the lesions. Sometimes examination with a special magnifying instrument or biopsy is done to evaluate suspicious lesions. HPV infection of the cervix is often detected on routine Pap tests. Special tests are now available to detect the presence of HPV infection and to distinguish among the more common strains of HPV, including those that cause most cases of cervical cancer.

Treatment focuses on reducing the number and size of warts. The currently available treatments do not eradicate HPV infection. Warts may be removed by cryosurgery (freezing), electrocautery (burning), or laser surgery. Direct applications of podophyllin or other cytotoxic acids may be used. Two treatments may be applied by patients at home: imiquimod, an immune system enhancer, and podofilox, a drug that destroys warts.

HPV infection often resolves on its own after a number of months, although this is unpredictable. Even after treatment and the disappearance of visible warts, the individual may continue to carry HPV in healthy-looking tissue and can probably still infect others. Anyone who has ever had HPV infection should inform all partners. Condoms should be used, even though they do not provide total protection. Because of the relationship between HPV and cervical cancer, women who have had genital warts should have Pap tests at least every 12 months.

## Genital Herpes

**Genital herpes** affects about 45 million people in the United States. It is a major factor in the transmission of HIV worldwide and may also interact with HPV infection to increase the risk of cervical cancer. Two types of herpes simplex viruses, HSV 1 and HSV 2, cause genital herpes and oral-labial herpes (cold sores). Genital herpes is most often caused by HSV 2, and oral-labial herpes is most often caused by HSV 1, although both virus types can cause either genital or oral-labial lesions. The proportion of U.S. genital herpes cases caused by HSV 1 has increased dramatically over the past several decades and now stands at about 20% of cases. Genital herpes due to HSV 1 is usually acquired through oral-genital contact. HSV can also cause rectal lesions, usually transmitted through anal sex. Infection with HSV is generally lifelong; after infection, the virus lies dormant in nerve cells and can reactivate at any time.

HSV 1 infection is so common that 50–80% of U.S. adults have antibodies to HSV 1 (indicating previous exposure to the virus); most were exposed to HSV 1 during childhood. HSV 2 infection usually occurs between ages 18 and 25. Approximately 22% of adults—nearly one in four—have antibodies to HSV 2; about a million are infected each year.

HSV 2 is almost always sexually transmitted. It is theoretically possible, but much less common, to become infected through contaminated clothing, towels, or other objects. The infection is more easily transmitted when people have active sores, but HSV 2 can be transmitted to a sex partner even when no obvious lesions are present. Because HSV is asymptomatic in 80–90% of people, the infection is often acquired from a person who has no awareness that he or she is infected. If you have ever had an outbreak of genital herpes, you must always consider yourself contagious and inform your partners. Avoid intimate contact when any sores are present, and use condoms during all sexual contact.

Newborns can occasionally be infected with HSV, usually during passage through the birth canal of an infected mother or due to HSV infection acquired by the mother during the third trimester of pregnancy. Without treatment, 65% of newborns with HSV will die, and most who survive will have some degree of brain damage. The risk of mother-to-child HSV transmission during pregnancy and delivery is low (less than 1%) in women with long-standing herpes infection. However, a woman who acquires the infection during pregnancy, especially in the third trimester, has a much higher risk of transmitting the infection to her infant. Infected pregnant women sometimes deliver by cesarean section if active lesions are present at the time of delivery. Fortunately, most babies born to mothers with a history of genital herpes do not acquire the infection, and most women are able to have normal vaginal deliveries.

**Symptoms** Up to 90% of people who are infected with HSV have no symptoms. Those that do develop symptoms often first notice them within 2–20 days of having sex with an infected partner. (However, it is not unusual for the first outbreak to occur months or even years after initial exposure.) The first episode of genital herpes frequently causes flulike symptoms in addition to genital lesions. The lesions usually heal within 3 weeks, but the virus remains alive in an inactive state within nerve cells. A new outbreak can occur at any time. On average, newly diagnosed people will experience five to eight outbreaks per year, with a decrease in the frequency of outbreaks over time. Recurrent episodes are usually less severe than the initial one, with fewer and less painful sores that heal more quickly. Outbreaks can be triggered by stress, illness, fatigue, sun exposure, sexual intercourse, and menstruation.

**Diagnosis and Treatment** Genital herpes is often diagnosed on the basis of symptoms. A new blood test that can determine if a person is infected with HSV 1 or HSV 2 is now available and may potentially alert many asymptomatic people to the fact that they are infected.

There is no cure for herpes. Once infected, a person carries the virus for life. Antiviral drugs such as acyclovir can be taken at the beginning of an outbreak to shorten the severity and duration of symptoms. People who have frequent outbreaks can take acyclovir or similar drugs on a daily basis to suppress outbreaks. A person on suppressive therapy can still transmit HSV to an uninfected partner, but the risk is probably reduced by about half. Support groups are available to help people learn to cope with herpes. Vaccines for genital herpes are currently in development.

## Hepatitis B

Hepatitis can cause serious and sometimes permanent damage to the liver, which can result in death in severe cases. One of the many types of hepatitis is caused by hepatitis B virus (HBV). HBV is somewhat similar to HIV; it is found in most body fluids, and it can be transmitted sexually, by injection drug use, and during pregnancy and delivery. However, HBV is much more contagious than HIV, and it can also be spread through nonsexual close contact. Hepatitis B is a potentially fatal disease with no cure, but fortunately there is an effective vaccine that is recommended for everyone under age 19 and for all adults at increased risk for hepatitis B.

Other forms of viral hepatitis can also be sexually transmitted. Hepatitis A is of particular concern for people who engage in anal sex; a vaccine is available and is recommended for all people at risk. Less commonly, hepatitis C can be transmitted sexually. Experts believe that traumatic sexual activity that causes tissue damage is most likely to transmit HCV.

**Transmission** HBV is found in all body fluids, including blood and blood products, semen, saliva, urine, and vaginal secretions. It is easily transmitted through any sexual activity that involves the exchange of body fluids, the use of contaminated needles, and any blood-to-blood contact, including the use of contaminated razor blades, toothbrushes, and eating utensils. The primary risk factors are sexual exposure and injection drug use; having multiple partners greatly increases risk. A pregnant woman can transmit HBV to her unborn child.

**Symptoms** Many people infected with HBV never develop symptoms; they have what are known as "silent" infections. Mild cases of hepatitis cause flulike symptoms such as fever, body aches, chills, and loss of appetite. As the illness progresses, there may be nausea, vomiting, dark-colored urine, abdominal pain, and jaundice.

People with hepatitis B sometimes recover completely, but they can also become chronic carriers of the virus, capable of infecting others for the rest of their life. Some chronic carriers remain asymptomatic, while others develop chronic liver disease. Chronic hepatitis can cause cirrhosis of the liver, liver failure, and a deadly form of liver cancer. Hepatitis kills some 5000 Americans each year; worldwide, the annual death toll exceeds 600,000.

**Diagnosis and Treatment** Blood tests can be used to diagnose hepatitis through analysis of liver function and detection of the specific organism causing the infection. There is no cure for hepatitis B; antiviral drugs may be used for cases of chronic HBV infection. For people exposed to HBV, treatment with hepatitis B immunoglobulin can provide protection against the virus.

**Prevention** Preventive measures for hepatitis B are similar to those for HIV infection: Avoid sexual contact that involves sharing body fluids, including saliva; use condoms during sexual intercourse; and don't share needles. If you choose to have tattooing or body piercing done, make sure all needles and equipment are sterile. The vaccine for hepatitis B is safe and highly effective.

### Syphilis

**Syphilis,** a disease that once caused death and disability for millions, can now be effectively treated with antibiotics. Each year, there are about 7000–10,000 new cases of early syphilis in the United States, and about 70,000 people are diagnosed at all stages of the disease. Studies have found an association between syphilis infection and use of the Internet as a means to meet sex partners among men who have sex with men. Another recent trend is an increase in the proportion of cases of syphilis from oral sex.

Syphilis is caused by a spirochete called *Treponema pallidum,* a thin, corkscrew-shaped bacterium. The disease is usually acquired through sexual contact, although infected pregnant women can transmit it to the fetus. The pathogen passes through any break or opening in the skin or mucous membranes and can be transmitted by kissing, vaginal or anal intercourse, or oral-genital contact.

**Symptoms** Syphilis progresses through several stages. *Primary syphilis* is characterized by an ulcer called a **chancre** that appears within 10–90 days after exposure. Chancres contain large numbers of bacteria and make the disease highly contagious when present; they are often painless and typically heal on their own within a few weeks. If the disease is not treated during the primary stage, about a third of infected individuals progress to chronic stages of infections.

*Secondary syphilis* is usually marked by mild, flulike symptoms and a skin rash that appears 3–6 weeks after the chancre. The rash may cover the entire body or only a few areas, but the palms of the hands and soles of the feet are usually involved. Areas of skin affected by the rash are highly contagious but usually heal within several weeks or months. If the disease remains untreated, the symptoms of secondary syphilis may recur over a period of several years. In about a third of cases of untreated secondary syphilis, the individual develops *late,* or *tertiary, syphilis.* Late syphilis can damage many organs of the body, possibly causing severe dementia, cardiovascular damage, blindness, and death.

In infected pregnant women, the syphilis bacterium can cross the placenta. If the mother is not treated, the probable result is stillbirth, prematurity, or congenital deformity. In many cases, the infant is also born infected *(congenital syphilis)* and requires treatment.

**Diagnosis and Treatment** Syphilis is diagnosed by examination of infected tissues and with blood tests. All stages can be treated with antibiotics, but damage from late syphilis can be permanent.

## OTHER STDS

Although less serious than the diseases already described, a few other diseases are transmitted sexually or linked to sexual activity.

Trichomoniasis, often called "trich," is a common STD, with about 5 million new cases per year. The single-celled organism that causes trich, *Trichomonas vaginalis,* thrives in warm, moist conditions, making women particularly susceptible to these infections in the vagina. Women who become symptomatic with trich develop a greenish, foul-smelling vaginal discharge and severe itching and irritation of the vagina and vulva. Treatment with metronidazole (Flagyl) is important because studies suggest that trich may increase the risk of HIV transmission and, in pregnant woman, premature delivery.

Bacterial vaginosis (BV) is the most common cause of abnormal vaginal discharge in women of reproductive age. BV involves a shift in the makeup of the bacteria that

**Terms**

VW

**syphilis** A sexually transmitted bacterial infection caused by the spirochete *Treponema pallidum.*

**chancre** The sore produced by syphilis in its earliest stage.

normally inhabit the vagina: Instead of *Lactobacillus* being most numerous, there is an overgrowth of anaerobic microorganisms and bacteria such as *Gardnerella vaginalis.* BV is clearly associated with sexual activity, but research on the degree to which BV is sexually transmitted is ongoing. Recent research suggests that a sexually transmitted virus that infects and kills *Lactobacillus* may be the underlying cause of BV. Douching also substantially increases the risk of BV. Topical and oral antibiotics are used to treat BV, but BV often recurs after treatment.

Symptoms of BV include a vaginal discharge with a fishlike odor and, in some cases, vaginal irritation; many women with BV have no symptoms. Some studies have shown an association between BV and increased risk of PID, HIV transmission, infection following childbirth or gynecological surgery (including abortion), and, in pregnant women, premature delivery. The CDC recommends that any pregnant woman who has symptoms of BV or who is at risk for premature delivery be screened and, if necessary, treated for BV.

Chancroid is a sexually transmitted bacterial infection caused by *Haemophilus ducreyi.* Prevalent in some parts of the world, chancroid is relatively uncommon in the United States, although there are periodic outbreaks. The infection is characterized by painful open sores in the genital area that may resemble the sores associated with herpes or syphilis. Chancroid is treated with antibiotics.

Pubic lice, commonly called "crabs," and scabies are highly contagious parasitic infestations. Treatment is generally easy, although repeat applications of medication may be needed.

## WHAT YOU CAN DO

You can take responsibility for your health and contribute to a general reduction in the incidence of STDs in three major areas: education, diagnosis and treatment, and prevention.

### Education

Education efforts targeted at increasing public awareness about AIDS through the media have included public service announcements, dramatic presentations, and support from well-known public figures. Colleges offer courses in human sexuality. Free pamphlets and other literature are available from public health departments, health clinics, physicians' offices, student health centers, and Planned Parenthood, and easy-to-understand books are available in libraries and bookstores. Several national hotlines have been set up to provide free, confidential information and referral services to callers anywhere in the country (see the For More Information section at the end of the chapter).

Although information about STDs is widely disseminated, learning about STDs is still up to every person individually. You must assume responsibility for learning about the causes and nature of STDs and their potential effects on you, the children you may have, and those with whom you have sexual relationships.

### Diagnosis and Treatment

Early diagnosis and treatment of STDs can help you and your sex partner(s) avoid unnecessary complications and help prevent the spread of STDs.

**Get Vaccinated** Every young, sexually active person should be vaccinated for hepatitis B. Men who have sex with men should also be vaccinated for hepatitis A. In the next 5–10 years, vaccines for HPV, HSV, and possibly even some strains of HIV may become available.

**Be Alert for Symptoms** If you are sexually active, be alert for any sign or symptom of disease, such as a rash, a discharge, sores, or unusual pain, and don't hesitate to have a professional examination if you notice such a symptom.

**Get Tested** Remember that almost all STDs—including HIV infection—can be completely asymptomatic for long periods of time. Sexually active young women should have pelvic exams and Pap tests at least once a year, with chlamydia and gonorrhea screening in most cases. Sexually active men, especially if they have had more than one partner, should receive periodic STD and HIV screening.

Men who have sex with men are at especially high risk for HIV and other STDs. The CDC currently recommends that sexually active men who have sex with men be screened for STDs every year—more often if they have multiple anonymous partners or inject drugs. All sexually active gay and bisexual men should be vaccinated for hepatitis A and B.

Testing for STDs is done through private physicians, public health clinics, community health agencies, and most student health services. If you are diagnosed as having an STD, you should begin treatment as quickly as possible. Inform your partner(s), and avoid any sexual activity until your treatment is complete and testing indicates that you are cured. If your partner tells you that he or she has contracted an STD, get tested immediately, even if you don't have any symptoms. Asymptomatic partners are often treated to ensure that an infection will not spread or recur.

**Inform Your Partners** Telling a partner that you have exposed him or her to an STD isn't easy. Despite the awkwardness and difficulty, it is crucial that your sex partner or partners be informed and urged to seek testing and/or treatment as quickly as possible. The responsibility of informing partners is an ethical task too important to shirk.

**Get Treated** With the exception of AIDS treatments, treatments for STDs are safe and generally inexpensive. If you are being treated, follow instructions carefully and complete all the medication as prescribed. Don't stop taking the medication just because you feel better or your symptoms have disappeared. Above all, don't give any of your medication to your partner or to anyone else. Being cured of an STD does not mean that you will not get it again, and exposure does not confer lasting immunity, nor does it prevent you from getting any other STD.

## Prevention

The only sure way to avoid exposure to STDs is to abstain from sexual activity. But if you do choose to be sexually active, the key is to think about prevention *before* you have a sexual encounter or find yourself in the "heat of the moment." Find out what your partner thinks before you become sexually involved. Remember, you can become infected with an STD from just one unprotected encounter.

All your good intentions are likely to fly out the window if you enter into a sexual situation when you are intoxicated. If you or your partner (or both of you) is drunk, you are likely to be less cautious about sex than you would be if you were sober. Many people use alcohol and drugs as a way to deal with their anxiety in social and sexual situations. However, being intoxicated leaves you vulnerable to sexual assault and greatly increases your risk of acquiring a serious STD.

Plan ahead for safer sex. Know what sexual behaviors are risky. Find out about your partner's sexual history and practices. Be honest, and ask your partner to do the same, but don't stake your health and life on assumptions about your partner's honesty. Even if your partner's past seems low-risk, still insist on using a condom every time you have sex (see the box "Talking About Condoms and Safer Sex" on p. 344). Many honest people are simply unaware that they have an STD.

Aside from abstinence, the next most effective approach to preventing STDs is having sex only with one mutually monogamous, uninfected partner. If you are sexually active, use a condom during every act of intercourse to reduce your risk of contracting a disease. Although not foolproof, a properly used condom provides an effective barrier against pathogens, including HIV. A disease can be transmitted if there is contact with an infected area that isn't protected by the condom, however. The use of a barrier over the cervix (diaphragm or cervical cap) in addition to a condom may provide women with some additional protection.

Approaches to STD prevention that do not work include urinating or douching after intercourse, engaging in oral sex, and genital play without full penetration. Birth control pills and sterilization protect you against conception and unwanted pregnancy but not against STDs.

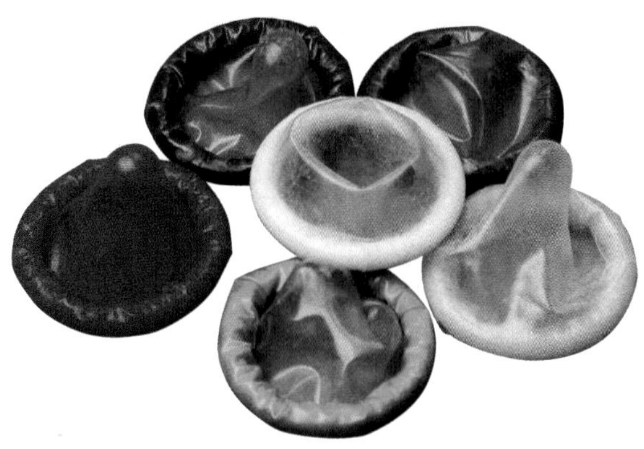

The use of condoms declined as more advanced methods of contraception, such as birth control pills and IUDs, became available. But condoms are once again gaining in popularity because of the protection they provide against STDs.

Caring about yourself and your partner means asking questions and being aware of signs and symptoms. It may be a bit awkward, but the temporary embarrassment of asking intimate questions is a small price to pay to avoid contracting or spreading disease. If your partner thinks less of you for being concerned, you may want to reconsider the relationship in terms of your personal values. Concern about STDs is part of a sexual relationship, not an intrusion into it, just as sexuality is part of life, not separate from it.

### Tips for Today

The immune system is a remarkable information network; it operates continuously on the cellular level to keep you well. You can support your immune system by practicing a wellness lifestyle—getting enough sleep, managing stress, eating well, exercising, and protecting yourself against infectious agents, including those that are sexually transmitted.

*Right now you can*

- Go wash your hands, and count out 20 seconds while doing so; you can estimate 20 seconds by singing "Twinkle, Twinkle, Little Star" slowly or "Happy Birthday" twice.
- Plan to move up your bedtime by 15 minutes, starting tonight.
- Put a small pack of tissues in your bag or coat pocket to use when you sneeze or cough, to avoid transmitting infection to others.
- Make an appointment with a school health clinic, Planned Parenthood, a public health department, or your personal physician if you are sexually active and have not recently been screened for STDs, including HIV.
- Resolve to discuss condom use with your partner if you are sexually active and are not already using condoms.

Take Charge

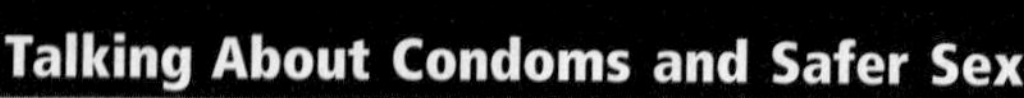

## Talking About Condoms and Safer Sex

The only sure way to prevent STDs, including HIV infection, is to abstain from sexual activity. If you choose to be sexually active, you should do everything possible to protect yourself from STDs. This includes good communication with your sex partner(s).

The time to talk about safer sex is before you begin a sexual relationship. However, even if you've been having unprotected sex with your partner, it is still worth it to start practicing safer sex now. If you're nervous about initiating a conversation about safer sex, rehearse what you will say first. Practice in front of a mirror or with a friend.

There are many ways to bring up the subject of safer sex and condom use with your partner. Be honest about your concerns and stress that protection against STDs means that you care about yourself and your partner. Here are a few suggestions:

- "I heard on the news that more and more people are buying and using condoms. I think it shows that people are being more responsible about sex. What do you think?"
- "I'm worried about the diseases we can get from having sex because so many don't have symptoms. I want to protect both of us by using condoms whenever we have sex."
- "I've been thinking about making love with you. But first we need to talk about how to have safer sex and be protected."

You may find that your partner shares your concerns and also wants to use condoms. He or she may be happy and relieved that you have brought up the subject of safer sex. However, if he or she resists the idea of using condoms, you may need to negotiate. Stress that you both deserve to be protected and that sex will be more enjoyable when you aren't worrying about STDs (see the suggestions to the right). If you and your partner haven't used condoms before, buy some and familiarize yourselves with how to use them. Once you feel more comfortable handling condoms, you'll be able to use them correctly and incorporate them into your sexual activity in fun ways. Consider trying the female condom.

If your partner still won't agree to use condoms, think carefully about whether you want to have a sexual relationship with him or her. Safer sex is part of a responsible, caring sexual relationship, and it's smart to say no to a partner who won't use a condom. It's up to you to protect yourself.

| If your partner says . . . | Try saying . . . |
|---|---|
| "They're not romantic." | "Worrying about AIDS isn't romantic, and with condoms we won't have to worry." OR "If we put one on together, a condom could be fun." |
| "You don't trust me." | "I do trust you, but how can I trust your former partners or mine?" OR "It's important to me that we're both protected." |
| "I don't have any diseases. I've been tested." | "I'm glad you've been tested, but tests aren't foolproof for all diseases. To be safe, I always use condoms." |
| "I forgot to bring a condom. But it's OK to skip it just this once." | "I'd really like to make love with you, but I never have sex without a condom. Let's go get some." |
| "I don't like the way they feel." | "They might feel different, but let's try." OR "Sex won't feel good if we're worrying about diseases." OR "How about trying the female condom?" |
| "I don't use condoms." | "I use condoms every time." OR "I don't have sex without condoms." |
| "But I love you." | "Being in love can't protect us from diseases." OR "I love you, too. We still need to use condoms." |
| "But we've been having sex without condoms." | "I want to start using condoms now so we won't be at any more risk." OR "We can still prevent infection or reinfection." |

SOURCE: Dialogue from San Francisco AIDS Foundation. 1988. *Condoms for Couples* (IMPACT AIDS, 3692 18th Street, San Francisco, CA 94110). 

## SUMMARY

- The step-by-step process by which infections are transmitted from one person to another includes the pathogen, its reservoir, a portal of exit, a means of transmission, a portal of entry, and a new host.
- The immune response is carried out by white blood cells that are continuously produced in the bone marrow. It has four stages: recognition of the invading pathogen; rapid replication of killer T cells and B cells; attack by killer T cells and macrophages; suppression of the immune response.
- Immunization is based on the body's ability to remember previously encountered organisms and retain its strength against them.
- Allergic reactions occur when the immune system responds to harmless substances as if they were dangerous antigens.
- Bacteria are single-celled organisms; some cause disease in humans. Bacterial infections include pneumonia, meningitis, strep throat, tuberculosis, Lyme disease, and ulcers; they can be treated with antibiotics.
- Viruses cannot grow or reproduce themselves; different viruses cause the common cold, influenza, measles,

mumps, rubella, chicken pox, cold sores, mononucleosis, encephalitis, hepatitis, polio, and warts.

- Other diseases are caused by certain types of fungi, protozoa, parasitic worms, and prions.
- Autoimmune diseases occur when the body identifies its own cells as foreign.
- HIV affects the immune system, making an otherwise healthy person less able to resist a variety of infections.
- HIV is carried in blood and blood products, semen, vaginal and cervical secretions, and breast milk. HIV is transmitted through the exchange of these fluids.
- There is currently no cure or vaccine for HIV infection. Drugs have been developed to slow the course of the disease and to prevent or treat certain secondary infections.
- Chlamydia and gonorrhea cause epididymitis and urethritis in men; in women, they can lead to PID and infertility if untreated.
- Pelvic inflammatory disease (PID) is an infection of the uterus and oviducts that may extend to the ovaries and pelvic cavity.
- Human papillomavirus (HPV) is the cause of both genital warts and cervical cancer. Treatment does not eradicate the virus, which can be passed on even by asymptomatic people.
- Genital herpes is a common incurable infection that can be fatal to newborns. After an initial infection, outbreaks may recur at any time.
- Hepatitis B is a viral infection of the liver transmitted through sexual and nonsexual contact.
- Syphilis is a highly contagious bacterial infection that can be treated with antibiotics. Untreated, it can lead to deterioration of the central nervous system and death.
- All STDs are preventable; the key is practicing responsible sexual behaviors. Those who are sexually active are safest with one mutually monogamous, uninfected partner. Using a condom properly with every act of sexual intercourse helps protect against STDs.

## Take Action

1. **Create an immunization record:** Find out from your parents or your health records which immunizations you have had, including when you last had a tetanus shot. Are your immunizations up to date? If they aren't, or if you're not sure, check with your school health center about its recommendations.

2. **Compare cold remedies:** Go to your local pharmacy and examine the cold and cough remedies. Exactly which symptoms does each one claim to alleviate, and with what active ingredient? If possible, ask the pharmacist which ones he or she recommends for various symptoms.

3. **Visit a health care provider:** If you have ever engaged in unprotected sex or another behavior that puts you at risk for STDs, talk with your health care provider about being screened for common STDs. What tests are available and useful for your situation?

## For More Information

### Books


Barry, J. 2005. *The Great Influenza: The Epic Story of the Deadliest Plague in History*. New York: Penguin. *A compelling account of the medical, social, and political aspects of the influenza epidemic of 1918–1919.*

McIlvenna, T. 2005. *The Complete Guide to Safer Sex*. Fort Lee, N.J.: Barricade Books. *Provides practical advice for STD prevention.*

Moore, E. A. 2004. *Encyclopedia of Sexually Transmitted Diseases*. Jefferson, N.C.: McFarland. *Includes a variety of information about STDs in an easy-to-use format.*

Preston, R. 2002. *The Demon in the Freezer*. New York: Random House. *A look at the recent history of smallpox, including its eradication in nature and its potential use as a bioweapon.*

Sompayrac, L. M. 2003. *How the Immune System Works*. 2nd ed. Malden, Mass.: Blackwell Science. *A highly readable overview of basic concepts of immunity.*


### VW Organizations, Hotlines, and Web Sites

*American Academy of Allergy, Asthma, and Immunology*. Provides information and publications; pollen counts are available from the hotline and Web site.

800-822-2762
http://www.aaaai.org

*American College of Allergy, Asthma, and Immunology*. Provides information for patients and physicians; Web site includes an extensive glossary of terms related to allergies and asthma.

http://www.acaai.org

*American Social Health Association (ASHA)*. Provides written information and referrals on STDs; sponsors support groups for people with herpes and HPV.

919-361-8488 (herpes hotline)
http://www.ashastd.org

*American Society for Microbiology*. Resources include a library of images and an introduction to microbes.

http://www.microbeworld.org (Microbe World online)
http://www.washup.org (Clean Hands Campaign)

*The Body/A Multimedia AIDS and HIV Information Resource*. Provides basic information about HIV—prevention, testing, treatment—and links to related sites.

http://www.thebody.com

*Bugs in the News!* Provides information about microbiology—allergies, antibodies, antibiotics, mad cow disease, and more—in easy-to-understand language.

http://people.ku.edu/~jbrown/bugs.html

*CDC National Center for Infectious Diseases*. Provides extensive information on a wide variety of infectious diseases.

http://www.cdc.gov/ncidod

*CDC National Immunization Program.* Information and answers to frequently asked questions about immunizations.
800-CDC-SHOT
877-FYI-TRIP (international travel information)
http://www.cdc.gov/nip; http://www.cdc.gov/travel

*CDC STD and AIDS Hotlines.* Callers can obtain information, counseling, and referrals for testing and treatment. The hotlines offer information on more than 20 STDs and include Spanish and TTY service.
800-342-AIDS or 800-227-8922
800-344-SIDA (Spanish); 800-243-7889 (TTY, deaf access)

*CDC National Prevention Information Network.* Provides extensive information and links on HIV/AIDS and other STDs.
800-458–5231
http://www.cdcnpin.org

*Cells Alive!* Includes micrographs of immune cells and pathogens at work.
http://www.cellsalive.com

*HIV InSite: Gateway to AIDS Knowledge.* Provides information about prevention, education, treatment, statistics, clinical trials, and new developments.
http://hivinsite.ucsf.edu

*Joint United Nations Programme on HIV/AIDS (UNAIDS).* Provides statistics and information on the international HIV/AIDS situation.
http://www.unaids.org

*Latex Love.* Sponsored by the makers of Trojan condoms, this site includes directions for condom use and sample dialogues for overcoming excuses for not using condoms.
http://www.trojancondoms.com/quizzes/safer_sex

*National Institute of Allergy and Infectious Diseases.* Includes fact sheets about many topics relating to allergies and infectious diseases, including tuberculosis and STDs.
http://www.niaid.nih.gov

*World Health Organization: Infectious Diseases.* Provides fact sheets about many emerging and tropical diseases as well as information about current outbreaks.
http://www.who.int/topics/en

See also the listings in Chapter 6 (contraception) and Chapter 9 (food safety).

## Selected Bibliography


American Association of Blood Banks. 2004. *Facts About Blood and Blood Banking* (http://www.aabb.org/All_About_Blood/FAQs/aabb_faqs.htm; retrieved December 2, 2004).

Andries, K., et al. 2005. A diarylquinoline drug active on the ATP synthetase of *Mycobacterium tuberculosis. Science* 307(5707): 223–227.

Brown, D. R., et al. 2005. A longitudinal study of genital human papillomavirus infection in a cohort of closely followed adolescent women. *Journal of Infectious Diseases* 191(2): 182–192.

Cashman, N. R., and B. Caughey. 2004. Prion diseases—Close to an effective therapy? *Nature Reviews: Drug Discovery* 3(12): 874–884.

Centers for Disease Control and Prevention. 2005. Antiretroviral postexposure prophylaxis after sexual, injection-drug use, or other nonoccupational exposure to HIV in the United States. *MMWR Recommendations and Reports* 54(RR02): 1–20.

Centers for Disease Control and Prevention. 2005. *West Nile Virus Statistics, Surveillance, and Control* (http://www.cdc.gov/ncidod/dvbid/westnile/surv&controlCaseCount04_detailed.htm; retrieved January 31, 2005).

Centers for Disease Control and Prevention. 2004. Bovine spongiform encephalopathy in a dairy cow—Washington state, 2003. *Morbidity and Mortality Weekly Report* 52(53): 1280–1285.

Centers for Disease Control and Prevention. 2004. Transmission of primary and secondary syphilis by oral sex. *Morbidity and Mortality Weekly Report* 53(41): 966–968.

Centers for Disease Control and Prevention. 2003. Internet use and early syphilis infection among men who have sex with men. *Morbidity and Mortality Weekly Report* 52(50): 1229–1232.

Centers for Disease Control and Prevention. 2003. HIV/STD risks in young men who have sex with men who do not disclose their sexual orientation. *Morbidity and Mortality Weekly Report* 52(5): 81–85.

Centers for Disease Control and Prevention. 2002. 2002 guidelines for treatment of sexually transmitted diseases. *MMWR Recommendations and Reports* 51(RR-6).

Crosby, R., and R. J. DiClemente. 2004. Use of recreational Viagra among men having sex with men. *Sexually Transmitted Infections* 80(6): 466–468.

Erbelding, E. J., and J. M. Zenilman. 2005. Toward better control of sexually transmitted diseases. *New England Journal of Medicine* 352(7): 720–721.

Fairweather, D., and N. R. Rose. 2004. Women and autoimmune diseases. *Emerging Infectious Diseases* 10(11): 2005–2011.

Fauci, A. S. 2004. Emerging infectious diseases: A clear and present danger to humanity. *Journal of the American Medical Association* 292(15): 1887–1888.

Hightow, L. B., et al. 2005. The unexpected movement of the HIV epidemic in the Southeastern United States: Transmission among college students. *Journal of Acquired Immune Deficiency Syndrome* 38(5): 531–537.

Ksiazek, T. G., et al. 2003. A novel coronavirus associated with severe acute respiratory syndrome. *New England Journal of Medicine* Online Article NEJMoa030781.

Levy, S. B., and B. Marshall. 2004. Antibacterial resistance worldwide: Causes, challenges, and responses. *Nature Medicine* 10(12 suppl): S122–S129.

Miller, W. C., et al. 2004. Prevalence of chlamydial and gonococcal infections among young adults in the United States. *Journal of the American Medical Association* 291(18): 2229–2236.

National Immunization Program. 2005. *Epidemiology and Prevention of Vaccine-Preventable Diseases,* 8th ed. Rev. Waldorf, Md.: Public Health Foundation.

National Immunization Program. 2005. *ACIP Recommends Meningococcal Vaccine for Adolescents and College Freshmen* (http://www.cdc.gov/nip/vaccine/meningitis/mcv4/mcv4_acip.htm; retrieved April 6, 2005).

Ness, R. B., et al. 2005. Douching, pelvic inflammatory disease, and incident gonococcal and chlamydial genital infection in a cohort of high-risk women. *American Journal of Epidemiology* 61(2): 186–195.

Prusiner, S. B. 2004. Detecting mad cow disease. *Scientific American,* July.

Snow, R. W., et al. 2005. The global distribution of clinical episodes of *Plasmodium falciparum* malaria. *Nature* 434: 214–217.

Tanaka, M., et al. 2003. Trends in pertussis among infants in the United States. *Journal of the American Medical Association* 290(22): 2968–2975.

World Health Organization. 2004. *Antiretroviral Drugs for Treating Pregnant Women and Preventing HIV Infection in Infants* (http://www.who.int/hiv/pub/mtct/en/arvdrugswomenguidelinesfinal.pdf; retrieved December 6, 2004).

World Health Organization. 2004. *WHO Guidelines for the Global Surveillance of Severe Acute Respiratory Syndrome (SARS), Updated Recommendations, October 2004.* Geneva: World Health Organization.

Zheng, J., et al. 2004. Ethanol stimulation of HIV infection of oral epithelial cells. *Journal of Acquired Immune Deficiency Syndromes* 37(4): 1445–1453.

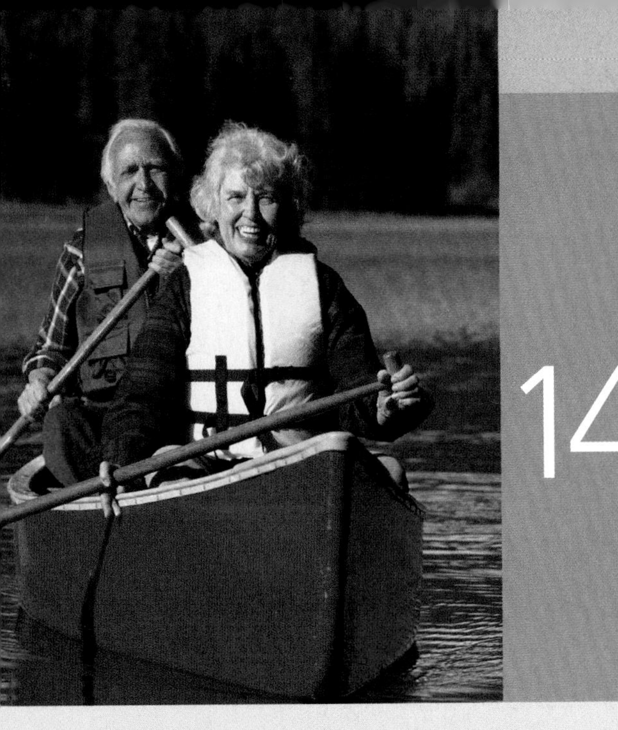

# 14

## Looking AHEAD

After reading this chapter, you should be able to

- List strategies for healthful aging
- Explain the physical, social, and mental changes that may accompany aging and discuss how people can best confront these changes
- Describe practical considerations of older adults and caregivers, including housing, finances, health care, communication, and transportation
- Understand personal considerations in preparing for death, including making a will, assessing choices for end-of-life care, and making arrangements for a funeral or memorial service
- Describe the experience of living with a life-threatening illness and list ways to support a person who is dying
- Explain the grieving process and how support can be offered to adults and children who have experienced a loss

# The Challenge of Aging

Many people would like to live for a long time and never grow old. When we see that old age has taken us in its grip, we're stunned. We regard old age as something foreign. But aging is a normal process of development that occurs over the entire lifetime. It happens to everyone, but at different rates for different people. Some people are "old" at 25, and others are still "young" at 75.

Learning to accept and deal with aging and death is a difficult but important part of life, a process that requires information, insight, and commitment. If you optimize wellness during young adulthood, you can exert great control over the physical and mental aspects of aging, and you can better handle your response to events that might be out of your control. With foresight and energy you can shape a creative, graceful, and even triumphant old age.

## GENERATING VITALITY AS YOU AGE

As we age, we experience both gains and losses. Physical and mental changes occur gradually, over a lifetime. Biological aging includes all the normal, progressive, irreversible changes to one's body that begin at birth and continue until death. Psychological aging and social aging usually involve more abrupt changes in circumstance and emotion: relocating, changing homes, losing a spouse and friends, retiring, having a lower income, and changing roles and social status. These changes represent opportunities for growth throughout life.

Successful aging requires preparation. People need to establish good health habits in their teens and twenties. During their twenties and thirties, they usually develop important relationships and settle into a particular lifestyle. By their mid-forties, they generally know how much money they need to support the lifestyle they've chosen. At this point, they must assess their financial status and perhaps adjust their savings in order to continue enjoying that lifestyle after retirement. In their mid-fifties, they need to reevaluate their health insurance plans and may want to think about retirement housing. In their seventies and beyond, they need to consider ways of sharing their legacy with the next generation. Throughout life, people should cultivate interests and hobbies they enjoy, both alone and with others, so they can continue to live an active and rewarding life in their later years.

**Visit the *Core Concepts in Health* Online Learning Center (www.mhhe.com/inselbrief10e) for study aids and many additional resources.**

In the News

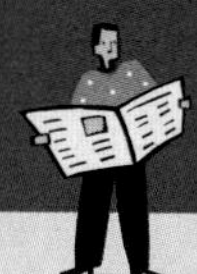

## Stem Cells

### What Are Stem Cells?

Nearly all the cells in our body are differentiated, meaning they are committed to specific functions. We have heart cells, skin cells, nerve cells—over 260 cell types in all. Stem cells, in contrast, are undifferentiated; they can renew themselves by continuing to divide in their undifferentiated state for long periods, and they can develop into specialized cells—a characteristic called *plasticity*. Stem cells theoretically could be used to generate replacement cells for a wide array of diseased or injured tissues and organs—for example, insulin-producing cells to treat type 1 diabetes, cardiac muscle cells for repair of a damaged heart, or healthy brain cells for people with Parkinson's disease.

### Embryonic Stem Cells

As their name suggests, embryonic stem cells are derived from embryos. About 4–5 days after fertilization, an embryo is a microscopic hollow ball of cells referred to as a blastocyst. The inner cell mass contains about 30 stem cells; researchers can remove these cells and grow them in culture for a fairly long period, producing millions of embryonic stem cells. Currently, most embryonic stem cells used in research are derived from eggs that have been fertilized in vitro and then donated for research purposes; they are not derived from embryos fertilized within a woman's body. Stem cells from embryos are *pluripotent,* that is, they can develop into virtually any cell type.

### Adult Stem Cells

Adult stem cells are rare—perhaps only 1 adult stem cell for every 100,000 specialized tissue cells in the body. Adult stem cells appear to have some degree of plasticity; for example, hematopoietic stem cells in bone marrow can differentiate into all the different types of blood cells. However, evidence that adult stem cells from one tissue can develop into fully functional cells of another type of tissue is limited.

The most studied type of adult stem cell, and the only type of stem cell widely used in clinical applications, is the hematopoietic stem cell. These cells are used in transplants to restore blood and immune components to the bone marrow of people being treated for cancer and other diseases.

Another avenue of stem cell research—and one possible way around the problem of rejection in organ transplants—is somatic cell nuclear transfer. In this technique, the nucleus from a somatic (body) cell is transferred into an egg from which the nucleus has been removed. The egg is then allowed to develop in the lab into a blastocyst, and the resulting stem cells are removed and cultured. This technique, also known as *therapeutic cloning,* produces a line of stem cells that are genetically matched to the cell donor; using these cells for transplant should eliminate problems with rejection. (This technique is distinct from so-called *reproductive cloning,* in which an embryo is created in the lab using somatic cell transfer but then implanted in a uterus and allowed to develop in order to produce an offspring who is genetically identical to the donor of the original somatic cell.)

### The Future: Potential and Controversy

Stem cell research is in its infancy, and both technical difficulties and major ethical questions remain. Many scientists believe that research into both embryonic and adult stem cells will be needed to advance the therapeutic potential of stem cell research. However, the use (and destruction) of human embryos for this research is controversial. Some people advocate a complete ban; others would permit the use of existing stem cell lines, the use of "extra" embryos produced by in vitro fertilization, and/or the use of embryos created specifically for research from eggs and sperm donated by volunteers.

In 2001, President Bush banned the use of federal funds for any research related to the creation of new embryonic stem cell lines, thus limiting research to a small number of existing cell lines. Researchers believe that there are problems with this limitation, highlighted by the announcement in 2005 that all existing stem cell lines may have become contaminated with nonhuman compounds via the technique used to maintain them. A number of private institutions and individual states are now providing funds for the creation of new embryonic stem cell lines.

## What Happens as You Age?

Many of the characteristics associated with aging are not due to aging at all. Rather, they are the result of neglect and abuse of our bodies and minds. These assaults lay the foundation for later problems like arthritis, heart disease, diabetes, hearing loss, and hypertension. We sacrifice our optimal health by smoking, having poor nutrition, overeating, abusing alcohol and drugs, bombarding our ears with excessive noise, and exposing our bodies to too much ultraviolet radiation from the sun. We also jeopardize our bodies through inactivity, and we endure abuse from the toxic chemicals in our environment.

But even with the healthiest behavior and environment, aging inevitably occurs. It results from biochemical processes we don't yet fully understand. Further research may help pinpoint the causes of aging and aid in the development of therapies to repair damage to aging organs (see the box "Stem Cells"). Figure 14-1 shows some of the changes that are a part of aging.

## Life-Enhancing Measures: Age-Proofing

You can prevent, delay, lessen, or even reverse some of the changes associated with aging through good habits. Simple things you can do daily will make a vast difference to your level of energy and vitality—your overall wellness. The following suggestions have been mentioned throughout this text. But because they are profoundly related to health in later life, we highlight them here.

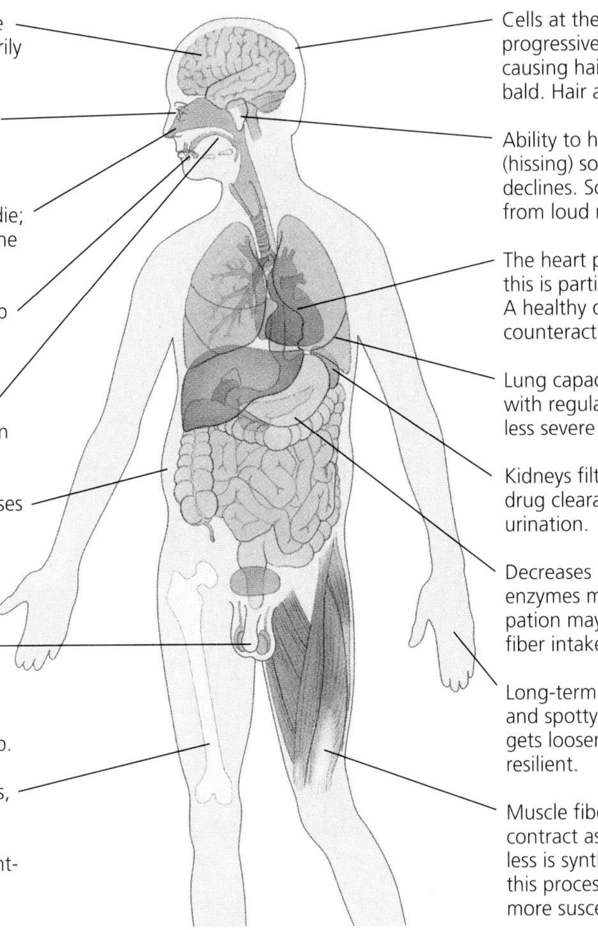


**Figure 14-1 Age-related changes in the body.** The body changes in predictable ways as we age. Many of these changes can be slowed by choices we make throughout our lives.

**Challenge Your Mind** Creativity and intelligence remain stable in healthy individuals. Develop interests and hobbies you can enjoy throughout your life. Staying involved in learning as a lifelong process can help you remain alert and keep your mental abilities.

**Develop Physical Fitness** Exercise significantly enhances both psychological and physical health. The positive effects of exercise include:

- Lower blood pressure and healthier cholesterol levels
- Better protection against heart attacks and an increased chance of survival should one occur
- Sustained capacity of the lungs
- Weight control through less accumulation of fat
- Maintenance of strength, flexibility, and balance
- Protection against osteoporosis and type 2 diabetes
- Increased effectiveness of the immune system
- Maintenance of mental agility and flexibility, response time, memory, and hand-eye coordination

The stimulus that exercise provides also seems to protect against the loss of fluid intelligence, the ability to find solutions when confronted with a new problem. Fluid intelligence depends on rapidity of responsiveness, memory, and alertness. Individuals who exercise regularly are also less susceptible to depression than those whose level of physical activity has declined.

Find a variety of activities that you enjoy and can do regularly. Accumulate at least 30–60 minutes of moderate-intensity physical activity every day, and begin a formal exercise program to develop cardiorespiratory endurance, muscular strength and endurance, and flexibility (see Chapter 10). It's never too late to start exercising. Even in people over 80, endurance and strength training can improve balance, flexibility, and physical functioning and reduce the potential for dangerous falls.

**Eat Wisely** Good health at any age is enhanced by eating a varied diet full of nutrient-rich foods. Follow the recommendations in the 2005 Dietary Guidelines for Americans to obtain adequate amounts of all essential nutrients while maintaining a healthy weight. Special guidelines for older adults include the following:

- Consume vitamin B-12 and extra vitamin D from fortified foods or supplements.
- To help control blood pressure, limit consumption of sodium to 1500 mg per day and consume adequate potassium (4700 mg per day).
- Consume foods rich in dietary fiber and adequate fluids to help prevent constipation, which may occur in up to 20% of older adults. A diet rich in whole grains, vegetables, and fruits can meet the recommended goals for fiber.
- Focus on nutrient-dense foods to obtain adequate nutrients while keeping energy intake at a level that doesn't lead to unhealthy weight gain.
- Pay special attention to food safety; older adults tend to be more susceptible to foodborne illness.

Refer to Chapter 9 for more on the Dietary Guidelines for Americans. Tufts University has developed a special Food Guide Pyramid for older adults (http://nutrition.tufts.edu).

**Maintain a Healthy Weight** Weight management is especially difficult if you have been overweight most of your life. A sensible program of expending more calories through exercise, cutting calorie intake, or a combination of both will work for most people who want to lose weight, but there is no magic formula. Obesity is not physically healthy, and it leads to premature aging.

**Control Drinking and Overdependence on Medications** Alcohol abuse ranks with depression as a common hidden mental health problem, affecting about 10% of older adults. (The ability to metabolize alcohol decreases with age.) The problem is often not identified because the effects of alcohol or drug dependence can mimic disease, such as Alzheimer's disease. Signs of potential alcohol or drug dependence include unexplained falls or frequent injuries, forgetfulness, depression, and malnutrition. Problems can be avoided by not using alcohol to relieve anxiety or emotional pain and not taking medication when safer forms of treatment are available.

**Don't Smoke** The average pack-a-day smoker can expect to live about 13–14 years less than a nonsmoker. Furthermore, smokers suffer more illnesses that last longer, and they are subject to respiratory disabilities that limit their total vigor for many years before their death. Premature balding, skin wrinkling, and osteoporosis have been linked to cigarette smoking.

**Schedule Physical Examinations to Detect Treatable Diseases** When detected early, many diseases, including hypertension, diabetes, and many types of cancer, can be successfully controlled by medication and lifestyle changes. Regular testing for **glaucoma** after age 40 can prevent blindness from this eye disease. Recommended immunizations, including those for influenza and pneumococcus, can protect you from preventable infectious diseases.

**Recognize and Reduce Stress** Stress-induced physiological changes increase wear and tear on your body. Cut down on the stresses in your life. Don't wear yourself out through lack of sleep, substance abuse or misuse, or overwork. Practice relaxation, using the techniques described in Chapter 2. If you contract a disease, consider it your body's attempt to interrupt your life pattern; reevaluate your lifestyle, and perhaps slow down.

## CONFRONTING THE CHANGES OF AGING

The changes that occur with aging have repercussions that must be grappled with and resolved. Just as you can act now to limit the physical changes of aging, you can also begin preparing yourself psychologically, socially, and financially for changes that may occur later in life.

### Planning for Social Changes

Retirement marks a major change in the second half of life. As the longevity of Americans has increased, people spend a larger proportion of their lives in retirement.

**Changing Roles and Relationships** Changes in social roles are a major feature of middle age. Children become young adults and leave home, putting an end to daily parenting. Parents experiencing this "empty nest syndrome" must adapt to changes in their customary responsibilities and personal identities. And although retirement may be a desirable milestone for most people, it may also be viewed as a threat to prestige, purpose, and self-respect—the loss of a valued or customary role—and will probably require a period of adjustment.

Retirement and the end of child rearing also bring about changes in the relationship between marriage partners. The amount of time a couple spend-together will increase and activities will change. Couples may need a period of adjustment, in which they get to know each other as individuals again. Discussing what types of activities each partner enjoys can help couples set up a mutually satisfying routine of shared and independent activities.

**Increased Leisure Time** Planning ahead for retirement is crucial. What kinds of things do you enjoy doing? How will you spend your days? If you have developed diverse interests, retirement can be a joyful and fulfilling period of your life. It can provide opportunities for

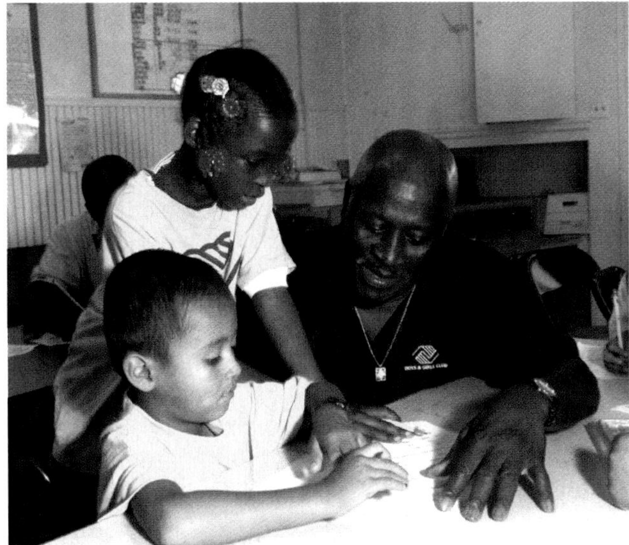

One of the challenges of aging is finding satisfying activities that provide meaningful connections with others. This retired man provides homework assistance and learning activities as part of an after school program.

expanding your horizons by giving you the chance to try new activities, take classes, and meet new people. Volunteering in your community can enhance self-esteem and allow you to be a contributing member of society (see the box "Help Yourself by Helping Others" on p. 352).

**The Economics of Retirement** Financial planning for retirement should begin early in life. People in their twenties and thirties should estimate how much money they need to support their standard of living, calculate their projected income, and begin a savings program. The earlier people begin such a program, the more money they will have at retirement.

Financial planning for retirement is especially critical for women. American women are much less likely than men to be covered by pension plans, reflecting the fact that many women have lower-paying jobs or work part-time during their childbearing years. They tend to have less money vested in other types of retirement plans as well. Although the gap is narrowing, women currently outlive men by about 5–6 years, and they are more likely to develop chronic conditions that impair their daily activities later in life. The net result of these factors is that older women are almost twice as likely as older men to live in poverty. Women should investigate their retirement plans and take charge of their finances to be sure they will be provided for as they get older.

## Adapting to Physical Changes

Some changes in physical functioning are inevitable, and successful aging involves anticipating and accommodating these changes. Decreased energy and changes in health mean that older people have to develop priorities for how to use their energy. Rather than curtailing activities to conserve energy, they need to learn how to generate energy. This usually involves saying yes to enjoyable activities and paying close attention to the need for rest and sleep. Adapting, rather than giving up, favorite activities may be the best strategy for dealing with physical limitations. For example, if **arthritis** interferes with playing an instrument, a person can continue to enjoy music by attending concerts or checking out music from the local library.

**Hearing Loss** The loss of hearing is a common physical change that can have a particularly strong effect on the lives of older adults. Hearing loss affects a person's ability to interact with others and can lead to a sense of isolation and depression. Hearing loss should be assessed and treated by a health care professional; in some cases, hearing can be completely restored by dealing with the underlying cause of hearing loss. In other cases, hearing aids may be prescribed.

**Vision Changes** Vision usually declines with age. For some individuals this can be traced to conditions such as glaucoma or **age-related macular degeneration (AMD)** that can be treated medically. Glaucoma is caused by increased pressure within the eye due to built-up fluid. The optic nerve can be damaged by this increased pressure, resulting in a loss of side vision and, if untreated, blindness. Medication can relieve the pressure by decreasing the amount of fluid produced or by helping it drain more efficiently. Laser and conventional surgery are other options. People over 60, African Americans over 40, and anyone with a family history of glaucoma are at risk.

AMD is a slow disintegration of the macula, the tissue at the center of the retina where fine, straight-ahead detail is distinguished. It is not known what causes the 85% of AMD cases known as "dry," in which usually one eye is gradually affected. About 15% of AMD cases are the more serious "wet" type, in which new blood vessels in the eye grow toward the macula and leak fluid, quickly causing serious damage. Risk factors for AMD are age, gender (women may be at higher risk than men), smoking, elevated cholesterol levels, and family history. Although dry AMD cannot be treated, it progresses so gradually that

### Terms

**glaucoma** A disease in which fluid inside the eye is under abnormally high pressure; can lead to the loss of peripheral vision and blindness.

**arthritis** Inflammation of a joint or joints, causing pain and swelling.

**age-related macular degeneration (AMD)** A deterioration of the macula (the central area of the retina) leading to blurred vision and sensitivity to glare; some cases can lead to blindness.

Mind/Body/Spirit

## Help Yourself by Helping Others

Choosing to help others—whether as a volunteer for a community organization or through spontaneous acts of kindness—can enhance emotional, social, spiritual, and physical wellness. In a national survey of volunteers from all fields, helpers reported the following benefits:

- "Helper's high"—physical and emotional sensations such as sudden warmth, a surge of energy, and a feeling of euphoria that occur immediately after helping
- Feelings of increased self-worth, calm, and relaxation
- A perception of greater physical health
- Fewer colds and headaches, improved eating and sleeping habits, and some relief from the pain of chronic diseases such as asthma and arthritis

Just how might helping benefit the health of the helper? By helping others, we may relieve our own distress and guilt over their problems. Helping others can be effective at banishing a bad mood or a case of the blues. Helping may block physical pain because we can pay attention to only a limited number of things at a given time. Helping others can also expand our perspective and enhance our appreciation for our own lives. Helping may benefit physical health by providing a temporary boost to the immune system and by combating stress and hostile feelings linked to the development of chronic diseases.

Helping others doesn't require a huge time commitment or a change of career. To get the most out of helping, keep the following guidelines in mind:

- *Make contact.* Choose an activity that involves personal contact.
- *Help as often as possible.*
- *Volunteer with others.* Working with a group enables you to form bonds with other helpers who can support your interests and efforts.
- *Focus on the process, not the outcome.* We can't always measure or know the results of our actions.
- *Practice random acts of kindness.* Smile, let people go ahead of you in line, pick up litter, and so on.
- *Adopt a pet.* Several studies suggest that pet owners enjoy better health, perhaps by feeling needed or by having a source of unconditional love and affection.
- *Avoid burnout.* Recognize your own limits, pace yourself, and try not to feel guilty or discouraged.

In addition to the benefits for you, volunteering has the added bonus of having a positive impact on the wellness of others. It fosters a sense of community and can provide some practical help for many of the problems facing our society today.

SOURCES: Shmotkin, D., T. Blumstein, and B. Modan. 2003. Beyond keeping active: Concomitants of being a volunteer in old-old age. *Psychological Aging* 18(3): 602–607; adapted with permission from Sobel, D. S., M.D., and R. Ornstein, Ph.D. 1996. *The Healthy Mind, Healthy Body Handbook.* Los Altos, Calif.: DRx.

many people can adjust to it. Some cases of wet AMD can be treated with laser surgery. Both glaucoma and AMD can be detected with regular screening.

Vision can also be affected by conditions that are products of aging. By the time they reach their forties, many people have developed **presbyopia,** a gradual decline in the ability to focus on objects close to them. This occurs because the lens of the eye no longer expands and contracts as readily. **Cataracts,** a clouding of the lens caused by lifelong oxidation damage (a by-product of normal body chemistry), may dim vision by the sixties.

**Arthritis** Half of all people over the age of 65 have some form of arthritis. This degenerative disease causes joint inflammation leading to chronic pain, swelling, and loss of mobility. There are more than 100 different types of arthritis; osteoarthritis (OA) is by far the most common. In a person with OA, the cartilage that caps the bones in joints wears away, forming sharp spurs. It most often affects the hands and weight-bearing joints of the body—knees, ankles, and hips. OA is second only to heart disease in disabling people so that they cannot work; 74% of those it affects are women.

Strategies for reducing the risk of arthritis and, for those who already have OA, for managing it include exercise, weight management, and avoidance of heavy or repetitive muscle use. Exercise lubricates joints and strengthens the muscles around them, protecting them from further damage. Swimming, walking, and tai chi are good low-impact exercises. Maintaining an appropriate weight is important to avoid placing stress on the hips, knees, and ankles.

If joints are severely damaged and activity is limited, surgery to repair or replace joints may be considered, but medication is usually the first treatment. Many people with OA take medication to relieve inflammation and reduce pain. Nonsteroidal anti-inflammatory drugs like ibuprofen can help but can irritate the digestive tract; prescription drugs that relieve pain without damaging the stomach have been found to have other dangerous side effects (see Chapter 15). Acetaminophen can also reduce pain without upsetting the stomach, but exceeding the recommended dosage can cause liver damage. Balancing the benefits and risks of medications is an important consideration for people at any age.

Recent studies suggest that two dietary supplements, glucosamine and chondroitin sulfate, do have a mild anti-inflammatory effect that eases some OA symptoms. Due to potential risks and side effects, a health care provider should be consulted before either compound is taken.

**Menopause** A special concern for women is the natural process of menopause and the changes accompanying it. During their forties or fifties, women's ovaries gradually stop functioning; estrogen levels drop, and eventually menstruation ceases. Several years before a woman stops menstruating, her periods usually become irregular. Hot flashes, vaginal dryness, sleep disturbances, and mood swings may start around this time.

During the 1990s, about one-third of menopausal women used hormone replacement therapy (HRT) to alleviate the symptoms of menopause and possibly prevent chronic diseases such as CVD and osteoporosis. Many experts believed that HRT would substantially reduce a woman's risk for CVD because estrogen has favorable effects on blood lipids and other risk factors. However, recent studies have shown that HRT may actually increase a woman's risk for CVD, as well as her risk for breast cancer, gallbladder disease, and blood clots. The risks are slight but significant, and experts now recommend that women use HRT only for the control of severe menopausal symptoms and for as brief a time as possible. HRT has been shown to significantly reduce the risk of fractures and to lower the risk of colon cancer. The bottom line is that decisions about HRT may be difficult and are best made by taking into account an individual woman's overall health. Other medications for menopausal symptoms are also available.

Lifestyle strategies to reduce menopause-related problems include many of the healthy habits discussed throughout the text: stop smoking, exercise, eat a healthy diet, lose excess weight, and perform relaxation techniques regularly.

**Osteoporosis** As described in Chapter 9, **osteoporosis** is a condition in which bones become dangerously thin and fragile over time. Problems associated with osteoporosis are fractures, loss of height, stooped posture, severe back and hip pain, and breathing problems.

Women are at greater risk than men for osteoporosis because they have 10–25% less bone in their skeleton, and bone loss accelerates in women during the first 5–10 years after the onset of menopause because of the drop in estrogen production. Black women have higher bone density and fewer fractures than white or Asian women. Other risk factors include a family history of osteoporosis, early menopause (before age 45), abnormal or irregular menstruation, a history of anorexia, and a thin, small frame. Thyroid medication, corticosteroid drugs for arthritis or asthma, and long-term use of the contraceptive Depo-Provera can also have a negative impact on bone mass.

Preventing osteoporosis requires building as much bone as possible during your young years and then maintaining it as you age. Diet and exercise play key roles; see Chapter 9 for recommendations for calcium, vitamin D, and vitamin K intake. Weight-bearing aerobic activities must be performed regularly throughout life to have lasting effects. Strength training improves bone density, muscle mass, strength, and balance, protecting against both bone loss and falls, a major cause of fractures. Even for people in their seventies, low-intensity strength training has been shown to improve bone density. It is also important to avoid tobacco use and manage depression and stress.

Bone mineral density testing can be used to gauge an individual's risk of fracture and help determine if any treatment is needed. Below-normal bone density may be classified as *osteopenia,* which is usually treated with exercise and nutrition. A greater loss of bone mass is classified as full-blown osteoporosis and is often treated with medications.

## Handling Psychological and Mental Changes

Many people associate old age with forgetfulness, and slowly losing one's memory was once considered an inevitable part of growing old. However, we now know that most older adults in good health remain mentally alert and retain their full capacity to learn and remember new information. Many people become smarter as they become older and more experienced.

**Dementia** Severe and significant brain deterioration in elderly individuals, termed **dementia,** affects about 7% of people under age 80 (the incidence rises sharply for people in their eighties and nineties). Early symptoms include slight disturbances in a person's ability to grasp the situation he or she is in. As dementia progresses, memory failure becomes apparent, and the person may forget conversations, the events of the day, or how to perform simple tasks. It is important to have any symptoms evaluated by a health care professional because some of the over 50 known causes of dementia are treatable. The two most common forms of dementia among older people—**Alzheimer's disease** and multi-infarct dementia—are

### Terms

VW

**presbyopia** The inability of the eyes to focus sharply on nearby objects, caused by a loss of elasticity of the lens that occurs with advancing age.

**cataracts** Opacity of the lens of the eye that impairs vision and can cause blindness.

**osteoporosis** The loss of bone density, causing bones to become weak, porous, and more prone to fractures.

**dementia** Deterioration of mental functioning (including memory, concentration, and judgment) resulting from a brain disorder; often accompanied by emotional disturbances and personality changes.

**Alzheimer's disease** A disease characterized by a progressive loss of mental functioning (dementia), caused by a degeneration of brain cells.

In Focus

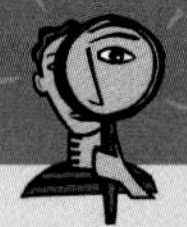

## Alzheimer's Disease

Alzheimer's disease (AD) is a fatal brain disorder that causes physical and chemical changes in the brain. As the brain's nerve cells are destroyed, the system that produces the neurotransmitter acetylcholine breaks down, and communication among parts of the brain deteriorates. Autopsies reveal that the interiors of the affected neurons are filled with clusters of proteins known as tangles: the spaces between the neurons are filled with protein deposits called amyloid plaques. More than 4 million Americans have Alzheimer's disease, and that number is expected to quadruple in the next 50 years, as more people live into their eighties and nineties. AD usually occurs in people over 60 but can occur in people as young as 40.

### Symptoms

The first symptoms of AD are forgetfulness and inability to concentrate. A person may have difficulty performing familiar tasks at home and work and have problems with abstract thinking. As the disease progresses, people experience severe memory loss, especially for recent events. They may vividly remember events from their childhood but be unable to remember the time of day or their location. Depression and anxiety are also common. In the later stages, people with AD are disoriented and may even hallucinate; some experience personality changes—becoming very aggressive or very docile. Eventually, they lose control of physical functioning and are completely dependent on caregivers. On average, a person will survive 8 years after the development of the first symptoms.

### Causes

Scientists do not yet know what causes Alzheimer's disease. Age is the main risk factor, although about 10% of cases seem tied to inherited gene mutations. Inherited familial AD generally strikes people before age 65, while the more common late-onset AD occurs in people 65 and older. Some evidence suggests that many of the same factors that affect heart disease risk also apply to AD. High blood pressure, excess body weight, inactivity, smoking, unhealthy cholesterol levels, high homocysteine and CRP levels, metabolic syndrome, diabetes, depression, stress, and diets high in saturated and trans fats all seem to be associated with increased risk for AD.

People who regularly take nonsteroidal anti-inflammatory drugs (NSAIDS) like ibuprofen (often to control arthritis) and people who regularly consume fish rich in omega-3 fatty acids appear to have lower rates of AD, indicating a possible protective effect of substances that reduce inflammation. Some studies indicate that vitamin E and other antioxidants may reduce risk for AD or slow the progress of the disease, suggesting that oxidative stress caused by free radicals may also play a role.

### Diagnosis and Treatment

Currently, the only certain way to diagnose AD is to examine brain tissue during an autopsy. In most cases, physicians use a combination of a medical history, neurological and psychological tests, physical exams, blood and urine tests, and a brain-imaging scan. Good early results have also been seen using a test that measures levels of a specific protein in spinal fluid. A behavior diary can also aid in diagnosis.

For people with mild to moderate AD, there are several drugs that provide modest improvements in memory. Several medications help maintain cognitive function by inhibiting the breakdown of the neurotransmitter acetylcholine but do not alter the course of the disease. These so-called cholinesterase inhibitors include Aricept (donepezil), Cognex (tacrine), Exelon (rivastigmine), and Reminyl (galantamine). People with AD may also be prescribed antidepressant or antianxiety medications. As scientists gain more insight into Alzheimer's disease, they hope to develop more effective treatments that will ease the burden of AD for both families and society.

---

irreversible. Alzheimer's disease is characterized by changes in brain nerve cells (see the box "Alzheimer's Disease"). Multi-infarct dementia results from a series of small strokes or changes in the brain's blood supply that destroy brain tissue.

Repeatedly telling stories about the past—something older people often do—doesn't necessarily indicate dementia. Reminiscence is a normal part of development and allows an older person to integrate life by making past events meaningful in the present. Reminiscing can be of great significance to members of the younger generations because it is a rich source of social, cultural, and family history.

**Grief** Another psychological and emotional challenge of aging is dealing with grief and mourning. Aging is associated with loss—the loss of friends, peers, physical appearance, possessions, and health. Grief is the process of getting through the pain of loss, and it can be one of the loneliest and most intense times in a person's life. It can take a year or two or more to completely come to terms with the loss of a loved one. Unresolved grief can have serious physical and psychological or emotional health consequences and may require professional help.

**Depression** Unresolved grief can lead to depression, a common problem in older adults (see Chapter 3). If you notice the signs of depression in yourself or someone you know, consult a mental health professional. Both professional treatment and support groups can help people deal successfully with major life changes, such as retirement, moving, health problems, or loss of a spouse. If someone refuses help, be reassuring and emphasize that treatment helps make people feel better.

Depression is probably the single most significant factor associated with suicidal behavior in older adults. Suicide is relatively common among the elderly—especially

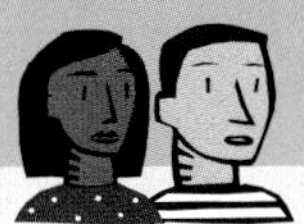

Gender Matters

## Why Do Women Live Longer?

Women live longer than men in most countries around the world, even in places where maternal mortality rates are high. In the United States, women on average can expect to live about 5 years longer than men (see table). Worldwide, among people over age 100, women outnumber men about 9 to 1.

The reason for the gender gap in life expectancy is not entirely understood but may be influenced by biological, social, and lifestyle factors. Estrogen production and other factors during a woman's younger years may protect her from early heart disease and from age-related declines in the pumping power of the heart. Women may have lower rates of stress-related illnesses because they cope more positively with stress by seeking social support.

The news for women is not all good, however, because not all their extra years are likely to be healthy years. They are more likely than men to suffer from chronic conditions like arthritis and osteoporosis. Women's longer life spans, combined with the facts that men tend to marry younger women and that widowed men remarry more often than widowed women, means there are many more single older women than men. Older men are more likely to live in family settings, whereas older women are more likely to live alone. Older women are also less likely to be covered by a pension or to have retirement savings, so they are more likely to be poor.

Increased male mortality can be traced in part to higher rates of behaviors such as smoking and alcohol and drug abuse. Testosterone production may be partly responsible in that it is linked to aggressive and risky behavior and to unhealthy cholesterol levels. Men have much higher rates of death than women from car crashes and other unintentional injuries, firearm-related deaths, homicide, suicide, AIDS, and early heart attack. Gender roles that promote risky behavior among young men are a factor in many of these causes of death. Indeed, among people who have made it to age 65, the gender longevity gap is smaller.

Social and behavioral factors may be more important than physiological causes in explaining the gender gap; for example, among the Amish, a religious sect that has strict rules against smoking and drinking, men usually live as long as women. This means that the longevity gap could be substantially narrowed through lifestyle changes.

**Life Expectancy**

| Year | Men | Women |
|---|---|---|
| **At birth:** | | |
| 1900 | 46.3 | 48.3 |
| 1950 | 65.6 | 71.1 |
| 2000 | 74.3 | 79.7 |
| 2050* | 79.7 | 84.3 |
| **At age 65:** | | |
| 1900 | 11.5 | 12.2 |
| 1950 | 12.8 | 15.0 |
| 2000 | 16.2 | 19.3 |
| 2050* | 20.3 | 22.4 |

**projected*

SOURCES: U.S. Census Bureau. 2005. *We the People: Women and Men in the United States*. Washington, D.C.: U.S. Census Bureau; Aging: The stronger sex. 2005. *Economist*, January 13; National Centers for Health Statistics. 2004. *Health, United States, 2004*. Hyattsville, Md.: National Center for Health Statistics; World Health Organization. 2003. *Gender, Health, and Aging*. Geneva: World Health Organization.

white males over the age of 65. One explanation for this is that because white men generally have greater power and status in our society, aging and retirement represent a relatively greater loss for them. Women, more accustomed to "secondary" status, are not as threatened by the loss of economic and social power. Another theory is that white men tend to have weaker social ties than women or than men from other cultural groups and as they retire their increasing social isolation leads to depression and suicide. Some cultural groups, particularly Latinos and African Americans, afford greater respect and status to older people, who are valued for their wisdom and experience. Cultural groups that emphasize family and social ties also seem to have lower rates of suicide.

One of the most important ways of dealing with the changes associated with aging is to adopt a flexible attitude toward whatever life brings you. Self-acceptance can help make the later years more meaningful and enjoyable. Accepting limitations, having an optimistic outlook, and having a sense of humor are tools that can help you cope with all of life's changes.

## LIFE IN AN AGING AMERICA

**Life expectancy** is the average length of time we can expect to live. It is calculated by averaging mortality statistics, the ages of death of a group of people over a certain period. Current life expectancy is 77.3 years for someone born in 2002, but those who reach age 65 can expect to live even longer—18 more years or longer—because they have already survived hazards to life in the younger years. Women have a longer life expectancy than men (see the box "Why Do Women Live Longer?").

As life expectancy increases, a larger proportion of the population will be in their later years. This change will necessitate new government policies and changes in our general attitudes toward older adults.

**Term**

**life expectancy** The average length of time a person is expected to live.

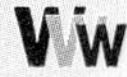

## America's Aging Minority

People over 65 are a large minority in the American population—over 35 million people, about 13% of the total population in 2000 (Figure 14-2). As birth rates drop, the percentage increases dramatically. The enormous increase in the over-55 population is markedly affecting our stereotypes of what it means to grow old. The misfortunes associated with aging—frailty, forgetfulness, poor health, isolation—occur in fewer people in their sixties and seventies and are shifting instead to burden the very old, those over 85.

In general, today's older adults are better off than they have ever been in the past. They have more money than they did 20 years ago. The poverty rate of the elderly has dropped from 28.5% to 10% since the 1960s, largely from the effects of Social Security payments and health care benefits from Medicare. About 81% of older Americans own their homes. Their living expenses are lower after retirement because they no longer support children and have fewer work-related expenses; they consume and buy less food. They receive greater amounts of assistance, such as Medicare, pay proportionately lower taxes, and have greater net worth from lifetime savings.

As the aging population increases proportionately, however, the number of older people who are ill and dependent rises. Health care remains the largest expense for older adults. Tens of thousands of older Americans live in poverty, particularly minorities and women living alone. These other elderly—poverty-stricken, isolated, lonely—are just as ignored as they ever were, and their numbers are increasing.

Retirement finds many older people with their incomes reduced to subsistence levels. The majority of older Americans live with fixed sources of income, such as pensions, that are eroded by inflation. Many Americans rely on Social Security payments as their only source of income; they are not covered by other types of retirement plans. **Social Security** was intended to serve as a supplement to personal savings and private pensions, not as a sole source of income. It is vital that people plan early for an adequate retirement income.

## Family and Community Resources for Older Adults

With help from friends, family members, and community services, people in their later years can remain active and independent. About 66% of noninstitutionalized older Americans live with a spouse or other family member; the other 34% live alone or with a nonrelative. Overall, only 4% live in nursing homes or other institutional settings at any point in time, but among those over age 85, about 20% live in a nursing home. In about three out of four cases, a grown daughter or daughter-in-law assumes a caregiving role for elderly relatives. Recent surveys

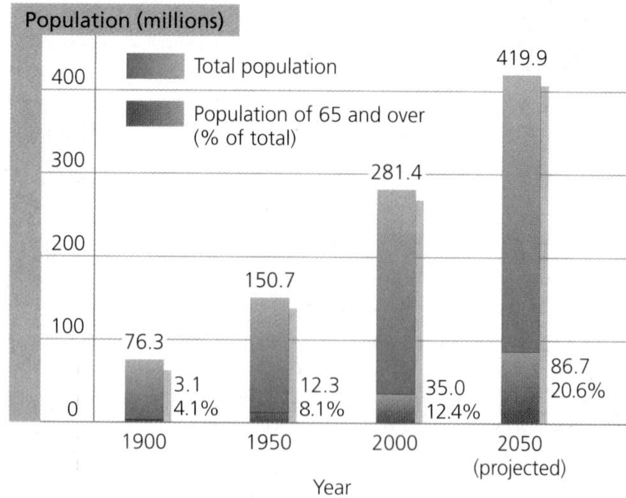

(a) Population growth over age 65 as a proportion of the total population.

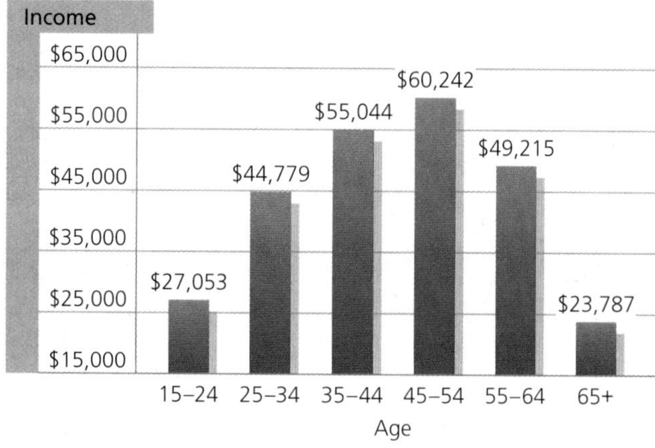

(b) Median household income by age of the household head.

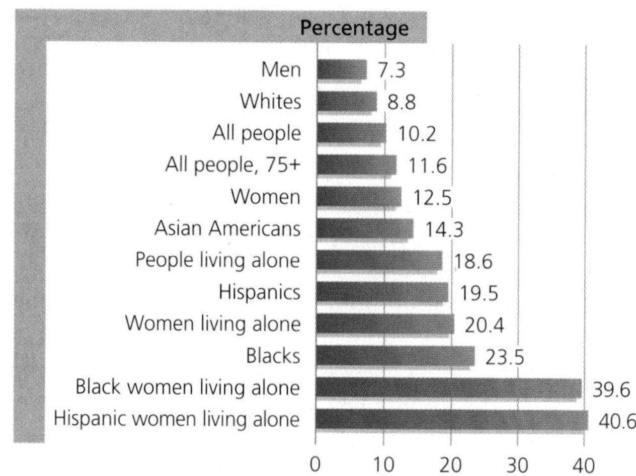

(c) Percentages of groups over age 65 below the poverty level.

VITAL STATISTICS

**Figure 14-2** A statistical look at older Americans. SOURCE: U.S. Bureau of the Census. U.S. Administration on Aging.

indicate that the average woman will spend about 17 years raising children and 18 years caring for an aging relative.

Caregiving can be rewarding, but it is also hard work. If the experience is stressful and long-term, family members may become emotionally exhausted. Caregivers should use available community services and consider their own needs for relaxation and relief from caregiving duties. Corporations are increasingly responsive to the needs of their employees who are family caregivers by providing services such as referrals, flexible schedules and leaves, and on-site adult care. Professional health care advice is another critical part of successful home care.

The best thing a family can do to prepare for the task of caring for aging parents is to talk frankly about the future. What does everyone expect will happen? What living and caring options are available, and which ones do family members prefer? What community resources are available? Planning ahead can reduce the stress on everyone involved and help ease difficult transitions.

### Government Aid and Policies

The federal government helps older Americans through several programs, such as food stamps, housing subsidies, Social Security, Medicare, and Medicaid. Social Security, the life insurance and old-age pension plan, has saved many from destitution, although it is intended not as a sole source of income but as a supplement to other income.

Medicare is a major health insurance program for the elderly and the disabled, paying about 30% of the medical costs of older Americans. It provides basic health care coverage for acute episodes of illness that require skilled professional care; it also pays for some preventive services. In the past, Medicare did not cover prescription drug costs, but programs involving discount cards and drug benefits are currently being phased in. Medicare pays less than 2% of nursing home costs, and private insurers pay less than 1%, creating a tremendous financial burden for nursing home residents and their families. Because of these gaps in coverage, many older people are joining managed health care plans to get more care for their money. When their financial resources are exhausted, people may apply for Medicaid, which provides medical insurance to low-income people of any age.

Health care policy planners hope that rising medical costs for older adults will dwindle dramatically through education and prevention. Health care professionals are beginning to practice preventive medicine and advise older people about how to avoid and, if necessary, how to manage disabilities. They try to instill an ethic of physical and psychological maintenance that will prevent chronic disease and enable older people to live long, healthy, vigorous lives.

There can be benefits to aging, but they don't come automatically. They require planning and wise choices earlier in life. One octogenarian, Russell Lee, founder of a medical clinic in California, perceived the advantages of aging as growth: "The limitations imposed by time are compensated by the improved taste, sharper discretion, sounder mental and esthetic judgment, increased sensitivity and compassion, clearer focus—which all contribute to a more certain direction in living. . . . The later years can be the best of life for which the earlier ones were preparation."

## WHAT IS DEATH?

From a tsunami devastating a fishing village in Southeast Asia to a man in a crowded restaurant having a heart attack to an elderly woman dying peacefully with her family close by, images of death pervade our consciousness. Nevertheless, very rarely do we think about the inevitability of death in our own lives. Accepting and dealing with death are important tasks that present unique challenges to our sense of self and relationship to others and our understanding of the meaning of life itself. Although times of pain and distress may accompany the dying process, facing death also presents opportunity for growth as well as affirmation of the preciousness of simple aspects of our daily lives.

Questions about the meaning of death and what happens when we die are central concerns of the great religions and philosophies. Some promise a better life after death. Others teach that everyone is evolving toward perfection or divinity, a goal reached after successive rounds of death and rebirth. There are also those who suggest that it is not possible to know what happens—if anything—after death, that any judgment about whether life is worth living must be made on the basis of satisfactions or rewards that we create for ourselves in this life.

### Defining Death

Traditionally, death has been defined as cessation of the flow of vital bodily fluids. This occurs when the heart stops beating and breathing ceases. These traditional signs are adequate for determining death in most cases. However, the use of respirators and other life-support systems in modern medicine allows some body functions to be artificially sustained. The concept of **brain death** has been developed to determine whether a person is alive or dead when the traditional signs are inadequate because of supportive medical technology.

#### Terms

**Social Security** A government program that provides financial assistance to people who are unemployed, disabled, or retired (and over a certain age); financed through taxes on businesses and workers.

**brain death** A medical determination of death as the cessation of brain activity indicated by various diagnostic criteria, including a flat EEG reading.

V w

According to the standards published in 1968 by a Harvard Medical School committee, brain death involves the following four characteristics: (1) lack of receptivity and response to external stimuli, (2) absence of spontaneous muscular movement and spontaneous breathing, (3) absence of observable reflexes, and (4) absence of brain activity, as signified by a flat **electroencephalogram (EEG).** The Harvard criteria require a second set of tests to be performed after 24 hours has elapsed, and they exclude cases of hypothermia (body temperature below 90°F), as well as situations involving central nervous system depressants, such as barbiturates.

In contrast to **clinical death,** which is determined by either the cessation of heartbeat and breathing or the criteria for establishing brain death, **cellular death** refers to a gradual process that occurs when heartbeat, respiration, and brain activity have stopped. It encompasses the breakdown of metabolic processes and results in complete nonfunctionality at the cellular level.

The way in which death is defined has potential legal and social consequences in a variety of areas, including criminal prosecution, inheritance, taxation, treatment of the corpse, and even mourning. It also affects the practice of organ transplantation, because some organs—hearts, most obviously—must be harvested from a human being who is legally determined to be dead.

### Learning About Death

Our understanding of death changes as we grow and mature, as do our attitudes toward it. Very young children view death as an interruption and an absence, but their lack of a mature time perspective means that they do not understand death as final and irreversible. A child's understanding of death evolves greatly from about age 5 to age 9. During this period, most children come to understand that death is final, universal, and inevitable. A child who consciously recognizes these facts is said to possess a mature understanding of death. This understanding of death is further refined during the years of adolescence and young adulthood by considering the impact of death on close relationships and contemplating the value of religious or philosophical answers to the enigma of death.

It is important to add, however, that individuals who possess a mature understanding of death commonly hold nonempirical ideas about it as well. Such nonempirical ideas—that is, ideas not subject to scientific proof—deal mainly with the notion that human beings survive in some form beyond the death of the physical body. What happens to an individual's "personality" after he or she dies? Does the self or soul continue to exist after the death of the physical body? If so, what is the nature of this "afterlife"? Developing personally satisfying answers to such questions is also part of the process of acquiring a mature understanding of death.

### Denying Versus Welcoming Death

Our ability to find meaning and comfort in the face of mortality depends not only on our having an understanding of the facts of death, but also on our attitudes toward it. Many people seek to avoid any thought or mention of death. The sick and old are often isolated in hospitals and nursing homes. Relatively few Americans have been present at the death of a loved one. Where the reality of death is concerned, "out of sight, out of mind" often appears to be the rule of the day. Instead of facing death directly, we tend to amuse ourselves with unrealistic portrayals on television and movie screens. The fictitious deaths of characters we barely know do not cause us to confront the reality of death as it is experienced in real life.

Although some commentators characterize the predominant attitude toward death in the United States as "death denying," others are reluctant to paint society as a whole with such a broad brush. Individuals often maintain conflicting or ambivalent attitudes toward death. Those who come to view death as a relief or release from insufferable pain may have at least a partial sense of welcoming death. Few people wholly avoid or wholly welcome death. Problems can arise, however, when avoidance or denial fosters the notion that death happens to others, but not to you or me. (For another perspective, see the box "Día de los Muertos: The Day of the Dead.")

## PLANNING FOR DEATH

Acknowledging the inevitability of death allows us to plan for it. Adequate planning can help ensure that a sudden, unexpected death is not made even more difficult for survivors. Although some decisions cannot be made until one is actually in a particular situation, many decisions relating to dying and death can be anticipated, considered, and discussed with close relatives and friends.

**Terms**

VW

**electroencephalogram (EEG)** A record of the electrical activity of the brain (brain waves).

**clinical death** A determination of death made according to accepted medical criteria.

**cellular death** The breakdown of metabolic processes at the level of the cell.

**will** A legal instrument expressing a person's intentions and wishes for the disposition of his or her property after death.

**estate** The money, property, and other possessions belonging to a person.

**testator** The person who makes a will.

**intestate** Referring to the situation in which a person dies without having made a legal will.

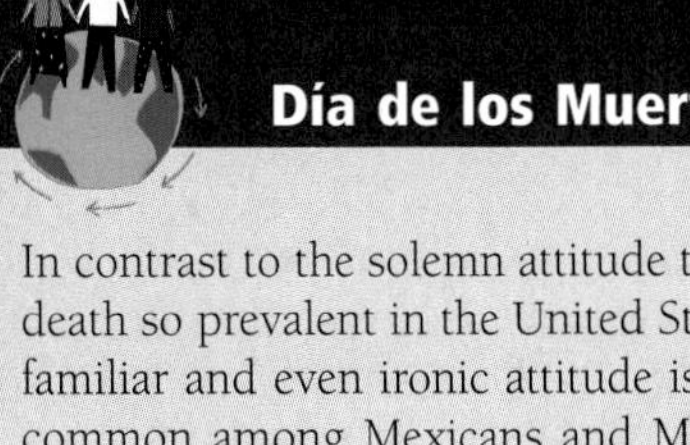

Dimensions of Diversity

## Día de los Muertos: The Day of the Dead

In contrast to the solemn attitude toward death so prevalent in the United States, a familiar and even ironic attitude is more common among Mexicans and Mexican Americans. In the Mexican worldview, death is another phase of life, and those who have passed into it remain accessible. Ancestors are not forever lost, nor is the past dead. This sense of continuity has its roots in the culture of the Aztecs, for whom regeneration was a central theme. When the Spanish came to Mexico in the sixteenth century, their beliefs about death, along with symbols such as skulls and skeletons, were absorbed into the native culture.

Mexican artists and writers confront death with humor and even sarcasm, depicting it as the inevitable fate that all—even the wealthiest—must face. At no time is this attitude toward death livelier than at the beginning of each November on the holiday known as Día de los Muertos, "the Day of the Dead." This holiday coincides with All Souls' Day, the Catholic commemoration of the dead, and represents a unique blending of indigenous ritual and religious dogma.

Festive and gay, the celebration in honor of the dead typically spans two days—one day devoted to dead children, one to adults. It reflects the belief that the dead return to Earth in spirit once a year to rejoin their families and partake of holiday foods prepared especially for them. The fiesta usually begins at midday on October 31, with flowers and food—candies, cookies, honey, milk—set out on altars in each house for the family's dead. The next day, family groups stream to the graveyards, where they have cleaned and decorated the graves of their loved ones, to celebrate and commune with the dead. They bring games, music, and special food—chicken with *mole* sauce, enchiladas, tamales, and *pan de muertos,* the "bread of the dead," sweet rolls in the shape of bones. People sit on the graves, eat, sing, and talk with the departed ones. Tears may be shed as the dead are remembered, but mourning is tempered by the festive mood of the occasion.

During the season of the dead, graveyards and family altars are decorated with yellow candles and yellow marigolds—the "flower of death." In some Mexican villages, yellow flower petals are strewn along the ground, connecting the graveyard with all the houses visited by death during the year.

Does this more familiar attitude toward death help people accept death and come to terms with it? Keeping death in the forefront of consciousness may provide solace to the living, reminding them of their loved ones and assuring them that they themselves will not be forgotten when they die. Yearly celebrations and remembrances may help people keep in touch with their past, their ancestry, and their roots. The festive atmosphere may help dispel the fear of death, allowing people to look at it more directly. Although it is possible to deny the reality of death even when surrounded by images of it, such practices as Día de los Muertos may help people face death with more equanimity.

SOURCES: Adapted from DeSpelder, L., and A. Strickland. 2005. *The Last Dance,* 7th ed. New York: McGraw-Hill; Azcentral. 2000. *Día de los Muertos* (http://www.azcentral.com/rep/dead; retrieved March 8, 2001); Puente, T. 1991. Día de los Muertos. *Hispanic,* October; Milne, J. 1965. *Fiesta Time in Latin America.* Los Angeles: Ward Ritchie Press.

## Making a Will

Surveys indicate that about seven out of ten Americans die without leaving a will. A **will** is a legal instrument expressing a person's intentions and wishes for the disposition of his or her property after death. It is a declaration of how one's **estate**—that is, money, property, and other possessions—will be distributed after death. During the life of the **testator** (the person making the will), a will can be changed, replaced, or revoked. Upon the testator's death, it becomes a legal instrument governing the distribution of the testator's estate.

When a person dies **intestate**—that is, without having left a valid will—property is distributed according to rules set up by the state. The failure to execute a will may result in a distribution of property that is not compatible with a person's wishes nor best suited to the interests and needs of heirs. If you haven't yet made a will, start thinking about how you'd like your property distributed in the case of your death. If you have a will, consider whether it needs to be updated in response to a key life event such as marriage, the birth of a child, or the purchase of a home. In making a will, it is generally advisable to involve close family members to prevent problems that can arise when actions are taken without the knowledge of those who will be affected.

## Considering Options for End-of-Life Care

If you were facing the prospect of dying soon, would you prefer to spend your last days or weeks at home, cared for by relatives and friends? Or would you rather have access to the sophisticated medical technologies available in a hospital? Currently, about 25% of Americans die at home, about 25% die in nursing facilities, and about 50% die in hospitals, including more than 20% in intensive care units. By becoming aware of our options, we and our families are empowered to make informed, meaningful choices.

**Home Care** Many people express a preference to be cared for at home during the end stage of a terminal illness. An obvious advantage of home care is the fact that the dying person is in a familiar setting, ideally in the company of family and friends. For home care to be an option, however, support generally must be provided not only by family and friends, but also by skilled, professional caregivers.

Mind/Body/Spirit

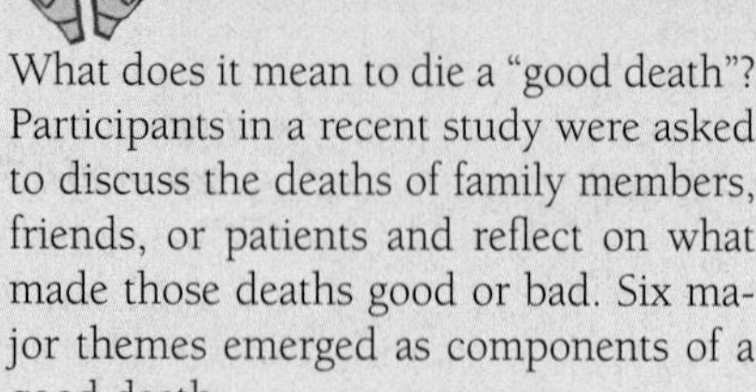

## In Search of a Good Death

What does it mean to die a "good death"? Participants in a recent study were asked to discuss the deaths of family members, friends, or patients and reflect on what made those deaths good or bad. Six major themes emerged as components of a good death.

The first component was pain and symptom management. Many people fear dying in pain, and portrayals of bad deaths usually included inadequate pain management. Every health care provider told regret-filled stories of patients who died in pain. Patients were concerned with both current and future pain control; when reassured that pain could be managed with drugs, they were less anxious.

The second major component of a good death was clear decision making. Both providers and families feared entering a medical crisis without knowledge of patient preferences. Patients and families who had good communication with health care providers and had discussed treatment decisions ahead of time felt empowered, and providers felt they were giving good care. Researchers noted that although all uncertainty about end-of-life decisions cannot be eliminated, tolerance for uncertainty may increase if values and preferences are clarified.

The third component was preparation for death. Patients expressed satisfaction when they had adequate time to prepare their wills and help plan the events that would follow their death, such as funeral arrangements. Many times, providers avoided end-of-life discussions to prevent their patients from losing hope, thus depriving them of the opportunity to plan ahead. Patients and families also wanted to know what to expect during the course of the illness and what physical and psychosocial changes would take place as death approached.

The fourth element was completion, the opportunity to review one's life, to resolve conflicts, to spend time with loved ones, and to say good-bye. Participants confirmed the deep importance of spirituality or meaningfulness at the end of life. Many times, patients were able to view their experience of dying as part of a broader life trajectory and thus continue to grow emotionally and spiritually in their last days. Issues of faith were often mentioned as important to healing.

The fifth component was contributing to others. Patients wanted to know that they still had something to offer to others, whether it was making someone laugh or lightening the load of someone closer to death. Many patients found that as they reflected on their lives, what they valued most was their personal relationships with family and friends, and they were anxious to impart this wisdom to others.

The last component of a good death was affirmation of the whole person. Patients appreciated empathic health care providers, and family members were comforted by those who treated their loved ones as unique and whole people, rather than as a "disease." The quality of dying is related to the acknowledgment that people die "in character," that is, as an extension of who they have been in their lives.

The study affirmed that most people think of death as a natural part of life, not as a "failure of technology." Although the biomedical aspects of end-of-life care are crucial, they merely provide a point of departure toward a good death. When pain is properly managed and the practical aspects of dying are taken care of, patients and their families have the opportunity to address the important emotional, psychological, and spiritual issues that all human beings face at the end of life.

SOURCE: Steinhauser, K. S., et al. 2000. In search of a good death: Observations of patients, families, and providers. *Annals of Internal Medicine* 132(10): 825–832.

**Hospital-Based Palliative Care** Although hospitals are primarily organized to provide short-term intensive treatment for acute injury and illness, they are also adopting the principles of **palliative care** for patients who require comprehensive care at the end of life. Unlike acute care, which involves taking active measures to sustain life, palliative care focuses on controlling pain and relieving suffering by caring for the physical, psychological, spiritual, and existential needs of the patient. Although the emphasis is generally placed on comfort care, palliative therapies can be combined with cure-oriented treatment approaches in some cases. In all cases, the goal of palliative care is to achieve the best possible quality of life for patients and their families.

**Hospice Programs** As a comprehensive program of care offering a set of services designed to support terminally ill patients and their families, **hospice** is a well-known form of palliative care. Although the term *hospice* sometimes refers to a freestanding medical facility to which terminally ill patients are admitted, most hospice care takes place in patients' homes with family members as primary caregivers. Hospice (and palliative care generally) seeks to provide state-of-the-art care to prevent or relieve pain and other distressing symptoms, as well as to offer emotional and spiritual support to both patient and family. The primary aim is to help people live as fully as possible until the end of their lives (see the box "In Search of a Good Death).

## Deciding to Prolong Life or Hasten Death

Modern medicine can keep the human organism alive despite the cessation of normal heart, brain, respiratory, or kidney function. But should a patient without any hope of recovery be kept alive by means of artificial life support? What if a patient has fallen into a **persistent vegetative state**, a state of profound unconsciousness, lacking any sign of normal reflexes and unresponsive to external stimuli, with no reasonable hope of improvement?

Ethical questions about the "right to die" have become prominent since the landmark case of Karen Ann Quinlan in 1975. At age 22, she was admitted in a comatose state to an intensive care unit. When she remained unresponsive in a persistent vegetative state, her parents asked that artificial respiration be discontinued. The request to withdraw treatment was eventually approved by the New Jersey Supreme Court.

Since then, courts have ruled on removing other types of life-sustaining treatment, including artificial feeding mechanisms that provide nutrition and hydration to permanently comatose patients who are able to breathe on their own. Most notable was the case of Nancy Beth Cruzan. As a result of injuries she received in 1983, Cruzan was in a persistent vegetative state. To provide nourishment, Nancy's physicians implanted a feeding tube, the only form of life support she was receiving.

In 1990, the U.S. Supreme Court ruled that the right to refuse unwanted treatment, even if it is life-sustaining, is constitutionally protected. However, the court said that states are justified in requiring that only the patient can decide to withdraw treatment. Because Nancy apparently had not provided a clear expression of her wishes prior to her injury, the state of Missouri was not bound to honor her parents' request for removal of the feeding tube. A few months later, however, in light of new testimony from several of Nancy's friends that she had expressed a wish "not to live like a vegetable," a state court ruled that the legal standard of "clear and convincing" evidence of Nancy's wishes had been met, and therefore permission was granted for removal of the feeding tube. The question of whether to remove an implanted feeding tube was also at the heart of the high-profile case of Terri Schiavo. These cases emphasized the importance of expressing one's preferences about life-sustaining treatment—preferably in writing—before the need arises.

### Withholding or Withdrawing Treatment

The right of a competent patient to refuse unwanted treatment is now generally established in both law and medical practice. The consensus is that there is no medical or ethical distinction between withholding (not starting) a treatment and withdrawing (stopping) a treatment once it has been started. The choice to forgo life-sustaining treatment involves refusing treatments that would be expected to extend life. The right to refuse treatment remains constitutionally protected even when a patient is unable to communicate. Although specific requirements vary, all of the states authorize some type of written advance directive to honor the decisions of individuals unable to speak for themselves but who have previously recorded their wishes in an appropriate legal document.

The practice of withholding or withdrawing a treatment that could potentially sustain life is sometimes termed **passive euthanasia**, although many people consider this term a misnomer because it tends to confuse the widely accepted practice of withholding or withdrawing treatment with the generally unacceptable and unlawful practice of taking active steps to cause death.

### Assisted Suicide and Active Euthanasia

In contrast to withdrawing or withholding treatment, assisted suicide and active euthanasia refer to practices that intentionally hasten the death of a person. Assisted suicide refers to providing someone with the means to commit suicide, knowing that the recipient intends to use them to end his or her life. In **physician-assisted suicide (PAS)**, a physician provides lethal drugs or other interventions—at the patient's explicit request—with the understanding that the patient plans to use them to end his or her life. The patient, not the doctor, administers the fatal dose.

In 1997, the Supreme Court reviewed two cases relating to physician-assisted suicide. The decisions in these cases (*Washington v. Glucksberg* and *Vacco v. Quill*) are important for several reasons. First, the Court upheld the distinction between, on the one hand, withholding or withdrawing treatment and, on the other hand, physician-assisted suicide. Second, the Court affirmed the rights of states to craft policy concerning physician-assisted suicide, either prohibiting it, as most states now do, or permitting it under some regulatory system, as is now happening in Oregon.

Oregon is currently the only state where PAS is permitted. The Death with Dignity Act, a ballot initiative, was passed by Oregon voters in 1994 and, after surviving judicial challenges, was reaffirmed in 1997. During its first 7 years of implementation, 208 people were reported to have legally committed suicide with the assistance of their physicians. These patients exhibited strong beliefs in personal autonomy and a determination to control the end of their lives. The decision to request a prescription for lethal medication was associated mainly with concerns about loss of autonomy and control.

A third finding of importance in the Supreme Court's 1997 rulings about PAS relates to the concept of double

### Terms

**palliative care** A form of medical care aimed at reducing the intensity or severity of a disease by controlling pain and other discomforting symptoms.

**hospice** A program of care for dying patients and their families.

**persistent vegetative state** A condition of profound unconsciousness in which a person lacks normal reflexes and is unresponsive to external stimuli, lasting for an extended period with no reasonable hope of improvement.

**passive euthanasia** The practice of withholding (not starting) or withdrawing (stopping) treatment that could potentially sustain a person's life, with the recognition that, without such treatment, death is likely to occur.

**physician-assisted suicide (PAS)** The practice of a physician intentionally providing, at the patient's request, lethal drugs or other means for a patient to hasten death with the understanding that the patient plans to use them to end his or her life.

effect in the medical management of pain. The doctrine of double effect states that a harmful effect of treatment, even if it results in death, is permissible if the harm is not intended and occurs as a side effect of a beneficial action. Sometimes the dosages of medication needed to relieve a patient's pain must be increased to levels that can cause respiratory depression, resulting in the patient's death. The Court said that such medication for pain, even if it hastens death, is not physician-assisted suicide if the intent is to relieve pain.

Unlike physician-assisted suicide, **active euthanasia** involves a deliberate act to end another person's life. Voluntary euthanasia (also known as voluntary active euthanasia, or VAE) is the intentional termination of life at the patient's request by someone other than the patient. In practice, this generally means that a competent patient requests direct assistance to die, and he or she receives assistance from a qualified medical practitioner. At present, active euthanasia has found greatest acceptance in the Netherlands, where physicians are permitted to give lethal injections to patients who request death. VAE is currently unlawful in the United States, and it is for this practice that Michigan physician Dr. Jack Kevorkian was convicted of second-degree murder in 1999. Taking active steps to end someone's life is a crime—even if the motive for doing so results from good intentions as an act of mercy.

## Completing an Advance Directive

To make your preferences known about medical treatment to health care providers and others who should be aware of them, it is important to document them through a written **advance directive.** Two forms of advance directives are legally important. First is the **living will,** which enables individuals to provide instructions about the kind of medical care they wish to receive if they become incapacitated or otherwise unable to participate in treatment decisions. The second important form of advance directive is the **health care proxy,** which is also known as a durable power of attorney for health care. This document makes it possible to appoint another person to make decisions about medical treatment if you become unable to do so. The proxy is expected to act in accordance with your wishes as stated in an advance directive or as otherwise made known.

For advance directives to be of value, you must do more than merely complete the paperwork. Discuss your wishes ahead of time with caregivers and family members as well as with your physician. (See Take Action at the end of the chapter for information on obtaining an advance directive form for your state.)

## Becoming an Organ Donor

Each day about 74 people receive an organ transplant while another 17 people on the waiting list die because not enough organs are available. There are currently over 85,000 Americans waiting for organ transplants, including more than 12,000 people under age 35. If you decide to become a donor, the first step is to indicate your wish by completing a **Uniform Donor Card** (Figure 14-3); alternatively, you can indicate your wish on your driver's license. Because relatives are called upon to make decisions about organ and tissue donation at the time of a loved one's death, your second step is to discuss your decision with your family.

## Planning a Funeral or Memorial Service

Just as people gather to commemorate other major transitions in a person's life, such as birth and marriage, funerals

### Terms

VW

**active euthanasia** A deliberate act intended to end another person's life; voluntary active euthanasia involves the practice of a physician administering—at the request of a patient—medication or some other intervention that causes death.

**advance directive** Any statement made by a competent person about his or her choices for medical treatment should he or she become unable to make such decisions or communicate them in the future.

**living will** A type of advance directive that allows individuals to provide instructions about the kind of medical care they wish to receive if they become unable to participate in treatment decisions.

**health care proxy** A type of advance directive that allows an individual to appoint another person as an agent in making health care decisions in the event he or she becomes unable to participate in treatment decisions; also known as a durable power of attorney for health care.

**Uniform Donor Card** A consent form authorizing the use of the signer's body parts for transplantation or medical research upon his or her death.

**embalming** The process of removing blood and other fluids and replacing them with chemicals to disinfect and temporarily retard deterioration of a corpse.

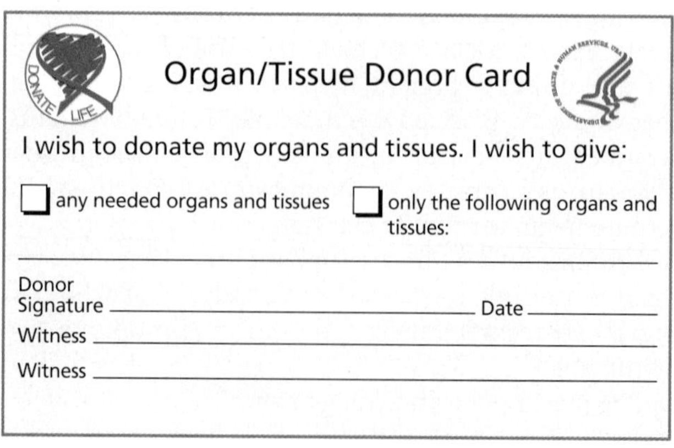

DONATE LIFE

Organ/Tissue Donor Card

I wish to donate my organs and tissues. I wish to give:

☐ any needed organs and tissues ☐ only the following organs and tissues:

Donor Signature ______ Date ______

Witness ______

Witness ______

**Figure 14-3 A sample organ/tissue donor card.** SOURCE: U.S. Department of Health and Human Services (http://www.organdonor.gov/signup1.html; retrieved February 15, 2005).

Take Charge

## Tasks for Survivors

Some of the following tasks must be attended to soon after a death occurs, whereas others take weeks or months to complete. Many of these tasks, especially those that need to be dealt with in the first hours and days following the death, can be taken care of by friends and relatives of the immediate survivors.

- Prepare a list of relatives, close friends, and business colleagues, and arrange to telephone them about the death as soon as possible. Friends can help with the notification process.
- Find out whether the deceased left instructions or made plans for disposition of the body or for a funeral or memorial service.
- If no prior plan exists, contact a mortuary or memorial society for help in making arrangements. Clergy, friends, and other family members can be asked to help decide what is most appropriate.
- If flowers are to be omitted from the funeral or memorial service, choose an appropriate charity or other memorial to which gifts can be made.
- Write the obituary. Include the deceased's age, place of birth, cause of death, occupation, academic degrees, memberships, military service record, accomplishments, names and relationships of nearest survivors, and an announcement of the time and place of the funeral or memorial service.
- Arrange for family members or close friends to take turns welcoming those who come to express their condolences in person and responding to those who telephone their condolences.
- Ask friends to help coordinate the supplying of meals for the first few days following the death, as well as the management of other household tasks and child care, if necessary.
- Arrange hospitality for relatives and friends who are visiting from out of town.
- If a funeral ceremony is planned, choose the individuals who are to be pallbearers, and notify them that you would like their participation.
- Notify the lawyer, accountant, and other personal representatives who will be helping to settle the deceased's estate.
- Send handwritten or printed notes of acknowledgment to the people who have provided assistance or who have sent flowers, contributions, or their condolences.
- With the help of a lawyer or an accountant, review all insurance policies as well as other sources of potential death benefits, such as Social Security, military service, fraternal organizations, and unions.
- Review all debts, mortgages, and installment payments. Some may carry clauses that cancel debt in the event of death. If payments must be delayed, contact creditors to arrange for a grace period.

and memorial services are rites of passage that commemorate a person's life in a community and acknowledge his or her passing from that community. Funerals and memorial services provide a framework that allows survivors to support one another as they cope with the fact of their loss and express their grief.

**Disposition of the Body** People generally have a preference about the final disposition of their body. For most Americans, the choice is either burial or cremation. *Burial* usually involves a grave dug into the soil or entombment in a mausoleum. *Cremation* involves subjecting a body to intense heat. Cremated remains can be buried, placed in a columbarium niche, put into an urn kept by the family or interred in an urn garden, or scattered at sea or on land. A body destined for burial or cremation may or may not be embalmed. If the body is to be viewed during a wake or will be present at the funeral, **embalming** is generally done.

**Arranging a Service** Although it is becoming more common for individuals and families to express a preference for no services, bereaved relatives and friends can derive important benefits from having an opportunity to honor the deceased and express their grief through ceremony. Decisions about your own last rites are ideally made with a view to the needs and wishes of your survivors. Religious and cultural or ethnic traditions play a major role in shaping the way people honor their dead. The diversity of life and death in the United States calls for a diversity of rites. A meaningful funeral or memorial service can be designed in many different ways.

Costs also may influence the choices people make for last rites. The typical cost of a funeral, not including cemetery costs, is about $5000–$7000. Less expensive options for disposal of the body include direct cremation or immediate burial, both of which involve no viewing and no funeral ceremony. Veterans are eligible for burial in a national cemetery, an option that can also reduce costs.

The bottom line is that a wide range of options is available to meet consumers' diverse needs. Making at least some plans ahead of time and discussing the options with family members can help reduce the burden on survivors who find themselves facing a number of decisions once death occurs (see the box "Tasks for Survivors").

## COPING WITH DYING

There is no one right way to live with or die of a life-threatening illness. Every disease has its own set of problems and challenges, and each person copes with these problems and challenges in his or her own way. Living with an illness that is life-threatening and incurable can be described as a "living-dying" experience. Hope and honesty are often delicately balanced—honesty to face reality as it is, hope for a positive outcome. The object of hope changes. The early hope that the symptoms are not really serious gives way to hope that a cure is possible. When the illness is deemed incurable, there is hope for more time. As time begins to run out, one hopes for a pain-free death, a "good death."

### The Tasks of Coping

In her 1969 book *On Death and Dying,* Elisabeth Kübler-Ross suggested that the response to an awareness of imminent death involves five psychological stages: denial, anger, bargaining, depression, and acceptance. The notion that these "five stages" occur in a linear progression has since become a kind of modern myth of how people *ought* to cope with dying. Unfortunately, this can lead to the idea that it is a person's "task" to move sequentially through these stages, one after another, and that if this is not accomplished, the person has somehow failed. In fact, however, Kübler-Ross said that individuals go back and forth among the stages during the course of an illness and different stages can occur simultaneously.

The notion of sequential stages, however, has been deemphasized in favor of highlighting the *tasks* that deserve attention in coping with a life-threatening illness. Charles Corr, for example, distinguishes four primary dimensions in coping with dying:

1. *Physical:* Satisfying bodily needs and minimizing physical distress
2. *Psychological:* Maximizing a sense of security, self-worth, autonomy, and richness in living
3. *Social:* Sustaining significant relationships and addressing the social implications of dying
4. *Spiritual:* Identifying, developing, or reaffirming sources of meaning and fostering hope

Contemplating these dimensions gives us a framework for considering the specific tasks that need to be addressed in coping with dying. However, we must remember that a person's death is as unique as his or her life. Each person's pathway through life-threatening illness is determined by factors such as the specific disease and its course, his or her personality, and the available supportive resources.

People who apparently cope best with life-threatening illness often exhibit a "fighting spirit" that views the illness not only as a threat, but also as a challenge. These people strive to inform themselves about their illness and take an active part in treatment decisions. They are optimistic and have a capacity to discover positive meaning in ordinary events. Holding to a positive outlook despite distressing circumstances involves creating a sense of meaning that is bigger than the threat. In the context of life-threatening illness, this encompasses a person's ability to comprehend the implications an illness has for the future, as well as for his or her ability to accomplish goals, maintain relationships, and sustain a sense of personal vitality, competence, and power.

### Supporting a Dying Person

People often feel uncomfortable in the presence of a person who is close to dying. What can we say? How should we act? It may seem that any attempt to be comforting could result only in words that are little more than stale platitudes. Yet we want to express concern and establish meaningful contact with the person who is facing death. In such circumstances, the most important gift we can bring is that of listening. Offering the dying person opportunities to speak openly and honestly about his or her experience can be crucial, even when such conversation is initially painful.

We tend to place dying people in a special category, but the reality is that their needs are not fundamentally different from anyone else's, although their situation is perhaps more urgent. Dying people need to know that they are valued, that they are not alone, that they are not being unfairly judged, and that those closest to them are also striving to come to terms with a difficult situation. As with any relationship, there are opportunities for growth on both sides.

## COPING WITH LOSS

Even if we have not experienced the death of someone close, we are all survivors of losses that occur in our lives because of changes and endings. The loss of a job, the ending of a relationship, transitions from one school or neighborhood to another—these are examples of the kinds of losses that occur in all our lives. Such losses are sometimes called "little deaths," and, in varying degrees, they all involve grief.

### Experiencing Grief

**Grief** is the reaction to loss. It encompasses thoughts and feelings, as well as physical and behavioral responses. Mental distress may involve disbelief, confusion, anxiety, disorganization, and depression. The emotions that can

Funeral or memorial services give friends and relatives of the deceased the opportunity to mark their grief through ritual and ceremony.

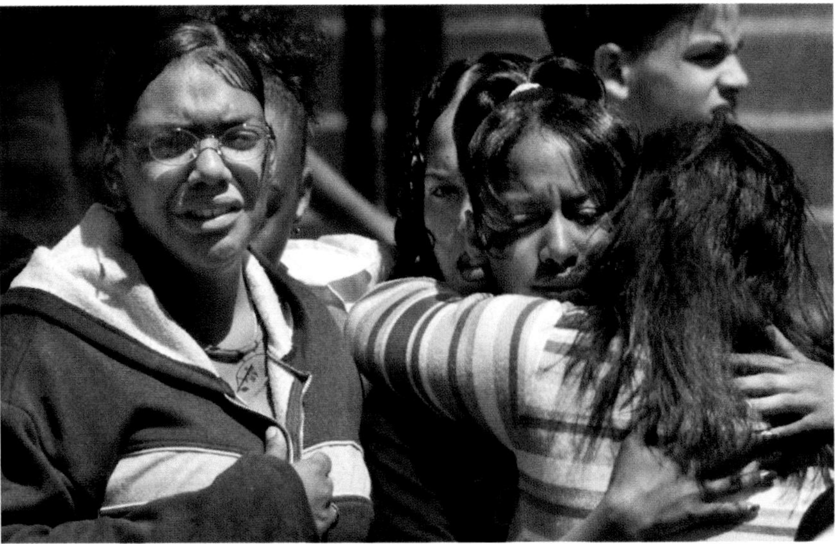

be present in normal grief include not only sorrow and sadness, but also relief, anger, and self-pity, among others. Common behaviors associated with grief include crying, "searching" for the deceased, and talking incessantly about the deceased and the circumstances of the death. Bereaved people may be restless, as if not knowing what to do with themselves. Physically, grief may involve frequent sighing, insomnia, and loss of appetite. Grief may also evoke a reexamination of religious or spiritual beliefs as a person struggles to make meaning of the loss. All such manifestations of grief can be present as part of one's total response to **bereavement**—that is, the event of loss.

**Mourning** is closely related to grief and is often used as a synonym for it. However, mourning refers not so much to the *reaction* to loss but to the *process* by which a bereaved person adjusts to loss and incorporates it into his or her life. How this process is managed is determined, at least partly, by cultural and gender norms for the expression of grief. Considered jointly, grief and mourning are the means to healing the pain of loss.

**Tasks of Mourning** Experiencing grief is part of the process by which a bereaved person integrates a significant loss into his or her life. Psychologist William Worden has identified four tasks that must be attended to:

1. *Accepting the reality* of the loss
2. *Working through the pain* of grief
3. *Adjusting to a changed environment* in which the deceased is absent
4. *Emotionally relocating the deceased and moving on with life*

Accomplishing the fourth task does not mean dishonoring the deceased's memory or denying normal feelings of connection that persist beyond death. Making the journey of grief and attending to the various tasks along the way, we come to a place where we learn how to keep a special place for the deceased in our hearts and memories while moving forward with our lives.

**The Course of Grief** Grieving, like dying, is highly individual. In the first hours or days following a death, a bereaved person is likely to experience overwhelming shock and numbness, as well as a sense of disbelief. Consider the ways in which people die: the aged grandmother, dying quietly in her sleep; the despondent executive who commits suicide; a young soldier killed in battle; the chronically ill person who dies a "lingering death." The cause or mode of death—natural, accidental, homicide, or suicide—has an impact on how grief is experienced. Even when a death is anticipated, grief is not necessarily diminished when the loss becomes real.

The sense of disorganization experienced by survivors during the early period of grief is set against the need to attend to decisions and actions surrounding the disposition of the deceased's body. As family and friends gather to offer mutual support, funeral ceremonies are held. Engaging in such activities promotes accepting the reality of the death and moving beyond the initial shock and numbness.

### Terms

VW

**grief** A person's reaction to loss as manifested physically, emotionally, mentally, and behaviorally.

**bereavement** The objective event of loss.

**mourning** The process whereby a person actively copes with grief in adjusting to a loss and integrating it into his or her life.

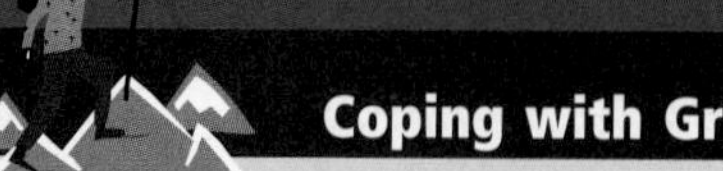

Take Charge

## Coping with Grief

- Recognize and acknowledge the loss.
- React to grief by accepting and expressing it.
- Take time for nature's process of healing.
- Know that powerful, overwhelming feelings will change with time.
- Review and remember the relationship with the deceased.
- Share your pain by accepting support from others.
- Surround yourself with life: plants, animals, friends.
- Make use of mementos to promote your mourning, not to live in the past.
- Avoid major decisions, if possible, and give yourself time to readjust.
- Adapt to a new world without forgetting the old.
- Prepare for change, new interests, new friends, creativity, and growth.
- Reinvest in life.

SOURCES: The Centre for Living with Dying (554 Mansion Park Dr., Santa Clara, CA 95054; 408-980-9801); Rando, T. A. 1993. *The Treatment of Complicated Mourning.* Champaign, Ill.: Research Press.

The middle phase of grief is characterized by anxiety, apathy, and pining for the deceased. The "pangs of grief" are felt as the bereaved person deeply experiences the pain of separation. There is often a sense of despair as a person repeatedly goes over the events surrounding the loss, perhaps fantasizing that somehow everything could be undone and be as it was before. During this period, the bereaved also begins looking toward the future and taking the first steps toward building a life without the deceased.

There is no predetermined timetable for completing this mourning process. The last phase of "active" grief involves coming to a sense of resolution. The acute pain and emotional turmoil of grief subside. Physical and mental balance is reestablished. The bereaved becomes increasingly reintegrated into his or her social world. Sadness doesn't go away completely, but it recedes into the background. Although reminders of the loss stimulate active grieving from time to time, the main focus is the present, not the past. Adjusting to loss may sometimes feel like a betrayal of the deceased loved one, but it is healthy to engage again in ongoing life and the future (see the box "Coping with Grief").

### Supporting a Grieving Person

In experiencing a significant loss, a person initially may feel and behave much like a frightened, helpless child. He or she may respond best to the kind of loving support that is given by a parent. A hug may be more comforting than any words. Also, because talking about a loss is an important way that survivors cope with the changed reality, simply listening can be very helpful. The key to being a good listener is to refrain from making judgments about whether the feelings expressed by a survivor are "right" or "wrong," "good" or "bad."

Funerals and other leave-taking ceremonies generally help survivors gain a sense of closure and begin to integrate a loss into their lives. For some, funerals are occasions of weeping and wailing; for others, stoic and subdued emotions are the rule. Different styles of mourning behavior can be equally valid and appropriate.

Social support is as critical during the later course of grief as it is during the first days after a loss. Besides the support from individuals who are part of their social network, bereaved people may want to share their stories and concerns through organized support groups.

Children tend to cope with loss in a healthier fashion when they are included as part of their family's experience of grief and mourning. In talking about death with children, the most important guideline is to be honest. Set the explanation you are offering at the child's level of understanding. A child's readiness for more details can usually be assessed by paying attention to his or her questions.

## COMING TO TERMS WITH DEATH

We may wish we could keep death out of view and not make a place for it in our lives. But this wish cannot be fulfilled. With the death of a beloved friend or relative, we are confronted with emotions and thoughts that relate not only to the immediate loss but also to our own mortality. Our encounters with dying and death teach us that relationships are more important than things and that life offers no guarantees. In discovering the meaning of death in our own lives, we find that life is both precious and precarious. Allowing ourselves to make room for death, we discover that it touches not only the dying or bereaved person and his or her family and friends, but also the wider community of which we are all part. We recognize that dying and death offer opportunities for extraordinary growth in the midst of loss. Denying death, it turns out, results in denying life.

**Tips for Today**

Cultivating physical and mental wellness in your earlier years can help you both to age gracefully and to develop a healthy attitude toward loss and death. Facing the natural processes of aging and dying, despite your fears and discomfort, can deepen your appreciation of life.

*Right now you can*

- Start a list of the books you'd like to read for pleasure and get one of them from the library or bookstore
- Get in the habit of volunteering by contacting a nonprofit group in your community and offering your time and talent; consider a literacy campaign, a soup kitchen, a youth mentoring program, or Habitat for Humanity
- Review your finances, and determine if you are saving as much as possible toward retirement.
- Think about whether you want to be an organ donor; if you do, look into filling out a donor card (see Take Action at the end of the chapter).
- Consider asking your parents or grandparents what their wishes are for end-of-life care and for funeral arrangements, if you don't already know.

## SUMMARY


- People who take charge of their health during their youth have greater control over the physical and mental aspects of aging.
- Age-proofing strategies include challenging your mind, exercising, eating wisely, maintaining a healthy weight, controlling drinking and medication overuse, avoiding tobacco use, recognizing and reducing stress, and obtaining regular screening tests.
- Retirement can be a fulfilling and enjoyable time of life for those who adjust to their new roles, enjoy participating in a variety of activities, and have planned ahead for financial stability.
- Slight confusion and forgetfulness are not signs of a serious illness; however, severe symptoms may indicate Alzheimer's disease or another form of dementia.
- Resolving grief and mourning and dealing with depression are important tasks for older adults.
- People over 65 form a large minority in the United States, and their status is improving.
- Family and community resources can help older adults stay active and independent.
- Government aid to the elderly includes food stamps, housing subsidies, Social Security, Medicare, and Medicaid.
- Dying and death are more than biological events; they have social and spiritual dimensions.
- The traditional criteria for determining death focus on vital signs such as breathing and heartbeat. Brain death is characterized by a lack of physical responses other than breathing and heartbeat.
- A will is a legal instrument that governs the distribution of a person's estate after death.
- End-of-life care may involve a combination of home care, hospital stays, and hospice or palliative care.
- The practice of withholding or withdrawing potentially life-sustaining treatment is sometimes termed passive euthanasia.
- Physician-assisted suicide occurs when a physician provides lethal drugs or other interventions, at a patient's request, with the understanding that the patient plans to use them to end his or her life.
- Advance directives, such as living wills and health care proxies, are used to express one's wishes about the use of life-sustaining treatment.
- People can donate their bodies or specific organs for transplantation and other medical uses after death.
- Bereaved people usually benefit from participating in a funeral or memorial service to commemorate a loved one's death.
- Coping with dying involves physical, psychological, social, and spiritual dimensions.
- In offering support to a dying person, the gift of listening can be especially important.
- Grief encompasses thoughts and feelings, as well as physical and behavioral responses.
- Mourning, the process by which a person integrates a loss into his or her life, is determined partly by social and cultural norms for expressing grief.


## Take Action

1. **Be a volunteer:** Develop a project that benefits you and a facility for the elderly in your community. For example, teach an older adult how to send an e-mail. Have an older adult teach you how to repair an old faucet or make bread. Organize a group of friends or coworkers to volunteer at a nursing home.

2. **Investigate cultural attitudes about aging:** Interview several people from different cultural backgrounds about their attitudes toward aging and older people. How do they view the aging process? How are elderly people treated or viewed in their culture? What family stories do they have about older members of the family? Do you notice any significant differences between their attitudes and stories and yours?

3. **Consider organ donation:** In most states, the Department of Motor Vehicles provides organ donor forms. You can also request a donor form or download one from the National Kidney Foundation (800-622-9010; http://www.kidney.org), the Coalition on Donation (800-355-7427; http://www.shareyourlife.org), or the Department of Health and Human

Services (http://www.organdonor.gov). When you receive your donor form, consider the advantages and disadvantages of becoming a donor. If you decide to be a donor, fill out the card and keep it with your driver's license. Discuss your decision with members of your family. If your state has an organ donor registry, sign up.

4. **Review an advance directive:** Obtain sample copies of advance directives that are appropriate for the state you live in. Check with your local hospital or health services organization for these forms, or request them from The National Hospice and Palliative Care Organization (800-658-8898; http://www.nhpco.org). Review the forms and consider the advantages and disadvantages of using them. If you decide to execute a living will or health care proxy, discuss your decision with members of your family and anyone else who might become involved in your health care.

5. **Visit a hospice:** Visiting a hospice or speaking with someone who works in a hospice is a good way to learn more about the process of death and dying and how such a setting can support patient and family in making a more peaceful and meaningful death where dignity and connection with loved ones is carefully preserved. To find a hospice close to you, visit the Web site for the National Hospice and Palliative Care Organization (www.nhpco.org). Click on "Find a Provider" and then "Hospice Program." After you enter your zip code, the site will provide contact information for the hospices nearest to you.

## For More Information

### Books


Batuello, J. T. 2003. *End of Life Decisions: A Practical Guide*. College Station, Tx.: Virtualbookworm. *A guide to end-of-life decisions, including those related to pain relief and palliative and hospice care.*

Colby, W. H. 2003. *Long Goodbye: The Deaths of Nancy Cruzan*. Carlsbad, Calif.: Hay House. *A close-up look at a key case that helped define medical and legal issues related to brain death.*

DeSpelder, L. A., and A. L. Strickland. 2005. *The Last Dance: Encountering Death and Dying,* 7th ed. New York: McGraw-Hill. *A comprehensive and readable text highlighting a broad range of topics related to dying and death.*

Lazarus, R. S., and B. N. Lazarus. 2005. *Coping with Aging*. New York: Oxford. *Explores the experience of aging from the standpoint of the individual.*

Vaillant, G. E. 2003. *Aging Well: Surprising Guideposts to a Happier Life from the Landmark Harvard Study of Adult Development*. New York: Little, Brown. *Provides information on quality-of-life issues from three longevity studies that followed people for more than 50 years.*


### WW Organizations and Web Sites

*AARP.* Provides information on all aspects of aging, including health promotion, health care, and retirement planning.
888-OUR-AARP
http://www.aarp.org

*Access America for Seniors.* A gateway to government resources on the Internet for older Americans.
http://www.seniors.gov

*Aging Well.* A practical resource for seniors that includes information on diet, exercise, safety, and medical care.
http://agingwell.state.ny.us

*Alzheimer's Association.* Offers tips for caregivers and patients and information on the causes and treatment of Alzheimer's disease.
800-272-3900
http://www.alz.org

*Arthritis Foundation.* Provides information about arthritis, including free brochures, referrals to local services, and research updates.
800-568-4045
http://www.arthritis.org

*Association for Death Education and Counseling (ADEC).* Provides resources for education, bereavement counseling, and care of the dying.
860-586-7503
http://www.adec.org

*Growth House.* Offers an extensive directory of Internet resources relating to life-threatening illness and end-of-life care.
http://www.growthhouse.org

*Longwood College Library: Doctor Assisted Suicide—A Guide to Web Sites and the Literature.* Information on physician-assisted suicide and links to related sites.
http://web.lwc.edu/administrative/library/suic.htm

*National Funeral Directors Association (NFDA).* Provides resources related to funerals and funeral costs, body disposition, and bereavement support.
800-228-6332
http://www.nfda.org

*National Hospice and Palliative Care Organization (NHPCO).* Provides information about hospice care and advance directives, including online national directory of hospices listed by state and city.
800-658-8898
http://www.nhpco.org

*National Institute on Aging.* Provides fact sheets and brochures on aging-related topics.
http://www.nih.gov/nia

*National Osteoporosis Foundation.* Provides information on the causes, prevention, detection, and treatment of osteoporosis.
http://www.nof.org

*NIH Senior Health.* Provides information on key senior health topics; accessible for people with low vision.
http://nihseniorhealth.gov

*Oregon Department of Health and Humans Services.* Provides information about Oregon's Death with Dignity Act.
http://egov.Oregon.gov/DHS/ph/pas

*U.S. Administration on Aging.* Provides fact sheets, statistical information, and Internet links to other resources on aging.
http://www.aoa.gov

*U.S. Department of Health and Human Services: Organ Donation.* Provides information and forms for organ donation.
http://www.organdonor.gov

# Selected Bibliography


Abbott, R. D., et al. 2004. Walking and dementia in physically capable elderly men. *Journal of the American Medical Association* 292(12): 1447–1453.

Abouna, G. M. 2003. Ethical issues in organ transplantation. *Medical Principles in Practice* 12(1): 54–69.

Americans over 50 at risk for bone fractures. 2005. *FDA Consumer,* January/February.

Anderson, K., et al. 2005. Depression and the risk of Alzheimer's disease. *Epidemiology* 16(2): 233–238.

Angus, D. C., et al. 2004. Use of intensive care at the end of life in the United States: An epidemiologic study. *Critical Care Medicine* 32(3): 638–643.

Annas, G. J. 2005. "Culture of life" politics at the bedside—the case of Terri Schiavo. *New England Journal of Medicine,* epub March 23.

Arthritis Foundation. 2004. *Alternative Therapies: Glucosamine and Chondroitin Sulfate* (http://www.arthritis.org/conditions/alttherapies/Glucosamine.asp; retrieved February 6, 2005).

Byock, I. 2000. Palliative care. In *On Our Own Terms: Moyers on Dying,* ed. Public Affairs Television, 10–11. New York: WNET.

Centers for Disease Control and Prevention. 2005. Racial/ethnic differences in the prevalence and impact of doctor-diagnosed arthritis—United States, 2002. *Morbidity and Mortality Weekly Report* 54(5): 119–123.

Congdon, N., et al. 2004. Causes and prevalence of visual impairment among adults in the United States. *Archives of Ophthalmology* 144(4): 477–485.

Curtis, L. H., et al. 2004. Inappropriate prescribing for elderly Americans in a large outpatient population. *Archives of Internal Medicine* 164(15): 1621–1625.

Kohara, H., et al. 2005. Sedation for terminally ill patients with cancer with uncontrollable physical distress. *Journal of Palliative Medicine* 8(1): 20–25.

Kübler-Ross, E. 1997. *On Death and Dying.* Reprint Edition. New York: Simon & Schuster.

Lanza, R., and N. Rosenthal. 2004. The stem cell challenge. *Scientific American,* June.

Martin, M. J., et al. 2005. Human embryonic stem cells express an immunogenic nonhuman sialic acid. *Nature Medicine* 11(2): 228–232.

National Hospice and Palliative Care Organization. 2004. *Hospice Facts and Figures* (http://www.nhpco.org; retrieved February 15, 2005).

National Institutes of Health. 2004. *Stem Cell Basics* (http://stemcells.nih.gov/info/basics; retrieved February 6, 2005).

Oregon Health Division. 2005. *Seventh Annual Report on Oregon's Death with Dignity Act* (http://egov.oregon.gov/DHS/ph/pas/ar-index.shtml; retrieved April 11, 2005).

Patel, K. 2004. Euthanasia and physician-assisted suicide policy in the Netherlands and Oregon: A comparative analysis. *Journal of Health and Social Policy* 19(1): 37–55.

Quill, T. E. 2005. Terri Schiavo—A tragedy compounded. *New England Journal of Medicine,* epub March 23.

Rosengren, A., et al. 2005. Body mass index, other cardiovascular risk factors, and hospitalization for dementia. *Archives of Internal Medicine* 165(3): 321–326.

Searight, H. R., and J. Gafford. 2005. Cultural diversity at the end of life: Issues and guidelines for family physicians. American Family Physician 71(3): 515–522.

Shadbolt, B., J. Barresi, and P. Craft. 2002. Self-rated health as a predictor of survival among patients with advanced cancer. *Journal of Clinical Oncology* 20(10): 2514–2519.

Speece, M. W., and S. B. Brent. 1996. The development of children's understanding of death. In *Handbook of Childhood Death and Bereavement,* ed. C. A. Corr and D. M. Corr. New York: Springer.

Tsang, W. W., and C. W. Hui-Chan. 2005. Comparison of muscle torque, balance, and confidence in older tai chi and healthy adults. *Medicine and Science in Sports and Exercise* 37(2): 280–289.

U.S. Department of Health and Human Services. 2004. *Bone Health and Osteoporosis: A Report of the Surgeon General.* Washington, D.C.: U.S. Department of Health and Human Services.

Weisman, A. D. 1984. *The Coping Capacity: On the Nature of Being Mortal.* New York: Human Sciences Press.

Wenrich, M. D., et al. 2003. Dying patients' need for emotional support and personalized care from physicians. Perspectives of patients with terminal illness, families, and health care providers. *Journal of Pain and Symptom Management* 25(3): 236–246.

Whitmer, R. A., et al. 2005. Midlife cardiovascular risk factors and risk of dementia in late life. *Neurology* 64(2): 277–281.

Wilson, R. S., et al. 2005. Proneness to psychological distress and risk of Alzheimer disease in a biracial community. *Neurology* 64(2): 380–382.

Yaffe, K., et al. 2004. The metabolic syndrome, inflammation, and risk of cognitive decline. *Journal of the American Medical Association* 292(18): 2237–2242.

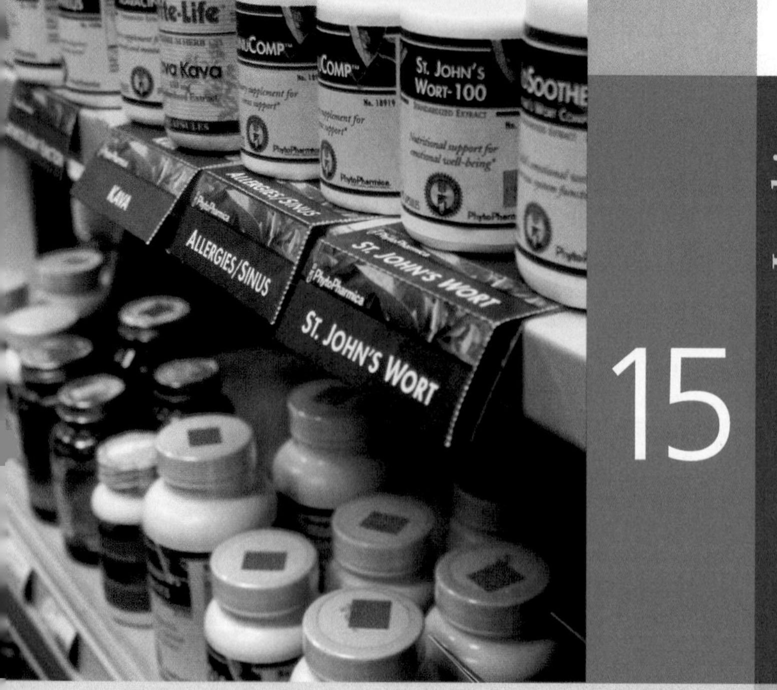


15

## Looking AHEAD

After reading this chapter, you should be able to

- Explain the self-care decision-making process and discuss options for self-treatment
- Describe the basic premises, practices, and providers of conventional medicine
- Describe the basic premises, practices, and providers of complementary and alternative medicine
- Explain how to communicate effectively with a health care provider and to evaluate different forms of treatment
- Discuss different types of health insurance plans

# Conventional and Complementary Medicine: Skills for the Health Care Consumer

Today, people are becoming more confident of their ability to solve personal health problems on their own. People who manage their own health care gather information and learn skills from physicians and other health care providers, friends, classes, books, Web sites, or self-help groups. They solicit opinions and advice, make decisions, and take action. They know how to practice safe, effective self-care, and they know how to make decisions about medical care, whether conventional Western medicine or complementary and alternative medicine. This chapter will help you develop the skills both to identify and manage medical problems and to make the health care system work effectively for you.

## SELF-CARE: MANAGING MEDICAL PROBLEMS

Effectively managing medical problems involves developing several skills. First, you need to learn how to be a good observer of your own body and assess your symptoms. You also must be able to decide when to seek professional advice and when you can safely deal with the problem on your own. You need to know how to safely and effectively self-treat common medical problems. Finally, you need to know how to develop a partnership with physicians and other health care providers and how to carry out treatment plans.

### Self-Assessment

Symptoms are often an expression of the body's attempt to heal itself. For example, a fever may be an attempt to make the body less hospitable to infectious agents, and a cough can help clear the airways. Carefully observing symptoms lets you identify those signals that suggest you need professional assistance. Begin by noting when the symptom began, how often and when it occurs, what makes it worse, what makes it better, and whether you have any associated symptoms. You can also monitor your body's vital signs, such as temperature and heart rate. Medical self-tests for such things as blood pressure, blood sugar, pregnancy detection, and urinary tract infections can also help you make a more informed decision about when to seek medical help and when to self-treat.

## Decision Making: Knowing When to See a Physician

In general, you should check with a physician for symptoms that are described as follows:

1. *Severe.* If the symptom is very severe or intense, medical assistance is advised. Examples include severe pains, major injuries, and other emergencies.
2. *Unusual.* If the symptom is peculiar and unfamiliar, it is wise to check it out with your physician. Examples include unexplained lumps, changes in a mole, problems with vision, difficulty swallowing, numbness, weakness, unexplained weight loss, and blood in sputum, urine, or stool.
3. *Persistent.* If the symptom lasts longer than expected, seek medical advice. Examples in adults include fever for more than 5 days, a cough lasting longer than 2 weeks, a sore that doesn't heal within a month, and hoarseness lasting longer than 3 weeks.
4. *Recurrent.* If a symptom tends to return again and again, medical evaluation is advised. Examples include recurrent headaches, stomach pains, and backache.

Sometimes a single symptom is not a cause for concern, but when the symptom is accompanied by other symptoms, the combination suggests a more serious problem. For example, a fever with a stiff neck suggests meningitis. If you think that you need professional help, you must decide how urgent the problem is. If it is a true emergency, you should go (or call someone to take you) to the nearest emergency room (ER). Emergencies include

- Major trauma or injury, such as head injury, suspected broken bone, deep wound, severe burn, eye injury, or animal bite
- Uncontrollable bleeding or internal bleeding, as indicated by blood in the sputum, vomit, or stool
- Intolerable and uncontrollable pain or severe chest pain
- Severe shortness of breath
- Persistent abdominal pain, especially if associated with nausea and vomiting
- Poisoning or drug overdose
- Loss of consciousness or seizure
- Stupor, drowsiness, or disorientation that cannot be explained
- Severe or worsening reaction to an insect bite or sting or to a medication, especially if breathing is difficult

If your problem is not an emergency but still requires medical attention, call your physician's office. Often you can be given medical advice over the phone without the inconvenience of a visit.

## Self-Treatment: Many Options

In most cases, your body itself can relieve your symptoms and heal the disorder. Patience and careful self-observation are often the best choices in self-treatment. Nondrug options are also often easy, inexpensive, safe, and highly effective. For example, massage, ice packs, and neck exercises may at times be more helpful than drugs in relieving headaches and other pains. Getting adequate rest, increasing exercise, drinking more water, eating more or less of certain foods, using humidifiers, changes in ergonomics when working at a desk, and so on are just some of the hundreds of nondrug options for preventing or relieving many common health problems. For a variety of disorders caused or aggravated by stress, the treatment of choice may be relaxation, visualization, humor, assertive communication, changing negative thoughts, or other stress-management strategies.

If these strategies aren't enough, you may decide to treat yourself with nonprescription or **over-the-counter (OTC) medications.** These are medicines that the Food and Drug Administration (FDA) has determined are safe for use without a physician's prescription. There are more than 100,000 OTC drugs on the market. About 60% of all medications are sold over the counter, and more than 600 products sold over the counter today use ingredients or dosage strengths available only by prescription 20 years ago.

Although many OTC products are effective, others are unnecessary or divert attention from better ways of coping. Many ingredients in OTC drugs—perhaps 70%—have not been proven to be effective. And any drug may have risks and side effects. Follow these simple guidelines to self-medicate safely:

1. Always read labels, and follow directions carefully. The information on most OTC drug labels now appears in a standard format developed by the FDA (Figure 15-1).

2. Do not exceed the recommended dosage or length of treatment unless you discuss it with your physician.

3. Use caution if you are taking other medications or supplements, because OTC and prescription drugs and herbs can interact. If you have questions about drug interactions, ask your physician or pharmacist *before* you mix medicines.

### Term

**over-the-counter (OTC) medication** A medication or product that can be purchased by the consumer without a prescription.

Vw

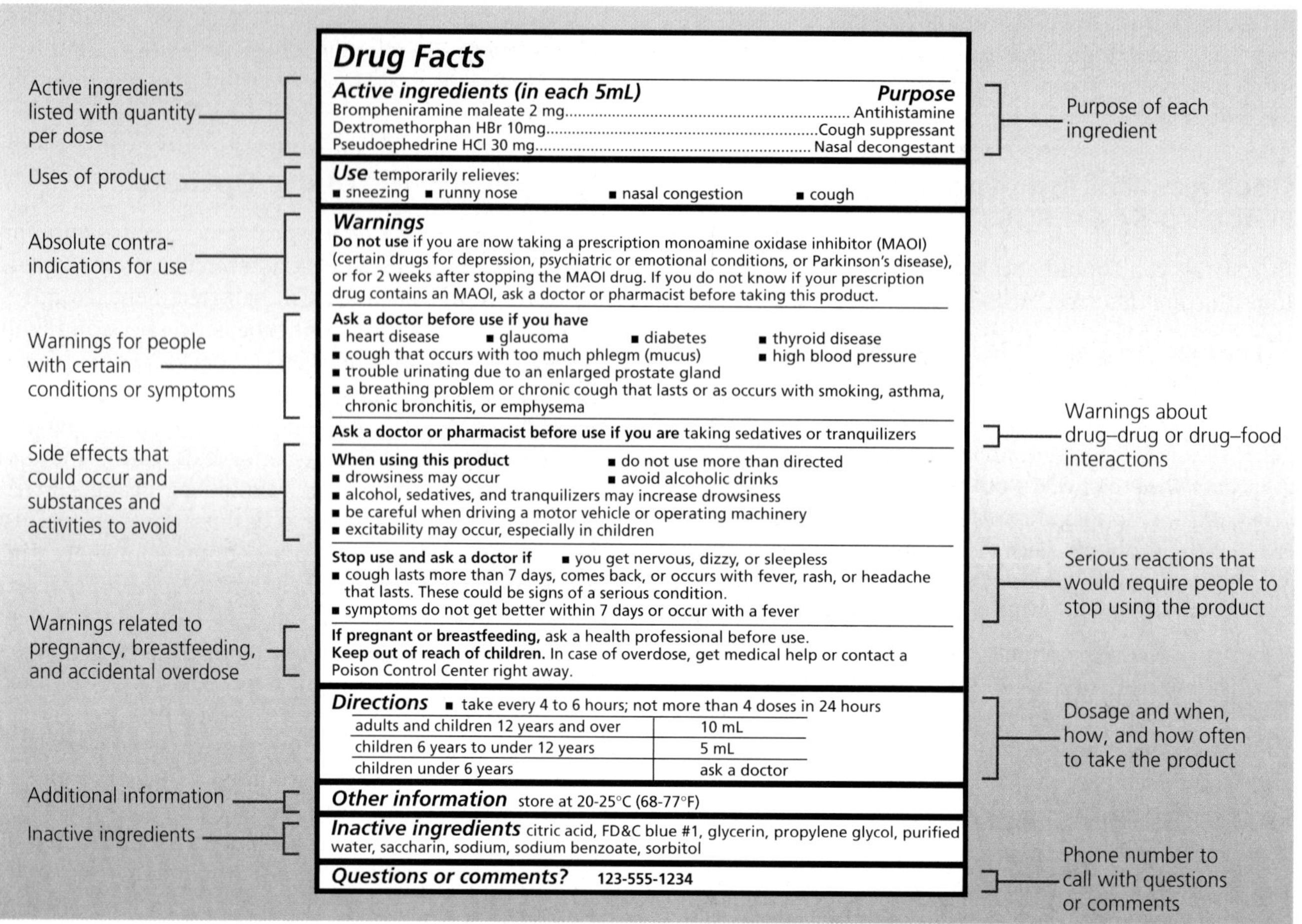


**Figure 15-1 Reading and understanding OTC drug labels.** SOURCE: Food and Drug Administration. 1999. Over-the-counter human drugs; labeling requirements; final rule. *Federal Register* 64, no. 51(17 March): 13254–13303.

4. Try to select medications with one active ingredient rather than combination ("all-in-one") products. A product with multiple ingredients is likely to include drugs for symptoms you don't even have.

5. When choosing medications, try to buy **generic drugs,** which contain the same active ingredient as the brand-name product but generally at a much lower cost.

6. Never use a drug from an unlabeled container or in the dark when you can't read what the label says.

7. If you are pregnant or nursing or have a chronic condition such as kidney disease, consult your physician before self-medicating.

8. The expiration date marked on many medications is an estimate of how long the *unopened* medication is likely to be potent. Once the package is opened, the medication will probably be potent for about a year if stored properly. Mark the date on the package when you open it, and dispose of it safely after a year by taking it to a pharmacy or hospital.

9. Store your medications in a cool, dry place—not the medicine cabinet in your bathroom—that is out of the reach of children.

10. Use special caution with aspirin. Because of an association with a rare but serious problem known as Reye's syndrome, aspirin should not be used by children or adolescents who may have the flu, chicken pox, or any other viral illness.

Only a few basic supplies are really needed in your home medicine cabinet; they include such items as adhesive bandages and antibacterial ointment for minor wounds; a thermometer for taking your temperature; ibuprofen, aspirin, or similar drugs for minor pain or fever; antihistamines for allergies; antacids for heartburn and indigestion; hydrocortisone cream for skin irritations; lozenges for sore throat; needle-nosed tweezers for splinters; elastic bandages, ice packs, and heating pads for sprains and strains; cough syrup for coughs; decongestant for nasal congestion; and sunscreen to prevent sunburn. Additional items depend on the particular health problems you or your family is likely to have.

## PROFESSIONAL MEDICAL AND HEALTH CARE: CHOICES AND CHANGE

When self-treatment is not appropriate or sufficient, you need to seek professional medical care, whether by going to a hospital emergency room, by scheduling an appointment with your physician, or by accessing some other part of the American medical and health care system. This system is a broad network of individuals and organizations, including independent practitioners, allied health care providers, hospitals, clinics, and public and private insurance programs.

In recent years, many Americans have also sought health care from practitioners of **complementary and alternative medicine (CAM),** defined as those therapies and practices that do not form part of conventional, or "mainstream," health care and medical practices as taught in most U.S. medical schools and offered in most U.S. hospitals. The most commonly used CAM therapies are relaxation techniques, herbal medicine, massage, and chiropractic (Table 15-1). People often use CAM therapies in addition to their conventional medical treatments, but many do not tell their physicians about it.

VITAL STATISTICS

**Table 15-1** Use of Complementary and Alternative Therapies in the United States

| | Percent Who Ever Used Therapy |
|---|---|
| Prayer | 55.3 |
| Natural products (nonvitamin, nonmineral) | 25.0 |
| Chiropractic care | 19.9 |
| Deep breathing exercises | 14.6 |
| Meditation | 10.2 |
| Massage | 9.3 |
| Yoga | 7.5 |
| Diet-based therapies | 6.8 |
| Progressive relaxation | 4.2 |
| Acupuncture | 4.0 |
| Megavitamin therapy | 3.9 |
| Homeopathic treatment | 3.6 |
| Guided imagery | 3.0 |
| Tai chi | 2.5 |
| Hypnosis | 1.8 |
| Energy healing therapy/Reiki | 1.1 |
| Biofeedback | 1.0 |
| **Any therapy** | **74.6** |

SOURCE: Barnes, P. M., et al. 2004. Complementary and alternative medicine use among adults: United States, 2002. *Advance Data from Vital and Health Statistics* No. 343. Hyattsville, Md.: National Center for Health Statistics.

Consumers turn to CAM for a large variety of purposes related to health and well-being, such as boosting their immune system, lowering their cholesterol levels, losing weight, quitting smoking, or enhancing their memory. There are indications that people with chronic conditions, including cancer, asthma, autoimmune diseases, and HIV infection, are particularly likely to try CAM therapies. Despite their growing popularity, many CAM practices remain controversial, and individuals need to be critically aware of safety issues. In the next sections of this chapter, we examine the principles and providers of both **conventional medicine**—the dominant medical system in the United States and Europe, also referred to as standard Western medicine or biomedicine—and of complementary and alternative medicine, with particular attention to consumer issues.

## CONVENTIONAL MEDICINE

Referring to conventional medicine as "standard Western medicine" draws attention to the fact that it differs from the various medical systems that have developed in China, Japan, India, and other parts of the world. Calling it "biomedicine" reflects conventional medicine's basis in the findings of a variety of biological sciences.

### Premises and Assumptions of Conventional Medicine

One of the important characteristics of Western medicine is the belief that disease is caused by identifiable physical factors. This belief can be traced back to Hippocrates, the Greek physician of the fourth century B.C. who is credited with placing the practice of medicine on a scientific footing. In Hippocrates' time, the causes of disease were thought to include the interplay of various forces and elements; today, Western medicine identifies the causes of disease as pathogens, such as bacteria and viruses, genetic factors, and unhealthy lifestyles that result in changes at the molecular and

**Terms**

**generic drug** A drug that is not registered or protected by a trademark; a drug that does not have a brand name.

**complementary and alternative medicine (CAM)** Therapies or practices that are not part of conventional or mainstream health care and medical practice as taught in most U.S. medical schools and available at most U.S. health care facilities; examples of CAM practices include acupuncture and herbal remedies.

**conventional medicine** A system of medicine based on the application of the scientific method; diseases are thought to be caused by identifiable physical factors and characterized by a representative set of symptoms; also called *biomedicine* or *standard Western medicine*.

cellular levels. In most cases, however, the focus is primarily on the physical causes of the illness rather than mental or spiritual imbalance.

Another feature that distinguishes Western biomedicine from other medical systems is the concept that every disease is defined by a certain set of symptoms and that these symptoms are similar in most patients suffering from this disease. Western medicine tends to treat illness as an isolated biological disturbance that can occur in any human being, rather than as integral in some way to the individual with the illness.

Related to the idea of illness as the result of invasion by outside factors is the strong orientation toward methods of destroying pathogens or preventing them from causing serious infection. The public health measures of the nineteenth and twentieth centuries—chlorination of drinking water, sewage disposal, food safety regulations, vaccination programs, education about hygiene, and so on—are an outgrowth of this kind of orientation. (As described in Chapter 1, these public health measures are largely responsible for the 25-year increase in life expectancy that Americans have experienced in the twentieth century.)

The implementation of public health measures is one way to control pathogens; another is the use of drugs. The discovery and development of sulfa drugs, antibiotics, and steroids in the twentieth century, along with advances in chemistry that made it possible to identify the active ingredients in common herbal remedies, paved the way for the current close identification of Western medicine with **pharmaceuticals** (medical drugs, both prescription and over-the-counter). Western medicine also relies heavily on surgery and on advanced medical technology to discover the physical causes of disease and to remove or destroy them.

Finally, Western medicine is based on scientific ways of obtaining knowledge and explaining phenomena. Scientific explanations have a blend of characteristics that set them apart from other types of explanation, such as those based on common sense, faith, belief, or authority. Scientific explanations are

- *Empirical*—they are based on the evidence of the senses and on objective and systematic observation, often carried out under carefully controlled conditions; they must be capable of verification by others.
- *Rational*—they follow the rules of logic and are consistent with known facts.
- *Testable*—either they are verifiable through direct observation or they lead to predictions about what should occur under conditions not yet observed.
- *Parsimonious*—they explain phenomena with the fewest number of assumptions.
- *General*—they have broad explanatory power.

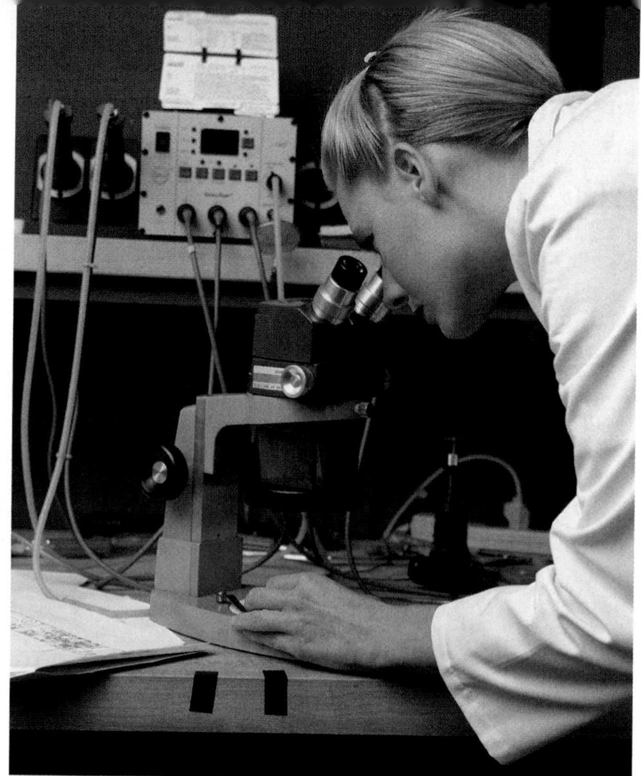

Conventional Western medicine is firmly grounded in scientific explanations resulting from the application of the scientific method to a question or problem. The identification of bacteria and other microorganisms as a key cause of disease led to many public health measures and treatments that reduced U.S. deaths from infectious diseases.

- *Rigorously evaluated*—they are constantly evaluated for consistency with the evidence and known principles, for parsimony, and for generality.
- *Tentative*—scientists are willing to entertain the possibility that their explanations are faulty.

Western medicine translates the scientific method into practice through the research process, a highly refined and well-established approach to exploring the causes of disease and ensuring the safety and efficacy of treatments. Research studies range from case studies—descriptions of a single patient's illness and treatment—to clinical trials conducted on large populations and carried out under carefully controlled conditions over a period of many years. The process of drug development is equally rigorous. Drugs are developed and tested through an elaborate course that begins with preliminary research in the lab and continues through trials with human participants, review and approval by the FDA, and monitoring of the drug's effects after it is on the market. The process may take 12 years or more, and only about 20% of drugs are eventually approved.

When results of research studies are published in medical journals, a community of scientists, physicians, researchers, and scholars has the opportunity to share the findings and enter a dialogue about the subject. Publication of research often prompts further research designed to replicate and confirm the findings, challenge the conclusions, or pursue a related line of thought or experiment. (For guidelines on how to interpret research when it is reported in the popular press, see the box "Evaluating Health News" on p. 376.)

## The Providers of Conventional Medicine

Conventional medicine is practiced by a wide range of health care professionals in the United States. Several kinds of professionals are permitted to practice medicine independently, including medical doctors, osteopaths, podiatrists, optometrists, and dentists.

- **Medical doctors** are practitioners who hold a doctor of medicine (M.D.) degree from an accredited medical school. In the United States, an education in medicine has several stages: 4 years of premedical education in a college or university, with an emphasis on the sciences; 4 years of medical school, which teaches basic medical skills and awards the M.D. degree; graduate medical study, called a residency and lasting from 3 to 8 years, during which a specialty is chosen and studied and a medical license is obtained; and continuing medical education to keep abreast of advances in medical science. Twenty-four medical specialties are currently approved by the American Board of Medical Specialties, each with its own rule-making and certifying body. The larger specialties are further divided into subspecialties; for example, internal medicine includes subspecialties such as cardiology and gastroenterology. Visit the Web site for the American Board of Medical Specialties (www.abms.org) for a complete list. Becoming a subspecialist generally requires several more years of formal training after the completion of a residency.
- **Doctors of osteopathic medicine** (D.O.) are graduates of osteopathic medical schools, which place special emphasis on musculoskeletal problems and manipulative therapy. M.D.s and D.O.s are the two types of "complete" physicians in the United States, meaning they are trained and licensed to perform surgery and prescribe medication.
- **Podiatrists** are practitioners who specialize in the medical and surgical care of the feet. They hold a doctor of podiatric medicine (D.P.M.) degree.
- **Optometrists** are practitioners trained to examine the eyes, detect eye diseases, and treat vision problems. They hold a doctor of optometry (O.D.) degree.
- **Dentists** specialize in the care of the teeth and mouth. They are graduates of 4-year dental schools and hold the doctor of dental surgery (D.D.S.) or doctor of medical dentistry (D.M.D.) degree.

In addition to these practitioners, there are millions of other trained health care professionals, known as **allied health care providers,** working in the United States. Some of them are licensed to work independently; others are permitted to work under medical supervision or medical referral. They include registered nurses (R.N.s), licensed vocational nurses (L.V.N.s), physical therapists, social workers, registered dietitians (R.D.s), physician assistants (P.A.s), nurse practitioners, and certified nurse midwives.

## Choosing a Primary Care Physician

Most experts believe it is best to have a primary care physician, someone who gets to know you, who coordinates your medical care, and who refers you to specialists when you need them. Primary care physicians include those certified in family practice, internal medicine, pediatrics, and obstetrics-gynecology. These physicians are able to diagnose and treat the vast majority of common health problems; they also provide many preventive health services. The best time to look for a physician is before you are sick.

To select a physician, begin by making a list of possible choices. If your insurance limits the health care providers you can see, check the plan's list first. Ask for recommendations from family, friends, coworkers, local medical societies, and the physician referral service at a local clinic or hospital. Once you have the names of a few physicians you might want to try, call their offices to find out information such as the following:

- Is the physician covered by your health plan and accepting new patients?
- What are the office hours, and when is the physician or office staff available? What do patients do if they need urgent care or have an emergency?

### Terms

Vw

**pharmaceuticals** Medical drugs, both prescription and over-the-counter.

**medical doctor** An independent practitioner who holds a doctor of medicine degree from an accredited medical school.

**doctor of osteopathic medicine** A medical practitioner who has graduated from an osteopathic medical school; osteopathy incorporates the theories and practices of scientific medicine but focuses on musculoskeletal problems and manipulative therapy.

**podiatrist** A practitioner who holds a doctor of podiatric medicine degree and specializes in the medical and surgical care of the feet.

**optometrist** A practitioner who holds a doctor of optometry degree and is trained to examine the eyes, detect eye diseases, and prescribe corrective lenses.

**dentist** A practitioner who holds a doctor of medical dentistry or doctor of dental surgery degree and who specializes in the prevention and treatment of diseases and injuries of the teeth, mouth, and jaws.

**allied health care providers** Health care professionals who typically provide services under the supervision or control of independent practitioners.

## Evaluating Health News



Health-related research is now described in popular newspapers and magazines rather than just medical journals, meaning that more and more people have access to the information. Greater access is certainly a plus, but news reports of research studies may oversimplify or exaggerate both the results and what those results mean to the average person. Researchers do not set out to mislead people, but they must often strike a balance between reporting promising preliminary findings to the public, thereby allowing people to act on them, and waiting 10–20 years until long-term studies confirm (or disprove) a particular theory.

All this can leave you in a difficult position. You cannot become an expert on all subjects, capable of effectively evaluating all the available health news. However, the following questions can help you better assess the health advice that appears in the popular media:

1. *Is the report based on research or on an anecdote?* Information or advice based on one or more carefully designed research studies has more validity than one person's experiences.

2. *What is the source of the information?* A study published in a respected peer-reviewed journal has been examined by editors and other researchers in the field, people who are in a position to evaluate the merits of a study and its results. Many journal articles also include information on the authors and funders of research, alerting readers to any possible conflicts of interest. Research presented at medical meetings should be considered very preliminary because the results have not yet undergone a thorough prepublication review; many such studies are never published. It is also wise to ask who funded a study to determine whether there is any potential for bias. Information from government agencies and national research organizations is usually considered fairly reliable.

3. *How big was the study?* A study that involves many subjects is more likely to yield reliable results than a study involving only a few people. Another important indication that a finding is meaningful is if several different studies yield the same results.

4. *Who were the participants involved in the study?* Research findings are more likely to apply to you if you share important characteristics with the participants of the study. For example, the results of a study on men over age 50 who smoke may not be particularly meaningful for a 30-year-old nonsmoking woman. Even less applicable are studies done in test tubes or on animals. Such research should be considered very preliminary in terms of its applicability to humans. Promising results from laboratory or animal research frequently cannot be replicated in human study subjects.

5. *What kind of study was it?* Epidemiological studies involve observation or interviews in order to trace the relationship among lifestyle, physical characteristics, and diseases. While epidemiological studies can suggest links, they cannot establish cause-and-effect relationships. Clinical or interventional studies or trials involve testing the effects of different treatments on groups of people who have similar lifestyles and characteristics. They are more likely to provide conclusive evidence of a cause-and-effect relationship. The best interventional studies share the following characteristics:

- *Controlled.* A group of people who receive the treatment is compared with a matched group of people who do not receive the treatment.
- *Randomized.* The treatment and control groups are selected randomly.
- *Double-blind.* Researchers and participants are unaware of who is receiving the treatment.
- *Multicenter.* The experiment is performed at more than one institution.

A third type of study, meta-analysis, involves combining the results of individual studies to get an overall view of the effectiveness of a treatment.

6. *What do the statistics really say?* First, are the results described as "statistically significant"? If a study is large and well designed, its results can be deemed statistically significant, meaning there is less than a 5% chance that the findings resulted from chance. Second, are the results stated in terms of relative or absolute risk? Many findings are reported in terms of relative risk—how a particular treatment or condition affects a person's disease risk. Consider the following examples of relative risk:

- According to some estimates, taking estrogen without progesterone can increase a postmenopausal woman's risk of dying from endometrial cancer by 233%.
- Giving AZT to HIV-infected pregnant women reduces prenatal transmission of HIV by about 90%.

The first of these two findings seems far more dramatic than the second—until one also considers absolute risk, the actual risk of the illness in the population being considered. The absolute risk of endometrial cancer is 0.3%; a 233% increase based on the effects of estrogen raises it to 1%, a change of 0.7%. Without treatment, about 25% of infants born to HIV-infected women will be infected with HIV; with treatment, the absolute risk drops to about 2%, a change of 23%. Because the absolute risk of an HIV-infected mother passing the virus to her infant is so much greater than a woman's risk of developing endometrial cancer (25% compared with 0.3%), a smaller change in relative risk translates into a much greater change in absolute risk.

7. *Is new health advice being offered?* If the media report new guidelines for health behavior or medical treatment, examine the source. Government agencies and national research foundations usually consider a great deal of evidence before offering health advice. Above all, use common sense, and check with your physician before making a major change in your health habits based on news reports.

SOURCES: Woloshin, S., and L. M. Schwartz. 2002. Press releases: Translating research into news. *Journal of the American Medical Association* 287(21): 2856–2858; Medicine and the media. 1999. *Harvard Women's Health Watch,* February; Medical hype: How to read between the lines. 1998. *Consumer Reports on Health,* October; Making sense of health research. 1998. *Healthline,* May.

- Which hospitals does the physician use?
- How many other physicians are available to "cover" when he or she isn't available, and who are they?
- How long does it usually take to get a routine appointment?
- Does the office send reminders about preventive tests such as Pap tests?
- Does the physician (or a nurse or physician assistant) give advice over the phone for common problems?

Finally, schedule a visit with the physician you think you would most like to use. During that first visit, you'll get a sense of how well matched you are and how well he or she might meet your medical needs. After the visit, consider whether you felt comfortable with the physician, felt listened to and respected, and understood what you were told. Although you may want to give the relationship some time to develop, you should trust your own reactions when deciding whether a particular health care provider is the right one for you.

## Getting the Most Out of Your Medical Care

The key to making the health care system work for you lies in good communication with your physician and other members of the health care team. Studies show that patients who are more active in interacting with physicians and ask more questions enjoy better health outcomes.

**The Physician-Patient Partnership** The physician-patient relationship is undergoing an important transformation. The image of the all-knowing physician and the passive patient is slowly fading. What is emerging is more of a physician-patient *partnership,* in which the physician acts more like a consultant and the patient participates more actively. You should expect your physician to be attentive, caring, and able to listen and clearly explain things to you. You also must do your part. You need to be assertive in a firm but not aggressive manner. You need to express your feelings and concerns, ask questions, and, if necessary, be persistent. If your physician is unable to communicate clearly with you despite your best efforts, you probably need to change physicians.

When you have an appointment, make a written list of your key concerns and questions, along with notes about your symptoms. Present your concerns at the beginning of the visit, to set the agenda. Be specific and concise about your symptoms, and be open and honest about your concerns. Let your physician know if you are taking any drugs, are allergic to any medications, are breastfeeding, or may be pregnant. At the end of the visit, briefly repeat the physician's diagnosis, prognosis, and instructions, and make sure you understand your next steps.

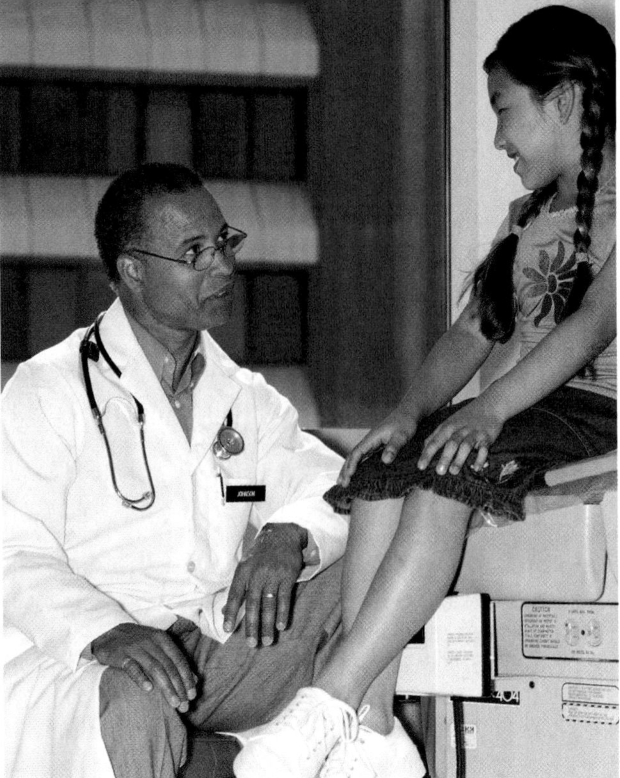

Good communication is a crucial factor in an effective physician-patient partnership.

**The Diagnostic Process** A key part of your appointment is the medical history, which includes your primary reason for the visit, your current symptoms, your past medical history, and your social history (job, family life, major stressors, living conditions, and health habits). Keeping up-to-date records of your medical history can help you provide your physician with key facts about your health.

The next step is the physical exam, which usually begins with a review of vital signs: blood pressure, heart rate (pulse), breathing rate, and temperature. Depending on your primary complaint, your physician may give you a complete physical, or the exam may be directed to specific areas, such as your ears, nose, and throat.

Finally, your physician may order medical tests to complete the diagnosis. Physicians can order X rays, biopsies, blood and urine tests, scans of various types, and a wide array of **endoscopies** to view, probe, or analyze almost any part of the body. If your physician orders a test for you, be sure you know why you need it, what the

**Term**

**endoscopy** A medical procedure in which a viewing instrument is inserted into a body cavity or opening. Specific procedures are named for the area viewed: inside joints (arthroscopy), inside airways (bronchoscopy), inside the abdominal cavity (laparoscopy), and inside the lower portion of the large intestine, or sigmoid colon (sigmoidoscopy).

risks and benefits of the test are for you, how you should prepare for it (for example, by fasting or discontinuing medications or herbal remedies), and what the test will involve. Also ask what the test results mean, because no test is 100% accurate—**false positives** and **false negatives** do occur—and interpretation of some tests is subjective.

**Medical and Surgical Treatments** Once the diagnosis is made, you and your physician can consider treatment options. Many conditions can be treated in a variety of ways; in some cases, lifestyle changes should be considered along with other options.

**PRESCRIPTION MEDICATIONS** Thousands of lives are saved each year by **antibiotics,** heart medications, insulin, and scores of other drugs, but we pay a price for having such powerful tools. A report from the Institute of Medicine (IOM) estimated that preventable medication errors result in more than 7000 deaths each year in hospitals alone, with tens of thousands more in outpatient facilities. Problems and issues related to prescription drug use include the following:

- **Medication errors:** Physicians may overprescribe drugs, sometimes in response to pressure by patients (see the box "Prescription Drug Use and Regulation: Lessons from Vioxx"). Adverse effects can occur if a physician prescribes the wrong drug or a dangerous combination of drugs; such problems are especially prevalent for older adults, who typically take more medications. At the pharmacy, patients may receive the wrong drug or may not be given complete information about drug risks, side effects, and interactions.
- **Off-label drug use:** Once a drug is approved by the FDA for one purpose, it can legally be prescribed (although not marketed) for purposes not listed on the label. Many off-label uses are safe and supported by some research, but both consumers and health care providers need to take special care with off-label use of medications.
- **Online pharmacies:** Although convenient, some online pharmacies may sell products or engage in practices that are illegal in the offline world, putting consumers at risk for receiving adulterated, expired, or counterfeit drugs. The FDA recommends that consumers avoid sites that prescribe drugs for the first time without a physical exam, sell prescription drugs without a prescription, or sell drugs not approved by the FDA. You should also avoid sites that do not provide access to a registered pharmacist to answer questions or that do not provide a U.S. address and phone number to contact if there's a problem. The National Association of Boards of Pharmacy sponsors a voluntary certification program for Internet pharmacies. To be certified, a pharmacy must have a state license and allow regular inspections.
- **Costs:** Spending on prescription drugs is rising faster than the rate of inflation and is now the fastest-growing portion of U.S. health care spending. Consumers may be able to lower their drug costs by using generic versions of medications; by joining a drug discount program sponsored by a company, organization, or local pharmacy; and by investigating mail-order or Internet pharmacies.

### Terms

**false positive** A test result that incorrectly detects a disease or condition in a healthy person.

**false negative** A test result that fails to correctly detect a disease or condition.

**antibiotic** A substance derived from a mold or bacterium that inhibits the growth of other microorganisms.

Patients also share some responsibility for problems with prescription drugs. Many people don't take their medications properly, skipping doses, taking incorrect doses, stopping too soon, or not taking the medication at all. An estimated 30–50% of the more than 3 billion prescriptions dispensed annually in the United States are not taken correctly and thus do not produce the desired results. Consumers can increase the safety and effectiveness of their treatment by asking the following questions:

- *Do I really need this prescription, or are there non-drug alternatives?*
- *What is the name of the medication, and what is it supposed to do, within what period of time?*
- *How and when do I take the medication, how much do I take, and for how long? What should I do if I miss a dose?*
- *What other medications, foods, drinks, or activities should I avoid?* Other drugs, including alcohol, herbs, and OTC drugs, can interact with medications, diminishing or increasing their effect. For example, certain antibiotics, including ampicillin and tetracycline, may prevent oral contraceptives from working. Others may increase the effects of sunlight on the skin.
- *What are the side effects, and what do I do if they occur?*
- *Can I take a generic drug rather than a brand-name one?* Generic drugs contain the same active ingredients as the original brand-name drug, but they may contain different inactive ingredients. They are usually substantially less expensive, but sometimes physicians have reasons for preferring a particular brand.
- *Is there written information about the medication?* There are many sources of information, including the FDA-approved inserts in drug packaging and books.

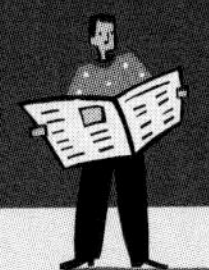

## Prescription Drug Use and Regulation: Lessons from Vioxx

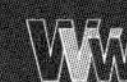

In February 2005, the FDA announced plans for changes designed to enhance its oversight of prescription drugs. Pressure on the agency had been growing following several high-profile problems with approved drugs. These cases included the risk of suicide associated with use of certain antidepressants among children and teenagers (see Chapter 3), and, more recently, the risk of heart problems among people taking certain anti-inflammatory drugs for arthritis.

### The Vioxx Story in Brief

Many people with arthritis take medications to reduce pain and inflammation. Traditional nonsteroidal anti-inflammatory drugs (NSAIDs) like aspirin and ibuprofen are effective, but they carry the risk of stomach irritation and even ulcers—especially if taken over long periods, as is common for a chronic condition like arthritis. Newer NSAIDs known as COX-2 inhibitors are designed to reduce pain and inflammation while causing less stomach irritation. COX-2 inhibitors include Vioxx (rofecoxib), Celebrex (celecoxib), and Bextra (valdecoxib).

Vioxx, approved in 1999, was heavily advertised and widely used. As early as 2000, studies began to find increased rates of cardiovascular problems among Vioxx users. Results of a large-scale study in 2004 found that Vioxx users were more likely to suffer a heart attack or sudden cardiac death than people using Celebrex or older NSAIDs. In response to this study, Vioxx was removed from the market. (Due to risks related to CVD and a serious skin condition, Bextra was pulled from the market in April 2005.)

The rise and fall of Vioxx has inspired debate on a number of issues relating to how drugs are marketed, prescribed, and regulated. Why weren't the risks identified before the drug was approved? Why didn't the FDA act earlier? Should such widespread drug marketing be allowed?

### New Drugs and Postapproval Monitoring

Although pharmaceutical companies carry out extensive preapproval trials on new drugs, even the most extensive studies involve just a few thousand people. A large natural experiment begins when the drug is approved and physicians start prescribing it to people in the general population. Side effects and risks that did not show up in studies often become apparent when more people begin taking a drug. Problems can also develop when certain drugs are used in combination with other drugs or dietary supplements.

Preapproval studies may exclude certain groups for safety reasons. For example, initial studies of Vioxx did not include people with preexisting heart conditions, who may have been more at risk for the problems identified after the drug was approved. In addition, the increased risk from Vioxx did not show up until people had been taking the drug for at least 18 months—a longer period than most preapproval drug studies.

Part of the FDA's 2005 proposal is for greater postapproval surveillance, including an independent review board and a Web site with emerging drug safety data accessible to both consumers and physicians. Consumers should be especially alert for adverse effects if they are taking a drug that is new to the market. Consider older, more widely used drugs first.

### Direct-to-Consumer Advertising

The pharmaceutical industry spends up to 20% of its marketing budget on direct-to-consumer (DTC) advertising, which has grown rapidly since 1995. Most of these ads are for a small number of the most popular drugs.

Proponents of DTC advertising claim that it enhances public health by providing educational information about underdiagnosed conditions such as diabetes, high cholesterol, and depression and by motivating people to seek care. DTC advertising may be particularly useful in getting health information to people who have no regular source of health care. It may also provide patients with an opportunity to discuss medical conditions that they might otherwise be hesitant to bring up, such as depression.

Opponents claim that DTC advertising is more promotional than educational, is misleading and omits important precautions, is designed to create consumer demand by creating problems and needs, and causes patients to pressure physicians to prescribe particular drugs. One recent study found that most DTC ads fail to provide information about how a drug works, its success rate, how long it must be taken, alternative treatments, or helpful lifestyle changes.

There is also concern that DTC advertising leads patients to request heavily advertised drugs when older, less expensive medications may be equally effective. Many people equate "newer" with "better," but that is not always the case. The COX-2 inhibitors were designed for people at risk for stomach irritation from traditional NSAIDs, but most people who used Vioxx were actually at low risk for problems from traditional NSAIDs. For most people, older NSAIDs, which have an established safety record, are just as effective as the newer drugs and much less expensive.

### Selective Publication of Study Results

Many drug studies are carried out by the pharmaceutical industry, which has little incentive to publish the results of trials in which medications are found to be *ineffective*. In the case of antidepressants, manufacturers did not publicize studies that raised safety questions and failed to show drugs were effective for treating pediatric depression. Selective publication provides an inaccurate picture of the risks and benefits of a particular drug.

In response to criticism, pharmaceutical companies have set up a voluntary Web-based clearinghouse that will contain both positive and negative research findings (www.clinicalstudyresults.org). Major medical journals have pledged not to publish results of any clinical trial that is not preregistered. That is, researchers must register all trials when they begin, so unflattering or conflicting findings cannot be covered up. The U.S. Congress has also proposed legislation on this issue.

### Balancing Risks and Benefits

All medications have risks and benefits. When choosing a particular medication, work with your physician to balance the risks and benefits of the drug to your own personal health. Apply critical thinking skills to drug ads, recognizing them for what they are, and use special caution when taking recently approved medications.

SOURCES: Food and Drug Administration. 2005. *FDA Improvements in Drug Safety Monitoring* (http://www.fda.gov/oc/factsheets/drugsafety.html; retrieved February 28, 2005); Beardsley, S. 2005. Avoiding another Vioxx. *Scientific American*, February; Kimmel, S. E., et al. 2005. Patients exposed to rofecoxib and celecoxib have different odds of nonfatal myocardial infarction. *Annals of Internal Medicine* 142(3): 157–164; Dai, C., R. S. Stafford, and G. C. Alexander. 2005. National trends in cyclooxygenase-2 inhibitor use since market release: Nonselective diffusion of a selectively cost-effective innovation. *Archives of Internal Medicine* 165(2): 171–177.

**SURGERY** Each year, more than 70 million operations and related procedures are performed. Some key questions include the following:

- *Why do I need surgery at this time?* Your physician should be able to explain the reason for the surgery and what is likely to happen if you don't have it. Getting a second opinion about surgery is recommended and may be required by your health insurance plan.
- *What are the risks and complications of the surgery?* Overall risk depends on the type of operation performed, the surgeon, and your general state of health. Ask about the *mortality rate* (risk of death) and the *morbidity rate* (risk of nonlethal complications).
- *Can the operation be performed on an outpatient basis?* Outpatient (ambulatory) surgery has many advantages, including lower costs and fewer opportunities for hospital-associated complications.
- *What can I expect before, during, and after surgery?* Knowing what to expect can help you prepare for the surgery and speed your recovery.

## COMPLEMENTARY AND ALTERNATIVE MEDICINE

Where conventional Western medicine tends to focus on the body, on the physical causes of disease, and on ways to eradicate pathogens in order to restore health, traditional medicine tends to focus on an integration of mind, body, and spirit and to seek ways to restore the whole person to harmony so that he or she can regain health. Where conventional medicine is based on science, traditional medicine tends to be based on accumulated experience. The NIH National Center for Complementary and Alternative Medicine (NCCAM) groups CAM practices into five domains: alternative medical systems, mind-body interventions, biological-based therapies, manipulative and body-based methods, and energy therapies (Figure 15-2). What follows is a general introduction to the types of CAM available and a brief description of some of the more widely used ones.

### Alternative Medical Systems

Many cultures elaborated complete systems of medical philosophy, theory, and practice long before the current biomedical approach was developed. The complete systems that are best known in the United States are probably traditional Chinese medicine (TCM), also known as traditional Oriental medicine, and homeopathy. Traditional medical systems have also been developed in many other regions of the world, including North, Central, and South America; the Middle East; India; Tibet; and Australia. In many countries, these medical approaches continue to be used today—frequently alongside Western medicine and quite often by physicians trained in Western medicine.

| Domain | Characteristics | Examples |
|---|---|---|
| Alternative Medical Systems | Involve complete systems of theory and practice that have evolved independently of and often long before the conventional biomedical approach | Traditional Chinese medicine; Kampo; Ayurveda (India); Native American, Aboriginal, African, Middle-Eastern, Tibetan, Central and South American medical systems; homeopathy; naturopathy |
| Mind-Body Interventions | Employ a variety of techniques designed to make it possible for the mind to affect bodily function and symptoms | Meditation, certain uses of hypnosis, prayer, mental healing |
| Biological-Based Therapies | Include natural and biologically based practices, interventions, and products, many of which overlap with conventional medicine's use of dietary supplements | Herbal, special dietary, orthomolecular*, and individual biological therapies |
| Manipulative and Body-Based Methods | Include methods that are based on manipulation and/or movement of the body | Chiropractic, osteopathy, massage therapy |
| Energy Therapies | Focus on energy fields within the body (biofields) or from other sources (electromagnetic fields) | Qi gong, Reiki, therapeutic touch, bioelectromagnetic-based therapies |

* Orthomolecular therapies are treatments of diseases with varying, but usually high, concentrations of chemicals, including minerals (e.g., magnesium), hormones (e.g., melatonin), or vitamins.

**Figure 15-2 The five domains of CAM practices.**

Alternative medical systems tend to have concepts in common. For example, the concept of life force or energy exists in many cultures. In traditional Chinese medicine, the life force contained in all living things is called *qi* (sometimes spelled chi). In ayurveda, the traditional medical system of India, the life force is called *prana*. Most traditional medical systems think of disease as a disturbance or imbalance not just of physical processes but also of forces and energies within the body, the mind, and the spirit. Treatment aims at reestablishing equilibrium, balance, and harmony. Because the whole patient, rather than an isolated set of symptoms, is treated in most comprehensive alternative medical systems, it is rare that only a single treatment approach is used. Most commonly, multiple techniques and methods are employed and are continually adjusted according to the changes in the patient's health status that occur naturally or are brought about by the treatment.

**Traditional Chinese Medicine** In **Traditional Chinese Medicine (TCM),** the free and harmonious flow of qi produces health—a positive feeling of well-being and vitality in body, mind, and spirit. Illness occurs when the flow of qi is blocked or disturbed. TCM works to restore and balance the flow of blocked qi; the goal is not only to treat illnesses but also to increase energy, prevent disease, and support the immune system.

Two of the primary treatment methods in TCM are herbal remedies and **acupuncture.** Chinese herbal remedies number about 5800 and include plant products, animal parts, and minerals. The use of a single medicinal botanical is rare in Chinese herbal medicine; rather, several different plants are combined in very precise proportions, often to make a tea or soup. For example, a remedy might include a primary herb that targets the main symptom, a second herb that enhances the effects of the primary herb, a third that lessens side effects, and a fourth that helps deliver ingredients to a particular body site.

Acupuncture works to correct disturbances in the flow of qi through the insertion of long, thin needles at appropriate points in the skin. Qi is believed to flow through the body along several meridians, or pathways, and there are approximately 360 acupuncture points located along these meridians. The points chosen for acupuncture are highly individualized for each patient, and they change over the course of treatment as the patient's health status changes.

The World Health Organization has compiled a list of over 40 conditions in which acupuncture may be beneficial. At a conference called by the National Institutes of Health (NIH), a panel of experts found evidence that acupuncture was effective in relieving nausea and vomiting after chemotherapy and pain after surgery, including dental surgery. They added, however, that there is not yet enough evidence to show conclusively that acupuncture is effective for headaches, menstrual cramps, tennis elbow, back pain,

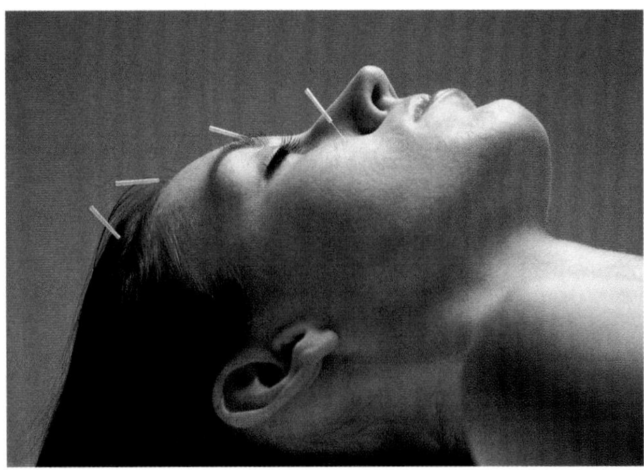

Acupuncture is one of the key treatment methods in traditional Chinese medicine. It involves the insertion of long, thin needles at appropriate points in the skin to restore balance to the flow of qi.

carpal tunnel syndrome, asthma, or other conditions. Western researchers typically use a different framework for understanding the effects of acupuncture. For example, they might explain pain relief not in terms of qi but in terms of stimulation of the nervous system and release of hormones and neurotransmitters.

Although more than 1 million Americans receive acupuncture each year, there have been few adverse events (negative effects) associated with it in the United States. Nonetheless, problems can occur from the improper insertion and manipulation of needles and from the use of unsterile needles. The FDA regulates acupuncture needles like other standard medical devices and requires that they be sterile. Most states require some form of licensing or credentialing for practitioners of acupuncture, but the requirements for licensure vary widely.

**Homeopathy** An alternative medical system of Western origin, **homeopathy** was developed about 200 years ago by the German physician Samuel Hahnemann (1755–1843) and is based on two main principles: "Like cures like," and remedies become more effective with greater dilution. "Like cures like" summarizes the concept

### Terms

VW

**Traditional Chinese medicine (TCM)** The traditional medical system of China, which views illness as the result of a disturbance in the flow of qi, the life force; therapies include acupuncture, herbal medicine, and massage.

**acupuncture** Insertion of long, thin needles into the skin at points along meridians, pathways through which qi is believed to flow; needles correct imbalances in qi; a practice common in traditional Chinese medicine.

**homeopathy** An alternative medical system of Western origin in which illnesses are treated by giving very small doses of drugs that in larger doses in a healthy person would produce symptoms like those of the illness.

Mind/Body/Spirit

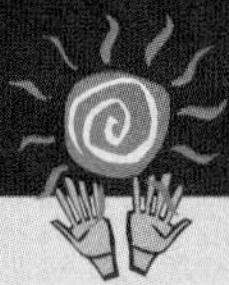

## The Power of Belief: The Placebo Effect

A placebo is a chemically inactive substance or ineffective procedure that a patient believes is an effective medical therapy for his or her condition. Researchers frequently give placebos to the control group in an experiment testing the efficacy of a particular treatment. By comparing the effects of the actual treatment with the effects of the placebo, researchers can judge whether the treatment is effective. The so-called placebo effect occurs when a patient improves after receiving a placebo. In such cases, the effect of the placebo on the patient cannot be attributed to the specific actions or properties of the drug or procedure.

Researchers have consistently found that 30–40% of all patients given a placebo show improvement. This result has been observed for a wide variety of conditions or symptoms, including coughing, seasickness, depression, migraines, and angina. For some conditions, placebos have been effective in up to 70% of patients. In some cases, people given a placebo even report having the side effects associated with an actual drug. Placebos are particularly effective when they are administered by a physician whom the patient trusts.

A clear demonstration of the placebo effect occurred in a recent study that examined the effectiveness of a drug used to treat benign enlargement of the prostate. The men who participated in the study were randomly assigned to one of two groups: One group received the medication; the other received a placebo, a look-alike dummy pill. More than half the men who got the placebo pills reported significant relief from their symptoms, including faster urine flow—despite the fact that men on the placebo actually experienced an *increase* in the size of their prostates. How did the men in the study experience fewer symptoms despite no improvement in their condition (prostate enlargement)? Researchers hypothesize that the patients' positive expectations of the medication's effects may have resulted in decreased nerve activity and muscle relaxation affecting the bladder, prostate, and urethra. Studies on patients with depression and people with Parkinson's disease have found that treatment with an inactive placebo results in changes in brain function. Such changes in the electrical or chemical activity of the brain may help explain the placebo effect.

The placebo effect can be exploited by unscrupulous people who sell worthless medical treatments to the scientifically unsophisticated public. But placebo power can also be harnessed for its beneficial effects. When a skilled and compassionate medical practitioner provides a patient with a sense of confidence and hope, the positive aspects of placebo power can boost the benefits of standard medical treatment. Whenever you swallow a pill, you swallow your expectations right along with the medication or herb; imagining how the pill is helping you can stimulate a positive placebo effect. Getting well, like getting sick, is a complex process. Anatomy, physiology, mind, emotions, and the environment are all inextricably intertwined. But the placebo effect does show that belief can have both psychological and physical effects.

SOURCES: Leuchter, A. F., et al. 2002. Changes in brain function of depressed subjects during treatment with placebo. *American Journal of Psychiatry* 159(1): 122–129; Nordenberg, T. 2000. The healing power of placebos. *FDA Consumer,* January/February; The powerful placebo: An effect without a cause. 2000. *Harvard Men's Health Watch,* June.

that a substance that produces the symptoms of an illness or disease in a healthy person can cure the illness when given in very minute quantities. Remedies containing very small quantities of a particular substance are obtained by repeatedly diluting the original solution. The extent of dilution varies, but the final extract is often so dilute that few, if any, of the original molecules are left in it. According to homeopathic thinking, such highly diluted extracts not only retain some form of biological activity but actually become more potent.

Over 1000 different substances (plant and animal parts, minerals, and chemicals) can be used to prepare homeopathic remedies, and each of these substances is thought to have different effects at different dilutions. That means a homeopath must not only choose the correct remedy for a particular patient but also decide on the specific dilution of that remedy in order to achieve the desired effect.

In order to assess a patient's condition, homeopaths generally spend quite a bit of time talking with a patient and assessing his or her physical and emotional health before deciding on the correct remedy at the proper dilution. This intensive interaction between the practitioner and the patient might play an important role in the success of the therapy. Indeed, critics of homeopathy often attribute its reported effectiveness to this nonspecific "placebo effect" (see the box "The Power of Belief: The Placebo Effect"). However, when the results of 185 homeopathic trials were analyzed recently, it was concluded that the clinical effects of homeopathy could not be completely explained by the placebo effect. At the same time, homeopathy was not found to be effective for any single clinical condition. Homeopathy remains one of the most controversial forms of CAM.

Because of the extremely dilute nature of homeopathic remedies, it is generally assumed that they are safe. To date, the FDA has not found any serious adverse events associated with the use of homeopathy, with the possible exception of situations in which a patient might have been successfully treated with standard medical approaches but chose to rely solely on homeopathy. The FDA regulates homeopathic remedies, but they are subject to many fewer restrictions than prescription or over-the-counter drugs. A few states require practitioners to have special licenses, but most providers practice homeopathy as a specialty under another medical license, such as medical doctor or nurse practitioner.

## Mind-Body Interventions

Mind-body interventions make use of the integral connection between mind and body and the effect each can have on the other. They include many of the stress-management techniques discussed in Chapter 2, including meditation, yoga, visualization, tai chi, and biofeedback. Psychotherapy, support groups, prayer, and music, art, and dance therapy can also be thought of as mind-body interventions. Obviously, there is no clear line between these forms of CAM and conventional medicine. The placebo effect is one of the most widely known examples of mind-body interdependence.

Some forms of **hypnosis** are considered to be CAM therapies, although the use of hypnotherapy for certain conditions was accepted more than 40 years ago by the American Medical Association. Hypnosis involves the induction of a state of deep relaxation during which the patient is more suggestible (more easily influenced). While the patient is in such a hypnotic trance, the practitioner tries to help him or her change unwanted behavior or deal with pain and other symptoms. Hypnosis is sometimes used in smoking cessation programs and as a nondrug approach to anxiety disorders such as phobias and chronic conditions such as irritable bowel syndrome.

Hypnosis can be used by medical professionals (M.D.s, D.O.s, D.D.S.s) but is also offered by hypnotherapists. Physicians are certified by their own associations; many states require hypnotherapists to be licensed, but the requirements for licensing vary substantially. There is little regulation of practitioners of other relaxation techniques, but it is very rare that adverse events result from such techniques. Many studies have shown that support groups, friendships, strong family relationships, and prayer can all have a positive impact on health.

## Biological-Based Therapies

**Biological-based therapies** consist primarily of herbal therapies or remedies, botanicals, and dietary supplements. Herbal remedies are a major component of all indigenous forms of medicine; prior to the development of pharmaceuticals at the end of the nineteenth century, people everywhere in the world relied on materials from nature for pain relief, wound healing, and treatment of a variety of ailments. Herbal remedies are also a common element in most systems of traditional medicine. Much of the **pharmacopoeia** of modern scientific medicine originated in the folk medicine of native peoples, and many drugs used today are derived from plants.

A majority of botanical products are sold as dietary supplements, that is, in the form of tablets, pills, capsules, liquid extracts, or teas. Like foods, dietary supplements must carry ingredient labels (see Chapter 9). As with food products, it is the responsibility of the manufacturers to ensure that their dietary supplements are safe and properly labeled prior to marketing. The FDA is responsible for monitoring the labeling and accompanying literature of dietary supplements and for overseeing their safety once they are on the market.

Well-designed clinical studies have been conducted on only a small number of botanicals. A few commonly used botanicals, their uses, and the evidence supporting their efficacy are presented in Table 15-2 on page 384. Participants in clinical trials with St. John's wort, ginkgo, and echinacea experienced only minor adverse events. However, most clinical trials of this type last for only a few weeks, so the tests did not indicate whether it is safe to take these botanicals for longer periods of time. They also didn't examine the effects of different dosages or how the botanicals interact with other drugs.

For the vast majority of other botanicals, there are almost no reliable research findings on efficacy or safety. That is extremely worrisome because, of all the CAM approaches, the consumption of botanical supplements has the greatest potential to result in serious and even life-threatening consequences (see the box "Herbal Remedies: Are They Safe?" on p. 385).

## Manipulative and Body-Based Methods

Touch and body manipulation are long-standing forms of health care. Manual healing techniques are based on the idea that misalignment or dysfunction in one part of the body can cause pain or dysfunction in another part; correcting these misalignments can bring the body back to optimal health.

Manual healing methods are an integral part of osteopathic medicine, now considered a form of conventional medicine. Other physical healing methods include massage, acupressure, Feldenkrais, Rolfing, and numerous other techniques. The most commonly accepted of the CAM manual healing methods is **chiropractic**, a method that focuses on the relationship between structure, primarily of joints and muscles, and function, primarily

### Terms

Vw

**hypnosis** The process by which a practitioner induces a state of deep relaxation in which an individual is more suggestible; commonly used in cases of pain, phobia, and addiction.

**biological-based therapies** CAM therapies that include natural and biologically based practices, interventions, and products; examples include herbal remedies and dietary supplements.

**pharmacopoeia** A collection of drugs and medicinal preparations.

**chiropractic** A system of manual healing most frequently used to treat musculoskeletal problems; the primary treatment is manipulation of the spine and other joints. Practitioners hold a doctor of chiropractic degree and are licensed.

## Table 15-2 Commonly Used Botanicals, Their Uses, Evidence for Their Effectiveness, and Contraindications

| Botanical | Use | Evidence | Examples of Adverse Effects and Interactions |
|---|---|---|---|
| Echinacea *(Echinacea purpurea, E. angustifolia, E. pallida)* | Stimulation of immune functions; to prevent colds and flulike diseases; to lessen symptoms of colds and flus | Some trials showed that it prevents colds and flus and helps patients recover from colds faster, but others found it ineffective | Might cause liver damage if taken over long periods of time (more than 8 weeks); since it is an immune stimulant, it is not advisable to take it with immune suppressants (e.g., corticosteroids) |
| Feverfew *(Tanacetum parthenium)* | Prevention of headaches and migraines | The majority of trials indicate that it is more effective than placebo, but the evidence is not yet conclusive | Should not be used by people allergic to other members of the aster family; has the potential to increase the effects of warfarin and other anticoagulants |
| Garlic *(Allium sativum)* | Reduction of cholesterol | Short-term studies have found a modest effect; long-term studies are needed | May interact with some medications, including anticoagulants, cyclosporine, and oral contraceptives |
| Ginkgo *(Ginkgo biloba)* | Improvement of circulation and memory | Improves cerebral insufficiency and slows progression of Alzheimer's disease and other types of senile dementia in some patients; improves blood flow in legs | Could increase bleeding time; should not be taken with nonsteroidal anti-inflammatory drugs or anticoagulants; gastrointestinal disturbance |
| Ginseng* *(Panax ginseng)* | Improvement of physical performance, memory, immune function, and glycemic control in diabetes; treatment of herpes simplex 2 | No conclusive evidence exists for any of these uses | Interacts with warfarin and alcohol in mice and rats, hence should probably not be used with these drugs; may cause liver damage |
| St. John's wort *(Hypericum perforatum)* | Treatment of depression | There is strong evidence that it is significantly more effective than placebo, is as effective as some standard antidepressants for mild to moderate depression, and causes fewer adverse effects | Known to interact with a variety of pharmaceuticals and should not be taken together with digoxin, theophylline, cyclosporine, indinavir, and serotonin-reuptake inhibitors |
| Saw palmetto *(Serenoa repens)* | Improvement of prostate health | Appears to be moderately effective, but the evidence is not yet considered conclusive | Has no known interactions with drugs, but should probably not be taken with hormonal therapies |

*There are two other species of ginseng, namely *Panax quinquefolium* (American ginseng) and *Eleutherococcus senticosus* (Siberian ginseng), but in clinical trials for cerebral insufficiency and dementia only *Panax ginseng* has been tested.

of the nervous system, to maintain or restore health. An important therapeutic procedure is the manipulation of joints, particularly those of the spinal column. However, chiropractors also use a variety of other techniques, including physical therapy, exercise programs, patient education and lifestyle modification, nutritional supplements, and orthotics (mechanical supports and braces) to treat patients. They do not use drugs or surgery.

Chiropractors, or doctors of chiropractic, are trained for a minimum of four full-time academic years at accredited chiropractic colleges and can go on to postgraduate training in many countries. Chiropractic is accepted by many health care and health insurance providers to a far greater extent than the other types of CAM therapies. Chiropractic has been shown to be effective for acute low-back pain; promising results have also been reported with the use of chiropractic techniques in neck pain and headaches. However, there are no well-controlled studies to support manipulation for asthma, gastrointestinal problems, infectious diseases, or other nonmechanical problems.

A caution is in order regarding chiropractic: Spinal manipulation performed by a person without proper chiropractic training can be extremely dangerous. There

### Terms

Vw

**energy therapies** Forms of CAM treatment that use energy fields originating either within the body or from outside sources to promote healing.

**qigong** A component of traditional Chinese medicine that combines movement, meditation, and regulation of breathing to enhance the flow of qi, improve blood circulation, and enhance immune function.

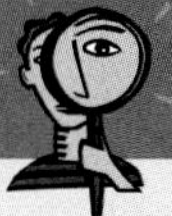

## Herbal Remedies: Are They Safe?

Consider the following research findings and FDA advisories:

- St. John's wort interacts with drugs used to treat HIV infection and heart disease; the herb may also reduce the effectiveness of oral contraceptives and many other drugs.
- Chinese herbs contaminated through a manufacturing error with the powerful carcinogen aristolochic acid caused kidney damage and bladder cancer in patients at a weight-loss clinic in Belgium.
- Supplements containing kava have been linked to severe liver damage, and anyone who has liver problems or takes medications that can affect the liver are advised to consult a physician before using kava-containing supplements.
- In a sample of ayurvedic herbal medicine products, 20% were found to contain potentially harmful levels of lead, mercury, and/or arsenic.

These findings highlight growing safety concerns about dietary supplements, which now represent annual sales of more than $15 billion in the United States.

### Drug Interactions

As in the case of St. John's wort, the chemicals in botanicals can interact dangerously with prescription and over-the-counter drugs. Botanicals may decrease the effects of drugs, making them ineffective, or increase their effects, in some cases making them toxic. Alarmingly, most patients fail to tell their physicians about their use of herbal substances. Botanicals can also interact with each other, and many manufacturers are offering new combinations of botanical preparations without scientific information about the interactions of the individual ingredients.

### Lack of Standardization

A related problem is the lack of standardization in the manufacturing of herbal products. The Dietary Supplement Health and Education Act of 1994 requires that dietary supplement labels list the name and quantity of each ingredient. However, confusion can result because different plant species may have the same common name. The content of herbal preparations is also variable. A 2003 study of echinacea supplements found that only about half contained the species and amount listed on the label; 10% of the samples contained no echinacea at all. Part of the reason for such variation is the difficulty of identifying the active ingredients in botanicals and isolating and standardizing their concentrations. The chemical composition of a supplement is also affected by the growing, harvesting, processing, and storage conditions of plants.

### Contamination and Toxicity

A variety of traditional Chinese and ayurvedic remedies contain heavy metals such as lead, mercury, and arsenic as part of the formula, all of which can be highly toxic and can cause irreversible damage. Some Chinese herbal remedies have been found to contain pharmaceutical drugs, including tranquilizers and steroids. Others contain herbs not listed on the label, sometimes substitute herbs that have toxic effects, as in the case of the weight-loss pills used in the Belgian clinic. Furthermore, many plants are poisonous or can cause damage to the liver or kidneys if taken over long periods of time. Experts have also advised against taking supplements that contain raw animal parts, particularly central nervous system tissue, out of concern that disease may be transmissible this way.

### The Role of Government

Some European governments assume greater responsibility in regulating botanicals than the U.S. government. In Germany, herbal medicine has a long history, but herbs are considered medicines rather than supplements; they are usually prescribed by physicians. Manufacturing is standardized so that content, quantity, quality, and purity are guaranteed. Botanicals do not have to be proven effective to be marketed, but they do have to be proven safe.

In the United States, because herbs are considered supplements rather than food or drug products, they do not have to meet FDA food and drug standards for safety or effectiveness, nor do they currently have to meet any manufacturing standards. The manufacturer is responsible for ensuring that a supplement is safe before it is marketed; the FDA has the power to restrict a substance if it is found to pose a health risk after it is on the market. Because U.S. manufacturers can put almost anything into an herbal supplement, American consumers are at risk for buying and using products that may be not just useless but harmful as well. Part of the reasoning behind this situation is that "natural" products are considered safer than conventional medicines. As the incidents with St. John's wort, aristolochic acid, kava, and ayurvedic products demonstrate, this is not always the case.

are several organizations, in particular the American Chiropractic Association, that can help you locate a licensed chiropractor near you.

## Energy Therapies

**Energy therapies** are forms of treatment that use energy fields originating either within the body (biofields) or from other sources (electromagnetic fields). Biofield therapies are based on the idea that energy fields surround and penetrate the body and can be influenced by movement, touch, pressure, or the placement of hands in or through the fields. **Qigong**, a component of traditional Chinese medicine, combines movement, meditation, and regulation of breathing to enhance the flow of qi, improve blood circulation, and enhance immune function.

**Therapeutic touch** is derived from the ancient technique of "laying-on of hands"; it is based on the premise that healers can identify and correct energy imbalances by passing their hands over the patient's body. **Reiki** is one form of therapeutic touch; it is intended to correct disturbances in the flow of life energy (ki is the Japanese form of the Chinese qi) and enhance the body's healing powers through the use of 13 specific hand positions on the patient.

Bioelectromagnetics is the study of the interaction between living organisms and electromagnetic fields, both those produced by the organism itself and those produced by outside sources. The recognition that the body produces electromagnetic fields has led to the development of many diagnostic procedures in Western medicine, including electroencephalography (EEG), electrocardiography (ECG), and nuclear magnetic resonance (NMR) scans. **Bioelectromagnetic-based therapies** involve the use of electromagnetic fields to manage pain and to treat conditions such as asthma. Although promising, the available research is still very limited and does not allow firm conclusions about the efficacy of these therapies. Most scientists believe that consumer products containing small magnets have no significant effect on the human body.

## Evaluating Complementary and Alternative Therapies

Because there is less information available about complementary and alternative therapies, as well as less regulation of associated products and providers, it is important for consumers to take an active role when they are thinking about using them (see the box "Avoiding Health Fraud and Quackery").

**Working with Your Physician** The NCCAM advises consumers not to seek complementary therapies without first visiting a conventional health care provider for an evaluation and diagnosis of their symptoms. It's usually best to discuss and try conventional treatments that have been shown to be beneficial for your condition. If you are thinking of trying any alternative therapies, it is critically important to tell your physician in order to avoid any dangerous interactions with conventional treatments you are receiving. Areas to discuss with your physician include the following:

- *Safety:* Is there something unsafe about the treatment in general or for you specifically? Are there safety issues you should be aware of, such as the use of disposable needles in acupuncture?
- *Effectiveness:* Is there any research about the use of the therapy for your condition?
- *Timing:* Is the immediate use of a conventional treatment indicated?
- *Cost:* Is the therapy likely to be very expensive, especially in light of the potential benefit?

If appropriate, schedule a follow-up visit with your physician to assess your condition and your progress after a certain amount of time using a complementary therapy. Keep a symptom diary to more accurately track your symptoms and gauge your progress. (Symptoms such as pain and fatigue are very difficult to recall with accuracy, so an ongoing symptom diary is an important tool.) If you plan to pursue a therapy against your physician's advice, you need to tell him or her.

For dietary supplements, pharmacists can also be an excellent source of information, especially if they are familiar with other medications you are taking.

**Questioning the CAM Practitioner** You can also get information from individual practitioners and from schools, professional organizations, and state licensing boards. Ask about education, training, licensing, and certification. If appropriate, check with local or state regulatory agencies or the consumer affairs department to determine if any complaints have been lodged against the practitioner. Some guidelines for talking with a CAM practitioner include the following:

- Ask the practitioner why he or she thinks the therapy will be beneficial for your condition. Ask for a full description of the therapy and any potential side effects.
- Describe in detail any conventional treatments you are receiving.
- Ask how long the therapy should continue before it can be determined if it is beneficial.
- Ask about the expected cost of the treatment. Does it seem reasonable? Will your health insurance pay some or all of the costs?

If anything an alternative practitioner says or recommends directly conflicts with advice from your physician, discuss it with your physician before making any major changes in any current treatment regimen or in your lifestyle.

### Terms

VW

**therapeutic touch** A CAM practice based on the premise that healers can identify and correct energy imbalances by passing their hands over the patient's body.

**Reiki** A CAM practice intended to correct disturbances in the flow of life energy and enhance the body's healing powers through the use of 13 hand positions on the patient.

**bioelectromagnetic-based therapies** CAM therapies based on the notion that electromagnetic fields can be used to promote healing and manage pain.

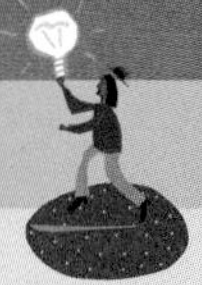

Critical Consumer

## Avoiding Health Fraud and Quackery

VW

According to the Federal Trade Commission, consumers waste billions of dollars on unproven, fraudulently marketed, and sometimes useless health care products and treatments.

The first rule of thumb for evaluating any health claim is that if it sounds too good to be true, it probably is. Also be on the lookout for the typical phrases and marketing techniques fraudulent promoters use to deceive consumers:

- The product is advertised as a quick and effective cure-all or diagnostic tool for a wide range of ailments.
- The promoters use words like *scientific breakthrough, miraculous cure, exclusive product, secret ingredient,* or *ancient remedy.* Also remember that just because a product is described as "natural" or unprocessed does not necessarily mean it's safe.
- The text is written in "medicalese"—impressive-sounding terminology to disguise a lack of good science.
- The promoter claims the government, the medical profession, or researchers have conspired to suppress the product.
- The advertisement includes undocumented case histories claiming amazing results.
- The product is advertised as in limited supply or available from only one source, and payment is required in advance.
- The promoter promises a no-risk "money-back guarantee." Be aware that many fly-by-night operators are not around to respond to your request for a refund.

To check out a particular product, talk to a physician or another health care professional and to family members and friends. Be wary of treatments offered by people who tell you to avoid talking to others. Check with the Better Business Bureau or local attorney general's office to see whether other consumers have lodged complaints about the product or the product's marketer. You can also check with the appropriate health professional group. For example, check with the American Diabetes Association or the National Arthritis Foundation if the products are promoted for diabetes or arthritis. Take special care with products and devices sold online; the broad reach of the Internet, combined with the ease of setting up and removing Web sites, makes online sellers particularly difficult to regulate.

If you think you have been a victim of health fraud or if you have an adverse reaction that you think is related to a particular supplement, you can report it to the appropriate agency:

- *False advertising claims:* Contact the FTC by phone (877-FTC-HELP), by mail (Consumer Response Center, Federal Trade Commission, Washington, DC 20580), or online (http://www.ftc.gov; click on File a Complaint). You can also contact your state attorney general's office, your state department of health, or the local consumer protection agency (check your local telephone directory).
- *False labeling on a product:* Contact the FDA district office consumer complaint coordinator for your geographic area. (The FDA regulates safety, manufacturing, and product labeling.)
- *Adverse reaction to a supplement:* Call a doctor or another health care provider immediately. You may also report your adverse reaction to FDA MedWatch by calling 800-FDA-1088 or by visiting the MedWatch Web site (http://www.fda.gov/medwatch).
- *Unlawful Internet sales:* If you find a Web site that you think is illegally selling drugs, medical devices, dietary supplements, or cosmetics, report it to the FDA. Problems can be reported to MedWatch or via the FDA Web site (http://www.fda.gov/oc/buyonline/buyonlineform.htm).

SOURCES: Meadows, M. 2005. Use caution buying medical products online. *FDA Consumer,* January/February; Federal Trade Commission. 2001. *"Miracle" Health Claims: Add a Dose of Skepticism* (http://www.ftc.gov/bcp/conline/pubs/health/frdheal.htm; retrieved December 14, 2002); Food and Drug Administration. 1999. *How to Report Adverse Reactions and Other Problems with Products Regulated by FDA* (http://www.fda.gov/opacom/backgrounders/problem.html; retrieved July 19, 2000); Kurtzweil, P. 1999. How to spot health fraud. *FDA Consumer,* November/December.

**Doing Your Own Research** You can investigate CAM therapies on your own by going to the library or doing research online, although caution is in order when using Web sites for the various forms of CAM. A good place to start is the Web sites of government agencies like the FDA or NCCAM and of universities and similar organizations that conduct government-sponsored research on CAM approaches (see For More Information on p. 391).

If possible, also talk to people with the same condition you have who have received the same treatment. Remember, though, that patient testimonials shouldn't be used as the sole criterion for choosing a therapy or assessing its safety and efficacy. Controlled scientific trials usually provide the best information and should be consulted whenever possible. Perhaps more so than for any other consumer products and services, the use of CAM calls for consumer skills, critical thinking, and caution.

Despite many profound and irreconcilable philosophical differences between conventional medicine and CAM, there are abundant opportunities for learning, collaborating, and providing parallel care. Conventional medicine has already adopted many principles prevalent in complementary and alternative disciplines, including the ideas of health promotion, of personal responsibility for health, and of wellness as a multidimensional ideal. At the same time, practitioners of CAM are looking to Western methods to modernize and optimize some of their practices, such as the preparation and standardization of herbal remedies. Within each is an enormous amount of time-tested information that has its own logic and use. In the future, greater understanding and collaboration across boundaries will certainly benefit the patient-consumer.

## PAYING FOR HEALTH CARE

The American health care system is one of the most advanced and comprehensive in the world, but it is also the most expensive. The United States currently spends more than $1.7 trillion on health care, or $6000 per person. Health care costs are expected to nearly double in the first decade of the twenty-first century, reaching $2.8 trillion, or about $9000 per person, by 2010 (Figure 15-3). Health care spending is growing faster than the rest of the U.S. economy.

Health care is currently financed by a combination of private and public insurance plans, patient out-of-pocket payments, and government assistance. Currently, private insurance and individual patients pay about 55% of the total; the government pays the remaining 45%, mainly through Medicare and Medicaid (discussed below). Most nonelderly Americans receive their health insurance through their employers.

Despite high spending, not everyone is included in this financing system. More than 40 million people, the vast majority of them employed, have no health care insurance at all (see the box "Who Are the Uninsured?").

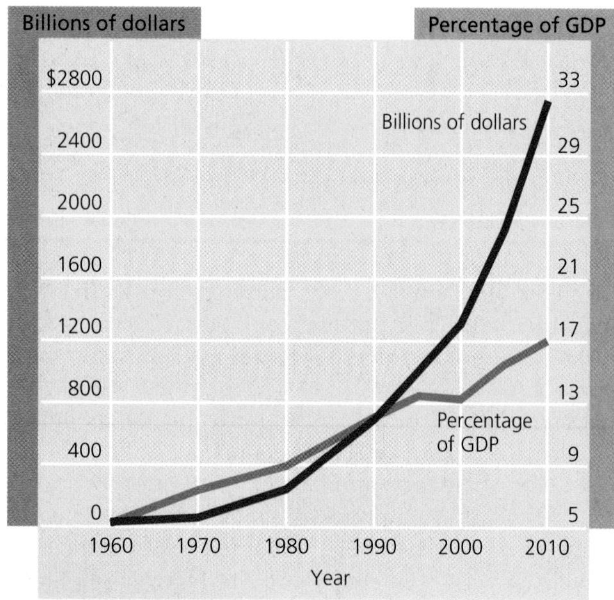


VITAL STATISTICS

**Figure 15-3 U.S. health care expenditures.** SOURCE: Centers for Medicare and Medicaid Services (http://cms.hhs.gov).

Many more are underinsured, meaning they may be uninsured for periods of time, have health insurance that does not cover all needed services, and/or have high out-of-pocket costs. People who are underinsured may skip physician visits and not take all prescribed medications. New government health insurance programs for children have reduced the number of Americans under age 18 who lack health insurance; however, the uninsured include almost 8 million children—10% of all American children—most in working, low-income families. Among Americans 18–64 years of age, about 18%, or nearly one in five, are without health insurance. Lack of insurance affects both access to care and quality of care.

### Health Insurance

Health insurance enables people to receive health care they might not otherwise be able to afford. Health insurance plans are either fee-for-service (or indemnity) or managed care. With both types the individual or the employer pays a basic premium, usually on a monthly basis; there are often other payments as well.

#### Traditional Fee-for-Service (Indemnity) Plans

In a fee-for-service, or indemnity, plan, you can use any medical provider (such as a physician or a hospital) you choose. You or the provider sends the bill to your insurance company, which pays part of it. Usually you have to pay a "deductible" amount each year, and then the plan will pay a percentage—often 80%—of what they consider the "usual and customary" charge for covered services.

**Managed-Care Plans** **Managed-care plans** have agreements with certain physicians, hospitals, and health care providers to offer a range of services to plan members at reduced cost. In general, you have lower out-of-pocket costs and less paperwork with a managed-care plan than with an indemnity plan, but you also have less freedom in choosing health care providers. Most Americans with job-based insurance are covered by managed-care plans, which may follow several different models:

- **Health maintenance organizations (HMOs)** offer members a range of services for a set monthly fee. You choose a primary care physician who manages your care and refers you to specialists if you need them.
- **Preferred provider organizations (PPOs)** are plans that have arrangements with physicians and other providers who have agreed to accept lower fees.
- **Point-of-service (POS) plans** are options offered by many HMOs in which you can see a physician outside the plan and still be partially covered.

Many managed-care plans try to reduce costs over the long term by paying for routine preventive care, such as

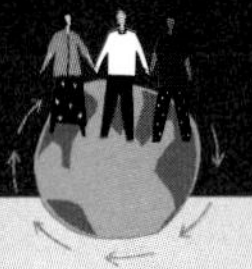

Dimensions of Diversity

## Who Are the Uninsured?

Despite high national levels of spending on health care, many Americans under age 65—about 17% or nearly 1 in 5—do not have health insurance. (Americans age 65 and over are often covered by government programs.) The overall statistic about the uninsured hides some important differences among groups (see table).

- *Low income:* The factor most closely associated with lack of health insurance is low income.
- *Age:* Younger adults may not be regularly employed and so may not be covered by an insurance plan through work.
- *Ethnicity:* Much of the ethnic variations are explained by socioeconomic status. However, other factors may also contribute, including language barriers, differing cultural attitudes toward medical care, and living in medically underserved communities.

People without health insurance receive less health care and lower quality of care. They have fewer physician visits and less preventive care. To help overcome the health gap between ethnic minorities and the general population, the U.S. Department of Health and Human Services sponsors "Take a Loved One to the Doctor Day." Held on the third Tuesday in September, this event is designed to encourage people to obtain preventive care. People are encouraged to make an appointment for themselves or for a friend or family member who hasn't seen a health care provider recently.

People who don't have a regular health care provider or who don't have health insurance can contact a local health department or local community center to find out more about free or low-cost care. For more information, visit the Closing the Health Gap Web site (www.healthgap.omhrc.gov).

| | Uninsured Americans Under Age 65 (Percent) |
|---|---|
| **Total** | **16.6** |
| Income (percent of poverty level) | |
| Below 100% | 31.4 |
| 100–149% | 32.8 |
| 150–199% | 25.6 |
| 200% or more | 10.9 |
| Age (years) | |
| Under 18 | 10.7 |
| 18–24 | 28.2 |
| 25–34 | 23.8 |
| 35–44 | 17.8 |
| 45–54 | 14.1 |
| 55–64 | 11.6 |
| Ethnicity | |
| White | 12.6 |
| Asian American | 17.2 |
| African American | 19.2 |
| Latino | 33.8 |
| American Indian/ Alaska Native | 38.7 |

SOURCES: Office of Minority Health Resource Center. 2005. *Fact Sheet: Take a Loved One to the Doctor Day 2005* (http://www.healthgap.omhrc.gov/2005factsheetdrday.htm; retrieved February 25, 2005); National Center for Health Statistics. 2004. *Health, United States, 2004.* Hyattsville, Md.: National Center for Health Statistics.

regular checkups and screening tests and prenatal care; they may also encourage prevention by offering health education and lifestyle modification programs for members. Other cost-cutting measures are less consumer-oriented. Consumers' choice of physicians is limited, and they may have to wait longer for appointments and travel farther to see participating doctors. If a patient violates the rules for obtaining services, the plan typically will not cover the cost of the services in question. Nonemergency visits to emergency rooms are also frequently not covered.

**Health Savings Accounts** **Health savings accounts (HSAs)** are a new form of health insurance coverage that became available in 2004. An HSA includes two parts: (1) a health plan with a high deductible, and (2) a tax-exempt personal savings account that is used for qualified medical expenses. The individual makes pre-tax contributions to the savings account, and latter uses these funds or other cash payments to cover medical expenses before the plan's deductible is met. Once the deductible is

### Terms

VW

**managed-care plan** A health care program that integrates the financing and delivery of services by using designated providers, utilization review, and financial incentives for following the plan's policies; HMOs, PPOs, and POS plans are examples of managed-care plans.

**health maintenance organization (HMO)** A prepaid health insurance plan in which patients receive health care from designated providers.

**preferred provider organization (PPO)** A prepaid health insurance plan in which providers agree to deliver services for discounted fees; patients can go to any provider, but using nonparticipating providers results in higher costs to the patient.

**point-of-service (POS) plan** A managed-care plan that covers treatment by an HMO physician but permits patients to seek treatment elsewhere with a higher copayment.

**health savings account (HSA)** Health insurance coverage that includes a health plan with a high deductible and a tax-exempt personal savings account that is used for qualified medical expenses.

met, the plan pays remaining medical costs according to the type of policy. The savings account can also be used for certain other types of expenses not covered by the plan. The benefit of an HSA is that it gives the consumer more control over health care spending; it can also potentially lower insurance premiums for some people because health plans with high deductibles tend to have lower premiums.

**Government Programs** Americans who are 65 or older and younger people with certain disabilities can be covered by **Medicare,** a federal health insurance program that helps pay for hospitalization, physician services, and prescription drugs. **Medicaid** is a joint federal-state health insurance program that covers some low-income people, especially children, pregnant women, and people with certain disabilities.

## Choosing a Policy

Choosing health insurance can be complicated; it's important to evaluate the coverage provided by different plans and decide which one is best for you. Consider the following questions:

- Is the plan accredited, and how is it rated for quality?
- Does the plan include the physicians and hospitals you want?
- Does the plan provide the benefits you need? Consider services such as prescription medications, physical therapy, well baby care, mental health services, eye care, home health care, and CAM therapies.
- Does the plan fit your budget? Include monthly premiums, annual deductibles, and copayments for appointments and medication.

Colleges typically provide medical services through a student health center; some require students to purchase additional insurance if they are not covered by family policies. It's usually economical to remain on a family policy as long as possible. After college, most people secure group coverage through their place of employment or through membership in an organization. If you are choosing insurance, consider a number of different plans and use your critical thinking skills to find the one that best suits your needs.

### Terms

VW

**Medicare** A federal health insurance program for people 65 or older and for younger people with certain disabilities.

**Medicaid** A federally subsidized state-run plan of health care for people with low income.

### Tips for Today

Most of the time, you can take care of yourself without consulting a health care provider. You can eat sensibly, get enough exercise, manage stress, minimize your chances of getting an infection, and so on. When you do need professional care, you can continue to take responsibility for yourself by making informed, reasoned decisions about the care you obtain, whether conventional or CAM.

*Right now you can*

- Make sure you have enough on hand of any prescription medication that you take and that your prescription is up to date.
- Make sure you have basic first aid supplies at home and prepare or buy a small first aid kit for your car or office.
- Research any alternative or complementary practice or product you are using, either at the library or online, to find out if it is considered safe.
- Sit back in your chair and practice relaxation through breathing: Inhale slowly and deeply, imagining warm air flowing to all parts of your body; exhale from your abdomen, imagining tension flowing out of your body; continue for 5 or 10 minutes or until you feel relaxed.

## SUMMARY


- Informed self-care requires knowing how to evaluate symptoms. It's necessary to see a physician if symptoms are severe, unusual, persistent, or recurrent.
- Self-treatment doesn't necessarily require medication, but OTC drugs can be a helpful part of self-care.
- Conventional medicine is characterized by a focus on the external, physical causes of disease; the identification of a set of symptoms for different diseases; the development of public health measures to prevent disease and of drugs and surgery to treat them; the use of rational, scientific thinking to understand phenomena; and a well-established research methodology.
- Conventional practitioners include medical doctors, doctors of osteopathic medicine, podiatrists, optometrists, and dentists, as well as allied health care providers.
- The diagnostic process involves a medical history, a physical exam, and medical tests. Patients should ask questions about medical tests and treatments recommended by their physicians.
- Safe use of prescription drugs requires knowledge of what the medication is supposed to do, how and when to take it, and what the side effects are.
- Complementary and alternative medicine (CAM) is defined as those therapies and practices that do not form part of conventional or "mainstream" health care and medical practice as taught in most U.S. medical schools and offered in most U.S. hospitals.

- CAM is characterized by a view of health as a balance and integration of body, mind, and spirit; and a body of knowledge based on accumulated experience and observations of patient reactions.
- Alternative medical systems such as traditional Chinese medicine and homeopathy are complete systems of medical philosophy, theory, and practice.
- Mind-body interventions include meditation, yoga, group support, hypnosis, and prayer.
- Biological-based therapies consist of herbal remedies, botanicals, and dietary supplements.
- Manipulative and body-based methods include massage and other physical healing techniques; the most commonly accepted is chiropractic.
- Energy therapies are designed to influence the flow of energy in and around the body; they include qigong, therapeutic touch therapies, and Reiki.
- Because there is less information available about CAM and less regulation of its practices and providers, consumers must be proactive in researching and choosing treatments, using critical thinking skills and exercising caution.
- Health insurance plans are usually described as either fee-for-service (indemnity) or managed-care plans. Government programs include Medicaid, for the poor, and Medicare, for those who are 65 and over or chronically disabled.

## Take Action

1. **Consider special health risks:** Ask your physician whether you have any medical condition that may require special attention in an emergency. If you do, complete a medical ID card for your wallet, or obtain a medical ID bracelet or necklace. More complete emergency service can be obtained by joining Medic Alert (800-ID-ALERT; www.medicalert.org).

2. **Compare supplements:** Visit a local drugstore and compare different brands of the same herbal remedy or dietary supplement. How similar are the supplements in terms of ingredients, recommended dosages, and price? What aspect of health do the supplements claim to benefit, and how do they make the claim? Research any unfamiliar ingredients using the resources listed in For More Information and in Chapter 9.

3. **Make a preventive-care appointment for yourself or someone you know:** Promote wellness in yourself and those around you by participating in "Take a Loved One to the Doctor Day." Make an appointment for preventive care for yourself or a friend or family member (see p. 389 for more information). If needed, help someone keep his or her appointment by volunteering to provide transportation or child care.

## For More Information

### Books


Brody, H. 2000. *The Placebo Response.* New York: Cliff Street Books. *Describes the placebo effect and how it may be used to benefit health.*

Committee on the Use of Complementary and Alternative Medicine by the American Public. 2005. *Complementary and Alternative Medicine in the United States.* Washington, D.C.: National Academy Press. *Outlines ways of integrating conventional and complementary therapies and proposes changes to dietary supplement laws.*

Howard Hughes Medical Institute, ed. 2000. *Exploring the Biomedical Revolution.* Baltimore: Johns Hopkins University Press. *Explores biomedical research and its impact on the fight against human disease.*

Medical Economics Staff. 2005. *PDR for Nonprescription Drugs and Dietary Supplements, 2005.* Montvale, N.J.: Medical Economics. *A reference covering the safety and efficacy of over-the-counter drugs and dietary supplements available today.*

Spencer, J. W., and J. Jacobs. 2003. *Complementary and Alternative Medicine: An Evidence-Based Approach.* St. Louis, Mo.: Mosby. *Provides background information and the current state of evidence for the efficacy of a wide variety of CAM therapies.*

Whorton, J. C. 2002. *Nature Cures: The History of Alternative Medicine in America.* New York: Oxford University Press. *Provides a history of alternative medicine in the United States, including background information on many CAM therapies.*


### WW Organizations, Hotlines, and Web Sites

*Agency for Healthcare Research and Quality (AHRQ).* Provides practical, evidence-based information on health care treatments and outcomes for consumers and practitioners.
http://www.ahrq.gov

*American Board of Medical Specialties.* Provides information on board certification, including information on specific physicians.
866-275-2267
http://www.abms.org

*American Chiropractic Association.* Provides information on chiropractic care, consumer tips, and a searchable directory of certified chiropractors.
http://www.amerchiro.org

*American Medical Association (AMA).* Provides information about physicians, including their training, licensure, and board certification.
http://www.ama-assn.org

*American Osteopathic Association.* Provides information on osteopathic physicians, including board certification.
800-621-1773
http://www.osteopathic.org

*ConsumerLab.com.* Provides information on the results of tests of dietary supplements, including information on actual ingredients and concentrations.
http://www.consumerlab.com

*Food and Drug Administration: Information for Consumers.* Provides materials on dietary supplements, foods, prescription and OTC drugs, and other FDA-regulated products.
888-INFO-FDA
http://www.fda.gov/opacom/morecons.html

*National Center for Complementary and Alternative Medicine (NCCAM).* Provides general information packets, answers to frequently asked questions about CAM, consumer advice for safer use of CAM, research abstracts, and bibliographies.
888-644-6226
http://nccam.nih.gov

*National Council Against Health Fraud.* Provides news and information about health fraud and quackery and links to related sites.
http://www.ncahf.org

*Quackwatch.* Provides information on health fraud, quackery, and health decision making.
http://www.quackwatch.org

See also the listings for Chapters 2 and 9; the box on dietary supplements in Chapter 9 (p. 222) suggests Web sites with more information on supplements.

## Selected Bibliography


Allais, G., et al. 2002. Acupuncture in the prophylactic treatment of migraine without aura: A comparison with flunarizine. *Headache* 42(9): 855–861.

American Medical Association. 2004. *Health Savings Accounts at a Glance.* Chicago: American Medical Association.

Bell, R. A., R. L. Kravitz, and M. S. Wilkes. 2000. Direct-to-consumer prescription drug advertising, 1989–1998. A content analysis of conditions, targets, inducements, and appeals. *Journal of Family Practice* 49(4): 329–335.

Bordens, K. S., and B. B. Abbott. 2005. *Research Design and Methods: A Process Approach,* 6th ed. New York: McGraw-Hill.

Bren, L. 2004. Study: U.S. generic drugs cost less than Canadian drugs. *FDA Consumer,* July/August.

Brobst, D. E., et al. 2004. Guggulsterone activates multiple nuclear receptors and induces CYP3A gene expression through the pregnane X receptor. *Journal of Pharmacology and Experimental Therapeutics* 310(2): 528–535.

Budetti, P. P. 2004. 10 years beyond the health security act failure: Subsequent developments and persistent problems. *Journal of the American Medical Association* 292(16): 2000–2006.

Centers for Disease Control and Prevention. 2004. Complementary and alternative medicine use among adults: United States, 2002. *Advance Data from Vital and Health Statistics* No. 343. Hyattsville, Md.: National Center for Health Statistics.

Centers for Medicare and Medicaid Services. 2004. *National Health Expenditures and Selected Economic Indicators, Levels and Average Annual Percent Change: Selected Calendar Years 1990–2013* (http://www.cms.hhs.gov/statistics/nhe/projections-2003/t1.asp; retrieved February 23, 2005).

Eisenberg, D. M. 1997. Advising patients who seek alternative medical therapies. *Annals of Internal Medicine* 127: 61–69.

Ernst, E. 2004. Prescribing herbal medications appropriately. *Journal of Family Practice* 53(12): 985–988.

Fontanarosa, P. B., D. Rennie, and C. D. DeAngelis. 2003. The need for regulation of dietary supplements—lessons from ephedra. *Journal of the American Medical Association* 289(12): 1568–1570.

Free rein for drug ads? 2003. *Consumer Reports,* February.

Gan, T. J., et al. 2004. A randomized controlled comparison of electro-acupoint stimulation or ondansetron versus placebo for the prevention of postoperative nausea and vomiting. *Anesthesia and Analgesia* 99(4): 1070–1075.

Gilroy, C. M., et al. 2003. Echinacea and truth in labeling. *Archives of Internal Medicine* 163.

Institute of Medicine, Committee on the Consequences of Uninsurance. 2003. *A Shared Destiny: Community Effects of Uninsurance.* Washington, D.C.: National Academy Press.

Kaiser Family Foundation. 2005. *Trends and Indicators in the Changing Health Care Marketplace.* Menlo Park, Calif.: Kaiser Family Foundation.

Linde, K., et al. 1998. Are the clinical effects of homeopathy placebo effects? A meta-analysis of placebo-controlled trials. *Lancet* 350(9081): 834–843.

Miller, F. G., et al. 2004. Ethical issues concerning research in complementary and alternative medicine. *Journal of the American Medical Association* 291(5): 599–604.

National Center for Health Statistics. 2005. Trends in health insurance and access to medical care for children under age 19 years. *Advance Data from Vital and Health Statistics* No. 355.

National Center for Complementary and Alternative Medicine. 2002. *Are You Considering Complementary and Alternative Therapies?* (http://nccam.nih.gov/health/decisions/index.htm; retrieved February 28, 2005).

Rados, C. 2004. FDA reiterates warning against online drug buying. *FDA Consumer,* September/October.

Rosenthal, M. B., et al. 2002. Promotion of prescription drugs to consumers. *New England Journal of Medicine* 346(7): 498–505.

Saper, R. B., et al. 2004. Heavy metal content of ayurvedic herbal medicine products. *Journal of the American Medical Association* 292(23): 2868–2873.

Solomon, P. R., et al. 2002. Ginkgo for memory enhancement: A randomized controlled trial. *Journal of the American Medical Association* 288(7): 835–840.

The uninsured: Americans at risk. 2004. *Consumer Reports,* January.

Taseng, C., et al. 2004. Cost-lowering strategies used by Medicare beneficiaries who exceed drug benefit caps and have a gap in drug coverage. *Journal of the American Medical Association* 292(8): 952–960.

Weissman, J. S., et al. 2003. *Health Affairs: Forum on Prescription Drug Promotion* (http://www.healthaffairs.org/WebExclusives/Pharma_Web_Excl_022603.htm; retrieved March 18, 2003).

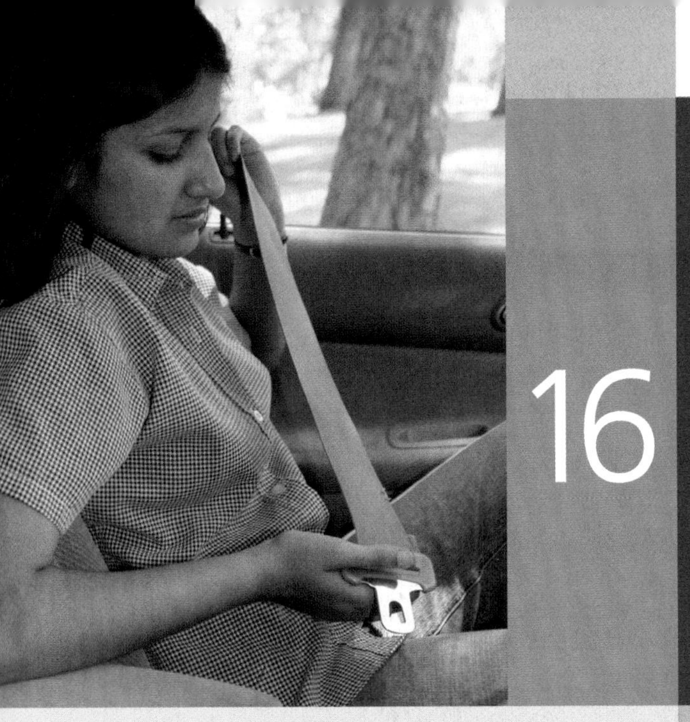

16

## Looking AHEAD

After reading this chapter, you should be able to

- List the most common types of unintentional injuries and strategies for preventing them
- Describe factors that contribute to violence and intentional injuries
- Discuss different forms of violence and how to protect yourself from intentional injuries
- List strategies for helping others in an emergency situation

# Personal Safety: Protecting Yourself from Unintentional Injuries and Violence

Each year, about 150,000 Americans die from injuries, and many more are disabled. An **intentional injury** is one that is purposely inflicted, by either oneself or another person; examples are homicide, suicide, and assault. If an injury occurs when no harm is intended, it is considered an **unintentional injury.** Motor vehicle crashes, falls, and fires often result in unintentional injuries. (Public health officials prefer not to use the word *accidents* to describe unintentional injuries because it suggests events beyond human control. *Injuries* are predictable outcomes of factors that can be controlled or prevented.) Although Americans tend to express more concern about intentional injuries, unintentional injuries are actually more common. The following occur on an average day in the United States:

- 45 homicides
- 85 suicides
- 280 deaths from unintentional injuries
- 1500 suicide attempts
- 20,000 interpersonal assaults
- 55,000 disabling injuries

Unintentional injuries are the fifth leading cause of death among all Americans and the leading cause of death and disability among children and young adults. Heart disease, cancer, stroke, and chronic lower respiratory diseases are responsible for more deaths each year than injuries, but because unintentional injuries are so common among people, they account for more **years of potential life lost** than any other cause of death. Suicide and homicide rank

### Terms

**intentional injury** An injury that is purposely inflicted, by either oneself or another person.

**unintentional injury** An injury that occurs without harm being intended.

**years of potential life lost** The difference between an individual's life expectancy and his or her age at death.

VW

VW Visit the *Core Concepts in Health* Online Learning Center (www.mhhe.com/inselbrief10e) for study aids and many additional resources.

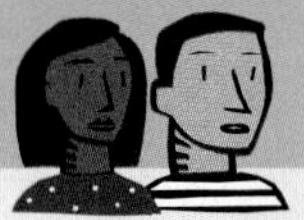

Gender Matters

## Injuries Among Young Men

Overall, rates of injury are highest among young adults and seniors over age 85. Except among the oldest group of adults, the nonfatal injury rate is substantially higher in males than in females—and it peaks among young adult males (Figure 1). Males also significantly outnumber females in injury deaths—whether unintentional or intentional (Figure 2).

Why do men, especially young men, have such high rates of injury? Gender roles may play a key role: Traditional gender roles for males may associate masculinity with risk-taking behavior and a disregard for pain and injury, and risk-taking behavior may be particularly common among young men. Men are more likely to drive dangerously, drink and drive, binge drink, and use aggressive behavior to control situations—all of which can lead to higher rates of fatal and nonfatal injury. Men may also have a lower perception of risk of dangerous behaviors compared with women.

Traditional gender roles may also make it more difficult for men to admit to injury or emotional vulnerability. Physical injuries may worsen or become chronic if care is not sought promptly. Untreated depression can lead to suicide.

In addition, men may have greater exposure to some injury situations. Compared with women, men may drive more miles, have greater access to firearms, and be more likely to ride motorcycles, operate machinery, and have jobs associated with high rates of workplace injuries. They may be more likely to be engage in sports and other recreational activities associated with high rates of injuries. Greater access and use of firearms plays a role in higher rates of deaths among men from assault and suicide; as described in Chapter 3, women are more likely than men to attempt suicide, but men are much more likely to succeed, primarily because they are more likely to use firearms.

Some researchers suggest that the male hormone testosterone may play a role in risky and aggressive behavior. Differences in brain structure and activity may also influence how men and women respond to stressors and how quickly and to what degree they become verbally or physical aggressive in response to anger.

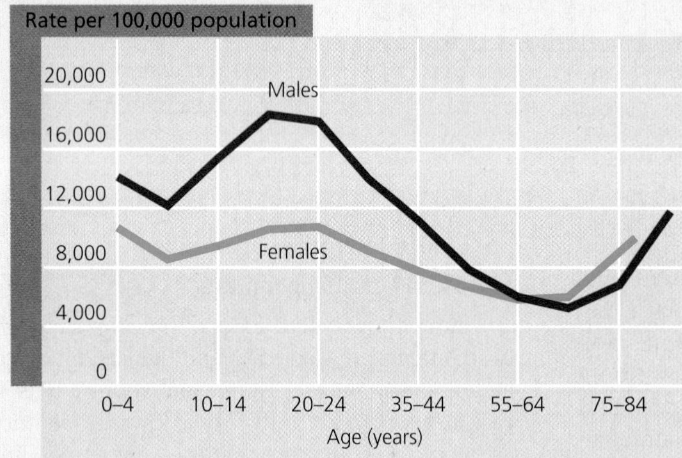


**Figure 1** Nonfatal injury rate by age and sex

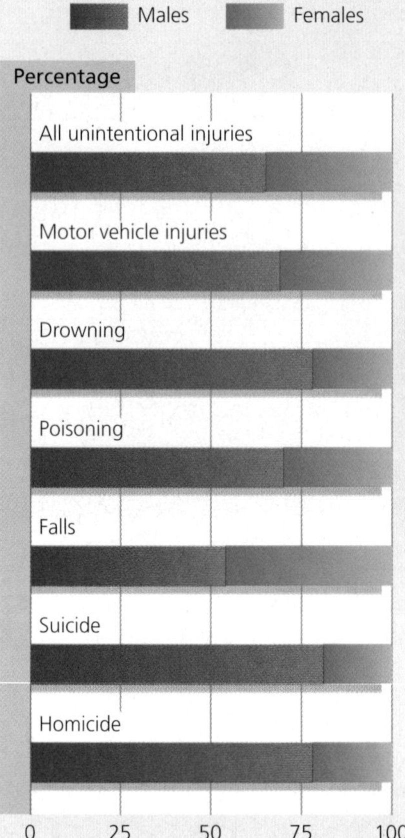


**Figure 2** Injury deaths: Percentage of victims by sex

Further studies are needed to identify all the factors underlying excessive risk-taking among men and how these risk behaviors can be changed to lower the rates of fatal and nonfatal injury among men.

SOURCES: Centers for Disease Control and Prevention. 2004. Surveillance for fatal and nonfatal injuries—United States, 2001. *MMWR Surveillance Summaries* 53(SS7): 1–57; World Health Organization. 2002. *Gender and Road Traffic Injuries*. Geneva: World Health Organization; Courtenay, W. 1998. College men's health: An overview and a call to action. *Journal of American College Health* 46(6): 279–290.

eleventh and sixteenth respectively on the list of leading causes of death among Americans; because they often affect young people, they also account for many years of potential life lost. Injuries affect all segments of the population, but they are particularly common among men, minorities, and people with low incomes, primarily due to social, environmental, and economic factors (see the box "Injuries Among Young Men").

## UNINTENTIONAL INJURIES

Injury situations are generally categorized into four general classes, based on where they occur: motor vehicle injuries, home injuries, leisure injuries, and work injuries (Table 16-1). In all of these arenas, the action you take can mean the difference between injury or death and no injury at all.

VITAL STATISTICS

**Table 16-1 Unintentional Injuries in the United States**

| | Deaths | Disabling Injuries |
|---|---|---|
| Motor vehicle | 44,800 | 2,400,000 |
| Home | 33,100 | 7,900,000 |
| Leisure | 21,300 | 7,100,000 |
| Work | 4,500 | 3,400,000 |
| All classes* | 101,500 | 20,700,000 |

*Deaths and injuries for the four separate classes total more than the "All classes" figures because of rounding and because some deaths and injuries are included in more than one class.

SOURCE: National Safety Council. 2004. *Injury Facts, 2004 Edition.* Itasca, Ill.: National Safety Council.

## Motor Vehicle Injuries

Motor vehicle crashes are the leading cause of death for Americans between the ages of 1 and 34. Worldwide, motor vehicle crashes kill 1.2 million and injure up to 50 million people each year, making motor vehicle injuries the eleventh leading cause of death overall. **Motor vehicle injuries** also result in the majority of cases of paralysis due to spinal injuries, and they are the leading cause of severe brain injury in the United States.

**Factors Contributing to Motor Vehicle Injuries** Common causes of motor vehicle injuries are speeding, aggressive driving, fatigue, inexperience, cell phones and other distractions, the use of alcohol and other drugs, and the incorrect use of safety belts and other safety devices.

**SPEEDING** Nearly 60% of all motor vehicle crashes are caused by bad driving, especially speeding. As speed increases, momentum and the force of impact increase, and the time allowed for the driver to react (reaction time) decreases. Speed limits are posted to establish the safest maximum speed limit for a given area under ideal conditions; if visibility is limited or the road is wet, the safe maximum speed may be considerably lower.

**AGGRESSIVE DRIVING** Speeding is also a hallmark of aggressive drivers—those who operate a motor vehicle in an unsafe and hostile manner. Other characteristics of aggressive driving include frequent, erratic, and abrupt lane changes; tailgating; running red lights or stop signs; passing on the shoulder; and blocking other cars trying to change lanes or pass. Aggressive drivers increase the risk of crashes for themselves and others; injuries may also occur if aggressive drivers stop their vehicles and confront each other following an incident.

**FATIGUE AND SLEEPINESS** Driving requires mental alertness and attentiveness. Studies have shown that sleepiness causes slower reaction time, reduced coordination and vigilance, and delayed information processing. Research shows that even mild sleep deprivation causes a deterioration in driving ability comparable to that caused by a 0.05% blood alcohol concentration—a level considered hazardous when driving.

**CELL PHONES AND OTHER DISTRACTIONS** Anything that distracts a driver—a bad mood, pets or children in the car—can increase the risk of a motor vehicle injury. Several common causes of crashes, including failing to yield and disregarding traffic signals, have been linked to driver distraction, and it is estimated that distraction is a contributing factor in 25–50% of all crashes. As the use of cell phones has spread, their potential to distract drivers has been recognized (see the box "Cellular Phones and Distracted Driving" on p. 396).

**ALCOHOL AND OTHER DRUGS** Alcohol is involved in about 40% of all fatal crashes. Alcohol-impaired driving is illegal in all states; the legal limit for blood alcohol concentration (BAC) is 0.08%, but people are impaired at much lower BACs. The combination of fatigue and alcohol use increases the risk even further. Because alcohol affects reason and judgment as well as the ability to make fast, accurate, and coordinated movements, a person who has been drinking will be less likely to recognize that he or she is impaired. Use of many over-the-counter and all psychoactive drugs is potentially dangerous if you plan to drive.

**SAFETY BELTS, AIR BAGS, AND CHILD SAFETY SEATS** Although some type of mandatory safety belt law is in effect in 49 states (excluding New Hampshire) and the District of Columbia, only about 80% of motor vehicle occupants use safety belts even though they are the single most effective way to reduce the risk of crash-related death. If you wear a combination lap and shoulder belt, your chances of surviving a crash are three to four times better than those of a person who doesn't wear one. And ask others in the vehicle to buckle up; unrestrained passengers increase the risk of injury and death to others in the car should a crash occur.

Some people think that if they are involved in a crash they are better off being thrown free of their vehicle. In fact, the chances of being killed are 25 times greater if you are thrown from a vehicle. Safety belts also provide protection from the "second collision." If a car is traveling

**Term**

**motor vehicle injuries** Unintentional injuries and deaths involving motor vehicles in motion, both on and off the highway or street; incidents causing motor vehicle injuries include collisions between vehicles and collisions with objects or pedestrians.

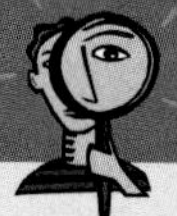

## In Focus: Cellular Phones and Distracted Driving

At any given moment, nearly 8% of drivers—about 1 in 12—are talking on a cell phone. In 2001, New York became the first state to ban the use of handheld cellular phones while driving; drivers there must use hand-free equipment or face fines of up to $100. In 2004, New Jersey and the District of Columbia passed similar bans, and many other states have bans under consideration. Around the world, many countries have laws against the use of handheld cell phones while driving.

Available evidence indicates that use of a cell phone while driving can increase the risk of motor vehicle crashes. In a study using a driver-training simulator, cell phone users were about 20% slower to respond to sudden hazards than were other drivers, and they were about twice as likely to rear-end a braking car in front of them. Among young adult drivers who used a cell phone, reaction time was reduced to the level of a 70-year-old driver who was not using a phone. Another study found a fourfold increase in the risk of collision among motorists who talk on the phone while driving. It is unclear, however, if bans such as those in New York will help reduce the risk: Studies have not found much, if any, benefit in the use of headsets. It appears that the mental distraction of talking is a factor in crashes rather than that one hand is holding the phone.

The safest strategy is not to use your phone while driving. For people who live in areas where cell phone use is legal while driving and who choose to use a phone, the following strategies may help increase safety:

- Be very familiar with your phone and its functions, especially speed dial and redial.
- Store frequently called numbers on speed dial so you can place calls without looking at the phone.
- Use a hands-free device so that you can keep both hands on the steering wheel.
- Let the person you are speaking to know you are driving and be prepared to end the call at any time.
- Don't place or answer calls in heavy traffic or hazardous weather conditions.
- Don't take notes or look up phone numbers while driving.
- Time calls so that you can place them when you are at a stop.
- Never engage in stressful or emotional conversations while on the road. If you are discussing a complicated or emotional matter, pull over to the side of the road or into a parking lot to complete your conversation.

Remember that, as a driver, your primary obligation is to pay attention to the road—for your own safety and the safety of others.

SOURCES: National Traffic Safety Administration. 2005. *Traffic Safety Facts Research Note: Driver Cell Phone Use in 2004—Overall Results.* Washington, D.C.: National Traffic Safety Administration; Strayer, D. L., and F. A. Drews. 2004. Profiles in driver distraction: Effects of cell phone conversations on younger and older drivers. *Human Factors* 46(4): 640–649; World of Wireless Communications. 2000. *Consumer Resources: Driving Safety Tips* (http://www.wow com/consumer/driving/safetyold.cfm; retrieved December 16, 2000); Redelmeier, D. A., and R. J. Tibshirani. 1997. Association between cellular-telephone calls and motor vehicle collisions. *New England Journal of Medicine* 336(7): 453–458.

at 65 mph and hits another vehicle, the car stops first; then the occupants stop because they are traveling at the same speed. The second collision occurs when the occupants of the car hit something inside the car, such as the steering column, dashboard, or windshield. The safety belt stops the second collision from occurring and spreads the stopping force of the collision over the body.

Since 1998, all new cars have been equipped with dual air bags—one for the driver and one for the front passenger. Many vehicles also offer optional side air bags, which further reduce the risk of injury. Although air bags provide supplementary protection in the event of a collision, most are useful only in head-on collisions. They also deflate immediately after inflating and therefore do not provide protection in collisions involving multiple impacts. Air bags are not a replacement for safety belts; everyone in a vehicle should buckle up.

Air bags deploy forcefully and can injure a child or short adult who is improperly restrained or sitting too close to the dashboard. To ensure that air bags work safely, always follow these basic guidelines: Place infants in rear-facing infant seats in the back seat, transport children age 12 and under in the back seat, always use safety belts or appropriate safety seats, and keep 10 inches between the air bag cover and the breastbone of the driver or passenger. If necessary, adjust the steering wheel or use seat cushions to ensure that an inflating air bag will hit a person in the chest and not in the face. Children who have outgrown child safety seats but are still too small for adult safety belts alone (usually age 4–8) should be secured using booster seats that ensure that the safety belt is positioned low across the waist.

In the rare event that a person cannot comply with air bag guidelines, permission to install an on-off switch that temporarily disables the air bag can be applied for from the National Highway Traffic Safety Administration (NHTSA). Air bags currently prevent far more injuries than they cause and are expected to save at least 3200 lives each year once they are installed in all vehicles.

**Preventing Motor Vehicle Injuries** About 75% of all motor vehicle collisions occur within 25 miles of home and at speeds lower than 40 mph. Strategies for preventing motor vehicle injuries include the following:

- Obey the speed limit. If you have to speed to get somewhere on time, you're not allowing enough time.
- Always wear a safety belt. Fasten the lap belt, even if the vehicle has automatic shoulder belts. The shoulder strap should cross the collarbone, and the lap belt should fit low and snug across the hips and pelvic area. Pregnant women should position the lap belt as low as possible on the pelvic area.
- Never drive under the influence of alcohol or other drugs. Never ride with a driver who has been drinking or using drugs.
- Keep your car in good working order. Regularly inspect the tires, oil and fluid levels, windshield wipers, spare tire, and so on.
- Always allow enough following distance. Use the "3-second rule": When the vehicle ahead passes a reference point, count out 3 seconds. If you pass the reference point before you finish counting, drop back and allow more following distance.
- Always increase your following distance and slow down if weather or road conditions are poor.
- Choose interstate highways rather than rural roads. Highways are much safer because of better visibility, wider lanes, fewer surprises, and other factors.
- Always signal when turning or changing lanes.
- Stop completely at stop signs. Follow all traffic laws.
- Take special care at intersections. Always look left, right, and then left again. Make sure you have plenty of time to complete your maneuver in the intersection.
- Don't pass on two-lane roads unless you're in a designated passing area and have a clear view ahead.
- Children under the age of 12 should ride in the back seat of a motor vehicle. Young children and infants should ride in approved child safety seats or booster seats appropriate for their age and size.

**Motorcycles and Mopeds** About one out of every ten traffic fatalities among people age 15–34 involves someone riding a motorcycle. Injuries from motorcycle collisions are generally more severe than those involving automobiles because motorcycles provide little, if any, protection. Moped riders face additional challenges. Mopeds usually have a maximum speed of 30–35 mph and have less power for maneuverability, especially in an emergency. Strategies for preventing motorcycle and moped injuries include the following:

- Maximize your visibility by wearing light-colored clothing, driving with your headlights on, and correctly positioning yourself in traffic.
- Develop the necessary skills. Lack of skill, especially when evasive action is needed to avoid a collision, is a major factor in motorcycle and moped injuries. Skidding from improper braking is the most common cause of loss of control.
- Wear a helmet. Helmets should be marked with the symbol DOT, certifying that they conform to federal safety standards established by the Department of Transportation. Helmet use is required by law in nearly half of the states.
- Protect your eyes with goggles, a face shield, or a windshield.
- Drive defensively, particularly when changing lanes and at intersections, and never assume that you've been seen by other drivers.

**Bicycles** Injuries to bicyclists and pedestrians are considered motor-vehicle-related because they are usually caused by motor vehicles. Bicycle injuries result primarily from riders not knowing or understanding the rules of the road, failing to follow traffic laws, not having sufficient skill or experience to handle traffic conditions, or being intoxicated. Bicycles are considered vehicles; bicyclists must obey all traffic laws that apply to automobile drivers, including stopping at traffic lights and stop signs.

Head injuries are involved in about two-thirds of all bicycle-related deaths. Wearing a helmet reduces the risk of head injury by 85%, but fewer than 50% of cyclists wear helmets (see the box "Choosing a Bicycle Helmet" on p. 398). Safe cycling strategies include the following:

- Wear safety equipment, including a helmet, eye protection, gloves, and proper footwear. Secure the bottom of your pant legs with clips, and secure your shoelaces so they don't get tangled in the chain.
- Maximize your visibility by wearing light-colored, reflective clothing. Equip your bike with reflectors, and use lights, especially at night or when riding in wooded or other dark areas.
- Ride with the flow of traffic, not against it, and follow all traffic laws. Use bike paths when they are available.
- Ride defensively; never assume that drivers have seen you. Be especially careful when turning or crossing at corners and intersections. Watch for cars turning right.
- Stop at all traffic lights and stop signs. Know and use hand signals.
- Continue pedaling at all times when moving (no coasting) to help keep the bike stable and to maintain your balance.
- Properly maintain the working condition of your bicycle.

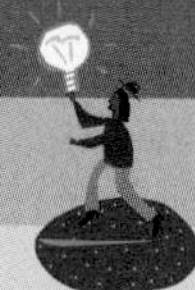

Critical Consumer

## Choosing a Bicycle Helmet

Wearing a bicycle helmet can help you avoid serious head injury, brain damage, or even death in the event of a collision or fall. Helmets have a layer of stiff foam, which absorbs shock and cushions a blow to your head, covered by a thin plastic shell that will "skid" along the ground. For maximum protection, it's important to select a correctly fitting helmet. When you go shopping, remember the four S's: size, strap, straight, and sticker.

- *Size:* Try on several different sizes before making your selection; it may take several tries before you find the most comfortable fit. The helmet should be very snug but not overly tight on your head. Pads are usually provided to help adjust the fit. A good salesperson can also help you get the right fit. When the helmet is strapped onto your head, it should not move more than an inch in any direction, and you should not be able to pull or twist it off no matter how hard you try.
- *Strap:* Be sure that the chin strap fits snugly under your chin and that the V in the strap meets under your ear; avoid thin straps. Check to be sure that the buckle is strong and won't pop open and that the straps are sturdy.
- *Straight:* The helmet should sit straight on your head, not tilted back or forward (see the figure). A rule of thumb is that the rim should be about two finger widths above your eyebrows (depending on the height of your forehead).
- *Sticker:* Since March 1999, helmets sold in the United States must meet uniform safety standards established by the U.S. Consumer Product Safety Commission (CPSC). Look for a sticker or label that says the helmet meets the CPSC standard. If a helmet does not have one, it does not meet federal safety standards and should not be used.

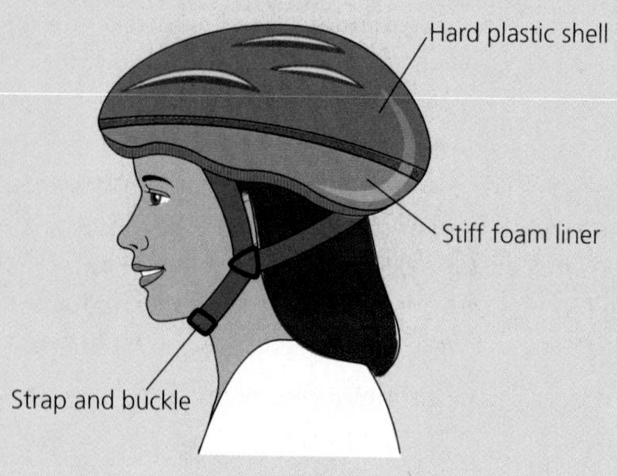


You are more likely to wear your helmet if it is comfortable, so be sure that vents on the helmet provide airflow to promote cooling and sweat control. You will be safer with a brightly colored helmet that makes you more visible to drivers, especially in rainy, foggy, or dark conditions. Reflective tape will also increase your visibility. Finally, a helmet is a good place to put emergency information (your name, address, and phone number, plus any emergency medical conditions and an emergency contact). Tape change inside the helmet for a phone call.

If you are involved in a crash, replace your helmet. Even if the helmet doesn't have any visible signs of damage, its ability to protect your head may be compromised. As the Bicycle Helmet Safety Institute says, "No one ever complains about the cost of their second bike helmet."

SOURCES: Bicycle Helmet Safety Institute. 2005. *A Consumer's Guide to Bicycle Helmets* (http://www.helmets.org/guide.htm; retrieved March 3, 2005); Bicycle Helmet Safety Institute. 2004. *How to Fit a Bicycle Helmet* (http://www.bhsi.org/fit.htm; retrieved December 10, 2004); National Safety Council. 2000. *Choose the Right Helmet for Your Favorite Summer Sport* (http://www.nsc.org/pubs/fsh/archive/summr00/helmet.htm; retrieved July 26, 2000).

## Home Injuries

A person's place of residence, whether a house, an apartment, a trailer, or a dormitory, is considered home. People spend a great deal of time at home and feel that they are safe and secure there. However, home can be a dangerous place. The most common fatal **home injuries** are the result of falls, fires, poisoning, suffocation, and unintentional shootings.

### Term

**home injuries** Unintentional injuries and deaths that occur in the home and on home premises to occupants, guests, domestic servants, and trespassers; falls, burns, poisonings, suffocations, unintentional shootings, drownings, and electrical shocks are examples.

**Falls** Most deaths occurring from falls involve falling on stairs or steps or from one level to another. Falls also occur on the same level, from tripping, slipping, or stumbling. Alcohol is a contributing factor in many falls. Strategies for preventing falls include the following:

- Install handrails and nonslip applications in the shower and bathtub.
- Keep floors, stairs, and outside areas clear of objects or conditions that could cause slipping or tripping, such as ice, snow, electrical cords, and toys.
- Put a light switch by the door of every room so no one has to walk across a room to turn on a light. Use night lights in bedrooms, halls, stairs, and bathrooms.
- When climbing a ladder, use both hands. Never stand higher than the third step from the top. When using a stepladder, make sure the spreader brace is

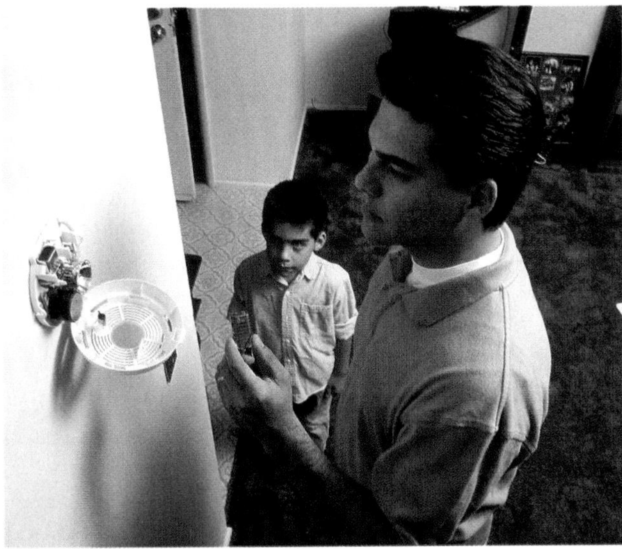

The risk of dying in a fire is reduced by half if you use a smoke detector. Install detectors on every floor, check them monthly, and replace the batteries at least once a year.

in the locked position. With straight ladders, set the base out 1 foot for every 4 feet of height. Don't use chairs to reach things.

- If there are small children in the home, place gates at the top and bottom of stairs. Never leave a baby unattended on a bed or table. Install window guards to prevent children from falling out of windows.

**Fires** A death caused by a residential fire occurs every 2 hours. Cooking is the leading cause of home fire injuries; careless smoking is the leading cause of fire deaths, followed by problems with heating equipment and arson. To prevent fires, it's important to dispose of all cigarettes in ashtrays and to never smoke in bed. Other strategies include proper maintenance of fireplaces, furnaces, heaters, chimneys, and electrical outlets, cords, and appliances. If you use a portable heater, keep it at least 3 feet away from curtains, bedding, or anything else that might catch fire. Never leave heaters on unattended.

It's important to be adequately prepared to handle fire-related situations. Plan at least two escape routes out of each room, and designate a location outside the home as a meeting place. For practice, stage a home fire drill; do it at night, as that's when most deadly fires occur.

Install smoke detectors on every level of your home. Your risk of dying in a fire is almost twice as high if you do not use them. Clean the detectors and check the batteries once a month, and replace the batteries at least once a year. More than 90% of U.S. homes have at least one smoke alarm, but about half are no longer functioning a year after installation, most commonly because batteries need to be replaced or dust and debris need to be cleaned out of the unit.

If a fire does occur, following these strategies can help prevent injuries:

- Get out as quickly as possible, and go to the designated meeting place. Don't stop for a keepsake or a pet. Never hide in a closet or under a bed. Once outside, count heads to see if everyone is out. If you think someone is still inside the burning building, tell the firefighters. Never go back inside a burning building.
- If you're trapped in a room, feel the door. If it is hot or if smoke is coming in through the cracks, don't open it; use the alternative escape route. If you can't get out of a room, go to the window and shout or wave for help.
- Smoke inhalation is the largest cause of death and injury in fires. To avoid inhaling smoke, crawl along the floor away from the heat and smoke. Cover your mouth and nose, ideally with a wet cloth, and take short, shallow breaths.
- If your clothes catch fire, don't run. Drop to the ground, cover your face, and roll back and forth to smother the flames. Remember: stop-drop-roll.

**Poisoning** More than 2.4 million poisonings and over 14,000 poison-related deaths occur every year in the United States. Poisons come in many forms, some of which are not typically considered poisons. For example, medications are safe when used as prescribed, but overdosing and incorrectly combining medications with another substance may result in poisoning. Other poisonous substances in the home include cleaning agents, petroleum-based products, insecticides and herbicides, cosmetics, nail polish and remover, and many houseplants. All potentially poisonous substances should be used only as directed and stored carefully, out of the reach of children.

The most common type of poisoning by gases is carbon monoxide poisoning. Carbon monoxide gas is emitted by motor vehicle exhaust and some types of heating equipment. The effects of exposure to this colorless, odorless gas include headache, blurred vision, and shortness of breath, followed by dizziness, vomiting, and unconsciousness. Carbon monoxide detectors similar to smoke detectors are available for home use. To prevent poisoning by gases, never operate a vehicle in an enclosed space, have your furnace inspected yearly, and use caution with any substance that produces potentially toxic fumes.

A key strategy for preventing serious poisoning injuries is to keep the national poison control hotline number (800-222-1222) in a convenient location. A call to the national hotline will be routed to a local Poison Control Center, which provides expert emergency advice 24 hours a day. If a poisoning does occur, it's important that you act quickly. Remove the poison from contact with the victim's eyes, skin, or mouth, or move the victim away from contact with poisonous gases. Call the Poison Control Center immediately for instructions; do not follow the emergency instructions on product labels because they may be incorrect; do not induce vomiting. If you are advised to go to an emergency room, take the poisonous substance or container with you.

**Suffocation and Choking** Suffocation accounts for about 3500 deaths annually in the United States. Children can suffocate if they put small items in their mouth, get tangled in their crib bedding, or get trapped in airtight appliances like old refrigerators. Keep small objects out of reach of children under age 3, and don't give them raw carrots, hot dogs, popcorn, gum, or hard candy. Examine toys carefully for small parts that could come loose; don't give plastic bags or balloons to small children.

Many choking victims can be saved with the **Heimlich maneuver** (refer to the inside back cover of your text). The American Red Cross recommends the Heimlich maneuver (also called "abdominal thrusts") as the easiest and safest thing to do when an adult is choking. Back blows administered in conjunction with abdominal thrusts are an acceptable procedure for dislodging an object from the throat of an infant.

**Firearms** About 40% of all unintended firearm deaths occur among people age 5–29. People who use firearms should remember the following:

- Never point a loaded gun at something you do not intend to shoot.
- Store unloaded firearms under lock and key, in a place separate from the ammunition.
- Always inspect firearms carefully before handling.
- Behave in the safe and responsible manner advocated in firearms safety courses.

Proper storage is critical. Do not assume that young children cannot fire a gun. About 25% of 3–4-year-olds and 70% of 5–6-year-olds have enough finger strength to pull a trigger. Every year, about 120 Americans are unintentionally shot to death by children under 6. About 8.3 million children live in households with unlocked guns, including 2.6 million who live in households where guns are stored loaded or with ammunition nearby.

Probably the best advice for anyone who picks up a gun is to assume it is loaded. Too many deaths and injuries occur when someone unintentionally shoots a friend while under the impression that the gun he or she is handling is not loaded. If you plan to handle a gun, you should also avoid the use of alcohol and drugs, which affect judgment and coordination. (Firearms and intentional injuries are discussed later in the chapter.)

## Leisure Injuries

Leisure activities encompass a large part of our free time, so it is not surprising that **leisure injuries** are a significant health-related problem in the United States. Specific safety strategies for activities associated with leisure injuries include the following:

- Don't swim alone, in unsupervised places, under the influence of alcohol, or for an unusual length of time; use caution when swimming in unfamiliar surroundings or in water colder than 70°F. Check the depth of water before diving. Make sure that residential pools are fenced and that children are never allowed to swim unsupervised.
- Always use a **personal flotation device** (life jacket) when on a boat.
- For all sports and recreational activities, make sure facilities are safe, follow the rules, and practice good sportsmanship. Develop adequate skill in the activity, and use proper safety equipment, including, where appropriate, a helmet, eye protection, correct footwear, and knee, elbow, and wrist pads.
- If using equipment such as skateboards, snowboards, inline skates, scooters, mountain bikes, or all-terrain vehicles, wear a helmet and other safety equipment, and avoid excessive speeds and unsafe stunts. Playground equipment should be used only for those activities for which it is designed.
- If you are active in excessively hot and humid weather, drink plenty of fluids, rest frequently in the shade, and slow down or stop if you feel uncomfortable. Danger signals of heat stress include excessive perspiration, dizziness, headache, muscle cramps, nausea, weakness, rapid pulse, and disorientation.
- Do not use alcohol or other drugs during recreational activities—such activities require coordination and sound judgment. To avoid choking, don't chew gum or eat while active.

## Work Injuries

Despite improvements, more than 3 million Americans suffer disabling injuries on the job each year, and certain types of **work injuries,** including skin disorders and repetitive strain injuries, are increasing. Although laborers make up less than half of the workforce, they account for more than 75% of all work-related injuries and illnesses. Most fatal occupational injuries involve crushing injuries, severe lacerations, burns, and electrocutions; among women, the leading cause of workplace injury deaths is homicide.

Back problems account for about 25% of work injuries; many of these could be prevented through proper lifting technique (Figure 16-1).

- Avoid bending at the waist. Remain in an upright position and crouch down if you need to lower yourself to grasp the object. Bend at the knees and hips.
- Place feet securely about shoulder-width apart; grip the object firmly.

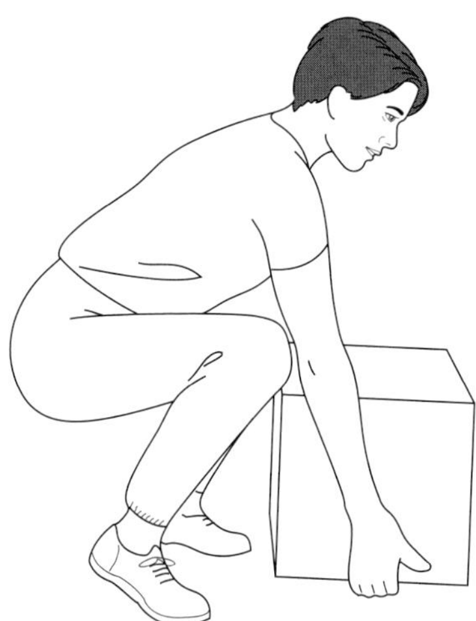

**Figure 16-1 Correct lifting technique.** Stay upright, bending at the knees and hips.

- Lift gradually, with straight arms. Avoid quick, jerky motions. Lift by standing up or pushing with your leg muscles. Keep the object close to your body.
- If you have to turn, change the position of your feet. Twisting is a common and dangerous cause of injury. Plan ahead so that your pathway is clear and turning can be minimized.
- Put the object down gently, reversing the rules for lifting.

Musculoskeletal injuries and disorders in the workplace include **repetitive strain injuries (RSIs).** RSIs are caused by repeated strain on a particular part of the body. Twisting, vibrations, awkward postures, and other stressors may contribute to RSIs. **Carpal tunnel syndrome** is one type of RSI that has increased in recent years due to increased use of computers, both at work and in the home (see the box "Carpal Tunnel Syndrome" on p. 402).

General strategies for preventing work-related injuries include following the safety instructions associated with the job, finding out where first aid equipment is located and knowing how to use it, watching for and reporting safety hazards, and using any safety equipment that is provided by the employer. Whatever the working conditions, employees should make a conscious effort to avoid hazardous situations.

## VIOLENCE AND INTENTIONAL INJURIES

Violence—the use of physical force with the intent to inflict harm, injury, or death upon oneself or another—is a major public health concern in the United States. More than 2 million Americans are victims of violent injury each year; about three violent crimes occur every minute. Worldwide, interpersonal violence is the third leading cause of death among people age 15–44.

In general, the overall U.S. violent crime rate increased between the 1950s and 1970s and then leveled off until the mid-1980s, when it again began to rise until 1992. The rate fell steadily from 1993 to 2000 and then rose slightly in 2001 and 2002—although it remained well below the 1992 rate and declined again in 2003. Possible factors cited for the general decline in violent crime include the aging of the population, reduced unemployment, the decline of the crack cocaine trade, law enforcement strategies to get guns off the street, violence prevention programs for youth, and longer prison sentences. In comparison to other industrialized countries, U.S. rates of violence are abnormally high in only two areas—homicide and firearm-related deaths. The U.S. homicide death rate is four to ten times that of similar countries, and the firearm death rate in the United States exceeds that of other developed countries eightfold.

### Factors Contributing to Violence

Everyone gets angry sometimes, but few people translate their angry and aggressive impulses into action. Most intentional injuries and deaths are associated with an argument or the committing of another crime. However, there are a great many forms of violence, and no single factor can explain all of them.

**Social Factors** Rates of violence are not the same throughout society; they vary by geographic region, neighborhood, socioeconomic level, and many other factors. In the United States, violence is highest in the

### Terms

**Heimlich maneuver** A maneuver developed by Henry J. Heimlich, M.D., to help force an obstruction from the airway.

**leisure injuries** Unintentional injuries and deaths that occur in public places or places used in a public way, not involving motor vehicles; includes most sports and recreation deaths and injuries; falls, drownings, burns, and heat and cold stress are examples.

**personal flotation device** A device designed to save a person from drowning by buoying up the body while in the water; also called a *life jacket.*

**work injuries** Unintentional injuries and deaths that arise out of and in the course of gainful work, such as falls, electrical shocks, exposure to radiation and toxic chemicals, burns, cuts, back sprains, and loss of fingers or other body parts in machines.

**repetitive strain injury (RSI)** A musculoskeletal injury or disorder caused by repeated strain on the hand, arm, wrist, or other part of the body; also called *cumulative trauma disorder (CTD).*

**carpal tunnel syndrome** Compression of the median nerve in the wrist, often caused by repetitive use of the hands, such as in computer use; characterized by numbness, tingling, and pain in the hands and fingers; can cause nerve damage.

In Focus

## Carpal Tunnel Syndrome

Carpal tunnel syndrome (CTS) is a repetitive strain injury characterized by pressure on the median nerve in the wrist. It is the most commonly reported work-related medical problem, accounting for about half of all work-related injuries. Women are about twice as likely as men to be affected by carpal tunnel syndrome.

The median nerve travels from the forearm to the hand through a tunnel in the wrist formed by the wrist bones (carpals) and associated tendons and covered by a ligament. The median nerve can become compressed for a variety of reasons, including swelling of the surrounding tendons caused by pregnancy, diabetes, arthritis, or repetitive wrist motions during activities such as typing, cutting, or carpentry work. Symptoms of CTS include numbness, tingling, burning, and/or aching in the hand, particularly in the thumb and the first three fingers. The pain may worsen at night and may shoot up from the hand as far as the shoulder.

Many cases of carpal tunnel syndrome clear up on their own or with minimal treatment. Modification of the movement that is causing the problem is critically important. For example, adjusting the height of a computer keyboard so that the wrists can be held straight during typing can help relieve pressure on the wrists. CTS is often first treated by immobilizing the wrist with a splint during the night. People may also be given anti-inflammatory drugs or injections of cortisone in the wrist to reduce swelling. In a small percentage of severe cases, surgery to cut the ligament and reduce the pressure on the nerve may be recommended.

If you engage in activities like typing or cutting that involve repetitive motions, there are some strategies you can try to reduce your risk of developing carpal tunnel syndrome. Begin by modifying your work environment to reduce the stress on your wrists. Alternate activities to avoid spending long stretches of time engaged in the same motion. Warm up your wrists before you begin any repetitive motion activity, and take frequent breaks to stretch and flex your wrists and hands:

- Extend your arms out in front of you and stretch your wrists by pointing your fingers to the ceiling; hold for a count of five. Then straighten your wrists and relax your fingers for a count of five.
- With arms extended, make a tight fist with both hands and then bend your wrists so your knuckles are pointed toward the floor; hold for a count of five. Then straighten your wrists and relax your fingers for a count of five.

Repeat these stretches several times, and finish by letting your arms hang loosely at your sides and shaking them gently for several seconds.

SOURCES: Ly-Pen, D., et al. 2005. Surgical decompression versus local steroid injection in carpal tunnel syndrome: A one-year, prospective, randomized, open, controlled clinical trial. *Arthritis and Rheumatism* 52(2): 612–619; Carpal tunnel syndrome. 2002. *Journal of the American Medical Association* 288(10): 1310; American Academy of Orthopaedic Surgeons. 2000. *Exercises to Do at Work to Prevent Carpal Tunnel Syndrome* (http://orthoinfo.aaos.org/fact/thr_report.cfm?Thread_ID=5&topcategory=Hand; retrieved March 11, 2001)

West, followed by the South, and among those who are disadvantaged in some way. Neighborhoods that are disadvantaged in status, power, and economic resources are typically the ones with the most violence. Rates of violence are highest among young people and minorities, groups that have relatively little power. People under age 25 account for nearly half the arrests for violent crime in the United States and about 40% of the arrests for homicide.

People who feel a part of society (have strong family and social ties), who are economically integrated (have a reasonable chance at getting a decent job), and who grow up in areas where there is a feeling of community (good schools, parks, and neighborhoods) are significantly less likely to engage in violence. American society, where more than one-third of all children live in poverty and where the gap between rich and poor keeps growing, should be expected to breed violence.

**Violence in the Media** The mass media play a major role in exposing audiences of all ages to violence as an acceptable and effective means of solving problems. Children may view as many as 10,000 violent acts on television and in movies each year. Computer and video games may also include many violent acts, and the concern is that children's exposure to violence will make them more accepting or tolerant of it. The consequences of violence, on both perpetrator and victim, are shown much less frequently.

A 2005 study linked TV viewing to bullying among children. Researchers found that the more hours per day that a 4-year-old spent watching TV, the more likely the child was to engage in bullying behavior in school in later years. Factors that reduced the rate of bullying included cognitive stimulation, such as parents reading to a child, and emotional support and attention. It is thought that emotional support from parents helps children develop empathy, social competence, and self-regulation—skills that make them better able to deal with peers without resorting to aggressive or bullying behavior.

The role of media violence in violent behavior is an area of controversy. However, it makes sense for parents to be aware of the potential influence of the media on their children. A child may not clearly understand the distinctions between the fantasy world portrayed in the media and the complexities of the real world. Parents should monitor the TV shows, movies, video games, music, and other forms of media to which children are exposed. Watching programs with children gives parents the opportunity to talk to children about violence and its consequences, to explain

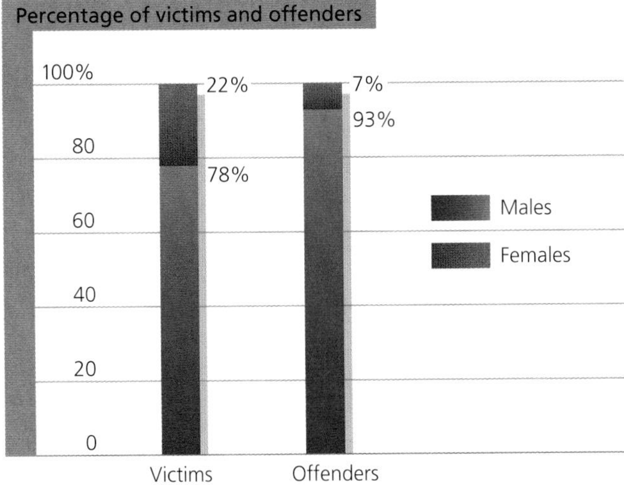

(a) Homicide victims and offenders by sex

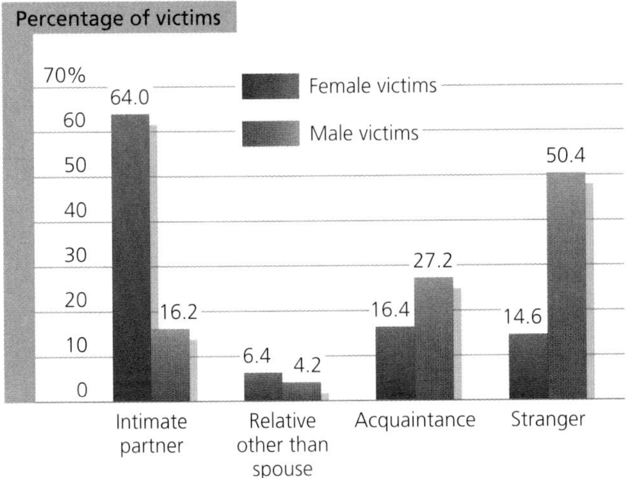

(b) Adult victims of violence by victim-offender relationship and sex of victim

VITAL STATISTICS

**Figure 16-2 Facts about violence in the United States.** SOURCES: Federal Bureau of Investigation. 2004. *Crime in the United States. Uniform Crime Reports, 2003.* Washington, D.C.: U.S. Department of Justice; Tjaden, P., and N. Thoennes. 2000. *Full Report of the Prevalence, Incidence, and Consequences of Violence Against Women.* Washington, D.C.: U.S. Department of Justice.

that violence is not the best way to resolve conflicts or solve problems, and to point out examples of positive behaviors such as kindness and cooperation.

**Gender** In most cases, violence is committed by men (Figure 16-2). Males are more than nine times more likely than females to commit murder, and three times more likely than females to be murdered. Some researchers have suggested that the male hormone testosterone is in some way linked to aggressive behavior. Others point to prevailing cultural attitudes about male roles (men as dominant and controlling) as an explanation for the high rate of violence among men. However, these theories do not explain why it is that violent men are more likely to live in the West, belong to minorities, be poor, and be young.

Women do commit acts of violence, including a small but substantial proportion of murders of spouses. This fact has been used to argue that women have the same capacity to commit violence as men, but most researchers note substantial differences. Men often kill their wives as the culmination of years of violence or after stalking them; they may kill their entire family and themselves at the same time. Women virtually never kill in such circumstances; rather, they kill their husbands after repeated victimization or while being beaten.

**Interpersonal Factors** Although most people fear attack from strangers, the majority of victims are acquainted with their attacker (see Figure 16-2). Approximately 60% of murders of women and 80% of sexual assaults are committed by someone the woman knows. In many cases, the people we need to fear the most live in our own household. Crime victims and violent criminals tend to share many characteristics—that is, they are likely to be young, male, in a minority, and poor.

**Alcohol and Other Drugs** Substance abuse and dependence are consistently associated with interpersonal violence and suicide. Intoxication affects judgment and may increase aggression in some people, causing a small argument to escalate into a serious physical confrontation. On college campuses, alcohol is involved in about 95% of all violent crimes.

**Firearms** Many criminologists feel that the high rate of homicide in the United States is directly related to the fact that we are the only industrialized country in which handguns are widespread and easily available. Simply put, most victims of assaults with other weapons don't die, but the death rate from assault by handgun is extremely high. The possession of a handgun can change a suicide attempt to a completed suicide and a violent assault to a murder. Every hour, guns are used to kill four people in the United States.

Over 100,000 deaths and injuries occur in the United States each year as a result of the use of firearms. Firearms are used in more than two-thirds of homicides, and studies reveal a strong correlation between the incidence of gun ownership and homicide rates for a given area of the country. Over half of all suicides involve a firearm, and people living in households in which guns are kept have a risk of suicide that is five or more times greater than that of people living in households without guns.

## Assault

Assault is the use of physical force by a person or persons to inflict injury or death on another; homicide, aggravated assault, and robbery are examples of assault. The victims of

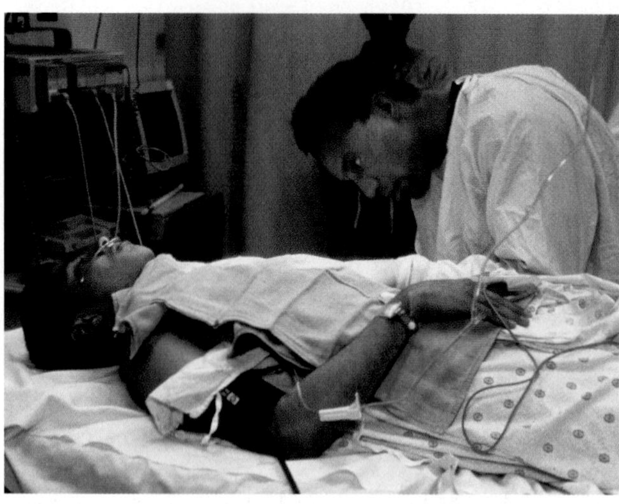

For every violent death that occurs in the United States, there are at least 100 nonfatal injuries caused by violence. The victims of most types of violence are statistically likely to be young (under 25 years), poor, in a minority, urban, and—except for rape and domestic violence—male.

assaultive injuries and their perpetrators tend to resemble one another in terms of ethnicity, educational background, psychological profile, and reliance on weapons. In many cases, the victim actually magnifies the confrontation through the use of a weapon.

## Homicide

Men, teenagers, young adults, and members of minority groups, particularly African Americans and Latinos, are most likely to be murder victims. Among black males, the rate of death from homicide is about six times higher than the rate for the U.S. population as a whole. Poverty and unemployment have been identified as key factors in homicide, and this may account for the high rates of homicide among blacks and other minority groups.

Most homicides are committed with a firearm, occur during an argument, and occur among people who know one another. Intrafamilial homicide, where the perpetrator and victim are related, accounts for about one out of every eight homicides. About 40% of family homicides are committed by spouses, usually following a history of physical and emotional abuse directed at the woman.

## Gang-Related Violence

Gangs are most frequently associated with large cities, but gang activity also extends to the suburbs and even to rural areas. It is estimated that more than 800,000 Americans belong to gangs; the average age for joining a gang is 14. Most gangs control a particular territory and will oppose other gangs, as well as police and community efforts to eliminate them. Gangs may be involved in illegal drug trade, extortion, and "protection" schemes. Gang members are more likely than non–gang members to possess weapons, and violence may result from conflicts over territory or illegal activities.

Gangs are more common in areas that are poor and suffer from high unemployment, population density, and crime. In these areas, an individual may feel that his or her hope of legitimate success in life is out of reach and know that involvement in the drug market makes some gang members rich. Often, gangs serve as a mechanism for companionship, self-esteem, support, and security; indeed, in some areas gang membership may be viewed as the only possible means of survival.

## Hate Crimes

When bias against another person's race or ethnicity, national origin, religion, sexual orientation, or disability motivates a criminal act, the offense is classified as a hate crime. Hate crimes may be committed against people or property. Those against people may include intimidation, assault, and even rape or murder. Crimes against property most frequently involve graffiti, the desecration of churches or synagogues, cross burnings, and other acts of vandalism or property damage.

About 7500 hate crimes are reported every year; many more go unreported. Crimes against people make up about 70% of all incidents; intimidation and assault are the most common offenses. Racial or ethnic bias was cited as the motivating bias in 51% of the hate crimes reported in 2003; national origin was cited in 14% of the cases, religion in 18%, and sexual orientation in 17%. Suspects frequently are not identified, but research indicates that a substantial number of hate crimes are committed by males under age 20. Hate crimes are frequently, but not always, associated with fringe groups that have extremist ideologies, such as the Ku Klux Klan and neo-Nazi groups. The Southern Poverty Law Center tracks more than 700 hate groups and group chapters currently active in the United States; the rapid growth of hate sites on the Internet is another area of concern.

To combat hate crimes, individuals and communities must foster tolerance, understanding, and an appreciation of differences among people.

## School Violence

Tragedies like the shootings at Columbine High School in Colorado and Red Lake Senior High School in Minnesota have brought national attention to the problem of school violence. According to the National School Safety Center, more than 400 school-associated violent deaths of students, faculty, and administrators have occurred since 1992. A majority of these deaths occurred in urban areas and involved use of a firearm; as with other types of violence, both victims and offenders were predominantly young men. Homicide and suicide are the most serious and least common types of violence in schools; an estimated 400,000 less serious incidents of violence and crime occur each year, including theft, vandalism, and fights not involving weapons.

Children are actually much safer at school than away from it. Less than 1% of all homicides among youths age 5–19 occur at school, and 90% of schools report no incidents of serious violence. Children and adolescents are far more likely to be killed by an adult in their own home or away from school than they are to die as a result of school-associated violence. According to the CDC, the overall number of violent incidents has decreased steadily since 1992; however, the number of multiple-victim events may have increased.

Characteristics associated with youths who have caused school-associated violent deaths include a history of uncontrollable angy outbursts, violent and abusive language and behavior, isolation from peers, depression and irritability, access to and preoccupation with weapons, and lack of support and supervision from adults. Being a victim of teasing, bullying, or social exclusion (rejection) may lead to aggressive behavior and violence. Recommendations for reducing school violence include offering classroom training in anger management, social skills, and improved self-control; providing mental health and social services for students in need; developing after-school programs that help students build self-esteem and make friends; and keeping guns out of the hands of children and out of schools.

## Workplace Violence

Each year U.S. workers experience an average of 1.5 million minor assaults, 400,000 serious assaults, 85,000 robberies, 50,000 sexual assaults, and 700 homicides. Police and corrections officers have the most dangerous jobs, followed by taxi drivers, security guards, bartenders, mental health professionals, and workers at gas stations and convenience and liquor stores. Most of the perpetrators of workplace violence are white males over 21 years of age. Firearms are used in more than 80% of workplace homicides, and the majority of these homicides occur during the commission of a robbery or other crime.

General crime prevention strategies, including use of surveillance cameras and silent alarms and limiting the amount of cash on hand, can help reduce workplace violence related to robberies. Clear guidelines about acceptable behavior and prompt action after any threats or incidents of violence can help control violence between acquaintances or coworkers. The OSHA Web site (www.osha.gov/SLTC/workplaceviolence) has violence prevention tips for workers in some of the jobs with high rates of workplace violence.

## Terrorism

In 2001, more Americans died as a result of terrorism than in any prior year; the attacks on September 11 killed more than 3000 people, including citizens of 78 countries. The FBI defines terrorism as the unlawful use of force or violence against persons or property to intimidate or coerce a government, the civilian population, or any segment thereof in furtherance of political or social objectives. Terrorism is one form of what the World Health Organization calls collective violence (see the box "Violence and Health: A Global View"). Terrorism can be either domestic, carried out by groups based in the United States, or international. It comes in many forms, including biological, chemical, nuclear, and cyber. Its intent is to promote helplessness by instilling fear of harm or destruction.

Most of the terrorism-prevention activities occur at the federal, state, and community levels. U.S. government efforts include close work with the diplomatic, law-enforcement, intelligence, economic, and military communities. The mission of the Department of Homeland Security is to help prevent, protect against, and respond to acts of terrorism on U.S. soil. It is coordinating efforts to protect electric and water supply systems, transportation, gas and oil, emergency services, the computer infrastructure, and other systems. The Patriot Act was designed to give law-enforcement agencies additional tools and improved interagency cooperation for the purpose of investigating and preventing terrorism.

One step individuals can take is to put together an emergency plan and kit for their family or household that can serve for any type of emergency or disaster (see the box "Emergency Preparedness" on p. 407). The impact of terrorism can extend beyond the attack itself; refer to Chapters 2 and 3 for advice on coping with the stress of terrorism and mass violence and for guidelines for recognizing and treating post-traumatic stress disorder.

## Family and Intimate Violence

Family violence generally refers to any rough and illegitimate use of physical force, aggression, or verbal abuse by one family member toward another. Such abuse may be physical and/or psychological in nature. Based on reported cases, an estimated 5–7 million women and children are abused each year in the United States.

**Battering** Studies reveal that 95% of domestic violence victims are women. Violence against wives or intimate partners, or battering, occurs at every level of society but is more common at lower socioeconomic levels. It occurs more frequently in relationships with a high degree of conflict—an apparent inability to resolve arguments through negotiation and compromise. About 25% of women report having been physically assaulted or raped by an intimate partner.

At the root of much of this abusive behavior is the need to control another person. Abusive partners are controlling partners. They not only want to have power over another person, but also believe they are entitled to it, no

Dimensions of Diversity

## Violence and Health: A Global View

In 2002, the World Health Organization (WHO) issued its *World Report on Violence and Health,* which examines the magnitude and impact of violence throughout the world. Each year, more than 1.6 million people die from violent acts: Suicide claims a life every 40 seconds, homicide every minute, and armed conflict every 2 minutes. Violence is among the leading causes of death for people age 15–44, accounting for 14% of deaths among males and 7% of deaths among females. Millions more victims of violence survive but are left with physical, psychological, and reproductive problems. Beyond individual misery, violence has devastating social and economic consequences.

### Interpersonal Violence

WHO defines *interpersonal violence* as the intentional use of physical force or power, threatened or actual, against another person that is likely to result in injury, death, psychological harm, or deprivation. Each year, more than 500,000 people die from interpersonal violence, and more than 60 million children and elderly adults are maltreated. It's estimated that 10–70% of women experience physical violence at the hands of an intimate partner during their lifetime; in addition, forced prostitution, child marriage, sexual trafficking, and female genital mutilation are prevalent in some areas of the world.

Worldwide, adolescents and young adults are the primary victims and perpetrators of interpersonal violence. Individual risk factors include being young, male, and poor; being intoxicated; and having easy access to firearms. At the community and social levels, risk factors include low social capital (norms and networks that promote coordination and cooperation), high crime rates, rapid social change, poverty, poor rule of law and corruption, gender inequality, firearm availability, and armed conflict. Rates of violence are particularly high among the poorest sectors of the population in countries with a wide gap between rich and poor.

### Collective Violence

WHO applies the term *collective violence* to violence inflicted by one group against another group to achieve political, economic, or social objectives. Collective violence includes armed conflict within or between states; genocide, repression, and other human rights abuses; terrorism; and organized violent crime. Characteristics of countries with increased risk of violent conflict include long-standing tensions between groups, a lack of democratic processes, unequal access to power, unequal distribution and control of resources, and rapid demographic changes.

In the twentieth century, an estimated 191 million people—well over half of them civilians—lost their lives directly or indirectly as a result of armed conflict, and many more were injured. In some conflicts, civilians were mutilated or raped as part of a deliberate strategy to humiliate and demoralize communities. In addition to directly causing deaths and injuries, collective violence destroys infrastructure and disrupts trade, food production, and vital services, thus setting the stage for famine, increased rates of infectious diseases, and mass movements of refugees. The resulting social turmoil also increases rates of interpersonal violence.

### What Can Be Done?

The WHO report emphasizes that violence is neither an inevitable part of the human condition nor an intractable social problem. Rather, the wide variation in violence within and among nations over time suggests that violence is the product of a complex but modifiable set of social and environmental factors. But only a global response can make the world a safer and healthier place for all. Potential strategies to reduce violence include the following:

- Individual and relationship approaches to encourage healthy attitudes and behaviors, such as training in social, parenting, and relationship skills.
- Community-based efforts to raise public awareness and address local social and material causes of violence, such as creating safe places for children to play and adopting community policing
- Societal approaches to change underlying cultural, social, and economic factors, such as policy changes to reduce poverty and inequality, efforts to change harmful social and cultural norms (for example, ethnic discrimination or gender inequality), and disarmament and demobilization programs in countries emerging from conflict

SOURCES: World Health Organization. 2002. *The World Health Report 2002: Reducing Risks, Promoting Healthy Life*. Geneva: World Health Organization; World Health Organization. 2002. *World Report on Violence and Health*. Geneva: World Health Organization.

matter what the cost to the other person. Abuse includes behavior that physically harms, arouses fear, prevents a person from doing what she wants, or compels her to behave in ways she does not freely choose. Early in a relationship, a person's tendency to be controlling may not be obvious. If you are concerned about whether a person you are dating has the potential to be abusive, review the guidelines in the box "Recognizing the Potential for Abusiveness in a Partner" on page 408.

In abusive relationships, the abuser (in most cases a man) usually has a history of violent behavior, traditional beliefs about gender roles, and problems with alcohol abuse. He has low self-esteem and seeks to raise it by dominating and imposing his will on another person. Research has revealed a three-phase cycle of battering, consisting of a period of increasing tension, a violent explosion and loss of control, and a period of contriteness in which the man begs forgiveness and promises it will never happen again. The batterer is drawn back to this cycle over and over again, but he never succeeds in changing his feelings about himself.

Battered women often stay in violent relationships for years. They may be economically dependent on their

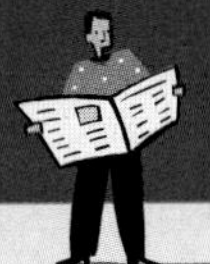

## Emergency Preparedness

Although you usually cannot predict when a disaster situation will occur, there are things you can do to be better prepared.

### Emergency Supplies

Your kit of emergency supplies should include everything you'll need to make it on your own for at least 3 days. You'll need nonperishable food, water, first aid supplies, essential medications, a battery-powered radio, toiletries, clothing, a flashlight or candles and matches, cash, keys, copies of important documents, and supplies for sleeping outdoors in any season/ weather (blankets, sleeping bags, tent, and so on). Don't forget about special-needs items for infants, seniors, and pets.

In the case of certain types of terrorist attacks or industrial disasters, you may need supplies to "shelter in place"—to create a barrier between yourself and any dangerous airborne materials. These supplies might include filter masks or folded cotton towels that can be placed over the mouth and nose. Plastic sheeting and duct tape can be used to seal windows and doors.

You may want to create several kits of emergency supplies. The primary one would contain supplies for home use. Put together a smaller, lightweight version that you can take with you if you are forced to evacuate your residence. Smaller kits for your car and your office are also recommended.

### A Family or Household Plan

You and your family or the members of your household may or may not be together when a disaster strikes. You should have a plan about where to meet and how to communicate. Choose at least two potential meeting places—one in your neighborhood and one or more in other areas. Your community may also have set locations for community shelters.

Where you go may depend on the circumstances of the emergency situation. Use your common sense, and listen to the radio or television to obtain instructions from emergency officials about whether to evacuate or stay in place. In addition, know all the transportation options in the vicinity of your home, school, and workplace; roadways and public transit may be affected, so a sturdy pair of walking shoes is a good item to keep in your emergency kit.

Everyone in the household should also have the same emergency contact person to call, preferably someone who lives outside the immediate area. Local phone service may be significantly disrupted, so long-distance calls may be more likely to go through. Everyone should carry the relevant phone numbers and addresses at all times.

It is also important to check into the emergency plans at any location where you or family members spend time, including schools and workplaces. For each location, know the safest place to be for different types of emergencies—for example, load-bearing interior walls during an earthquake or the basement during a tornado. Also know how to turn off water, gas, and electricity in case of damaged utility lines; keep the needed tools next to the shutoff valves.

Other steps you can take to help prepare for emergencies include taking a first aid class and setting up an emergency response group in your neighborhood or building. More complete information is available from the American Academy of Pediatrics (www.aap.org); the American Red Cross (www.redcross.org); the Federal Emergency Management Agency (www.fema.gov); and the U.S. Department of Homeland Security (www.ready.gov).

SOURCES: U.S. Department of Homeland Security. 2005. *Ready America* (http://www.ready.gov/index.html; retrieved March 4, 2005); Your preparedness guide for any emergency. 2004. *Consumer Reports*, September.

partners, feel trapped or fear retaliation if they leave, believe their children need a father, or have low self-esteem themselves. They may love or pity their husband, or they may believe they'll eventually be able to stop the violence. They usually leave the relationship only when they become determined that the violence must end. Battered women's shelters offer physical protection, counseling, support, and other assistance.

**Stalking and Cyberstalking** Battering is closely associated with **stalking,** characterized by harassing behaviors such as following or spying on a person and making verbal, written, or implied threats. In the United States, it is estimated that 1 million women and 400,000 men are stalked each year; about 87% of stalkers are men. About half of female victims are stalked by current or former intimate partners; of these, 80% had been physically or sexually assaulted by that partner during the relationship. A stalker's goal may be to control or scare the victim or to keep her or him in a relationship. Most stalking episodes last a year or less, but victims may experience social and psychological effects long after the stalking ends.

The use of the Internet, e-mail, chat rooms, and other electronic communications devices to stalk another person is known as **cyberstalking.** As with offline stalking, the majority of cyberstalkers are men, and the majority of victims are women, although there have been same-sex cyberstalking incidents. Cyberstalkers may send harassing or threatening e-mails or chat room messages to the victim, or they may encourage others to harass the victim—for

### Terms

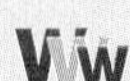

**stalking** Repeatedly harassing or threatening a person through behaviors such as following a person, appearing at a person's residence or workplace, leaving written messages or objects, making harassing phone calls, or vandalizing property; frequently directed at a former intimate partner.

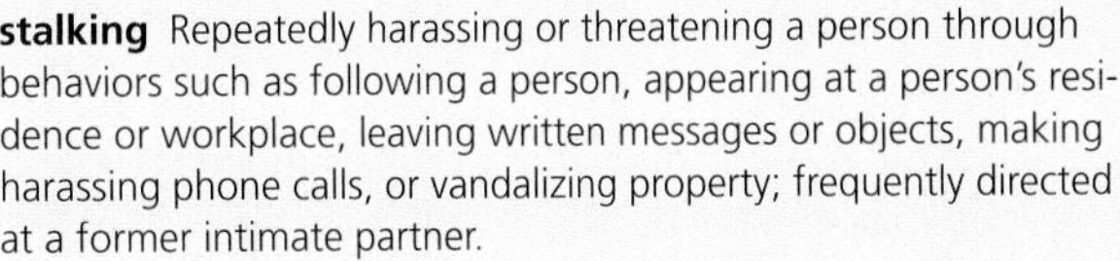

**cyberstalking** The use of e-mail, chat rooms, bulletin boards, or other electronic communications devices to stalk another person.

Take Charge

## Recognizing the Potential for Abusiveness in a Partner

There are no sure ways to tell whether someone will become abusive or violent toward an intimate partner, but there are warning signs that you can look for. (Remember that, although most abusive relationships involve male violence directed at a woman, women can also be abusive, as can partners in a same-sex relationship. Because most abusers are male, the following material refers to the abuser as "he.") If you are concerned that a person you are involved with has the potential for violence, observe his or her behavior, and ask yourself these questions:

- What is this person's attitude toward women? How does he treat his mother and his sister? How does he work with female students, female colleagues, or a female boss? How does he treat your women friends?
- What is his attitude toward your autonomy? Does he respect the work you do and the way you do it? Or does he put it down, tell you how to do it better, or encourage you to give it up? Does he tell you he'll take care of you?
- How self-centered is he? Does he want to spend leisure time on your interests or his? Does he listen to you? Does he remember what you say?
- Is he possessive or jealous? Does he want to spend every minute with you? Does he cross-examine you about things you do when you're not with him?
- What happens when things don't go the way he wants them to? Does he blow up? Does he always have to get his way?
- Is he moody, mocking, critical, or bossy? Do you feel as if you're "walking on eggshells" when you're with him?
- Do you feel you have to avoid arguing with him?
- Does he drink too much or use drugs?
- Does he refuse to use condoms or take other precautions for safer sex?

Listen to your own uneasiness, and stay away from any man who disrespects women, who wants or needs you intensely and exclusively, and who has a knack for getting his own way almost all the time.

If you are in a serious relationship with a controlling person, you may already have experienced abuse. Consider the questions on the following list:

- Does your partner constantly criticize you, blame you for things that are not your fault, or verbally degrade you?
- Does he humiliate you in front of others?
- Is he suspicious or jealous? Does he accuse you of being unfaithful or monitor your mail or phone calls?
- Does he "track" all your time? Does he discourage you from seeing friends and family?
- Does he prevent you from getting or keeping a job or attending school? Does he control your shared resources or restrict your access to money?
- Has he ever pushed, slapped, hit, kicked, bitten, or restrained you? Thrown an object at you? Used a weapon on you?
- Has he ever destroyed or damaged your personal property or sentimental items?
- Has he ever forced you to have sex or to do something sexually you didn't want to do?
- Does he anger easily when drinking or taking drugs?
- Has he ever threatened to harm you or your children, friends, pets, or property?
- Has he ever threatened to blackmail you if you leave?

If you answered yes to one or more of these questions, you may be experiencing domestic abuse. If you believe you or your children are in imminent danger, look in your local telephone directory for a women's shelter, or call 9-1-1. If you want information, referrals to a program in your area, or assistance, contact one of the organizations listed in For More Information at the end of the chapter.

SOURCES: Family Violence Prevention Fund. 1996. *Take Action Against Domestic Violence.* San Francisco, Calif.: Family Violence Prevention Fund; How to tell if you're in an abusive situation. 1994. *San Francisco Chronicle,* 24 June; Jones, A. 1994. *Next Time She'll Be Dead.* Boston: Beacon Press.

example, by impersonating the victim and posting inflammatory messages and personal information on bulletin boards or in chat rooms. Guidelines for staying safe online include the following:

- Never use your real name as an e-mail username or chat room nickname. Select an age- and gender-neutral identity.
- Avoid filling out profiles for accounts related to e-mail use or chat room activities with information that could be used to identify you.
- Do not share personal information in public spaces anywhere online or give it to strangers.
- Learn how to filter unwanted e-mail messages.
- If you do experience harassment online, do not respond to the harasser. Log off or surf elsewhere.

If you receive unwanted online contact, make it clear to that person that you want all contact to stop. If harassment continues, contact the harasser's Internet service provider (ISP) by identifying the domain of the stalker's account (after the "@" sign); most ISPs have an e-mail address for complaints. Often, an ISP can try to stop the conduct by direct contact with the harasser or by closing his or her account. Save all communications for evidence, and contact your ISP and your local police department.

Battering and stalking are related forms of intimate violence, often involving verbal or physical abuse directed at controlling another person. Education, counseling, and support can help the victims of family violence. This college workshop helps people identify the signs of battering and the reasons why people may stay in abusive relationships.

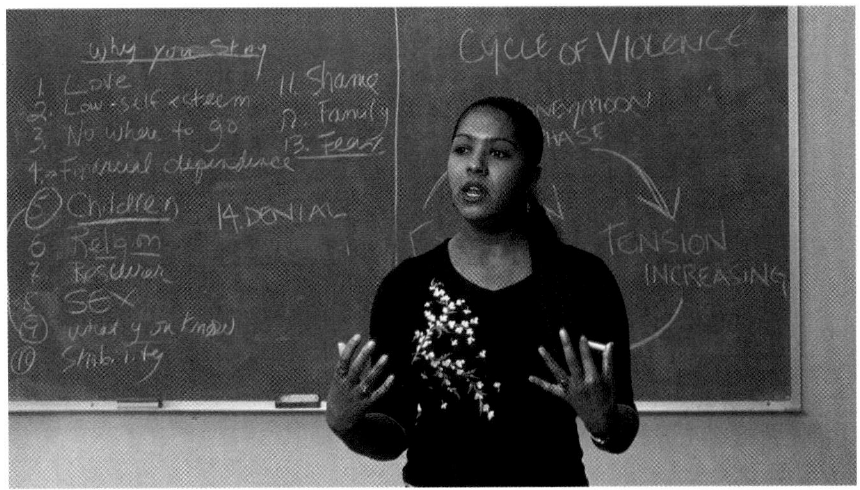


**Violence Against Children** Every year, at least 1 million American children are physically abused by their parents, and another 1 to 2 million are victims of neglect. Parental violence is one of the five leading causes of death for children age 1–18. Parents who abuse children tend to have low self-esteem, to believe in physical punishment, to have a poor marital relationship, and to have been abused themselves (although many people who were abused as children do not grow up to abuse their own children). Poverty, unemployment, and social isolation are characteristics of families in which children are abused. Single parents, both men and women, are at especially high risk for abusing their children. Very often one child, whom the parents consider different in some way, is singled out for violent treatment.

**Elder Abuse** Each year, at least 500,000 older persons are abused; only one in six incidents is reported. Most abusers are family members who are serving as caregivers. Elder abuse can take different forms: physical, sexual, or emotional abuse; financial exploitation; neglect; or abandonment. Neglect is the most common form of abuse, accounting for about 55% of reported cases. Physical abuse accounts for about 15% of reported cases, and financial exploitation for about 13%. Abuse often occurs when caring for a dependent adult becomes too stressful for the caregiver, especially if the elder is incontinent, has suffered mental deterioration, or is violent. Abuse may become an outlet for frustration. Many believe that the solution to elder abuse is support in the form of greater social and financial assistance, such as adult day-care centers and education and public care programs.

## Sexual Violence

The use of force and coercion in sexual relationships is one of the most serious problems in human interactions. The most extreme manifestation of sexual coercion—forcing a person to submit to another's sexual desires—is rape, but sexual coercion occurs in many subtler forms.

**Sexual Assault: Rape** Sexual coercion that relies on the threat and use of physical force or takes advantage of circumstances that render a person incapable of giving consent (such as when drunk) constitutes **sexual assault** or **rape.** When the victim is younger than the legally defined "age of consent," the act constitutes **statutory rape,** whether or not coercion is involved. Coerced sexual activity in which the victim knows or is dating the rapist is often referred to as **date rape** (or acquaintance rape). Most victims know their assailant, but less than one-third of all sexual crimes are reported.

Any woman—or man—can be a rape victim. It is estimated that more than 3.5 million women are raped each year and that 1 in 6 women and 1 in 33 men has experienced an attempted or completed rape at some point in their lives. A study of college students found that between 1 in 4 and 1 in 5 college women experience a completed or attempted rape during their college years. The majority of male victims of rape are not in prison.

WHO COMMITS RAPE? Men who commit rape may be any age and come from any socioeconomic group. Some rapists are exploiters in the sense that they rape on the spur of the moment and mainly want immediate gratification. Some attempt to compensate for feelings of sexual inadequacy and an inability to obtain satisfaction otherwise. Others are more hostile and sadistic and are primarily interested not in sex but in hurting and humiliating a particular woman or women in general.

### Terms

**sexual assault** or rape The use of force to have sex with someone against that person's will.

**statutory rape** Sexual interaction with someone under the legal age of consent.

**date rape** Sexual assault by someone the victim knows or is dating; also called *acquaintance rape.*

Most women are in much less danger of being raped by a stranger than of being sexually assaulted by a man they know or date. Surveys suggest that as many as 25% of women have had experiences in which the men they were dating persisted in trying to force sex despite pleading, crying, screaming, or resisting. Surveys have also found that more than 60% of all rape victims were raped by a current or former spouse, boyfriend, or date.

Most cases of date rape are never reported to the police, partly because of the subtlety of the crime. Usually no weapons are involved, and direct verbal threats may not have been made. Rather than being terrorized, the victim usually is attracted to the man at first. Victims of date rape tend to shoulder much of the responsibility for the incident, questioning their own judgment and behavior rather than blaming the aggressor.

**FACTORS CONTRIBUTING TO DATE RAPE** One factor in date rape appears to be the double standard about appropriate sexual behavior for men and women. Although the general status of women in society has improved, it is still a commonly held cultural belief that nice women don't say yes to sex (even when they want to) and that real men don't take no for an answer.

There are also widespread differences between men and women in how they perceive romantic encounters and signals. In one study, researchers found that men tend to interpret women's actions on dates, such as smiling or talking in a low voice, as indicating an interest in having sex, whereas the women interpreted the same actions as just being "friendly." Men's thinking about forceful sex also tends to be unclear. One psychologist reports that men find "forcing a woman to have sex against her will" more acceptable than "raping a woman," even though the former description is the definition of rape.

**DATE-RAPE DRUGS** Recently there has been an increase in the reported use of "date-rape drugs" other than alcohol. The drugs used in date-rape situations include flunitrazepam (Rohypnol), gamma hydroxybutyrate (GHB), and ketamine hydrochloride ("Special K"). As described in Chapter 7, these drugs have a variety of effects, including sedation and anterograde amnesia, meaning victims have little memory of what happens while they are under the influence of the drug. The Drug-Induced Rape Prevention and Punishment Act of 1996 adds up to 20 years to the prison sentence of any rapist who uses a drug to incapacitate a victim. Strategies such as the following can help ensure that your drink is not tampered with at a bar or party:

- Check with campus or local police to find out if drug-facilitated sexual assault has occurred in your area and, if so, where.
- Drink moderately and responsibly. Avoid group drinking and drinking games.
- Be wary of opened beverages—alcoholic or nonalcoholic—offered by strangers. When at an unfamiliar bar, watch the bartender pour your drink.
- Let your date be the first to drink from the punchbowl at a bar, club, or rave.
- If an opened beverage tastes, looks, or smells strange, do not drink it. If you leave your drink unattended, such as when you dance or use the restroom, obtain a fresh drink when you return to your table.
- If you go to a party, club, or bar, go with friends. Have a prearranged plan for checking on each other visually and verbally. If you feel giddy or lightheaded, get assistance.

Both males and females can take actions that will reduce the incidence of acquaintance rape; see the box "Preventing Date Rape" for specific suggestions.

**DEALING WITH A SEXUAL ASSAULT** Experts disagree about whether a woman who is faced with a rapist should fight back or give in quietly to avoid being injured or to gain time in the hope of escaping. Some rapists say that if a woman had screamed or resisted loudly, they would have run; others report they would have injured or killed her. (If a rapist is carrying a weapon, most experts advise against fighting unless absolutely necessary.) A woman who is raped by a stranger is more likely to be physically injured than a woman raped by someone she knows. Each situation is unique, and a woman should respond in whatever way she thinks best. If a woman chooses not to resist, it does not mean that she has not been raped.

If you are threatened by a rapist and decide to fight back, here is what Women Organized Against Rape (WOAR) recommends:

- Trust your gut feeling. If you feel you are in danger, don't hesitate to run and scream. It is better to feel foolish than to be raped.
- Yell—and keep yelling. It will clear your head and start your adrenaline going; it may scare your attacker and also bring help. Don't forget that a rapist is also afraid of pain and afraid of getting caught.
- If an attacker grabs you from behind, use your elbows for striking his neck, his sides, or his stomach.
- Try kicking. Your legs are the strongest part of your body, and your kick is longer than his reach. Kick with your rear foot and with the toe of your shoe. Aim low to avoid losing your balance.
- His most vulnerable spot is his knee; it's low, difficult to protect, and easily knocked out of place. Don't try to kick a rapist in the crotch; he has been protecting this area all his life and will have better protective reflexes there than at his knees.
- Once you start fighting, keep it up. Your objective is to get away as soon as you can.

Take Charge

## Preventing Date Rape

### Guidelines for Women

- Believe in your right to control what you do. Set limits, and communicate these limits clearly, firmly, and early. Say no when you mean no.
- Be assertive with someone who is sexually pressuring you. Men often interpret passivity as permission.
- If you are unsure of a new acquaintance, go on a group date or double date. If possible, provide your own transportation.
- Remember that some men assume sexy dress and a flirtatious manner mean a desire for sex.
- Remember that alcohol and drugs interfere with clear communication about sex.
- Use the statement that has proven most effective in stopping date rape: "This is rape, and I'm calling the police."

### Guidelines for Men

- Be aware of social pressure. It's OK not to "score."
- Understand that no means no. Don't continue making advances when your date resists or tells you she wants to stop. Remember that she has the right to refuse sex.
- Don't assume sexy dress and a flirtatious manner are invitations to sex, that previous permission for sex applies to the current situation, or that your date's relationships with other men constitute sexual permission for you.
- Remember that alcohol and drugs interfere with clear communication about sex.

- Remember that ordinary rules of behavior don't apply. It's OK to vomit, act "crazy," or claim to have a sexually transmitted disease.

If you are raped, tell what happened to the first friendly person you meet. Call the police, tell them you were raped, and give your location. Try to remember as many facts as you can about your attacker; write down a description as soon as possible. Don't wash or change your clothes, or you may destroy important evidence. The police will take you to a hospital for a complete exam; show the physician any injuries. Tell the police simply, but exactly, what happened. Be honest, and stick to your story.

If you decide that you don't want to report the rape to the police, be sure to see a physician as soon as possible. You need to be checked for pregnancy and STDs.

**THE EFFECTS OF RAPE** Rape victims suffer both physical and psychological injury. For most, physical wounds heal within a few weeks. Psychological pain may endure and be substantial. Even the most physically and mentally strong are likely to experience shock, anxiety, depression, shame, and a host of psychosomatic symptoms after being victimized. These psychological reactions following rape comprise rape trauma syndrome, which is characterized by fear, nightmares, fatigue, crying spells, and digestive upset. (Rape trauma syndrome is a form of post-traumatic stress disorder; see Chapter 3.) Self-blame is very likely; society has contributed to this tendency by perpetuating the myths that women can actually defend themselves and that no one can be raped if she doesn't want to be. Fortunately, these false beliefs are dissolving in the face of evidence to the contrary.

Many organizations offer counseling and support to rape victims. Look in the telephone directory under Rape or Rape Crisis Center for a hotline number to call. Your campus may have counseling services or a support group.

**Child Sexual Abuse** Child sexual abuse is any sexual contact between an adult and a child who is below the legal age of consent. Adults and older adolescents are able to coerce children into sexual activity because of their authority and power over them. Threats, force, or the promise of friendship or material rewards may be used to manipulate a child. Sexual contacts are typically brief and consist of genital manipulation; genital intercourse is much less common. One highly traumatic form of sexual abuse is **incest**, sexual activity between people too closely related to legally marry.

Sexual abusers are usually male, heterosexual, and known to the victim. The abuser may be a relative, a friend, a neighbor, or another trusted adult acquaintance. Child abusers are often pedophiles, people who are sexually attracted to children. They may have poor interpersonal and sexual relationships with other adults and feel socially inadequate and inferior.

Child sexual abuse is often unreported. Surveys suggest that as many as 27% of women and 16% of men were sexually abused as children. An estimated 150,000–200,000 new cases of child sexual abuse occur each year. It can

**Term**

**incest** Sexual activity between close relatives, such as siblings or parents and their children.

Vw

leave lasting scars; victims are more likely to suffer as adults from low self-esteem, depression, anxiety, eating disorders, self-destructive tendencies, sexual problems, and difficulties in intimate relationships.

If you were a victim of sexual abuse as a child and feel it may be interfering with your functioning today, you may want to address the problem. A variety of approaches can help, such as joining a support group of people who have had similar experiences, confiding in a partner or friend, or seeking professional help.

**Sexual Harassment** Unwelcome sexual advances, requests for sexual favors, and other verbal, visual, or physical conduct of a sexual nature constitute **sexual harassment** if such conduct explicitly or implicitly affects academic or employment decisions or evaluations; interferes with an individual's academic or work performance; or creates an intimidating, hostile, or offensive academic, work, or student living environment.

Extreme cases of sexual harassment occur when a manager, professor, or other person in authority uses his or her ability to control or influence jobs or grades to coerce people into having sex or to punish them if they refuse. A hostile environment can be created by conduct such as sexual gestures, displaying of sexually suggestive objects or pictures, derogatory comments and jokes, sexual remarks about clothing or appearance, obscene letters, and unnecessary touching or pinching.

If you have been the victim of sexual harassment, you can take action to stop it. Be assertive with anyone who uses language or actions you find inappropriate. If possible, confront your harasser either in writing, over the telephone, or in person, informing him or her that the situation is unacceptable to you and you want the harassment to stop. Be clear. "Do not *ever* make sexual remarks to me" is an unequivocal statement. If assertive communication doesn't work, assemble a file or log documenting the harassment, noting the details of each incident and information about any witnesses. You may discover others who have been harassed by the same person, which will strengthen your case. Then file a grievance with the harasser's supervisor or employer.

If your attempts to deal with the harassment internally are not successful, you can file an official complaint with your city or state Human Rights Commission or Fair Employment Practices Agency, or with the federal Equal Employment Opportunity Commission. You may also wish to pursue legal action under the Civil Rights Act or under local laws prohibiting employment discrimination. Very often, the threat of a lawsuit or other legal action is enough to stop the harasser.

### What You Can Do About Violence

It is obvious that violence in our society is not disappearing and that it is a serious threat to our collective health and well-being. This is especially true on college campuses, which in a sense are communities in themselves but sometimes lack the authority to tackle the issue of violence directly (see the box "Staying Safe on Campus"). Although government and law enforcement agencies are working to address the problem of violence, individuals must take on a greater responsibility to bring about change.

Reducing gun-related injuries may require changes in the availability, possession, and lethality of the 8–12 million firearms sold in the United States each year. As part of the Brady gun control law, computerized instant background checks are performed for most gun sales to prevent purchases by convicted felons, people with a history of mental instability, and certain other groups. In some states, waiting periods are required in addition to the background checks. Some groups advocate a complete ban on the sale of all handguns.

Safety experts also advocate the adoption of consumer safety standards for guns, including features such as childproofing and indicators to show if a gun is loaded. Technologies are now available to personalize handguns to help prevent unauthorized use. Education about proper storage is also important. Surveys indicate that in about 23% of gun-owning households, the weapon is stored loaded, and in 28% the gun is kept hidden but not locked. To be effective, any approach to firearm injury prevention must have the support of law enforcement and the community as a whole.

## PROVIDING EMERGENCY CARE

A course in **first aid** can help you respond appropriately when someone is injured. One important benefit of first aid training is learning what *not* to do in certain situations. For example, a person with a suspected neck or back injury should not be moved unless other life-threatening conditions exist. A trained person can assess emergency situations accurately before acting.

Emergency rescue techniques can save the lives of people who are choking, who have stopped breathing, or whose hearts have stopped beating. As described earlier, the Heimlich maneuver is used when a victim is choking. Pulmonary resuscitation (also known as rescue breathing, artificial respiration, or mouth-to-mouth resuscitation) is used when a person is not breathing. **Cardiopulmonary resuscitation (CPR)** is used when a pulse cannot be found. Training is required before a person can perform CPR. Courses are offered by the American Red Cross and the American Heart Association. A new feature of some of these courses is training in the use of automatic external defibrillators (AEDs), which monitor the heart's rhythm and, if appropriate, deliver an electrical shock to restart the heart. Because of the importance of early use of defibrillators in saving heart attack victims, these devices are being installed in public places, including casinos and airports.

Take Charge

## Staying Safe on Campus

College campuses can be the site of criminal activity and violence just as any other environment or living situation can be—and so they require the same level of caution and awareness that you would use in other situations. Two key points to remember: 80% of campus crimes are committed by a student against a fellow student, and alcohol or drug use is involved in 90% of campus felonies. Drinking or drug use can affect judgment and lower inhibitions, so be aware if you or another person is under the influence. Here are some suggestions for keeping yourself safe on campus:

- Don't travel alone after dark. Many campuses have shuttle buses that run from spots on campus such as the library and the dining hall to residence halls and other locations. Escorts are often available to walk with you at night.
- Be familiar with well-lit and frequently traveled routes around campus if you do need to walk alone.
- If you have a car, follow the usual precautions about parking in well-lit areas, keeping the doors locked while you are driving, and never picking up hitchhikers.
- Always have your keys ready as you approach your residence hall, room, and car. Don't lend your keys to others.
- Let friends and family members know your schedule of classes and activities to create a sort of buddy system.
- Be sure the doors and windows of your dorm room have sturdy locks, and use them.
- Don't prop open doors or hold doors open for nonstudents or nonresidents trying to enter your dorm. Be aware of nonresidents around your dorm. If someone says that he or she is meeting a friend inside, that person should be able to call the friend from outside the building.
- Keep valuables and anything containing personal information—credit cards, wallets, jewelry, and so on—hidden. Secure expensive computer and stereo equipment with cables so that it can't be easily stolen. Use a quality U-shaped lock whenever you leave a bicycle unattended.
- Be alert when using an ATM, and don't display large amounts of cash.
- Stay alert and trust your instincts. Don't hesitate to call the police or campus security if something doesn't seem or feel right.

The Jeanne Clery Disclosure of Campus Security Policy and Campus Crime Statistics Act, named for a Lehigh University student who was murdered in her residence hall in 1986, requires colleges and universities to collect and report campus crime statistics. You can now review this information online at the Crime Statistics Web site of the U.S. Department of Education's Office of Postsecondary Education (http://ope.ed.gov/security/Search.asp).

SOURCES: Security on Campus, Inc. 2001. *Campus Safety: Tips and Evaluation Brochure* (http://www.campussafety.org/students/tips.html; retrieved December 16, 2002); U.S. Department of Education, Office of Postsecondary Education. 2000. *Campus Security* (http://www.ed.gov/offices/OPE/PPI/security.html; retrieved December 16, 2000).

As a person providing assistance, you are the first link in the **emergency medical services (EMS) system.** Your responsibility may be to render first aid, provide emotional support for the victim, or just call for help. It is important to remain calm and act sensibly. The basic pattern for providing emergency care is check-call-care:

- *Check the situation:* Make sure the scene is safe for both you and the injured person.
- *Check the victim:* Conduct a quick head-to-toe examination. Assess the victim's signs and symptoms, such as level of responsiveness, pulse, and breathing rate. Look for bleeding and any indications of broken bones or paralysis.
- *Call for help:* Call 9-1-1 or a local emergency number. Identify yourself and give as much information as you can about the condition of the victim and what happened.
- *Care for the victim:* If the situation requires immediate action (no pulse, shock, etc.), provide first aid if you are trained to do so.

Like other kinds of behavior, preventing injuries and acting safely involve choices you make every day. You can motivate yourself to act in the safest way possible by increasing your knowledge and level of awareness,

### Terms

V w

**sexual harassment** Unwelcome sexual advances, requests for sexual favors, and other conduct of a sexual nature that affects academic or employment decisions or evaluations; interferes with an individual's academic or work performance; or creates an intimidating, hostile, or offensive academic, work, or student living environment.

**first aid** Emergency care given to an ill or injured person until medical care can be obtained.

**cardiopulmonary resuscitation (CPR)** An emergency first aid procedure that combines artificial respiration and artificial circulation; used in first aid emergencies where breathing and blood circulation have stopped.

**emergency medical services (EMS) system** A system designed to network community resources for providing emergency care.

by examining your attitudes to see if they're realistic, by knowing your capacities and limitations, by adjusting your responses when environmental hazards exist, and, in general, by taking responsibility for your actions. You can't eliminate all risks and dangers from your life—no one can do that—but you can improve your chances of avoiding injuries and living to a healthy, ripe old age.

**Tips for Today**

Although people worry about violence, unintentional injuries—such as those resulting from car crashes, falls, and fires—are much more common. In fact, unintentional injuries are the leading cause of death for people under the age of 35. To protect yourself from injuries, learn to incorporate sensible safety precautions into your daily life.

*Right now you can*

- Pick up anything on the floor of your home that could cause tripping or slipping.
- Make sure the electrical outlets in your home are not overloaded and that extension cords do not run under rugs or where people walk.
- Test the batteries in the smoke detectors in your home and replace them if they aren't working.
- Check your bike helmet to make sure it fits properly and meets the requirements described in the box "Choosing a Bicycle Helmet." Wear it the next time you go for a ride.

## SUMMARY

- Key factors in motor vehicle injuries include aggressive driving, speeding, a failure to wear safety belts, alcohol and drug intoxication, fatigue, and distraction.
- Motorcycle, moped, and bicycle injuries can be prevented by developing appropriate skills, driving or riding defensively, and wearing proper safety equipment.
- Most fall-related injuries are a result of falls at floor level, but stairs, chairs, and ladders are also involved in a significant number of falls.
- Careless smoking and problems with cooking or heating equipment are common causes of home fires. Being prepared for fire emergencies means planning escape routes and installing smoke detectors.
- The home can contain many poisonous substances, including medications, cleaning agents, plants, and fumes from cars and appliances.
- Performing the Heimlich maneuver can prevent someone from dying from choking.
- The proper storage and handling of firearms can help prevent injuries; assume that a gun is loaded.
- Many injuries during leisure activities result from the misuse of equipment, lack of experience, use of alcohol, and a failure to wear proper safety equipment.
- Most work-related injuries involve extensive manual labor; back problems are most common. Newer problems include repetitive strain injuries.
- Factors contributing to violence include poverty, the absence of strong social ties, the influence of the mass media, cultural attitudes about gender roles, problems in interpersonal relationships, alcohol and drug abuse, and the availability of firearms.
- Types of violence include assault, homicide, gang-related violence, hate crimes, school violence, workplace violence, and terrorism.
- Battering and child abuse occur at every socioeconomic level. The core issue is the abuser's need to control other people.
- Most rape victims are women, and most know their attackers. Factors in date rape include different standards of appropriate sexual behavior for men and women and different perceptions of actions.
- Sexual harassment is unwelcome sexual advances or other conduct of a sexual nature that affects academic or employment performance or evaluations or that creates an intimidating, hostile, or offensive academic, work, or student living environment.
- Steps in giving emergency care include making sure the scene is safe for you and the injured person, conducting a quick examination of the victim, calling for help, and providing emergency first aid.

## Take Action

1. **Take a course:** Contact the American Red Cross or American Heart Association in your area, and ask about first aid and CPR classes. These courses are usually given frequently and at a variety of times and locations. They can be invaluable in saving lives. Consider taking one or both of the courses.

2. **Investigate local resources:** Find out what resources are available on your campus or in your community for victims of rape, hate crimes, or other types of violence. Does your campus sponsor any violence prevention programs or activities? If so, consider participating in one.

3. **Prepare for a fire:** Contact your local fire department and obtain a checklist for fire safety procedures. What would you do if a fire started in your home? What types of evacuation procedures would be necessary? Carry out a practice fire drill at home to see what problems might arise in a real emergency.

## Behavior Change Strategy

### Adopting Safer Habits

For the next 7–10 days, keep track of any mishaps you are involved in or injuries you receive, recording them on a daily behavior record like the one shown in Chapter 1. Count each time you cut, burn, or injure yourself, fall down, run into someone, or have any other potentially injury-causing mishap, no matter how trivial. Also record any risk-taking behaviors, such as failing to wear your safety belt or bicycle helmet, drinking and driving, exceeding the speed limit, putting off home repairs, and so on. For each entry (injury or incidence of unsafe behavior), record the date, the time, what you were doing, who else was there and how you were influenced by him or her, what your motivations were, and what you were thinking and feeling at the time.

At the end of the monitoring period, examine your data. For each incident, determine both the human factors and the environmental factors that contributed to the injury or unsafe behavior. Were you tired? Distracted? Did you not realize this situation was dangerous? Did you take a chance? Did you think this incident couldn't happen to you? Was visibility poor? Were you using defective equipment? Then consider each contributing factor carefully, determining why it existed and how it could have been avoided or changed. Finally, consider what preventive actions you could take to avoid such incidents or to change your behaviors in the future.

As an example, let's say that you usually don't use a safety belt when you run local errands in your car and that several factors contribute to this behavior: You don't really think you could be involved in a crash so close to home, you only go on short trips, you just never think to use it, and so on. One of the contributing factors to your unsafe behavior is inadequate knowledge. You can change this factor by obtaining accurate information about auto crashes (and their usual proximity to a victim's home) from this chapter and from library or Internet research. Just acquiring information about auto crashes and safety belt use may lead you to examine your beliefs and attitudes about safety belts and motivate you to change your behavior.

Once you're committed, you can use behavior change techniques described in Chapter 1, such as completing a contract, asking family and friends for support, and so on, to build a new habit. Put a note or picture reminding you to buckle up in your car where you can see it clearly. Recruit a friend to run errands with you and to remind you about using your safety belt. Once your habit is established, you may influence other people—especially people who ride in your car—to use safety belts all the time. By changing this behavior, you have reduced the chances that you or your passengers will suffer a serious injury or even die in a vehicle crash.

4. **Prepare for a poisoning injury:** Post the number for the national poison control hotline (800-222-1222) near your telephone. Obtain information on poisonings from a Poison Control Center, and read it carefully so you know what to do in case of poisoning.

5. **Volunteer in your neighborhood or community:** Contact your local police or civic organization to find out about setting up a neighborhood watch or emergency response team. Talk with your neighbors to find out more about what you can do to help prevent crime and prepare for emergencies.

## For More Information

### Books

*Home Emergency Guide.* 2003. New York: DK. *Provides background information on first aid and flowcharts with advice for dealing with many emergency situations.*

Lindquist, S. 2000. *The Date Rape Prevention Book: The Essential Guide for Girls and Women.* Naperville, Ill.: Sourcebooks. *How to avoid problem situations and what to do when confronted with danger.*

MacPherson, J. 2003. *AAA Auto Guide: Driving Survival. How to Stay Safe on the Road.* Heathrow, Fl: AAA Publishing. *Provides helpful strategies for choosing and maintaining a safe vehicle and for handling a variety of driving situations.*

McGrew, J. 2005. *Think Safe: Practical Measures to Increase Security at Home, at Work, and Throughout Life.* Hilton Head Island, S.C.: Cameo Publications. *A general guide to safety and crime and violence prevention.*

World Health Organization *World Reports. Visit the WHO Web site* (www.who.int) *to review the recent* World Reports *focusing on violence (2002) and motor vehicle injuries (2004).*

### Organizations, Hotlines, and Web Sites

*American Automobile Association Foundation for Traffic Safety.* Provides consumer information about all aspects of traffic safety; Web site has online quizzes and extensive links.
800-305-SAFE
http://www.aaafts.org

*American Bar Association: Domestic Violence.* Provides information on statistics, research, and laws relating to domestic violence.
http://www.abanet.org/domviol/home.html

*Consumer Product Safety Commission.* Provides information and advice about safety issues relating to consumer products.
http://www.cpsc.gov

*CyberAngels.* Provides information on online safety and help and advice for victims of cyberstalking.
http://www.cyberangels.org

*National Center for Injury Prevention and Control.* Provides consumer-oriented information about unintentional injuries and violence.
http://www.cdc.gov/ncipc

*National Highway Traffic Safety Administration.* Supplies materials about reducing deaths, injuries, and economic losses from motor vehicle crashes.
888-327-4236
http://www.nhtsa.dot.gov

*National Safety Council.* Provides information and statistics about preventing unintentional injuries.
630-285-1121
http://www.nsc.org

*National Violence Hotlines.* Provide information, referral services, and crisis intervention.
800-799-SAFE (domestic violence); 800-422-4453 (child abuse); 800-656-HOPE (sexual assault)

*Prevent Child Abuse America.* Provides statistics, information, and publications relating to child abuse, including parenting tips.
http://www.preventchildabuse.org

*Rape, Abuse, and Incest National Network (RAINN).* Provides guidelines for preventing and dealing with sexual assault and abuse.
http://www.rainn.org

*SafeUSA.* Provides information about safety at home, in schools, at work, on the road, and in communities.
http://www.safeusa.org

The following sites provide statistics and background information on violence and crime in the United States:

*Bureau of Justice Statistics:* http://www.ojp.usdoj.gov/bjs
*Federal Bureau of Investigation:* http://www.fbi.gov
*Justice Information Center:* http://www.ncjrs.org

## Selected Bibliography


Browne, K. D., and C. Hamilton-Giachritsis. 2005. The influence of violent media on children and adolescents: A public-health approach. *Lancet* 365(9460): 702–710.

Centers for Disease Control and Prevention. 2004. Impact of primary laws on adult use of safety belts—United States, 2002. *Morbidity and Mortality Weekly Report* 53(12): 257–260.

Centers for Disease Control and Prevention. 2004. Surveillance for fatal and nonfatal injuries—United States, 2001. *MMWR Surveillance Summaries* 55(SS7): 1–57.

Centers for Disease Control and Prevention. 2004. Violence-related behaviors among high school students—United States, 1991–2003. *Morbidity and Mortality Weekly Report* 53(29): 651–655.

Centers for Disease Control and Prevention. 2005. Unintentional non-fire-related carbon monoxide exposures—United States, 2001–2003. *Morbidity and Mortality Weekly Report* 54(2): 36–39.

Cummings, P., and F. P. Rivara. 2004. Car occupant death according to the restraint use of other occupants. *Journal of the American Medical Association* 291(3): 343–349.

D'Ovidio, R. D., and J. Doyle. 2003. A study on cyberstalking: Understanding investigative hurdles. *FBI Law Enforcement Bulletin* 72(3): 10–17.

Federal Bureau of Investigation. 2004. *Crime in the United States. Uniform Crime Reports, 2003.* Washington, D.C.: U.S. Department of Justice.

Federal Bureau of Investigation. 2004. *Hate Crime Statistics, 2003.* Washington, D.C.: U.S. Department of Justice.

Graffunder, C. M., et al. 2004. Through a public health lens. Preventing violence against women: An update from the U.S. Centers for Disease Control and Prevention. *Journal of Women's Health* 13(1): 5–15.

Gray-Vickrey, P. 2004. Combating elder abuse. *Nursing* 34(10): 47–51.

Grossman, D. C., et al. 2005. Gun storage practices and risk of youth suicide and unintentional firearm injuries. *Journal of the American Medical Association* 293(6): 707–714.

Iudice, A., et al. 2005. Effects of prolonged wakefulness combined with alcohol and hands-free cell phone divided attention tasks on simulated driving. *Human Psychopharmacology* 20(2): 125–132.

Johnson, J. G., et al. 2002. Television viewing and aggressive behavior during adolescence and adulthood. *Science* 295(5564): 2468–2471.

Kilpatrick, D. 2004. Interpersonal violence and public policy: What about the victims? *Journal of Law, Medicine, and Ethics* 32(1): 73–81.

McGwin, G., et al. 2003. The association between occupant restraint systems and risk of injury in frontal motor vehicle collisions. *Journal of Trauma* 54: 1182–1187.

Miller, M., D. Azrael, and D. Hemenway. 2002. Rates of household firearm ownership and homicide across U.S. regions and states. *American Journal of Public Health* 92(12).

National Center for Injury Prevention and Control. 2005. *Sexual Violence Fact Sheet* (http://www.cdc.gov/ncipc/factsheets/svfacts.htm; retrieved April 16, 2005).

National Center for Injury Prevention and Control. 2004. *Intimate Partner Violence Fact Sheet* (http://www.cdc.gov/ncipc/factsheets/ipvfacts.htm; retrieved January 26, 2005).

National Safety Council. 2004. *Injury Facts.* Itasca, Ill.: National Safety Council.

National School Safety Center. 2005. *Report on School Associated Violent Deaths* (http://www.nssc1.org/savd/savd.pdf; retrieved March 2, 2005).

National Traffic Safety Administration. 2005. *Traffic Safety Facts Research Note: Driver Cell Phone Use in 2004—Overall Results.* Washington, D.C.: National Traffic Safety Administration.

Quinlan, K. P., et al. 2005. Alcohol-impaired driving among U.S. adults, 1993–2002. *American Journal of Preventive Medicine* 28(4): 346–350.

Rosenfeld, R. 2004. The case of the unsolved crime decline. *Scientific American,* February.

Silverman, J. G., A. Raj, and K. Clements. 2004. Dating violence and associated sexual risk and pregnancy among adolescent girls in the United States. *Pediatrics* 114(2): e220–225.

World Health Organization. 2004. *World Report on Road Traffic Injury Prevention.* Geneva: World Health Organization.

Zimmerman, F. J., et al. 2005. Early cognitive stimulation, emotional support, and television watching as predictors of subsequent bullying among grade-school children. *Archives of Pediatrics and Adolescent Medicine* 59(4): 384–388.

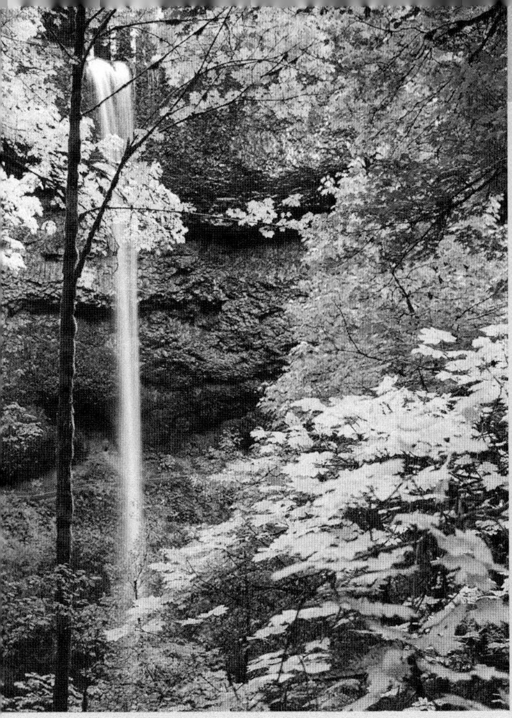

17

## Looking AHEAD

After reading this chapter, you should be able to

- Describe the methods used to deal with the classic environmental concerns of clean water and waste disposal
- Discuss the effects of rapid increases in human population and list factors that may limit or slow world population growth
- Describe the short- and long-term effects of air, chemical, and noise pollution and exposure to radiation
- Outline strategies that individuals, communities, and nations can take to preserve and restore the environment

# Environmental Health

Environmental health has historically focused on preventing infectious diseases spread by water, waste, food, rodents, and insects. Although these problems still exist, the focus of environmental health has expanded and become more complex, for several reasons. First, we now recognize that environmental pollutants contribute not only to infectious diseases but to many chronic diseases as well. In addition, technological advances have increased our ability to affect and damage the environment. And finally, rapid population growth, which has resulted partly from past environmental improvements, means that far more people are consuming and competing for resources than ever before, magnifying the effect of humans on the environment.

**Environmental health** is therefore seen as encompassing all the interactions of humans with their environment and the health consequences of these interactions. Fundamental to this definition is a recognition that we hold the world in trust for future generations and for other forms of life. Our responsibility is to pass on to the next generation an environment no worse, and preferably better, than the one we enjoy today (see the box "Nature and the Human Spirit" on p. 418). Although many environmental problems are complex and seem beyond the control of the individual, there are ways that people can make a difference in the future of the planet.

## CLASSIC ENVIRONMENTAL HEALTH CONCERNS

The field of environmental health originally grew out of efforts to control communicable diseases. Discoveries led to the development of practices such as systematic garbage collection, sewage treatment, filtration and chlorination of drinking water, and food inspection. These successful efforts to control communicable diseases changed the health profile of the developed world.

In the United States, a huge, complex, public health system is constantly at work behind the scenes. Any time this system is disrupted, danger recurs—whether after a natural disaster such as the 2004 Asian tsunami or a manmade disaster such as a terrorist attack—and prompt restoration of basic health services becomes crucial to human survival. And every time we venture beyond the boundaries of our everyday world, whether traveling to a less-developed country or camping in a wilderness area, we are reminded of the importance of these basics: clean

**Term**

**environmental health** The collective interactions of humans with the environment and the short-term and long-term health consequences of those interactions.

VVW

Mind/Body/Spirit

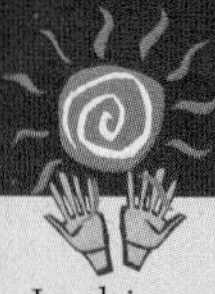

## Nature and the Human Spirit

In this excerpt from her book *The Sense of Wonder,* noted scientist and author Rachel Carson affirms the nurturing power of the natural world and urges us to appreciate the deep relationship between nature and the human spirit.

> What is the value of preserving and strengthening this sense of awe and wonder, this recognition of something beyond the boundaries of human existence? Is the exploration of the natural world just a pleasant way to pass the golden hours of childhood or is there something deeper?
>
> I am sure there is something much deeper, something lasting and significant. Those who dwell, as scientists or laymen, among the beauties and mysteries of the earth are never alone or weary of life. Whatever the vexations or concerns of their personal lives, their thoughts can find paths that lead to inner contentment and to renewed excitement in living. Those who contemplate the beauty of the earth find reserves of strength that will endure as long as life lasts. There is symbolic as well as actual beauty in the migration of the birds, the ebb and flow of the tides, the folded bud ready for spring. There is something infinitely healing in the repeated refrains of nature—the assurance that dawn comes after night, and spring after the winter.

SOURCE: Carson, R. 1956. *The Sense of Wonder.* New York: Harper & Row. 

water, sanitary waste disposal, safe food, and insect and rodent control.

## Clean Water

Few parts of the world have adequate quantities of safe, clean drinking water, and yet few things are as important to human health. Many cities rely at least in part on wells that tap local groundwater, but often it is necessary to find lakes and rivers to supplement wells. Because such surface water is more likely to be contaminated with both organic matter and pathogenic microorganisms, it is purified in water-treatment plants before being piped into the community.

In most areas of the United States, water systems have adequate, dependable supplies, are able to control waterborne disease, and provide water without unacceptable color, odor, or taste. However, problems do occur. In 1993, more than 400,000 people became ill and 100 died when Milwaukee's drinking water was contaminated with the bacterium *Cryptosporidium.* The Centers for Disease Control and Prevention (CDC) estimate that 1 million Americans become ill and 900–1000 die each year from microbial illnesses from drinking water. Pollution by hazardous chemicals from manufacturing, agriculture, and household wastes is another concern. Water shortages are also a problem. Some parts of the United States are experiencing rapid population growth that outstrips the ability of local systems to provide adequate water to all.

### What You Can Do to Protect the Water Supply

- Take showers, not baths, to minimize your water consumption. Don't let water run when you're not actively using it while brushing your teeth, shaving,

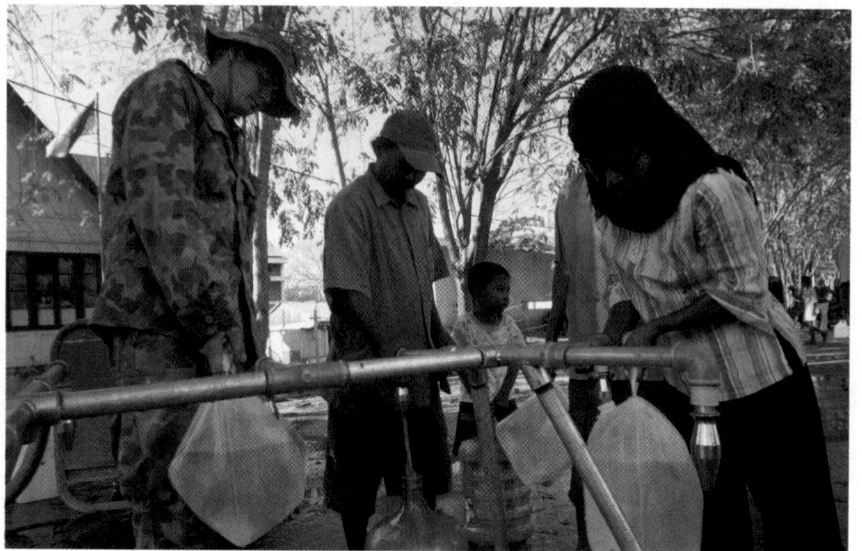

We often take for granted the well-organized system responsible for environmental health in our society, but natural disasters remind us of its fragility. In addition to forcing people from their homes, flooding such as that caused by the 2004 Asian tsunami can cause widespread disruption in essential services such as the delivery of electricity, gas, and clean drinking water, which increases the probability of disease transmission.

or hand-washing clothes. Don't run a dishwasher or washing machine until you have a full load.

- Install sink faucet aerators and water-efficient shower heads, which use two to five times less water with no noticeable decrease in performance.
- Purchase a water-saver toilet, or put a displacement device in your toilet tank to reduce the amount of water used with each flush.
- Fix any leaky faucets in your house. Leaks can waste thousands of gallons of water per year.
- Use organic rather than chemical fertilizers, and don't overfertilize your lawn or garden; the extra could end up in the groundwater.
- Don't pour toxic materials such as cleaning solvents, bleach, or motor oil down the drain. Store them until you can take them to a hazardous waste collection center.
- Replant your lawn and garden with plants requiring less water. Avoid watering your lawn during the hottest part of the day to minimize evaporation.

## Waste Disposal

Humans generate large amounts of waste, which must be handled in an appropriate manner if the environment is to be safe and sanitary.

**Sewage** Most cities have sewage-treatment systems that separate fecal matter from water in huge tanks and ponds and stabilize it so that it cannot transmit infectious diseases. Once treated and biologically safe, the water is released back into the environment. The sludge that remains behind is often contaminated with **heavy metals** and is handled as hazardous waste; if not contaminated, sludge may be used as fertilizer. Many cities have now begun expanded sewage-treatment measures to remove heavy metals and other hazardous chemicals. This action has resulted from many studies linking exposure to chemicals such as mercury, lead, and **polychlorinated biphenyls (PCBs)** with long-term health consequences, including cancer and damage to the central nervous system.

**Solid Waste** The bulk of the organic food garbage produced in American kitchens is now dumped in the sewage system by way of the mechanical garbage disposal. The garbage that remains is not very hazardous from the standpoint of infectious disease because there is very little food waste in it, but it does represent an enormous disposal and contamination problem.

**WHAT'S IN OUR GARBAGE?** The biggest single component of household trash by weight is paper products, including junk mail, glossy mail-order catalogs, and computer

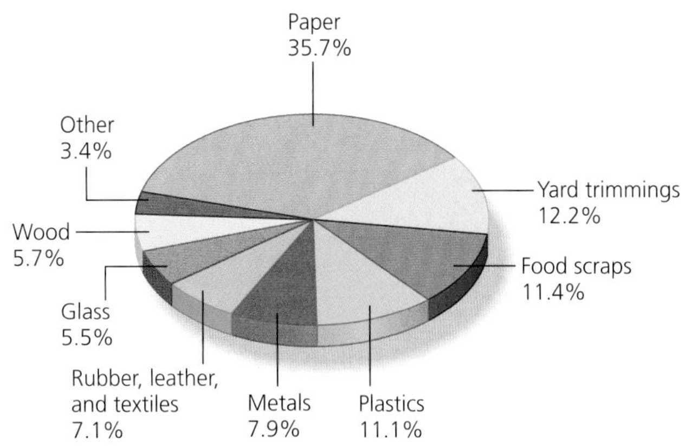


VITAL STATISTICS

**Figure 17-1 Components of municipal solid waste, by weight.** The total amount of trash produced by U.S. residences, businesses, and institutions is the equivalent of 4.4 pounds of waste per person, per day, up from 2.7 pounds in 1960. SOURCE: Environmental Protection Agency. 2004. *Municipal Solid Waste: Basic Facts* (http://www.epa.gov/epaoswer/non-hw/muncpl/facts.htm; retrieved March 6, 2005).

printouts (Figure 17-1). About 1% of the solid waste is toxic; a new source of toxic waste is the disposal of computer components in both household and commercial waste. Burning, as opposed to burial, reduces the bulk of solid waste, but it may release hazardous material into the air. Manufacturing, mining, and other industries all produce large amounts of potentially dangerous materials that cannot simply be dumped.

**DISPOSING OF SOLID WASTE** Since the 1960s, much solid waste has been buried in **sanitary landfill** disposal sites. Layers of solid waste are covered with thin layers of dirt until the site is filled. Some communities then plant grass and trees and convert the site into a park. Landfill is relatively stable; almost no decomposition occurs in the solidly packed waste. But burying solid waste in sanitary landfills has several disadvantages. Much of this waste contains chemicals, ranging from leftover pesticides to nail polish remover to paints and oils, which should not be released indiscriminately into the environment. Despite precautions, buried contaminants do leak into the surrounding soil and groundwater. Burial is also expensive and requires huge amounts of space.

Industrial toxic waste poses an even greater disposal problem. In 1980, Congress enacted the Superfund

### Terms

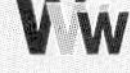

**heavy metal** A metal with a high specific gravity, such as lead, copper, or tin.

**polychlorinated biphenyl (PCB)** An industrial chemical used as an insulator in electrical transformers and linked to certain human cancers.

**sanitary landfill** A disposal site where solid wastes are buried.

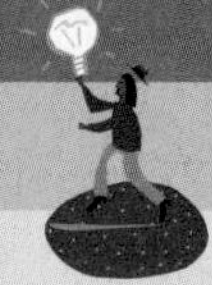

Critical Consumer

## How to Be a Green Consumer

You can quickly and easily develop habits that direct your consumer dollar toward environmentally friendly products.

- Remember the four Rs of green consumerism:
  *Reduce* the amount of trash and pollution you generate by consuming and throwing away less.
  *Reuse* as many products as possible—either yourself or by selling them or donating them to charity.
  *Recycle* all appropriate materials and buy recycled products whenever possible.
  *Respond* by educating others about reducing waste and recycling, by finding creative ways to reduce waste and toxicity, and by making your preferences known.
- Choose products packaged in refillable, recycled, reusable containers or in readily recyclable materials, such as paper, cardboard, aluminum, or glass. Don't buy products that are excessively packaged or wrapped.
- Look for products made with the highest possible content of recycled paper, metal, glass, plastic, and other materials.
- Choose simple products containing the lowest amounts of bleaches, dyes, and fragrances. Look for organically grown foods and clothes made from organically grown cotton or Fox Fibre or another naturally colored type of cotton.
- Buy high-quality appliances that have an Energy Star seal from the EPA or some other type of certification indicating that they are energy- and water-efficient.
- Get a reusable cloth shopping bag. Don't bag items that don't need to be bagged. If you forget to bring your bag to the store, it doesn't matter much if you use a paper or plastic bag to carry your purchases home. What's important is that you reuse whatever bag you get.
- Don't buy what you don't need—borrow, rent, or share. Take good care of the things you own, repair items when they break, and replace them with used rather than new items whenever possible. Sell or donate used items rather than throwing them out.
- Walk or bike to the store. If you must drive, do several errands at once to save energy and cut down on pollution.
- Look beyond the products to the companies that make them. Support those with good environmental records. If some of your favorite products are overpackaged or contain harmful ingredients, write to the manufacturer.
- Keep in mind that doing something is better than doing nothing. Even if you can't be a perfectly green consumer, doing your best on any purchase *will* make a difference.

SOURCES: U.S. Environmental Protection Agency. 2002. *Reduce, Reuse, and Recycle* (http://www.epa.gov/epaoswer/non-hw/reduce/catbook/the4.htm; retrieved March 6, 2005); Makower, J., J. Elkington, and J. Hailes. 1993. *The Green Consumer.* New York: Penguin Books; Madigan, C. O., and A. Elwood. 1995. *Life's Big Instruction Book.* New York: Warner Books.

program to clean up inactive hazardous waste sites that are a threat to human health and the environment. By 2004, cleanup was complete at 60% of priority sites, but further action was still needed at about 600 priority sites and nearly 10,000 other sites.

Because of the expense and potential chemical hazards of any form of solid waste disposal, many communities today encourage individuals and businesses to recycle their trash. Some cities offer curbside pickup of recyclables; others have recycling centers to which people can bring their waste. Recycling programs have been successful in reducing the proportion of solid waste sent to landfills. In 1980, 81% went to landfills; in 2000, about 55%.

### What You Can Do to Reduce Garbage

- Buy products with the least amount of packaging you can, or buy products in bulk (see the box "How to Be a Green Consumer"). Buy products packaged in glass, paper, or metal containers; avoid plastic and aluminum (unless it's recycled). Reuse glass containers to store products bought in bulk or other nontoxic household items.
- Buy recycled or recyclable products. Avoid disposables; instead, use long-lasting or reusable products such as refillable pens and rechargeable batteries.
- Avoid using foam or paper cups and plastic stirrers by bringing your own china coffee mug and metal spoon to work or wherever you drink coffee or tea. Pack your lunch in reusable containers, and use a cloth or plastic lunch sack or a lunch box.
- To store food, use glass jars and reusable plastic containers rather than foil and plastic wrap.
- Recycle your newspapers, glass, cans, paper, and other recyclables. If you receive something packaged with foam pellets, take them to a commercial mailing center that accepts them for recycling.
- Do not throw items such as computers, televisions, VCRs, cell phones, microwave ovens, digital cameras, household batteries, or fluorescent lights into the trash. Take all these to state-approved recycling centers; check with your local disposal service for more information.
- Start a compost pile for your organic garbage (nonanimal food and yard waste) if you have a yard. If

you live in an apartment, you can create a small composting system using earthworms, or take your organic wastes to a community composting center.

- Stop junk mail. To cancel your junk mail, send a request to Mail Preference Service, Direct Marketing Association, P.O. Box 643, Carmel, NY 10512 (http://www.dmaconsumers.org).

## Food Inspection

Many agencies inspect food at various points in production. On the federal level, the U.S. Department of Agriculture (USDA) inspects grains and meats, and the U.S. Food and Drug Administration (FDA) is responsible for ensuring the wholesomeness of foods and regulating the chemicals that can be used in foods, drugs, and cosmetics. On the state level, public health departments inspect dairy herds, milking barns, storage tanks, tankers that transport milk, and processing plants. Local health departments inspect and license restaurants.

Overall, the food distribution system in the United States is safe and efficient, but cases of foodborne illness do occur. Many cases of foodborne illness can be prevented through the proper storage and preparation of food. (For guidelines on avoiding foodborne illness and information on other food safety issues, see Chapter 9.)

## Insect and Rodent Control

A great number of illnesses can be transmitted to humans by animal and insect vectors. In recent years, we have seen outbreaks of encephalitis transmitted by mosquitoes; Lyme disease from ticks in the Northeast, Midwest, and West; Rocky Mountain spotted fever from another type of tick in the Southeast; bubonic plague from fleas on wild mammals in the West; and West Nile virus transmitted by mosquitoes. Rodents carry forms of hantavirus, tapeworms, and *Salmonella*. Disability and death from these diseases can be prevented by spraying insecticides when necessary, wearing protective clothing, and exercising reasonable caution in infested areas (see Chapter 13).

# POPULATION GROWTH

Throughout most of history, humans have been a minor pressure on the planet. About 300 million people were alive in the year A.D. 1; by the time Europeans were settling in the United States 1600 years later, the world population had increased gradually to a little over 500 million. But then it began rising exponentially—zooming to 1 billion by about 1800, more than doubling by 1950, and then doubling again in just 40 years (Figure 17-2).

The world's population, currently about 6.5 billion, is increasing at a rate of about 78 million per year—150 people every minute. The United Nations projects that world population will reach 9.1 billion by 2050 and will continue to increase until it levels off above 10 billion in 2200. Virtually all of this increase is taking place in less-developed regions. This rapid expansion of population, particularly in the past 50 years, is generally believed to be responsible for most of the stress humans put on the environment.

No one knows how many people the world can support, but most scientists agree that there is a limit. The primary factors that may eventually put a cap on human population are likely to be the limits of the earth's resources—land, water, energy, and food. The mass media have exposed the entire world to the American lifestyle and raised people's expectations of living at a comparable level. But such a lifestyle is supported by levels of energy consumption that the earth cannot support worldwide. The United States has about 5% of the world's population but uses 25% of the world's energy.

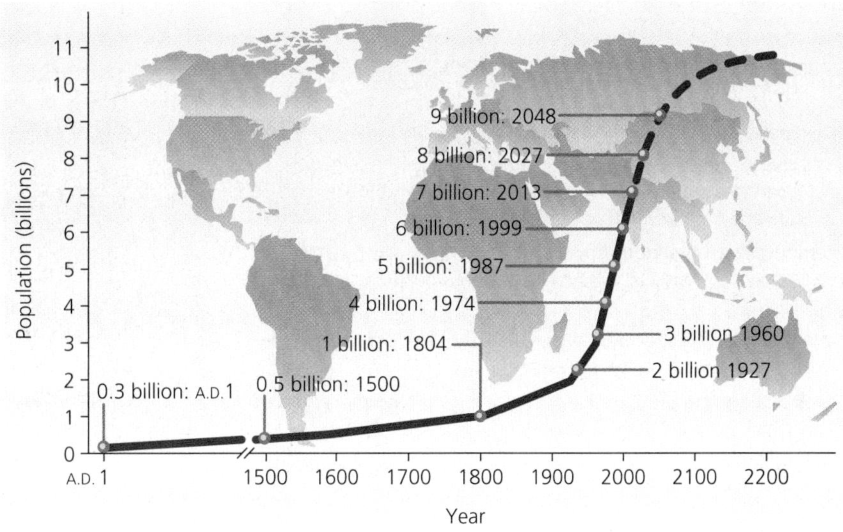


VITAL STATISTICS

**Figure 17-2 World population growth.** The United Nations estimates that the world's population will continue to increase dramatically until it stabilizes above 10 billion people in 2200. SOURCES: United Nations Population Division. 2005. *World Population Prospects: The 2004 Revision.* New York: United Nations; U.S. Bureau of the Census.

Although it is apparent that population growth must be controlled, population trends are difficult to influence and manage. A variety of interconnecting factors fuel the current population explosion, including high fertility rates, lower death rates, and lack of family planning resources. Increasing death rates through disease, famine, or war might slow population growth, but few people would argue in favor of these as methods of population control. (The latest United Nations population estimates already project that there will be 344 million fewer people alive in 2050 than there would have been without the effect of deaths from HIV/AIDS.)

To be successful, population management must change the condition of people's lives, especially poverty, to remove the pressures for having large families. Research indicates that the combination of improved health, better education, and increased literacy and employment opportunities for women works together with family planning to decrease fertility rates. Unfortunately, in the fastest-growing countries, the needs of a rapidly increasing population use up financial resources that might otherwise be used to improve lives and ultimately slow population growth.

## POLLUTION

The term *pollution* refers to any unwanted contaminant in the environment that may pose a health risk.

### Terms

VW

**Air Quality Index (AQI)** A measure of local air quality and what it means for health. Concentrations of five major pollutants are measured and assigned index values between 0 and 500, with values above 100 considered unhealthy; the highest of the five values becomes the overall AQI for the day. Health warnings and recommendations may be issued when AQI values exceed 100.

**fossil fuels** Buried deposits of decayed animals and plants that are converted into carbon-rich fuels by exposure to heat and pressure over millions of years; oil, coal, and natural gas are fossil fuels.

**smog** Hazy atmospheric conditions resulting from increased concentrations of ground-level ozone and other pollutants. Smog most commonly occurs when oxides of nitrogen and hydrocarbons, primarily from motor vehicle exhaust, react in the presence of sunlight; also known as *photochemical smog*. (The term was first used to describe the combination of smoke and fog in early-twentieth-century London.)

**temperature inversion** A weather condition in which a cold layer of air is trapped by a warm layer so that pollutants cannot be dispersed.

**greenhouse effect** A warming of the earth due to a buildup of carbon dioxide and certain other gases.

**global warming** An increase in the earth's atmospheric temperature when averaged across seasons and geographical regions.

**ozone layer** A layer of ozone molecules ($O_3$) in the upper atmosphere that screens out UV rays from the sun.

### Air Pollution

Air pollution is not a human invention or even a new problem. The air is "polluted" naturally with every forest fire, pollen bloom, and dust storm, as well as with countless other natural pollutants. To these natural sources, humans contribute the by-products of their activities.

**Air Quality and Smog** Air pollution can cause illness and death if pollutant levels are high; young children, older adults, and people with chronic health conditions are particularly at risk. The EPA uses a measure called the **Air Quality Index (AQI)** to indicate whether air pollution levels pose a health concern. The AQI is used for five major air pollutants: carbon monoxide, sulfur dioxide, nitrogen dioxide, particulate matter, and ground-level ozone. A major source of these pollutants is the burning of **fossil fuels** by vehicles and power plants. AQI values run from 0 to 500; the higher the AQI, the greater the level of pollution and associated health danger. Information on the AQI in your area is often available in newspapers, on television and radio, on the Internet, and from state and local telephone hotlines.

The term **smog** was first used in the early 1900s in London to describe the combination of smoke and fog. What we typically call smog today is a mixture of pollutants, with ground-level ozone being the key ingredient. Major smog occurrences are linked to the combination of several factors. Heavy motor vehicle traffic, high temperatures, and sunny weather can increase the production of ozone. Pollutants are also more likely to build up in areas with little wind and/or where a topographic feature such as a mountain range or valley prevents the wind from pushing out stagnant air.

A weather event called a **temperature inversion** also contributes to smog buildup. A temperature inversion occurs when there is little or no wind and a layer of warm air traps a layer of cold air next to the ground. Normally, the sun heats the earth, making the air closest to the ground warmer than that just above it. Warm air rises and is replaced by cooler air, which in turn is warmed and rises, thereby producing a natural circulation. This circulation, combined with horizontal wind circulation, prevents pollutants from reaching dangerous levels. When there is a temperature inversion, this replacement and cleansing action cannot occur. The effect is like covering an area with a dome that traps all the pollutants and prevents vertical dispersion. If this condition persists for several days, the buildup of pollutants may reach dangerous levels and threaten people's health.

**The Greenhouse Effect and Global Warming** The temperature of the earth's atmosphere depends on the balance between the amount of energy the planet absorbs from the sun (mainly as high-energy ultraviolet radiation) and the amount of energy radiated back into

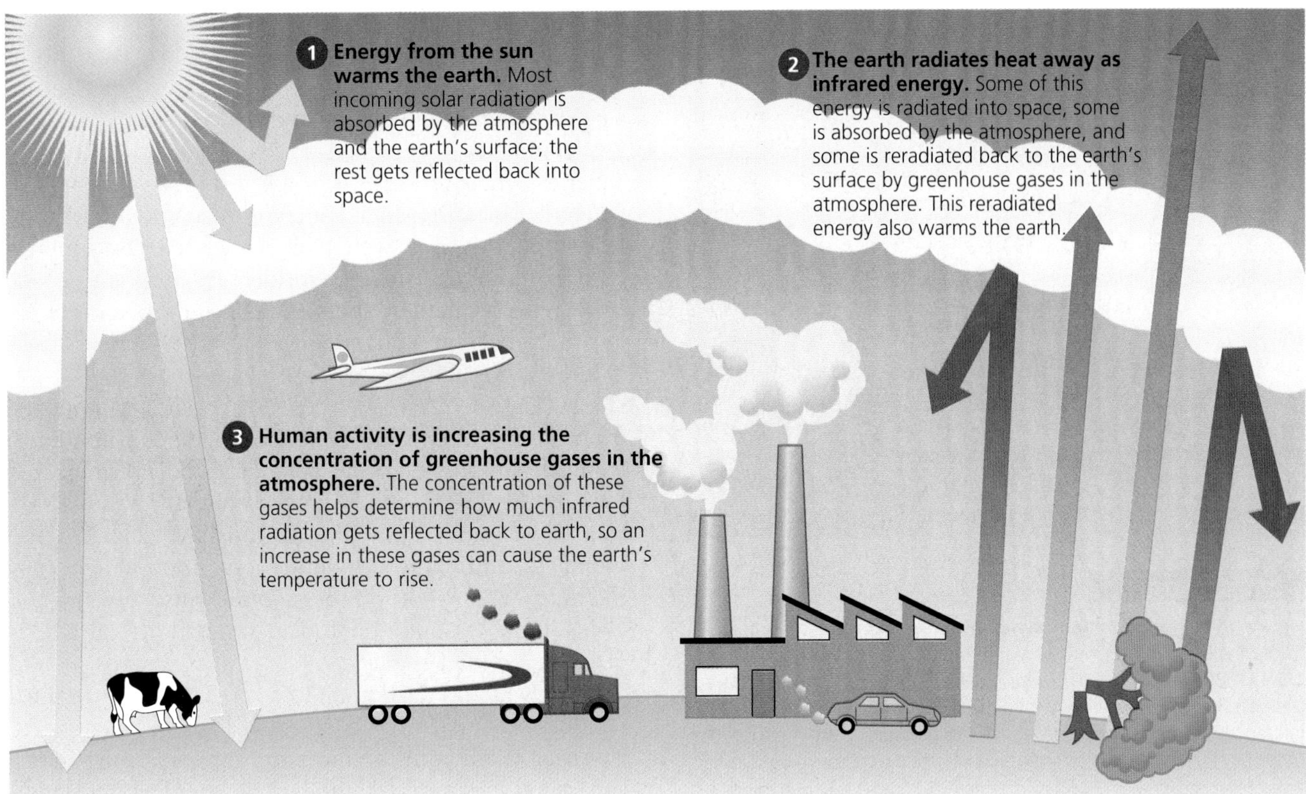


**Figure 17-3 The greenhouse effect.**

space as lower-energy infrared radiation. Key components of temperature regulation are carbon dioxide, water vapor, methane, and other "greenhouse gases"—so named because, like a pane of glass in a greenhouse, they let through visible light from the sun but trap some of the resulting infrared radiation and reradiate it back to the earth's surface. This reradiation causes a buildup of heat that raises the temperature of the lower atmosphere, a natural process known as the **greenhouse effect.** Without it, the atmosphere would be far cooler and much more hostile to life.

Human activity may be tipping this balance toward **global warming** (Figure 17-3). The concentration of greenhouse gases is increasing because of human activity, especially the combustion of fossil fuels. Carbon dioxide levels in the atmosphere have increased rapidly since the onset of the Industrial Revolution, and current levels are higher than at any time in the past 160,000 years. Deforestation, often by burning, also sends carbon dioxide into the atmosphere and reduces the number of trees available to convert carbon dioxide into oxygen. But energy use in the developed world is the primary cause of increases in the concentrations of greenhouse gases. The United States alone is responsible for one-third of the world's total emissions of carbon dioxide.

According to a 2001 report from the United Nations–sponsored Intergovernmental Panel on Climate Change, the average global temperature will likely increase by about 2.5–10.4°F (1.4–5.8°C) by 2100, with a corresponding significant rise in sea level. Although the full implications of climate change are unknown, possible consequences include the following:

- Increased rainfall and flooding in some regions, increased drought in others. Coastal zones, where half the world's people live, would be severely affected.
- Increased mortality from heat stress, urban air pollution, and tropical diseases (due to the spread of disease-carrying organisms like mosquitoes). Severe weather events such as hurricanes, tornadoes, droughts, and floods may also increase, along with associated deaths.
- A poleward shift of about 50–350 miles (150–550 km) in the location of vegetation zones, affecting crop yields, irrigation demands, and forest productivity.

Since record-keeping began in the mid-1800s, 9 of the 10 hottest years have occurred since 1990, the 3 hottest since 1997 (Figure 17-4). Data from tree rings, ice cores, and other sources suggest that recent temperatures are the warmest in 1000 years. For more on global warming, see the box "Climate Change: Politics and Science" on page 425.

**Thinning of the Ozone Layer** A second air pollution problem is the thinning of the **ozone layer** of the atmosphere, a fragile, invisible layer about 10–30 miles

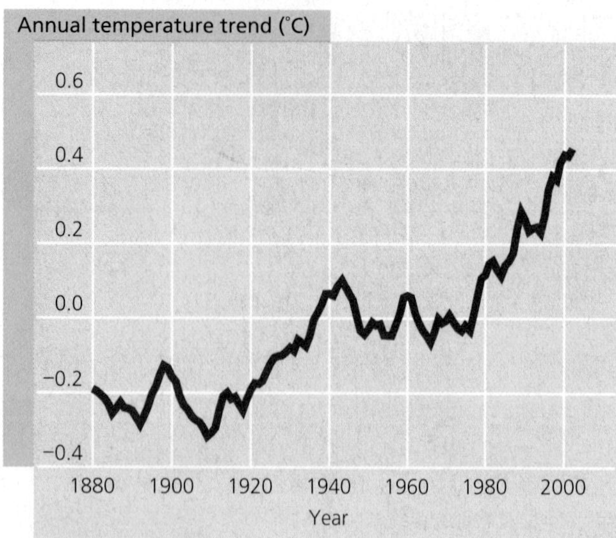


VITAL STATISTICS

**Figure 17-4 Trend in annual mean temperature.** This graph traces the trend in the annual mean temperature relative to the 1951–1980 mean value. There has been a strong warming trend over the past 30 years; variability within the overall trend is caused by such influences as large volcanic eruptions and periodic changes in ocean patterns (El Niño). SOURCE: NASA Goddard Institute for Space Studies. 2005. *Global Temperature Trends: 2004 Summation* (http://www.giss.nasa.gov/data/update/gistemp/2004; retrieved March 5, 2005).

above the earth's surface that shields the planet from the sun's hazardous ultraviolet (UV) rays. Since the mid-1980s, scientists have observed the seasonal appearance and growth of a "hole" in the ozone layer over Antarctica. More recently, thinning over other areas—including Canada, Scandinavia, the northern United States, Russia, Australia, and New Zealand—has been noted.

The ozone layer is being destroyed primarily by **chlorofluorocarbons (CFCs)**, industrial chemicals used as coolants in refrigerators and in home and automobile air conditioners; as foaming agents in some rigid foam products, including insulation; as propellants in some kinds of aerosol sprays (most such sprays were banned in 1978); and as solvents. When CFCs rise into the atmosphere, winds carry them toward the polar regions and chemical reactions occur that destroy ozone.

Since 1979, about 15% of Antarctic ozone has been destroyed, although locally and seasonally up to 95% of the ozone disappears (forming the "hole"). The size and shape of the hole are affected by meteorological factors as well as by the presence of ozone-destroying chemicals. The largest and deepest hole to date occurred in late 2000 over Antarctica. It extended over populated areas of South America, where residents were advised to stay indoors and take other measures to avoid UV exposure. (UV radiation levels under the hole were high enough to cause sunburn within 7 minutes.) In the Northern Hemisphere, ozone levels have declined by about 10% since 1980, and certain areas may be temporarily depleted in late winter and early spring by as much as 40%.

The loss of ozone is of concern because without the ozone layer to absorb the sun's UV radiation, life on Earth would be impossible. The potential effects of increased long-term exposure to UV light for humans include skin cancer, wrinkling and aging of the skin, cataracts and blindness, and reduced immune response. UV light may interfere with photosynthesis and cause lower crop yields; it may also kill phytoplankton and krill, the basis of the ocean food chain.

Worldwide production and use of CFCs have declined rapidly since the danger to the ozone layer was recognized. However, CFCs persist in the atmosphere for long periods, and scientists estimate that the ozone layer will not significantly recover until about 2050.

### Acid Precipitation

A by-product of many industrial processes, **acid precipitation** occurs when atmospheric pollutants combine with moisture in the air and fall to earth as highly acidic rain, snow, sleet, or hail. It occurs especially when coal containing large amounts of sulfur is burned and chemicals are released into the atmosphere. Acidification of lakes and streams due to acid precipitation has completely eradicated fish and other aquatic species in some areas. Trees are also affected because acid precipitation damages leaves, strips the soil of key nutrients, and releases toxic substances such as heavy metals from the soil. Acid precipitation also corrodes metals and damages stone and paint on buildings, monuments, and cars. The areas most affected are Canada, Scandinavia, parts of central Europe, and, in the United States, the Adirondacks, the mid-Appalachian highlands, the upper Midwest, and high elevations in the West.

### Energy Use and Air Pollution

Americans are the biggest energy consumers in the world (Table 17-1, p. 426). About 85% of the energy we use comes from fossil fuels—oil, coal, and natural gas. The remainder comes from nuclear power and renewable energy sources (such as hydroelectric, wind, and solar power). Energy consumption is at the root of many environmental problems, especially those relating to air pollution. Automobile exhaust and the burning of oil and coal by industry and by electricity-generating plants are primary causes of smog, acid precipitation, and the greenhouse effect. The mining of coal and the extraction

## Terms

**chlorofluorocarbons (CFCs)** Chemicals used as spray-can propellants, refrigerants, and industrial solvents, implicated in the destruction of the ozone layer.

**acid precipitation** Rain, snow, sleet, or hail with a low pH (acid), caused by atmospheric moisture combining with products of industrial combustion to form acids such as sulfur dioxide; harmful to forests and lakes, which cannot tolerate changes in acidity/alkalinity.

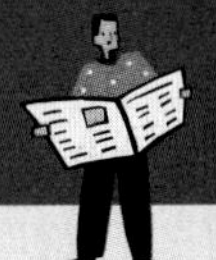

## Climate Change: Politics and Science

On February 16, 2005, the Kyoto Protocol to the United Nations Convention on Climate Change took effect. The protocol requires participating nations to reduce emissions of greenhouse gases by an average of 5.2% below 1990 levels by 2008–2012. Countries that miss their targets will be penalized with bigger cuts when the next set of emissions targets is set in 2012.

The pact was signed in 1997, but it could not take effect until countries accounting for at least 55% of global greenhouse emissions signed on; this hurdle was met when Russia ratified the protocol in 2004. The major industrialized countries that are *not* participating are the United States and Australia. If the United States had ratified the accord, it would have been required to reduce emissions by 6% below 1990 levels; U.S. emissions have actually increased significantly since 1990, including a more than 15% increase in carbon dioxide emissions.

### Kyoto: Controversial but Critical?

Key areas of controversy relating to the Kyoto protocol include the following:

- *The science of climate change:* Critics of Kyoto, including the U.S. government, have argued that scientific knowledge regarding global warming is incomplete and it is therefore premature to set mandatory emissions cuts. However, as described in the next section, scientific consensus on the human contribution toward climate change has been growing.
- *Kyoto's actual impact:* Even proponents acknowledge that the Kyoto protocol will have a relatively small impact. Current estimates have the Kyoto accord cutting just 0.1°C off the 1.4–5.8°C increase forecasted by 2100. However, supporters believe that the pact is a crucial first step and that it sets up a framework for more significant efforts in the future; its greatest immediate value may be symbolic.
- *The role of developing countries:* Developing countries were exempt from the Kyoto accord to give them an opportunity to pursue economic development and alleviate widespread poverty. These nations currently have far lower per-capita energy use and greenhouse gas production than the United States. However, the combination of large population size and rapid industrial development means that any increase in greenhouse gas production in countries like India and China will have a substantial impact on worldwide emissions.
- *Economic costs:* The U.S. government argues that stiff limits on emissions would hurt economic growth; it favors voluntary cuts in emissions and investment in cleaner technologies. The Kyoto protocol does have mechanisms by which wealthy countries can, essentially, pay to pollute. It allows countries to meet their emission reduction goals through emissions trading, meaning they can buy credits from other countries that are surpassing their targets. Countries that invest in clean technologies would thus be able to sell emissions credits to other countries.

### A Growing Scientific Consensus

The idea that human production of greenhouse gasses could lead to global warming was originally proposed in the 1890s, but the first major review of the evidence was not undertaken until the 1988 formation of the United Nations Intergovernmental Panel on Climate Change (IPCC). Based on complex climate models, the IPCC concluded that global temperatures are, indeed, increasing, and that human activity is responsible for a significant proportion of this increase. These conclusions have been supported by individual research and other agencies and organizations, including the National Academy of Sciences. Current scientific study and debate now appears to be focused not on whether human activity is causing global warming but rather on just how much human-caused warming will occur.

Where does the evidence for global warming come from? Firm world temperature data exists for the period since 1880, and that data shows a clear increase. For earlier periods, scientists use a variety of data sources, including tree rings and ice cores, to estimate past temperatures. Based on these data, temperatures are currently higher than at any point in the past 1000 years. Greenhouse gases are also at record-high concentrations in the atmosphere.

Researchers have also been able to measure declining amounts of infrared radiation escaping into space—and more trapped radiation leads to heating of the atmosphere. Another key piece of evidence was announced in early 2005, when researchers reported that computer climate models based on human-produced warming predicted with 95% accuracy actual changes seen in ocean temperatures throughout the world over the past 40 years.

We may already be seeing some of the early effects of global warming, ranging from earlier flowering of plants to increases in severe weather events. The Arctic is heating up nearly twice as fast as the rest of the planet, and problems related to thawing permafrost have already been reported—including the collapse of buildings and the destabilization of oil pipelines, roads, and airports. Glaciers and ice sheets are melting, with corresponding increases in sea level.

### What Next?

Scientists continue to develop new and better climate models and to map the impacts of climate change. One key goal is to produce better models of how overall trends may affect specific regions. For example, 2003 was the third hottest year on record overall, but Europe experienced its hottest summer in 500 years, with about 30,000 deaths due to heat.

On the policy front, some European leaders have vowed to step up the campaign to involve the countries that have the greatest impact on greenhouse gas emissions. The United States, the European Union, Canada, Russia, Japan, China, and India together emit 75% of the world's greenhouse gasses. Proposals for involving developing countries include financial incentives and technology transfers to help them limit emissions without impacting their efforts to reduce poverty.

Despite the official U.S. position, some states are taking steps to limit greenhouse emissions on their own. For example, California is requiring stiff reductions in vehicle emissions, and several states in the Northeast are setting up an emissions trading system similar to that in the Kyoto accord. Individuals can also take steps to limit their contributions to global warming; try some of the lifestyle changes suggested in the sections on reducing air pollution and energy use.

SOURCES: United Nations. 2005. *United Nations Convention on Climate Change: Essential Background* (http://unfccc.int/essential_background/items/2877.php; retrieved March 6, 2005); Scripps Institution. 2005. *Scripps Researchers Find Clear Evidence of Human-Produced Warming in World's Oceans* (http://scrippsnews.ucsd.edu/article_detail.cfm?article_num=666; retrieved March 6, 2005); National Research Council. 2001. *Climate Change Science: An Analysis of Some Key Questions*. Washington, D.C.: National Academy Press; Intergovernmental Panel on Climate Change. 2001. *Climate Change 2001: Impacts, Adaptation, and Vulnerability*. Geneva: Intergovernmental Panel on Climate Change.

VITAL STATISTICS

**Table 17-1 Energy Use in Selected Countries, 2002**

| | Per Capita Energy Use (million Btu) |
|---|---|
| United States | 339 |
| Australia | 286 |
| Russia | 191 |
| France | 184 |
| Japan | 172 |
| United Kingdom | 162 |
| South Africa | 101 |
| Mexico | 65 |
| China | 33 |
| India | 13 |

SOURCE: Energy Information Administration. 2004. *International Total Primary Energy and Related Information* (http://www.eia.doe.gov/emeu/international/total.html; retrieved March 7, 2005).

and transportation of oil cause pollution on land and in the water; coal miners often suffer from serious health problems related to their jobs. Nuclear power generation creates hazardous wastes and carries the risk of dangerous releases of radiation.

Two key strategies for controlling energy use are conservation and the development of nonpolluting, renewable sources of energy. Although the use of renewable energy sources has increased in recent years, renewables still supply only a small proportion of our energy. Despite recent increases in U.S. consumer gas prices, more than 70% of commuters drive alone to work, and low-fuel-economy sport utility vehicles (SUVs) remain popular. Every gallon of gas burned puts about 20 pounds of carbon dioxide into the atmosphere. The International Center for Technology Assessment estimates that the actual price of gasoline—including tax breaks, government subsidies, and environmental, health, and social costs of gas usage—is as high as $15.14 per gallon. A more positive U.S. trend has been the introduction of hybrid electric vehicles (HEVs), which combine a conventional internal combustion engine with an electric motor, resulting in about twice the fuel economy of conventional vehicles.

**Indoor Air Pollution** Although most people associate air pollution with the outdoors, your home may also harbor potentially dangerous pollutants. Some of these compounds trigger allergic responses, and others have been linked to cancer. Common indoor pollutants include environmental tobacco smoke; carbon monoxide and other combustion by-products from wood stoves, fireplaces, kerosene heaters and lamps, and gas ranges; formaldehyde gas from resins used in particle board, plywood paneling, and some carpeting and upholstery; and biological pollutants, including bacteria, dust mites, mold, and animal dander.

### What You Can Do to Prevent Air Pollution

- Cut back on driving. Ride your bike, walk, use public transportation, or carpool in a fuel-efficient vehicle.
- Keep your car tuned up and well maintained. Use only unleaded gas, and keep your tires inflated at recommended pressures. To save energy when driving, avoid quick starts, stay within the speed limit, limit the use of air conditioning, and don't let your car idle unless absolutely necessary. Have your car's air conditioner checked and serviced by a station that uses environmentally friendly refrigerants (car air conditioners made before 1994 are a major source of CFCs).
- Buy energy-efficient appliances, and use them only when necessary. Run the washing machine, dryer, and dishwasher only when you have full loads, and do laundry in warm or cold water instead of hot; don't overdry your clothes. Clean refrigerator coils and clothes dryer lint screens frequently. Towel or air-dry your hair rather than using an electric dryer.
- Replace incandescent bulbs with compact fluorescent bulbs (not fluorescent tubes). Although they cost more initially, they'll save you money over the life of the bulb.
- Make sure your home is well-insulated with ozone-safe agents; use insulating shades and curtains to keep heat in during winter and out during summer. Seal any openings that produce drafts. In cold weather, put on a sweater and turn down the thermostat. In hot weather, wear lightweight clothing and, whenever possible, use a fan instead of an air conditioner to cool yourself.
- Plant and care for trees in your own yard and neighborhood. Because they recycle carbon dioxide, trees work against global warming. They also provide shade and cool the air, so less air conditioning is needed.
- Before discarding a refrigerator, air conditioner, or humidifier, check with the waste hauler or your local government to ensure that ozone-depleting refrigerants will be removed prior to disposal. If you use a metered-dose inhaler, ask your physician if an ozone-safe inhaler is available for your medication.
- To prevent indoor air pollution, keep your house adequately ventilated, and buy some houseplants; they have a natural ability to rid the air of harmful pollutants.
- Keep paints, cleaning agents, and other chemical products in their original, tightly sealed containers.

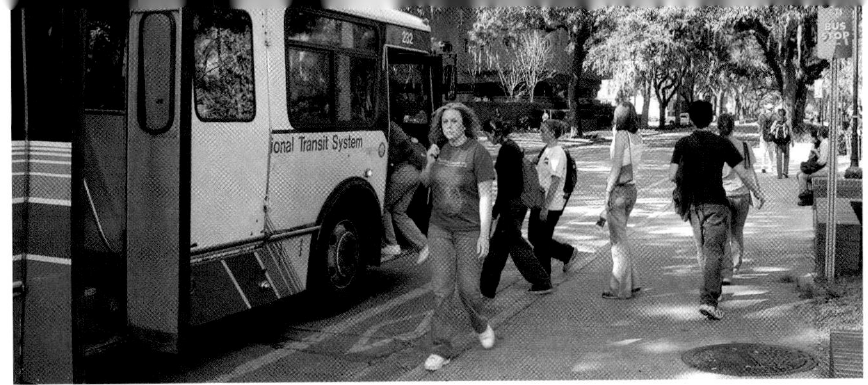

A key strategy for reducing air pollution and greenhouse gas emissions is to reduce energy consumption. Most people drive alone to commute to work or school; try to cut back on your solo driving time by riding your bike, walking, carpooling, or using public transportation.

- Don't smoke, and don't allow others to smoke in your room, apartment, or home. If these rules are too strict for your situation, limit smoking to a single, well-ventilated room.
- Clean and inspect chimneys, furnaces, and other appliances regularly. Install carbon monoxide detectors.

## Chemical Pollution

Chemical pollution is by no means a new problem, but today, new chemical substances are constantly being created and introduced into the environment—as pesticides, herbicides, solvents, cleaning fluids, flame retardants, and hundreds of other products. We have many more chemicals, in more concentrated forms and in wider use, and larger numbers of people are exposed and potentially exposed to them than ever before. The following are brief descriptions of just a few current problems.

**Asbestos** A mineral-based compound, asbestos was widely used for fire protection and insulation in buildings until the late 1960s. Microscopic asbestos fibers can be released into the air when this material is applied or when it later deteriorates or is damaged. These fibers can lodge in the lungs, causing **asbestosis,** lung cancer, and other serious lung diseases. Similar conditions expose workers to risk in the coal mining industry, from coal and silica dust (black lung disease), and in the textile industry, from cotton fibers (brown lung disease).

**Lead** Lead poisoning continues to be a serious problem, particularly among children living in older buildings and adults who are exposed to lead in the workplace. When lead is ingested or inhaled, it can damage the central nervous system, cause mental impairment, hinder oxygen transport in the blood, and create digestive problems. Severe lead poisoning may cause coma or even death. Lead damage to the brain can start even before birth if a pregnant woman has elevated levels of lead in her body.

The CDC estimates that as many as 500,000 children under age 6 may have unsafe lead levels in their blood. Many of these children live in poor, inner-city areas (see the box "Poverty and Environmental Health" on p. 428). Young children can easily ingest lead from their environment by picking up dust and dirt on their hands and then putting their fingers in their mouth. Lead-based paints are believed to be the chief culprit in lead poisoning of children. They were banned from residential use in 1978, but as many as 57 million American homes still contain lead paint. The use of lead in plumbing is now also banned, but some old pipes and faucets contain lead that can leach into drinking water.

Lead gets into the air from industrial and vehicle emissions, from tobacco smoke and paint dust, and from the burning of solid wastes that contain lead. Levels of lead in the air have dropped sharply as leaded gas use has declined, but many vehicles still use leaded fuel. Other sources of lead are foods stored or served in lead-glazed pottery or lead crystal and processed foods sold in lead-soldered cans.

**Pesticides** **Pesticides** are used primarily for two purposes: to prevent the spread of insectborne diseases and to maximize food production by killing insects that eat crops. Both uses have risks as well as benefits. Most pesticide hazards to date have been a result of overuse, but there are concerns about the health effects of long-term exposure to small amounts of pesticide residues in foods, especially for children.

**Mercury** A naturally occurring metal, mercury is a toxin that affects the nervous system and may damage the brain, kidneys, and gastrointestinal tract; increase blood pressure, heart rate, and heart attack risk; and cause cancer. Mercury slows fetal and child development and causes irreversible deficits in brain function. A 2005 study estimated that the economic cost of the impact of mercury on children's brain development is $8.7 billion annually. Coal-fired power plants are the largest producers

### Terms

**asbestosis** A lung condition caused by inhalation of microscopic asbestos fibers, which inflame the lung and can lead to lung cancer.

**pesticides** Chemicals used to prevent the spread of diseases transmitted by insects and to maximize food production by killing insects that eat crops.

Dimensions of Diversity

## Poverty and Environmental Health

Residents of poor and minority communities are often exposed to more environmental toxins than residents of wealthier communities, and they are more likely to suffer from health problems caused or aggravated by pollutants. Poor neighborhoods are often located near highways and industrial areas that have high levels of air and noise pollution; they are also common sites for hazardous waste production and disposal. Residents of substandard housing are more likely to come into contact with lead, asbestos, carbon monoxide, pesticides, and other hazardous pollutants associated with peeling paint, old plumbing, poorly maintained insulation and heating equipment, and attempts to control high levels of pests such as cockroaches and rodents. Poor people are more likely to have jobs that expose them to asbestos, silica dust, and pesticides, and they are more likely to catch and consume fish contaminated with PCBs, mercury, and other toxins.

The most thoroughly researched and documented link among poverty, the environment, and health is lead poisoning in children. Many studies have shown that children of low-income black families are much more likely to have elevated levels of lead in their blood than white children. One survey found that two-thirds of urban African American children from families earning less than $6000 a year had elevated lead levels. The CDC and the American Academy of Pediatrics recommend annual testing of blood lead levels for all children under age 6, with more frequent testing for children at special risk.

Asthma is another health threat that appears to be linked with both environmental and socioeconomic factors. The number of Americans with asthma has grown dramatically in the past 20 years; most of the increase has occurred in children, with African Americans and the poor hardest hit. Researchers are not sure what accounts for this increase, but suspects include household pollutants, pesticides, air pollution, cigarette smoke, and allergens like cockroaches. These risk factors are likely to cluster in poor urban areas where inadequate health care may worsen asthma's effects.

A new push for research on the health effects of exposure to toxins on low-income communities is being called for by the environmental justice movement. New studies are investigating the links between environmental factors and respiratory problems, skin diseases, and cancer. While health researchers seek to quantify the health impacts, neighborhood activists continue to fight against the "dumping" of pollution in poor communities.

of mercury; other sources include mining and smelting operations and the disposal of consumer products containing mercury.

Mercury persists in the environment, and, like pesticides, it is bioaccumulative. In particular, large, long-lived fish may carry high levels of mercury. The FDA recommends that pregnant women, women of childbearing age who may become pregnant, women who are breastfeeding, and young children not consume shark, swordfish, king mackerel, and tilefish and limit total fish consumption to 12 ounces per week. Chapter 9 includes more information on safe fish consumption; see the box "Gender and Environmental Health" for more on issues affecting pregnant women.

The list of real and potential chemical pollution problems may well be as long as the list of known chemicals. As mentioned earlier, hazardous wastes are also found in the home and should be handled and disposed of properly. They include automotive supplies (motor oil, antifreeze, transmission fluid), paint supplies (turpentine, paint thinner, mineral spirits), art and hobby supplies (oil-based paint, solvents, acids and alkalis, aerosol sprays), insecticides, batteries, computer and electronic components, and household cleaners containing sodium hydroxide (lye) or ammonia. Many cities provide guidelines about approved disposal methods and have hazardous waste collection days. Look in the government pages of your phone book under Environmental Health or Hazardous Waste.

### What You Can Do to Prevent Chemical Pollution

- When buying products, read the labels, and try to buy the least toxic ones available. Choose non-toxic nonpetrochemical cleansers, disinfectants, polishes, and other personal and household products.
- Dispose of your household hazardous wastes properly. If you are not sure whether something is hazardous or don't know how to dispose of it, contact your local environmental health office or health department. Don't burn trash.
- Buy organic produce or produce that has been grown locally. Wash, scrub, and, if appropriate, peel fruits and vegetables. Consider eating less meat; animal products require more pesticides, fertilizer, water, and energy to produce.
- If you must use pesticides or toxic household products, store them in a locked place where children and pets can't get to them. Don't measure chemicals with food-preparation utensils, and wear gloves whenever handling them.
- If you have your house fumigated for pest control, be sure to hire a licensed exterminator. Keep everyone, including pets, out of the house while the crew works and, if possible, for a few days after.

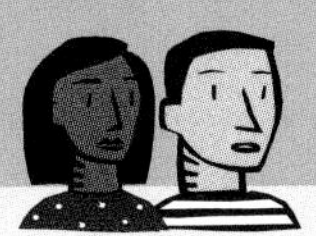

Gender Matters

## Gender and Environmental Health

Although many environmental health risks are shared by all, some risks and impacts disproportionately affect women or men. Women and men often have different roles and responsibilities with respect to family, community, and the workforce. These differences can have an impact on the types of environmental hazards that individuals are exposed to and on what the potential risks of those exposures are.

In many societies, women are more often involved in day-to-day activities associated with the environment, including food preparation, agricultural work, and tasks around the home. These activities can expose women to greater levels of indoor air pollution, water pollution, foodborne pathogens, agricultural chemicals, and waste contamination. Indoor pollutants, especially soot from burning wood, charcoal, and other solid fuels used for home heating and cooking, are a particular risk for women. Exposure to this particulate pollution increases the risk of respiratory diseases, lung cancer, and reproductive problems.

All humans are exposed to chemicals in air, food, and drinking water, and we all carry a body "load" of chemicals. Some of these chemicals bioaccumulate in our bones, blood, or fatty tissues. Women are smaller than men, on average, and have a higher percentage of body fat; so chemicals that accumulate in fatty tissue may pose a relatively greater risk for women. On the other hand, men may be more likely to work in industries that involve significant occupational exposures to disease-related toxins; for example, coal miners have an increased risk of lung cancer (black lung disease).

Although any chemical exposure can be a concern for health, women face the added risk of passing pollutants to a developing fetus during pregnancy or to an infant through breast feeding. Even relatively low exposure to pollutants can result in a significant chemical body load in an infant or young child because of their small body size. And because infants and children are still developing, the effects of chemical exposure can be significant and devastating. It is not unusual for dangerous environmental toxin exposures to be first recognized through noticeable effects on infants or children.

Reproductive risks are not limited to women and infants in developing parts of the world. Even in industrialized countries with strong environmental laws, infants and children are impacted by such chemicals as lead and mercury. In 2005, scientists announced that they had found elevated levels of the rocket fuel chemical perchlorate in human breast milk in amounts above the safe dose set by the National Academy of Sciences. Many other chemicals, including PCBs and pesticides, have already been found in breast milk.

Studies are ongoing to identify and reduce environmental hazards in the United States and throughout the world. However, many of the people most directly affected by environmental health problems—women, children, and people living in poor communities—have limited economic, social, and political power. It is important that everyone impacted by environmental problems be given a voice in determining environmental policies.

SOURCES: Kirk, A. B., et al. 2005. Perchlorate and iodide in dairy and breast milk. *Environmental Science and Technology,* Web release, February 22; McCally, M., ed. 2002. *Life Support: The Environment and Human Health.* Cambridge, Mass.: MIT Press; Population Reference Bureau. 2002. *Women, Men, and Environmental Change: The Gender Dimensions of Environmental Policies and Programs.* Washington, D.C.: Population Reference Bureau.

## Radiation

**Radiation** can come in different forms, such as ultraviolet rays, microwaves, or X rays, and from different sources, such as the sun, uranium, and nuclear weapons. Of most concern to health are gamma rays produced by radioactive sources such as nuclear weapons, nuclear energy plants, and radon gas; these high-energy waves are powerful enough to penetrate objects and break molecular bonds. Although gamma radiation cannot be seen or felt, its effects at high doses can include **radiation sickness** and death; at lower doses, chromosome damage, sterility, tissue damage, cataracts, and cancer can occur. Other types of radiation can also affect health; for example, exposure to UV radiation from the sun or from tanning salons can increase the risk of skin cancer.

Nuclear weapons pose a health risk of the most serious kind to all species. Reducing these stockpiles is a challenge and a goal for the twenty-first century. Power-generating plants that use nuclear fuel also pose health problems. When **nuclear power** was first developed as an alternative to oil and coal, it was promoted as clean, efficient, inexpensive, and safe. In general, this has proven to be the case. However, despite all the built-in safeguards and regulating agencies, accidents in nuclear power plants do happen, and the consequences of such accidents are far more serious than those of similar accidents in other types of power-generating plants. An additional, enormous problem is disposing of the radioactive wastes these plants generate. To date, no storage method has been devised that can provide infallible, infinitely durable shielding for nuclear waste.

Another area of concern is the use of radiation in medicine, primarily the X ray. From a personal health point of view, individuals should never have a "routine" X ray examination; each such exam should have a definite

### Terms

**radiation** Energy transmitted in the form of rays, waves, or particles.

**radiation sickness** An illness caused by excess radiation exposure, marked by low white blood cell counts and nausea; possibly fatal.

**nuclear power** The use of controlled nuclear reactions to produce steam, which in turn drives turbines to produce electricity.

Vw

...e, and its benefits and risks should be carefully weighed. Recently, there has been concern about electromagnetic radiation associated with common modern devices such as microwave ovens, computer monitors, cellular telephones, and even high-voltage power lines. These forms of radiation do have effects on health, but research results are inconclusive.

Another recent area of concern is **radon,** a naturally occurring radioactive gas found in certain soils, rocks, and building materials. When the breakdown products of radon are inhaled, they cling to lungs and bombard sensitive tissue with radioactivity. Radon can enter a home by rising through the soil into the basement through dirt floors, cracks, and other openings. In 2005, the Surgeon General issued a national health advisory on radon, recommending that Americans test their homes for radon every 2 years, and retest any time they move, make structural changes to a home, or occupy a previously unused level of a residence. If elevated levels of radon are found (4 pCi/L or more), the problem should be dealt with as soon as possible through such measures as sealing cracks or installing basement ventilation systems. More information is available at the EPA Web site or by calling 1-800-SOS-RADON.

### What You Can Do to Avoid Radiation

- If your physician orders an X ray, ask why it is necessary. Only get X rays that you need, and keep a record of the date and location of every X ray exam.
- Follow the Surgeon General's recommendations for radon testing.
- Find out if there are radioactive sites in your area. If you live or work near such a site, form or join a community action group to get the site cleaned up.

## Noise Pollution

We are increasingly aware of the health effects of loud or persistent noise in the environment. Concerns focus on two areas: hearing loss and stress. Prolonged exposure to sounds above 80–85 **decibels** (a measure of the intensity of a sound wave) can cause permanent hearing loss.

### Terms

VW

**radon** A naturally occurring radioactive gas emitted from rocks and natural building materials that can become concentrated in insulated homes, causing lung cancer.

**decibel** A unit for expressing the relative intensity of sounds on a scale from 0 for the average least perceptible sound to about 120 for the average pain threshold.

**tinnitus** Ringing in the ears, a condition that can be caused by excessive noise exposure.

Whispering has an intensity of about 30 decibels; normal conversation, 50–60 decibels; heavy traffic, 90 decibels; a rock concert, 120 decibels; and a jet engine, 150 decibels. The Occupational Safety and Health Administration (OSHA) sets legal standards for noise in the workplace, but no laws exist regulating noise levels at rock concerts, which often exceed OSHA standards for the workplace.

Most hearing loss occurs in the first 2 hours of exposure, and hearing usually recovers within 2 hours after the noise stops. But if exposure continues or is repeated frequently, hearing loss may be permanent. The employees of a club where rock music is played loudly are at greater risk than the patrons of the club, who might be exposed for only 2 hours at a time. Another possible effect of exposure to excessive noise is **tinnitus,** a condition of more or less continuous ringing or buzzing in the ears.

Excessive noise is also an environmental stressor, producing the typical stress response described in Chapter 2: faster heart rate, increased respiration, higher blood pressure, and so on. A chronic and prolonged stress response can have serious effects on health.

### What You Can Do to Avoid Noise Pollution

- Wear ear protectors when working around noisy machinery.
- When listening to music on a headset with a volume range of 1–10, keep the volume no louder than 4; your headset is too loud if you are unable to hear people around you speaking in a normal tone of voice.
- Avoid loud music. Don't sit or stand near speakers or amplifiers at a rock concert, and don't play a car radio or stereo so high that you can't hear the traffic.
- Avoid exposure to painfully loud sounds, and avoid repeated exposure to any sounds above 80 decibels.

# HEALING THE ENVIRONMENT

Faced with a vast array of confusing and complex environmental issues, you may feel overwhelmed and conclude that there isn't anything you can do about global problems. But this is not true. If everyone made individual changes in his or her life, the impact would be tremendous. At the same time, it is important to recognize that large corporations and manufacturers are the ones primarily responsible for environmental degradation. To influence them, people have to become educated, demand changes in production methods, and elect people to office who consider environmental concerns along with sound business incentives.

Large-scale changes and individual actions complement each other. What you do every day *does* count. Following the suggestions in the What You Can Do sections throughout this chapter will help you make a difference

Take Charge

## Making Your Letters Count

It takes only a few minutes to write to an elected official, but it can make a difference on an environmental issue you care about. When elected officials receive enough letters or e-mails on an issue, it does influence their vote—they want to be re-elected, and your vote counts! To give your letter the greatest possible impact, use these guidelines:

- Use your own words and your own stationery.
- Be clear and concise. Keep your letter to one or two paragraphs, never more than one page.
- Focus on only one subject in each letter, and identify it clearly. Refer to legislation by its name or number.
- Request a specific action—vote a particular way on a piece of legislation, request hearings, cosponsor a bill—and state your reasons for your position.
- If you live or work in the legislator's district, say so.
- Courteous letters work best. Don't be insulting or unnecessarily critical.

You can send letters via regular mail; however, increased security screenings often delay delivery. You can e-mail the president or vice president at the following addresses:

president@whitehouse.gov

vice-president@whitehouse.gov

To locate the contact information for your United States senators and representatives, visit the following Web sites:

Senate: www.senate.gov

House of Representatives: www.house.gov/writerep

in the environment. In addition, you can become a part of larger community actions to work for a healthier world:

- Share what you learn about environmental issues with your friends and family.
- Join, support, or volunteer your time to organizations working on environmental causes that are important to you.
- Contact your elected representatives and communicate your concerns. For guidelines on how to be heard, see the box "Making Your Letters Count."

Tips for Today

Environmental health involves protecting ourselves from environmental dangers and protecting the environment from the dangers we ourselves create. The two are intimately connected, and both require that we take responsibility for our actions every day.

*Right now you can*

- Turn off the lights in any unoccupied rooms.
- Plan to buy compact fluorescent lightbulbs to replace your incandescent ones.
- Turn down the heat a few degrees and put on a sweater, or turn off the air conditioner and change into shorts.
- Make an appointment to have your car checked if it's not running well or needs a tune-up.
- Check your trash can for recyclable items—soda cans, plastic water bottles, white paper, magazines—and put aside any you find for recycling or put them in your recycling bins.

## SUMMARY

- Environmental health encompasses all the interactions of humans with their environment and the health consequences of those interactions.
- Concerns with water quality focus on pathogenic organisms and hazardous chemicals from industry and households, as well as on water shortages.
- Sewage treatment prevents pathogens from contaminating drinking water; it often must also deal with heavy metals and hazardous chemicals.
- The amount of garbage is growing all the time; paper is the biggest component. Recycling can help solid waste disposal problems.
- The world's population is increasing rapidly, especially in the developing world.
- Increased amounts of air pollutants are especially dangerous for children, older adults, and people with chronic health problems.
- Factors contributing to the development of smog include heavy motor vehicle traffic, hot weather, stagnant air, and temperature inversion.
- Carbon dioxide and other natural gases act as a "greenhouse" around the earth, increasing the temperature of the atmosphere. Levels of these gases are rising through human activity; as a result, the world's climate could change.
- The ozone layer that shields the earth's surface from the sun's UV rays has thinned and developed holes in certain regions.
- Acid precipitation occurs when certain atmospheric pollutants combine with moisture in the air.

- [En]vironmental damage from energy use can be limited through energy conservation and the development of nonpolluting, renewable sources of energy.
- Indoor pollutants can trigger allergies and illness in the short term and cancer in the long term.
- Potentially hazardous chemical pollutants include asbestos, lead, pesticides, mercury, and many household products. Proper handling and disposal are critical.
- Radiation can cause radiation sickness, chromosome damage, and cancer, among other health problems.
- Loud or persistent noise can lead to hearing loss and/or stress.
- The impact of personal changes made by every concerned individual could be tremendous.

## Take Action

1. **Inventory household hazardous waste:** Find out what hazardous chemicals you have in your household. Read the labels for disposal instructions. If there aren't any instructions, call your local health department and ask how to dispose of specific chemicals. Also ask if there are hazardous waste disposal sites in your community or special pickup days. If possible, get rid of some or all of the hazardous wastes in your home.

2. **Identify recycling resources:** Investigate the recycling facilities in your community. Find out how materials are recycled and what they are used for in their recycled state. If recycling isn't available in your community, contact your local city hall to find out how a recycling program can be started.

3. **Track your trash output:** Keep track of exactly how many bags (or gallons) of trash your household produces per week. Is it more or less than the national weekly average of 6.73 bags (87.5 gallons) per three-person household? In either case, try to reduce it by recycling, composting, and buying and using fewer disposable products.

4. **Organize a cleanup day:** With a group of fellow students or coworkers, participate in an environmental cleanup event in your community. Depending on where you live, you might clean up trash along a beach, a river, a public park, or a roadside. You can tie your event to Earth Day or International Cleanup Day, or simply choose a day that works for your group.

## For More Information

### Books


Getis, J. 1999. *You Can Make a Difference: Be Environmentally Responsible,* 2nd ed. New York: McGraw-Hill. *Describes environmental problems and suggestions for individual action.*

McCally, M., ed. 2002. *Life Support: The Environment and Human Health.* Cambridge, Mass.: MIT Press. *Describes how humans affect the environment and how environmental problems impact health.*

Cunningham, W. P., et al. 2004. *Environmental Science: A Global Concern.* 8th ed. New York: McGraw-Hill. *A nontechnical survey of basic environmental science and key concern.*

Maslin, M., 2005. *Global Warming: A Very Short Introduction.* New York: Oxford University Press. *A survey of the science and politics of global warming.*


Useful annual or biennial publications include the following:


National Wildlife Federation. 2005. *2005 Conservation Directory.* Washington, D.C.: National Wildlife Federation.

World Resources Institute. 2003. *World Resources 2002–2004.* Washington, D.C.: World Resources Institute.

Worldwatch Institute. 2005. *Vital Signs 2005.* New York: Norton.


### WW Organizations, Hotlines, and Web Sites

*CDC National Center for Environmental Health.* Provides brochures and fact sheets on a variety of environmental issues.
http://www.cdc.gov/nceh/default.htm

*The Earth Times.* An international online newspaper devoted to global environmental issues.
http://www.earthtimes.org

*Ecological Footprint.* Calculates your personal "ecological footprint" based on your diet, transportation patterns, and living arrangements.
http://www.myfootprint.org

*Energy Efficiency and Renewable Energy Network (EREN). U.S. Department of Energy.* Provides information about alternative fuels and tips for saving energy at home and in your car.
http://www.eere.doe.gov

*Fuel Economy.* Provides information on the fuel economy of cars made since 1985 and tips on improving gas mileage.
http://www.fueleconomy.gov

*Indoor Air Quality Information Hotline.* Answers questions, provides publications, and makes referrals.
800-438-4318

*National Lead Information Center.* Provides information packets and specialist advice.
800-LEAD-FYI

*National Oceanic and Atmospheric Administration (NOAA): Climate.* Provides information on a variety of issues related to climate, including global warming, drought, and El Niño and La Niña.
http://www.noaa.gov/climate.html

*National Safety Council Environmental Health Center.* Provides information on lead, radon, indoor air quality, hazardous chemicals, and other environmental issues.
http://www.nsc.org/ehc.htm

*Student Environmental Action Coalition (SEAC).* A coalition of student and youth environmental groups; the Web site has contact information for local groups.
215-222-4711
http://www.seac.org

*United Nations.* Several U.N. programs are devoted to environmental problems on a global scale; the Web sites provide information on current and projected trends and on international treaties developed to deal with environmental issues.

http://www.un.org/popin (Population Division)

http://www.unep.org (Environment Programme)

*U.S. Environmental Protection Agency (EPA).* Provides information about EPA activities and many consumer-oriented materials. The Web site includes special sites devoted to global warming, ozone loss, pesticides, and other areas of concern.

http://www.epa.gov

*Worldwatch Institute.* A public policy research organization focusing on emerging global environmental problems and the links between the world economy and the environment.

http://www.worldwatch.org

There are many national and international organizations ing on environmental health problems. A few of the largest a best known are listed below:

*Greenpeace:* 800-326-0959; http://www.greenpeace.org
*National Audubon Society:* 212-979-3000; http://www.audubon.org
*National Wildlife Federation:* 800-822-9919; http://www.nwf.org
*Nature Conservancy:* 800-628-6860; http://www.tnc.org
*Sierra Club:* 415-977-5500; http://www.sierraclub.org

## Selected Bibliography


American Council for an Energy-Efficient Economy. 2005. *Green Book: Market Trends* (http://www.greenercars.org/gctext.html; retrieved March 1, 2005).

Bell, M. L., et al. 2004. Ozone and short-term mortality in 95 U.S. urban communities, 1987–2000. *Journal of the American Medical Association* 292(19): 2372–2378.

CDC National Center for Environmental Health. 2004. *Children's Blood Lead Levels in the United States* (http://www.cdc.gov/nceh/lead/research/kidsBLL.htm; retrieved March 6, 2005).

Centers for Disease Control and Prevention. 2004. Adult blood lead epidemiology and surveillance. *Morbidity and Mortality Weekly Report* 53(26): 578.

Donohoe, M. 2003. Causes and health consequences of environmental degradation and social injustice. *Social Science and Medicine* 56(3): 573–587.

Energy Information Administration. 2005. *Impacts of Modeled Recommendations of the National Commission on Energy Policy.* Washington, D.C.: U.S. Department of Energy.

Environmental Protection Agency. 2004. *Superfund National Accomplishments Summary Fiscal Year 2004* (http://www.epa.gov/superfund/action/process/numbers04.htm; retrieved March 6, 2005).

Environmental Protection Agency. 2005. *Municipal Solid Waste: Basic Facts* (http://www.epa.gov.epaoswer/non-hw/muncpl/facts.htm; retrieved March 1, 2005).

Environmental Protection Agency. 2005. *The Particle Pollution Report: Current Understanding of Air Quality and Emissions through 2003* (http://www.epa.gov/airtrends/pm.html; retrieved March 1, 2005).

Gauderman, W. J., et al. 2004. The effect of air pollution on lung development from 10 to 18 years of age. *New England Journal of Medicine* 351(11): 1057–1067.

Intergovernmental Panel on Climate Change. 2001. *Climate Change 2001: Impacts, Adaptation and Vulnerability.* Geneva: Intergovernmental Panel on Climate Change.

Ivanov, V. K., et al. 2003. Thyroid cancer incidence among adolescents and adults in the Bryansk region of Russia following the Chernobyl accident. *Health Physics* 84(1): 46–60.

Kunzli, N., et al. 2005. Ambient air pollution and atherosclerosis in Los Angeles. *Environmental Health Perspectives* 113(2): 201–206.

NASA Goddard Institute for Space Studies. 2005. *Global Temperature Trends: 2004 Summation* (http://www.giss.nasa.gov/data/update/gistemp/2004; retrieved March 5, 2005).

National Oceanic and Atmospheric Administration. 2005. *Billion Dollar U.S. Weather Disasters, 1980–2004* (http://www.ncdc.noaa.gov/oa/reports/billionz.html; retrieved March 1, 2005).

National Oceanic and Atmospheric Administration. 2005. *Northern Hemisphere Winter Summary* (http://www.cpc.ncep.noaa.gov/products/stratosphere/winter_bulletins/nh_03-04/index.html; retrieved March 1, 2005).

Parmesan, C., G. Yohe. 2003. A globally coherent fingerprint of climate change impacts across natural systems. *Nature* 421(6918): 37–42

Parker, J. D., et al. 2005. Air pollution and birth weight among term infants in California. *Pediatrics* 115(1): 121–128.

Pope, C. A., et al. 2002. Lung cancer, cardiopulmonary mortality, and long-term exposure to fine particulate air pollution. *Journal of the American Medical Association* 287(9): 1132–1141.

Trasande, L., P. J. Landrigan, and C. Schechter. 2005. Public health and economic consequences of methylmercury toxicity to the developing brain. *Environmental Health Perspectives* online, February 28.

United Nations Population Division. 2005. *World Population Prospects: The 2004 Revision.* New York: United Nations.

U.S. Department of Health and Human Services. 2005. *Surgeon General Releases National Health Advisory on Radon* (http://www.surgeongeneral.gov/pressreleases/sg01132005.html; retrieved January 24, 2005).

Uysal, N., and R. M. Shapira. 2003. Effects of ozone on lung function and lung diseases. *Current Opinion in Pulmonary Medicine* 9(2): 144–150.

Virtanen, J. K., et al. 2005. Mercury, fish oils, and risk of acute coronary events and cardiovascular disease, coronary heart disease, and all-cause mortality in men in eastern Finland. *Arteriosclerosis, Thrombosis, and Vascular Biology* 25(1): 228–233.

World Health Organization. 2005. *International Decade for Action: Water for Life 2005–2015* (http://www.who.int/water_sanitation_health/2005advocguide/en/index1.html; retrieved March 6, 2005).

Worldwatch Institute. 2004. *Vital Signs 2004.* New York: Norton.

# Nutritional Content of Popular Items from Fast-Food Restaurants

## Arby's

| | Serving size | Calories | Protein | Total fat | Saturated fat | Total carbohydrate | Sugars | Fiber | Cholesterol | Sodium | Vitamin A | Vitamin C | Calcium | Iron | % calories from fat |
|---|---|---|---|---|---|---|---|---|---|---|---|---|---|---|---|
| | g | | g | g | g | g | g | g | mg | mg | (% RDI) | | | | |
| Regular roast beef | 154 | 320 | 21 | 13 | 6 | 34 | 5 | 2 | 45 | 950 | 0 | 0 | 6 | 20 | 34 |
| Super roast beef | 241 | 440 | 22 | 19 | 7 | 48 | 11 | 3 | 45 | 1130 | 2 | 2 | 8 | 25 | 39 |
| Junior roast beef | 125 | 270 | 16 | 9 | 4 | 34 | 5 | 2 | 30 | 740 | 0 | 0 | 6 | 15 | 33 |
| Chicken fingers (4 pack) | 192 | 640 | 31 | 38 | 8 | 42 | 0 | 3 | 70 | 1590 | 0 | 0 | 2 | 15 | 55 |
| Market Fresh® Ultimate BLT | 293 | 780 | 23 | 46 | 9 | 75 | 18 | 6 | 50 | 1570 | 15 | 30 | 15 | 25 | 53 |
| Market Fresh® Roast Turkey & Swiss | 357 | 720 | 45 | 27 | 6 | 74 | 16 | 5 | 90 | 1790 | 8 | 4 | 35 | 30 | 35 |
| Market Fresh® Low Carbys™ Southwest chicken wrap | 259 | 550 | 35 | 30 | 9 | 45 | 1 | 30 | 75 | 1690 | 10 | 10 | 40 | 10 | 49 |
| Martha's Vineyard™ salad (w/o dressing) | 291 | 250 | 26 | 8 | 4.5 | 23 | 23 | 4 | 60 | 490 | 60 | 40 | 20 | 10 | 28 |
| Raspberry vinaigrette | 57 | 172 | 0 | 12 | 1.5 | 16 | 14 | 0 | 0 | 344 | 0 | 4 | 0 | 0 | 63 |
| Santa Fe™ salad (w/o dressing) | 328 | 520 | 27 | 29 | 9 | 40 | 6 | 5 | 60 | 1120 | 130 | 45 | 25 | 20 | 50 |
| Curly fries – medium | 128 | 410 | 5 | 22 | 3 | 47 | N/A | 5 | 0 | 950 | 8 | 10 | 6 | 10 | 49 |
| Jalapeno Bites® – regular (5) | 110 | 310 | 5 | 19 | 7 | 29 | 3 | 2 | 30 | 530 | 15 | 0 | 4 | 6 | 55 |

SOURCE: Arby's © 2005, Arby's, Inc. (http://www.arbysrestaurant.com). Used with permission of Arby's, Inc.

## Burger King

| | Serving size | Calories | Protein | Total fat | Saturated fat | Trans fat | Total carbohydrate | Sugars | Fiber | Cholesterol | Sodium | Vitamin A | Vitamin C | Calcium | Iron | % calories from fat |
|---|---|---|---|---|---|---|---|---|---|---|---|---|---|---|---|---|
| | g | | g | g | g | g | g | g | g | mg | mg | % Daily Value | | | | |
| Original WHOPPER® | 291 | 700 | 31 | 42 | 13 | 1 | 52 | 8 | 4 | 85 | 1020 | 20 | 15 | 10 | 30 | 54 |
| Original WHOPPER® w/o mayo | 270 | 540 | 30 | 24 | 10 | 1 | 52 | 8 | 4 | 75 | 900 | 10 | 15 | 10 | 30 | 40 |
| Original DOUBLE WHOPPER® w/cheese | 399 | 1060 | 56 | 69 | 27 | 2.5 | 53 | 9 | 4 | 185 | 1540 | 25 | 15 | 30 | 45 | 59 |
| Original WHOPPER JR.® | 158 | 390 | 17 | 22 | 7 | 0.5 | 31 | 5 | 2 | 45 | 550 | 10 | 6 | 8 | 15 | 51 |
| BK VEGGIE® Burger* | 215 | 420 | 23 | 16 | 3 | 0 | 46 | 7 | 7 | 10 | 1090 | 20 | 10 | 10 | 20 | 34 |
| Original chicken sandwich | 204 | 560 | 25 | 28 | 6 | 2 | 52 | 5 | 3 | 60 | 1270 | 8 | 0 | 6 | 15 | 45 |
| CHICKEN TENDERS® (8 pieces) | 123 | 340 | 22 | 19 | 5 | 3.5 | 20 | 0 | <1 | 50 | 840 | 2 | 0 | 2 | 4 | 50 |
| French fries (medium, salted) | 117 | 360 | 4 | 18 | 5 | 4.5 | 46 | <1 | 4 | 0 | 640 | 0 | 15 | 2 | 4 | 45 |
| Onion rings (medium) | 91 | 320 | 4 | 16 | 4 | 3.5 | 40 | 5 | 3 | 0 | 460 | 0 | 0 | 10 | 0 | 45 |
| Chili (w/o cheese or crackers) | 217 | 190 | 13 | 8 | 3 | 0 | 17 | 5 | 5 | 25 | 1040 | 25 | 60 | 8 | 8 | 38 |
| Fire-grilled chicken caesar salad (w/o dressing or toast) | 286 | 190 | 25 | 7 | 3 | 0 | 9 | 1 | 1 | 50 | 900 | 85 | 40 | 15 | 8 | 33 |
| CROISSAN'WICH® w/bacon, egg, and cheese | 126 | 340 | 14 | 20 | 7 | 1.5 | 26 | 7 | <1 | 200 | 920 | 8 | 0 | 15 | 10 | 53 |
| HERSHEY®'S sundae pie | 79 | 300 | 3 | 18 | 10 | 1.5 | 31 | 23 | 1 | 10 | 190 | 2 | 0 | 4 | 6 | 54 |
| Chocolate Shake (medium) | 397 | 600 | 10 | 18 | 11 | 0 | 97 | 94 | 2 | 70 | 470 | 15 | 6 | 45 | 8 | 27 |

* Burger King Corporation makes no claim that the BK VEGGIE® Burger or any of its products meets the requirements of a vegan or vegetarian diet.

SOURCE: BURGER KING® nutritional information used with permission from Burger King Brands, Inc.

## Domino's Pizza

(1 serving = 2 of 8 slices or ¼ of 14-inch pizza; 2 of 8 slices or ¼ of 12-inch pizza; 1 6-inch pizza)

| | Serving size | Calories | Protein | Total fat | Saturated fat | Total carbohydrate | Sugars | Fiber | Cholesterol | Sodium | Vitamin A | Vitamin C | Calcium | Iron | % calories from fat |
|---|---|---|---|---|---|---|---|---|---|---|---|---|---|---|---|
| | g | | g | g | g | g | g | g | mg | mg | % Daily Value | | | | |
| 14-inch lg. hand-tossed cheese | 219 | 516 | 21 | 15 | 7 | 75 | 6 | 4 | 32 | 1080 | 18 | 0 | 26 | 23 | 26 |
| 14-inch lg. thin crust cheese | 148 | 382 | 17 | 17 | 7 | 43 | 6 | 2 | 32 | 1172 | 18 | 0 | 32 | 8 | 40 |
| 14-inch lg. deep dish cheese | 256 | 677 | 26 | 30 | 11 | 80 | 9 | 5 | 41 | 1575 | 21 | <1 | 33 | 31 | 40 |
| 12-inch med. hand-tossed cheese | 159 | 375 | 15 | 11 | 5 | 55 | 5 | 3 | 23 | 776 | 13 | 0 | 19 | 17 | 26 |
| 12-inch med. thin crust cheese | 106 | 273 | 12 | 12 | 5 | 31 | 4 | 2 | 23 | 835 | 13 | 0 | 23 | 5 | 40 |
| 12-inch med. deep dish cheese | 181 | 482 | 19 | 22 | 8 | 56 | 6 | 3 | 30 | 1123 | 15 | <1 | 24 | 22 | 41 |
| Toppings: pepperoni | * | 98 | 5 | 9 | 3 | <1 | <1 | <1 | 20 | 364 | <1 | <1 | <1 | 2 | 83 |
| ham | * | 31 | 5 | 2 | <1 | <1 | <1 | <1 | 12 | 292 | <1 | <1 | <1 | 1 | 58 |
| Italian sausage | * | 110 | 5 | 9 | 3 | 3 | <1 | <1 | 22 | 342 | <1 | <1 | 2 | 3 | 74 |
| bacon | * | 153 | 8 | 13 | 4 | <1 | <1 | <1 | 22 | 424 | 0 | 15 | <1 | 2 | 77 |
| beef | * | 111 | 6 | 10 | 4 | <1 | <1 | <1 | 21 | 309 | <1 | 0 | <1 | 3 | 81 |
| anchovies | * | 45 | 9 | 2 | <1 | <1 | <1 | <1 | 18 | 791 | <1 | 0 | 5 | 6 | 40 |
| extra cheese | * | 68 | 6 | 6 | 3 | <1 | <1 | <1 | 15 | 228 | 6 | 0 | 12 | <1 | 79 |
| cheddar cheese | * | 71 | 5 | 6 | 3 | <1 | <1 | <1 | 18 | 110 | 4 | 0 | 13 | <1 | 76 |
| Barbeque buffalo wings (1 piece) | 25 | 50 | 6 | 2 | <1 | 2 | 1 | <1 | 26 | 175 | <1 | <1 | <1 | 2 | 36 |
| Buffalo chicken kickers™ (1 piece) | 24 | 47 | 4 | 2 | <1 | 3 | <1 | <1 | 9 | 163 | 0 | 0 | <1 | 0 | 38 |
| Blue cheese sauce | 42 | 223 | 1 | 23 | 4 | 2 | 2 | <1 | 20 | 417 | 1 | 0 | 2 | <1 | 93 |
| Breadsticks (1 stick) | 37 | 116 | 3 | 4 | <1 | 18 | 1 | 1 | 0 | 152 | <1 | <1 | <1 | 5 | 31 |
| Double cheesy bread | 43 | 142 | 4 | 6 | 2 | 18 | <1 | 1 | 6 | 183 | 2 | <1 | 5 | 5 | 38 |

* Topping information is based on minimal portioning requirements for one serving of a 14-inch large pizza; add the values for toppings to the values for a cheese pizza. The following toppings supply fewer than 15 calories per serving: green and yellow peppers, onion, olives, mushrooms, pineapple.

SOURCE: Domino's Pizza, 2005 (http://www.dominos.com). © Domino's Pizza, 2004. Reproduced with permission from Domino's Pizza LLC.

## Jack in the Box

| | Serving size | Calories | Protein | Total fat | Saturated fat | Trans fat | Total carbohydrate | Sugars | Fiber | Cholesterol | Sodium | Vitamin A | Vitamin C | Calcium | Iron | % calories from fat |
|---|---|---|---|---|---|---|---|---|---|---|---|---|---|---|---|---|
| | g | | g | g | g | g | g | g | g | mg | mg | % Daily Value | | | | |
| Breakfast Jack® | 129 | 305 | 13 | 14 | 4 | 0.5 | 34 | 3 | 0 | 205 | 715 | N/A | N/A | N/A | N/A | 41 |
| Supreme croissant | 155 | 475 | 16 | 27 | 8.5 | 3.5 | 41 | 4 | 1 | 220 | 815 | N/A | N/A | N/A | N/A | 51 |
| Hamburger | 119 | 310 | 17 | 14 | 5 | 0 | 30 | 6 | 0 | 45 | 590 | N/A | N/A | N/A | N/A | 41 |
| Jumbo Jack® w/cheese | 306 | 695 | 24 | 41.5 | 16 | 1 | 55 | 11 | 2 | 70 | 1305 | N/A | N/A | N/A | N/A | 54 |
| Sourdough Jack® | 246 | 715 | 26 | 51 | 18 | 2.5 | 36 | 7 | 2 | 75 | 1165 | N/A | N/A | N/A | N/A | 64 |
| Chicken fajita pita | 247 | 315 | 22 | 9 | 4 | 0 | 33 | 4 | 0 | 65 | 1080 | N/A | N/A | N/A | N/A | 26 |
| Sourdough grilled chicken club | 249 | 505 | 29 | 27 | 6.5 | 1.5 | 35 | 4 | 2 | 75 | 1220 | N/A | N/A | N/A | N/A | 48 |
| Deli Trio Pannido™ | 271 | 645 | 30 | 34 | 8.5 | 0 | 53 | 4 | 2 | 95 | 2530 | N/A | N/A | N/A | N/A | 47 |
| Jack's Spicy Chicken® | 270 | 615 | 24 | 30.5 | 5.5 | 2.5 | 62 | 7 | 3 | 50 | 1090 | N/A | N/A | N/A | N/A | 45 |
| Monster taco | 110 | 240 | 8 | 14 | 5 | 2 | 20 | 4 | 3 | 20 | 390 | N/A | N/A | N/A | N/A | 53 |
| Egg rolls (3) | 198 | 445 | 14 | 19 | 6 | 3 | 55 | 10 | 6 | 15 | 1080 | N/A | N/A | N/A | N/A | 0 |
| Chicken breast strips (5) | 226 | 630 | 35 | 38 | 8 | 6 | 39 | 1 | 3 | 90 | 1470 | N/A | N/A | N/A | N/A | 54 |
| Stuffed jalapeños (7) | 168 | 530 | 15 | 30 | 13 | 4.5 | 51 | 5 | 4 | 45 | 1600 | N/A | N/A | N/A | N/A | 51 |
| Barbeque dipping sauce | 28 | 45 | 0 | 0 | 0 | 0 | 11 | 4 | 0 | 0 | 330 | N/A | N/A | N/A | N/A | 0 |
| Seasoned curly fries (medium) | 125 | 400 | 6 | 23 | 5 | 7 | 45 | 1 | 5 | 0 | 890 | N/A | N/A | N/A | N/A | 52 |
| Onion rings | 119 | 500 | 6 | 30 | 6 | 10 | 51 | 3 | 3 | 0 | 420 | N/A | N/A | N/A | N/A | 54 |
| Side salad | 164 | 155 | 5 | 7.5 | 2.5 | 0.5 | 16 | 3 | 0 | 10 | 290 | N/A | N/A | N/A | N/A | 44 |
| Ranch dressing | 71 | 390 | 1 | 41 | 6 | 0 | 4 | 2 | 0 | 30 | 590 | N/A | N/A | N/A | N/A | 95 |
| Oreo® cookie ice-cream shake (small) | 301 | 670 | 11 | 33 | 19 | 3 | 81 | 62 | 1 | 110 | 350 | N/A | N/A | N/A | N/A | 45 |

N/A: not available.

SOURCE: Jack in the Box, Inc. 2005 (http://www.jackinthebox.com). The following trademarks are owned by Jack in the Box, Inc.: Breakfast Jack,® Jumbo Jack,® Sourdough Jack,® Jack in the Box.® Reproduced with permission from Jack in the Box, Inc.

## ..C

| | Serving size | Calories | Protein | Total fat | Saturated fat | Trans fat | Total carbohydrate | Sugars | Fiber | Cholesterol | Sodium | Vitamin A | Vitamin C | Calcium | Iron | % calories from fat |
|---|---|---|---|---|---|---|---|---|---|---|---|---|---|---|---|---|
| | g | | g | g | g | g | g | g | g | mg | mg | % Daily Value | | | | |
| Original Recipe® breast | 161 | 380 | 40 | 19 | 6 | 2.5 | 11 | 0 | 0 | 145 | 1150 | 0 | 0 | 0 | 6 | 45 |
| Original Recipe® thigh | 126 | 360 | 22 | 25 | 7 | 1.5 | 12 | 0 | 0 | 165 | 1060 | 0 | 0 | 0 | 6 | 63 |
| Extra Crispy™ breast | 162 | 460 | 34 | 28 | 8 | 4.5 | 19 | 0 | 0 | 135 | 1230 | 0 | 0 | 0 | 8 | 55 |
| Extra Crispy™ thigh | 114 | 370 | 21 | 26 | 7 | 3 | 12 | 0 | 0 | 120 | 710 | 0 | 0 | 0 | 6 | 63 |
| Hot & Spicy breast | 179 | 460 | 33 | 27 | 8 | N/A | 20 | 0 | 0 | 130 | 1450 | 0 | 0 | 0 | 6 | 53 |
| Hot & Spicy thigh | 128 | 400 | 22 | 28 | 8 | N/A | 14 | 0 | 0 | 125 | 1240 | 0 | 0 | 0 | 8 | 63 |
| Tender Roast® sandwich w/sauce | 196 | 390 | 31 | 19 | 4 | 0.5 | 24 | 0 | 1 | 70 | 810 | 0 | 0 | 4 | 10 | 44 |
| Tender Roast® sandwich w/o sauce | 177 | 260 | 31 | 5 | 1.5 | 0.5 | 23 | 0 | 1 | 65 | 690 | 0 | 0 | 4 | 10 | 17 |
| Hot Wings™ (6) | 134 | 450 | 24 | 29 | 6 | 4 | 23 | 1 | 1 | 145 | 1120 | 6 | 6 | 8 | 10 | 58 |
| Colonel's Crispy Strips® (3) | 151 | 400 | 29 | 24 | 5 | 4.5 | 17 | 0 | 0 | 75 | 1250 | 0 | 6 | 0 | 10 | 54 |
| Popcorn chicken (large) | 170 | 650 | 29 | 43 | 10 | 7 | 38 | 0 | 0 | 70 | 1530 | 0 | 4 | 4 | 35 | 60 |
| Chicken pot pie | 423 | 770 | 33 | 40 | 15 | 14 | 70 | 2 | 5 | 115 | 1680 | 200 | 0 | 0 | 20 | 47 |
| Corn on the cob (5.5") | 162 | 150 | 5 | 3 | 1 | 0 | 26 | 10 | 7 | 0 | 10 | 0 | 10 | 6 | 6 | 18 |
| Mashed potatoes w/gravy | 136 | 130 | 2 | 4.5 | 1 | 0.5 | 18 | 1 | 1 | 0 | 380 | 2 | 4 | 0 | 2 | 34 |
| Baked beans | 136 | 230 | 8 | 1 | 1 | 0.25 | 46 | 22 | 7 | 0 | 720 | 8 | 6 | 15 | 30 | 4 |
| Cole slaw | 130 | 190 | 1 | 11 | 2 | 0.25 | 22 | 13 | 3 | 5 | 300 | 25 | 40 | 4 | 0 | 52 |
| Biscuit (1) | 57 | 190 | 2 | 10 | 2 | 3.5 | 23 | 1 | 0 | 1.5 | 580 | 0 | 0 | 0 | 4 | 47 |
| Potato salad | 128 | 180 | 2 | 9 | 1.5 | 0.25 | 22 | 5 | 1 | 5 | 470 | 0 | 10 | 0 | 2 | 45 |

SOURCE: KFC Corporation, 2005. Nutritional information provided by KFC Corporation from its website www.kfc.com as of April 2005 and subject to the conditions listed therein. KFC and related marks are registered trademarks of KFC Corporation. Reproduced with permission from Kentucky Fried Chicken Corporation.

## McDonald's

| | Serving size | Calories | Protein | Total fat | Saturated fat | Trans fat | Total carbohydrate | Sugars | Fiber | Cholesterol | Sodium | Vitamin A | Vitamin C | Calcium | Iron | % calories from fat |
|---|---|---|---|---|---|---|---|---|---|---|---|---|---|---|---|---|
| | g | | g | g | g | g | g | g | g | mg | mg | % Daily Value | | | | |
| Hamburger | 105 | 260 | 13 | 9 | 3.5 | 0.5 | 33 | 7 | 1 | 30 | 530 | 2 | 2 | 15 | 15 | 31 |
| Quarter Pounder® | 171 | 420 | 24 | 18 | 7 | 1 | 40 | 8 | 3 | 70 | 730 | 2 | 2 | 15 | 25 | 46 |
| Quarter Pounder® w/cheese | 199 | 510 | 29 | 25 | 12 | 1.5 | 43 | 9 | 3 | 95 | 1150 | 10 | 2 | 30 | 25 | 43 |
| Big Mac® | 219 | 560 | 25 | 30 | 10 | 1.5 | 46 | 8 | 3 | 80 | 1010 | 8 | 2 | 25 | 25 | 48 |
| Big N' Tasty® | 232 | 520 | 24 | 29 | 9 | 1.5 | 41 | 8 | 3 | 80 | 730 | 8 | 10 | 15 | 25 | 50 |
| Filet-O-Fish® | 141 | 400 | 14 | 18 | 4 | 1 | 42 | 8 | 1 | 40 | 640 | 2 | 0 | 15 | 10 | 40 |
| McChicken® | 147 | 420 | 15 | 22 | 4.5 | 1 | 41 | 5 | 1 | 45 | 760 | 0 | 2 | 15 | 15 | 48 |
| Medium French Fries | 114 | 350 | 4 | 16 | 3 | 4 | 47 | 0 | 5 | 0 | 220 | 0 | 10 | 2 | 6 | 43 |
| Chicken McNuggets® (6 pieces) | 96 | 250 | 15 | 15 | 3 | 1.5 | 15 | 0 | 0 | 35 | 670 | 2 | 2 | 2 | 4 | 52 |
| Chicken Select® Premium Breast Strips (5 pieces) | 221 | 630 | 39 | 33 | 6 | 4.5 | 46 | 0 | 0 | 90 | 1550 | 0 | 6 | 4 | 8 | 48 |
| Tangy Honey Mustard Sauce | 43 | 70 | 1 | 2 | 0 | 0 | 13 | 9 | 1 | 0 | 160 | 0 | 0 | 0 | 1 | 29 |
| Bacon Ranch Salad w/Grilled Chicken (w/o dressing) | 288 | 240 | 31 | 9 | 4 | 0 | 11 | 4 | 3 | 85 | 940 | 90 | 50 | 15 | 10 | 33 |
| Caesar Salad w/Crispy Chicken (w/o dressing) | 284 | 300 | 24 | 14 | 4.5 | 1.5 | 22 | 3 | 3 | 50 | 910 | 90 | 50 | 20 | 10 | 40 |
| California Cobb Salad (w/o chicken and dressing) | 214 | 150 | 11 | 9 | 4 | 0 | 7 | 4 | 3 | 85 | 400 | 100 | 45 | 15 | 8 | 53 |
| Newman's Own® Ranch Dressing (2 oz) | 56 | 170 | 1 | 15 | 2.5 | 0 | 9 | 4 | 0 | 20 | 530 | 0 | 0 | 4 | 0 | 76 |
| Egg McMuffin® | 138 | 290 | 17 | 11 | 4.5 | 0 | 30 | 2 | 2 | 235 | 850 | 10 | 2 | 30 | 15 | 34 |
| Sausage Biscuit w/Egg | 162 | 500 | 18 | 32 | 10 | 5 | 36 | 2 | 1 | 250 | 1080 | 6 | 0 | 8 | 20 | 58 |
| Hotcakes (2 pats margarine & syrup) | 228 | 600 | 9 | 17 | 4 | 4 | 102 | 45 | 2 | 20 | 620 | 8 | 0 | 15 | 15 | 27 |
| Fruit 'n Yogurt Parfait | 149 | 160 | 4 | 2 | 1 | 0 | 31 | 21 | <1 | 5 | 85 | 0 | 15 | 15 | 4 | 13 |
| Chocolate Triple Thick® Shake (16 oz) | 448 | 580 | 13 | 14 | 8 | 1 | 102 | 84 | <1 | 50 | 250 | 20 | 0 | 45 | 10 | 21 |

SOURCE: McDonald's Corporation, 2005 (http://www.mcdonalds.com). Used with permission from McDonald's Corporation.

## Subway

Based on standard formulas with 6-inch subs on Italian or wheat bread

| | Serving size | Calories | Protein | Total fat | Saturated fat | Trans fat | Total carbohydrate | Sugars | Fiber | Cholesterol | Sodium | Vitamin A | Vitamin C | Calcium | Iron | % calories from fat |
|---|---|---|---|---|---|---|---|---|---|---|---|---|---|---|---|---|
| | g | | g | g | g | g | g | g | g | mg | mg | % Daily Value | | | | |
| Italian BMT® | 243 | 450 | 23 | 21 | 8 | 0 | 47 | 8 | 4 | 55 | 1790 | 8 | 30 | 15 | 25 | 42 |
| Meatball Marinara | 377 | 560 | 24 | 24 | 11 | 1 | 63 | 13 | 7 | 45 | 1610 | 15 | 50 | 20 | 40 | 39 |
| Subway® Seafood Sensation | 250 | 450 | 16 | 22 | 6 | 0.5 | 51 | 8 | 5 | 25 | 1150 | 8 | 30 | 15 | 25 | 44 |
| Cheese steak | 250 | 360 | 24 | 10 | 4.5 | 0 | 47 | 9 | 5 | 35 | 1090 | 8 | 30 | 15 | 45 | 25 |
| Subway® melt | 320 | 450 | 36 | 14 | 6 | 0 | 51 | 9 | 4 | 70 | 2330 | 8 | 30 | 15 | 30 | 28 |
| Classic tuna | 250 | 530 | 22 | 31 | 7 | 0 | 45 | 7 | 4 | 45 | 1030 | 8 | 30 | 10 | 30 | 53 |
| Sweet onion chicken teriyaki | 281 | 370 | 26 | 5 | 1.5 | 0 | 59 | 19 | 4 | 50 | 1220 | 6 | 40 | 8 | 25 | 12 |
| Roast beef | 224 | 290 | 19 | 5 | 2 | 0 | 45 | 8 | 4 | 20 | 920 | 4 | 30 | 6 | 30 | 16 |
| Turkey breast | 224 | 280 | 18 | 4.5 | 1.5 | 0 | 46 | 7 | 4 | 20 | 1020 | 4 | 30 | 4 | 25 | 14 |
| Veggie Delite® | 167 | 230 | 9 | 3 | 1 | 0 | 44 | 7 | 4 | 0 | 520 | 4 | 30 | 6 | 25 | 12 |
| Turkey breast deli | 152 | 210 | 13 | 3.5 | 1.5 | 0 | 36 | 4 | 3 | 15 | 730 | 4 | 15 | 10 | 25 | 15 |
| Chicken Bacon Ranch Wrap (w/cheese) | 256 | 440 | 41 | 27 | 10 | 0 | 18 | 1 | 9 | 90 | 1670 | 10 | 15 | 30 | 15 | 55 |
| Turkey breast wrap | 184 | 190 | 24 | 6 | 1 | 0 | 18 | 2 | 9 | 20 | 1290 | 4 | 10 | 10 | 15 | 28 |
| Bacon and egg breakfast sandwich on Deli round | 123 | 320 | 15 | 15 | 4.5 | n/a | 34 | 3 | 3 | 190 | 520 | 6 | 6 | 8 | 25 | 42 |
| Grilled chicken & baby spinach salad (w/o dressing) | 300 | 140 | 20 | 3 | 1 | 0 | 11 | 4 | 4 | 50 | 450 | 200 | 80 | 10 | 20 | 19 |
| Tuna (w/cheese) salad (w/o dressing) | 404 | 360 | 16 | 29 | 6 | 0.5 | 12 | 5 | 4 | 45 | 600 | 70 | 50 | 15 | 15 | 73 |
| New England clam chowder | 240 | 110 | 5 | 3.5 | 0.5 | n/a | 16 | 1 | 1 | 10 | 990 | 2 | 2 | 10 | 4 | 29 |
| Chili con carne | 240 | 240 | 15 | 10 | 5 | 0 | 23 | 14 | 8 | 15 | 860 | 15 | 0 | 6 | 10 | 38 |
| Sunrise refresher (small) | 341 | 120 | 1 | 0 | 0 | 0 | 29 | 28 | 1 | 0 | 20 | 4 | 210 | 2 | 0 | 0 |
| Choclate chip cookie | 45 | 210 | 2 | 10 | 4 | 1 | 30 | 18 | 1 | 15 | 160 | 4 | 0 | 0 | 6 | 43 |

SOURCE: Subway U.S. Nutrition Info as found on http://www.subway.com, 4/5/2005. Reprinted by permission of Subway.

## Taco Bell

| | Serving size | Calories | Protein | Total fat | Saturated fat | Trans fat | Total carbohydrate | Sugars | Fiber | Cholesterol | Sodium | Vitamin A | Vitamin C | Calcium | Iron | % calories from fat |
|---|---|---|---|---|---|---|---|---|---|---|---|---|---|---|---|---|
| | g | | g | g | g | g | g | g | g | mg | mg | % Daily Value | | | | |
| Taco | 78 | 170 | 8 | 10 | 4 | 0.5 | 13 | 1 | 1 | 25 | 350 | 4 | 2 | 6 | 6 | 53 |
| Taco Supreme® | 113 | 220 | 9 | 14 | 7 | 1 | 14 | 2 | 1 | 35 | 360 | 8 | 6 | 8 | 6 | 57 |
| Soft taco, beef | 99 | 210 | 10 | 10 | 4 | 1 | 21 | 2 | 1 | 25 | 620 | 4 | 2 | 10 | 8 | 43 |
| Gordita Supreme,® steak | 153 | 290 | 16 | 13 | 5 | 0.5 | 28 | 7 | 2 | 35 | 520 | 6 | 6 | 10 | 15 | 37 |
| Gordita Baja,® chicken | 153 | 320 | 17 | 15 | 3.5 | 0 | 29 | 7 | 2 | 40 | 690 | 6 | 6 | 10 | 10 | 42 |
| Gordita Baja,® chicken "Fresco Style" | 153 | 230 | 15 | 6 | 1 | 0 | 29 | 7 | 2 | 25 | 570 | 6 | 10 | 6 | 10 | 23 |
| Chalupa Supreme, beef | 153 | 390 | 14 | 24 | 10 | 3 | 31 | 4 | 1 | 35 | 600 | 8 | 6 | 15 | 8 | 55 |
| Chalupa Supreme, chicken | 153 | 370 | 17 | 20 | 8 | 3 | 30 | 4 | 1 | 45 | 530 | 6 | 8 | 10 | 6 | 49 |
| Bean burrito | 198 | 370 | 14 | 10 | 3.5 | 2 | 55 | 4 | 8 | 10 | 1200 | 10 | 8 | 20 | 15 | 24 |
| Burrito Supreme,® chicken | 248 | 410 | 21 | 14 | 6 | 2 | 50 | 5 | 5 | 45 | 1270 | 15 | 15 | 20 | 15 | 31 |
| Grilled stuffed burrito, beef | 325 | 720 | 27 | 33 | 11 | 3.5 | 79 | 6 | 7 | 55 | 2090 | 15 | 6 | 35 | 25 | 41 |
| Tostada | 170 | 250 | 11 | 10 | 4 | 5 | 29 | 2 | 7 | 15 | 710 | 10 | 8 | 15 | 8 | 36 |
| Zesty Chicken Border Bowl™ w/dressing | 418 | 730 | 23 | 42 | 9 | 4 | 65 | 5 | 12 | 45 | 1640 | 20 | 15 | 15 | 20 | 52 |
| Fiesta taco salad | 548 | 870 | 31 | 47 | 16 | 9 | 80 | 10 | 12 | 65 | 1780 | 20 | 20 | 40 | 35 | 49 |
| Steak quesadilla | 184 | 540 | 26 | 31 | 14 | 2 | 40 | 4 | 3 | 70 | 1370 | 15 | 2 | 50 | 15 | 52 |
| Nachos Supreme | 195 | 450 | 13 | 26 | 9 | 5 | 42 | 3 | 5 | 35 | 810 | 8 | 8 | 10 | 10 | 58 |
| Nachos BellGrande® | 308 | 780 | 20 | 43 | 13 | 10 | 80 | 5 | 11 | 35 | 1300 | 8 | 8 | 20 | 15 | 50 |
| Pintos 'n cheese | 128 | 180 | 10 | 7 | 3.5 | 1 | 20 | 1 | 6 | 15 | 700 | 10 | 6 | 15 | 6 | 35 |
| Mexican rice | 131 | 210 | 6 | 10 | 4 | 1.5 | 23 | 1 | 3 | 15 | 740 | 20 | 8 | 10 | 10 | 43 |

SOURCE: Taco Bell Corporation, 2005 (http://www.tacobell.com). Reproduced courtesy of Taco Bell Corporation.

## ndy's

| | Serving size | Calories | Protein | Total fat | Saturated fat | Trans fat | Total carbohydrate | Sugars | Fiber | Cholesterol | Sodium | Vitamin A | Vitamin C | Calcium | Iron | % calories from fat |
|---|---|---|---|---|---|---|---|---|---|---|---|---|---|---|---|---|
| | g | | g | g | g | g | g | g | g | mg | mg | % Daily Value | | | | |
| Classic Single® w/everything | 218 | 410 | 25 | 19 | 7 | 1 | 37 | 8 | 2 | 70 | 910 | N/A | N/A | N/A | N/A | 42 |
| Big Bacon Classic® | 282 | 580 | 33 | 29 | 12 | 1.5 | 45 | 11 | 3 | 95 | 1430 | N/A | N/A | N/A | N/A | 45 |
| Jr. hamburger | 117 | 270 | 15 | 9 | 3.5 | 0.5 | 34 | 7 | 2 | 30 | 610 | N/A | N/A | N/A | N/A | 30 |
| Jr. bacon cheeseburger | 165 | 380 | 20 | 19 | 7 | 1 | 34 | 6 | 2 | 55 | 830 | N/A | N/A | N/A | N/A | 45 |
| Ultimate Chicken Grill Sandwich | 225 | 360 | 31 | 7 | 1.5 | 0 | 44 | 11 | 2 | 75 | 1100 | N/A | N/A | N/A | N/A | 18 |
| Spicy Chicken Fillet Sandwich | 225 | 510 | 29 | 19 | 3.5 | 1.5 | 57 | 8 | 2 | 55 | 1480 | N/A | N/A | N/A | N/A | 34 |
| Homestyle Chicken Fillet Sandwich | 230 | 540 | 29 | 22 | 4 | 1.5 | 57 | 2 | 2 | 55 | 1320 | N/A | N/A | N/A | N/A | 37 |
| Caesar side salad (no toppings or dressing) | 99 | 70 | 6 | 4.5 | 2 | 0 | 2 | 1 | 1 | 10 | 190 | N/A | N/A | N/A | N/A | 58 |
| Chicken BLT salad (no toppings or dressing) | 376 | 360 | 34 | 19 | 9 | 0.5 | 10 | 4 | 4 | 95 | 1140 | N/A | N/A | N/A | N/A | 48 |
| Taco Supremo salad (no toppings or dressing) | 495 | 360 | 27 | 16 | 8 | 1 | 29 | 8 | 8 | 65 | 1090 | N/A | N/A | N/A | N/A | 40 |
| Creamy ranch dressing | 64 | 230 | 1 | 23 | 4 | 0.5 | 5 | 3 | 0 | 15 | 580 | N/A | N/A | N/A | N/A | 90 |
| Reduced fat creamy ranch dressing | 64 | 100 | 1 | 8 | 1.5 | 0 | 6 | 3 | 1 | 15 | 550 | N/A | N/A | N/A | N/A | 72 |
| Biggie® fries | 159 | 440 | 5 | 19 | 3.5 | 5 | 63 | 0 | 7 | 0 | 380 | N/A | N/A | N/A | N/A | 39 |
| Baked potato w/broccoli & cheese | 411 | 440 | 10 | 15 | 3 | 0 | 70 | 6 | 9 | 10 | 540 | N/A | N/A | N/A | N/A | 31 |
| Baked potato w/bacon & cheese | 380 | 560 | 16 | 25 | 7 | 0 | 67 | 6 | 7 | 35 | 910 | N/A | N/A | N/A | N/A | 40 |
| Chili, small, plain | 227 | 200 | 17 | 5 | 2 | 0 | 21 | 5 | 5 | 35 | 870 | N/A | N/A | N/A | N/A | 23 |
| Chili, large w/cheese | 357 | 370 | 29 | 13 | 6.5 | 0 | 32 | 7 | 7 | 65 | 1420 | N/A | N/A | N/A | N/A | 32 |
| Crispy Chicken Nuggets™ (5) | 75 | 220 | 10 | 14 | 3 | 1.5 | 13 | 0 | 0 | 35 | 490 | N/A | N/A | N/A | N/A | 57 |
| Barbecue sauce (1 packet) | 28 | 40 | 1 | 0 | 0 | 0 | 10 | 5 | 0 | 0 | 160 | N/A | N/A | N/A | N/A | 0 |
| Frosty,™ medium | 298 | 430 | 10 | 11 | 7 | 0 | 74 | 55 | 0 | 45 | 200 | N/A | N/A | N/A | N/A | 23 |

SOURCE: Wendy's International, Inc., 2004 (http://www.wendys.com). Reproduced with permission from Wendy's International, Inc. The information contained in Wendy's Nutritional Information is effective as of March, 2005. Wendy's International, Inc., its subsidiaries, affiliates, franchisees and employees do not assume responsibility for a particular sensitivity or allergy (including peanuts, nuts or other allergies) to any food product provided in our restaurants. We encourage anyone with food sensitivities, allergies, or special dietary needs to check on a regular basis with Wendy's Consumer Relations Department to obtain the most up-to-date information.

Information on additional foods and restaurants is available online; see the Web sites listed with the tables in this appendix and the following additional sites: **Hardees:** http://www.hardees.com **White Castle:** http://www.whitecastle.com

# Index

Page references in boldface refer to pages on which terms are defined.


AA (Alcoholics Anonymous), 158–159, 175, 176–177
abortion, 116, **131**, 131–137
abstinence, 94, **125–126**, 127, 335
abusive behavior, 406, 408
academic stressors, 32
Acceptable Macronutrient Distribution Ranges (AMDRs), 198–199, 230
acceptance, 46–47
accidents. *See* unintentional injuries
acculturation stress, 34
acid precipitation, **424**
acquaintance (date) rape, **409**, 409–411
acquired immunity, 317
acquired immunodeficiency syndrome (AIDS)
  defined, **329**
  diagnosis of, 331, 333–334
  statistics on, 319, 329, 330, 332
  transmission of, 331–332, 335–336, 339
  treatment of, 155, 333–335
  *See also* human immunodeficiency virus (HIV) infection
acrylamide, 305
ACSM (American College of Sports Medicine), 237, 238–239
ACTH (adrenocorticotropic hormone), **24**, 25
active euthanasia, **362**
active immunity, 318
acupuncture, **381**
added sugars, 200–201, 211, 215, 217
addiction. *See* addictive behaviors, alcohol use, nicotine, psychoactive drugs
addictive behaviors, **140**–143
Adequate Intake (AI), 206, 228
adipose tissue, 254. *See also* body fat
adolescence, 48, 59
adoption, 136
adrenal androgens, 245
adrenal glands, **24**, 25, 88, **89**
adrenaline (epinephrine), **24**, 25, 29, 319
adrenocorticotropic hormone (ACTH), **24**, 25
adult identity, 48
advance directives, **362**
advertising
  body image and, 270
  by food industry, 209
  of pharmaceuticals, 379
  tobacco use and, 179
  *See also* media
AED (automated external defibrillators), 289, 412
aerobic (cardiorespiratory endurance) exercise, **238**, 239, 241–242, 246
AFP (alpha-fetoprotein), 103
African Americans
  AIDS in, 332
  alcohol use by, 176–177
  asthma in, 428
  body image in, 270
  breast cancer in, 297
  cardiovascular disease in, 284, 285
  cervical cancer in, 300
  depression in, 53
  diabetes in, 259
  drug use by, 157
  glaucoma in, 351
  health concerns of, 8
  hypertension in, 280
  lead poisoning in, 428
  obesity in, 261
  prostate cancer in, 299, 309
  sickle-cell disease in, 7, 104
  single-parent families of, 81
  sodium intake by, 211
  tobacco use by, 179, 181
  *See also* ethnicity
age-related macular degeneration (AMD), **351**, 351–352
aging, 347–369
  adapting to physical changes, 351–353
  age-proofing measures, 348–350
  cardiovascular disease and, 283, 284
  changes in the body, 348–349
  elder abuse, 409
  exercise and, 235
  fertility and, 98
  government aid and policies, 357, 389
  human sexuality and, 91
  income and, 356
  nutrition and, 219–220, 350
  psychological and mental changes, 353–355
  social changes, 350–351
  statistics on, 356
  successful, 347–348
  susceptibility to STDs and, 339
  vitamin B-12 and, 207, 220
agoraphobia, **52**, 53
AIDS. *See* acquired immunodeficiency syndrome
air bags, 396
air pollution, 422–427
  acid precipitation, 424
  energy use and, 424–426
  greenhouse effect and global warming, 422–424
  indoor, 426
  ozone layer thinning, 423–424
  preventing, 426–427
Air Quality Index (AQI), **422**
Al-Anon, 175
alarm reaction, 29
Alaska Natives
  alcohol use by, 177
  drug use by, 157
  health concerns of, 8
  obesity in, 261
  *See also* ethnicity
alcohol
  absorption of, 165
  calories in, 194
  chemistry of, 164–165
  defined, 164, **165**
  metabolism and excretion of, 165–167
  violence and, 403
  *See also* alcohol use
alcohol abuse, **172**, 173–175
alcohol dependence, **172**, 174
Alcoholics Anonymous (AA), 158–159, 175, 176–177
alcoholism, 172, **173**, 173–175
alcohol poisoning, 168
alcohol-related neurodevelopmental disorder (ARND), **171**
alcohol use, 164–177
  alcohol abuse, 172, 173–175
  binge drinking, 169, 172–173
  blood alcohol concentration, 166–167, 169, 395
  cancer and, 165, 171, 297, 305
  cardiovascular disease and, 283, 293
  chronic effects of, 170–171
  driving and, 169–170, 394
  drugs combined with, 168
  ethnic differences and, 175–177
  gender differences in, 7, 175–177
  hangovers, 167–168
  health benefits of, 171–172
  immediate effects of, 167–169, 350
  injuries and, 168, 398
  pregnancy and, 106, 107, 171
  responsibility in, 176
  sexual decision making and, 97, 168–169, 335
  spirituality and, 146
  statistics on, 141, 173, 175
  stress and, 41
allergens, **318**, 318–319
allergies, 224, **318**, 318-319, 325
allied health care providers, **375**
allostatic load, 29
alpha-fetoprotein (AFP), 103
alpha-linolenic acid, 197, 230
altered states of consciousness, **154**, 155
alternative medicine. *See* complementary and alternative medicine
Alzheimer's disease (AD), **353**, 353–354
AMD (age-related macular degeneration), **351**, 351–352
AMDRs (Acceptable Macronutrient Distribution Ranges), 198–199, 230
amenorrhea, **258**
American Cancer Society (ACS), 296
American College of Sports Medicine (ACSM), 237, 238–239
American Heart Association (AHA), 278, 284, 293, 311
American Indians
  alcohol use by, 177
  diabetes in, 8, 259
  drug use by, 157
  health concerns of, 8
  obesity in, 261
  *See also* ethnicity
American Psychiatric Association (APA), 142, 143, 144
amino acids, **195**, 245
amniocentesis, **103**
amniotic sac, 102, **103**
amoebic dysentery, 326
amphetamines, 150, 152–153
amyloid plaques, 354
anabolic steroids, **245**
analgesics, 323
anal intercourse, 95, 331, 335-336, 337, 340
anaphylaxis, **318**, 319
androgens, 88, **89**
anemia, **204**
aneurysms, 290, **291**
anger, 51–52, 72, 282–283
angina pectoris, **288**
anorexia nervosa, 256, **271**
anterograde amnesia, 151, 410
anthrax, 328
antianxiety agents, 149
antibiotic resistance, 322, 327
antibodies, **316**, 317, 318
antidepressants
  action of, 56–57
  advertising for, 379
  for eating disorders, 273
  examples of, 58
  in young people, 59
antigens, **316**
antihistamines, 319, 323
antioxidants, **202**, 204–205, **306**, 354
antipsychotics, 58
antivirals, 333, 340
anxiety, defined, **52**
anxiety disorders, 52–55, 57
anxiolytics, 58
aorta, 278, **279**

…urysm, 182
…ar scores, **108**, 109–110
Arby's, A-1
aristolochic acid, 385
arousal, sexual, 91–92
arrhythmias, **288**
arteries, 278–279, **279**
arthritis, 236, 316, 328, **351**, 352
arthroscopy, 377
artificial insemination, 98
artificial sweeteners, 263
asbestos, 427
asbestosis, **427**
Asian Americans
  alcohol use in, 166, 177
  drug metabolism in, 53
  drug use in, 53, 157
  health concerns of, 8
  obesity in, 261
  *See also* ethnicity
Asian flu, 324
aspirin, 288, 294, 297, 323
assault, 403–404. *See also* sexual assault
assertiveness, **50**, 51
assisted reproductive technology (ART), 99
asthma, 186, 236, 319, 428
atherosclerosis, 30, **280**, 282, 286–287
athletes
  female athlete triad, 258
  injuries in, 248–249
  nutrition in, 220
  sudden death in, 291
Atkins diet, 267
atria (*singular,* atrium), **277**, 279
attachment, **67**, 111
attention-deficit/hyperactivity disorder, 153
authenticity, **47**
autoeroticism, 94, **95**
autoimmune disease, **316**, 328
automated external defibrillators (AED), 289, 412
automobile safety, alcohol and, 169–170
autonomic nervous system, **24**
autonomy, **47**
avian influenza A(H5N1), 324
ayurvedic herbal medicines, 385

bacteria (*singular,* bacterium)
  antibiotic-resistant, 322, 327
  defined, **321**
  diseases from, 306, 320–322
  in water supplies, 418
bacterial vaginosis (BV), 341–342
Baha'i faith, on tobacco use, 178
balloon angioplasty, 288–289
barbiturates, 149–150
barrier methods of contraception
  cervical caps, 124, 125
  contraceptive sponges, 121, 124–125
  diaphragms with spermicide, 123–124, 127
  female condoms, 121, 122–123, 127
  Lea's shield, 124
  male condoms, 119–121, 127
  principles of, 114
Bartholin's glands, 337
basal cell carcinoma, **301**
battering, 405–407. *See also* abuse
B cells, **316**, 316–317
BDD (body dysmorphic disorder), 269
beans (legumes), **195**, 195–196, 216–217
behavioral therapy, 61
behavior change strategies
  adopting safer habits, 415
  changing one's drug habits, 162
  choosing healthy beverages, 225
  dealing with social anxiety, 63
  dealing with test anxiety, 43
  kicking the tobacco habit, 191
  modifying diets for heart health and cancer prevention, 311
  motivation for change, 13–16, 20
  personal contracts, 18
  personal exercise program plans, 251
  personalized plans for wellness, 16–19
  weight-management programs, 275
benign tumors, **294**, 294–295
Benson, Herbert, 38–39
benzodiazepines, 149–151
benzo(a)pyrene, 182, 186
bereavement, **365**, 365–366. *See also* death and dying
beta-carotene, 306
beverages, healthy, 225
Bextra (valdecoxib), 379
bicycle safety, 397–398
bidis, 185
Billings method of contraception, 126–127
binge drinking, 169, 172–173, **173**
binge-eating disorder, **271**, 272
binge eating, stress and, 41
bioelectromagnetic-based therapies, **386**
bioengineering, benefits of, 12. *See also* genetically modified (GM) organisms
biological-based therapies, 380, **383**
biomedicine, **373**. *See also* conventional medicine
biopsies, **294**, 295
bioterrorism, 328
bipolar disorder, **57**
birth. *See* childbirth
birth control. *See* contraception
birth defects,103, 105,106, 107, 171, 204
bisexuality, defined, 94
black lung disease, 429
Blacks. *See* African Americans
blastocysts, 102, **103**, 348
blended families, 82
blood. *See* cardiovascular system
blood alcohol concentration (BAC), 166–167, **167**, 169, 395
blood pressure
  cardiovascular disease and, 294
  classification of, 280
  exercise and, 236
  measurement of, 279–280
  metabolic syndrome and, 286
  *See also* high blood pressure
BMI (body mass index), **255**, 255–256
body-based healing methods, 380, **383**, 383–385
body composition, **232**, 233, 254–256. *See also* body fat
body dysmorphic disorder (BDD), 269
body fat
  cancer and, 306
  cardiovascular disease and, 281–282
  classification of, 257
  diabetes and, 259
  distribution of, 257, 281–282
  essential *vs.* nonessential, 254, 255
  excess, 256–257
  genetic factors in, 260
  very low levels of, 258
  *See also* weight management
body image
  acceptance and change, 270–271
  defined, **257**
  dissatisfaction with, 257–258
  ethnicity and, 270
  exercise, self-esteem and, 264
  gender differences in, 270
  severe problems with, 269–270
  weight management and, 257–258
body mass index (BMI), **255**, 255–256
body piercing, 325, 331
bone marrow, 296, **297**, 348
bone marrow transplants, 308
bone mass, 206, 234, 353. *See also* osteoporosis
borderline disordered eating, 272
*Borrelia burgdorferi,* 321
botanicals. *See* herbal products
bovine spongiform encephalopathy (BSE), 213, 326
brain, 30, 147, 167, 170, 171, 235
brain attacks. *See* strokes
brain death, **357**, 357–358
Braxton Hicks contractions, **100**
BRCA1 (breast cancer gene 1), 304
breast cancer, 297–299
  alcohol use and, 171–172
  detection of, 298, 309
  risk factors in, 297–298, 304, 305
  treatment and prevention of, 298–299
breastfeeding, 110–111, 331, 429
breast self-examination (BSE), 298, 309
breathing for relaxation, 39–40
broken heart syndrome, 284
BSE (bovine spongiform encephalopathy), 213, 326
BSE (breast self-examination), 298, 309
bubonic plague, 421
Buddhism, 49, 178
bulimia nervosa, **271**, 271–272
buprenorphine, 158
bupropion (Zyban), 189
Burger King, A-1
burial, 363
burnout, **33**
BV (bacterial vaginosis), 341–342

CAD (coronary artery disease), **183**, **286**, 287. *See also* coronary heart disease
caffeine, 106, 153, 162
calcium, 90, 205, 206, 229, 293
calendar method of contraception, 126
calories
  in alcohol, 165
  in the American diet, 209
  cardiovascular disease risk and, 293
  daily requirements, 216
  defined, 194, **195**
  discretionary calorie allowance, 217
  energy density, 262
  in nutrient classes, 195
  weight management and, 208, 210, 262
CAM. *See* complementary and alternative medicine
cancer, 294–310, 328
  alcohol use and, 165, 171, 297, 305
  benign *vs.* malignant tumors, 294–295
  breast, 171–172, 297–299, 304–305, 309
  cervical, 184, 300, 309, 338–339
  colon, 91, 197, 297, 305, 309
  defined, **294**
  diagnosing and treating, 155, 296, **297**, 308–309
  dietary factors in, 305–306
  exercise and, 234, 297–298, 306
  genetics and, 303–305
  Kaposi's sarcoma, 306, 324, 333
  leukemia, 295, 296
  liver, 306, 319, 341
  lung, 182–183, 186, 296–297, 427
  metastasis in, 294, 295
  oral, 184–185, 303, 305
  ovarian, 300–301
  pancreatic, 305
  prevention of, 309–310, 311
  prostate, 299–300, 305, 309

rectal, 297, 309
skin, 296, 301–303
smoking and, 182–183, 296, 297, 300
statistics on, 295, 305
stomach, 306
testicular, 93, 301, 303–304
types of, 295–296
uterine (endometrial), 300, 309
warning signs of, 308
*Candida albicans,* 92, 326
*Cannabis sativa* (marijuana), 41, 98, 150, 154–155
capillaries, 278, **279**
carbohydrates
calories in, 194
cardiovascular disease risk and, 293
defined, **199**
glycemic index, 200, 286
low-carbohydrate diets, 267
premenstrual syndrome and, 90
recommended intake of, 199, 200–201, 210, 211, 230
simple *vs.* complex, 199–200
weight management and, 263
carbon dioxide, 423
carbon monoxide, 186, 399
carcinogens
defined, **297**
in the environment, 306–308
lung cancer and, 296
in tobacco smoke, 180–181, 182, 185–187, 305
carcinomas, 296. *See also* cancer
cardiac arrest, 288, 289
cardiac defibrillation, 288
cardiac myopathy, **171**
cardiopulmonary resuscitation (CPR), **288**, 412–413, **413**
cardiorespiratory endurance, **232**, 234
cardiorespiratory endurance exercise, **238**, 239, 241–242, 246
cardiovascular disease (CVD), 277–294
aging and, 283
alcohol consumption and, 283, 293
aspirin and, 288, 294
atherosclerosis, 280, 282, 286–287
cholesterol and, 280–281, 294
congenital heart disease, 291
congestive heart failure, 291
defined, **235**, **277**
detecting and treating, 288–289
diabetes and, 282, 284, 285
dietary factors in, 292–293, 311
ethnicity and, 284–285
exercise and, 234, 281, 293
gender differences in, 283–284
heart attacks, 284, 287–289
heart valve disorders, 292
heredity and, 283
high blood pressure and, 279–280
metabolic syndrome and, 285–286
obesity and, 281–282
physical inactivity and, 281
preventing, 292–294, 311
psychological and social factors in, 282–283
pulmonary heart disease, 182
rheumatic heart disease, 292
smoking and, 182, 278–279, 293
statistics on, 287
stress and, 28, 30, 282, 294
strokes, 285, 288, 289–291
triglyceride levels and, 282
cardiovascular system, 170–171, 277–278
caregivers, 357
carotenoids, 205, **306**
carpal tunnel syndrome, **401**, 402
Carson, Rachel, 418
cataracts, 352, **353**
Caucasians
cystic fibrosis in, 7, 104
drug use by, 157
skin cancer in, 301
testicular cancer in, 303
CD4 T cells, **329**, 331
Celebrex (celecoxib), 379
celibacy, 94, **95**
cell phones, 308, 395–396, 430
cellular death, **358**
central nervous system (CNS), **149–151**, 152–153, 177
cerebral cortex, **181**
cerebrovascular accidents (CVA). *See* strokes
cervical cancer, 184, 300, 309, 338–339
cervical caps, 124, **125**
cervical dysplasia, 300, 338
cervix, 86, **87**
cesarean section, **110**
CFCs (chlorofluorocarbons), **424**, 426
chancres, **341**
chancroid, 342
CHD. *See* coronary heart disease
check-call-care system, 413
chemotherapy, 155, 296, **297**
chewing tobacco, 184–185. *See also* tobacco use
chicken pox, 324
childbirth, 107–111
children
adoption of, 136
advertising aimed towards, 209
aspirin use and, 323, 372
attachment styles and, 67
diabetes in, 259
divorce and, 79
environmental tobacco smoke and, 186
firearm safety and, 400
gender role learning by, 67
lead poisoning in, 427
mercury poisoning in, 427–428
school violence and, 404–405
sexual abuse of, 411–412
sunburns in, 301
television violence and, 402–403
violence against, 404–405, 409, 411–412
*See also* infants and newborns
child safety seats, 396
chiropractic, **383**, 383–385
chlamydia, 336–337, **337**
*Chlamydia pneumoniae,* 321
*Chlamydia trachomatis,* 336–337
chlorofluorocarbons (CFCs), **424**, 426
choking, 400
cholera, 327
cholesterol
cardiovascular disease and, 279, 280–281
defined, **197**
metabolic syndrome and, 286
recommended blood levels of, 281, 294
recommended intake of, 292
sources of, 211
chorionic villus sampling (CVS), **103**
Christianity, 49, 178
chromium picolinate, 245
chromosomes, **304**
chronic bronchitis, **183**
chronic diseases, defined, **2**, 3
chronic hostility, 282–283
chronic obstructive lung disease (COLD), 183
Cialis (tadalafil), 93
cigarette smoking. *See* smoking
cigarette tar, **181**, 182
cigars, 185. *See also* tobacco use
cilia, 315
circumcision, 86–87, **87**
cirrhosis, 170, **171**
civil unions, 77
CJD (Creutzfeldt-Jacob disease), 213, 326
climate change (global warming), **422**, 422–424, 425
clinical death, **358**
clitoris, 86, **87**
clonidine, 189
cloning, **98**, 99, 348
clove cigarettes, 185
club drugs, 151
cluster headaches, 7, 31
CMV (cytomegalovirus), 324
CNS. *See* central nervous system
coarctation of the aorta, 291
cocaine, 150, **152**
codependency, **159**, 159–160
cognitive distortions, **50**
cognitive techniques, in stress management, 37–38
cognitive therapy, 61–62
cohabitation, **75**
coitus, **95**
coitus interruptus, 127
COLD (chronic obstructive lung disease), 183
colds, 323
cold sores, 324, 339. *See also* herpesviruses
collective violence, 405, 406
college students
binge drinking among, 172–173, 174
campus safety, 413
choosing mental health professionals, 62
dietary challenges for, 218–219
eating disorders in, 271
health insurance for, 390
meningitis in, 321
nontraditional, 32
stress and, 27–28, 32
test anxiety, 43
colon cancer, 91, 197, 297, 305, 309
colostrum, **110**
commercial sex, 95–96
commitment, 68–69, 78–79
common colds, 323
communication
about contraception, 131
conflict and conflict resolution, 72–74
gender and, 71–72, 73
guidelines for, 72
health care and, 9
nonverbal, 71
online relationships, 76
psychological health and, 51
on sexual behavior, 96
skills for, 71
stress and, 36
competitiveness, in relationships, 69–70, 71
complementary and alternative medicine (CAM), 380–388
alternative medical systems, 380–382
bioelectromagnetic-based therapies, 386
biological-based therapies, 380, 383
defined, **373**
depression treated by, 60
energy therapies, 380, 384, 385–386
evaluating, 386–388
manipulative and body-based methods, 380, 383–385
mind-body interventions, 380, 383
complex carbohydrates, 199–200, 293
compulsions, 54, **55**. *See also* obsessive-compulsive disorder
compulsive gambling, 142–143
compulsive overeaters, 272

...d tomography (CT) scans, 290–291, **291**, 307, 308
conception, **97**, 97–98
condoms, female, 121, 122–123, 127
condoms, male, **119**, 119–121, 127, 330, 335–336, 338, 344
congenital heart disease, **291**
congenital malformations, **105**
congestive heart failure, **291**
consumer guidelines
alternative remedies for depression, 60
avoiding health fraud and quackery, 387
common cold treatments, 323
dietary supplement labels, 222
dietary supplements and PMS, 90
exercise footwear, 247
fat and sugar substitutes, 263
food labels, 221
health information evaluation, 14, 376
HIV tests, 334
how to be a green consumer, 420
mental health professionals, 62
over-the-counter contraceptives, 121
smoking cessation products, 189
sunscreens and sun-protective clothing, 302
tattoos and body piercing, 325
weight-loss diets, 267
contagious disease, defined, 323. *See also* infectious diseases
continuation rate, **115**
contraception, 114–131
abstinence, 125–126
cervical caps, 124, 125
choosing methods, 121, 129, 131
communicating about, 96, 131
contraceptive implants, 117–118
contraceptive skin patches, 116–117
contraceptive sponges, 121, 124–125
diaphragms with spermicide, 123–124, 127
effectiveness of methods, 128
emergency, 118–119
fertility awareness method, 126–127
injectable contraceptives, 118
intrauterine devices, 116, 119
Lea's shield, 124
men's involvement in, 122
oral contraceptives, 115–116
principles of, 114–115
risks from, 116
sterilization, 126, 127–129
vaginal contraceptive rings, 117
vaginal spermicides, 125
withdrawal method, 127
contraceptive behavior, 114, **115**
contraceptive failure rate, **115**
contraceptive implants, 117–118
contraceptive skin patch, 116–117
contraceptive sponges, 121, 124–125, **125**
contractions, **108**
conventional medicine, 373–380
cool-down periods, 241–242
coping strategies
after terrorism, mass violence, or natural disasters, 35
counterproductive, 40–41
defense mechanisms, 49–50
for dying, 364
for grief, 365–366
for weight management, 264
*See also* stress management
coronary angiograms, 288
coronary artery disease (CAD), **183**, **286**, 287. *See also* coronary heart disease
coronary bypass surgery, 289
coronary heart disease (CHD), 182, 279, **286**, 287, 293
coronary thrombosis, **286**, 287
corpus luteum, 88–89, **89**
cortisol, stress and, **24**, 25, 29, 329
Cowper's glands, 86
COX-2 inhibitors, 379
CPR (cardiopulmonary resuscitation), **288**, 412–413, **413**
"crabs," 342
crack cocaine, 150, 152
C-reactive protein (CRP), 284–285
creatine monohydrate, 245
creativity, 47
cremation, 363
Creutzfeldt-Jacob disease (CJD), 213, 326
cross-training, **249**, 249–250
cruciferous vegetables, 206–207, **207**, 311
Cruzan, Nancy Beth, 361
crystal methamphetamine, 335
CT (computed tomography) scans, 290–291, **291**, 307, 308
cultural differences
health care and, 9
psychological disorders and, 53
stress and, 27
*See also* ethnicity
cunnilingus, **95**
CVA (cerebrovascular accidents). *See* strokes
CVD. *See* cardiovascular disease
CVS (chorionic villus sampling), **103**
cyberfriends, 76
cyberstalking, **407**, 407–408
Cycle-Beads™, 126
cystic fibrosis, 7, 104
cytokines, 316–318, 329
cytomegalovirus (CMV), 324

Daily Values, **208**
dairy products, 104, 210, 217, 224
DASH (Dietary Approaches to Stop Hypertension) diet plan, 208, 280, 293
date rape, 149–150, **409**, 409–411
date-rape drugs, 149–151, 410
dating, 75. *See also* intimate relationships
Day of the Dead, 359
death and dying, 357–366
advance directives, 362
coming to terms with, 366
coping with dying, 364–366
death defined, **357**, 357–358
depression and, 354–355
end-of-life care, 359–360
funerals and memorial services, 362–363
grief, 354
prolonging or hastening, 360–362
tasks for survivors, 363
wills, 358–359
death, causes of
acquired immunodeficiency syndrome, 328–329
alcohol use, 168, 170, 171, 174
cancer, 295, 296
cardiovascular disease, 281, 286
environmental pollution, 306–307
gender differences in, 7
homicides, 401, 403, 404–405
infant mortality, 108
infectious diseases, 319
injuries, 393–394, 395, 401
lack of exercise, 234
leading causes in U.S., 3, 4
smoking, 182–183
suicide, 56
Death with Dignity Act of 1994 (Oregon), 361
decibels, **430**
decongestants, 323
deep breathing, 39
DEET, 302, 322
defense mechanisms, **49**, 49–50
Defense of Marriage Act (DOMA), 77
delusions, 59
dementia, **353**, 353–354
demoralization, 49, 55
dendritic cells, **316**, 316–317
dentists, **375**
Department of Homeland Security, 405
depersonalization, **154**
Depo-Provera, 118, 353
depressants, **149**, 149–152. *See also* alcohol use
depression, 55–57
aging and, 354–355
alternative remedies for, 60
cardiovascular disease and, 282
defined, **55**
gender differences in, 7, 57
helping others with, 55–56
postpartum, 110–111
symptoms of, 55
treatment for, 56–57, 59
in young people, 59
DES (diethylstilbestrol), 98, 301, 303
designated drivers, 169
dexfenfluramine (Redux), 269
DHEA (dehydroepiandrosterone), 245
diabetes
caffeine and, 153
cardiovascular disease and, 282, 284, 285
cholesterol levels and, 294
ethnicity and, 8
excess body fat and, 257
exercise and, 233, 234, 236, 259
gestational, 105, 259
insulin resistance and, 258–259
lifestyle and, 11
nutritional needs in, 202, 220
pre-diabetes, 259
prevention and treatment of, 259
rise in, 254
symptoms of, 258, 259
types of, 258, 259
Día de los Muertos, 359
diaphragms with spermicide, **123**, 123–124, 127
diastole, 278, 279–280
diet. *See* nutrition
diet aids, 265–266
dietary fiber, defined, **201**. *See also* fiber
Dietary Guidelines for Americans, **207**, 208–212
Dietary Reference Intakes (DRIs), 206–208, **207**, 214, 228–230
dietary supplements
labels on, 220, 222
during and before pregnancy, 105
premenstrual syndrome and, 90
regulation of, 220, 385
for strength training, 244
for weight management, 265–266
*See also* herbal products
Dietary Supplement Verification Program (DSVP), 222
diet books, 265
dieter's teas, 266
diethylstilbestrol (DES), 98, 301, 303
diets
DASH plan, 208, 280, 293
for diabetes, 259
diet books, 265
low-carbohydrate, 267
low-fat, 267

MyPyramid food guidance system, 212, 214–217
obesity and, 260–261, 262–263
Therapeutic Lifestyle Changes, 294
vegetarian, 217–218
weight-loss, 267, 275
digestion, 30, 170, 194, **195**, 200
dilation and evacuation (D & E), **136**
direct-to-consumer (DTC) advertising, 379
disabilities, people with, 8, 236
disaster preparedness, 407
discretionary calorie allowance, 215, 217
discrimination, 9, 34, 76, 285
disease. *See* genetic diseases and disorders; infectious diseases; sexually transmitted diseases
distilling, 165
distress, **29**
disulfiram (Antabuse), 166, 175
diversity issues
in contraceptive use, 130
Día de los Muertos, 359
in discrimination and stress, 34
in drug use, 157
exercise for people with special health concerns, 236
in genetic diseases, 104
in health disparities, 9
in HIV infection around the world, 330
interfaith and intrafaith partnerships, 74
in lack of health insurance, 389
in metabolism of alcohol, 166
in overweight and obesity, 261
in poverty and environmental health, 428
in psychological disorders, 53
stereotyping, 5–6
in stress, 34
in violence and health, 406
in wellness goals, 6–10
*See also* ethnicity
diverticulitis, **202**
DNA (deoxyribonucleic acid), **304**, 304–305, 329
doctors of osteopathic medicine (D. O.), **375**
DOMA (Defense of Marriage Act), 77
domestic violence, 403, 405–409
Domino's Pizza, A–1
dose-response function, 148, **149**, 169, 234
douche, **125**
Down syndrome, 103
drinking water, 418–419
DRIs (Dietary Reference Intakes), 206–208, **207**, 214, 228–230
driving
aggressive, 395
alcohol use and, 169–170, 394
cell phone use during, 395–396
fatigue and, 395
safety strategies, 396–397
Drug-Induced Rape Prevention and Punishment Act, 151, 410
drugs, defined, **140**. *See also* drug use and abuse, medications, psychoactive drugs
drug testing, 158
drug use and abuse
alcohol combined with, 168
cardiovascular disease and, 283
defined, 143–144
economic cost of, 157
effects on the body, 147–149
ethnicity and, 157
gender differences in, 145
injection drug users, 147, 330, 331–332, 336
legal consequences of, 147
legalizing drugs, 158
physical dependence, 144, 145
preventing drug abuse, 160
reasons for, 146–147
risk factors for dependence, 147
role of drugs in your life, 160–162
sexual decision making and, 97
spirituality and, 146
stress and, 41
treatment for dependence, 158–160
trends in, 156–161
users, 144–146, 148
*See also* medications; prescription drugs; psychoactive drugs
DSVP (Dietary Supplement Verification Program), 222
DTs (delirium tremens), **173**
durable power of attorney for health care, 362
dysthymic disorder, 55

"Eat 5 to 9 a Day for Better Health," 209, 218
eating disorders, 256, **271**, 271–273
Ebola hemorrhagic fever (EHF), 327
ECG (electrocardiograms), 240, **241**, **288**
eclampsia, **107**
*E. coli,* 327
economic status. *See* poverty; socioeconomic status
ecstasy (MDMA), 150–151, 156
ectopic pregnancy, **107**, 336
educational attainment
cardiovascular disease and, 285
cervical cancer and, 300
health concerns and, 8–9
EEG (electroencephalograms), **358**
ejaculation, 86, **120**
EKG (electrocardiograms), 240, **241**, **288**
elder abuse, 409
electrical impedance analysis, 256
electrocardiograms (ECG or EKG), 240, **241**, **288**
electroconvulsive therapy (ECT), 56, **57**
electroencephalograms (EEG), **358**
electromagnetic fields, 386
electromagnetic radiation, 430
electron-beam computed tomography (EBCT), 288
ELISA (enzyme-linked immunosorbent assay), **333**
embalming, **362**, 363
embolus, 290, **291**
embryonic stem cells, 348
embryos, 99, 102, **103**
emergency contraception, 118–119, 121
emergency medical services (EMS) system, **413**.
emergency preparedness, 405, 407
emerging infectious diseases, 326–328
emotional wellness, 1–2. *See also* wellness
emotions
cardiovascular disease and, 30
gender differences in, 73
immune system and, 29–30
weight management and, 264
emphysema, **183**
empty nest syndrome, 350
enabling behaviors, 159–160
encephalitis, 326–327
endemic, defined, **321**
endocrine glands, **87**
endocrine system, **24**, 24–26, 29–30, 87–88
end-of-life care, 359–360. *See also* death and dying
endometrial (uterine) cancer, 300, 309
endometriosis, 92–93, 98
endometrium, 89, **97**
endorphins, **24**, 25, **235**
endoscopies, **377**, 377–378
endurance exercise, 234, **238**, 239, 241–242, 246
endurance, muscular, **232**, 242–243
energy balance, 208, 210, 255, 267, 275
energy density in foods, 262
energy expenditure, in physical activity, 237
energy therapies, 380, **384**, 385–386
energy use, air pollution and, 424–426
environmental health, 417–433
acid precipitation, 424
air pollution, 422–427
chemical pollution, 427–428
clean water supply, 418–419
defined, **417**
emerging diseases and, 327
energy use and, 424–426
food inspection, 421
gender differences and, 429
greenhouse effect and global warming, 422–424
healing the environment, 420, 430–431
industrial pollution, 206–207
insect and rodent control, 421
noise pollution, 430
ozone layer thinning, 423–424
population growth, 421–423
poverty and, 427, 428
pregnancy and, 105–106
radiation, 307–308, 429–430
waste disposal, 419–421
environmental tobacco smoke (ETS), 164, **165**, **185**, 185–187, 279, 296, 300
environmental wellness, 2
ephedra/ephedrine, 245, 265–266
epidemics, 324, **325**
epidemiological studies, 376
epididymis, 86
epididymitis, 337
epinephrine, **24**, 25, 29, 319
Epstein-Barr virus, 306, 324
erectile dysfunction, 93
erogenous zones, **91**
erotic fantasy, 94, **95**
erythropoietin (EPO), 245
essential fat, 254, **255**
essential nutrients, 194, **195**. *See also* nutrition
estates, **358**, 359
estradiol, 89
estrogens
breast cancer and, 297
as cancer promoters, 305
cardiovascular disease and, 284
defined, **89**
in hormone replacement therapy, 91, 253, 284, 297
life expectancy and, 355
in the menstrual cycle, 88–89
in oral contraceptives, 115
ethnicity
alcohol use and, 175–177
asthma and, 319
attitudes towards death and dying, 359
body image and, 270
bone density and, 353
breast cancer and, 297
cardiovascular disease and, 284–285, 287
cervical cancer and, 300
contraceptive use and, 130
diabetes and, 259
discrimination and stress and, 34
drug use and, 157
genetic diseases and, 7–8, 104
health disparities and, 9
health insurance coverage and, 389
overweight and obesity and, 261
prostate cancer and, 299
psychological disorders and, 53
skin cancer and, 301
stress and, 27
suicide rates and, 56, 355
testicular cancer and, 303
wellness goals and, 6–8
*See also* diversity issues; *specific ethnic groups*

. ee environmental tobacco smoke
.agenol, 185
euphoria, **149**
European Americans. *See* Caucasians
eustress, **29**
euthanasia, 361–362
exercise, 231–252
aging and, 349, 352
benefits of, 233–235, 259, 349
cancer and, 234, 297–298, 306
cardiorespiratory endurance, 238–239, 241–242, 246
cardiovascular disease and, 234, 281, 293
cross-training, 249–250
defined, 237
drugs and supplements for, 244–245
injuries from, 248–249
lifestyle approach to, 237–240
mental functioning and, 235
physical fitness and, 232–233
prenatal, 106–107
recommended amounts of, 238–239
resistance, 233, 242–244, 293
self-esteem and, 264
stress and, 34
target heart range in, 241–242
warm-up and cool-down, 241–242
weight management and, 210, 236–237, 263–264
*See also* exercise programs
exercise programs
basic principles of, 240–241, 248–250, 251
cardiorespiratory endurance exercise, 238–239, 241–242, 246
eating and drinking and, 246–247
FITT exercise principles, 239, 240, 245–246
flexibility training, 239, 244–245
footwear for, 247
lifestyle physical activity, 237–240
medical clearance for, 240
for people with special health concerns, 236
physical activity pyramid, 239
during pregnancy, 106–107
selecting instructors, equipment, and facilities, 243, 246
for specific skills, 245
strength training, 239, 242–244, 246, 293
exercise testing, 288

fallopian tubes, 86, **97**
falls, 398–399
false negatives, **378**
false positives, **378**
FAM (fertility awareness method), **126**, 126–127
families
caregiving for older adults in, 356–357
deciding to become a parent, 79–80
drug use and, 157
family life cycle, 81
parenting styles, 80–81
single-parent, 81–82
stepfamilies, 82
stress and, 36
successful, 82
violence in, 403, 404, 405–409
FAS (fetal alcohol syndrome), 106, **107**, **171**
fast-food restaurants, 219, A-1 to A-4
fat, body. *See* body fat
fathers, pregnancy tasks for, 102
fatigue, driving and, 395
fats, dietary
calories in, 194, 262
cancer and, 297–298, 305, 311
cardiovascular disease and, 292, 311
fat substitutes, 264
health effects of, 197–198
low-fat diets, 267
oils, 217
recommended intake of, 197–199, 211, 215, 230, 262, 292
reducing saturated and trans, 212, 292, 311
triglycerides, 196, 281, 282, 286
types, 196–197
weight management and, 262
*See also* cholesterol
FDA (Food and Drug Administration), 220, 222, 385
fecal occult blood test (FOBT), 309
feedback, in relationships, 71
fellatio, **95**
female athlete triad, **258**
female sex organs, 86
fenfluramine (Pondimin), 269
fertility, 97–99, **115**
fertility awareness method (FAM), **126**, 126–127
fertilization, **97**
fertilized egg, **97**
fetal alcohol syndrome (FAS), 106, **107**, **171**
fetal development, 101–103
fetus, **98**, 99. *See also* pregnancy
fevers, 318
fiber, dietary
cancer risk and, 305–306
defined, **201**
recommended intake of, 202, 230, 292–293
sources of, 202
types of, 201–202
weight management and, 266
fight-or-flight reaction, **24**, 25–26
financial planning, 351
firearms, 394, 400, 403, 406, 412
fires, injuries from, 399
first aid, 412–413, **413**
automated external defibrillators, 289, 412
cardiopulmonary resuscitation, 288, 412–413
check-call-care system, 413
choking, 400
dealing with an alcohol emergency, 168
for exercise injuries and discomforts, 248–249
for heart attack or stroke victims, 288–289
poisoning, 399–400
fish, 197, 105, 211, 213, 293, 305, 428
fitness, physical, **232**, 234, 349
FITT exercise principles, 239, 240, 245–246
flashbacks, **156**
flexibility, defined, **232**
flexibility training, 239, 244–245
flu. *See* influenza
fluid intelligence, 349
flunitrazepam (Rohypnol), 410
fluoxetine (Prozac), 59, 273
flushing syndrome, 166
folic acid (folate), 203
cancer risks and, 306
cardiovascular disease risks and, 293
homocysteine levels and, 286
recommended intake of, 105, 207, 228
follicles, 89, **97**
follicle-stimulating hormone (FSH), 88–89
food
energy density in, 262
genetically modified, 223–224
groups, 214–217
ingested chemicals in, 306
organic, 223
*See also* nutrition
food additives, 223
food allergies, **224**
Food and Drug Administration (FDA), 220, 222, 385
food inspection, 421
food intolerances, 104, 210, **224**
food irradiation, **223**
food safety, 105, 212–213, 327, 421
footwear, exercise, 247
foreplay, 95
fortified wines, 165
fossil fuels, **422**, 424–426, 427
fraternal twins, **98**
free radicals, **204**, 204–205, 234, **306**
fried foods, cancer and, 305
friendships, 36, 67–68
fruits, 210, 215, 216, 306, 311
FSH (follicle-stimulating hormone), 88–89
functional fiber, **202**
funerals, 362–363
fungi, diseases from, 320, 326, **327**

GAD (generalized anxiety disorder), 54, **55**
gambling, compulsive, 142–143
gamete intrafallopian transfer (GIFT), 98–99
gamma globulin, 318
gamma hydroxybutyrate (GHB), 149–151, 410
gamma radiation, 429
gang-related violence, 404
garbage disposal, 419–421
*Gardnerella vaginalis,* 342
garlic supplements, 220
GAS (general adaptation syndrome), 28–29, **29**
gastric bypass surgery, 269
gay, lesbian, and bisexual people. *See* sexual orientation
gender, defined, **6**
gender differences
in alcohol metabolism, 166
in alcohol use, 7, 175–176
in body image, 270
in cancer, 295
in cardiovascular disease, 283–284
in causes of death, 4
in communication, 71–72, 73
in contraception involvement, 122
in depression and anxiety, 57
in drug use and abuse, 145
in environmental health, 429
in headaches, 7, 31
in injuries, 394
in life expectancy, 7, 355
in love and sex, 69
in muscular strength, 243
in nutritional needs, 218
in obesity, 261
in sexually transmitted diseases, 339
in stress responses, 7, 27–28
in suicide rates, 56
in tobacco use, 184
in violence, 403
in wellness factors, 7
gender roles, 27, **67**
general adaptation syndrome (GAS), 28–29, **29**
generalized anxiety disorder (GAD), 54, **55**
generic drugs, 372, **373**
genes, 10–**11**, 12, 104, **304**–305. *See also* genetics and heredity
genetically modified (GM) organisms, **223**, 223–224
genetic diseases
diagnosing during pregnancy, 103
ethnicity and, 7–8, 104
genome and, 10–11
heart diseases, 292–293
*See also under specific genetic diseases*
genetics and heredity
alcoholism and, 175
breast cancer and, 297

cardiovascular disease and, 283, 285
colon and rectal cancer and, 297
in conception, 97
genetically modified foods, 223–224
intracytoplasmic sperm injection defects, 99
obesity and, 260
prostate cancer and, 299
role of DNA in cancer, 304–305
wellness and, 10–11
genital herpes, 300, **338**, 339–340
genital warts, **338**
genome, 10–11, **11**
germ cells, **85**
gestational diabetes, 105, 259
GHB (gamma hydroxybutyrate), 149–151, 410
giardiasis, 326
GIFT (gamete intrafallopian transfer), 98–99
glans, 86–87, **87**
glaucoma, 350, **351**, 351–352
global warming, **422**, 422–424, 425
glucose, 200, **201**, 257
glycemic index, 200, **201**
glycogen, 200, **201**
gonads, **85**
gonorrhea, 95, 322, **337**
grains, 200–201, 214, 215
greenhouse effect, **422**, 422–423, 425
grief, 354, 364–366, **365**
gun control, 412

HAART (highly active antiretroviral therapy), 333, 334
*Haemophilus ducreyi*, 342
Hahnemann, Samuel, 381
hallucinations, 59
hallucinogens, 150–151, **154**, 155–156
hand washing, 315, 323
hangovers, 167–168
hantavirus pulmonary syndrome (HPS), 327
harassment, 407–408, 412, **413**
hardiness, 27
hard liquors, 165
harm reduction strategies, 159
hate crimes, 404
hatha yoga, 39–40
HAV (hepatitis A), 324–325, 342
hazardous wastes, 419–420, 428
HBV (hepatitis B), 306, 324–325, 340–342
HCG (human chorionic gonadotropin), 89, 100, 103
HCV (hepatitis C), 147, 306, 324–325, 340
HDL. *See* high-density lipoproteins
headaches, 7, 31
health care
access disparities in, 9, 11
choosing primary care physicians, 375, 377
complementary and alternative medicine, 380–388
conventional medicine, 373–380
evaluation of health information, 14
paying for, 388–390
physician-patient relationship, 377
self-care, 370–372
when to consult a professional, 61, 371
health care proxies, **362**
health disparities, 4–5, 9
health fraud, 387
health insurance, 388–390
health journals, 16–17
health maintenance organizations (HMOs), 388, **389**
health news, evaluating, 376
health savings accounts (HSAs), **389**, 389–390
*Healthy People 2010*, 4–6, 218, 300
hearing problems, 349, 351, 430
heart, 232, 234, 241–242, 277–279
heart attacks, 7, 284, **286**, 287–289. *See also* cardiovascular disease; heart disease
heart disease
alcohol consumption and, 293
congenital, 291
congestive heart failure, 291
detecting and treating, 288–289
exercise and, 234, 236, 281, 293
heart attacks, 284, 287–289
heart valve disorders, 292
personality types and, 26
pulmonary, 182
rheumatic, 292
smoking and, 182, 278–279, 293, 296
*See also* cardiovascular disease
heart valve disorders, 292
heavy metals, **419**, 427–428
Hegar's sign, 100
height-weight charts, 255
Heimlich maneuver, 400, **401**, 412
*Helicobacter pylori*, 306, 321
helmets, 397–398, 400
helper T cells, **316**, 316–317, 328
helping others
with alcohol problems, 168, 177
with depression, 55–56
with drug problems, 159
with eating disorders, 273
helping yourself by, 352
supporting dying persons, 364
supporting grieving persons, 366
hematopoietic stem cells, 348
hemochromatosis, 104
hemophilia, **331**
hemorrhagic strokes, **288**, 289–290
hepatitis, **325**. *See also specific types*
hepatitis A (HAV), 324–325, 342
hepatitis B (HBV), 306, 324, 325, 340–342
hepatitis C (HCV), 147, 306, 324, 325, 340
herbal products
for depression, 56, 60
safety of, 385
table of commonly used, 384
in Traditional Chinese Medicine, 381
for weight management, 265–266
*See also* dietary supplements
heredity. *See* genetics and heredity
heroin, 149–150, 158
herpes simplex virus (HSV) types 1 and 2, 324, 339–340
herpesviruses, 8, 300, 306, 324, **325**, 338, 339–340
heterosexuality, defined, **75**, 94
HHV-8 (human herpesvirus 8), 306, 324
hierarchy of needs, 46–47
"high," 148, **149**
high blood pressure
in African Americans, 284, 285
caffeine and, 153
cardiovascular disease and, 279–280, 294
classification of, 280
exercise and, 236
prehypertension, 280
sodium and potassium intake and, 211–212, 293
strokes and, 290
high-density lipoproteins (HDL), 197, 279, **280–281**, 286
highly active antiretroviral therapy (HAART), 333, 334
Hinduism, on tobacco use, 178
Hispanics. *See* Latinos/Latinas
histamine, **316**, 319
HIV (human immunodeficiency virus), **329**. *See also* human immunodeficiency virus (HIV) infection
HIV antibody tests, **333**
HIV infection. *See* human immunodeficiency virus (HIV) infection
HIV-positive, **333**
HIV RNA assay, 332, **333**, 334
HMOs (health maintenance organizations), 388, **389**
Hodgkin's disease, 306
home injuries, **398**, 398–400
homeopathy, **381**, 381–382
homeostasis, **26**
homicides, 401, 403, 404–405
homocysteine, 286
homophobia, 76
homosexuality, defined, **75**, 94. *See also* sexual orientation
honesty, 69
hormonal methods of contraception
contraceptive implants, 117–118
contraceptive skin patch, 116–117
emergency contraception, 118–119, 121
injectable contraceptives, 118
oral contraceptives, 115–116
principles of, 114
vaginal contraceptive rings, 117
hormone replacement therapy (HRT), 91, 284, 297, 353
hormones
aging and, 91
in contraceptives, 114–119
defined, **24**
hormone replacement therapy, 91, 253, 284, 297
reproductive life cycle and, 87–91
*See also under specific hormones*
hospice programs, 360, **361**
HPV. *See* human papillomavirus
HRT (hormone replacement therapy), 91, 284, 297, 353
HSV (herpes simplex virus) types 1 and 2, 324, 339–340. *See also* herpesviruses
human chorionic gonadotropin (HCG), 89, 100, 103
human herpesvirus 8 (HHV-8), 306, 324
human immunodeficiency virus (HIV) infection
defined, **329**, 331
hemophilia and, 331
in injection drug users, 147, 331
phases of, 330–331
populations of special concern for, 96, 330, 332
pregnancy and, 106, 331, 333–334
preventing, 96–97
statistics on, 329, 330, 332
symptoms and diagnosis of, 332–334
transmission of, 95, 96, 331–332, 335–336, 339
treatment of, 333–335
tuberculosis and, 321
*See also* acquired immunodeficiency syndrome
humanistic therapy, 62
human papillomavirus (HPV), 300, 309, 325-326, **338**, 338–339
humor, stress and, 38
hydrocodone, 149–150
hydrocortisone (cortisol), **24**, 25, 29, 329
hydrogenation, 196–197, **197**
hydrostatic weighing, 256
*Hypericum perforatum* (St. John's wort), 56, 60, 220, 384, 385
hyperinsulinemia, 285
hypertension, defined, **279**. *See also* high blood pressure
hypertrophic cardiomyopathy (HCM), **291**
hypnosis, **383**
hypnotics, 58
hypothalamus, **24**, 25, 88, **89**
hysterectomy, **129**

[illegible]en, 352, 354
[illegible]SI (intracytoplasmic sperm injection), 99
identical twins, **98**
identity, adult, 48
IDUs (injection drug users), 147, 330, 331–332, 336
IgE (immunoglobulin E), 319
imagery, 39. *See also* visualization
immigrants and refugees, 9, 34, 285
immune response, 316–317
immune system
  allergies and, 318–319
  chain of infection and, 314–315
  exercise and, 235
  gender differences in, 7
  HIV infection and, 329, 331
  immune response, 316–317
  immunization and, 318
  intimate relationships and, 79
  personality type and, 27
  physical and chemical barriers to infection, 315
  stress and, 29–30, 328–329
  supporting, 328
  white blood cells in, 315–317
immunity, **316**, 317
immunization, 318. *See also* vaccines
immunoglobulin E (IgE), 319
immunotherapy, 319
Implanon, 118
impotence, 93
incest, **411**
incomplete proteins, 195
incubation, **318**
indoor air pollution, 426
industrial pollution, 206–207, 419–420
infants and newborns
  environmental tobacco smoke and, 186
  herpesviruses in, 340
  infections in, 331, 333–334, 337, 340, 341
  infant mortality, 108
  premature, 108
  vitamin K in, 208
infatuation, 68
infections, 314–315, **315**
infectious diseases
  bacterial, 320–322
  cancer and, 306
  chain of infection, 314–315
  defined, **2**
  emerging, 326–328
  fungal, 320, 326
  from parasitic worms, 320, 326, 327
  protozoal, 320, 326, 327
  statistics on, 319
  table of pathogens and, 320
  viral, 320, 323–326
infertility, 93, **98**, 98–99, 337
inflammation, 234, 284–285, 287, 315, 316, 319, 329, 337–338, 352
inflammatory response, 315, 316, 319
influenza, **323**, 323–324
inhalants, 150, 156
injectable contraceptives, 118
injection drug users (IDUs), 147, 330, 331–332, 336
injuries, intentional. *See* violence
injuries, unintentional, 393–401
  alcohol-related, 168, 398
  exercise-related, 235, 248–249
  home, 398–400
  leisure, 400, 401
  motor vehicle, 395–397
  preventing, 396–397
  providing emergency care for, 412–414
  statistics on, 393, 394, 395
  stress and, 30
  in young men, 394
inner-directed, **47**
insect control and repellents, 302, 322
insomnia, stress and, 30, 35
insulin resistance, 233–234, 258–259, 285–286. *See also* diabetes
intellectual wellness, 2
intentional injuries, **393**, 401–412. *See also* violence
interfaith and intrafaith partnerships, 74
interferons, 316
interleukins, 316
Internet
  addiction to, 143
  cyberstalking, 407–408
  evaluating health information on, 14
  fitness programs on, 246
  online pharmacies, 378
  online relationships, 76
  virtual social networks, 33
  weight-loss programs on, 268
interpersonal stressors, 32
interpersonal therapy, 62
interpersonal violence, 406. *See also* violence
interpersonal wellness, 2
intestate, **358**, 359
intimate relationships, 66–84
  abusiveness in, 405–408
  capacity for, 47, 48
  challenges in, 69–70
  choosing a partner, 74
  communication in, 71–74
  conflict and conflict resolution in, 72–74
  dating, 75
  ending, 71
  family life, 79–82
  friendships, 67–68
  health and, 79
  interfaith and intrafaith partnerships, 74
  living together, 75
  love and, 68–69
  marriage, 78–79
  online relationships, 76
  same-sex partnerships, 75–77
  self-concept and self-esteem and, 66–67
  singlehood and, 76–78
  successful, 70
  unhealthy, 70–71
intoxication, **140**, 147
intracerebral hemorrhage, 290
intracytoplasmic sperm injection (ICSI), 99
intrauterine devices (IUDs), 116, **119**, 127
intrauterine insemination, 98
introverts, 54
in vitro fertilization (IVF), 98–99
iron, 104, 205, 229
irradiation of food, **223**
ischemic strokes, **288**, 289–290
Islam, 49, 178
isometric (static) exercises, 242–243, **243**
isotonic (dynamic) exercises, **243**
IUDs (intrauterine devices), 116, **119**, 127
IVF (in vitro fertilization), 98–99

Jack in the Box, A-1
Japan, social phobias in, 53
jealousy, 70
Jewish people
  alcohol metabolism in, 166
  Judaism, 49, 178
  Tay-Sachs disease in, 7, 104
Johnson, Virginia, 92
journals
  emotional release through, 60
  headache journals, 31
  health journals, 16–17
  humor journals, 38
  stress management and, 37
Judaism, 49, 178
junk mail, 421

Kaposi's sarcoma, 306, 324, 333
Kegel exercises, 107
ketamine hydrochloride, 150–151, 410
Kevorkian, Dr. Jack, 362
KFC, A-2
killer T cells, **316**, 316–317
kilocalories, defined, 194, **195**. *See also* calories
Kübler-Ross, Elisabeth, 364
Kyoto Protocol, 425

labels
  on dietary supplements, 220, 222
  on food, 201, 220–221
  on over-the-counter medications, 371–372
labor, **108**, 108–110
lactation, **110**
lacto-ovo-vegetarians, **218**
lactose intolerance, 104, 210, 224
lacto-vegetarians, **218**
landfills, 419–420
laparoscopy, 128–129, **129**, 338, 377
Latinos/Latinas
  AIDS in, 332
  alcohol use by, 177
  body image in, 270
  cardiovascular disease in, 285
  diabetes in, 8, 259, 286
  drug use by, 157
  health concerns of, 8
  obesity in, 261
  sickle-cell disease in, 104
  single-parent families of, 81
  *See also* ethnicity
LDL (low-density lipoproteins), **197**, 279–281, **280**
lead poisoning, 427, 428
Lea's shield, 124
legumes, **195**, 195–196, 216–217
leisure injuries, 400, **401**
leisure time, aging and, 350–351
lesbian, gay, and bisexual (LGB) partnerships, 75–76. *See also* sexual orientation
leukemia, 295, 296
leukoplakia, 184
Levitra (vardenafil), 93
life expectancy
  chronic alcohol use and, 171
  defined, **355**
  gender differences in, 7, 355
  public health achievements and, 3, 374
  quality of life and, 5
  tobacco use and, 183
lifestyle
  exercise and, 237–240
  health disparities and, 9
  high blood pressure and, 280
  leading causes of death and, 4, 5
  obesity and, 11, 260–261
  Therapeutic Lifestyle Changes, 294
  wellness and, 19–20
lifestyle physical activity, 237–240. *See also* exercise programs
lifting techniques, 401
lightening, in pregnancy, 100
lineoleic acid, 197, 230
lipids, 196. *See also* fats, dietary
listening skills, 71–72
*Listeria monocytogenes,* 105
lithium carbonate, 57–58

liver cancer, 306, 319, 341
liver disease (cirrhosis), 170, **171**
living together, 75
living wills, **362**
locus of control, **15**, 47
loneliness, 51
love, in intimate relationships, 68–69
low-back pain, exercise and, 235
low birth weight (LBW), **107**, 107–108
low-carbohydrate diets, 267
low-density lipoproteins (LDL), **197**, 279–281, **280**
low-fat diets, 267
LSD, 150–151, 155–156
Lunelle, 118
lung cancer, 296–297
  asbestos and, 427
  detection and treatment of, 296–297
  gender differences in, 184
  risk factors for, 296
  smoking and, 182–183, 184, 186
lupus, 316, 328
luteinizing hormone (LH), 88–89
lycopene, 306
Lyme disease, 321, 421
lymphatic system, **294**, 295, 314, **315**, 316–317
lymph nodes, 316
lymphocytes, 29, 315–317, **316**
lymphomas, 296. *See also* cancer

macrophages, **315**, 315–317, 329
mad cow disease, 213, 326
magnesium, 90, 205, 229
magnetic resonance imaging (MRI), 308, 325
*ma huang* (ephedra), 245, 265
mainstream smoke, **186**
malaria, 319
male condoms. *See* condoms, male
male sex organs, 86–87
malignant tumors, **294**, 294–295
mammograms, 298, **299**, 309
managed-care plans, 388–389, **389**
mania, **57**
manipulative and body-based methods, 380, **383**, 383–385
manual healing methods, 383–385
manual vacuum aspiration (MVA), **135**
margarine, 196
marijuana, 41, 98, 150, 154–155
marriage
  benefits of, 78
  interfaith and intrafaith, 74
  issues in, 78
  role of commitment in, 78–79
  same-sex, 75–76, 77
  separation and divorce, 79
  statistics on, 78
  *See also* intimate relationships
Maslow, Abraham, 46–47
Master Settlement Agreement (MSA) of 1998, 187
Masters, William, 92
masturbation, **93**, 93–95
maximal oxygen consumption ($VO_{2max}$), 241
McDonald's, A-2
MDMA (ecstasy), 150–151, 156
meat, 197, 215, 217, 297, 305, 306
media
  advertising in, 179, 209, 270, 379
  body image and, 270
  tobacco use in, 179
  violence in, 402–403
Medicaid, 9, 357, **390**
medical doctors (M. D.), 371, **375**
medical marijuana, 155
Medicare, 356, 357, **390**
medications
  advertising for, 379
  aging and, 350
  for alcohol treatment, 175
  antibiotics, 322, 327
  antidepressants, 56–59, 273, 379
  antivirals, 333, 340
  during childbirth, 110
  in conventional medicine, 374, 378–379
  costs of, 378
  development of, 374, 379
  for drug treatment, 158
  errors in, 378
  generic, 372, 373
  for infertility, 98
  metabolism of, 53
  off-label drug use, 378
  over-the-counter, 323, 371–372
  placebo effect and, 382
  for psychological disorders, 56, 58, 59
  questions to ask about, 378, 380
  for tobacco cessation, 189
  for weight loss, 268–269
  *See also* drug use and abuse
meditation, **39**
melanoma, **301**, 303
memorial services, 362–363
memory T and B cells, **316**, 317
men
  aging in, 91
  alcohol use by, 176
  cardiovascular disease in, 283–284
  communication by, 73
  in date rape prevention, 411
  drug use and abuse by, 145
  infertility in, 98
  injuries in young, 394
  involvement in contraception, 122
  muscular strength in, 243
  nutritional needs in, 218
  sex organs in, 86–87
  sexual maturation in, 91
  suicide in, 57
  vasectomies in, 128, 129
  violence in, 403
  *See also* gender differences
menarche, 88
meningitis, 319, **321**
menopause, **91**, 284, 353
menstrual cycle, 88–91, **89**, 184, 258, 353
mental health professionals, 61–62
menthol cigarettes, 181
mercury poisoning, 427–428
mescaline, 150, 156
metabolic rate. *See metabolism*
metabolic syndrome, 259, 285–286
metabolism
  of alcohol, 165–167
  defined, **165**
  exercise and, 234
  of medications, 53
  resting metabolic rate, 260
metastasis, **294**, 295
methadone, 158, 159
methamphetamine, 150, 152–153, 335
MI (myocardial infarction), **286**. *See also* heart attacks
microbes, cancer and, 306
microbicides, 335
mifepristone (RU-486), 132, 135–136
migraines, 31
milk, 104, 210, 216–217, 224
mind-body interventions, 380, **383**
mind/body/spirit
  anger, hostility, and heart disease, 283
  exercise and the mind, 235
  exercise, body image, and self-esteem, 264
  healthy connections, 36
  helping oneself by helping others, 352
  immunity and stress, 329
  intimate relationships and health, 79
  nature and the human spirit, 418
  paths to spiritual wellness, 49
  placebo effect, 382
  in search of a good death, 360
  sexual decision making, 94
  spirituality and drug abuse, 146
  stress and the brain, 30
  tobacco use and religion, 178
  warning signs of wellness, 3
minerals, **204**, 204–206, 229
miscarriages, **107**, 131
mitral valve prolapse (MVP), **292**
Moderation Management, 175
monosodium glutamate (MSG), 223
monounsaturated fats, 196–198, **197**
mood disorders, 55–57, 58. *See also* depression
morphine, 149–150
mosquitoborne infections, 319, 322, 326–327, 421
  motivation, 13–16, 20, 180, 249, 275
motorcycle safety, 397
motor vehicle injuries, **395**, 395–397
mourning, **365**, 365–366
MRI (magnetic resonance imaging), 308, 325
MSG (monosodium glutamate), 223
mucus method of contraception, 126–127
multi-infarct dementia, 353–354
murder, 401, 403, 404–405
muscle dysmorphia, 269–270
muscular endurance, **232**, 242–243
muscular strength, **232**, 239, 242–244, 246, 293
music, stress management and, 40
mutagens, 304
mutations, cancer and, 304–305, 307
mycoplasmas, 320, 321
myocardial infarction (MI), **286**. *See also* heart attacks
myotonia, 92, **93**
  MyPyramid, 212, 214–217

naltrexone, 175
narcotics, 149
Narcotics Anonymous (NA), 158–159
National Cholesterol Education Program (NCEP), 281, 292, 294
National Weight Control Registry, 267
Native Americans. *See* American Indians
Native Hawaiians, 8, 157. *See also* ethnicity
natural disasters, coping strategies after, 35
natural killer cells, **316**, 316–317
necrotizing fascitis, 321
*Neisseria gonorrhoeae*, 337
neoplasms (malignant tumors), **294**, 294–295
nervous system, stress and, 24–26, 29–30
neural tube defects, 103, 105
neuropeptides, 29
neurotransmitters, 24, **235**
neutrophils, **315**
niacin, 203, 228
nicotine
  addiction to, 177–179
  cardiovascular disease and, 278–279
  in cigars, 185
  defined, 164, **165**
  in spit tobacco, 184
  toxic properties of, 180
  *See also* tobacco use
nicotine replacement therapy, 184, 189
nitrates, 306

[illegible]es, 306
noise pollution, 430
nonessential (storage) fat, 254, **255**
nonoxynol-9, 120, 331, 336
nonsteroidal anti-inflammatory drugs (NSAIDS), 354, 379
nontraditional college students, 32
nonverbal communication, 71
norepinephrine (noradrenaline), **24**, 29
normality, **45**
Norplant contraceptive implant, 117–118
NSAIDS (nonsteroidal anti-inflammatory drugs), 354, 379
nuclear power, **429**
nuclear transfer, 99
nuclear weapons, 429
nurses, 375
nutrition, 194–230
  aging and, 219–220, 319–320, 349–350
  antioxidants, 202, 204–205, 306, 354
  in athletes, 220
  cancer risk and, 297–298, 305–306
  carbohydrates, 194, 199–201, 211, 230
  cardiovascular disease prevention and, 292–294
  in college students, 218–219
  colon cancer and, 197, 297, 305
  Daily Values, 208
  defined, **195**
  Dietary Guidelines for Americans, 208–212
  Dietary Reference Intakes, 206–208, 214, 228–230
  dietary supplements, 105, 206–208, 220, 222
  exercise programs and, 246–247
  in fast-food restaurants, A-1 to A-4
  fats, 194, 196–199, 211–212, 230, 311
  fiber, 201–202, 230
  fish consumption, 105, 197, 211, 213, 293
  food allergies and intolerances, 104, 210, 224
  food and supplement labels, 201, 220–222
  food irradiation, 223
  genetically modified foods, 223–224
  *Healthy People 2010*, 4–6, 218, 300
  minerals, 204–206
  MyPyramid, 212, 214–217
  organic foods, 223
  phytochemicals, 206, 207, 306, 311
  portion sizes, 214–217, 262
  prenatal, 105
  proteins, 194, 195–196, 199, 230
  stress and, 35
  vegetarian diets, 217–218
  vitamins, 202–204, 228–229
  water, 204
NuvaRing, 117

obesity
  cancer and, 305, 306
  cardiovascular disease and, 281
  contributing factors, 11, 254, 260–261
  ethnicity and, 261
  exercise and, 236
  genetic factors in, 260
  health risks of, 256–257, 259
  metabolic syndrome and, 286
  self-esteem and, 264
  statistics on, 253–254
  surgery for, 269
  treatment of, 254, 269
  *See also* weight management
obituaries, 363
obsessions, 54, **55**
obsessive-compulsive disorder (OCD), 54, **55**, 57
OC. *See* oral contraceptives
occupational injuries, 400–401
off-label drug use, 378
oils, 217. *See also* fats, dietary
Olestra (Olean), 263
omega-3 fatty acids, **197**, 198, 211, 293, 305, 354
omega-6 fatty acids, 198, 305
oncogenes, **304**
online pharmacies, 378
online relationships, 76
online weight-loss programs, 268
opioids, **149**, 150
opportunistic infections, 333
optometrists (O.D.), **375**
oral cancer, 184–185, 303, 305
oral contraceptives (OC), **115–116**, 184, 220, 278, 284, 297, 337
oral sex, 95, 331, 335, 337, 340
Orasure test, 334
organ donors, 362
organic foods, **223**
organ transplants, 348, 358
orgasmic dysfunction, 93
orgasms, 92, **93**
orlistat (Xenical), 268
Ornish diet, 267
osteoarthritis (OA), 352
osteopaths, **375**
osteopenia, 353
osteoporosis
  aging and, 91, 353
  defined, **204**, **353**
  exercise and, 234, 236
  nutrition and, 206
  smoking and, 184
OTC (over-the-counter) medications, 121, 323, 371–372
other-directed, **47**
ovarian cancer, 300–301
ovaries, 86, **87**, 88, **97**
Overeaters Anonymous (OA), 268
over-the-counter (OTC) medications, 121, 323, 371–372
overweight
  body composition and, 255
  cardiovascular disease and, 281
  ethnicity and, 261
  statistics on, 253
  *See also* obesity
oviducts, 86, **97**
ovulation, 88–89, 114
oxycodone, 149–150
oxytocin, 28
ozone layer, **422**, 423–424

Pacific Islander Americans, 8, 157. *See also* ethnicity
palliative care, 360, **361**
pancreas, 170, 257
pancreatic cancer, 305
pandemics, 324, **325**
panic disorder, **52**, 53, 57
Pap tests, 116, **117**, 300, **301**, 309
parasitic worms, 320, 326, **327**
parasympathetic division, **24**
parenting styles, 80–81
parents
  adoption by, 136
  decision to become, 79–80
  family life cycle, 81
  parenting styles, 80–81
  pregnancy tasks for fathers, 102
  single, 81–82
  *See also* families
Parkinson's disease, 382
Partial Birth Abortion Ban Act of 2004, 132
partial vegetarians, **218**
Partnership for Healthy Weight Management, 268
passion, 69
passive euthanasia, **361**
passive immunity, 318
pathogens, 314, **315**. *See also* infectious diseases
pathological gambling, 142–143
PCBs (polychlorinated biphenyls), **419**
PCP, 150, 156
pedophiles, 411
peer counseling, 60–61, 158–159
pelvic inflammatory disease (PID), 93, 98, 107,115,119, 336, **337–338**
penis, 86, **87**
PEP (postexposure prophylaxis), 333
peptic ulcers, 183
percent body fat, 166, **255**, 257, 258, 260
perchlorate, 429
performance-enhancing drugs, 245
perinatal HIV transmission, 331
peripheral arterial disease, 287
permethrin, 322
persistent vegetative state, 360–361, **361**
personal contract for behavior change, 18
personal flotation devices, 400, **401**
personality, **26**, 26–27, 282
personalized plan for wellness, 16–19
personal plan for stress management, 41–42
personal safety, 393–416
  adopting safer habits, 415
  on campus, 413
  food safety, 105, 212–213, 327
  at home, 398–400
  injury statistics, 394, 395
  during leisure activities, 400, 401
  in motor vehicles, 395–397
  providing emergency care, 412–414
  safer sex, 96–97, 335–336, 343–344
  at school, 404–405
  in the workplace, 400–401, 405
  *See also* injuries, violence
pertussis (whooping cough), 319
pescovegetarians, **218**
pesticides, **427**
pharmaceuticals, 374, **375**. *See also* medications
pharmacological properties of drugs, 148, **149**
pharmacopoeia, **383**
phenylpropanolamine, 245, 266
phobias, **52**, 52–53
phosphorus, 205, 229
photochemical smog, 422
physical activity
  declining, 231, 261
  exercise compared with, 237
  recommended amounts of, 238–239
  weight management and, 266, 275
  *See also* exercise
physical activity pyramid, 239
physical dependence, 144, **145**, 147
physical fitness, **232**, 234, 349
physical wellness, 1
physician-assisted suicide (PAS), **361**, 361–362
physicians, when to see, 371
phytochemicals, 206, **207**, **306**, 311
PID. *See* pelvic inflammatory disease
piercings, 325, 331
pinworms, 326
pipe smoking, 185. *See also* tobacco use
pituitary gland, **24**, 25, 88–89, **89**
placebo effect, 59, 60, **61**, 148, **149**, 382–383
placenta, 102, **103**, 109–110
Plan B, 118–119
planetary wellness, 2
plant stanols and sterols, 293, 294
plaques, **286**, 286–287
platelets, **279**, 281

PMDD (premenstrual dysphoric disorder), **89**, 89–90
PMS (premenstrual syndrome), **89**, 89–90
*Pneumocystis carinii*, 333
pneumonia, 319, 320–321, **321**, 333
PNI (psychoneuroimmunology), **29**, 29–30
podiatrists (D. P. M.), **375**
point-of-service (POS) plans, 388, **389**
poisoning, 399–400
pollution
  air, 422–427
  cancer and, 306–307
  chemical, 427–428
  gender differences and, 429
  industrial, 306–307
  noise, 430
  *See also* environmental health
polychlorinated biphenyls (PCBs), **419**
polyunsaturated fats, 196–198, **197**
population growth, 421–423
pornography, 95
portion sizes, 214–217, 262
POS (point-of-service) plans, 388, **389**
postexposure prophylaxis (PEP), 333
postpartum depression, **110**, 111
postpartum period, **110**, 110–111
post-traumatic stress disorder (PTSD), 30, 35, 54–**55**, 57, 411
potassium, 205, 212, 230, 285, 293
poverty
  environmental health and, 427, 428
  health concerns and, 8–9, 327
  health insurance coverage and, 389
  in older Americans, 356
  self-rated health status and, 9
  *See also* socioeconomic status
pre-diabetes, 259, 285
preeclampsia, **107**
preferred provider organizations (PPOs), 388, **389**
pregnancy, 99–108
  alcohol use in, 106, 107, 171
  childbirth classes, 107, 110
  complications during, 107–108
  drug use in, 57, 148, 152–154
  ectopic, 107, 336
  exercise during, 106–107
  fetal development, 101–103
  gestational diabetes, 105, 259
  HIV infection during, 106, 331, 333–334
  nutrition during, 105
  pollution exposures during, 429
  pregnancy tasks for fathers, 102
  prenatal care, 103–107
  smoking and, 106, 187
  termination of (*See* abortion)
  weight gain during, 100
pregnancy tests, 100
prehypertension, 280
premature ejaculation, 93
premature infants, 108
premenstrual dysphoric disorder (PMDD), **89**, 89–90
premenstrual syndrome (PMS), **89**, 89–90
premenstrual tension, **89**
prenatal care, 103–107
presbyopia, 352, **353**
prescription drugs. *See* medications
Preven, 118–119
primary care physicians, 375, 377
prions, 320, 326, **327**
problem-solving, 37–38
prodromal period, **318**
progesterone, 88–89, **89**, 91, 115
progestins, 88, **89**, 117
progressive overload, 240
proof value, **165**
prostate cancer, 299–300, 305, 309
prostate gland, 86
prostate-specific antigen (PSA) blood test, **299**, 309
prostatitis, 93
prostitution, 95–96
proteins, dietary, 194, 195–197, 199, 230, 245, 263
protozoa, diseases from, 320, 326, **327**
Prozac (fluoxetine), 59, 273
PSA (prostate-specific antigen) blood test, **299**, 309
pscyhotherapy, 61–62
psychiatrists, 61
psychoactive drugs, 140–163
  abuse of, 143–147
  club drugs, 151
  defined, **140**
  dependence on, 144, 145
  depressants, 149–152
  effects on the body, 147–149
  hallucinogens, 150–151, 154, 155–156
  inhalants, 150, 156
  injection drug users, 147, 330, 331–332, 336
  opioids, 149
  sexually transmitted diseases and, 335
  statistics on, 141
  stimulants, 150–151, 152–153, 177
  table of, 150
  users of, 144–146, 148
  *See also* drug use and abuse
psychodynamic therapy, 62
psychological disorders, 52–60
  alcoholism and, 174
  anxiety disorders, 52–55, 57
  ethnicity and culture and, 53
  mood disorders, 55–57
  professional help for, 61–62
  schizophrenia, 53, 58–60
  self-help for, 60–61
  treatment for, 55, 56–58
psychological health, 45–65
  achieving self-esteem, 48–49
  anger management, 51–52
  communication and, 51
  defense mechanisms, 49–50
  growing up psychologically, 47–48
  loneliness and, 51
  Maslow's hierarchy of needs, 46–47
  optimism and, 50–51
  *See also* psychological disorders
psychoneuroimmunology (PNI), **29**, 29–30
PTSD. *See* post-traumatic stress disorder
puberty, 88, **89**, 91
pubic lice, 342
public health, 3, 327, 374
pulmonary circulation, 277, 279
pulmonary edema, 291
pulmonary heart disease, 182
purging, **271**

qi, 381
qigong, **384**, 385–386
quackery, 387
Quinlan, Karen Ann, 360–361

racism, 9, 404
radiation
  cancer from, 307–308
  as cancer treatment, 296, 308
  defined, **429**
  gamma, 429
  infrared, 425
  for irradiated foods, 223
  from radon, 307–308, 430
  ultraviolet, 301–302, 424
  X rays, 307, 308, 429–430
radiation sickness, **429**
radioactive waste disposal, 429
radon, 307–308, **430**
raloxifene, 299
rape, 409–411. *See also* sexual assault
rape trauma syndrome, 411
Rational Recovery, 175
realism, 46
recessive genes, 104
Recommended Dietary Allowances (RDAs), 206–208, **207**, 228
rectal cancer, 297, 309
recycling programs, 420–421
refined carbohydrates, 200
refractory period, 92
Reiki, **386**
reinforcement, in addiction, 141
relative risk, 376
relaxation response, 38, **39**
relaxation techniques, 38–40, 110, 329
religion
  interfaith and intrafaith partnerships, 74
  paths to spiritual wellness, 49
  psychological health and, 60
  same-sex marriage and, 77
  stress and, 37
  tobacco use and, 178
  *See also* mind/body/spirit; spirituality
remission, **297**
repetitive strain injuries (RSIs), **401**, 402
reproduction
  conception, 97–98
  hormones and reproductive life cycle, 87–91
  sex organs, 86–87
  sexual maturation, 88–91
  *See also* pregnancy
reproductive cloning, 348
reproductive technology, 99
rescue breathing, 412
research, evaluating, 376
resistance exercise, 233, 239, 242–244, 243, 246, 293
respiratory system, 182–183, 315
restenosis, 289
resting metabolic rate (RMR), 260, **261**
retirement, economics of, 351, 356
Reye's syndrome, 323, 372
rheumatic fever, **292**
rheumatoid arthritis, 316, 328
Rh factor, 105
R-I-C-E principle, 249
Ritalin, 150, 153
RMR (resting metabolic rate), 260, **261**
Rocky Mountain spotted fever, 421
rodent control, 421
*Roe v. Wade* (1973), 131–132, 133
Rohypnol, 151–152
role models, 15
RSIs (repetitive strain injuries), **401**, 402
RU-486 (mifepristone), 132, 135–136
rubella virus, 105

SAD (seasonal affective disorder), 56–57, **57**
safer sex, 96–97, 335–336, 343–344
safety. *See* personal safety
safety belts, 395–396, 415
salt intake. *See* sodium (salt)
same-sex partnerships, 75–76, 77
sanitary landfills, **419**
sarcomas, 296. *See also* cancer
SARS (severe acute respiratory syndrome), 327
saturated fats,196, **197**,198, 292, 311

[Scha]vo, Terri, 361
schizophrenia, 53, 58–59, **59**
school violence, 404–405
scientific explanations, characteristics of, 374
scrapie, 326
scrotum, 86, **87**
seasonal affective disorder (SAD), 56–57, **57**
Seasonale, 115
secondhand smoke. *See* environmental tobacco smoke
sedation, **149**
sedative-hypnotics, **149**, 151
selective estrogen-receptor modulators (SERMs), 299
selective serotonin reuptake inhibitors (SSRIs), 59, 90
selenium, 205, 229
self-actualization, 46–47, **47**
self-assessments. *See the Study Guide*
self-care, 370–372
self-concept, 46–48, **47**, 66–67
self-disclosure, 71
self-efficacy, **15**
self-esteem, 46, 48–49, 66–67, 264
self-help for psychological disorders, 60
self-help groups, 158–159
self-image (self-concept), 46–48, **47**, 66–67
self-talk, 15, 50, 54, 62–63
Selye, Hans, 28–29
semen, 86, 92, **93**
seminal vesicles, 86
semivegetarians, **218**
September 11, 2001 terrorist attacks, 35, 405
seroconversion, **334**
seropositive, **333**
serotonin, exercise and, 235
severe acute respiratory syndrome (SARS), 327
sewage, 419
sex, defined, **6**. *See also* sexual behavior; sexual functioning; sexuality
sex hormones, 88
sex therapy, 93–94
sexual anatomy, 85–87
sexual assault, 409–411
  AIDS and, 339
  binge-drinking and, 169
  child sexual abuse, 411–412
  date rape, 409–411
  dealing with, 410–411
  defined, **409**
  effects of, 411
  men who commit, 409–410
  postexposure prophylaxis after, 333
sexual behavior
  abstinence, 94, 125–126, 127, 335
  anal intercourse, 95, 331, 335, 340
  atypical and problematic, 95
  celibacy, 94–95
  foreplay, 95
  HIV transmission and, 331, 335–336
  in intimate relationships, 68–69
  oral sex, 95, 331, 335, 337, 340
  responsible, 96–97
  sexual decision making, 94, 168–169
  sexual intercourse, 95, 335
sexual decision making, 94, 168–169
sexual dysfunctions, 92, **93**
sexual functioning, 91–94, 170. *See also* sexual behavior; sexuality
sexual harassment, 412, **413**
sexual intercourse, **95**, 335
sexuality
  aging and, 91
  communicating about, 96
  defined, **85**
  sexual anatomy, 85–87
  sexual dysfunctions, 92–94
  sexual maturation, 88–91
  sexual response cycle, 92
  sexual stimulation, 91–92
  *See also* sexual behavior; sexual functioning
sexually transmitted diseases (STDs), 328–344
  anal intercourse and, 95, 331, 335–337, 340
  bacterial vaginosis, 341–342
  cervical cancer and, 300, 309
  chancroid, 342
  chlamydia, 321, 336–337
  circumcision and, 87
  condoms and, 120–121, 127, 330, 335–336, 338
  contraceptive methods and, 127
  defined, **115**, **329**
  diagnosis and treatment of, 342–343
  diaphragms and, 123
  gender differences in, 7
  genital herpes, 300, 338, 339–340
  gonorrhea, 95, 322, 337
  hepatitis B, 324–325, 340–341
  human papillomavirus, 300, 309, 338–339
  informing partners, 342
  male-to-female transmission of, 339
  preventing, 96–97, 335–336, 342–344
  pubic lice, 342
  statistics on, 328
  syphilis, 95, 335, 341
  transmission of, 331–332, 335–336, 339
  trichomoniasis, 326, 341
  in women, 339
  *See also* human immunodeficiency virus (HIV) infection
sexual orientation
  defined, **75**, 94
  health concerns and, 8, 10
  HIV infection and, 332, 335, 342
  same-sex partnerships and, 75–76
sexual privacy, 96
sexual response cycle, 92
sexual stimulation, 91–92
sexual violence. *See* sexual assault
shingles, 324
shoes, athletic, 247
shopping, compulsive, 143
shyness, 54, 63
sibutramine (Meridia), 268
sickle-cell disease, 7, 12, 104
sidestream smoke, **186**
SIDS (sudden infant death syndrome), **108**
sigmoidoscopy, 297, 309, 377
simple carbohydrates, 199–200
simple (specific) phobias, **52**
singlehood, 76–78
sinus node, 278
skin, as barrier to infection, 315
skin cancer, 296, 301–303
skinfold measurements, 256
sleepiness, driving and, 395
sleep, stress and, 35
smog, **422**
smoke detectors, 399
smokeless (spit) tobacco, 184–185. *See also* tobacco use
smoking
  additives in cigarettes, 181
  beta-carotene and, 306
  cancer and, 182–183, 296, 297, 300
  cardiovascular disease and, 278–279, 284, 293
  contraceptives and, 116, 117
  gender differences in, 184
  health effects of, 181–184
  life expectancy and, 350
  light and low-tar cigarettes, 181
  menthol cigarettes, 181
  pregnancy and, 106, 187
  quitting, 188–190
  vitamin C and, 207
  *See also* tobacco use
smoking cessation products, 189–190
snuff, 184–185. *See also* tobacco use
social phobias, **52**, 53–54, 57, 63
Social Security, 356, **357**
social stressors, 33
social support
  cardiovascular disease and, 282
  friendships, 36, 67–68
  stress and, 34, 36
  support groups, 60–61, 158–159
social wellness, 2
socioeconomic status
  cardiovascular disease and, 282, 285
  cervical cancer and, 300
  contraceptive use and, 130
  health concerns and, 8–9
  obesity and, 261
  *See also* poverty
sodium (salt)
  in African Americans, 285
  blood pressure and, 280, 285
  functions of, 205
  premenstrual problems and, 90
  recommended intake of, 211–212, 230, 280, 293
solid waste disposal, 419–421
somatic cell nuclear transfer, 348
somatic nervous system, **26**
sonograms, **103**
sore throats, 292, 318, 321, 323
soy foods, 195, 217, 218, 293
specificity of exercise, 240
spending, compulsive, 143
sperm cells, 97
spermicides, **120**, 121, 123–124, 125, 127, 331, 336
SPF (sun protection factor), 302
sphygmomanometers, 279
spirituality
  alcohol treatment and, 177
  drug use and, 146, 156
  spiritual wellness, 2, 49
  stress and, 37
  tobacco use and, 178
  *See also* mind/body/spirit; religion
spiritual wellness, 2, 49
spit tobacco, 184–185, 303. *See also* tobacco use
sponges, contraceptive, 121, 124–125, **125**
spontaneous abortion (miscarriage), **107**, 131
squamous cell carcinoma, **301**
SSRIs (selective serotonin reuptake inhibitors), 59, 90
stages of change model, 16
stalking, **407**, 407–408
standard Western medicine, **373**. *See also* conventional medicine
stanols, 293, 294
staphylococcus bacteria, **321**
state dependence, **152**, 153
statistics
  on abortions, 134
  on alcohol abuse and dependence, 173, 175
  on annual mean temperature, 424
  on cancer, 295, 305
  on cardiovascular disease, 287
  on complementary and alternative therapy use, 373
  on energy use, 426

on health care costs, 388
on HIV infection, 330, 332
on infectious diseases, 319
on injuries, 394, 395
on leading causes of death in U.S., 3, 4, 5
on marital status, 78
on nonmedical drug use, 141
on older Americans, 356
on overweight and obesity, 253
on population growth, 421
on quality *vs.* quantity of life, 5
significance in, 376
on smokers, 181
on suicide rates, 56
on violence, 403
on waste disposal, 419
statutory rape, **409**
STDs. *See* sexually transmitted diseases
stem cells, 12, 348
stepfamilies, 82
stereotyping diversity, 5–6, 34
sterilization, **126**, 127–129
Sternberg, Robert, 68–69
sterols, 293, 294
stimulants, 150–151, **152**, 152–153, 177
St. John's wort *(Hypericum perforatum)*, 56, 60, 220, 384, 385
stomach cancer, 306
strength. *See* muscular strength
strength training, 239, 242–244, 246, 293. *See also* resistance exercise
strep throat, 292, **321**
streptococcus bacteria, **321**
*Streptococcus pneumoniae*, 321
stress, 23–44
acculturation, 34
aging and, 350
allostatic load, 29
cardiovascular disease and, 28, 30, 282, 294
college-related, 32
common sources of, 31–33
defined, **24**
discrimination and, 34
emotional and behavioral responses to, 26–28
gender differences in, 7, 27–28
general adaptation syndrome, 28–29
immune system and, 29–30, 328–329
job-related, 32–33
marital, 79
noise pollution and, 430
physical response to, 24–26, 28, 30
premenstrual problems and, 90
psychoneuroimmunology, 29–30
test anxiety, 43
*See also* stress management
stress cardiomyopathy, 284
stress management, 33–42
cognitive techniques, 37–38
counterproductive coping strategies, 40–41
exercise and, 34
getting help, 42
nutrition and, 35
personal plan for, 41–42
relaxation techniques, 38–40
sleep and, 35
social support and, 34
spirituality and, 37
time management and, 32, 36–37
weight management and, 266
writing and, 37
stressors, **24**, 31–33, 41
stress response, **24**
stretching exercises, 233, 241, 244–245
strokes, **288**, 289–291
structure-function claims, 222
subarachnoid hemorrhage, 290
substance abuse, defined, 143–144, **144**. *See also* alcohol use; drug use and abuse; psychoactive drugs; tobacco use
substance dependence, 144, **145**
Subway, A-3
suction curettage, **135**
sudden cardiac death, **288**
sudden death in athletes, 291
sudden infant death syndrome (SIDS), **108**
suffocation, 400
sugar. *See* added sugars, carbohydrates
sugar substitutes, 263
suicide
gender differences in, 7, 57
myths about, 58
in older adults, 354–355
physician-assisted, 361–362
warning signs of, 55
sulforaphane, 306
sun protection factor (SPF), 302
sun-protective clothing, 302
sunscreens, 302
Superfund program, 419–420
supplements. *See* dietary supplements
support groups, 60–61, 158–159
supportive influences
in behavior change, 15
in intimate relationships, 70, 79
stress and, 34, 36
suppressor T cells, **316**, 316–317
Supreme Court. *See* U. S. Supreme Court decisions
surgery
cancer, 296, 297, 298–299
contraception, 114
conventional medicine and, 378, 380
coronary bypass, 289
gastric bypass, 269
questions to ask about, 380
surrogate motherhood, 99
swimming safety, 400
sympathetic division, **24**
syndrome X (metabolic syndrome), 259, 285–286
synesthesia, **154**, 155
syphilis, 95, 219, 319, 335, **341**
syringe exchange programs (SEPs), 147, 159
systemic circulation, 277
systemic infections, 314
systole, 278, 279–280

Taco Bell, A-3
taijiquan, 40–41
tamoxifen, 299, 307
tanning salons, 301, 302
tapeworms, 326
target behaviors, **13**
target heart range, 241–242
tattoos, 325, 331
Tay-Sachs disease, 7, 103, 104
TB (tuberculosis), 319, **321**, 322, 333
T cells, **316**, 316–317, 328, 329
temperature inversions, **422**
temperature method of contraception, 126
tend-or-befriend response, 7, 28
tension headaches, 31
teratogens, **105**
terrorism, 35, 405, 407
test anxiety, 43
testators, **358**, 359
testes (*singular,* testis), 86, **87**, **97**
testicle self-examination, 304
testicular cancer, 93, 301, 303–304
testosterone, 28, 88, **89**, 91, 243, 355, 394, 4
tetanus, 319
thalassemia, 104
THC (tetrahydrocannabinol), 154–155
therapeutic cloning, 348
Therapeutic Lifestyle Changes (TLC), 294
therapeutic touch, **386**
therapists, finding, 61–62
thrombotic strokes, 290
thrombus, 290, **291**
thyroid medication, 353
TIA (transient ischemic attacks), 290, **291**
tickborne diseases, 321–322, 421
time-action function of drugs, 148, **149**
time management, 32, 36–37, 238
tinnitus, **430**
tobacco, defined, 164, **165**
tobacco use, 177–190
action against, 187–188
additives in cigarettes, 181
cancer and, 296, 300, 305, 306
cardiovascular disease and, 278–279, 284, 293
costs to society, 187
environmental tobacco smoke, 164–165, 182, 185–187
gender differences in, 184
immediate effects of, 181
life expectancy and, 184, 350
light and low-tar cigarettes, 181
long-term effects of, 181–184
menthol cigarettes, 181
nicotine addiction, 177–179, 184, 189, 278–279
oral contraceptives and, 116–117
in pregnancy, 106, 187
premenstrual problems and, 90
quitting, 180, 188–190, 191
reasons for starting, 179–180
religion and, 178
spit tobacco, 184–185
statistics on, 141, 181
stress and, 40
tobacco, defined, 164, **165**
toxic components, 180–181
vitamin C and, 207
Tolerable Upper Intake Level (UL), 207, 228
tolerance, 144, **145**, 173, 178
total fiber, **202**
toxic shock syndrome (TSS), **123**, 124–125, **321**
toxic wastes, 419–420
Traditional Chinese Medicine (TCM), **381**
tranquilizers, **149**, 151
trans fatty acids, 196–198, **197**, 212, 311
transient ischemic attacks (TIA), 290, **291**
transition, in labor, **108**, 109
transmissible spongiform encephalopathies (TSEs), 326
transmission, of pathogens, 314
trichomoniasis, 92, 326, 341
triglycerides, 196, 281, 282, 286
trimesters, **98**, 99, 102–103
triple marker screen (TMS), **103**
trypanosomiasis, 326
TSEs (transmissible spongiform encephalopathies), 326
tubal blockages, 98
tubal (ectopic) pregnancy, **107**, 336
tubal sterilization, 128–129, **129**
tuberculosis (TB), 319, **321**, 322, 333
tumors, 294–295. *See also* cancer
12-step programs, 158–159, 175–177
twins, **98**
type 1 diabetes, 258, 259. *See also* diabetes
type 2 diabetes, 233, 234, 258–259. *See also* diabetes

lerable Upper Intake Level), 207, 228
cerative colitis, 297
ulcers, 321
ultrasonography, **103**, 298, **299**, 308
ultraviolet A (UVA), 301–302
ultraviolet B (UVB), 301–302
Ultraviolet Protection Factor (UPF), 302
ultraviolet (UV) radiation, **301**, 301–302, 424
umbilical cord, 102, **103**
underwater weighing, 256
undescended testicles, 301, 303
Uniform Donor Card, **362**
unintentional injuries, 394–401
  bicycle, 397–398
  defined, **393**
  from firearms, 400
  home, 398–400
  leisure, 400, 401
  motor vehicle, 395–397
  work, 400–401
United Nations
  Intergovernmental Panel on Climate Change, 425
  World Health Organization, 188, 381, 406
United States Pharmacopeia (USP), 222
unsaturated fats, 196–197
urethritis, 337
urinary tract infections (UTIs), 87
USDA MyPyramid, 206, **207**, 212–217, 218
USP-DSVP mark, 222
U.S. Supreme Court decisions
  on abortion, 131–132, 133
  on right to die, 361
uterine cancer, 300, 309
uterus, 86, **87**, **97**
UV Index, 302
UV (ultraviolet) radiation, **301**, 301–302, 424

vaccines, **318**, 321, 324, 335
*Vacco v. Quill* (1997), 361
vacuum aspiration, **135**
vagina, 86, **87**
Vaginal Contraceptive Film (VCF™), 125
vaginal contraceptive rings, 117
vaginal spermicides, 125
vaginal yeast infections, 333
vaginismus, 93
vaginitis, 92
values, personal, 48
varicella-zoster virus, 324
vasa deferentia (*singular,* vas deferens), 86, 128, **129**
vasectomy, 128, **129**
vasocongestion, 92, **93**
VCF™ (Vaginal Contraceptive Film), 125
vegans, **217**, 217–218
vegetables, 206, 207, 210, 214–216, 306, 311
vegetarian diets, 196
veins, 278–279, **279**
vena cava, **277**, 279
ventricles, **277**, 279
ventricular fibrillation, 288
vertical transmission, 331
Viagra (sildenafil citrate), 93, 335
violence, 401–412
  alcohol-related, 168
  armed conflict, 406
  assault, 403–404
  child sexual abuse, 411–412
  coping strategies after, 35
  drug use and, 157
  factors contributing to, 168, 401–403
  family, 403, 405–409
  gang-related, 404
  hate crimes, 404
  homicide, 401, 403, 404–405
  interpersonal *vs.* collective, 406
  mass, 35
  in the media, 402–403
  rape, 409–411
  school, 404–405
  terrorism, 35, 405
  what to do about, 412
  workplace, 405
Vioxx (rofecoxib), 379
viruses
  defined, **323**
  diseases from, 320, 323–327
  immune response to, 316–317
  treatment of, 326, 421
  *See also specific diseases*
vision, aging and, 349, 351–352
visualization, 15, 36, 38–39, **39**
vitamins, **202**, 202–204, 228–229
vitamin A, 203–204, 228, A-1 to A-4
vitamin B-6, 203–204, 228, 286, 293
vitamin B-12, 203, 204, 207, 220, 228, 286, 293, 350
vitamin C, 203, 207, 228, 306
vitamin D, 203, 206, 208, 228
vitamin E, 90, 203, 228, 354
vitamin K, 203, 206, 208, 229
voluntary active euthanasia (VAE), **362**
vulva, 86, **87**

waist circumference, 257, 261
warm-up periods, 241–242
warts, 325–326, 338–339
*Washington v. Glucksberg* (1997), 361
waste disposal, 419–421
water
  clean water supply, 418–419
  recommended intake of, 204, 246–247
weight-loss programs, 268, 275
weight management, 253–276
  aging and, 350
  body composition and, 254–255
  body fat distribution, 257, 281–282
  body image and, 257–258, 269–271
  body mass index, 255–256
  determining appropriate weight, 210, 258–260
  diabetes and, 259
  diet and eating habits, 262–263
  *Dietary Guidelines for Americans* and, 208–210
  dietary supplements and diet aids, 265–266
  diet books, 265
  diets, 208, 267, 275, 280, 293
  eating disorders, 271–273
  energy balance and, 208, 210, 255
  excess body fat, 256–257
  exercise and, 210, 236–237, 263–264
  genetic factors, 260
  lifestyle factors, 260–261
  prescription drugs in, 268–269
  psychosocial factors in, 261–262
  resting metabolic rate and, 260
  statistics on, 253–254
  strategies for, 265–266, 275
  surgery for, 269
  weight-loss programs, 268, 275
weight training. *See* resistance exercise
Weight Watchers, 267
wellness, 1–22
  defined, **1**
  dimensions of, 1–2
  diversity and, 5–10
  ethnicity and, 6–9
  factors in, 10–12
  *Healthy People 2010* goals for, 4–5
  intimate relationships and, 79
  lifestyle changes, 19–20
  personalized plans for, 16–19
  self-efficacy in, 15
  sex and gender and, 6–7
  spiritual, 2, 49
wellness continuum, 2
wellness profile, 11–12
Wendy's, A-4
Western blot, **333**
Western medicine, **373**. *See also* conventional medicine
West Nile virus, 322, 326–327, 421
white blood cells, 315–317
Whites. *See* Caucasians
WHO (World Health Organization), 188, 381, 406
whole grains, 200–201, **201**, 210, 215
whooping cough (pertussis), 319
wills, **358**, 359
withdrawal (coitus interruptus), 127
withdrawal (from addictions), 144, **145**, 173, 178–179
women
  aging in, 91
  alcohol use by, 176
  body fat distribution in, 257
  cardiovascular disease in, 283–284
  communication by, 73
  date rape prevention, 411
  depression in, 52, 56, 57
  drug use and abuse by, 145
  environmental health and, 429
  family violence against, 405–407
  female athlete triad, 258
  HIV infection in, 332
  infertility in, 98
  menopause in, 91, 353
  muscular strength in, 243
  nutritional needs of, 218
  osteoporosis in, 353
  psychological disorders in, 52
  puberty in, 88
  sex organs in, 86
  sexually transmitted diseases in, 339
  sexual maturation in, 88–91
  stress in, 28
  suicide in, 57
  tend-or-befriend response in, 7, 28
  tobacco use by, 184
  tubal sterilization of, 128–129
  violence by, 403
  *See also* gender differences
Worden, William, 365
work injuries, 400–401, **401**
workplace
  job-related stressors, 32–33
  noise regulations, 430
  sexual harassment, 412, 413
  violence in, 405
World Health Organization (WHO), 188, 381, 406
writing, 37, 38

X rays, 307, 308, 429–430

years of potential life lost, **393**, 393–394
yeast infections, 92
yoga, 39–40

zinc, 205, 229
Zone diet, 267
zygote intrafallopian transfer (ZIFT), 98–99

# CHAPTER 1
# Taking Charge of Your Health

## Multiple Choice

1. An out-of-date definition of health is
   a. fulfillment of personal potential.
   b. personal wellness.
   c. absence of disease.
   d. multidimensional.

2. All of the following are dimensions of wellness described in the book EXCEPT
   a. planetary wellness.
   b. emotional wellness.
   c. interpersonal wellness.
   d. socioeconomic wellness.

3. Self-acceptance is most representative of
   a. physical wellness.
   b. emotional wellness.
   c. intellectual wellness.
   d. spiritual wellness.

4. The leading cause of death among Americans is
   a. heart disease.
   b. infection.
   c. cancer.
   d. stroke.

5. The *Healthy People 2010* report includes all of the following EXCEPT
   a. a goal of increasing quality and years of healthy life.
   b. a goal of eliminating health disparities among Americans.
   c. specific objectives in different focus areas related to wellness.
   d. specific budget goals for all federally funded health programs.

6. The most important contributor to wellness for most people is
   a. health behavior.
   b. health care.
   c. heredity.
   d. environment.

7. Which of the following behaviors is linked with the greatest number of the top ten leading causes of death in the United States?
   a. overconsumption of alcohol
   b. poor diet
   c. cigarette smoking
   d. physical inactivity

8. A target behavior may best be described as
   a. a risky behavior of a loved one that you would like to see changed.
   b. a risky behavior of your own that you would like to change.
   c. a healthy behavior that you would like to adopt.
   d. a reward you give yourself for achieving a goal.

9. Probably the LEAST effective health behavior change strategy is
   a. changing several behaviors at once.
   b. charting health behaviors.
   c. setting up short-term reward systems.
   d. selecting a simple behavior as the first target for change.

10. People in the ________ stage of change intend to take action to change a target behavior within 6 months.
   a. precontemplation
   b. contemplation
   c. preparation
   d. action



## True or False

T F 1. Wellness requires learning about and protecting yourself from environmental hazards.

T F 2. Personal wellness is defined primarily by a high level of cardiovascular fitness.

T F 3. A major *Healthy People 2010* objective is to increase years of healthy life among Americans.

T F 4. A healthy person has learned how to manage stress effectively.

T F 5. The human genome varies dramatically from person to person.

T F 6. An external locus of control is an advantage for behavior change.

T F 7. Some health behaviors are difficult or impossible to change without outside assistance.

T F 8. A good role model is a person who has reached the goal you are striving for.

T F 9. You are more likely to succeed if you pursue your behavior change program without telling friends or family members.

T F 10. Personal health contracts tend to set people up for failure by creating expectations that cannot be filled.

ANSWERS: Multiple Choice: 1. c (p. 1); 2. d (pp. 1–2); 3. b (p. 1); 4. a (p. 4, Table 1-1); 5. d (pp. 4–5); 6. a (p. 10); 7. c (p. 4, Table 1-1); 8. b (p. 13); 9. a (p. 13); 10. b (p. 16). True or False: 1. T (p. 2); 2. F (p. 1); 3. T (p. 4); 4. T (p. 11); 5. F (p. 10); 6. F (p. 15); 7. T (p. 13); 8. T (p. 15); 9. F (p. 18); 10. F (p. 18).

Name ____________________ Section ______________ Date ______________

## WELLNESS WORKSHEET S1

### Evaluate Your Lifestyle

All of us want optimal health. But many of us do not know how to achieve it. Taking this quiz, adapted from one created by the U.S. Public Health Service, is a good place to start. The behaviors covered in the test are recommended for most Americans. (Some of them may not apply to people with certain diseases or disabilities or to pregnant women, who may require special advice from their physicians.) After you take the quiz, add up your score for each section.

| | Almost always | Sometimes | Never |
|---|---|---|---|
| **Tobacco Use** | | | |
| If you never use tobacco, enter a score of 10 for this section and go to the next section. | | | |
| 1. I avoid using tobacco. | 2 | 1 | 0 |
| 2. I smoke only low-tar-and-nicotine cigarettes *or* I smoke a pipe or cigar *or* I use spit tobacco. | 2 | 1 | 0 |
| Tobacco Score: | ______ | | |
| **Alcohol and Other Drugs** | | | |
| 1. I avoid alcohol *or* I drink no more than 1 (women) or 2 (men) drinks a day. | 4 | 1 | 0 |
| 2. I avoid using alcohol or other drugs as a way of handling stressful situations or problems in my life. | 2 | 1 | 0 |
| 3. I am careful not to drink alcohol when taking medications, such as for colds or allergies, or when pregnant. | 2 | 1 | 0 |
| 4. I read and follow the label directions when using prescribed and over-the-counter drugs. | 2 | 1 | 0 |
| Alcohol and Other Drugs Score: | ______ | | |
| **Nutrition** | | | |
| 1. I eat a variety of foods each day, including seven or more servings of fruits and vegetables. | 3 | 1 | 0 |
| 2. I limit the amount of total fat and saturated and trans fat in my diet. | 3 | 1 | 0 |
| 3. I avoid skipping meals. | 2 | 1 | 0 |
| 4. I limit the amount of salt and sugar I eat. | 2 | 1 | 0 |
| Nutrition Score: | ______ | | |
| **Exercise/Fitness** | | | |
| 1. I engage in moderate exercise for 20–60 minutes, 3–5 times a week. | 4 | 1 | 0 |
| 2. I maintain a healthy weight, avoiding overweight or underweight. | 2 | 1 | 0 |
| 3. I do exercises to develop muscular strength and endurance at least twice a week. | 2 | 1 | 0 |
| 4. I spend some of my leisure time participating in physical activities such as gardening, bowling, golf, or baseball. | 2 | 1 | 0 |
| Exercise/Fitness Score: | ______ | | |

*(over)*

| **Emotional Health** | Almost always | Sometimes | Never |
|---|---|---|---|
| 1. I enjoy being a student, and I have a job or do other work that I like. | 2 | 1 | 0 |
| 2. I find it easy to relax and express my feelings freely. | 2 | 1 | 0 |
| 3. I manage stress well. | 2 | 1 | 0 |
| 4. I have close friends, relatives, or others I can talk to about personal matters and call on for help. | 2 | 1 | 0 |
| 5. I participate in group activities (such as church and community organizations) or hobbies that I enjoy. | 2 | 1 | 0 |
| Emotional Health Score: | ________ | | |

| **Safety** | | | |
|---|---|---|---|
| 1. I wear a safety belt while riding in a car. | 2 | 1 | 0 |
| 2. I avoid driving while under the influence of alcohol or other drugs. | 2 | 1 | 0 |
| 3. I obey traffic rules and the speed limit when driving. | 2 | 1 | 0 |
| 4. I read and follow instructions on the labels of potentially harmful products or substances, such as household cleaners, poisons, and electrical appliances. | 2 | 1 | 0 |
| 5. I avoid smoking in bed. | 2 | 1 | 0 |
| Safety Score: | ________ | | |

| **Disease Prevention** | | | |
|---|---|---|---|
| 1. I know the warning signs of cancer, diabetes, heart attack, and stroke. | 2 | 1 | 0 |
| 2. I avoid overexposure to the sun and use sunscreens. | 2 | 1 | 0 |
| 3. I get recommended medical screening tests (such as blood pressure checks and Pap tests), immunizations, and booster shots. | 2 | 1 | 0 |
| 4. I practice monthly breast/testicle self-exams. | 2 | 1 | 0 |
| 5. I am not sexually active *or* I have sex with only one mutually faithful, uninfected partner *or* I always engage in safer sex (using condoms) *and* I do not share needles to inject drugs. | 2 | 1 | 0 |
| Disease Prevention Score: | ________ | | |

**What Your Scores Mean**

**Scores of 9 and 10** Excellent! Your answers show that you are aware of the importance of this area to wellness. More important, you are putting your knowledge to work for you by practicing good health habits. As long as you continue to do so, this area should not pose a serious health risk. It's likely that you are setting an example for your family and friends to follow. Since you earned a very high test score on this part of the test, you may want to focus on other areas where your scores indicate room for improvement.

**Scores of 6–8** Your health practices in this area are good, but there is room for improvement. Look again at the items you answered with a "Sometimes" or "Never." What changes can you make to improve your score? Even a small change can often help you achieve better health.

**Scores of 3–5** Your health risks are showing! You may need more information about the risks you are facing and about why it is important for you to change these behaviors. Perhaps you need help in deciding how to successfully make the changes you desire.

**Scores of 0–2** Your answers show that you may be taking serious and unnecessary risks with your health. Perhaps you are not aware of the risks and what to do about them. You can easily get the information and help you need to improve, if you wish. The next step is up to you.

To see how your health habits affect your longevity potential, take the quiz at http://www.livingto100.com.

CHAPTER 2
# Stress: The Constant Challenge



## Multiple Choice

1. The division of our nervous system that triggers the stress response is the ____________ division.
   a. autonomic
   b. parasympathetic
   c. sympathetic
   d. somatic

2. The fight-or-flight reaction produces
   a. bronchial constriction.
   b. blood sugar reduction.
   c. increased digestion.
   d. increased blood cell production.

3. Which of the following is a brain chemical that helps to inhibit pain?
   a. cortisol
   b. epinephrine
   c. norepinephrine
   d. endorphin

4. Our behavioral responses to stressors are managed by our
   a. autonomic nervous system.
   b. parasympathetic nervous system.
   c. sympathetic nervous system.
   d. somatic nervous system.

5. Which of the following characteristics is most closely associated with the Type A personality?
   a. tolerance
   b. cynicism
   c. sense of inner purpose
   d. optimism

6. Eustress might be triggered by
   a. getting a bad grade.
   b. winning the lottery.
   c. being physically attacked.
   d. experiencing homeostasis.

7. Which of the following is one of the stages of the general adaptation syndrome?
   a. alarm
   b. ambivalence
   c. anger
   d. anxiety

8. All of the following are effective techniques for managing stress EXCEPT
   a. exercising regularly.
   b. meditating.
   c. drinking caffeine.
   d. prioritizing tasks.

9. All of the following are strategies for overcoming insomnia EXCEPT
   a. keeping to a regular schedule.
   b. avoiding alcohol before bedtime.
   c. exercising just before bedtime.
   d. having a snack just before bedtime.

10. Another term for imagery is
    a. progressive relaxation.
    b. visualization.
    c. meditation.
    d. biofeedback.

## True or False

T F 1. Stressors are events or situations that trigger the stress response.

T F 2. The two body systems that control the physical responses to stressors are the nervous system and the endocrine system.

T F 3. The parasympathetic division of the nervous system triggers the fight-orflight reaction.

T F 4. The fight-or-flight reaction occurs only when physical action is required to deal with a stressor.

T F 5. A person with a Type A personality who tends to be hostile and cynical has an increased risk of heart disease.

T F 6. A high level of stress can impair the immune system, thereby increasing one's risk for colds and allergy attacks.

T F 7. Exercise can help you manage stress only if performed at least four times a week.

T F 8. Blood pressure and heart rate increase during the relaxation response.

T F 9. Progressive relaxation involves focusing on a single word and taking deep breaths.

T F 10. Keeping a stress journal will help you identify and cope with daily stressors.

ANSWERS: Multiple Choice: 1. c (p. 24); 2. d (p. 25); 3. d (p. 25); 4. d (p. 26); 5. b (p. 26); 6. b (p. 29); 7. a (p. 29); 8. c (p. 35); 9. c (p. 35); 10. b (p. 38). True or False: 1. T (p. 24); 2. T (p. 24); 3. F (p. 24); 4. F (p. 26); 5. T (p. 26); 6. T (p. 30); 7. F (p. 34); 8. F (p. 38); 9. F (p. 38); 10. T ( p. 41).

Name ______________________ Section ______________ Date ______________

# WELLNESS WORKSHEET S2

## Identify Your Stress Level and Your Key Stressors

Vw

### How High Is Your Stress Level?

Many symptoms of excess stress are easy to self-diagnose. To help determine how much stress you experience on a daily basis, answer the following questions.

| Yes | No | | Yes | No | |
|---|---|---|---|---|---|
| | ____ | 1. How many of the symptoms of excess stress listed below do you experience frequently? Circle the appropriate symptoms. | ____ | ____ | 8. Do you often feel as if you have less energy than you need to finish the day? |
| ____ | ____ | 2. Are you easily startled or irritated? | ____ | ____ | 9. Do you have recurrent stomachaches or headaches? |
| ____ | ____ | 3. Are you increasingly forgetful? | ____ | ____ | 10. Is it difficult for you to find satisfaction in simple life pleasures? |
| ____ | ____ | 4. Do you have trouble falling or staying asleep? | ____ | ____ | 11. Are you often disappointed in yourself and others? |
| ____ | ____ | 5. Do you continually worry about events in your future? | ____ | ____ | 12. Are you overly concerned with being liked or accepted by others? |
| ____ | ____ | 6. Do you feel as if you are constantly under pressure to produce? | ____ | ____ | 13. Have you lost interest in intimacy or sex? |
| ____ | ____ | 7. Do you frequently use tobacco, alcohol, or other drugs to help you relax? | ____ | ____ | 14. Are you concerned that you do not have enough money? |

Experiencing some of the stress-related symptoms or answering "yes" to a few questions is normal. However, if you experience a large number of stress symptoms or you answered "yes" to a majority of the questions, you are likely experiencing a high level of stress. Take time out to develop effective stress-management techniques. Many coping strategies that can aid you in dealing with your college stressors are described in this chapter. Additionally, your school's counseling center can provide valuable support.

### Symptoms of Excess Stress

| Physical Symptoms | Emotional Symptoms | Behavioral Symptoms |
|---|---|---|
| Dry mouth | Anxiety or edginess | Crying |
| Excessive perspiration | Depression | Disrupted eating habits |
| Frequent illnesses | Fatigue | Disrupted sleeping habits |
| Gastrointestinal problems | Hypervigilance | Harsh treatment of others |
| Grinding of teeth | Impulsiveness | Increased use of tobacco, alcohol, or other drugs |
| Headaches | Inability to concentrate | Problems communicating |
| High blood pressure | Irritability | Sexual problems |
| Pounding heart | Trouble remembering things | Social isolation |
| Stiff neck or aching lower back | | |

*(over)*

## WELLNESS WORKSHEET S2—continued

### Weekly Stress Log

Now that you are familiar with the signals of stress, complete the weekly stress log to map patterns in your stress levels and identify sources of stress. Enter a score for each hour of each day according to the ratings listed below.

| | A.M. | | | | | | | P.M. | | | | | | | | | | | | | |
|---|---|---|---|---|---|---|---|---|---|---|---|---|---|---|---|---|---|---|---|---|---|
| | 6 | 7 | 8 | 9 | 10 | 11 | 12 | 1 | 2 | 3 | 4 | 5 | 6 | 7 | 8 | 9 | 10 | 11 | 12 | *Average* |
| Monday | | | | | | | | | | | | | | | | | | | | |
| Tuesday | | | | | | | | | | | | | | | | | | | | |
| Wednesday | | | | | | | | | | | | | | | | | | | | |
| Thursday | | | | | | | | | | | | | | | | | | | | |
| Friday | | | | | | | | | | | | | | | | | | | | |
| Saturday | | | | | | | | | | | | | | | | | | | | |
| Sunday | | | | | | | | | | | | | | | | | | | | |
| *Average* | | | | | | | | | | | | | | | | | | | | |

**Ratings**

1 = No anxiety; general feeling of well-being
2 = Mild anxiety; no interference with activity
3 = Moderate anxiety; specific signal(s) of stress present
4 = High anxiety; interference with activity
5 = Very high anxiety and panic reactions; general inability to engage in activity

To identify daily or weekly patterns in your stress level, average your stress rating for each hour and each day. For example, if your scores for 6:00 A.M. are 3, 3, 4, 3, and 4, with blanks for Saturday and Sunday, your 6:00 A.M. rating would be 17 ÷ 5, or 3.4 (moderate to high anxiety). Finally, calculate an average weekly stress score by averaging your daily average stress scores. Your weekly average will give you a sense of your overall level of stress.

### Identifying Sources of Stress

*External stressors:* List several people, places, or events that caused you a significant amount of discomfort this week. ____________________

____________________

____________________

____________________

*Internal stressors:* List any recurring thoughts or worries that produced feelings of discomfort this week.

____________________

____________________

____________________

____________________

# CHAPTER 3
# Psychological Health



## Multiple Choice

1. Which of the following best describes psychological health?
   a. being psychologically normal
   b. having no symptoms of mental disorders
   c. achieving self-actualization
   d. conforming to social demands

2. Self-actualized people are
   a. critical.
   b. verbal.
   c. realistic.
   d. self-absorbed.

3. Spiritual wellness can be promoted by
   a. creating art.
   b. participating in organized religion.
   c. spending time in nature.
   d. all of the above.

4. Achieving healthy self-esteem involves all of the following EXCEPT
   a. developing a positive self-concept.
   b. meeting challenges to self-esteem.
   c. developing defense mechanisms.
   d. learning to deal with anger.

5. An example of negative self-talk is
   a. I overdid it last night. Next time I'll make different choices.
   b. It may not be the best speech I'll ever give, but it was good enough to earn a grade of "B."
   c. I wonder why my boss wants to see me? I'll just have to wait and see.
   d. I got a bad grade on this paper because I'm incompetent at everything.

6. Shyness is
   a. a form of social anxiety.
   b. relatively uncommon among Americans.
   c. due to environmental factors rather than heredity.
   d. seldom outgrown.

7. A phobia is
   a. a persistent fear of a specific thing.
   b. a heart attack symptom.
   c. a common response to stress.
   d. a mood disorder.

8. A key symptom of post-traumatic stress disorder is
   a. reexperiencing a trauma in dreams.
   b. having recurrent, unwanted thoughts.
   c. experiencing sudden surges in anxiety.
   d. hearing voices when no one is present.

9. Which of the following may be symptomatic of depression?
   a. poor appetite
   b. insomnia
   c. restlessness
   d. all of the above

10. Characteristics of schizophrenia include all of the following EXCEPT
    a. disorganized thoughts.
    b. increased social activity.
    c. delusions.
    d. auditory hallucinations.

## True or False

T F 1. Normality is a key component of psychological health.

T F 2. Self-acceptance is a prerequisite for positive psychological health.

T F 3. Developing an adult identity is easier in a culture where many roles are possible.

T F 4. Expecting perfection is a pattern of realistic self-talk that helps people cope with challenges.

T F 5. A pessimistic outlook is typically learned during childhood.

T F 6. Psychologically healthy people always express their anger rather than suppress it.

T F 7. Fear of public speaking is an example of a social phobia.

T F 8. There is a strong association between severe depression and suicide.

T F 9. St. John's wort is an effective treatment for severe depression.

T F 10. Schizophrenia is a very rare disorder.

ANSWERS: Multiple Choice: 1. c (p. 46); 2. c (p. 46); 3. d (p. 49); 4. c (pp. 48–51); 5. d (p. 50); 6. a (p. 54); 7. a (p. 52); 8. a (p. 55); 9. d (p. 55); 10. b (p. 59).
True or False: 1. F (p. 45); 2. T (p. 46); 3. F (p. 48); 4. F (p. 50); 5. T (p. 50); 6. F (p. 51); 7. T (p. 53); 8. T (p. 55); 9. F (p. 60); 10. F (p. 58).

Name ______________________ Section ______________ Date ________________

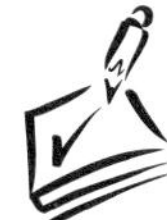

# WELLNESS WORKSHEET S3

## Recognizing Signs of Mood and Anxiety Disorders

Ww

Study Guide

### Part I. Depression and Bipolar Disorder

You should get evaluated by a professional if you've had five or more of the following symptoms for more than 2 weeks or if any of these symptoms cause such a big change that you can't keep up your usual routine.

**When You're Depressed:**

____ You feel sad or cry a lot, and it doesn't go away.

____ You feel guilty for no reason; you feel you're no good; you've lost your confidence.

____ Life seems meaningless, or you think nothing good is ever going to happen again.

____ You have a negative attitude a lot of the time, or it seems as if you have no feelings.

____ You don't feel like doing a lot of the things you used to like—music, sports, being with friends, going out, and so on—and you want to be left alone most of the time.

____ It's hard to make up your mind. You forget lots of things, and it's hard to concentrate.

____ You get irritated often. Little things make you lose your temper; you overreact.

____ Your sleep pattern changes: You start sleeping a lot more or you have trouble falling asleep at night; or you wake up really early most mornings and can't get back to sleep.

____ Your eating pattern changes: You've lost your appetite or you eat a lot more.

____ You feel restless and tired most of the time.

____ You think about death or feel as if you're dying or have thoughts about committing suicide.

**When You're Manic:**

____ You feel high as a kite . . . like you're on top of the world.

____ You get unrealistic ideas about the great things you can do . . . things that you really can't do.

____ Thoughts go racing through your head, you jump from one subject to another, and you talk a lot.

____ You're a nonstop party, constantly running around.

____ You do too many wild or risky things—with driving, with spending money, with sex, and so on.

____ You're so "up" that you don't need much sleep.

____ You're rebellious or irritable and can't get along at home or school or with your friends.

If you are concerned about depression in yourself or a friend, or if you are thinking about hurting or killing yourself, talk to someone about it and get help immediately. There are many sources of help: a good friend; an academic or resident adviser; the staff at the student health or counseling center; a professor, coach, or adviser; a local suicide or emergency hotline (get the phone number from the operator or directory) or the 911 operator; or a hospital emergency room.

### Part II. Are You Overly Anxious?

The self-test below was developed to help screen for common anxiety disorders. Answer "yes" or "no" for each question based on your experiences *during the past month.*

**Yes No**

**Panic disorder**

____ ____ 1. Did you experience a sudden unexplained attack of intense fear, anxiety, or panic for no apparent reason? (If "yes," continue with questions a–c; if "no," go to question 2.)

____ ____ a. Were you afraid you might have more of these attacks?

____ ____ b. Were you worried that these attacks could mean you were losing control, having a heart attack, or "going crazy"?

____ ____ c. Did these attacks cause changes or avoidance patterns in your behavior?

*(over)*

**Yes No**

____ ____ 2. Have you been afraid of not being able to get help or not being able to escape in certain situations, such as being on a bridge, in a crowded store, or in similar situations?

____ ____ 3. Have you been afraid or unable to travel alone?

**Generalized anxiety disorder**

____ ____ 4. Have you persistently worried about several different things, such as work, school, family, and money?

____ ____ 5. Did you find it difficult to control your worrying?

____ ____ 6. Did persistent worrying or nervousness cause problems with your work or your dealings with people?

**Obsessive-compulsive disorder**

____ ____ 7. Did you have persistent, senseless thoughts you could not get out of your head, such as thoughts of death, illnesses, aggression, sexual urges, contamination, or others?

____ ____ 8. Did you spend more time than necessary doing things over and over again, such as washing your hands, checking things, or counting things?

____ ____ 9. Did you spend more than one hour a day involved in your senseless thoughts or your needless checking, washing, or counting?

**Social phobia**

____ ____ 10. Were you afraid to do things in front of people, such as public speaking, eating, performing, or teaching?

____ ____ 11. Did you avoid or feel very uncomfortable in situations involving people, such as parties, weddings, dating, dances, and other social events?

**Post-traumatic stress disorder**

____ ____ 12. Have you ever had an extremely frightening, traumatic, or horrible experience—such as being the victim of a violent crime, being seriously injured in a car crash, being sexually assaulted, seeing someone seriously injured or killed, or being the victim of a natural disaster? (If "yes," continue with questions a—e.)

____ ____ a. Did you relive the experience through recurrent dreams, preoccupations, or flashbacks?

____ ____ b. Did you seem less interested in important things, not "with it," or unable to experience or express emotions?

____ ____ c. Did you have problems sleeping, concentrating, or keeping your temper?

____ ____ d. Did you avoid anything that reminded you of the original horrible event?

____ ____ e. Did you have some of the above problems for more than 1 month?

Consider seeking professional assistance if your daily functioning is impaired or if you are significantly troubled by any of the areas in which you answered "yes."

SOURCES: Part I from National Institute of Mental Health. 1999. *Let's Talk About Depression* (http://www.nimh.nih.gov/publicat/letstalk.cfm; retrieved August 31, 2000). Part II adapted with permission from Freedom from Fear. 1998. *Anxiety Disorders Screening Day Questionnaire.* New York: Freedom from Fear. Freedom from Fear is a national nonprofit mental illness advocacy organization. The organization's mission is to impact, in a positive way, the lives of all those affected by anxiety, depressive, and other related disorders through advocacy, education, research, and community support.

## CHAPTER 4
## Intimate Relationships and Communication



### Multiple Choice

1. Our gender role is defined for us by our
   a. genes.
   b. culture.
   c. decisions.
   d. sexual experiences.

2. All of the following are associated with long-term love relationships EXCEPT
   a. loyalty.
   b. idealization of the other person.
   c. respect.
   d. interest in the other person.

3. Jealousy
   a. proves the existence of commitment in a relationship.
   b. is associated with high self-esteem.
   c. is more closely related to insecurity than to love.
   d. secures a relationship by putting strict controls on the partners.

4. A destructive way to deal with anger is to
   a. suppress it.
   b. talk about your feelings.
   c. give yourself some space until your anger subsides.
   d. negotiate and explore alternatives.

5. First attraction is usually based on
   a. easily observable characteristics.
   b. personality traits.
   c. basic values.
   d. future aspirations.

6. Keys to good communication in a relationship include all of the following EXCEPT
   a. listening.
   b. feedback.
   c. competitiveness.
   d. self-disclosure.

7. An egalitarian partnership not based on traditional gender roles is a common characteristic of
   a. long-term marriages.
   b. cohabitating couples.
   c. relationships that have just begun.
   d. gay and lesbian relationships.

8. Which one of the following statements about marriage is TRUE?
   a. About 25% of marriages in the United States end in divorce.
   b. The primary functions and benefits of marriage are very different from other types of personal relationships.
   c. People are marrying at younger ages than in the past.
   d. Today, people tend to marry for personal, emotional reasons rather than for practical or economic reasons.

9. About _____ of all children under 18 live with only one parent.
   a. 5%
   b. 15%
   c. 25%
   d. 50%

10. Which of the following tends to be TRUE about strong families?
    a. They are without problems.
    b. They are likely to seek counseling about difficult problems that arise.
    c. They avoid talking about disagreements.
    d. They know they care for one another without having to show it.

## True or False

T F 1. Successful intimate relationships are more likely for people who have high self-esteem.

T F 2. Intimate partnerships tend to last longer and be more stable than friendships.

T F 3. For most people, love sustains a relationship and sex intensifies a relationship.

T F 4. Nonverbal communication is only a small part of the overall communication that occurs between two people.

T F 5. Men and women approach communication and conversation differently.

T F 6. Extensive use of the Internet is associated with more social contacts.

T F 7. About 50–55% of all American marriages end in divorce.

T F 8. Couple who cohabit before marriage are less likely to get divorced than those who do not cohabit.

T F 9. Marital satisfaction usually declines after children have left home.

T F 10. Healthy stepfamilies are less cohesive and more adaptable than healthy primary families.

ANSWERS: Multiple Choice: 1. b (p. 67); 2. b (p. 68); 3. c (p. 70); 4. a (p. 72); 5. a (p. 74); 6. c (p. 71); 7. d (p. 65); 8. d (p. 78); 9. c ( p. 81); 10. b (p. 82).
True or False: 1. T (p. 66); 2. F (p. 68); 3. T (p. 68); 4. F (p. 71); 5. T (pp. 71–73); 6. F (p. 76); 7. T (p. 79); 8. F (p. 75); 9. F (p. 81); 10. T (p. 82).

Name ______________________ Section ______________ Date ______________

## WELLNESS WORKSHEET S4

Intimate Relationships

Ww

### Part I. Love Maps Questionnaire

Emotionally intelligent couples have richly detailed "love maps"—they know about each other's history, major goals and beliefs, and day-to-day struggles. To assess the quality of your current love maps, answer each of the following questions with "true" or "false."

**T F** 1. I can name my partner's best friends.

**T F** 2. I can tell you what stresses my partner is currently facing.

**T F** 3. I know the names of some of the people who have been irritating my partner lately.

**T F** 4. I can tell you some of my partner's life dreams.

**T F** 5. I am very familiar with my partner's religious beliefs and ideas.

**T F** 6. I can tell you about my partner's basic philosophy of life.

**T F** 7. I can list the relatives my partner likes the least.

**T F** 8. I know my partner's favorite music.

**T F** 9. I can list my partner's three favorite movies.

**T F** 10. My partner is familiar with my current stresses.

**T F** 11. I know the three most special times in my partner's life.

**T F** 12. I can tell you the most stressful thing that happened to my partner as a child.

**T F** 13. I can list my partner's major aspirations and hopes in life.

**T F** 14. I know my partner's major current worries.

**T F** 15. My partner knows who my friends are.

**T F** 16. I know what my partner would want to do if he or she suddenly won the lottery.

**T F** 17. I can tell you in detail my first impressions of my partner.

**T F** 18. Periodically, I ask my partner about his or her world right now.

**T F** 19. I feel that my partner knows me pretty well.

**T F** 20. My partner is familiar with my hopes and aspirations.

***Scoring:*** Give yourself one point for each "true" answer.

***10 or above:*** This is an area of strength in your relationship. You have a fairly detailed map of your partner's everyday life, hopes, fears, and dreams. If you maintain this level of knowledge and understanding of each other, you'll be well equipped to handle any problem areas that crop up in your relationship.

***Below 10:*** Your relationship could stand some improvement in this area. By taking the time to learn more about your partner now, you'll find your relationship becomes stronger.

*(over)*

 

## WELLNESS WORKSHEET S4—continued

### Part II. Rate Your Family's Strengths

This Family Strengths Inventory was developed by researchers who studied the strengths of over 3000 families. To assess your family (either the family you grew up in or the family you have formed as an adult), circle the number that best reflects how your family rates on each strength. A number 1 represents the lowest rating and a number 5 represents the highest.

| | Low | | | | High |
|---|---|---|---|---|---|
| 1. Spending time together and doing things with each other | 1 | 2 | 3 | 4 | 5 |
| 2. Commitment to each other | 1 | 2 | 3 | 4 | 5 |
| 3. Good communication (talking with each other often, listening well, sharing feelings with each other) | 1 | 2 | 3 | 4 | 5 |
| 4. Dealing with crises in a positive manner | 1 | 2 | 3 | 4 | 5 |
| 5. Expressing appreciation to each other | 1 | 2 | 3 | 4 | 5 |
| 6. Spiritual wellness | 1 | 2 | 3 | 4 | 5 |
| 7. Closeness of relationship between spouses | 1 | 2 | 3 | 4 | 5 |
| 8. Closeness of relationship between parents and children | 1 | 2 | 3 | 4 | 5 |
| 9. Happiness of relationship between spouses | 1 | 2 | 3 | 4 | 5 |
| 10. Happiness of relationship between parents and children | 1 | 2 | 3 | 4 | 5 |
| 11. Extent to which spouses make each other feel good about themselves (self-confident, worthy, competent, and happy) | 1 | 2 | 3 | 4 | 5 |
| 12. Extent to which parents help children feel good about themselves | 1 | 2 | 3 | 4 | 5 |

***Scoring:*** Add the numbers you have circled. A score below 39 indicates below-average family strengths. Scores between 39 and 52 are in the average range. Scores above 53 indicate a strong family. Low scores on individual items identify areas that families can profitably spend time on. High scores are worthy of celebration but shouldn't lead to complacency. Like gardens, families need loving care to remain strong.

What do you think is your family's major strength? What do you like best about your family?

What about your family would you most like to change?

SOURCE: Part I from Gottman, J. M., and N. Silver. 1999. *The Seven Principles for Making Marriage Work.* New York: Three Rivers Press. Used by permission of Crown Publishers, a division of Random House. Part II from Stinnett, N., and J. DeFrain. 1986. *Secrets of Strong Families.*  To purchase copies of this book, please call 1-800-759-0190.

# CHAPTER 5
## Sexuality, Pregnancy, and Childbirth



### Multiple Choice

1. The male germ cell(s) is (are) the
   a. sperm.
   b. penis.
   c. testes.
   d. scrotum.

2. Puberty is first marked by
   a. the development of differentiated genitalia.
   b. achievement of emotional maturity.
   c. an ability to reproduce.
   d. the development of secondary sex characteristics.

3. A strategy for relieving symptoms of premenstrual syndrome is
   a. limit salt intake to minimize bloating.
   b. use alcohol for muscle relaxation.
   c. avoid exercise to minimize fatigue.
   d. increase intake of red meat to increase levels of iron.

4. The phase of the sexual response cycle unique to men is
   a. resolution.
   b. plateau.
   c. refractory period.
   d. excitement.

5. If the egg is not fertilized, it lasts about ____ hours after it reaches the uterus and then disintegrates.
   a. 2
   b. 12
   c. 24
   d. 48

6. In which of the following techniques for overcoming infertility are eggs and sperm surgically placed into the oviducts prior to fertilization?
   a. in vitro fertilization
   b. gamete intrafallopian transfer
   c. nuclear transfer
   d. zygote intrafallopian transfer

7. Pregnancy tests seek to detect the presence of
   a. human chorionic gonadotropin.
   b. prostaglandins.
   c. estrogen.
   d. progesterone.

8. Which method of prenatal testing analyzes hormone levels to determine the probability of fetal abnormalities?
   a. ultrasonography
   b. amniocentesis
   c. chorionic villus sampling
   d. triple screen marker

9. All of the following are characteristic of fetal alcohol syndrome EXCEPT
   a. unusual facial characteristics.
   b. mental impairments.
   c. heart defects.
   d. spina bifida.

10. During the second stage of labor
    a. the amniotic sac ruptures.
    b. contractions become more intense during transition.
    c. the baby moves through the birth canal.
    d. the placenta is expelled.

## True or False

T F 1. The function of the scrotum is to keep the testes at a lower temperature than the rest of the body.

T F 2. Worldwide, most male infants are circumcised.

T F 3. The final phase of the sexual response cycle is the orgasmic phase.

T F 4. Most forms of sexual dysfunction are treatable.

T F 5. Complications from sexually transmitted diseases are a primary cause of female infertility.

T F 6. Women of normal weight gain an average of 18–25% of their initial weight during pregnancy.

T F 7. The triple marker screen is used to determine the sex of the fetus.

T F 8. Adequate intake of folate before and during pregnancy reduces the risk of having a baby with spina bifida.

T F 9. Putting babies on their backs to sleep lowers their risk for sudden infant death syndrome (SIDS).

T F 10. About 1 in 10 babies born in the United States is delivered by cesarean section.

ANSWERS: Multiple Choice: 1. a (p. 85); 2. d (p. 88); 3. a (p. 90); 4. c (p. 92); 5. c (p. 97); 6. b (p. 98); 7. a (p. 100); 8. d (p. 103); 9. d (p. 106); 10. c. (p. 109). True or False: 1. T (p. 86); 2. F (p. 87); 3. F (p. 92); 4. T (p. 93); 5. T (p. 98); 6. T (p. 100); 7. F (p. 103); 8. T (p. 105); 9. T (p. 108); 10. F (p. 110).

Name ______________________ Section ______________ Date ______________

## WELLNESS WORKSHEET S5

### Creating a Detailed Family Health History and Tree

Ww

Study Guide

Knowing that a specific disease runs in your family allows you to watch closely for the early warning signs and get appropriate screening tests. It can also help you target important health habits to adopt. You can put together a simple family health tree by compiling key facts on your primary relatives: siblings, parents, aunts and uncles, and grandparents. If possible, have your primary relatives fill out a family health history record like the one below.

**Family Health History**

Name: ______________________ Ethnicity: __________ Date of birth: __________

Blood and Rh type: ______________ Occupation: ______________________

Please note any serious or chronic diseases you have experienced, with special attention to the following:

______ Alcoholism

______ Allergies

______ Arthritis

______ Asthma

______ Blood diseases (hemophilia, sickle-cell disease, thalassemia, hemochromatosis)

______ Cancer (breast, colon, ovarian, skin, stomach, etc.)

______ Cystic fibrosis

______ Diabetes

______ Epilepsy

______ Familial high blood cholesterol levels

______ Hearing defects

______ Heart defects

______ Huntington's disease

______ Hypertension (high blood pressure)

______ Learning disabilities (dyslexia, attention-deficit/hyperactivity disorder, autism)

______ Liver disease (particularly hepatitis)

______ Lupus

______ Mental illness (bipolar disorder, schizophrenia)

______ Mental impairment (Down syndrome, fragile X, etc.)

______ Migraine headaches

______ Miscarriages or neonatal deaths

______ Multiple sclerosis

______ Muscular dystrophy

______ Myasthenia gravis

______ Obesity

______ Phenylketonuria (PKU)

______ Respiratory disease (emphysema, bacterial pneumonia)

______ Rh disease

______ Skin disorders (particularly psoriasis)

______ Thyroid disorders

______ Tay-Sachs disease

______ Tuberculosis

______ Visual disorders (dyslexia, glaucoma, retinitis pigmentosa)

______ Other (please list):

*(over)*

## WELLNESS WORKSHEET S5—continued

List any important health-related behaviors (including tobacco use, dietary and exercise habits, and alcohol use):

Please note names of your relatives below, along with indications of any illnesses, such as those listed on the previous page, which affected them. If they are deceased, list age and cause. Also make note of their lifestyle habits such as smoking.

Father: ______________________________

______________________________

______________________________

Mother: ______________________________

______________________________

______________________________

Brothers and sisters: ______________________________

______________________________

______________________________

Children of brothers and sisters: ______________________________

______________________________

______________________________

If you don't have enough information on past generations, you can get clues by requesting death certificates from state health departments or medical records from relatives' physicians or hospitals where they died. Once you've collected the information you want, plug it into a tree format and look for patterns. In general, the more relatives you have with a particular condition and the closer they are to you, the greater your risk. Nongenetic factors such as health habits also play a role. Signs of a strong hereditary influence include appearance of a disease largely on one side of the family, developing the disease despite good health habits, and early onset of the disease. If you note clear patterns, you may want to discuss your health tree with your physician or a genetic counselor. (An online version of a family health tree is available at http://www.generationalhealth.com.)

## CHAPTER 6
## Contraception and Abortion



### Multiple Choice

1. Oral contraceptives prevent pregnancy by
   a. acting as a sperm barrier.
   b. causing spontaneous abortion.
   c. preventing ovulation.
   d. killing sperm.

2. Which of the following methods of contraception is most effective at preventing pregnancy?
   a. male condom
   b. oral contraceptives
   c. diaphragm with spermicide
   d. withdrawal

3. OrthoEvra is administered
   a. by skin patch.
   b. by injection.
   c. by implantation.
   d. orally.

4. Which of the following does NOT damage latex when used as a lubricant with condoms?
   a. Vaseline
   b. baby oil
   c. K-Y jelly
   d. hand lotion

5. Which of the following methods of contraception provides the most protection against HIV infection?
   a. latex male condom
   b. Depo-Provera injections
   c. diaphragm with spermicide
   d. oral contraceptives

6. Which of the following is NOT an advantage of diaphragm use?
   a. Its use is limited to times of sexual activity.
   b. It has few side effects.
   c. It decreases risk for toxic shock syndrome.
   d. It decreases risk for human papillomavirus infection.

7. The fertility awareness method is NOT recommended for any woman
   a. for whom pregnancy would be a serious problem.
   b. who has very irregular menstrual cycles.
   c. who needs protection against STDs.
   d. all of the above.

8. The *Roe v. Wade* decision
   a. made abortion legal during the first trimester of pregnancy but illegal during the second and third trimesters.
   b. made abortion legal during the first two trimesters but gave states the right to regulate certain factors.
   c. gave states the right to regulate abortion as long as they do not impose an undue burden on women seeking the procedure.
   d. required physicians to test a fetus for viability if the fetus is estimated to be 20 weeks or older.

9. Approximately what percentage of abortions are done after the 12th week of gestation?
   a. 5%
   b. 10%
   c. 25%
   d. 50%

10. The abortion method used in about 90% of all U.S. abortions is
    a. suction curettage.
    b. dilation and evacuation.
    c. manual vacuum aspiration.
    d. mifepristone.

## True or False

T F 1. The active ingredients in oral contraceptives are progesterone and testosterone.

T F 2. The contraceptive skin patch must be changed daily.

T F 3. The vaginal contraceptive ring can be left in place during intercourse.

T F 4. Hormonal emergency contraception works by inhibiting or delaying ovulation.

T F 5. Lambskin condoms provide good protection against STDs.

T F 6. It's okay to keep condoms in a pocket or wallet.

T F 7. The surgical risks associated with female and male sterilization are about equal.

T F 8. The case of *Webster v. Reproductive Health Services* legalized abortion.

T F 9. The number of abortions performed in the United States has increased steadily since the *Roe v. Wade* decision.

T F 10. Medical abortion with mifepristone is approved for use up to 49 days after the last menstrual period.

ANSWERS: Multiple Choice: 1. c (p. 115); 2. b (pp. 115, 128); 3. a (p. 116); 4. c (p. 120); 5. a (p. 120); 6. c (p. 123); 7. d (p. 127); 8. b (p. 131); 9. b (p. 134); 10. a (p. 135). True or False: 1. F (p. 115); 2. F (p. 116); 3. T (p. 117); 4. T (p. 118); 5. F (p. 120); 6. F (p. 121); 7. F (p. 128); 8. F (p. 131); 9. F (pp. 134–135); 10. T (p. 135).

Name ______________________ Section ______________ Date ______________

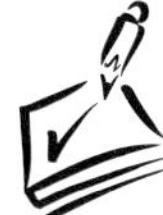

# WELLNESS WORKSHEET S6

## Contraception and Abortion

Ww

Study Guide

### Part I. Which Contraceptive Method Is Right for You and Your Partner?

If you are sexually active, you need to use the contraceptive method that will work best for you. A number of factors may be involved in your decision. The following questions will help you sort out these factors and choose an appropriate method. Answer yes (Y) or no (N) for each statement as it applies to you and, if appropriate, your partner.

Y or N

______ 1. I like sexual spontaneity and don't want to be bothered with contraception at the time of sexual intercourse.

______ 2. I need a contraceptive immediately.

______ 3. It is very important that I do not become pregnant now.

______ 4. I want a contraceptive method that will protect me and my partner against STDs.

______ 5. I prefer a contraceptive method that requires the cooperation and involvement of both partners.

______ 6. I have sexual intercourse frequently.

______ 7. I have sexual intercourse infrequently.

______ 8. I am forgetful or have a variable daily routine.

______ 9. I have more than one sexual partner.

______ 10. I have heavy periods with cramps.

______ 11. I prefer a method that requires little or no action or bother on my part.

______ 12. I am a nursing mother.

______ 13. I want the option of conceiving immediately after discontinuing contraception.

______ 14. I want a contraceptive method with few or no side effects.

If you answered yes to the numbers of statements listed on the left, the method on the right might be a good choice for you:

| | |
|---|---|
| 1, 3, 6, 10, 11, 12* | Oral contraceptives |
| 1, 3, 6, 8, 10, 11 | Contraceptive patch, vaginal ring |
| 1, 3, 6, 8, 10, 11, 12* | Contraceptive injections |
| 1, 3, 6, 8, 11, 12, 13 | IUD |
| 2, 4, 5, 7, 8, 9, 12, 13, 14 | Condoms (male and female) |
| 5, 7, 12, 13, 14 | Diaphragm with spermicide and cervical cap |
| 2, 5, 7, 8, 12, 13, 14 | Vaginal spermicides and sponge |
| 5, 7, 13, 14 | FAM and withdrawal |

12* Progestin-only hormonal contraceptives (the minipill and Depo-Provera injections) are safe for use by nursing mothers; contraceptives that include estrogen are not usually recommended.

Your answers may indicate that more than one method would be appropriate for you. To help narrow your choices, circle the numbers of the statements that are *most* important for you. Before you make a final choice, talk with your partner(s) and your physician. Consider your own lifestyle and preferences as well as characteristics of each method (effectiveness, side effects, costs, and so on). For maximum protection against pregnancy and STDs, you might want to consider combining two methods.

*(over)*

**Part II. Your Position on the Legality and Morality of Abortion**

To help define your own position on abortion, answer the following series of questions.

| | Agree | Disagree |
|---|---|---|
| 1. The fertilized egg is a human being from the moment of conception. | _____ | _____ |
| 2. The rights of the fetus at any stage take precedence over any decision a woman might want to make regarding her pregnancy. | _____ | _____ |
| 3. The rights of the fetus depend upon its gestational age: further along in the pregnancy, the fetus has more rights. | _____ | _____ |
| 4. Each individual woman should have final say over decisions regarding her health and body; politicians should not be allowed to decide. | _____ | _____ |
| 5. In cases of teenagers seeking an abortion, parental consent should be required. | _____ | _____ |
| 6. In cases of married women seeking an abortion, spousal consent should be required. | _____ | _____ |
| 7. In cases of late abortion, tests should be done to determine the viability of the fetus. | _____ | _____ |
| 8. The federal government should provide public funding for abortion to ensure equal access to abortion for all women. | _____ | _____ |
| 9. The federal government should not allow states to pass their own abortion laws; there should be uniform laws for the entire country. | _____ | _____ |

10. Does a woman's right to choose whether or not to have an abortion depend upon the circumstances surrounding conception or the situation of the mother? In which of the following situations, if any, would you support a woman's right to choose to have an abortion (check where appropriate)?

_____ An abortion is necessary to maintain the woman's life or health.

_____ The pregnancy is a result of rape or incest.

_____ A serious birth defect has been detected in the fetus.

_____ The pregnancy is a result of the failure of a contraceptive method or device.

_____ The pregnancy occurred when no contraceptive method was in use.

_____ A single mother, pregnant for the fifth time, wants an abortion because she feels she cannot support another child.

_____ A pregnant 15-year-old high school student feels having a child would be too great a disruption in her life and keep her from reaching her goals for the future.

_____ A pregnant 19-year-old college student does not want to interrupt her education.

_____ The father of the child has stated he will provide no support and is not interested in helping raise the child.

_____ Parents of two boys wish to terminate the mother's pregnancy because the fetus is male rather than female.

CHAPTER 7

# The Use and Abuse of Psychoactive Drugs

## Multiple Choice

1. Which of the following characteristics is commonly associated with addictive behaviors?
   a. strong compulsion
   b. loss of control
   c. escalating use
   d. all of the above

2. Which of the following is most closely associated with physical dependence on a drug?
   a. poor performance at work or school
   b. withdrawal symptoms
   c. escalating use of a drug
   d. expressing a desire to cut down on drug use

3. The method of drug use that significantly increases the user's risk for hepatitis and HIV infection is
   a. inhalation.
   b. ingestion.
   c. injection.
   d. absorption through the skin.

4. If a person responds to an inert substance as if it were an active drug, he or she is experiencing
   a. a placebo effect.
   b. state dependence.
   c. synesthesia.
   d. altered states of consciousness.

5. Opioids
   a. relieve pain.
   b. stimulate activity.
   c. induce alertness.
   d. cause hallucinations.

6. Which of the following is a central nervous system depressant?
   a. alcohol
   b. heroin
   c. marijuana
   d. LSD

7. The most likely physical reaction to amphetamine ingestion is
   a. sedation.
   b. fatigue.
   c. delirium.
   d. alertness.

8. The most widely used illegal drug in the United States is
   a. ecstasy.
   b. crack cocaine.
   c. heroin.
   d. marijuana.

9. The active ingredient in marijuana is
   a. ephedrine.
   b. psilocybin.
   c. tetrahydrocannabinol.
   d. benzodiazepine.

10. Significant physical withdrawal symptoms can occur in users of all of the following EXCEPT
    a. amphetamines.
    b. alcohol.
    c. caffeine.
    d. LSD.

## True or False

T F 1. Addictive behaviors are associated exclusively with psychoactive drugs.

T F 2. Two symptoms of drug dependence are tolerance and withdrawal.

T F 3. Most GHB available as a street drug is produced in pharmaceutical labs and tested to assure purity.

T F 4. Oxycodone is an opioid.

T F 5. Cocaine is a central nervous system stimulant.

T F 6. There are no known long-term effects of marijuana use.

T F 7. Substances in marijuana have some potential medical uses.

T F 8. Inhalants are present in many legal, seemingly harmless products.

T F 9. People whose jobs do not involve hazards cannot legally be tested for drugs.

T F 10. Medication-assisted treatment for drug abuse is losing favor because of its relatively high cost.

ANSWERS: Multiple Choice: 1. d (p. 141); 2. b (p. 144); 3. c (p. 147); 4. a (p. 148); 5. a (p. 149); 6. a (p. 149); 7. d (p. 152); 8. d (p. 154); 9. c (p. 154); 10. d (p. 155). True or False: 1. F (p. 140); 2. T (p. 144); 3. F (p. 151); 4. T (p. 149); 5. T (p. 152); 6. F (p. 154); 7. T (p. 155); 8. T (p. 156); 9. F (p. 158); 10. F (p. 158).

Name ______________________ Section ______________ Date ________________

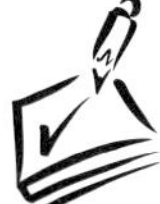

# WELLNESS WORKSHEET S7

Addictive Behaviors

**Part I. General Addictive Behavior Checklist**

Choose an activity or a behavior in your life that you feel may be developing into an addiction. Ask yourself the following questions about it, and answer yes (Y) or no (N).

Activity/behavior: ____________________________________________

_____ 1. Do you engage in the activity on a regular basis?

_____ 2. Have you engaged in the activity over a long period of time?

_____ 3. Do you currently engage in this activity more than you used to?

_____ 4. Do you find it difficult to stop or to avoid the activity?

_____ 5. Have you tried and failed to cut down on the amount of time you spend on the activity?

_____ 6. Do you turn down or skip social/recreational events in order to engage in the activity?

_____ 7. Does your participation in the activity interfere with your attendance and/or performance at school and/or work?

_____ 8. Have friends or family members spoken to you about the activity and indicated they think you have a problem?

_____ 9. Has your participation in the activity affected your reputation?

_____ 10. Have you lied to friends or family members about the amount of time, money, and other resources that you put into the activity?

_____ 11. Do you feel guilty about the resources that you put into the activity?

_____ 12. Do you engage in the activity when you are worried, frustrated, or stressed or when you have other painful feelings?

_____ 13. Do you feel better when you engage in the activity?

_____ 14. Do you often spend more time engaged in the activity than you plan to?

_____ 15. Do you have a strong urge to participate in the activity when you are away from it?

_____ 16. Do you spend a lot of time planning for your next opportunities to engage in the activity?

_____ 17. Are you often irritable and restless when you are away from the activity?

_____ 18. Do you use the activity as a reward for all other accomplishments?

*(over)*

**Part II. Checklist for Drug Dependency**

If you wonder whether you are becoming dependent on a drug, ask yourself the following questions. Answer yes (Y) or no (N).

_____ 1. Do you take the drug regularly?

_____ 2. Have you been taking the drug for a long time?

_____ 3. Do you always take the drug in certain situations or when you're with certain people?

_____ 4. Do you find it difficult to stop using the drug? Do you feel powerless to quit?

_____ 5. Have you tried repeatedly to cut down or control your use of the drug?

_____ 6. Do you need to take a larger dose of the drug in order to get the same high you're used to?

_____ 7. Do you feel specific symptoms if you cut back or stop using the drug?

_____ 8. Do you frequently take another psychoactive substance to relieve withdrawal symptoms?

_____ 9. Do you take the drug to feel "normal"?

_____ 10. Do you go to extreme lengths or put yourself in dangerous situations to get the drug?

_____ 11. Do you hide your drug use from others? Have you ever lied about what you're using or how much you use?

_____ 12. Do people close to you ask you about your drug use?

_____ 13. Are you spending more and more time with people who use the same drug as you?

_____ 14. Do you think about the drug when you're not high, figuring out ways to get it?

_____ 15. If you stop taking the drug, do you feel bad until you can take it again?

_____ 16. Does the drug interfere with your ability to study, work, or socialize?

_____ 17. Do you skip important school, work, social, or recreational activities in order to obtain or use the drug?

_____ 18. Do you continue to use the drug despite a physical or mental disorder or despite a significant problem that you know is worsened by drug use?

_____ 19. Have you developed a mental or physical condition or disorder because of prolonged drug use?

_____ 20. Have you done something dangerous or that you regret while under the influence of the drug?

**Evaluation**

On each of these checklists, the more times you answer yes, the more likely it is that you are developing an addiction. If your answers suggest abuse or dependency, talk to someone at your school health clinic or to your physician about taking care of the problem before it gets worse.

## CHAPTER 8
## Alcohol and Tobacco



### Multiple Choice

1. If a beverage is 100 proof, it contains ___ alcohol.
   a. 10%
   b. 25%
   c. 50%
   d. 100%

2. To help a person who has been drinking and is unconscious, you should
   a. wake the person up and give her or him a beverage with caffeine.
   b. leave the person alone to sleep it off.
   c. get the person on her or his feet to walk around.
   d. place the person on her or his side and watch for breathing problems.

3. Women generally have higher BACs than men after consuming the same amount of alcohol because they
   a. drink more.
   b. are less experienced drinkers.
   c. have a higher percentage of body fat.
   d. don't eat when they drink.

4. For women, binge drinking is defined as having ___ drinks in a row.
   a. 2
   b. 4
   c. 6
   d. 8

5. Which of the following statements comparing college students who binge drink with non-binge drinkers is FALSE?
   a. Binge drinkers are more likely to drink and drive.
   b. Binge drinkers are more likely to consider themselves problem drinkers.
   c. Binge drinkers are more likely to engage in unplanned, unprotected sex.
   d. Binge drinkers are less likely to keep up with their schoolwork.

6. The addictive drug in cigarettes is
   a. benzo(a)pyrene.
   b. formaldehyde.
   c. tar.
   d. nicotine.

7. The immediate effects of smoking a cigarette include which of the following?
   a. increased blood pressure
   b. improved sense of taste
   c. decreased heart rate
   d. increased appetite

Study Guide

8. Smoke exhaled by a smoker is referred to as
   a. mainstream smoke.
   b. sidestream smoke.
   c. primary smoke.
   d. secondary smoke.

9. Smoking causes a condition called ________, in which air sacs in the lungs are gradually destroyed.
   a. asthma
   b. aortic aneurysm
   c. chronic bronchitis
   d. emphysema

10. Which of the following smoking cessation products is available without a prescription?
    a. nicotine nasal spray
    b. bupropion
    c. nicotine lozenge
    d. nicotine inhaler

## True or False

T F 1. Alcohol is the leading cause of death among people between 15 and 24.

T F 2. The rate of alcohol metabolism cannot be accelerated.

T F 3. People can usually drive safely with a BAC of up to 0.20%.

T F 4. The consumption of alcohol in any amount has beneficial effects on the cardiovascular system.

T F 5. Children with fetal alcohol syndrome are born impaired, but they usually catch up with their peers both physically and mentally by age 5.

T F 6. Most alcoholics need professional help to stop drinking.

T F 7. Use of low-tar and "light" cigarettes reduces the risk of developing smoking-related illnesses.

T F 8. Due to increased rates of smoking among women, lung cancer has surpassed breast cancer as the leading cause of cancer death among women.

T F 9. Spit tobacco products deliver a dose of nicotine comparable to that provided by cigarettes.

T F 10. Clove cigarettes are a safe alternative to regular cigarettes.

ANSWERS: Multiple Choice: 1. c (p. 165); 2. d (p. 168); 3. c (p. 166); 4. b (p. 172); 5. b (p. 172); 6. d (p. 177); 7. a (p. 181); 8. a (p. 186); 9. d (p. 183); 10. c (p. 189). True or False: 1. T (p. 164); 2. T (p. 166); 3. F (p. 169); 4. F (pp. 170–171); 5. F (p. 171); 6. T (p. 175); 7. F (p. 181); 8. T (p. 182); 9. T (p. 184); 10. F (p. 185).

Name ______________________ Section ______________ Date ______________

# WELLNESS WORKSHEET S8

Alcohol and Tobacco

Ww



## Part I. Do You Have a Problem with Alcohol?

To determine if you may have a drinking problem, complete the following two screening tests.

### A. CAGE Screening Test

Answer yes or no to the following questions:

Have you ever felt you should . . . . . . . Cut down on your drinking?
Have people . . . . . . . . . . . . . . . . . . . Annoyed you by criticizing your drinking?
Have you ever felt bad or . . . . . . . . . . Guilty about your drinking?
Have you ever had an . . . . . . . . . . . . . Eye-opener (a drink first thing in the morning to steady your nerves or get rid of a hangover)?

One "yes" response suggests a possible alcohol problem. If you answered yes to more than one question, it is highly likely that a problem exists. In either case, it is important that you see your physician or other health care provider right away to discuss your responses to these questions.

### B. AUDIT Screening Test

For each question, choose the answer that best describes your behavior. Then total your scores.

| Questions | Points | | | | | Your Score |
|---|---|---|---|---|---|---|
| | 0 | 1 | 2 | 3 | 4 | |
| 1. How often do you have a drink containing alcohol? | Never | Monthly or less | 2–4 times a month | 2–3 times a week | 4 or more times a week | ____ |
| 2. How many drinks containing alcohol do you have on a typical day when you are drinking? | 1 or 2 | 3 or 4 | 5 or 6 | 7 to 9 | 10 or more | ____ |
| 3. How often do you have 6 or more drinks on one occasion? | Never | Less than monthly | Monthly | Weekly | Daily or almost daily | ____ |
| 4. How often during the last year have you found that you were not able to stop drinking once you had started? | Never | Less than monthly | Monthly | Weekly | Daily or almost daily | ____ |
| 5. How often during the last year have you failed to do what was normally expected because of drinking? | Never | Less than monthly | Monthly | Weekly | Daily or almost daily | ____ |
| 6. How often during the last year have you needed a first drink in the morning to get yourself going after a heavy drinking session? | Never | Less than monthly | Monthly | Weekly | Daily or almost daily | ____ |
| 7. How often during the last year have you had a feeling of guilt or remorse after drinking? | Never | Less than monthly | Monthly | Weekly | Daily or almost daily | ____ |
| 8. How often during the last year have you been unable to remember what happened the night before because you had been drinking? | Never | Less than monthly | Monthly | Weekly | Daily or almost daily | ____ |
| 9. Have you or has someone else been injured as a result of your drinking? | No | Yes, but not in the last year (2 points) | | Yes, during the last year (4 points) | | ____ |
| 10. Has a relative, friend, doctor, or other health worker been concerned about your drinking or suggested you cut down? | No | Yes, but not in the last year (2 points) | | Yes, during the last year (4 points) | | ____ |
| | | | | | **Total** | ____ |

A total score of 8 or more indicates a strong likelihood of hazardous or harmful alcohol consumption.

Even if you answered no to all four items in the CAGE screening test and scored below 8 on the AUDIT screening test, if you are encountering drinking-related problems with your academic performance, job, relationships, or health, or with the law, you should consider seeking help.

*(over)*

**Part II. Nicotine Dependence: Are You Hooked?**

Answer each question in the list below, giving yourself the appropriate points.

______ 1. How soon after you wake up do you have your first cigarette?

a. within 5 minutes (3)

b. 6–30 minutes (2)

c. 31–60 minutes (1)

d. After 60 minutes (0)

______ 2. Do you find it difficult to refrain from smoking in places where it is forbidden, such as the library, a theater, or a doctor's office?

a. yes (1)

b. no (0)

______ 3. Which cigarette would you most hate to give up?

a. the first one in the morning (1)

b. any other (0)

______ 4. How many cigarettes a day do you smoke?

a. 10 or less (0)

b. 11–20 (1)

c. 21–30 (2)

d. 31 or more (3)

______ 5. Do you smoke more frequently during the first hours after waking than during the rest of the day?

a. yes (1)

b. no (0)

______ 6. Do you smoke if you are so ill that you are in bed most of the day?

a. yes (1)

b. no (0)

______ TOTAL

A total score of 7 or greater indicates that you are very dependent on nicotine and are likely to experience withdrawal symptoms when you stop smoking. A score of 6 or less indicates low to moderate dependence.

SOURCES: CAGE test: National Institute on Alcohol Abuse and Alcoholism. 1996. *Alcoholism: Getting the Facts.* NIH Publication No. 96-4153; AUDIT test: Saunders, J. B., et al. 1993. Development of the Alcohol Use Disorders Identification Test (AUDIT): WHO collaborative project on early detection of persons with harmful alcohol consumption—II. *Addiction.* 88: 791–804, June. Reprinted with permission from Carfax Publishing, a division of Taylor & Francis Ltd. http://www.tandf.co.uk. Nicotine dependence test: Heatherton, T. F., et al. 1991. The Fagerstrom Test for Nicotine Dependence: A revision of the Fagerstrom Tolerance Questionnaire. *British Journal of Addictions* 86(9): 1119–1127.

# CHAPTER 9
# Nutrition Basics



## Multiple Choice

1. On average, adults need to consume about ___ calories per day.
   a. 1200
   b. 1500
   c. 2000
   d. 2500

2. The building blocks of protein are called
   a. soluble fiber.
   b. complex carbohydrates.
   c. amino acids.
   d. fatty acids.

3. If you consume more protein than you need, the excess will be
   a. excreted in urine.
   b. expired during respiration.
   c. stored as fat.
   d. stored as muscle.

4. Which of the following contains trans fat?
   a. partially hydrogenated oil
   b. olive oil
   c. safflower oil
   d. fish oil

5. A good source of omega-3 fatty acids is
   a. bread.
   b. rice.
   c. vegetables.
   d. fish.

6. Health experts recommend that most fat in the diet be
   a. saturated.
   b. unsaturated.
   c. trans.
   d. hydrogenated.

7. Increasing intake of which of the following would be a beneficial dietary change for most Americans?
   a. refined carbohydrates
   b. protein
   c. fat
   d. whole grains

*(over)*

8. The leading source of calories in the American diet is
   a. regular soft drinks.
   b. french fries.
   c. pizza.
   d. hamburgers.

9. According to MyPyramid, a person consuming 2000 calories a day should eat about ___ of fruits and vegetables daily?
   a. 1 cup.
   b. 2½ cups.
   c. 4½ cups.
   d. 6 cups.

10. For dietary supplements, which of the following is currently regulated by the FDA?
    a. potency
    b. effectiveness
    c. purity
    d. labels on packaging

## True or False

T F 1. A gram of carbohydrate supplies more calories than a gram of fat.

T F 2. Meat and fish are sources of incomplete proteins.

T F 3. Carbohydrate intake should represent 45–65% of total daily calories.

T F 4. Hydrogenation is a process that makes fats healthy for consumption.

T F 5. A high-fiber diet can help reduce the risk of type 2 diabetes.

T F 6. Vitamins are needed by the body to initiate or regulate chemical reactions.

T F 7. Free radicals prevent the damage caused to the body by antioxidants.

T F 8. A 3-ounce serving of meat or chicken is about the same size as a small paperback book.

T F 9. The recommended daily limit for sodium consumption is equivalent to 1 tablespoon of salt.

T F 10. Women need to consume nutrient-dense foods because they have higher calorie needs than men.

ANSWERS: Multiple Choice: 1. c (p. 194); 2. c (p. 195); 3. c (p. 196); 4. a (p. 196); 5. d (p. 197); 6. b (p. 198); 7. d (p. 200); 8. a (p. 209); 9. c (pp. 214–215); 10. d (p. 220). True or False: 1. F (p. 194); 2. F (p. 195); 3. T (p. 200); 4. F (p. 196); 5. T (p. 202); 6. T (p. 202); 7. F (p. 205); 8. F (p. 216); 9. F (p. 211); 10. F (p. 218).

Name ______________________ Section ______________ Date ______________

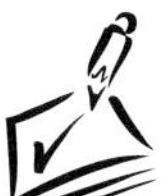

## WELLNESS WORKSHEET S9

### Your Daily Diet Versus MyPyramid Recommendations



1. **Keep a food record:** Keep a record of everything you eat on a typical day.
2. **Compare your intake to MyPyramid recommendations:** Complete the chart below using your food record. To determine the recommended number of servings for your calorie intake, refer to the MyPyramid chart in your text or visit MyPyramid.gov.

| Food Group | Recommended Daily Amounts/Servings for Your Energy Intake | Your Actual Daily Intake (Amounts/Servings) | Serving Sizes and Equivalents |
|---|---|---|---|
| **Grains (total)** | | | 1 oz equivalents = 1 slice of bread; 1 small muffin; 1 cup ready-to-eat cereal flakes; or ½ cup cooked cereal, rice, grains, pasta |
| *Whole grains* | | | |
| *Other grains* | | | |
| **Vegetables (total)** | | | ½ cup or equivalent (1 serving) = ½ cup raw or cooked vegetables; 1 cup raw leafy salad greens; or ½ cup vegetable juice |
| *Dark-green** | | | |
| *Deep-yellow** | | | |
| *Legumes** | | | |
| *Starchy** | | | |
| *Other** | | | |
| **Fruits** | | | ½ cup or equivalent (1 serving) = ½ cup fresh, canned, or frozen fruit; ½ cup fruit juice; 1 small whole fruit; or ¼ cup dried fruit |
| **Milk** | | | 1 cup or equivalent = 1 cup milk or yogurt; 1½ oz natural cheese; or 2 oz processed cheese |
| **Meat and beans** | | | 1 oz equivalents = 1 oz lean meat, poultry, or fish; ¼ cup cooked dry beans or tofu; 1 egg; 1 tablespoon peanut butter; ½ oz nuts or seeds |
| **Oils** | | | 1 teaspoon or equivalent = 1 teaspoon vegetable oil; 1 tablespoon mayonnaise or salad dressing |
| **Solid fats** | | | |
| **Added sugars** | | | |

* Compare your daily intake with the approximate daily intake derived from the weekly pattern given in MyPyramid.

It may be difficult to track values for added sugars and, especially, oils and fats, but be as accurate as you can. Check food labels for information on fat and sugar. (Note: For a more complete and accurate analysis of your diet, keep food records for three days and then average the results.)

*(over)*

3. **Further evaluate your food choices within the groups:** Based on the data you collected and what you learned in the chapter, what were the especially healthy choices you made (for example, whole grains and citrus fruits) and what were your less healthy choices? Identify the foods in the latter category by putting a checkmark next to them on your food record; these are areas where you can make changes to improve your diet. In particular, you may want to limit your intake of the following: processed, sweetened grains; high-fat meats and poultry skin; deep-fried fast foods; full-fat dairy products; regular sodas, sweetened teas, fruit drinks; alcohol beverages; other foods that primarily provide sugar and fat and few other nutrients. A significant proportion of the calories from these foods would be counted toward the discretionary calorie allowance for your level of energy intake; cutting back on these foods can help make room for greater amounts of healthier choices, including fruits, vegetables, and whole grains.

4. **Make healthy changes:** Bring your diet in line with MyPyramid recommendations by adding servings of food groups and subgroups for which you fall short of the recommendations. To maintain a healthy weight, you may need to balance these additions with reductions in other areas—by eliminating some of the fats, oils, sweets, and alcohol you consume; by cutting extra servings from food groups for which your intake is more than adequate; or by making healthier choices within the foods groups. Make a list of foods to add and a list of foods to limit or eliminate:

| *Foods to add:* | *Foods to limit or eliminate:* |
|---|---|
| ______________________________ | ______________________________ |
| ______________________________ | ______________________________ |
| ______________________________ | ______________________________ |
| ______________________________ | ______________________________ |

For a more detailed analysis of your current diet and physical activity level, complete the interactive online assessments at MyPyramid.gov.

CHAPTER 10

# Exercise for Health and Fitness



## Multiple Choice

1. Which of the following is NOT an element of health-related fitness?
   a. body composition
   b. muscular strength
   c. cardiorespiratory endurance
   d. speed

2. Flexibility is best described as
   a. the ability to move without pain during exercise.
   b. the ability to move the joints through their full range of motion.
   c. sustained motion without resistance.
   d. the ability to move rapidly during exercise.

3. Healthy body composition is characterized by a
   a. high proportion of fat tissue and a low proportion of fat-free mass.
   b. low proportion of fat tissue and a low proportion of fat-free mass.
   c. low proportion of fat tissue and a high proportion of fat-free mass.
   d. high proportion of fat tissue and a high proportion of fat-free mass.

4. Regular exercise does all the following EXCEPT
   a. raise metabolic rate.
   b. decrease levels of high-density lipoproteins.
   c. build bone density.
   d. protect cells from free radicals.

5. Which of the following is LEAST beneficial for developing cardiorespiratory endurance?
   a. jogging
   b. cycling
   c. weight lifting
   d. swimming

6. Cardiorespiratory endurance exercise intensity is measured according to the
   a. duration of a workout.
   b. heart rate.
   c. distance traveled.
   d. number of exercise sessions per week.

7. In order to improve cardiorespiratory endurance, a person should perform a minimum of ___ minutes of continuous or intermittent aerobic activity, 3-5 days per week.
   a. 10
   b. 20
   c. 45
   d. 60

8. For general fitness, the recommended number of repetitions for exercises in a strength training program is
   a. 2–4.
   b. 6–8.
   c. 8–12.
   d. 15–20.

9. To build flexibility, the American College of Sports Medicine recommends that you hold each stretch for
   a. 5–10 seconds.
   b. 10–30 seconds.
   c. 30–60 seconds.
   d. 1–2 minutes.

10. Which strategy will contribute to the success of your fitness program?
    a. Be sure to have water or commercial sports drinks on hand.
    b. Buy one pair of shoes that you can use for all of your fitness activities.
    c. If joining a health club, sign a long-term contract.
    d. Add protein supplements to your diet.

## True or False

T F 1. Muscular strength is the ability to contract a muscle over and over again.

T F 2. Exercise increases the efficiency of the body's metabolism.

T F 3. Weight-bearing exercise can help prevent osteoporosis.

T F 4. Regular exercise can improve mood, lessen depression, and boost creativity.

T F 5. To improve cardiorespiratory endurance, it is best to exercise at your maximum heart rate.

T F 6. Isometric exercise involves applying muscular force with movement.

T F 7. In a weight training program, use of a light weight and a high number of repetitions develops endurance more than strength.

T F 8. Most women develop large, bulky muscles from a regular, moderate program of resistance exercise.

T F 9. Ballistic stretching develops a high degree of flexibility with little risk of injury.

T F 10. The proper treatment for a strained muscle includes resting the affected area, applying ice until the swelling subsides, compressing the area with an elastic bandage, and elevating the affected body part.

ANSWERS: Multiple Choice: 1. d (pp. 232–233); 2. b (p. 232); 3. c (p. 233); 4. b (p. 234); 5. c (p. 241); 6. b (p. 241); 7. b (p. 241); 8. c (p. 244); 9. b (p. 244); 10. a (p. 247). True or False: 1. F (p. 232); 2. T (p. 234); 3. T (p. 234); 4. T (p. 235); 5. F (p. 241); 6. F (p. 242); 7. T (p. 244); 8. F (p. 243); 9. F (p. 244); 10. T (p. 249).

Name ____________________ Section ______________ Date ______________

# WELLNESS WORKSHEET S10

## Assessing and Developing Physical Fitness

Ww

Study Guide

Once you've decided whether you should obtain medical clearance before making a change in your exercise program, the next step is to assess your current level of physical fitness. The test presented here will allow you to make a relatively simple assessment of cardiorespiratory endurance.

### Part I. Assessing Cardiorespiratory Endurance

#### 1.5-Mile Run-Walk Test

Don't attempt this test unless you have completed at least 6 weeks of some type of conditioning activity. You may want to practice pacing yourself prior to taking the test to avoid going too fast at the start and becoming fatigued before you finish. Allow yourself a day or two to recover from your practice run before taking the test. Before beginning this test, warm up with some walking, easy jogging, and stretching exercises.

1. Ask someone with a stopwatch, clock, or watch with a second hand to time you.
2. Take the test on a running track or course that is flat and provides measurements of up to 1.5 miles. Cover the distance as fast as possible, at a pace that is comfortable for you. You can run or walk the entire distance or use some combination of running and walking.
3. Note the time it takes you to complete the 1.5-mile distance.

   Your time: ____ : ____ (minutes:seconds)
4. Cool down by walking or jogging slowly for about 5 minutes.
5. Determine the rating for your score by consulting the table below. If you are unable to complete the entire 1.5 miles, consider yourself very poor in CRE.

*Standards for the 1.5-Mile Run-Walk Test (minutes:seconds)*

| *Women* | *Superior* | *Excellent* | *Good* | *Fair* | *Poor* | *Very Poor* |
|---|---|---|---|---|---|---|
| Age: 18–29 | 11:00 or less | 11:15–12:45 | 13:00–14:15 | 14:30–15:45 | 16:00–17:30 | 17:45 or more |
| 30–39 | 11:45 or less | 12:00–13:30 | 13:45–15:15 | 15:30–16:30 | 16:45–18:45 | 19:00 or more |
| 40–49 | 12:45 or less | 13:00–14:30 | 14:45–16:30 | 16:45–18:30 | 18:45–20:45 | 21:00 or more |
| 50–59 | 14:15 or less | 14:30–16:30 | 16:45–18:30 | 18:45–20:30 | 20:45–23:00 | 23:15 or more |
| 60 and over | 14:00 or less | 14:15–17:15 | 17:30–20:15 | 20:30–22:45 | 23:00–24:45 | 25:00 or more |
| *Men* | | | | | | |
| Age: 18–29 | 9:15 or less | 9:30–10:30 | 10:45–11:45 | 12:00–12:45 | 13:00–14:00 | 14:15 or more |
| 30–39 | 9:45 or less | 10:00–11:00 | 11:15–12:15 | 12:30–13:30 | 13:45–14:45 | 15:00 or more |
| 40–49 | 10:00 or less | 10:15–11:45 | 12:00–13:00 | 13:15–14:15 | 14:30–16:00 | 16:25 or more |
| 50–59 | 10:45 or less | 11:00–12:45 | 13:00–14:15 | 14:30–15:45 | 16:00–17:45 | 18:00 or more |
| 60 and over | 11:15 or less | 11:30–13:45 | 14:00–15:45 | 16:00–17:45 | 18:00–20:45 | 21:00 or more |

SOURCES: Formula for maximal oxygen consumption taken from McArdle, W. D., F. I. Katch, and V. L. Katch. 1991. *Exercise Physiology: Energy, Nutrition, and Human Performance.* Philadelphia: Lea & Febiger, pp. 225–226. Ratings based on norms from the Cooper Institute for Aerobics Research, Dallas, Texas, *The Physical Fitness Specialist Manual,* revised 2000. Used with permission.

*(over)*

**Part II. Personal Fitness Program Plan and Contract**

A. I, ______________________ (name), am contracting with myself to follow a physical fitness program to work toward the following goals:

1. ______________________
2. ______________________
3. ______________________

B. My program plan is as follows:

| Activities | Components (Check ✓) | | | | | Frequency (Check ✓) | | | | | | | Intensity | Time |
|---|---|---|---|---|---|---|---|---|---|---|---|---|---|---|
| | CRE | MS | ME | F | BC | M | Tu | W | Th | F | Sa | Su | | |
| | | | | | | | | | | | | | | |
| | | | | | | | | | | | | | | |
| | | | | | | | | | | | | | | |
| | | | | | | | | | | | | | | |
| | | | | | | | | | | | | | | |

C. My program will begin on __________ (date). My program includes the following schedule of minigoals. For each step in my program, I will give myself the reward listed.

______________________ (minigoal 1) __________ (date) __________ (reward)

______________________ (minigoal 2) __________ (date) __________ (reward)

______________________ (minigoal 3) __________ (date) __________ (reward)

D. I will use the following tools to monitor my program and my progress toward my goals:

______________________ (list any charts, graphs, or journals you plan to use)

______________________

I sign this contract as an indication of my personal commitment to reach my goal.

______________________ (your signature) __________ (date)

I have recruited a helper who will witness my contract and ______________________

______________________ (list any way your helper will participate in your program)

______________________ (witness's signature) __________ (date)

CHAPTER 11

# Weight Management



## Multiple Choice

1. The most important factor in assessing a person's body composition is
   a. total body weight.
   b. body weight relative to age.
   c. proportion of body weight that is fat.
   d. body weight relative to height.

2. Which of the following elements in the energy-balance equation is under an individual's control?
   a. energy for food digestion
   b. energy for resting metabolism
   c. energy for basic body functions
   d. energy intake from food

3. People are at greater risk for heart disease if they tend to gain weight in the
   a. thighs.
   b. hips.
   c. abdomen.
   d. buttocks.

4. Body image is determined by
   a. one's own thinking.
   b. hydrostatic weighing.
   c. height-weight charts.
   d. calculation of body mass index.

5. Resting metabolic rate is
   a. the energy required to maintain basic body functions.
   b. the sum of all the processes by which food energy is used by the body.
   c. the body's total daily energy expenditure.
   d. the energy required to digest food.

6. A woman with a body mass index of 24.2 would be classified as
   a. underweight.
   b. normal weight.
   c. overweight.
   d. obese.

7. A person with diabetes or pre-diabetes might benefit from all of the following EXCEPT
   a. decreased intake of full-fat dairy products.
   b. weight loss.
   c. increased physical activity.
   d. increased intake of refined carbohydrates.

8. All of the following are good strategies for managing weight EXCEPT
   a. measuring portion sizes with a food scale.
   b. eating more quickly.
   c. planning your meals and snacks.
   d. serving food in small bowls or plates.

9. Bulimia nervosa is characterized by
   a. refusal to eat enough food to maintain normal, healthy body weight.
   b. high fat intake and low level of physical activity.
   c. alternating binging and purging.
   d. normal food consumption interrupted by episodes of binge eating.

10. To lose 1 pound in 1 week, you would need to create a daily negative energy balance of ______ calories.
    a. 100
    b. 250
    c. 500
    d. 1000

## True or False

T F 1. The range for healthy percent body fat is lower for women than for men.

T F 2. Obesity is a risk factor for cancer.

T F 3. Height-weight charts directly measure body fat.

T F 4. Most cases of type 2 diabetes are due to uncontrollable environmental factors.

T F 5. Fat stored in the hips is less of a health risk than fat stored in the abdomen.

T F 6. Most people can accurately estimate their total food intake.

T F 7. Intake of refined carbohydrates is linked to large shifts in blood glucose levels.

T F 8. Most participants in the National Weight Control Registry successfully lost weight using a low-carbohydrate, high-fat diet.

T F 9. Prescription drugs for weight loss are a good choice for people who need to lose less than 15 pounds.

T F 10. For an obese person, losing small amounts of weight can significantly improve physical and emotional health.

ANSWERS: Multiple Choice: 1. c (pp. 254–255); 2. d (p. 255); 3. c (p. 257); 4. a (p. 257); 5. a (p. 260); 6. b (p. 256); 7. d (p. 259); 8. b (p. 266); 9. c (p. 271); 10. c (p. 275). True or False: 1. F (p. 254); 2. T (p. 256); 3. F (p. 255); 4. F (p. 259); 5. T (p. 257); 6. F (p. 262); 7. T (p. 263); 8. F (p. 263); 9. F (p. 269); 10. T (p. 271).

Name ____________ Section ____________ Date ____________

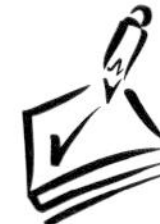

# WELLNESS WORKSHEET S11

## What Triggers Your Eating?

Ww

This test is designed to provide you with a score for five factors that describe many people's eating. This information will put you in a better position to manage your eating behavior and control your weight. Circle the number that indicates to what degree each situation is likely to make you start eating.

| Social | Very Unlikely | | | | | | | | | Very Likely |
|---|---|---|---|---|---|---|---|---|---|---|
| 1. Arguing or having a conflict with someone | 1 | 2 | 3 | 4 | 5 | 6 | 7 | 8 | 9 | 10 |
| 2. Being with others when they are eating | 1 | 2 | 3 | 4 | 5 | 6 | 7 | 8 | 9 | 10 |
| 3. Being urged to eat by someone else | 1 | 2 | 3 | 4 | 5 | 6 | 7 | 8 | 9 | 10 |
| 4. Feeling inadequate around others | 1 | 2 | 3 | 4 | 5 | 6 | 7 | 8 | 9 | 10 |
| **Emotional** | | | | | | | | | | |
| 5. Feeling bad, such as being anxious or depressed | 1 | 2 | 3 | 4 | 5 | 6 | 7 | 8 | 9 | 10 |
| 6. Feeling good, happy, or relaxed | 1 | 2 | 3 | 4 | 5 | 6 | 7 | 8 | 9 | 10 |
| 7. Feeling bored or having time on my hands | 1 | 2 | 3 | 4 | 5 | 6 | 7 | 8 | 9 | 10 |
| 8. Feeling stressed or excited | 1 | 2 | 3 | 4 | 5 | 6 | 7 | 8 | 9 | 10 |
| **Situational** | | | | | | | | | | |
| 9. Seeing an advertisement for food or eating | 1 | 2 | 3 | 4 | 5 | 6 | 7 | 8 | 9 | 10 |
| 10. Passing by a bakery, cookie shop, or other enticement to eat | 1 | 2 | 3 | 4 | 5 | 6 | 7 | 8 | 9 | 10 |
| 11. Being involved in a party, celebration, or special occasion | 1 | 2 | 3 | 4 | 5 | 6 | 7 | 8 | 9 | 10 |
| 12. Eating out | 1 | 2 | 3 | 4 | 5 | 6 | 7 | 8 | 9 | 10 |
| **Thinking** | | | | | | | | | | |
| 13. Making excuses to myself about why it's OK to eat | 1 | 2 | 3 | 4 | 5 | 6 | 7 | 8 | 9 | 10 |
| 14. Berating myself for being so fat or unable to control my eating | 1 | 2 | 3 | 4 | 5 | 6 | 7 | 8 | 9 | 10 |
| 15. Worrying about others or about difficulties I am having | 1 | 2 | 3 | 4 | 5 | 6 | 7 | 8 | 9 | 10 |
| 16. Thinking about how things should or shouldn't be | 1 | 2 | 3 | 4 | 5 | 6 | 7 | 8 | 9 | 10 |
| **Physiological** | | | | | | | | | | |
| 17. Experiencing pain or physical discomfort | 1 | 2 | 3 | 4 | 5 | 6 | 7 | 8 | 9 | 10 |
| 18. Experiencing trembling, headache, or light-headedness associated with not eating or having too much caffeine | 1 | 2 | 3 | 4 | 5 | 6 | 7 | 8 | 9 | 10 |
| 19. Experiencing fatigue or feeling overtired | 1 | 2 | 3 | 4 | 5 | 6 | 7 | 8 | 9 | 10 |
| 20. Experiencing hunger pangs or urges to eat, even though I've eaten recently | 1 | 2 | 3 | 4 | 5 | 6 | 7 | 8 | 9 | 10 |

*(over)*

### Scoring

Total your scores for each category, and enter them below. Then rank the scores by marking the highest score 1, next highest score 2, and so on. Focus on the highest ranked categories first, but any score above 24 is high and indicates that you need to work on that category.

| Category | Total Score | Rank Order |
|---|---|---|
| Social (Items 1–4) | ______ | ______ |
| Emotional (Items 5–8) | ______ | ______ |
| Situational (Items 9–12) | ______ | ______ |
| Thinking (Items 13–16) | ______ | ______ |
| Physiological (Items 17–20) | ______ | ______ |

### What Your Score Means

**Social** A high score here means you are very susceptible to the influence of others. Work on better ways to communicate more assertively, handle conflict, and manage anger. Challenge your beliefs about the need to be polite and the obligations you feel you must fulfill.

**Emotional** A high score here means you need to develop effective ways to cope with emotions. Work on developing skills in stress management, time management, and communication. Practicing positive but realistic self-talk can help you handle small daily upsets.

**Situational** A high score here means you are especially susceptible to external influences. Try to avoid external cues to eat and respond differently to those you cannot avoid. Control your environment by changing the way you buy, store, cook, and serve food. Anticipate potential problems, and have a plan for handling them.

**Thinking** A high score here means that the way you think—how you talk to yourself, the beliefs you hold, your memories, and your expectations has a powerful influence on your eating habits. Try to be less self-critical, less perfectionistic, and more flexible in your ideas about the way things ought to be. Recognize when you're making excuses or rationalizations that allow you to eat.

**Physiological** A high score here means that the way you eat, what you eat, or medications you are taking may be affecting your eating behavior. You may be eating to reduce physical arousal or deal with physical discomfort. Try eating three meals a day, supplemented with regular snacks if needed. Avoid too much caffeine. If any medication you're taking produces adverse physical reactions, switch to an alternative, if possible. If your medications may be affecting your hormone levels, discuss possible alternatives with your physician.

SOURCE: Adapted from Nash, J. D. 1997. *The New Maximize Your Body Potential.* Palo Alto, Calif.: Bull Publishing. Reprinted with permission from Bull Publishing Company.

CHAPTER 12

# Cardiovascular Disease and Cancer

## Multiple Choice

1. The type of blood vessel that delivers nutrients to the tissues and picks up waste-carrying blood is the
   a. artery.
   b. capillary.
   c. ventricle.
   d. vein.

2. Smoking affects the cardiorespiratory system in which one of the following ways?
   a. It decreases blood pressure.
   b. It increases the amount of oxygen available to the heart.
   c. It reduces levels of HDL in the bloodstream.
   d. It reduces blood clotting.

3. Which of the following diastolic blood pressure readings would be typical for a healthy adult?
   a. 50
   b. 75
   c. 110
   d. 150

4. A type of chest pain that may be a sign of heart disease is
   a. arrhythmia.
   b. thrombosis.
   c. aneurysm.
   d. angina.

5. Dietary changes that can protect against cardiovascular diseases include all of the following EXCEPT
   a. decreasing fiber intake.
   b. decreasing trans fat intake.
   c. replacing animal proteins with soy proteins.
   d. increasing fish consumption.

6. Metastasis occurs when
   a. cancer cells break off and invade other parts of the body.
   b. cancer cells begin to divide rapidly within an organ.
   c. a tumor grows big enough to interfere with body functions.
   d. a nonmalignant group of cells grows slowly.

7. Cancers of the blood-forming cells are
   a. carcinomas.
   b. leukemias.
   c. lymphomas.
   d. sarcomas.

8. The most common cause of cancer death in the United States is
   a. breast cancer.
   b. prostate cancer.
   c. lung cancer.
   d. colon cancer.

9. Which of the following types of cancer is caused by a sexually transmitted disease?
   a. ovarian cancer
   b. testicular cancer
   c. prostate cancer
   d. cervical cancer

10. Using a sunscreen with an SPF rating of 15 means that you
   a. can stay in the sun for 15 minutes without getting burned.
   b. can stay in the sun 15 times longer without getting burned than if you didn't use it.
   c. are protected against the full range of ultraviolet radiation.
   d. can remain in the sun as long as the UV index is below 15.

## True or False

T F 1. A low level of high-density lipoproteins in beneficial for heart health.

T F 2. Chronic hostility and anger increase one's risk of heart attack.

T F 3. Insulin resistance is a risk factor associated with metabolic syndrome.

T F 4. Hypertension usually has no symptoms.

T F 5. Hemorrhagic strokes are the most common type of stroke.

T F 6. The primary risk factor for lung cancer is smoking.

T F 7. Age is a key risk factor for both colon and prostate cancer.

T F 8. One woman in 20 will develop breast cancer.

T F 9. Oral cancers can be linked to the use of spit tobacco and alcohol.

T F 10. Estrogen is a cancer promoter.

ANSWERS: Multiple Choice: 1. b (p. 278); 2. c (p. 279); 3. b (p. 279); 4. d (p. 288); 5. a (p. 292); 6. a (p. 295); 7. b (p. 296); 8. c (p. 296); 9. d (p. 300); 10. b (p. 302). True or False: 1. F (p. 281); 2. T (p. 282); 3. T (p. 285); 4. T (p. 280); 5. F (p. 290); 6. T (p. 296); 7. T (pp. 297, 299); 8. F (p. 297); 9. T (p. 303); 10. T (p. 305).

Name ______________________ Section ______________ Date ______________

# WELLNESS WORKSHEET S12

## Cardiovascular Disease and Cancer

Ww

### Part I. Are You at Risk for Cardiovascular Disease?

Your risk for CVD depends on a variety of factors, many of which are under your control. To help identify your risk factors, circle the response for each risk category that best describes you.

1. Gender and Age
   - 0 Female age 55 or younger; male age 45 or younger
   - 2 Female over age 50 or male over age 45
2. Heredity
   - 0 Neither parent suffered a heart attack or stroke before age 60.
   - 3 One parent suffered a heart attack or stroke before age 60.
   - 7 Both parents suffered a heart attack or stroke before age 60.
3. Smoking
   - 0 Never smoked
   - 3 Quit more than 2 years ago and lifetime smoking is less than 5 pack-years*
   - 6 Quit less than 2 years ago and/or lifetime smoking is greater than 5 pack-years*
   - 8 Smoke less than 1/2 pack per day
   - 13 Smoke more than 1/2 pack per day
   - 15 Smoke more than 1 pack per day
4. Environmental Tobacco Smoke
   - 0 Do not live or work with smokers
   - 2 Exposed to ETS at work
   - 3 Live with smoker
   - 4 Both live and work with smokers
5. Blood Pressure
   The average of the last three readings:
   - 0 120/80 or below
   - 1 121/81 to 130/85
   - 3 Don't know
   - 5 131/86 to 150/90
   - 9 151/91 to 170/100
   - 13 Above 170/100
6. Total Cholesterol
   - 0 Lower than 190
   - 1 190 to 210
   - 2 Don't know
   - 3 211 to 240
   - 4 241 to 270
   - 5 271 to 300
   - 6 Over 300
7. HDL Cholesterol
   - 0 Over 60 mg/dl
   - 1 55 to 60
   - 2 Don't know HDL
   - 3 45 to 54
   - 5 35 to 44
   - 7 25 to 34
   - 12 Lower than 25
8. Exercise
   - 0 Exercise three times a week
   - 1 Exercise once or twice a week
   - 2 Occasional exercise less than once a week
   - 7 Rarely exercise
9. Diabetes
   - 0 No personal or family history
   - 2 One parent with diabetes
   - 6 Two parents with diabetes
   - 9 Type 1 diabetes
   - 13 Type 2 diabetes
10. Body Mass Index (kg/m$^2$)
   - 0 <23.0
   - 1 23.0–24.9
   - 2 25.0–28.9
   - 3 29.0–34.9
   - 5 35.0–39.9
   - 7 ≥40
11. Stress
   - 0 Relaxed most of the time
   - 1 Occasional stress and anger
   - 2 Frequently stressed and angry
   - 3 Usually stressed and angry

| **Total Score** | **Estimated Risk of Early Heart Attack or Stroke** |
|---|---|
| Less than 20 | Low risk |
| 20–29 | Moderate risk |
| 30–45 | High risk |
| Over 45 | Extremely high risk |

*Pack-years can be calculated by multiplying the number of packs you smoked per day by the number of years you smoked. For example, if you smoked a pack and a half a day for 5 years, you would have smoked the equivalent of 1.5 × 5 = 7.5 pack-years.

*(over)*

**Part II. Skin Cancer Risk Assessment**

Skin cancer is the most common cancer of all when cases of the highly curable forms are included in the count. Your risk of skin cancer from the ultraviolet radiation in sunlight depends on several factors. Take the quiz below to see how sensitive you are. The higher your UV-risk score, the greater your risk of skin cancer—and the greater your need to take precautions against too much sun. Score 1 point for each true statement:

____ 1. I have blond or red hair.
____ 2. I have light-colored eyes (blue, gray, green).
____ 3. I freckle easily.
____ 4. I have many moles.
____ 5. I had two or more blistering sunburns as a child.
____ 6. I spent lots of time in a tropical climate as a child.
____ 7. I have a family history of skin cancer.
____ 8. I work outdoors.
____ 9. I spend a lot of time in outdoor activities.
____ 10. I like to spend as much time in the sun as I can.
____ 11. I sometimes go to a tanning parlor or use a sunlamp.

____ **Total score**

| Score | Risk of skin cancer from UV radiation |
|---|---|
| 0 | Low |
| 1–3 | Moderate |
| 4–7 | High |
| 8–11 | Very high |

**Part III. Do You Eat Enough Cancer Fighters?**

Track your diet for 3 days, putting a mark ("1" for day 1, "2" for day 2, "3" for day 3) next to any food you eat:

____ Orange and yellow vegetables and (some) fruits, including apricots, cantaloupe, carrots, corn, papaya, pumpkin, red and yellow peppers, sweet potatoes, and winter squash

____ Dark green leafy vegetables, including chard; kale; romaine and other dark lettuces; spinach; and beet, collard, dandelion, mustard, and turnip greens

____ Cruciferous vegetables, including bok choy, broccoli, brussels sprouts, cabbage, cauliflower, and turnips

____ Citrus fruits, including grapefruit, lemon, lime, orange, and tangerine

____ Whole grains, including whole-grain bread, cereal, and pasta and brown rice

____ Legumes, including peas; lentils; and fava, navy, kidney, pinto, black, and lima beans

____ Berries, including strawberries, raspberries, blackberries, blueberries

____ Garlic and other allium vegetables, including onions, leeks, chives, scallions, and shallots

____ Soy products, including tofu, tempeh, soy milk, miso, and soybeans

____ Other cancer-fighting fruits: apples, cherries, grapes, kiwifruit, plums, prunes, raisins, watermelon

____ Other cancer-fighting vegetables: asparagus, beets, chili peppers, green peppers, radishes, tomatoes

Total average daily servings: ____ (day 1) + ____ (day 2) + ____ (day 3) = ____ ÷ 3 = ____

Try to eat at least five servings of cancer-fighting foods a day; the more servings, the better (as long as you maintain a healthy weight). (*Note:* Research is ongoing, and this list of cancer fighters is not comprehensive. Remember, nearly all fruits, vegetables, and whole-grains are healthy, disease-fighting dietary choices.)

# CHAPTER 13
# Immunity and Infection



## Multiple Choice

1. An organism that causes disease is a (an)
   a. allergen.
   b. pathogen.
   c. viral agent.
   d. parasite.

2. The release of histamines causes
   a. infection.
   b. illness.
   c. contamination.
   d. inflammation.

3. A reaction by the body's immune system to a harmless substance such as dust is
   a. acquired immunity.
   b. an antigen.
   c. an allergy.
   d. a vector.

4. Antibiotics are most effective against
   a. bacteria.
   b. parasites.
   c. viruses.
   d. colds.

5. Colds and influenza are caused by
   a. bacteria.
   b. protozoa.
   c. prions.
   d. viruses.

6. Which of the following STDs is curable with current treatments?
   a. herpes
   b. genital warts
   c. syphilis
   d. HIV infection

7. In untreated HIV infection, the average amount of time between the initial infection and the onset of symptoms is
   a. 1 year.
   b. 6 years.
   c. 11 years.
   d. 16 years.

8. Which of the following STDs is often asymptomatic among women?
   a. chlamydia
   b. gonorrhea
   c. hepatitis B
   d. all of the above

9. A leading cause of infertility among young women is
   a. human papillomavirus infection.
   b. HIV infection.
   c. syphilis.
   d. pelvic inflammatory disease.

10. Unlike HIV, hepatitis B is often transmitted through
    a. sexual intercourse.
    b. nonsexual close contact.
    c. injection drug use.
    d. contact during childbirth.

## True or False

T F 1. Lymphocytes travel in both the bloodstream and the lymphatic system.

T F 2. Acquired immunity is the ability of lymphocytes to "remember" previous infections.

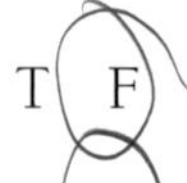

T F 3. West Nile virus is usually transmitted by contaminated food.

T F 4. Viruses cause only mild, short-term illness.

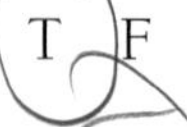

T F 5. Hand washing can prevent the transmission of pathogens.

T F 6. A woman with HIV infection is more likely to transmit the infection to a male sexual partner during intercourse than vice versa.

T F 7. HIV is not spread through casual contact.

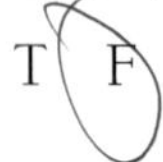

T F 8. The customary treatment for pelvic inflammatory disease is over-the-counter medication.

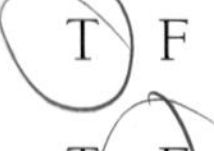

T F 9. Genital warts have been linked with cervical cancer.

T F 10. Use of lubricants containing nonoxynol-9 is an effective strategy for STD prevention.

ANSWERS: Multiple Choice: 1. b (p. 314); 2. d (p. 316); 3. c (p. 318); 4. a (p. 322); 5. d (p. 323); 6. c (p. 328); 7. c (p. 331); 8. d (pp. 337, 341); 9. d (p. 337); 10. b (p. 340). True or False: 1. T (p. 316); 2. T (p. 317); 3. F (p. 327); 4. F (pp. 323–325); 5. T (p. 328); 6. F (p. 331); 7. T (p. 331); 8. F (p. 338); 9. T (p. 338); 10. F (pp. 331, 336).

Name ______________________ Section ______________ Date ________________

**WELLNESS WORKSHEET S13**

## Checklist for Avoiding Infection

Ww

Study Guide

The best thing you can do to prevent an infection is to limit your exposure to pathogens. The next best thing is to keep your immune system as strong as possible. Read through the following list of statements and check whether each is mostly true or mostly false for you.

**True False**

**Exposure to Pathogens**

___ ___ I receive drinking water from a clean supply.

___ ___ The area in which I live has adequate sewage treatment.

___ ___ I frequently wash my hands with soap and warm water for at least 10-20 seconds.

___ ___ I avoid close contact with people who are infectious with diseases transmitted via the respiratory route (e.g., influenza, chicken pox, and tuberculosis).

___ ___ I do not inject drugs.

**When Outdoors**

___ ___ When hiking or camping, I do not drink water from streams, rivers, or lakes without first purifying it.

___ ___ I avoid contact with ticks, mosquitoes, rodents, bats, and other disease carriers.

___ ___ When hiking in the woods or playing in a yard in an area where Lyme disease or other tickborne infections have been reported, I take appropriate precautions:

- ___ Wear light-colored clothing: long pants, a long-sleeved shirt, and closed shoes.
- ___ Tuck my pants into my socks, shoes, or boots.
- ___ Tuck my shirt into my pants.
- ___ Wear light-colored, tightly woven fabrics.
- ___ Wear a hat.
- ___ Stay near the center of trails.
- ___ Check myself daily for ticks.
- ___ Shower and shampoo after each outing.
- ___ Wash clothes and check equipment after each outing
- ___ Use an insect repellant containing DEET, picaridan, or oil of lemon eucalyptus on my skin and/or a spray containing permethrin on my clothing.

___ ___ If I discover a tick attached to my skin, I remove it immediately in an appropriate manner (fill in): ________________________________

________________________________________

________________________________________

________________________________________

(over)

**True False**

**In a Sexual Relationship**

____ ____ I am in a monogamous relationship with a mutually faithful, uninfected partner.

____ ____ I use condoms.

____ ____ I discuss STDs and prevention with new partners.

____ ____ I avoid engaging in high-risk behaviors with any person who might carry HIV.

**In the Kitchen**

____ ____ I wash my hands thoroughly with warm soapy water before and after handling food.

____ ____ I don't let groceries sit in a warm car.

____ ____ I avoid buying food in containers that leak, bulge, or are severely dented.

____ ____ I use separate cutting boards for meat and for foods that will be eaten raw.

____ ____ I thoroughly clean all equipment (cutting boards, counters, utensils) before and after use.

____ ____ I rinse and scrub fresh fruits and vegetables carefully to remove all dirt.

____ ____ I cook all foods thoroughly, especially beef, poultry, fish, pork, and eggs.

____ ____ I verify that hamburgers are cooked to 160°F (71°C) with a food thermometer.

____ ____ I store foods below 40°F (5°C).

____ ____ I do not leave cooked or refrigerated foods at room temperature for more than 2 hours.

____ ____ I thaw foods in the refrigerator or microwave.

____ ____ I use only pasteurized milk and juice.

____ ____ I avoid coughing or sneezing over foods, even when I'm healthy.

____ ____ I cover any cuts on my hands when handling food.

**To Keep Your Immune System Healthy**

____ ____ I eat a balanced diet, following the guidelines presented in the Dietary Guidelines for Americans.

____ ____ I maintain a healthy weight.

____ ____ I get enough sleep, 6–8 hours per night.

____ ____ I exercise regularly.

____ ____ I don't smoke, and I drink alcohol only in moderation.

____ ____ I wash my hands frequently.

____ ____ I have effective ways of coping with stress.

____ ____ I get all recommended immunizations and booster shots.

____ ____ *For people with heart valve disorders that place them at increased risk of infection.* I check with my health care provider about antibiotic use before dental or surgical procedures and before body piercing.

False answers indicate areas where you could change your behavior to help avoid infectious diseases. Consider creating a behavior change strategy for any statement you checked false.

## CHAPTER 14
## The Challenge of Aging



### Multiple Choice

1. Which of the following remains most stable as you age?
   a. intelligence
   b. hearing
   c. eyesight
   d. flexibility

2. Which of the following statements about aging is TRUE?
   a. Requirements for vitamins and minerals are significantly lower for people over age 65.
   b. Glaucoma always leads to blindness.
   c. The ability to hear high-pitched sounds increases with age.
   d. Alcohol and drug dependence are common problems among the elderly.

3. The decline in the ability to focus on close objects that occurs in many people beginning in their forties is called
   a. cataracts.
   b. glaucoma.
   c. presbyopia.
   d. dendrite.

4. As birth rates drop, the percentage of elderly people will
   a. increase.
   b. decrease.
   c. stay the same.
   d. fluctuate.

5. Most older Americans live
   a. alone.
   b. with a relative.
   c. with a nonrelative.
   d. in a nursing home.

6. Which of the following is NOT a characteristic of brain death?
   a. unresponsivity
   b. incoherence
   c. flat EEG
   d. no movements or breathing

7. The testator of a will is the
   a. attorney.
   b. person making the will.
   c. closest living relative.
   d. beneficiary of the will.

8. In 1990 in the case of Nancy Beth Cruzan, the Supreme Court ruled that
   a. life support can only be removed from a vegetative patient if he or she has completed a living will making such a request.
   b. the right to refuse unwarranted treatment is constitutionally protected.
   c. physician-assisted suicide is illegal.
   d. there is no medical or ethical difference between withholding and withdrawing a treatment.

9. A legal document that allows one person to act as the agent of another in making medical decisions is a
   a. living will.
   b. Uniform Donor Card.
   c. will.
   d. durable power of attorney for health care.

10. All of the following are stages in Elisabeth Kübler-Ross's stages of dying theory EXCEPT
    a. denial.
    b. adjusting.
    c. depression.
    d. bargaining.

## True or False

T F 1. Older women are more likely to live in poverty than older men.

T F 2. Adult stem cells exhibit more plasticity than embryonic stem cells.

T F 3. Alzheimer's disease is an incurable form of dementia.

T F 4. Males born in the year 2000 have a longer life expectancy than females born in the same year.

T F 5. Most older Americans live in a nursing home at some point in their lives.

T F 6. Our attitudes toward death are formed in childhood and do not change much as we grow older.

T F 7. About one-third of Americans die without leaving a will.

T F 8. Palliative care focuses on relieving pain in a patient not expected to recover.

T F 9. Increasing a patient's pain medication to the point where, in addition to controlling pain, it also hastens death is considered physician-assisted suicide.

T F 10. Acceptance is the final stage in Kübler-Ross's model of the psychological stages that a dying person experiences.

ANSWERS: Multiple Choice: 1. a (p. 349); 2. d (p. 350); 3. c (p. 352); 4. a (p. 356);
5. b (p. 356); 6. b (p. 358); 7. b (p. 359); 8. b (p. 361); 9. d (p. 362); 10. b (p. 364).
True or False: 1. T (p. 351); 2. F (p. 348); 3. T (pp. 353–354); 4. F (p. 335);
5. F (p. 356); 6. F (p. 358); 7. F (p. 359); 8. T (p. 360); 9. F (p. 362); 10. T (p. 364).

Name ______________ Section ______________ Date ______________

## WELLNESS WORKSHEET S14

Are You Prepared for Aging?

Ww

### Assess Your Current Behaviors

Are you doing everything you can now to enhance the quality of your life as you age? Read through the following list of statements and check the answer that best describes your current behavior.

**Yes No**

____ ____ I exercise regularly.

____ ____ I eat wisely.

- ____ I eat meals low in fat and added sugars and high in essential nutrients and fiber (fresh fruits and vegetables, whole-grain cereals and breads, brown rice, pasta).
- ____ I limit saturated and trans fats and get protein from fish, skinless poultry, and plant sources.
- ____ I use fat free or low-fat dairy products.
- ____ I consume the recommended amount of calcium, vitamin D, and vitamin B-12.
- ____ I limit the amount of sodium I consume and consume adequate potassium.

____ ____ My weight is in the recommended range.

____ ____ I drink alcohol in moderation, if at all.

____ ____ I don't use tobacco in any form.

____ ____ I recognize the stressors in my life and take appropriate steps to control and deal with stress.

____ ____ I perform appropriate self-examinations.

____ ____ I have regular physical examinations that include appropriate screening tests.

____ ____ I participate in activities that keep my mind sharp and active.

### Thinking About Aging

Have you thought seriously about the changes that aging can bring? To help you begin thinking now about your life as you grow older, answer the following questions.

1. What things come to mind when you think of an older person? Can you imagine those things applying to you? What do you think you will be like when you are 70 years old?

2. What do you most look forward to as you grow older?

*(over)*

3. What do you most fear as you grow older?

4. How long would you like to keep working? What would you like to do after you retire? What hobbies or volunteer opportunities would you pursue?

5. Have you considered the loss of income that retirement often brings? What can you do now to help meet your economic needs in the future?

6. Older people often find themselves alone more frequently (due to the death of a spouse and/or close friends). Can you think of activities you enjoy doing alone?

7. If when you are older you are no longer able to care for yourself, what living and care arrangements would you prefer?

8. What would you do if your parents were no longer able to care for themselves?

9. List five positive and five negative things about aging.

## CHAPTER 15
## Conventional and Complementary Medicine: Skills for the Health Care Consumer



### Multiple Choice

1. All of the following symptoms or conditions require emergency medical care EXCEPT
   a. loss of consciousness.
   b. recurrent stomach pain.
   c. severe shortness of breath.
   d. steadily worsening reaction to an insect bite.

2. If you have a cough that lasts longer than 2 weeks, you should
   a. go to a hospital emergency room.
   b. call your primary physician to see if you should schedule an appointment.
   c. monitor your condition for another 1–2 weeks before contacting your physician.
   d. ask your pharmacist to recommend an over-the-counter or prescription medication.

3. The best choice in self-treatment is often
   a. contacting your physician to see what medications you should be taking.
   b. using prescription medications from the last time you had something similar.
   c. waiting for your body to heal itself.
   d. using a medical self-test kit to determine how serious your condition is.

4. Conventional Western medicine might identify all of the following as factors contributing to or causing illness or disease EXCEPT
   a. a streptococcal infection.
   b. a genetic tendency to obesity.
   c. a spiritual imbalance.
   d. a diet high in saturated fats and cholesterol.

5. Primary care physicians routinely do all of the following EXCEPT
   a. provide psychiatric care.
   b. provide pediatric care.
   c. provide preventive health services, such as immunizations and cancer screening tests.
   d. provide gynecological and obstetrical care.

6. The most successful patient-physician relationship appears to be one in which
   a. the patient relies exclusively on the physician's medical knowledge and expertise.
   b. the physician protects his or her time by discouraging or dismissing questions.
   c. the patient participates actively in decisions and the physician acts as a consultant.
   d. the physician protects the patient from confusing or distressing information and makes the important decisions about the patient's care.

7. A principle of homeopathy is
   a. a substance that causes a disease can cure the disease in small amounts.
   b. illnesses are caused by disturbances in the flow of qi.
   c. energy fields surrounding the body can be influenced by touch and movement.
   d. mind and body are connected and changing one can change the other.

8. The manipulation of joints in the spinal column is an important procedure in
   a. homeopathy.
   b. chiropractic.
   c. acupuncture.
   d. qigong.

9. If you are thinking of trying a complementary and alternative treatment for a medical condition, you should first discuss it with your conventional health care provider for all of the following reasons EXCEPT
   a. the treatment might interact dangerously with a conventional treatment you are receiving.
   b. there may be a beneficial conventional treatment for your condition.
   c. you may need a conventional treatment immediately.
   d. conventional treatments are the only effective treatments.

10. An advantage of fee-for-service insurance plans over managed-care plans is
    a. it is less expensive.
    b. it allows consumers more choice in health care providers.
    c. it is provided by the government.
    d. it is easier to get into a plan.

## True or False

T F 1. The FDA guarantees the safety and effectiveness of all medications on the market, both over-the-counter and prescription.

T F 2. Generic drugs have the same active ingredient as brand-name drugs.

T F 3. For a cold, the best medication is an all-in-one product that will treat many symptoms simultaneously.

T F 4. In conventional Western medicine, each person with a particular set of symptoms is treated in a basically similar way.

T F 5. In the United States the two types of physicians fully trained and licensed to perform surgery and prescribe medication are osteopaths and homeopaths.

T F 6. The goal of complementary and alternative medicine is to rid the body of disease-causing pathogens.

T F 7. Acupuncture has been found to be effective in relieving pain after surgery.

T F 8. Hypnosis can be performed only by a licensed medical doctor.

T F 9. Because herbal remedies and botanicals are derived from plants and other naturally occurring materials, they can be assumed to be very safe.

T F 10. In a health maintenance organization, you choose a primary care physician who manages your health care and refers you to specialists if you need them.

ANSWERS: Multiple Choice: 1. b (p. 371); 2. b (p. 371); 3. c (p. 371); 4. c (p. 374); 5. a (p. 375); 6. c (p. 377); 7. a (p. 382); 8. b (p. 384); 9. d (p. 386); 10. b (p. 388). True or False: 1. F (p. 371); 2. T (p. 372); 3. F (p. 372); 4. T (p. 374); 5. F (p. 375); 6. F (p. 380); 7. T (p. 381); 8. F (p. 383); 9. F (p. 385); 10. T (p. 388).

Name ______________________ Section ______________ Date ________________

## WELLNESS WORKSHEET S15

### Your Personal Health Profile

Ww

Complete as much as possible of this personal health profile and keep it up to date.

**General Information**

Age: ________

Height: ________

Weight: ________

Are you currently trying to _____ gain or _____ lose weight? (check if appropriate)

Blood pressure: ____ / ____

Blood lipid levels:

Total cholesterol: ________

HDL: ________

LDL: ________

Triglycerides: ________

Blood glucose level: ________

**Medical Conditions**

Check any of the following that apply to you and add other conditions that might affect your health and well-being.

____ heart disease

____ lung disease

____ diabetes

____ allergies

____ asthma

____ back pain

____ arthritis

____ other injury or joint problem

____ substance abuse problem

____ depression, anxiety, or another psychological disorder

____ eating disorder

____ other: ______________

____ other: ______________

List any conditions or diseases that are common in your family and/or ethnic group.

______________________________ ______________________________

______________________________ ______________________________

______________________________ ______________________________

**Medications/Treatments**

List any medications or supplements you are taking or any medical treatments you are undergoing. Include the name of the substance or treatment and its purpose. Include both prescription and over-the-counter drugs and any vitamin, mineral, or other dietary supplement you are taking.

| Medication/treatment | Condition/purpose |
|---|---|
| | |
| | |
| | |
| | |
| | |
| | |

*(over)*

### Screening Tests and Vaccinations

To ensure that you are getting the most out of your medical care, keep a record of your screening tests and vaccinations; see Chapters 12–13 for more information on these. Fill in any additional tests and vaccinations that are appropriate for your age, gender, and medical history.

| Screening test/immunization | Date last performed |
|---|---|
| Blood pressure check | |
| STD screening | |
| Cholesterol measurement | |
| Vision test | |
| Dental exam | |
| Pelvic exam and Pap test (women only) | |
| Clinical breast exam (women only) | |
| Other: | |
| Other: | |
| Other: | |
| Other: | |
| Tetanus/diphtheria vaccination | |
| Influenza vaccination | |
| Other: | |
| Other: | |

### Health Care Providers

Primary care physician: name __________ phone __________

Specialist physician: name __________ phone __________

Condition treated: __________

Other health care provider: name __________ phone __________

Condition treated: __________

Pharmacy: name __________ phone __________

Dentist: name __________ phone __________

Optometrist/ophthalmologist: name __________ phone __________

Health insurance provider: name __________ phone __________

Policy number: __________

Dental insurance provider: name __________ phone __________

Policy number: __________

Vision care insurance provider: name __________ phone __________

Policy number: __________

## CHAPTER 16
## Personal Safety: Protecting Yourself from Unintentional Injuries and Violence



### Multiple Choice

1. The leading cause of motor vehicle injuries is
   a. fatigue from long drives.
   b. cell phones.
   c. bad driving, especially speeding.
   d. poor vehicle maintenance.

2. Which of the following statements about the safe use of air bags is TRUE?
   a. Children younger than 12 should ride in the front seat.
   b. Riders should sit as close as possible to the passenger-side dashboard.
   c. If a car has air bags, wearing safety belts isn't necessary.
   d. The seat and steering wheel should be adjusted so that the air bag will deploy in front of the driver's chest rather than face.

3. All of the following are strategies for preventing bicycle injuries EXCEPT
   a. riding against the flow of traffic.
   b. wearing light-colored clothing.
   c. stopping at all traffic lights.
   d. using bicycle paths.

4. ______ is the leading cause of home fire deaths.
   a. Arson
   b. Cooking
   c. Burning of trash
   d. Smoking

5. Smoke detector batteries should be checked every
   a. week.
   b. month.
   c. 6 months.
   d. year.

6. The Heimlich maneuver is used in cases of
   a. poisoning.
   b. choking.
   c. burns.
   d. heart attack.

7. Carpal tunnel syndrome affects the
   a. eyes.
   b. wrists.
   c. back.
   d. skin.

8. In comparison to rates in other industrialized countries, U.S. rates of violence are abnormally high in which two areas?
   a. aggravated assault and homicide
   b. rape and robbery
   c. homicide and firearm-related deaths
   d. battering and rape

9. Which is TRUE regarding school violence?
   a. Students are less safe in school than away from school.
   b. Murder is the most common type of school violence.
   c. Victims of school violence are predominantly female.
   d. The majority of acts of school violence occur in urban areas.

10. Which of the following statements about date rape is FALSE?
    a. The double standard about appropriate sexual behavior for men and women is a factor in date rape.
    b. As many as 25% of women have had experiences in which a date tried to force sex.
    c. Most cases of date rape are reported to the police.
    d. Victims of date rape often feel responsible for the incident.

## True or False

T F 1. Suicide is an example of an unintentional injury.

T F 2. More Americans die from unintentional injuries each year than from intentional injuries.

T F 3. Automobile air bags cause more injuries than they prevent.

T F 4. Carbon monoxide gas has a strong, distinctive odor.

T F 5. When picking up a heavy object, it is better to bend at the hips and knees than to bend at the waist.

T F 6. About 10% of people killed in armed conflict in the twentieth century were civilians.

T F 7. Rates of violent crime are highest among people under age 25.

T F 8. Men and women are about equally likely to be victims of homicide.

T F 9. Violence against children by parents is one of the five leading causes of death for children age 1–18.

T F 10. Making sexual jokes or displaying sexually suggestive pictures can be considered sexual harassment.

ANSWERS: Multiple Choice 1. c (p. 395); 2. d (p. 396); 3. a (p. 397); 4. d (p. 399); 5. b (p. 399); 6. b (p. 400); 7. b (p. 401); 8. c (p. 401); 9. d (p. 404); 10. c (p. 409).
True or False: 1. F (p. 393); 2. T (p. 393); 3. F (p. 396); 4. F (p. 399); 5. T (p. 400); 6. F (p. 406); 7. T (p. 402); 8. F (p. 403); 9. T (p. 409); 10. T (p. 412).

Name ______________________ Section ______________ Date ________________

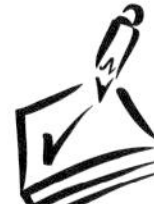

# WELLNESS WORKSHEET S16

## Personal Safety Checklist

Ww

Study Guide

Are you doing all you can to protect yourself from violence and injuries? The following statements relate to intentional injury incidents that can occur in a variety of settings. Put a check next to those statements that are true for you.

**At Home**

_____ My home has good lighting.

_____ Doors are secured with effective locks (deadbolts).

_____ All unused doors and windows are securely locked.

_____ I always lock all windows and doors when I go out.

_____ I have a dog and/or post "Beware of Dog" signs.

_____ Landscaping around the home doesn't provide opportunities for concealment.

_____ Keys are hidden in a secure, nonobvious place.

_____ I do not give anyone the opportunity to duplicate my keys.

_____ The front door has a peephole.

_____ I do not open my door to strangers or allow them into my home or yard.

_____ I ask to see ID or call to verify that repair and utility workers are legitimate.

_____ I use my initials in phone directory listings.

_____ My answering machine message does not imply that I live alone or am not home.

_____ Everyone in the household knows how to call for help.

_____ My neighbors and I have a system for alerting one another in case of an emergency.

_____ I participate in a neighborhood watch program.

**On the Street**

_____ I avoid walking alone, especially at night or in less-populous areas.

_____ I dress in clothing that allows freedom of movement.

_____ I walk purposefully, in an alert and confident manner.

_____ I walk on the outside of the sidewalk, facing traffic.

_____ I check routes to my destination before leaving so as not to appear lost.

_____ I never hitchhike.

_____ I carry valuables in a secure or concealed location and take special care at ATMs.

_____ I have my keys ready when I approach my vehicle or home.

_____ I carry change for a telephone call, fare for public transportation, and a whistle to blow if I am attacked or harassed.

_____ I keep alert for suspicious behavior, and I keep at least two arm lengths between myself and strangers.

*(over)*

## WELLNESS WORKSHEET S16—continued

**In My Car**

_____ My car is in good working condition.

_____ I carry emergency supplies in my car.

_____ I keep my gas tank at least half full.

_____ When driving, I keep doors locked and windows rolled up at least three-quarters of the way.

_____ I park my car in well-lighted areas or parking garages.

_____ I lock my car when I leave it.

_____ I check the interior of my car before unlocking it and getting in.

_____ I don't pick up strangers.

_____ I note the location of emergency call boxes, or I have a cellular phone in my car.

_____ I use caution if my car breaks down or if I am involved in a minor crash or bumped intentionally

_____ When I stop at a light or stop sign, I stop far enough behind the car in front to allow room to maneuver in case of emergency.

_____ I do not get into arguments with drivers of other vehicles.

**On Public Transportation**

_____ I wait in populated, well-lighted areas.

_____ I sit near the driver or conductor.

_____ I sit in a single seat or an outside seat.

_____ I check routes and times in advance, and confirm before boarding that the bus, subway, or train is bound for my destination.

**On Campus**

_____ Door and window locks are secure.

_____ Halls and stairwells have adequate lighting.

_____ Dorm doors are not left unlocked or propped open.

_____ I do not give dorm or residence keys to others.

_____ I keep my door locked.

_____ I do not allow strangers into my room.

_____ I do not walk, jog, or exercise alone at night.

_____ I use campus escort services or walk with friends.

_____ I know the areas that security guards patrol and stay where they can see or hear me if possible.

Your answers here can help you identify behaviors that you should change. Consider planning a behavior change strategy to alter one or more of your risky behaviors.

## CHAPTER 17
## Environmental Health

### Multiple Choice

1. Historically, the highest priority in environmental health was controlling
   a. infectious diseases.
   b. air pollution.
   c. population growth.
   d. energy waste.

2. In 2005, world population was about
   a. 500 million.
   b. 1.5 billion.
   c. 6.5 billion.
   d. 12.5 billion.

3. Which of the following is a disadvantage of landfill?
   a. It becomes unstable when decomposition occurs.
   b. Buried chemicals leak into the soil.
   c. It is often a breeding ground for infectious diseases.
   d. All of the above.

4. The increase in the concentrations of greenhouse gases is primarily the result of
   a. the release of CFCs.
   b. energy use in the developed world.
   c. heavy metal contamination.
   d. temperature inversions.

5. The ozone layer protects the earth from excessive
   a. radon exposure.
   b. nuclear radiation.
   c. ultraviolet radiation.
   d. chlorofluorocarbons.

6. Which one of the following is a major source of acid precipitation pollutants?
   a. air conditioners
   b. lead-based paints
   c. synthetic building materials
   d. industrial combustion of coal

7. Lead poisoning is a serious problem among children who
   a. live in older buildings.
   b. had low birth weights.
   c. have not been vaccinated.
   d. have poor diets.

8. All the following strategies can help reduce chemical pollution and its health effects EXCEPT
   a. burning your trash.
   b. buying locally grown and/or organic produce.
   c. eating less meat.
   d. trying to buy the least toxic products available.

9. A radioactive gas found in certain soils and rocks is
   a. lead.
   b. asbestos.
   c. ozone.
   d. radon.

10. Which of the following is NOT a possible effect of exposure to excessive noise?
   a. higher blood pressure
   b. higher blood cholesterol
   c. deafness
   d. tinnitus



## True or False

T F 1. You can minimize your water consumption by taking baths instead of showers.

T F 2. The bulk of our food garbage ends up in the sewage system.

T F 3. Plastic waste is the largest component (by weight) of household trash.

T F 4. The world's population is currently growing by about 25 people per minute.

T F 5. Increased mortality from tropical diseases is a possible result of global warming.

T F 6. Damage to the ozone layer should reverse itself as soon as CFC production declines.

T F 7. The population growth rate is higher in developed countries than in developing countries.

T F 8. Using compact fluorescent bulbs instead of incandescent bulbs reduces air pollution.

T F 9. Exposure to asbestos can cause lung cancer.

T F 10. Prolonged exposure to sounds above 80–85 decibels can cause permanent hearing loss.

ANSWERS: Multiple Choice: 1. a (p. 417); 2. c (p. 421); 3. b (p. 419); 4. b (p. 423); 5. c (p. 424); 6. d (p. 424); 7. a (p. 427); 8. a (p. 428); 9. d (p. 430); 10. b (p. 430); True or False: 1. F (p. 418); 2. T (p. 419); 3. F (p. 419); 4. F (p. 421); 5. T (p. 423); 6. F (p. 424); 7. F (p. 421); 8. T (p. 426); 9. T (p. 427); 10. T (p. 430).

Name ______________________ Section ______________ Date ______________

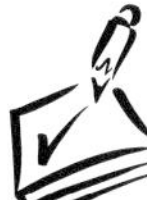

# WELLNESS WORKSHEET S17

## Environmental Health Checklist

Ww

The following list of statements relates to your impact on the environment. Put a check next to the statements that are true for you.

**Conserving Energy and Improving the Air**

_____ I ride my bike, walk, use public transportation, or carpool in a fuel-efficient vehicle whenever possible.

_____ I keep my car tuned up and well maintained.

_____ My vehicle is fuel efficient (city: _____ MPG; highway: _____ MPG).

_____ My car tires are inflated at the proper pressure.

_____ I avoid quick starts and drive within the speed limit.

_____ I don't use my car's air conditioner when opening the window would suffice.

_____ My residence is well insulated.

_____ Where possible, I use compact fluorescent bulbs instead of incandescent bulbs.

_____ I turn off lights and appliances when they are not in use.

_____ I avoid turning on heat or air conditioning whenever possible.

_____ I run the washing machine, dryer, and dishwasher only when they have full loads.

_____ I dry my hair with a towel rather than a hair dryer.

**Saving the Ozone Layer**

_____ I keep my car's air conditioner in good working order and have it serviced by a service station that recycles, rather than releases, CFCs.

_____ I check labels on aerosol cans and avoid those that contain CFCs.

_____ I avoid products containing methyl chloroform (1,1,1-trichloroethane).

_____ I don't have a halon fire extinguisher.

_____ I have an energy-efficient refrigerator, which I keep in good working order.

**Reducing Garbage**

_____ When shopping, I choose products with the least amount of packaging.

_____ I choose recycled and recyclable products and those sold in bulk.

_____ I avoid products packaged in plastic and unrecycled aluminum.

_____ I store food in glass jars and reusable plastic containers rather than using plastic wrap.

_____ I take my own bag along when I go shopping.

_____ Whenever possible, I use long-lasting or reusable products (such as refillable pens and rechargeable batteries).

_____ I use a ceramic mug and metal spoon for coffee and tea rather than disposable cups and stirrers.

_____ I recycle newspapers, glass, cans, paper, and other materials.

_____ I have a compost pile or bin for my organic garbage, or I take my organic garbage to a community composting center.

*(over)*

**Reducing Chemical Pollution and Toxic Wastes**

_____ When shopping, I read labels and try to buy the least toxic products available.

_____ I don't pour toxic materials (bleach, motor oil, etc.) down the sink.

_____ If I am unsure of the proper way to dispose of something, I contact my local health department or environmental health office.

_____ Whenever possible, I buy organic produce or produce that is in season and has been grown locally.

**Saving Water**

_____ I take showers instead of baths.

_____ I take short showers and switch off the water when I'm not actively using it.

_____ I do not run the water while brushing my teeth, shaving, or hand-washing clothes or dishes.

_____ My sinks have aerators installed in them.

_____ My shower has a low-flow showerhead.

_____ I have a water-saving toilet, or I have a water-displacement device in my toilet.

_____ I fix any faucets that leak.

**Preserving Wildlife and the Natural Environment**

_____ I snip or rip plastic six-pack rings before discarding them.

_____ I don't buy products made from endangered species.

_____ When hiking or camping, I never leave anything behind.

Statements that you have not checked can help you identify behaviors that you can change to improve environmental health. Consider planning a behavior change activity to alter one or more of your behaviors. To change some of the items listed, you may need the cooperation of your family and/or roommate(s). If there are environmental issues that are important to you, you can go beyond individual action by informing others, joining and volunteering your time to organizations working on environmental problems, and contacting your elected representatives.